drug
information

A GUIDE FOR
PHARMACISTS

Notice

Medicine is an ever-changing science. As new research and clinical experience broaden our knowledge, changes in treatment and drug therapy are required. The authors and the publisher of this work have checked with sources believed to be reliable in their efforts to provide information that is complete and generally in accord with the standards accepted at the time of publication. However, in view of the possibility of human error or changes in medical sciences, neither the authors nor the publisher nor any other party who has been involved in the preparation or publication of this work warrants that the information contained herein is in every respect accurate or complete, and they disclaim all responsibility for any errors or omissions or for the results obtained from use of the information contained in this work. Readers are encouraged to confirm the information contained herein with other sources. For example and in particular, readers are advised to check the product information sheet included in the package of each drug they plan to administer to be certain that the information contained in this work is accurate and that changes have not been made in the recommended dose or in the contraindications for administration. This recommendation is of particular importance in connection with new or infrequently used drugs.

drug
information

A GUIDE FOR PHARMACISTS

fourth edition

Editors

Patrick M. Malone, PharmD, FASHP
Associate Dean of Internal Affairs and
 Professor of Pharmacy Practice
College of Pharmacy
The University of Findlay
Findlay, Ohio

Karen L. Kier, PhD, MSc, RPh
Professor of Clinical Pharmacy
Director of Assessment
Raabe College of Pharmacy
Ohio Northern University
Ada, Ohio

John E. Stanovich, RPh
Assistant Professor of Pharmacy Practice
Assistant Dean for External Programs
College of Pharmacy
The University of Findlay
Findlay, Ohio

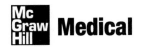

New York • Chicago • San Francisco • Lisbon • London • Madrid • Mexico City • Milan
New Delhi • San Juan • Seoul • Singapore • Sydney • Toronto

The *McGraw·Hill* Companies

Drug Information: A Guide for Pharmacists, Fourth Edition

Previous editions copyright © 2006, 2001 by The McGraw-Hill Companies, Inc., and copyright © 1996 by Appleton & Lange.

1 2 3 4 5 6 7 8 9 0   DOC/DOC   15 14 13 12 11

ISBN 978-0-07-162495-4
MHID 0-07-162495-3

This book was set in Century Old Style by Cenveo Publisher Services.
The editors were Michael Weitz and Robert Pancotti.
The production supervisor was Catherine H. Saggese.
Project management was provided by Manisha Singh, Cenveo Publisher Services.
The cover designer was Lashae V. Ortiz.
Cover photo credit: B. Busco.
RR Donnelley was printer and binder.

This book is printed on acid-free paper.

Library of Congress Cataloging-in-Publication Data

Drug information : a guide for pharmacists / editors, Patrick M. Malone,
Karen L. Kier, John E. Stanovich.—4th ed.
     p. ; cm.
   Includes bibliographical references and index.
   ISBN 978-0-07-162495-4 (pbk. : alk. paper)   1. Pharmacy—Information services.
  2. Drugs.   I. Malone, Patrick M., PharmD.   II. Kier, Karen L.   III. Stanovich, John E.
   [DNLM: 1. Drug Information Services.   2. Pharmacy
Administration—methods. QV 737]
   RS56.2.D78 2012
   615′.1—dc22   2011012143

International Edition ISBN 978-0-07-176819-1; MHID 0-07-176819-X. Copyright © 2012. Exclusive rights by The McGraw-Hill Companies, Inc., for manufacture and export. This book cannot be re-exported from the country to which it is consigned by McGraw-Hill. The International Edition is not available in North America.

McGraw-Hill books are available at special quantity discounts to use as premiums and sales promotions, or for use in corporate training programs. To contact a representative please e-mail us at bulksales@mcgraw-hill.com.

Contents

Chapter Four. Literature Evaluation I: Controlled Clinical Trial Evaluation 111

Michael Kendrach, Maisha Kelly Freeman, Terri M. Wensel, and Peter J. Hughes

Chapter Five. Literature Evaluation II: Beyond the Basics 193

Patrick J. Bryant, Karen P. Norris, Cydney E. McQueen, and Elizabeth A. Poole

Chapter Six. Pharmacoeconomics 269
James P. Wilson and Karen L. Rascati

Chapter Ten. Legal Aspects of Drug Information Practice 505
Martha M. Rumore

Chapter Eleven. Ethical Aspects of Drug
Information Practice 563
Linda K. Ohri

Chapter Twelve. Pharmacy and Therapeutics Committee **595**
Patrick M. Malone, Nancy L. Fagan, Mark A. Malesker, and Paul J. Nelson

Chapter Thirteen. Drug Evaluation Monographs **655**
Patrick M. Malone, Nancy L. Fagan, Mark A. Malesker,
Paul J. Nelson, and Linda K. Ohri

Chapter Fourteen. Quality Improvement and the
                 Medication Use Process **687**
Mark A. Ninno and Sharon Davis Ninno

Chapter Fifteen. Medication Misadventures I: Adverse Drug Reactions **733**

Philip J. Gregory and Zara Risoldi Cochrane

Chapter Sixteen. Medication Misadventures II: Medication and Patient Safety **757**

Kathryn A. Crea

Contributors

Elaine Blythe, PharmD
Adjunct, University of Florida College of
  Pharmacy
Associate Professor of Veterinary
  Pharmacology
St. Matthew's University, School of
  Veterinary Medicine
Grand Cayman Island, BWI
Veterinary Pharmacist, National Veterinary
  Response Team (NVRT)
Consultant Pharmacist, Micro Beef
  Technology
Omaha, Nebraska
Chapter 3

Patrick J. Bryant, PharmD, FSCIP
Clinical Professor of Pharmacy Practice
Director, Drug Information Center
University of Missouri–Kansas City
  School of Pharmacy
Kansas City, Missouri
Chapter 5

Karim Anton Calis, PharmD, MPH,
  FASHP, FCCP
Clinical Investigator
Program in Developmental Endocrinology
  and Genetics
Eunice Kennedy Shriver National Institute of
  Child Health and Human Development

National Institutes of Health
Clinical Professor
University of Maryland
Clinical Professor
Virginia Commonwealth University
Richmond, Virginia
Bethesda, Maryland
Chapter 2

Zara Risoldi Cochrane, PharmD
Assistant Professor of Pharmacy Practice
Creighton University
School of Pharmacy and Health Professions
Omaha, Nebraska
Chapter 15

Kathryn A. Crea, PharmD, BCPS
Professor of Pharmacy Practice
University of Findlay
Patient Safety Officer
Riverside Methodist Hospital
Columbus, Ohio
Chapter 16

Jean E. Cunningham, PharmD, BCPS
Assistant Professor of Pharmacy Practice
College of Pharmacy
The University of Findlay
Findlay, Ohio
Chapter 22

Lindsay E. Davison, PharmD
Regulatory Pharmaceutical Fellow in Drug
  Information
College of Pharmacy
Purdue University
West Lafayette, Indiana
Chapter 22

Stacie Krick Evans, PharmD
Pharmacy Educator
Orlando Health
Orlando, Florida
Chapter 18

Nancy L. Fagan, PharmD
Assistant Professor of Pharmacy Practice
Creighton University
School of Pharmacy and Health Professions
Omaha, Nebraska
Chapters 12 and 13

**Maisha Kelly Freeman, PharmD, MS,
  BCPS, FASCP**
Associate Professor of Pharmacy Practice
Samford University
McWhorter School of Pharmacy
Birmingham, Alabama
Chapter 4

Mary Lea Gora-Harper, PharmD, FASHP
Independent Pharmacist Consultant in Drug
  Information
Lexington, Kentucky
Chapter 1

Philip J. Gregory, PharmD
Assistant Professor of Pharmacy Practice
Creighton University
School of Pharmacy and Health Professions
Omaha, Nebraska
Chapter 15

**Bambi Grilley, RPh, RAC, CCRP,
  CCRC, CIP**
Director, Clinical Protocol Research and
  Regulatory Affairs
Texas Children's Cancer Center
Center for Cell and Gene Therapy
Associate Professor of Pediatrics
Baylor College of Medicine
Houston, Texas
Chapter 17

Peter J. Hughes, PharmD
Drug Information Specialist
Samford University
McWhorter School of Pharmacy
Birmingham, Alabama
Chapter 4

**Michael G. Kendrach, PharmD,
  BSPharm, FASHP**
Associate Dean for Academic Affairs
Professor, Department of Pharmacy Practice
McWhorter School of Pharmacy
Samford University
Birmingham, Alabama
Chapter 4

Karen L. Kier, PhD, MSc, RPh, BCPS
Professor of Clinical Pharmacy
Director of Assessment
Raabe College of Pharmacy
Ohio Northern University
Ada, Ohio
Chapter 8

**Mark A. Malesker, PharmD, FCCP,
  FASHP, BCPS**
Professor of Pharmacy Practice and Medicine
Creighton University Medical Center
Omaha, Nebraska
Chapters 12 and 13

Meghan J. Malone, PharmD
Ambulatory Care Resident
Duquesne University
Mylan School of Pharmacy
Pittsburgh, Pennsylvania
Chapter 9

Patrick M. Malone, PharmD, FASHP
Associate Dean of Internal Affairs and
    Professor of Pharmacy Practice
College of Pharmacy
The University of Findlay
Findlay, Ohio
Chapters 9, 12, and 13

**Patricia A. Marken, PharmD, FCCP,
    BCPP**
Associate Dean for Student Affairs
Professor of Pharmacy Practice and
    Administration
Professor of Medicine University of
    Missouri–Kansas City Schools of
    Pharmacy and Medicine
Kansas City, Missouri
Chapter 20

J. Russell May, PharmD, FASHP
Clinical Professor
College of Pharmacy
University of Georgia
Augusta, Georgia
Chapter 1

Cydney E. McQueen, PharmD
Clinical Associate Professor, Pharmacy
    Practice
University of Missouri–Kansas City School
    of Pharmacy
Kansas City, Missouri
Chapter 5

Kevin G. Moores, PharmD
Associate Professor (Clinical)
Director, Division of Drug Information
    Service
College of Pharmacy
The University of Iowa
Iowa City, Iowa
Chapter 7

Paul J. Nelson, MD
Maple Hill Medical Plaza
Omaha, Nebraska
Chapters 12 and 13

Mark A. Ninno, PharmD
Pharmacy Implementation Manager
VHA Performance Services
Oviedo, Florida
Chapter 14

Sharon Davis Ninno, PharmD
Corporate Medication Safety Coordinator
Orlando Health
Orlando, Florida
Chapter 14

Karen P. Norris, PharmD
Principal/Owner, Medical Writing
    Consultant
ApotheComm, LLC
Overland Park, Kansas
Chapter 5

Linda K. Ohri, PharmD, MPH
Associate Professor of Pharmacy Practice
Creighton University
School of Pharmacy and Health
    Professions
Omaha, Nebraska
Chapters 11 and 13

Debra L. Parker, PharmD
Assistant Professor of Pharmacy Practice
College of Pharmacy
The University of Findlay
Findlay, Ohio
Chapter 19

Elizabeth A. Poole, PharmD
Pharmacist
University of Pittsburgh Medical Center
Poison and Drug Information Center
Pittsburgh, Pennsylvania
Chapter 5

Karen L. Rascati, PhD
Professor, Pharmacy Practice and
  Administration Division
College of Pharmacy
University of Texas
Pharmacy Practice and Administration
  Division
Austin, Texas
Chapter 6

**Martha M. Rumore, PharmD, JD, LLM,
  FAPhA**
Clinical Manager, Drug Information
New York Presbyterian Hospital
Professor, Pharmacy & Health Outcomes
Touro College of Pharmacy
New York, New York
Chapter 10

Amy Heck Sheehan, PharmD
Associate Professor of Pharmacy Practice
College of Pharmacy
Purdue University
Drug Information Specialist
Indiana University Health
Indianapolis, Indiana
Chapter 2

Kelly M. Shields, PharmD
Associate Professor of Pharmacy Practice
Assistant Dean
Director of Pharmacy Student Services
Raabe College of Pharmacy
Ohio Northern University
Ada, Ohio
Chapter 3

**Kelly M. Smith, PharmD, BCPS,
  FASHP, FCCP**
Associate Dean, Academic and Student
  Affairs
Associate Professor, Department of
  Pharmacy Practice and Science
College of Pharmacy
University of Kentucky
Lexington, Kentucky
Chapter 21

Morgan L. Sperry, PharmD
Clinical Assistant Professor
Assistant Director, Drug Information
  Center
University of Missouri-Kansas City School
  of Pharmacy
Kansas City, Missouri
Chapter 20

Ryan W. Walters, MS
Research Analyst and Instructor
Division of Clinical Research and Evaluative
  Sciences
Department of Medicine
Creighton University Medical Center
Omaha, Nebraska
Chapter 8

Terri Wensel, PharmD, BCPS
Drug Information Specialist
Samford University
McWhorter School of Pharmacy
Birmingham, Alabama
Chapter 4

James P. Wilson, PharmD, PhD
Associate Professor
College of Pharmacy
University of Texas
Pharmacy Practice and Administration
  Divisions
Austin, Texas
Chapter 6

Preface

Ever since the publication of the first edition of this book in 1996, there has been an increasing realization of the importance of information. Much of this can be related to the increased availability of Internet information sources throughout society, along with the ever increasing ease by which material can be located and used. This increased emphasis on information has had an effect on both the healthcare professional, who uses the material, and the patient, who may look up material directly and even bring it in to talk about with a pharmacist or physician. The ability to obtain, manage, evaluate, and use information has become an important core skill for the professional.

This book was originally written to provide training in information management. In this fourth edition, the goal of this book continues to be to educate both students and practitioners on how to efficiently research, interpret, evaluate, collate, and disseminate information in the most usable form. Although there is no single correct method to perform these professional responsibilities, proven methods are presented and demonstrated. Also, seldom-addressed issues are covered, such as the legal and ethical considerations of providing information. In addition, besides normal updating of topics, many new topics and features have been added.

NEW TO THIS EDITION

- A series of Key Concepts have been placed at the beginning of each chapter, which are then identified throughout the chapter.
- The main areas outlined in the Learning Objectives for each chapter have now been highlighted throughout the chapter.
- Most chapters have Case Studies, in which a situation that might be faced by a practitioner is described, with a series of discussion points presented.

- In each chapter, a set of multiple-choice Self-Assessment Questions are presented and many chapters provide Suggested Readings for further information on topics.
- The drug literature evaluation chapters have been updated and expanded to cover newer concepts such as adaptive clinical trials.
- The chapter on statistics has been completely rewritten and greatly expanded to provide further information that allows the reader to determine whether appropriate statistical tests were conducted to evaluate data derived from clinical studies.
- The chapter that previously covered both adverse drug reactions and medication errors has been divided into two separate chapters, with an expansion of patient safety information.
- At the end of the book, five new chapters have been added. Drug information specialists are commonly involved in all of these new areas, as are many practicing pharmacists.
  - The first new chapter is on policy development, project design, and implementation. This chapter expands on the policy and procedure information in the chapter on professional writing and explores new areas.
  - Following this chapter, there are two new chapters that address the need for the ambulatory pharmacist to provide information; this topic expands to areas other than institutional practice, which tended to be the focus in previous editions. One chapter covers pharmacist practice needs in the area of drug information and the other chapter discusses dealing with patients and their information needs.
  - Following these chapters, there is a new chapter on what is necessary for training individuals in drug information.
  - Finally, in a continued effort to expand information into newer areas, there is a chapter on drug information in both the pharmaceutical manufacturers' realm and regulatory affairs (i.e., United States Food and Drug Administration). Drug information practitioners in those two areas address similar topics, but from different viewpoints. This chapter provides information on both viewpoints.

With the veritable flood of drug, medical, and pharmacy information available, much of which is complex, pharmacists have an increasing need for information management skills. This book will assist pharmacists or students with improvement of skills in drug information and will allow individuals to evolve into new roles for the advancement of the profession of pharmacy and patient care. We hope that you enjoy your journey toward expertise in information management.

1

Chapter One

Introduction to the Concept of Medication Information

Mary Lea Gora-Harper • J. Russell May

Learning Objectives

● *After completing this chapter, the reader will be able to*

- Define the term *drug information,* used in different contexts, and relate it to the term *medication information.*
- Describe the importance of drug information centers in the evolution of pharmacy practice.
- Identify the services provided by drug information centers.
- Describe the skills needed by pharmacists to perform medication information functions.
- Identify major factors that have influenced the ability of pharmacists to provide medication information.
- Describe practice opportunities for a medication information specialist.

Key Concepts

❶ Medication information may be either patient-specific or relative to a group of patients, such as in the development of a therapeutic guideline, coordination of an adverse drug event reporting and analysis program, publication of an electronic newsletter, or updating a Web site.

2 Several factors have been influential in the evolution of the pharmacist's role as a medication information provider in the last 50 years including the changing philosophy of practice, the emphasis on medication safety, integration of new information technology, changes in the health care environment with focus on evidence-based medicine and evaluation of outcomes, the sophistication of medication therapy, and the self-care movement.

3 A properly configured medical record provides decision support, facilitates workflow, and enables the routine collection of data for performance feedback in an effort to help improve efficiency and quality of care, including patient safety. This offers opportunities for pharmacists, and in particular medication information specialists, to take a leadership role in planning and implementing computerized intervention programs that automatically educate at the point of prescribing.

4 It is important not only that pharmacists keep up with medication use concepts, but that they also stay abreast of developments in the area of information technology in an effort to integrate new and valuable systems in a timely and efficient manner.

5 The focus of evidence-based medicine in health care has strengthened the need for pharmacists to have a solid understanding of medication information concepts and skills. Pharmacists need to be able to evaluate the medication use issues for a group of patients; search, retrieve, and critically evaluate the scientific literature; and apply the information to a targeted group of patients.

6 There are opportunities for drug information specialists to provide leadership in contract drug information centers, medical informatics, health maintenance organizations (HMOs), pharmacy benefit management organizations (PBMs), managed care organizations (MCOs), scientific writing and medical communications, poison control, pharmaceutical industry, and academia.

Introduction

The provision of medication information is among the most fundamental responsibilities of pharmacists. **1** *The information may be either patient-specific or relative to a group of patients, such as in the development of a therapeutic guideline, coordination of an adverse drug event reporting and analysis program, publication of an electronic newsletter, or updating a Web site.* The pharmacist can serve as a resource for issues regarding cost-effective medication selection and use, medication policy decisions (drug benefits), medication information resource selection, or practice-related issues. Medication information opportunities are developing and expanding with changes in the health care environment. With national efforts to expand access to care while reducing health care costs, the advent of consumerism, and the integration of new technologies (e.g., computerized physician order entry (CPOE), communication across settings of care), medication information opportunities are growing in several areas including MCOs, pharmaceutical industry, medical and specialty care clinics, scientific writing and medical communication companies, and the insurance industry.

The term drug information may have different meanings to different people depending on the context in which it is used. If asked to define this term, one could describe it as information in a reference or verbalized by an individual that pertains to medications. In many cases, individuals put this term in different contexts by associating it with other words that include

Specialist/practitioner/pharmacist/provider
Center/service/practice
Functions/skills

The first group of words implies a specific individual, the second group implies a place, and the third implies activities and abilities of individuals. The term "drug information" will be used in these different contexts to describe the beginnings and evolution of this area of practice. Relative to current practice, the term medication information is used in place of drug information to convey the management and use of information on medication therapy and to signify the broader role that all pharmacists take in information provision. These terms may refer to either the provision of information for a specific patient or in the context of addressing medication use issues for a population (i.e., a group of individuals defined by a set of common characteristics, such as in a set of policies and procedures on medication use developed by health professionals working in the emergency department of a hospital).

Drug informatics is another term used to describe the evolving roles of the medication information specialist. Drug informatics emphasizes the use of technology as an integral tool in effectively organizing, analyzing, managing, and communicating information on medication use in patients. With the growing integration of electronic health records and CPOE, there is greater opportunity to provide information on medications for individual patients at the point of care, and to be able to assess outcomes more readily in a population of patients.[1] The impact of new technologies and opportunities in drug informatics in current and future practice will be discussed later in the chapter.

The goals of this chapter are to describe how the role of the pharmacist has evolved in providing medication information, to discuss factors contributing to that evolution, and to describe opportunities for the use of medication information skills, either as a generalist or in a specialty practice. This chapter provides the foundation for understanding the pharmacist's need to have proficiency in the knowledge and skills discussed in this book.

The Beginning

The term *drug information* arose in the early 1960s when used in conjunction with the word *center* and *specialist*. In 1962, the first drug information center was opened at the University of Kentucky Medical Center.[2] An area separated from the pharmacy was dedicated to provide drug information. The center was to be "a source of selected, comprehensive drug information for staff physicians and dentists to evaluate and compare drugs"[2] as well as provide for the drug information needs of nurses. An important role was to be a resource for the evaluation of adverse drug reactions. The center was expected to take an active role in the education of health professional students including medicine, dentistry, nursing, and pharmacy. A stated goal was to influence pharmacy students in developing their role as drug consultants. Several other drug information centers were established shortly thereafter. Different approaches to providing drug information services included decentralizing pharmacists in the hospital, offering a clinical consultation service, and providing services for a geographic area through a regional center. The first formal survey, conducted in 1973, identified 54 pharmacist-operated centers in the United States.[3]

The individual responsible for operation of the center was called the drug information specialist. The expectation was that drug information would be stored in the center and retrieved, selected, evaluated, and disseminated by the specialist. Information would be disseminated to specific questions, to assist in the evaluation of drugs for use in the hospital, or to inform others, through newsletters, of current developments related to drugs. These and other functions, as listed in Table 1–1, have evolved over a period of years. A drug information center or specialist may be involved in one or all of these functions. Detailed information regarding these activities is provided in subsequent chapters.

To develop some perspective for the reader on why the development of drug information centers and specialists was important, consider four of the 15 summary points in a congressional review of a survey by the National Library of Medicine on The Nature and Magnitude of Drug Literature, published in 1963.[4]

1. "Drug literature is vast and complex. The very problem of defining what constitutes the literature is difficult."
2. "Drug literature is growing rapidly in size. It is also increasingly complex, i.e., interdisciplinary and interprofessional in nature. Thus, drug information 'sprawls across' many professional journals of the most varied types."
3. "Literature on clinical experience with drugs is sizable and is growing. Its effective use by the practitioner offers many difficulties."
4. "Competent evaluation of masses of drug information is particularly necessary."

● TABLE 1–1. MEDICATION INFORMATION SERVICES

• Supporting clinical services with medication information	• Coordinating formulary management initiatives
• Answering questions regarding medications	• Developing criteria/guidelines for medication use
• Coordinating pharmacy and therapeutics committee activity	• Analyzing the clinical and economic impact of drug policy decisions
• Developing medication use policies	• Managing medication usage evaluation/ medication use evaluation
• Publishing or editing information on appropriate medication use through newsletters, journal columns, Web sites, etc.	• Providing education (e.g., in-services, classes, experiential education) for health professionals, students, and consumers
• Managing investigational medication use (e.g., institutional review board activities, information for practitioners)	• Coordinating of adverse drug event reporting and analysis programs, e.g., adverse medication reactions
• Providing poison information	

Interestingly, these statements still seem applicable even today when given the figures that in 2008, PubMed, the most widely used service for biomedical information in the world, included over 18 million citations from over 5300 journals from MEDLINE and other life-science journals.[5] This number does not include all journals published either electronically (i.e., e-journal or electronic journal) on the Web or in print. This number does not consider the 17,000 textbooks published annually in the biomedical field.[6] Training in computer and information technology was considered one of the five core areas of focus for health professionals education in an Institute of Medicine report published in April 2003.[7] It is also one of the primary objectives identified by the American Society of Health-System Pharmacists (ASHP) to improve the practice of pharmacy in the health systems. Listed in the ASHP 2015 initiatives is to "increase the extent to which health-system pharmacists actively apply evidence-based methods to the improvement of medication therapy."[8] Clearly, the functions performed by pharmacists providing medication information are as important today as, if not more important than, at the beginning of the drug information concept.

In the 1960s, the availability of new drugs (e.g., neuromuscular blockers, first-generation cephalosporins) provided challenges for practitioners to keep abreast and make appropriate decisions for their patients. Part of the problem was finding a way to effectively communicate the wealth of information to those needing it. The information environment relied heavily on the print medium for the storage, retrieval, and dissemination of information. MedLARS (Medical Literature Retrieval and Analysis System) was developed by the National Library of Medicine in the early 1960s.[9] Although it provided a computerized form of searching, requests for searches were submitted and results were returned by mail. The ability to transmit such information over telephone lines (online technology) was not available until 1971 when MEDLINE was introduced and was limited to libraries. During this time, the drug information specialist was viewed as a person who could bridge the gap and effectively communicate drug information.[10] Of course, methods for accessing information have evolved greatly with the creation of the World Wide Web and the integration of the electronic medical record.

Early reports that examine the requirements for training of a drug information specialist recommended that the following courses be added or strengthened in the pharmacy school curricula: biochemistry, anatomy, physiology, pathology, and biostatistics and experimental design (with some histology, embryology, and endocrinology incorporated into other courses).[11] Such topics were either not incorporated or not emphasized in curricula of the 1960s. In today's pharmacy curricula, most of these topics receive considerable emphasis. Pharmacists today use knowledge and skills to make clinical decisions about medication use in specific patients or a group of patients in conjunction with other health professionals. Pharmacists may be principal or coinvestigators in research involving a variety of therapeutic topics including medication use, optimal dose, drug interactions, or adverse effects of new or existing medications. Likewise, pharmacists, sometimes with support of the pharmacy professional organizations, frequently author publications in the area of therapeutic guidelines, drug policy initiatives, or outcome analyses.

The development of drug information centers and drug information specialists was the beginning of the clinical pharmacy concept. It laid the groundwork for pharmacists to demonstrate the ability to assume more responsibility in providing input on patient drug therapy. Pharmacists were provided the opportunity to extend their patient-care contribution by taking a more active role in the clinical aspects of the decision-making process as it related to medication therapy. By using their extensive drug knowledge and expanding their background in certain areas, pharmacists could offer their expertise as a consultant on medication therapy. The tool the pharmacist would use to function in this capacity was the clinical drug literature. This role of consultant has expanded for all pharmacists and is discussed in more detail later.

The Evolution

It is useful to look at the evolution of drug information practice from the perspective of drug information centers and of practicing pharmacists. In 2004, one report describes the decline in the number of drug information centers nationally, with the number of drug information pharmacists and other personnel being the lowest in 30 years.[12-14]

In this survey,[13] 151 institutions were identified as having an organized drug information center, which was defined as "a center that regularly accepts a broad scope of requests from health care professionals, regardless of the location or affiliation of those professionals." The mailing list was compiled from several sources (e.g., previously published directory, the *Drug Topics Red Book* list of DICs). A total of 81 centers returned a completed survey. These numbers appear to be low. Some existing centers are missing from this list, and there has been controversy at meetings of drug information practitioners regarding centers being excluded because of the definition used to describe drug information centers.[13] Another source of drug information center locations, the 2008 *Physicians' Desk Reference*, lists a total of 100 centers nationally.[15] Calculating accurate numbers is difficult. The centers are identified for these two sources through various listings that have developed over the years, but no agency or organization is responsible for maintaining a list. Well-defined criteria are not established for using the titles of drug information center/ service. Some centers have specialized in a particular area of drug information, and their name may reflect that specific function (e.g., center of drug policy). In this case, their practice may be limited to only a particular site based on their source of funding. Likewise, these lists only address drug information centers listed in the United States (including Puerto Rico), and not most of those that have been created internationally. They also exclude centers/services provided by the pharmaceutical industry or those only available via the Internet. Therefore, depending on how one would define a drug information center, the numbers are certainly higher. When examining the availability of a drug information center specifically in the hospital environment, a 2007 survey[16] that examined over 500 U.S. hospitals, found that 8.1% used a formal drug information center as their source to provide objective drug information. Interestingly, this has almost doubled (4.1%) from a similar survey of hospitals conducted 5 years earlier.[17] The availability of a formal drug information center was more prevalent in larger hospitals.[16] For instance, when examining a subset of the hospitals with more than 400 beds, 28.2% of hospitals reported that they had a formal drug information center. This information supports the resurgence of the concept of a formal drug information center affiliated with hospitals. This change may be secondary to the emphasis on cost containment and quality standards through drug policy initiatives.

Drug information pharmacists working in centers appear to be better trained than in the past, and a larger percentage have a doctor of pharmacy degree (71% in 2003 and 42% in 1986 and 1992).[13] The number of individuals who have completed a drug information residency, fellowship, or master of science (MS) degree program in drug information has also increased in recent years (11% in 1992 and 29% in 2003).

In addition to the responsibility of answering questions, the most commonly reported services in 2003 were preparation of newsletters (80%) and participation in pharmacy and therapeutics committee activities (79%).[13] Teaching students appears to be a growing area of responsibility. Forty-one percent of respondents considered education to be their primary goal. There was an increase in the percentage of drug information centers that participated in any type of residency program training (83% in 2003). This is compared to 1976, 1980, 1986, and 1992 in which the number of centers that participated in any residency program ranged from 54% to 66%. There was also a larger number of drug information centers used for experiential training as part of a doctor of pharmacy program (95% in 2003 compared to 59% in 1992).[13] One college described their need to increase resources in their drug information center because of the growing number of students requiring experiential drug information education during their experiential training.[18] In one survey of U.S. colleges of pharmacy, 58% of respondents felt they had an inadequate number of drug information training sites.[19]

A few studies have described the economic benefit of maintaining a drug information center or related activity in an academic institution or hospital. One such study examined the economic impact of drug information services responding to patient-specific requests. The resultant benefit-to-cost ratio was found to be 2.9:1 to 13.2:1. Most of the cost savings resulted from a decreased need for monitoring (e.g., laboratory tests) or a decreased need for additional treatment related to an adverse effect.[20] Another study examined the drug cost avoidance and revenue associated with the provision of investigational drug services, which was not part of drug information centers in this study, but may be the responsibility of a drug information center. The annualized drug cost avoidance plus revenue was $2.6 million.[21] Studies of this nature are becoming increasingly important in an era of cost containment.

DRUG INFORMATION—FROM CENTERS TO PRACTITIONERS

The responsibilities of individual pharmacists regarding the provision of medication information have changed substantially over the years. Impetus for this change was provided not only by the development of drug information centers and the clinical pharmacy concept, but also by the Study Commission on Pharmacy.[22] This external group was established to review the state of the practice and education of pharmacists and report its findings. One of the findings and recommendations stated that

> …among deficiencies in the health care system, one is the unavailability of adequate information for those who consume, prescribe, dispense and administer drugs. This deficiency has resulted in inappropriate drug use and an unacceptable frequency of drug-induced disease. Pharmacists are seen as health professionals who could make an important contribution to the health care system of the future by providing information about drugs to consumers and health professionals. Education and training of pharmacists now and in the future must be developed to meet these important responsibilities.

The report of the Commission was issued in 1975, and since that time drug informa-tion practice has changed for both drug information centers and individual pharmacists. The development of clinical pharmacy has helped move pharmacy forward in recognizing its capabilities to contribute to the care of patients. Clinical pharmacy was thought of pri-marily as an institutional patient-care process and did not gain widespread acceptance outside of hospitals. Over time, the activity of the pharmacist as a medication expert for patients has gained acceptance in a variety of practice settings including community phar-macies, nursing homes, and primary and specialty practices in medicine. Pharmacists who provide patient-specific information with a goal of improving patient outcomes use the medical literature to support their choices.[23,24]

Pharmacists involved in patient-care areas (e.g., hospitals, clinics, long-term care, home health care) now frequently answer drug information questions, participate in eval-uating patients' drug therapy, and conduct medication usage evaluation activities. In one survey of more than 500 hospitals, approximately 95% have staff pharmacists routinely answer drug information questions.[16] The provision of medication information may be on a one-on-one basis or may occur using a more structured approach, such as a presentation to a class of diabetic patients or a group of nurses in the practice facility. In either case, the pharmacist educates those who are the beneficiaries of the medication information. Phar-macists may also participate in precepting students in patient care or pharmacy environ-ments. In any of these roles, the pharmacist must use appropriate information retrieval and evaluation skills to make sure that the most current and accurate information is pro-vided to make decisions about medication use for those they are serving. This role of pharmacists as providers of medication information continues to be an important compo-nent of the educational outcomes developed by the Center for the Advancement of Phar-maceutical Education (CAPE). These outcomes are initiated and maintained by the American Association of Colleges of Pharmacy (AACP) to help transform the pharmacy curriculum to support education of the future.[25] There is a well-described systematic approach to answering drug information questions (see Chapter 2). It is important to obtain the necessary background information including pertinent patient factors, disease factors, and medication-related factors to determine the true question. Good problem-solving skills are required to fully assess the situation, develop a search strategy, evaluate the information, then formulate and communicate a response. Good communication skills are essential to respond in a clear and concise manner, using terminology that is con-sistent with the patients', caregivers', or health professionals' level of understanding. Table 1–2 lists the medication information skills a pharmacist should possess when con-fronted with a medication information need.

Opportunities continue to grow for pharmacist participation in the continuum of care including home health care and long-term care that require a solid therapeutic knowl-edge base, an understanding of the medical literature, and the ability to communicate the

● TABLE 1–2. **MEDICATION INFORMATION SKILLS**

1. Assess available information and gather situational data needed to characterize question or issue
2. Formulate appropriate question(s)
3. Use a systematic approach to find needed information
4. Evaluate information critically for validity and applicability
5. Develop, organize, and summarize response for question or issue
6. Communicate clearly when speaking or writing, at an appropriate level of understanding
7. Anticipate other information needs

information through either verbal or written consultation. Pharmacists in community settings counsel patients, answer medication information questions, review patient medication regimens for potential problems, and participate in helping patients manage chronic diseases.

Opportunities for pharmacists are also available in the area of veterinary pharmacy. Both the animal owner and the veterinarian need information. A pharmacist may need to practically apply information from veterinary resources (e.g., *Veterinary Drug Handbook*, *Textbook of Veterinary Internal Medicine, National Animal Poison Control Center*) for the benefit of an animal.

FACTORS INFLUENCING THE EVOLUTION OF THE PHARMACIST'S ROLE AS A MEDICATION INFORMATION PROVIDER

❷ *In addition to the changing philosophy of practice, several other factors are influential in the evolution of the pharmacist's role as a medication information provider. These include the emphasis on medication safety, integration of new information technology, changes in the health care environment with focus on evidence-based medicine and evaluation of outcomes, the sophistication of medication therapy, and the self-care movement.*

Adverse Drug Events (ADEs)

The 1999 Institute of Medicine (IOM) report, *To Err Is Human: Building a Safer Health Care System,*[26] generated a great deal of discussion in the medical community and legislature because of the impact of ADEs on patient health and well-being, and because of economic implications. Despite efforts to decrease the frequency of medical errors after this report, many consumers are still dissatisfied with the quality of health care in the United States. In a recent survey,[27] 40% of respondents believed that the quality of health care has gotten worse in the past 5 years, while only 17% said that it has improved. Thirty-four percent of respondents said that they or a family member had experienced a medical error at some point in their life. Efforts are ongoing to lobby for additional funding for initiatives to decrease the risk of medical errors in the United States. Because of the pharmacist's role in helping to identify and prevent ADEs in patients, this could have future implications.

As mentioned earlier in this chapter, one of the primary roles for drug information specialists in the beginning was collecting and evaluating adverse drug reactions.[2] Pharmacists perform this function in institutional health systems, managed care, or the pharmaceutical industry. To illustrate how a central area for reporting ADEs, such as a drug information center in an institutional health system, can be beneficial, consider the following unpublished example from an academic medical center. The drug information center received three reports of patients developing methemoglobinemia within a 2-week period. The offending agent was suspected to be benzocaine spray. Upon investigation, the drug information pharmacist recognized that all reports had one thing in common: the administering nurse. The pharmacist witnessed the administration of the drug by the nurse the next time it was ordered for a patient. Instead of a single brief spray as directed by the prescribing information, several sprays were used, resulting in a potentially toxic dose of drug. The drug information pharmacist developed a series of in-services for nurses. No reports of benzocaine-induced methemoglobinemia have occurred since. In managed care settings, the same benefit could be achieved on an even larger scale.

The role of the drug information specialist in the pharmaceutical industry as it relates to reporting ADEs is especially important in postmarketing surveillance activities. Because of the specific definition of a study population using inclusion and exclusion criteria in a new drug trial, many ADEs go undetected until the agent is commercially available and used in a broader population. Patient safety may be improved by quickly identifying potential problems and communicating them to health care professionals. The training and expertise of drug information specialists qualifies them to play a major role in this process.

Integration of New Health Information Technologies

Computer technology has changed drastically, but positively, the ability to store and access information. Even though the amount of literature is much larger today than previously, it is more manageable. The World Wide Web (WWW) allows the user to easily access the scientific literature, government publications, items in the news, and many other items, frequently without cost to the clinician or the consumer. Handheld devices (e.g., smartphones) allow practitioners to have a full range of applications (decision-support tools, medical references) that can be available at the point of care. These devices offer the convenience of collecting and accessing information from a unit that can be carried in a user's pocket. In certain situations, these systems can be used more conveniently than a desktop computer for online searching, calculations, patient tracking, laboratory order entry, and results checking; to provide medication profiles and set appointments; and as a time-management tool and to search drug information databases (e.g., general drug information texts, medical specialty reference books, drug interaction resources). Patients and health care practitioners can find information on nearly every disease and treatment, and virtual health communities and forums provide a mutually supportive environment for patients, family, and friends. The use of Twitter, Facebook, e-mail, Web forums, and blogs has simplified the way in which peers can exchange news and share opinions. Several professional organizations (e.g., ASHP; http://www.ashp.org) have used technology to maintain awareness of important news affecting pharmacy and the health care environment (e.g., regulatory and health policy issues), drug shortages, and awareness of their meetings. Live continuing education is offered at a pharmacist's computer desktop through Webinars. A pharmacist working in a community pharmacy can obtain information about a foreign medication found only in a resource obtained from another country as easily as he or she can communicate with health care professionals locally. In one recent survey, an estimated 98% of pharmacists responded that they had access to the Internet at their practice site.[16] Although the Internet has been used to transfer information instantaneously to clinicians and researchers, its value as a patient-care resource and professional education tool is only starting to be tested. One of the concerns in using the Internet for transfer of patient information is confidentiality.[28-30]

There is an increasing need by health professionals, as well as the consumer, to get more information about medications sooner. Information is needed quickly when a new medication becomes commercially available because of the potential for health and cost implications, when a product is withdrawn from the market for safety reasons, or when data from a new study is released that could have an impact on how common ailments are treated. The lag time that occurs with the print format may not be acceptable for many direct patient-care issues. The Internet allows medical information to be available sooner to both health care professionals and the public. The availability of e-journals and e-texts has minimized the need to travel to a library. Online repositories for articles, such as BioMed Central (http://www.biomedcentral.com) and PubMed (http://www.pubmedcentral.nih. gov), have allowed individuals to access millions of articles quickly, easily, and free of charge. The site freemedicaljournals.com (http://www.freemedicaljournals.com) provides a comprehensive list of medical journals that are also free of charge. The majority of printed medical textbooks with an online version require a subscription; however, there are exceptions (e.g., http://www.merck.com, where eight editions of Merck Manuals can be viewed and searched for free). Registries of ongoing clinical trials, such as ClinicalTrials.gov (http://www.ClinicalTrials.gov), provide information on the purpose and criteria for participation in an ongoing clinical trial. This has allowed pharmacists to anticipate new therapies and perhaps help their patients receive medications not yet approved by the U.S. Food and Drug Administration (FDA) through enrollment in a clinical trial.

In addition to health professionals, patients are also accessing information on the Web, using sites that are sponsored by a variety of companies and individuals with diverse interests. In a recent survey, 85% of physician respondents had experienced a patient bringing Internet information to a visit.[31] Information that is either incomplete or inaccurate may result in harmful behavior, such as discontinuing medication or increasing the doses.[32] There is some effort toward helping consumers accurately assess the quality of information on the Internet. Health on the Net (http://www.hon.ch) is a nonprofit, nongovernment organization that uses criteria to assess the quality of a Web site. The organization will give a seal of approval to those sites that apply and meet the quality criteria. If misinformation or inaccurate information is found on the Web, organizations exist to monitor fraud (e.g., Quackwatch; http://www.quackwatch.com). One site that may be helpful in providing patients with information on a range of medical conditions and management is healthfinder (http://www.healthfinder.gov).

Drug information centers have created their own Web sites to post information about their center and services, provide links to related sites considered to be of acceptable quality, to accept adverse drug reaction reports, and as a convenient means of receiving and answering drug information questions and providing information regarding formulary changes, institution-specific therapeutic guidelines, and drug policy initiatives.[33] The advantage of having a request form for answering drug information questions or reporting adverse drug reactions on the Web is that physicians, pharmacists, or other health professionals can access computers at their practice site. This information is typically accessible only through an institution's intranet.[34] An intranet is a network that belongs to an organization and is designed to be accessible only by the organization's members, employees, or others with authorization. The Web site looks and acts just like other Web sites, but has a firewall surrounding it, and therefore the center can provide easy access to their primary patrons without receiving extraneous questions from outside their defined clientele.[35-37]

There is a massive effort nationally to modernize health care by making all medical records standardized and electronic.[38] This is considered to be the cornerstone for improvements in quality of care, patient safety, and efficiencies, all leading to an economic benefit. For example, the use of technology-based interventions may help reduce the risk of recurrent exposure to medications to which patients have a known allergy, especially with a real-time clinical decision-support system.[39] Overall, 41% of hospitals had one or more components of the medical record (e.g., medication administration record [MAR], clinical documentation, vital signs, CPOE, laboratory or radiology results, progress notes) in electronic form.[16] However, only 9.2% of hospitals with components of an electronic medical record (EMR) had a complete EMR system and did not use patient charts. Overall, 84.6% of hospitals provided pharmacists access to medication-relevant portions of the EMR for the purpose of managing medication therapy. The actual physician order was sent to the pharmacy by a variety of methods. Digital image capture was used by 32.7% of hospitals, followed by fax (23.7%) and electronic receipt through CPOE (5.1%). Although in another recent study of 1125 hospitals, a total of 220 (19.6%) had CPOE systems.[40] This discrepancy between the two surveys is probably secondary to the types of hospitals that were assessed.

❸ *A properly configured medical record provides decision support, facilitates workflow, and enables the routine collection of data for performance feedback in an effort to help improve efficiency and quality of care, including patient safety.*[41] *This offers opportunities for pharmacists, and in particular medication information specialists, to take a leadership role in planning and implementing computerized intervention programs that automatically educate at the point of prescribing.* The use of computer-based clinical support systems that provide patient information with recommendations based on the best evidence have proven to be valuable in the patient-care setting, including a reported decrease in length of hospital stay.[42,43] In one study that examined the value of using a decision-support program to assist physicians in using antiinfective agents, the length of hospital stay of patients who used the recommendations was compared with a group of patients who did not always use the recommendations, and was compared against a group of patients who were admitted to the unit 2 years before the intervention program. The length of hospital stay was statistically different with an average of 10 days, 16.7 days, and 12.9 days, respectively.[40]

Although technology affords remote-site access to medication information sources, it is critical that pharmacists have the skills to perceive, assess, and evaluate the information, and apply the information to the situation. One of the most rapidly changing technologies in health care is information technology. ❹ *It is important not only that pharmacists keep up with medication use concepts, but that they also stay abreast of developments in the area of information technology in an effort to integrate new and valuable systems in a timely and efficient manner.* The need for this type of training is emphasized in a recent IOM report.[7]

Focus on Evidence-Based Medicine and Drug Policy Development

Pharmacists' ability to apply their medication information skills to drug policy decisions will be of growing importance in this changing health care environment. This can be done by identifying trends of inappropriate medication use in a group of patients and providing supporting scientific evidence to help change behavior. Continued growth in national health expenditures has raised the concern of government, insurance agencies, health care providers, and the public in identifying strategies to control spending while maintaining access to quality health care. The United States spent more than $275 billion on prescription drugs in 2006.[44] Growth in prescription expenditures in 2007 was strongly influenced by several factors including the Medicare Part D benefit and increased spending on biologics. The Center for Medicare and Medicaid Services (CMS) estimates that total outpatient prescription drug costs was expected to increase by 8% in 2009.[44] Likewise, the IOM recently completed a 3-year study of the uninsured with a recommendation that universal health insurance coverage be available in the United States by 2010,[45] which at least is partially addressed by laws passed in 2010. In 2001, uninsured Americans received $35 billion in uncompensated medical care; $30 billion was ultimately paid for with tax dollars.[45] Although a list of insurance benefits has not been defined, it will be created based on evidence of improved patient care. Because drug expenditures are the largest component of the pharmacy operating budget and a significant portion of the entire health-system budget, the pharmacy budget frequently attracts significant attention from leadership. In recent years, there has been a shift from a fee-for-service inpatient focus to a capitated, managed care, ambulatory focus.[46] Managed care—a process seeking to manage the delivery of high-quality health care in order to improve cost-effectiveness—is consuming an ever-increasing portion of health care delivery. Today, providers are relying less on impressions of what *may* be happening in a practice setting and more on data that are actually being collected in that same group of patients (e.g., number of patients receiving appropriate dose of drugs). Goals are set for a particular group of patients (e.g., all patients receive beta-blocker therapy after a myocardial infarction) based on evidence found in the scientific literature. This connection of applying the scientific information to the patient-care setting is made through evidence-based medicine. Evidence-based medicine is an approach to practice and teaching that integrates current clinical research evidence with pathophysiologic rationale, professional expertise, and patient preferences to make decisions for a population.[47] ❺ *This has strengthened the need for pharmacists to have a solid understanding of medication information concepts and skills. Pharmacists need to be able to evaluate the medication use issues for a group of patients; search, retrieve, and critically evaluate the scientific literature; and apply the information to the targeted group of patients.*

Evidence-based medicine techniques are used in health care organizations in the development and implementation of a variety of quality assurance tools (e.g., therapeutic guidelines, clinical pathways, medication use evaluations, and disease state management) in an effort to improve patient outcomes and decrease costs across the health care system. The goal is to support the appropriate use of medications including correcting the overuse, underuse, or misuse of medicines. In the United States, the IOM designated evidence-based, patient-centered health care delivery as a key feature of high-quality medical care.[48] All of these situations require pharmacists to use medication information skills and to have various kinds of medication information support at the practice site or easily accessible at a remote site. The process of evidence-based medicine requires that systems be developed to measure and report processes and outcomes that can be used to drive quality improvement efforts. Data can be collected and analyzed by a medication information specialist using scientific methods to support the decision-making process in an MCO.

Outcomes research can be used to identify the effectiveness of pharmaceutical products and services in achieving desired health outcomes and, especially in light of the integration of the electronic medical record, will likely prove valuable in detecting problems and benefits.[49] Likewise, the branch of outcomes research, pharmacoeconomics, provides tools to assess cost, consequences, and efficiency (see Chapter 8).[50] Evidence-based medicine should include rigorously designed observational studies that include a full range of health outcomes (e.g., quality of life, patient functionality, and patient preferences). This will be discussed more fully in Chapter 8.

Sophistication of Medication Therapy

The sophisticated level of medication therapy that occurs today provides pharmacists much more opportunity to lend their expertise in assessing the medication information needs of professionals, patients, or family members, and providing literature to help choose the best medication to use within a class, to convey the appropriate information to help patients correctly and safely use the more potent medications, and to address administration and delivery problems. It is increasingly difficult for physicians and other health professionals to keep up with all of the developments in medication therapy, as well as keep abreast of the other information required for their practice. It is estimated that over 2000 compounds are in various stages of drug development.[51] A record 633 are new biotechnology medicines.[52] Several of the drugs in the different stages of development could have a substantial impact on clinical practice and drug expenditures once they are commercially available. For instance, it is anticipated that at least 750 of these medications are anticancer agents, which could have an impact on life expectancy, quality of life, and the related expenses associated with the potential need for increased ancillary care, additional physician office visits, or hospitalization.[51,52] It is important that drugs in the pipeline be monitored by pharmacists to provide adequate time to identify the patient population that will most benefit from the new drug and to help anticipate the cost of treating these patients compared to traditional therapy.[52,53]

There is also a trend toward individualization of health care using pharmacogenomic profiling to determine potential drug effectiveness.[54] Patients may be tested for genomic patterns, and their drug therapy will be altered accordingly. There are several potential benefits of using this pharmacogenomic technique: New, effective treatments for a variety of medical conditions could be identified faster and in smaller samples, computer modeling can help eliminate the medications that do not work, and because this technique can help identify the best candidates for a particular drug, it can help patients become more productive sooner.[55]

The Self-Care Movement

Finally, consumers have a continually growing desire for information about their medications. The growth of the self-care movement, the increase in focus on health care costs, and the improved accessibility of health information are some of the factors that have influenced patients to participate more fully in health care decisions, including the selection and use of medications. Based on these needs, direct-to-consumer advertising (DTCA) campaigns have appeared in virtually all mediums including magazines, television ads, Web-based ads, and radio reports. The potential negative impact of this information is the increased use of advertised drugs when alternatives may be more appropriate, resulting in increases in drug spending and utilization.[56]

E-marketing (marketing through digital media such as Web, e-mail, and wireless media) also continues to grow. More consumers are going on the Internet for health information. A 2008[57] Harris poll found that 81% (150 million consumers) of Internet users search for health information on the Web, compared to 1998 when the number of consumers was reported to be only 54 million. Today, 66% of all adults and 81% of those who are online use the Internet for health information. Likewise, 25% of respondents claimed that they searched for health information frequently (an average of 4.8 times per month) and believe that they were both successful in their search (89%) and found reliable information (86%). Just under half (47%) have discussed the information they obtained online with their physicians, and approximately half (49%) of those have gone back online to look for information as a result of that discussion.

Because a single individual is able to serve as author, editor, and publisher of a Web site, there is no safeguard on the quality of information available on the Internet. The end result may be a highly informed or perhaps misinformed consumer.[58-60] When patients find information about medications that they are either considering to start taking or are currently taking, from either the Internet, through the lay press, or by DTCA, a pharmacist can help them critically assess the medication information that they find and add to the information based on specific patient-related needs.

The need to critically assess information regarding complementary and alternative medicine (CAM) has become increasingly important, with approximately 38% of U.S. adults aged 18 years and over and approximately 12% of children using some form of CAM.[61]

There is a trend toward integrating CAM with conventional medicine. In a survey of over 6400 U.S. hospitals, approximately 37% offered some sort of CAM options. This is increased from 26.5% in 2005.[62,63] Eighty-four percent and 67% of respondents claimed that patient demand and clinical effectiveness, respectively, were the primary rationale for offering CAM services. This area presents a challenging situation for pharmacists because of the need to assess relevant outcomes data from well-designed clinical trials. Consumers are increasingly interested in finding reliable information regarding these products; pharmacists are in an excellent position to help provide such information. One drug information center describes its experience with a devoted telephone line to provide information regarding herbal supplements.[64] There was an increased demand for the service over time based on a higher call volume. This is consistent with the growing use of CAM nationally. It also described the challenges and limitations of finding reliable information on herbal products. Several resources are available that have information on herbal products.[65] It is just as important that the pharmacist provide information from reliable sources, as well as identify information that is lacking in regard to a particular product.

Groups like the National Council on Patient Information and Education (NCPIE) encourage patients to seek information when they have questions. The experience with some medication information hotlines that have been established for public access has indicated the public desire and need for information.[66] Such hotlines, often established by pharmacists, are intended to enhance the relationships between pharmacists, physicians, and patients.

The changing environment affords the pharmacist many opportunities to use the full spectrum of medication information skills. Factors such as the integration of new technologies, the focus on evidence-based medicine and drug policy development, the sophistication of medication therapy, and the advent of consumerism require that all pharmacists have a strong foundation in medication information concepts.

EDUCATING FOR THE NEED

The education of pharmacists continues to evolve in scope and depth. Many of the areas identified earlier as needed by the drug (medication) information specialist are now incorporated into pharmacy curricula and taught to all pharmacists. In 1991, a consensus conference in New Mexico was held to define a set of objectives for didactic and experiential training in drug information for the year 2000.[67] Twenty-three educators and practitioners participated in the conference. Several key concepts were developed including that (1) drug information should be a required component of the pharmacy curriculum and include both didactic and competency-based experiential components; (2) drug information concepts and skills should be spread throughout the curriculum, beginning the day the students enter pharmacy school; and (3) problem-solving should be a major technique in drug information education, with the goal of developing self-directed learners. Developing these skills should provide the foundation for the pharmacist to be a lifelong learner and problem solver. Based on the work of this conference, as well as changes in the health care system and the movement toward outcome-based education, colleges of pharmacy are redesigning their curricula to provide a more comprehensive and integrated approach to teaching medication information concepts and skills.[68,69] The CAPE outcomes, which are guidelines used for pharmacy education, continue to include medication information skills for all pharmacy students.[25] In a recent survey, all pharmacy schools offered didactic drug information education to first-professional-year students either as a stand-alone course (70%) or integrated throughout the professional curriculum.[70] Fifty-one of the 60 colleges offered an advanced pharmacy practice experience in drug information, and 62% of these had it as an elective. However, 58% of respondents felt that they had an inadequate number of drug information training sites. Communication skills are taught formally to facilitate the pharmacist's ability to transmit information to both health professionals and patients. Medication information and policy development are integrated throughout the three goal areas addressed in the pharmacy practice residency standards. Currently, there are 15 ASHP-accredited specialty practice (PGY-2) residencies in medication information with a total of 19 available positions (http://www.ashp.org/directories/residency). Many other advanced training opportunities exist in the pharmaceutical industry.

Opportunities in Specialty Practice

As the role of the practicing pharmacist has changed regarding medication information activities, so has the role of the specialist. The role of the medication information specialist has changed from an individual who specifically answers questions to one who focuses on the development of medication policies and provides information on complex medication information questions. ❻ *A specialist in medication information can provide leadership in a contract drug information center, medical informatics, health maintenance organizations (HMOs), pharmacy benefit management organizations (PBMs), managed care organizations (MCOs), scientific writing and medical communications, poison control, pharmaceutical industry, and academia.* In a survey that examined the career paths of pharmacists who completed a drug information specialty residency in 2000 or 2001, the types of careers were diverse. However, the most common positions were in industry (32%), academia (21%), medical writing (12%), and as a specialist in an institution (9%).[71] A specialist in medication information can be involved in multiple activities in practice settings listed in the following.

CONTRACT DRUG INFORMATION CENTER (FEE-FOR-SERVICE)

The need for accurate information pertaining to drug therapy is more acute today than ever before in the history of health care. One estimate suggests that outpatient prescription drug expenditures will increase at an average rate of 3%-5% in 2010.[72] Within the next decade health care costs will increase at an alarming rate, with total expenditures reaching the $2.1 trillion mark. A majority of these costs will be shouldered by the private sector, with a significant increase in prescription drug costs. Drug information practitioners are in an enviable position to provide a service that will improve patient outcomes and decrease health care costs through the provision of unbiased information that supports rational, cost-effective, and patient- and disease-specific drug therapy. One of the best ways to deliver such information is by contracting with a drug information service with formally trained health care professionals. Potential clients include managed care groups, contract pharmacy services, federal or state government, pharmacy benefits managers, buying groups, attorneys, pharmaceutical industry, small rural hospitals, chain pharmacies, and independent pharmacies. In one survey, 31% of MCOs contracted with a drug information center.[73] Several different fee structures have been used. A client may be charged a simple fee per question, or may be offered a detailed menu of services (e.g., written medication evaluations, continuing education programs, and guideline development for particular diseases) with the final cost being dependent on the number and types of services chosen by the contracting party.

Services provided within these contracts may include providing answers to drug information requests, preparation of new drug evaluation monographs, formulary drug class reviews, development of medication use evaluation criteria, providing journal reprints, pharmacoeconomics evaluations, writing a pharmacotherapy publication (e.g., Web site, blog, newsletter), and providing continuing education programming. Additional services the center may make available are access to online resources, access to in-house question files for sharing of information on commonly asked questions, and direct access to the center's Internet home page for review of medical use evaluations, formulary reviews, and newsletters.[74] One center reports providing information on drug shortages to the American Society of Health-System Pharmacists through a grant.[75] Frequently, the contracting drug information center also has responsibilities for pharmacy services (drug information, drug policy) as part of an entire health system, or is based in a college of pharmacy.

MEDICAL INFORMATICS IN A HEALTH SYSTEM

With the growth and development of new technologies (e.g., information systems), there are tremendous opportunities for an informatics specialist—an individual who has advanced medication information skills with a keen understanding of computer and information technology. This individual can help support patient-care activities by improving the efficiency of workflow and increasing access to patient-specific information and the medical literature through technology by remote site availability. This individual may also be involved in the area of institutional drug policy management. As the integration of electronic medical records and CPOE continues to expand, data that were only accessible through a paper record will be available for those professionals who understand the type of data that are needed for quality improvement efforts, and are able to get information efficiently out of the system and into the hands of clinicians at the point of care.[76] In a recent survey on technology, 42.9% and 17.8% of U.S. hospitals had one or more components of the medical record (e.g., medication administration record, clinical documentation) available electronically and in a CPOE system, respectively. Of those hospitals with

CPOE, 67.2% had clinical decision-support systems (CDSSs) to help direct prescribers toward evidence-based drug therapy.[77] As database designs evolve and become user-friendlier and computer systems become more sophisticated, there are increasing opportunities for applying computer technology, using CDSSs, to enhance many aspects of the medication use process. CDSSs can integrate patient-specific information, perform complex evaluations, and provide this information to a clinician at the point of care. These systems can be used to support initiatives with decisions on adverse drug reaction reporting and analysis programs, formulary management, continuous quality improvement effort, and clinical practice guidelines that provide feedback to the prescriber at the time the order is written.[77]

HMOS, PBMS, AND MCOS

A key opportunity that was identified in a strategic planning meeting in 1994 by the Consortium for the Advancement of Medication Information, Policy, and Research (CAMIPR) was the growing role for medication information specialists in the area of medication policy development/research and technology.[78] With total U.S. drug expenditures for pharmaceuticals increasing annually (e.g., $287 billion in 2006), this offers tremendous opportunities for the medication information specialist to provide leadership in the development and implementation of mechanisms to support the cost-effective selection and use of medications in HMOs, PBMs, and MCOs.[53,79] Potential activities may include the provision of medication use evaluation assessments, encouraging the use of cost-effective alternatives, managing formularies, providing information to support formulary guidelines (counter-detailing), and developing disease management programs.[80]

Medical and pharmacy outcomes research has been an increasing interest among health care providers, payers, and regulatory agencies. With the appropriate training (e.g., specialized residency in medication information practice or managed care experience) and expertise, opportunities are growing for the medication information specialist in the insurance industry, HMOs, MCOs, PBMs, state and national government agencies (e.g., Medicaid, Medicare), as well as other groups interested in the cost-efficient use of medications. Prior to approval by the FDA, drugs undergo testing in a limited number of patients. Once approved, experience in patients escalates and previously unrecognized, rare adverse events may be identified. The drug may also be found useful for conditions not described in the labeling. Perhaps one of the most important functions of postmarketing surveillance is in the area of adverse drug reaction reporting. This type of analysis can answer questions about drug interactions, identify potential new indications for the product, and study patients in a broader population. Organizations with a relatively large patient population offer opportunities to study these issues under the leadership of a medication information specialist.

Opportunities also exist to establish guidelines for selected disease states (e.g., management of patients with diabetes mellitus) or classes of drugs (e.g., selection of appropriate antibiotic for surgical prophylaxis). Practice guidelines are becoming an increasingly important part of the biomedical literature. These clinical guidelines are systematically developed to assist practitioners and patients with decisions about health care in an effort to improve the quality and consistency of health care while minimizing costs and liability.[81] Evidence-based practice guidelines are developed through systematic reviews of the literature appropriately adapted to local circumstances and values. Key questions to consider when reviewing a practice guideline have been proposed.[82] These questions primarily rely on how accurately the guideline reflects the research used to produce it. More information on therapeutic guidelines can be found in Chapter 7.

POISON CONTROL

Poison information is a specialized area of medication information, with the practitioner typically practicing in an accredited poison information center or an emergency room. Similar to the mission of traditional drug information centers, poison information centers exist to provide accurate and timely information to enhance the quality of care of patients. There are, however, several differences between a traditional drug information center and a poison control center. Health professionals generate most consultations received in drug information centers, whereas in a poison control center, most are generated from the public. Poison information centers must be prepared to provide information on the management of any poison situation, including household products, poisonous plants and animals, medications, and other chemicals. Because of the type of information that the specialist provides, nearly all requests for information to a poison control center are urgent, with an average response time of 5 minutes, compared to anywhere from 30 minutes to days for drug information centers, depending on the urgency of the call and complexity of information required.

Specialists in poison information require expertise in clinical toxicology to be able to obtain a complete history that correctly assesses the potential severity of exposure. They need to know where and how to search for this type of information and be able to develop an appropriate plan for intervention. Also, they need to be able to communicate the plan in a comprehensive, concise, and accurate manner to a consumer at an appropriate level of understanding. Because of the unique expertise of this type of specialist, a national certification examination is offered through the American Association of Poison Control Centers (AAPCC; http://www.aapcc.org/).

In addition to a poison control center providing information regarding individual patients, centers in the United States also contribute data to a larger program through the

National Poison Data System (NPDS; formerly the Toxic Exposure Surveillance System [TESS]). These data can be used to compare safety profiles for similar products to develop risk assessment guidelines for specific substances, to target national prevention programs, and to conduct postmarketing surveillance on products (e.g., chemicals). In 2007, 60 of the nation's 61 U.S. Poison Centers uploaded case data automatically.[83] Data were provided for over 4.2 million calls nationally. Despite the impact that regional poison control centers have on reducing morbidity and mortality with poison exposures, they are also facing increasing emphasis on economic justification. One study used a decision analysis to compare the cost-effectiveness of treating poison exposures with the services of a regional poison control center to treatment without access to any poison control center.[84] The average cost per patient treated with the services of a poison control center was almost half of that achieved without the services of a poison control center. These results were consistent regardless of exposure type, average inpatient and emergency department costs, and clinical outcome probabilities. Another study examined the public health cost savings by preventing the unnecessary utilization of emergency department services by providing home management by a regional poison control center.[85] On average, 70% of requests for poison information can be managed at home that would otherwise need to be handled in an emergency room environment. It is estimated that a median of $33 million (range $18 million to $45 million) in unnecessary health care charges were prevented by home management by a regional poison information center in 2007. A median of approximately $36 in unnecessary health care charges were prevented for each dollar of state funding the regional poison control center received. This is a large cost savings to residents compared to dollars received in state support.

PHARMACEUTICAL INDUSTRY

The pharmaceutical industry provides many career opportunities for pharmacists in a variety of areas including drug discovery, product development, information technology, training and development, scientific communications, health outcomes research, regulatory affairs, professional affairs, medical information services, and clinical research.[86,87] Within the area of medical information services, the pharmacist participates in typical types of activities such as answering drug information questions, reporting and monitoring adverse drug reactions, and providing information support to other departments. Other positions in medication information services include disease specialist, health outcomes associate, labeling associate, and medical or scientific writer. As a medical liaison, a pharmacist can help educate health professionals about a particular group of products or provide academic support or partnership for educational initiatives. In addition to providing written information on the drug product produced by the manufacturer, there are opportunities to provide additional information at pharmacy and therapeutics committees or state drug use review (DUR) boards. Pharmaceutical companies have extensive scientific data on their products, some of which is not available through other published sources or may require a formal FOI (freedom of information) request. Medication information specialists may also serve as reviewers for journal articles, evidence-based guidelines, and published drug monographs. Medication information specialists may interact with sales and marketing, participate with regulatory affairs issues, and handle product complaints. Regulatory affairs specialists help ensure that drugs under development meet the state and federal regulations that have been developed to protect the public. Pharmacists may be called on to review adverse effects identified in clinical studies and communicate this and other information to the appropriate research and development team.

Pharmacists with specialized training can take a leadership role in evaluating current research, serving as an associate in managing ongoing research or designing studies to help answer questions about new indications for future use of the product. The impact of new medications on the health care environment is also felt within the pharmaceutical industry. The area of health outcomes research is a growing area that offers tremendous opportunity for pharmacists to share their knowledge of the health care environment, research design, technology, and economics from the perspective of the pharmaceutical industry. As the sophistication of drug products and information management (e.g., electronic new drug applications [NDAs]) has increased, so have the opportunities for pharmacists to practice in the pharmaceutical industry and focus on using the skills of a medication information specialist.

ACADEMIA

The medication information specialist has the opportunity to provide leadership in the pharmacy curriculum, including both didactic and experiential training.[88] In addition to teaching medication information skills that are required across practice sites, the specialist also serves as a collaborator with other faculty on cases and activity designed to reinforce drug information skills for students. Approximately one-third of drug information centers are funded by a college of pharmacy.[13] This environment allows the student to be prepared to efficiently and accurately provide information to the appropriate audience, while emphasizing both didactic and competency-based experiential training. New academic opportunities for medication information training include the recently ACPE-required Introductory Pharmacy Practice Experiences or IPPEs (http://www.acpe-accredit. org). Students in their first 3 years of pharmacy school are now required to gain exposure to patient-care services prior to the last year of advanced pharmacy practice experiences

(APPEs). Answering real questions from patients and about patients may be one way to satisfy this requirement and prepare students for the challenging future.

SCIENTIFIC WRITING AND MEDICAL COMMUNICATION

Medical education and communication companies may provide educational programming to meet continuing education needs (e.g., symposia, workshops, monographs), or nonaccredited or promotional activities (e.g., sales training, publication planning, journal articles). Over 180 companies were providing this service in 2001.[89] In addition to having good writing skills, the pharmacist also needs to have scientific expertise and literature evaluation skills.[90] More than 77% of medical education and communication companies employ at least one licensed health care professional. These professionals may have several positions including director and scientific writer. Pharmacists in this capacity would work closely with editors, graphic designers, meeting planners, and computer programmers. This type of information may be communicated in a variety of ways including orally, in print format, and electronically on the Web (e.g., e-Medicine).

Summary and Directions for the Future

All pharmacists must be effective medication information providers regardless of their practice. As defined by the New Mexico Conference, an effective provider perceives, assesses, and evaluates medication information needs and retrieves, evaluates, communicates, and applies data from the published literature and other sources as an integral component of patient care. If the profession is to be successful in accepting patient-care responsibilities, all pharmacists must have a certain minimum level of skill to survive in the changing practice environment. Developing the skills of an effective medication information provider is the foundation for the pharmacist to be a lifelong learner and problem solver. The literature is a valuable component of both of these processes and will allow the individual pharmacist to adapt to the needs of a continually changing health care system.

Opportunities abound for pharmacists to use medication information skills in all practice settings either as a generalist or a specialist practitioner. There is still the need for the practitioner to have support from drug information centers to meet special information needs, to serve as a resource on effective medication use, and to assist pharmacy practitioners as well as others in solving medication therapy situations. Individuals with special training as medication information specialists will still be needed to operate the centers, and to provide leadership in the areas of drug informatics, institutional drug policy, poison control, pharmaceutical industry, medical writing, and in academia.

Self-Assessment Questions

1. In current practice, "medication information" is used in place of "drug information"
   a. To convey the management and use of information on medication therapy
   b. To prevent confusion with information on drugs of abuse
   c. To signify the broader role that all pharmacists take in information provision
   d. a and b
   e. a and c

2. The first drug information center was opened in 1962 at
   a. The University of Iowa
   b. The Ohio State University
   c. The University of Kentucky
   d. Misr International University in Cairo, Egypt
   e. None of the above

3. Which one of the following is *not* true?
   a. There are approximately 1700 textbooks published annually in the biomedical field.
   b. In 2008, PubMed included over 18 million citations from over 5300 journals.
   c. In the 2003 IOM report, training in computer and information technology was one of the five core areas of focus for health care professionals education.
   d. The ASHP 2015 initiatives include increasing pharmacists' application of evidence-based methods to improve medication therapy.
   e. The provision of medication information by pharmacists is at least as important today as it was in 1962.

4. The primary tool pharmacists use as a consultant on medication therapy is
   a. Physical assessment
   b. Clinical drug literature
   c. Pathophysiology
   d. Pharmaceutical calculations
   e. Medicinal chemistry

5. The number of formal Drug Information Centers listed in the 2008 *Physicians' Desk Reference* is
   a. 75
   b. 200
   c. 300
   d. 100
   e. 500

6. Regarding the level of training for drug information pharmacists practicing in centers,
   a. The percentage with PharmD degrees has decreased since the 1990s.
   b. The percentage with PharmD degrees has remained stable since the 1990s.
   c. The percentage with postgraduate training in drug information has increased since the 1990s.
   d. The percentage with postgraduate training in drug information has remained stable since the 1990s.
   e. Both b and c are correct.

7. In a recent study, the benefit-cost ratio of drug information services related to patient-specific requests was found to be 2.9:1 to 13.2:1. Most savings resulted from
   a. Decreasing the books in the library by increasing the use of electronic sources.
   b. Decreasing the need for drug monitoring.
   c. Decreasing the need for additional treatment related to an adverse event.
   d. Preventing adverse drug reactions.
   e. Both b and c are correct.

8. Factors influential in the evolution of the pharmacist's role as a medication information provider include
   a. Medication safety.
   b. Integration of new information technology.
   c. Focus on evaluation of outcomes.
   d. Both a and b are correct.
   e. All of the above.

9. One Web site that contains eight editions of medical manuals is
   a. http://www.CDC.gov
   b. http://www.merck.com
   c. http://www.freemedicaltextbooks.com
   d. http://www.fda.gov
   e. http://www.healthcareconsultant.edu

10. The nonprofit, nongovernmental organization that uses criteria to assess the quality of a Web site is
    a. Health on the Net
    b. Internet Health Watch
    c. Quality on the Net
    d. Health Net Quality Watch
    e. None of the above

11. Medication information specialists' primary leadership role(s) in the move to computerized intervention programs that automatically educate at the point of prescribing should be
    a. Testing the programs once they are in place
    b. Planning and implementing the programs
    c. Providing feedback to programmers on effectiveness
    d. Developing quality improvement programs for these systems
    e. None of the above

12. For pharmacies in organized health care settings, the largest component in the pharmacy operating budget is
    a. Personnel
    b. The Drug Information Center
    c. Clerical supplies
    d. Drugs
    e. IV Room equipment

13. A recent poll showed that what percentage of lay public Internet users search for health information on the Web?
    a. 99%
    b. 30%
    c. 81%
    d. 61%
    e. 27%

14. The most common career path for someone completing a drug information specialty residency program is
    a. Hospital drug information practice
    b. Medical writing
    c. Academia
    d. Poison control
    e. Industry

15. What percentage of pharmacy schools offer didactic drug information education as either a stand-alone course or integrated throughout the curriculum?
    a. 100%
    b. 90%
    c. 80%
    d. 75%
    e. 70%

REFERENCES

1. Hing HS, Burt CW, Woodwell DA. Electronic health record use by office-based physicians and their practices: United States, 2006. Advanced data from vital and health statistics (DHHS Publication no. (PHS) 2008-1250). No 393. Hyattsville (MD): National Center for Health Statistics; October 26, 2007. p. 1-7.
2. Parker PF. The University of Kentucky drug information center. Am J Hosp Pharm. 1965;22:42-7.
3. Amerson AB, Wallingford DM. Twenty years' experience with drug information centers. Am J Hosp Pharm. 1983;40:1172-8.
4. Walton CA. The problem of communicating clinical drug information. Am J Hosp Pharm. 1965;22:458-63.
5. National Libraries of Medicine [Internet]. Washington (DC): c1998-2009 [updated 2009 Mar 3; cited 2009 Jan 1]. Medline/PubMed Resource Guide. List of Journals Indexed for Medline. Available from: http://www.nlm.nih.gov/tsd/serials/lsiou.html.
6. Lowe HJ, Barnett GO. Understanding and using the Medical Subject Headings (MESH) vocabulary to perform literature searches. JAMA. 1994;271:1103-8.
7. Institute of Medicine. Health Professions Education: A Bridge to Quality. Washington (DC): National Academy Press; 2003.
8. American Society of Health-System Pharmacists [Internet]. Washington (DC):c1997-2008. [updated 2008 Mar; cited 2009 Jan 1]. 2015 ASHP Health System Pharmacy initiative. Available from: http://www.ashp.org/s_ashp/docs/files/2015_Goals_Objectives_0508.pdf.
9. Mehnert RB. A world of knowledge for the nation's health: the U.S. National Library of Medicine. Am J Hosp Pharm. 1986;43:2991-7.
10. Walton CA. Education and training of the drug information specialist. Drug Intel Clin Pharm. 1967;1:133-7.
11. Francke DE. The role of the pharmacist as a drug information specialist. Am J Hosp Pharm. 1966;23:49.
12. Koumis T, Cicero LA, Nathan JP, Rosenberg JM. Directory of pharmacist-operated drug information centers in the United States-2003. Am J Health Syst Pharm. 2004;61:2033-42.
13. Rosenberg JM, Koumis T, Nathan JP, Cicero LA, McGuire H. Current status of pharmacist-operated drug information centers in the United States. Am J Health Syst Pharm. 2004;61: 2023-32.
14. Koumis T, Rosenberg J. Update of directory of drug information centers. Am J Health Syst Pharm. 2005;62:1348.
15. Physicians' Desk Reference, 62nd ed. Montvale (NJ): Thomson Healthcare; 2008.
16. Pedersen CA, Schneider PJ, Scheckelhoff DJ. ASHP national survey of pharmacy practice in hospital settings: prescribing and transcribing—2007. Am J Health Syst Pharm. 2008;65:827-843.
17. Pedersen CA, Schneider PJ, Scheckelhoff DJ. ASHP national survey of pharmacy practice in hospital settings: dispensing and administration—2002. Am J Health Syst Pharm. 2003; 60:52-68.

18. Wilson AF, Moores KG, Bartels CL, Ohri LK, Malone PM. Expansion of drug information services in response to an increased clerkship teaching load. Am J Health Syst Pharm. 2005;62:2514-6.

19. Wang FEI, Troutman WG, Seo T, Peak A. Rosenberg JM. Drug information education in doctor of pharmacy programs. Am J Pharm Educ. 2006;70:51.

20. Kinky DE, Erush SC, Laskin MS, Gibson GA. Economic impact of a drug information service. Ann Pharmacother. 1999;33:11-6.

21. LaFleur J, Tyler LS, Sharma RR. Economic benefits of investigational drug services at an academic institution. Am J Health Syst Pharm. 2004;61:27-32.

22. Study Commission on Pharmacy. Pharmacists for the Future. Ann Arbor (MI): Health Administration Press; 1975:139.

23. Hepler CD, Strand LM. Opportunities and responsibilities in pharmaceutical care. Am J Hosp Pharm. 1990;47:533-50.

24. American Society of Health-System Pharmacists. ASHP Guidelines on the provision of medication information by pharmacists. Am J Health Syst Pharm. 1996;53:1843-5.

25. American Association of Colleges of Pharmacy [Internet]. Washington (DC): [updated 2004 May; cited 2009 Jan 1]. Center for the Advancement of Pharmaceutical Education. Available from: http://www.aacp.org/resources/education/Documents/CAPE2004.pdf. Accessed January 1, 2009.

26. Kohn LT, Corrigan JM, Donaldson MS. To Err Is Human: Building a Safer Health Care System. Washington (DC): National Academy Press; 1999.

27. Wachter RM. The end of the beginning: patient safety five years after 'To err is human'. Health Aff. 2004; Nov 30 [cited 2009 Jan 1]. Available from: http://content.healthaffairs.org/cgi/content/ full/hlthaff.w4.534/DC1.

28. Rind DM, Kohane IS, Szolovits P, Safran C, Chueh HC, Barnett GO, et al. Maintaining the confidentiality of medical records shared over the Internet and World Wide Web. Ann Intern Med. 1997;127:138-44.

29. Frisse ME. What is the Internet learning about you while you are learning about the Internet? Acad Med. 1996;71:1064-107.

30. Giacalone RP, Cacciatore GG. HIPAA and its impact on pharmacy practice. Am J Health Syst Pharm. 2003;60:433-45.

31. Murray E, Pollack L, Donelan K, Catania J, Lee K, Zapert K, et al. The impact of health information on the Internet on health care and the physician–patient relationship: national U.S. survey among 1,050 U.S. physicians. J Med Internet Res. 2003;5:e17.

32. Berland GK, Elliott MN, Morales LS, Algazy JI, Kravitz RL, Broder MS, et al. Health information on the Internet: accessibility, quality, and readability in English and Spanish. JAMA. 2001;285:2612-21.

33. Belgado Bernadette S. Drug information centers on the Internet. J Am Pharm Assoc. 2001;41:631-2.

34. Costerison EC, Graham AS. Developing and promoting an intranet site for a drug information service. Am J Health Syst Pharm. 2008;65:639-43.

35. Dugas M, Weinzierl S, Pecar A, Hasford J. An intranet database for a university hospital drug information center. Am J Health Syst Pharm. 2001;58:799-802.

36. Ruppelt SC, Vann R. Marketing a hospital-based drug information center. Am J Health Syst Pharm. 2001;58;1040.

37. Erbele SM, Heck AM, Blankenship CS. Survey of computerized documentation system use in drug information centers. Am J Health Syst Pharm. 2001;58:695-7.

38. www.money.cnn.com [Internet] cc 2009. [updated 2009 Jan 12; cited 2009 Jan 1]. Obama's big idea: digital health records. Available from: http://money.cnn.com/2009/01/12/technology/stimulus_health_care/.

39. Cresswell KM, Sheikh A. Information technology–based approaches to reducing repeat drug exposure in patients with known allergies. J Allergy Clin Immunol. 2008;121:1112-7.

40. Bond CA, Raehl CL. 2006 national clinical pharmacy services survey: clinical pharmacy services, collaborative drug management, medication errors, and pharmacy technology. Pharmacotherapy. 2008;28:1-13.

41. Elson RB, Connelly DP. Computerized medical records in primary care their role in mediating guideline-driven physician behavior change. Arch Fam Med. 1995;4:698-705.

42. Evans RS, Pestotnik SL, Classen DC, Clemmer TP, Weaver LK, Orme JF, et al. A computer-assisted management program for antibiotics and other anti-infective agents. N Engl J Med. 1998;338:232-8.

43. Hunt DL, Haynes RB, Hanna SE, Smith K. A computer-assisted management program for antibiotics and other anti-infective agents. JAMA. 1998;280;1339-46.

44. Poisal JS, Truffer C, Smith S, Sisko A, Cowan C, Keehan S, et al. Health spending projections through 2016: modest changes obscure Part D impact. Health Aff. 2007;26:242-53.

45. Institute of Medicine. Insuring America's Health: Principles and Recommendations. Washington (DC): Institute of Medicine; Jan. 2004.

46. APhA Special Report. Opportunities for the Community Pharmacist in Managed Care. Washington (DC): American Pharmaceutical Association; 1994.

47. Ellrodt G, Cook DJ, Lee J, Cho M, Hunt D, Weingarten S. Evidence-based disease management. JAMA. 1997;278:1687-92.

48. Committee on Quality of Health Care in America, Institute of Medicine. Crossing the Quality Chasm: A New Health System for the 21st Century. Washington (DC): National Academic Press; 2001.

49. Avorn J. In defense of pharmacoepidemiology—embracing the yin and yang of drug research. N Engl J Med. 2007;357(22):2219-21.

50. Vermeulen LC, Beis SJ, Cano SB. Applying outcomes research in improving the medication-use process. *Am J Health Syst Pharm.* 2000;57;2277-82.

51. Top 10 areas of research: report on the most popular fields of drug development. Med Ad News. 2003;137;S22.

52. Pharmaceutical research and manufacturers association (PHRMA) [Internet]. Washington (DC): cc 2008 [updated 2008 July 31; cited 2009 Jan 1]. Biotechnology research continues to bolster arsenal against disease with 633 medicines in development. 2008 Report. Medicines in Development. Available from: http://www.phrma.org/files/Biotech%202008.pdf.

53. Hoffman JM, Nilan D, Shah ND, Vermeulen LC, Doloresco F, Martin PK, et al. Projecting future drug expenditures—2009. Am J Health Syst Pharm. 2009;66:237-57.

54. Emilien G, Ponchon M, Caldas C, Isacson O, Maloteaux JM. Impact of genomics on drug discovery and clinical medicine. Q J Med. 2000;93:391-423.

55. Epler GR, Laskaris LL. Individualization health care and the pharmaceutical industry. Am J Health Syst Pharm. 2001;58:1042.

56. U.S. Government Accountability Office (GAO) report number GAO-07-54 entitled "Prescription Drugs: Improvements Needed in FDA's Oversight of Direct-to-Consumer Advertising," which was released on December 14, 2006. Available from: http://www.gao.gov/htext/d0754.html. Accessed February 15, 2010.

57. Harrisinteractive.com [Internet]. Rochester (NY): cc 2008 [updated 2008 July 29; cited 2009 Jan 1]. Number of "Cyberchondriacs"—Adults Going Online for Health Information—Has Plateaued or Declined. Available from: http://www.harrisinteractive.com/harris_poll/index.asp?PID=937.

58. Larner AJ. Use of Internet medical websites and of NHS direct by neurology outpatients before consultation Int J Clin Pract. 2002;56:219-21.

59. Silberg W, Lundberg GD, Musacchio RA. Assessing, controlling, and assuring the quality of medical information on the Internet. JAMA. 1997;277:1244-5.

60. Wyatt J. Measuring quality and impact on the World Wide Web. BMJ. 1997;314:1879-81.

61. National Institutes of Health, National Center for Complementary and Alternative Medicine [Internet]. Washington, DC: [updated 2008 Dec; cited 2009 Jan 1]. 2007 Statistics on CAM Use in the United States. Available from: http://nccam.nih.gov/news/camstats/2007/camsurvey_fs1.htm.

62. American Hospital Association [Internet]. Washington (DC): cc 2006-2009 [updated 2008 Sept 15; cited 2009 Jan 1]. Latest survey shows more hospitals offering complementary and alternative medicine services. Available from: http://nccam.nih.gov/news/camstats.htm.

63. Ananth S, Martin W. Health Forum 2005 Complementary and Alternative Medicine Survey of Hospitals: Summary of Results. Chicago: Health Forum LLC; 2006.

64. West PM, Lodolce AE, Johnston AK. Telephone service for providing consumers with information on herbal supplements. Am J Health Syst Pharm. 2001;58:1842-46.

65. Shields KM, McQueen CE, Bryant PJ. National survey of dietary supplement resources at drug information centers. J Am Pharm Assoc. 2004;44:36-40.

66. Meade V. Patient medication information hotlines multiply. Am Pharm. 1991;NS31:569-71.

67. Troutman WG. Consensus-derived objectives for drug information education. Drug Inform J. 1994;28:791-6.

68. Ferrill MJ, Norton LL. Drug information to biomedical informatics: a three-tier approach to building a university system for the twenty-first century. Am J Pharm Edu. 1997;61:81-6.

69. Gora-Harper ML, Brandt B. An educational design to teach drug information across the curriculum. Am J Pharm Edu. 1997;61:296-302.

70. Wang F, Troutman WG, Seo T, Peak A, Rosenberg JM. Drug information in doctor of pharmacy programs. Am J Pharm Educ. 2006;70:51.

71. Miller S, Clarke A. Impact of postdoctoral specialty residencies in drug information on graduates' career paths. Am J Health Syst Pharm. 2002;59:961-3.

72. Hoffman JM, Doloresco F, Vermeulen LC, Shah ND, Matusiak L, Hunkler RJ, Schumock GT. Projecting future expenditures—2010. Am J Health Syst Pharm. 2010;67:919-28.

73. McCloskey WW, Vogenberg FR. Drug information resources in managed care organizations. Am J Health Syst Pharm. 1998;55:2007-9.

74. Foresster LP, Scoggin JA, Valle RD. Pharmacy management company-negotiated contract for drug information services. Am J Health Syst Pharm. 1995;52:1074-7.

75. Fox ER, Tyler LS. Managing drug shortages: seven years' experience at one health system. Am J Health Syst Pharm. 2003;60:245-53.

76. Woodruff AE, Hunt CA. Involvement in medical informatics may enable pharmacists to expand their consultation potential and improve the quality of healthcare. Ann Pharmacother. 1992;26:100-4.

77. Pedersen CA, Gumpper KF. ASHP national survey on informatics: assessment of the adoption and use of pharmacy informatics in U.S. hospitals—2007. Am J Health Syst Pharm. 2008;65:2244-64.

78. Vanscoy GJ, Gajewski LK, Tyler LS, Gora-Harper ML, Grant KL, May JR. The future of medication information practices: a concensus. Ann Pharmacother. 1996;30:876-81.

79. Warren PN. Pharmacists to the fore. Managed Healthcare News. 1997;13:20H-20I.

80. Taniguchi R. Pharmacy benefit management companies. Am J Health Syst Pharm. 1995;52:1915-7.

81. Zinberg S. Practice guidelines—a continuing debate. Clin Obstet Gynecol. 1998;41:343-7.

82. Field JM, Lohr KN, eds. Guidelines for Clinical Practice: From Development to Use. Washington (DC): National Academy Press; 1992.

83. Bronstein AC, Spyker DA, Cantilena LR. 2007 Annual Report of the American Association of Poison Control Centers National Poison Data System (NPDS), 25th annual report. Clin Toxicol. 2008;46:927-1057.

84. Harrison MAJ, Draugalis JR, Slack MK, Langley PC. Cost-effectiveness of regional poison control centers. Arch Intern Med. 1996;156:2601-8.

85. Lovecchio F, Curry S, Waszolek K, Klemens J, Hovseth K, Glogan D. Poison control centers decrease emergency healthcare utilization costs. J Med Toxicol. 2008;4:221-4.

86. Gong SD, Millares M, VanRiper KB. Drug information pharmacists at health-care facilities, universities, and pharmaceutical companies. Am J Hosp Pharm. 1992;49:1121-30.

87. Riggins JL. Pharmaceutical industry as a career choice. Am J Health Syst Pharm. 2002;59: 2097-8.

88. Bernknopf AC, Karpinski JP, McKeever AL, Peak AS, Smith KM, Smith WD, et al. Drug information: from education to practice. Pharmacotherapy. 2009;29:331-46.

89. Overstreet KM. Medical education and communication companies: career options for pharmacists. Am J Health Syst Pharm. 2003;60:1896-7.

90. Moghadam RG. Scientific writing: a career for pharmacists. Am J Health Syst Pharm. 2003;60:1899-900.

SUGGESTED READINGS

1. Pedersen CA, Gumpper KF. ASHP national survey on informatics: assessment of the adoption and use of pharmacy informatics in U.S. hospitals—2007. Am J Health Syst Pharm. 2008;65:2244-64.
2. Hoffman JM, Shah ND, Vermeulen LC, Doloresco F, Grim P, Hunkler RJ, et al. Projecting future drug expenditures—2008. Am J Health Syst Pharm. 2008;65:234-53.
3. Hing HS, Burt CW, Woodwell DA. Electronic health record use by office-based physicians and their practices: United States, 2006. Advanced Data from Vital and Health Statistics (DHHS Publication no. (PHS) 2008-1250). No 393. Hyattsville (MD): National Center for Health Statistics; October 26, 2007. p. 1-7.
4. Bernknopf AC, Karpinski JP, McKeever AL, Peak AS, Smith KM, Smith WD, et al. Drug information: from education to practice. Pharmacotherapy. 2009;29:331-46.
5. Costerison EC, Graham AS. Developing and promoting an intranet site for a drug information service. Am J Health Syst Pharm. 2008;65:639-43.
6. Wang F, Troutman WG, Seo T, Peak A, Rosenberg JM. Drug information in doctor of pharmacy programs. Am J Pharm Educ. 2006;70:51.

Chapter Two

Formulating Effective Responses and Recommendations: A Structured Approach

Karim Anton Calis • Amy Heck Sheehan

Learning Objectives

After completing this chapter, the reader will be able to

- Develop strategies to overcome the impediments that prevent pharmacists from providing effective responses and recommendations.
- Outline the steps that are necessary to identify the actual drug information needs of the requestor.
- List and describe the four critical factors that should be considered and systematically evaluated when formulating a response.
- Define analysis and synthesis and explain how they are employed in the process of formulating responses and recommendations.
- List the elements and characteristics of effective responses to medication-related queries.

Key Concepts

1. Health care professionals can promote rational pharmacotherapy by ensuring that drug information is appropriately interpreted and correctly applied.

2. Absence of sufficient background information and pertinent patient data greatly diminishes the ability to provide effective responses.

3. Critical information that defines the problem and elucidates the context of the question is not readily volunteered but must be expertly elicited.

④ Providing responses and offering recommendations without knowledge of pertinent patient information, the context of the request, or how the information will be applied is unacceptable and potentially dangerous.

⑤ Formulating a response involves the use of a structured, organized approach whereby critical factors are systematically considered and thoroughly evaluated.

⑥ Responses to drug information queries often must be synthesized by integrating data from diverse sources through the use of logic and deductive reasoning.

Pharmacists are asked to provide responses to a variety of drug information questions every day. Although the type of requestor, query, and setting can vary, the process of formulating responses remains constant. This chapter introduces an organized, structured approach for formulating effective responses and recommendations.

As the medical literature expands, access to drug information resources by health care professionals and the public continues to grow. Yet many professionals and consumers lack the necessary skills to use this information effectively. This presents an opportunity and a challenge for pharmacists who wish to become bona fide drug therapy experts and assume a broader role in health care.

Regardless of specialty or practice site, pharmacists must strive to become pharmacotherapy specialists. Whether in a community pharmacy, outpatient clinic, or at the hospital bedside or other practice site, pharmacists can apply their knowledge to the care of patients. Pharmacists should not be relegated to the role of information dispenser or gatekeeper. Pharmacists must extend their knowledge of drugs and therapeutics to the clinical management of individual patients or the care of large populations. ❶ *Moreover, they must promote rational pharmacotherapy by ensuring that drug information is appropriately interpreted and correctly applied.*

Accepting Responsibility and Eliminating Barriers

Pharmacists should recognize that their responsibility extends beyond simply providing an answer to a question. Rather, it is to assist in resolving therapeutic dilemmas or managing patients' medication regimens. Knowledge of pharmacotherapy alone does not ensure success. Moreover, isolated information is not sufficient for formulating responses to questions or ensuring proper patient management. In fact, it is uncommon to find comprehensive answers in the literature that completely and effectively address specific situations or circumstances that clinicians encounter in their daily practices. Responses and recommendations must often be thoughtfully synthesized using information and knowledge gathered from a number of diverse sources. To effectively manage the care of patients and resolve complex situations, pharmacists also need added skills and competence in problem solving and direct patient care.

For pharmacists to provide meaningful responses and effective recommendations to drug information questions, real or perceived impediments must first be overcome. One such impediment is the false perception that many drug information questions do not pertain to specific patients. Another is the perception that the seemingly casual interactions with requestors and the lack of formal, written consultation somehow preclude the need for in-depth analysis and extensive involvement in patient management. Pharmacists sometimes oversimplify their interactions with requestors and fail to identify the context of the question or recognize its significance. Absence of sufficient background information and pertinent patient data greatly diminishes the ability of pharmacists to provide effective responses.

Identifying the Genuine Need

Historically, the approach to answering drug information queries has centered on the use of a systematic method first described by Watanabe and subsequently modified by others.[1,2] This simple approach relied on the collection of basic information to document and categorize the request and to subsequently develop an organized strategy for formulating cogent responses. Although this structure remains theoretically useful from a training standpoint, if strictly applied without proper context and guidance, it has the potential to artificially fragment the process and disrupt the natural exchange of information. A documentation form (see Appendix 2–1) may be useful to guide the process of data collection and ensure that all relevant information is considered. However, ultimately success will depend largely on maintaining the flow of information with minimal distractions and unnecessary or ill-timed questions. The goal should be to remove obstacles when communicating with clinicians so as to reveal the actual informational needs. This is particularly relevant in clinical settings where most queries are not purely academic or general in nature. In fact, it is rational to assume that queries from health care providers will invariably involve specific patients and unique clinical circumstances. For example, a physician who asks about the association of liver toxicity with lovastatin is probably not asking this question whimsically or out of curiosity. The physician most likely is caring for a patient who has developed signs or symptoms of hepatic impairment possibly associated with the use of this medication. Of course, other reasonable scenarios, albeit less likely, could have prompted such a question, but it, nonetheless, would be prudent to consider the possibility of a drug-induced liver injury in a specific patient.

Even questions that are not related to patient care (refer to Case Study 2–1 as an example) must be viewed in their proper context. Requestors of information are typically vague in verbalizing their needs and will generally provide adequate information only when specifically asked or thoughtfully prompted. Although these requestors may seem confident about their perceived needs, they may be less certain after further probing. Requestors, regardless of background, are often uncertain about what the pharmacist needs to know in order to assist them optimally. Therefore, critical information that defines the problem and elucidates the context of the question is not readily volunteered, but must be expertly elicited using effective questioning strategies (asking logical questions in a logical sequence) and other means. Such information may be essential for formulating informed responses. Failure of the requestor to disclose critical information or clarify the question does not obviate the need for such information or relieve the pharmacist of the duty to collect it. Although it is easy to assign blame to the requestor for failing to provide needed information, pharmacists must understand that it is their responsibility to obtain it completely and efficiently.

Good communication skills (both listening and questioning) are essential for enabling the pharmacist to gather relevant information and understand the real question (often referred to as the ultimate request) and the genuine needs of the requestor. Providing responses without knowledge of pertinent patient information, the context of the request, or how the information will be applied can be potentially dangerous. For assistance in identifying some of the questions to ask, please refer to Appendix 2–2. Even well-equipped drug information centers with trained staff are not immune to this problem. A study of the quality of pharmacotherapy consultations provided by formal drug information centers in the United States found that the centers generally failed to obtain pertinent patient data, thereby risking incorrect responses and inappropriate recommendations.[3]

Before attempting to formulate responses, pharmacists must consider several important questions to ensure that they understand the context of the query and the scope of the issue or problem (Table 2–1). ❷ *Without this information, pharmacists risk providing general responses that do not address the needs of the requestor.* More concerning, however, is that the information provided can be misinterpreted or misapplied. This not only compromises the pharmacist's credibility, but also can jeopardize patient care. Pharmacists must recognize the value and potential benefits of their contributions as members of the health care team. Lack of confidence in communicating with requestors can be a limiting factor. Because a telephone call or visit from a physician may not be perceived as a formal request for a consult, the significance of such apparently informal daily interactions easily can be overlooked.

TABLE 2–1. QUESTIONS TO CONSIDER BEFORE FORMULATING A RESPONSE

Is the requestor's name, profession, and affiliation known?

Does the question pertain to a specific patient?

Is there a clear understanding of the question or problem?

Is the correct question being asked?

Why is the question being asked? Why now?

Are the requestor's expectations understood?

Has pertinent patient history and background information been obtained?

What are the unique circumstances that generated the query?

What information is actually needed?

When is the information needed and in what format (e.g., verbal, written)?

How will the information provided be used or applied?

How has the problem or situation been managed to date?

Are there alternative explanations or management options that should be explored?

Pharmacists should understand that interactions with physicians and other clinicians present valuable opportunities for direct involvement in patient care. The lesson often missed is that there is a fine line between a simple, seemingly general drug information question and a meaningful pharmacotherapy consult. ❸ *Knowing the context of the question, obtaining the pertinent patient data and background information, and understanding the true needs of the requestor often can be the difference.*

Some pharmacists are quick to attempt to answer questions without adequately understanding the context or unique circumstances from which they evolved. They focus exclusively on the answer and ignore or fail to obtain key information needed to establish the framework of the question. In essence, this can result in a "correct" response being provided to address an "incorrect" question. For example, in a question about the dose of an antibiotic, an incorrect response can be formulated and inappropriate recommendations made if one fails to consider such factors as the patient's age, sex, condition being treated, end-organ function, weight and body composition, concomitant diseases (e.g., cystic fibrosis), possible drug interactions, site of infection, spectrum of activity of the antimicrobial, resistance patterns, or other factors such as pregnancy, dialysis, and other extracorporeal procedures.

In the absence of information that provides the proper context, a question about the half-life of a medication appears rather simple. However, if the question were posed for the purpose of assisting the requestor in determining a sufficient washout period for a crossover study, one would be remiss if factors other than the half-life of the parent compound were not considered. Proper determination of a washout period also would mandate consideration of other factors such as the activity and half-lives of known metabolites; the presence of potentially interacting medications; the effects of age, illness, or end-organ dysfunction; the persistence of pharmacodynamic effects of the medication beyond its detection in the plasma (e.g., omeprazole); and the effect of administration route on the apparent half-life (e.g., transdermally administered fentanyl).

The case studies in this chapter (see the following) emphasize the importance of looking beyond the initial question and recognizing that the requestor's needs often go well beyond a superficial answer to the primary question. Pharmacists should always anticipate additional questions or concerns, including those that are not directly asked or addressed by the requestor. These questions nonetheless must be considered if a clinical situation is to be managed optimally. In Case Study 2–4, as an example, a question is posed about ranitidine as a possible cause of thrombocytopenia. Although the requestor may neglect to pose additional clarifying questions, the pharmacist must anticipate and consider related issues and questions that will be critical in determining the success or failure of the response (Table 2–2). Failure to address these questions will undoubtedly result in an incorrect or inadequate response.

Pharmacists must learn to rely on their patient care skills, problem-solving skills, insight, and professional judgment. Computer databases and other specialized information sources can assist the pharmacist in identifying critical data, but overreliance on such resources without careful attention to pertinent background information and patient data can mislead even the most experienced clinician.

TABLE 2–2. IMPORTANT QUESTIONS NOT POSED BY THE REQUESTOR

Initial query posed by requestor: Can ranitidine cause thrombocytopenia?

What is the incidence of ranitidine-induced thrombocytopenia?

Are there any known predisposing factors?

Is the pathogenesis of this adverse effect understood?

How does the thrombocytopenia typically present?

Are there any characteristic subjective or objective findings?

Does thrombocytopenia due to ranitidine differ from that caused by other histamine-2 (H_2)-receptor antagonists, other medications, or other etiologies?

Is the thrombocytopenia dose related?

How severe can it become?

How soon after discontinuing the drug does it reverse?

How is it usually managed?

What is the likelihood of cross-reactivity with other H_2-receptor antagonists?

How risky is rechallenge with ranitidine?

Are there treatments available that can be used in place of ranitidine?

Are there alternative explanations for the thrombocytopenia in this patient (including other medications, medication combinations, or underlying medical conditions)?

What complications, if any, can be expected?

Formulating the Response

BUILDING A DATABASE AND ASSESSING CRITICAL FACTORS

Formulating a response involves a series of steps that must be performed completely, objectively, and in a logical sequence. This mandates the use of a structured, organized approach whereby critical factors are systematically considered and thoughtfully evaluated. The steps in this process include assembling and organizing a database of the patient information, gathering information about relevant disease states, collecting medication information, obtaining pertinent background information, and identifying other relevant factors and special circumstances. Table 2–3 outlines in detail the specific types of information that may need to be considered for each factor depending on the nature of the query. A more thorough list of possible background questions is found in Appendix 2–2. It should be noted that only some of this information might be pertinent for a given query or case scenario.

For patient-related questions, development of a patient-specific database is one of the first steps in preparing a response. This requires the collection of pertinent information from the patient, caregivers, health care providers, medical chart, and other patient records. A comprehensive medication history obtained by a pharmacist also is essential. This database invariably includes information that overlaps with the medical and nursing databases. Because physicians, nurses, patients, and others often lack a clear understanding of the type of information needed for effective pharmacotherapy consultations, pharmacists must be able to identify and efficiently extract pivotal patient information from diverse sources.

Once these data are collected and carefully assembled, they must be critically analyzed and evaluated in the proper context before final responses and recommendations are synthesized. Background reading on topics related to the query (e.g., diseases, medications, and laboratory tests) is often essential (see Chapter 3). This process also often involves careful evaluation of the literature (Chapters 4 and 5). To effectively perform the steps outlined previously, one must begin with a broad perspective (i.e., see the "big picture") to avoid losing sight of important information. ❹ *Approaching the problem haphazardly or with tunnel vision, and prematurely focusing on isolated details can misdirect even the most skilled clinician and can be very dangerous.*

ANALYSIS AND SYNTHESIS

❺ *Analysis and synthesis of information are among the most critical steps in formulating responses and recommendations.* Together they assist in forming opinions, arriving at judgments, and ultimately drawing conclusions. Analysis is the critical assessment of the nature, merit, and significance of individual elements, ideas, or factors. Functionally, it

TABLE 2–3. **FACTORS TO BE CONSIDERED WHEN FORMULATING A RESPONSE**

Patient Factors

Demographics (e.g., name, age, height, weight, gender, race/ethnic group, and setting)

Primary diagnosis and medical problem list

Allergies/intolerances

End-organ function, immune function, nutritional status

Chief complaint

History of present illness

Past medical history (including surgeries, radiation exposure, immunizations, psychiatric illnesses, and so forth)

Family history and genetic makeup

Social history (e.g., alcohol intake, smoking, substance abuse, exposure to environmental or occupational toxins, employment, income, education, religion, travel, diet, physical activity, stress, risky behavior, and compliance with treatment regimen)

Review of body systems

Medications (prescribed, over the counter, and complementary/alternative)

Physical examination

Laboratory tests

Diagnostic studies or procedures

Disease Factors

Definition

Epidemiology (including incidence and prevalence)

Etiology

Pathophysiology (for infectious diseases consider site of infection, organism susceptibility, resistance patterns, and so forth)

Clinical findings (signs and symptoms, laboratory tests, diagnostic studies)[a]

Diagnosis

Treatment (medical, surgical, radiation, biologic and gene therapies, other)

Prevention and control

Risk factors

Complications

Prognosis

Medication Factors

Name of medication or substance (proprietary, nonproprietary, other)

Status and availability (investigational, over-the-counter, prescription, orphan, foreign, complementary/alternative)

Physicochemical properties

Pharmacology and pharmacodynamics

Pharmacokinetics (liberation, absorption, distribution, metabolism, and elimination)

Pharmacogenetics

Indications (Food and Drug Administration [FDA] approved and unlabeled)

Uses (diagnosis, prevention, replacement, or treatment)

Adverse effects

continued

TABLE 2–3. **FACTORS TO BE CONSIDERED WHEN FORMULATING A RESPONSE (*Continued*)**

Medication Factors

Allergy
Cross-allergenicity or cross-reactivity
Contraindications and precautions
Effects of age, organ system function, disease, pregnancy, extracorporeal circulation, or other conditions or environments
Mutagenicity and carcinogenicity
Effect on fertility, pregnancy, and lactation
Acute or chronic toxicity
Drug interactions (drug–drug or drug–food)
Laboratory test interference (analytical or physiologic effects)
Administration (routes, methods)
Dosage and schedule
Dosage forms, formulations, preservatives, excipients, product appearance, delivery systems
Monitoring parameters (therapeutic or toxic)
Product preparation (procedures, methods)
Compatibility and stability

Pertinent Background Information, Special Circumstances, and Other Factors

Setting
Context
Sequence and time frame of events
Rationale for the question
Event(s) prompting the question
Unusual or special circumstances (including medical errors)
Acuity and time constraints
Scope of question
Desired detail or depth of response
Limitations of available information or resources
Completeness, sufficiency, and quality of the information
Applicability and generalizability of the information

[a]Factors such as disease or symptom onset, duration, frequency, severity, and so forth must always be carefully assessed.

involves separating the information into its isolated parts so that each can be critically assessed. Analysis requires thoughtful review and evaluation of the quality and overall weight of available evidence. Although this process requires consideration of all relevant positive findings, pertinent negative findings should not be overlooked.

Once the information has been carefully analyzed, synthesis can begin. Synthesis is the careful, systematic, and orderly process of combining or blending varied and diverse elements, ideas, or factors into a coherent response through the use of logic and deductive reasoning. This process relies not only on the type and quality of the data gathered, but also on how they are organized, viewed, and evaluated. Synthesis, as it relates to pharmacotherapy, involves the careful integration of critical information about the patient, disease, and medication along with pertinent background information to arrive at a judgment or conclusion. Synthesis can give existing information new meaning and, in effect, create new knowledge. ❻ *The use of analysis and synthesis to formulate a response is much like assembling a jigsaw puzzle.* If the pieces are identified and then grouped, organized, and assembled correctly, the picture will be comprehensible. However, if too many of the pieces are missing—as may be the case, for example, if patient information or if supporting evidence is incomplete or absent—or are not arranged logically (e.g., when information is not evaluated, interpreted, or applied correctly), providing an answer may prove difficult or altogether impossible. On occasion, only a partial response is possible and this caveat must be carefully explained to the requester.

RESPONSES AND RECOMMENDATIONS

An effective response obviously must answer the question. Other characteristics of effective responses and recommendations are outlined in Table 2–4. The response to a question must include a restatement of the request and clear identification of the problems, issues, and circumstances. The response should begin with an introduction to the topic and systematically present the specific findings. Pertinent background information and patient data should be succinctly addressed. Conclusions and recommendations are also included in the response along with pertinent reference citations from the literature. The format of responses (verbal or written) is discussed in Chapter 9. In formulating responses, pharmacists should disclose all available information that is relevant to the question. They should also present all reasonable options and explanations along with an evaluation of each. Specific recommendations must be scientifically sound, clearly justified, and well-documented.

TABLE 2–4. DESIRED CHARACTERISTICS OF A RESPONSE

Timely
Current
Accurate
Complete
Concise
Supported by the best available evidence
Well-referenced
Clear and logical
Objective and balanced
Free of bias or flaws
Applicable and appropriate for specific circumstances
Answers important related questions
Addresses specific management of patients or situations

A careful written record of the response must be maintained for follow-up and legal reasons. The records may be maintained in a patient's chart or simply in the provider's secure files.

FOLLOW-UP

When recommendations are made, follow-up always should be provided in a timely manner. Follow-up is required for outcomes assessment and, when necessary, to reevaluate the recommendations and make appropriate modifications. Also, it is a hallmark of a true professional and demonstrates the pharmacist's commitment to patient care. Furthermore, follow-up allows pharmacists to know if their recommendations were accepted and promptly implemented. Finally, follow-up also allows pharmacists to receive valuable feedback from other clinicians and to learn from the overall experience.

Case Study 2–1

■ INITIAL QUESTION

What is the molecular weight of enalapril?

■ POTENTIAL RESPONSE IN THE ABSENCE OF RELEVANT BACKGROUND INFORMATION

Enalapril is an oral angiotensin-converting enzyme (ACE) inhibitor that is indicated for the management of hypertension, symptomatic congestive heart failure, and asymptomatic left ventricular dysfunction.[4,5] The molecular weight of enalapril is 376.45.[6]

■ PERTINENT BACKGROUND INFORMATION

The requestor is a basic scientist who is conducting an *in vitro* experiment to evaluate the pharmacologic effects of enalapril. She would like to know the molecular weight of enalapril so that she can perform appropriate calculations specified for this experiment.

■ PERTINENT PATIENT FACTORS

N/A

■ PERTINENT DISEASE FACTORS

N/A

■ PERTINENT MEDICATION FACTORS

Enalapril is a prodrug that is converted *in vivo* to the pharmacologically active form, enalaprilat.[4,5] Both enalapril and enalaprilat are commercially available for use in the United States.

■ ANALYSIS AND SYNTHESIS

Considering that enalapril is a prodrug that must be converted to a pharmacologically active compound *in vivo*, and given that this researcher wishes to conduct an *in vitro* study, the researcher should use the active form of the drug in their experiment. Therefore, they should have requested the molecular weight of enalaprilat.

■ RESPONSE AND RECOMMENDATIONS

Enalapril is an oral angiotensin-converting enzyme inhibitor that is indicated for the management of hypertension, symptomatic congestive heart failure, and asymptomatic left ventricular dysfunction. Because enalapril is a prodrug that requires conversion to the active form, the requestor was advised to consider using enalaprilat in the experiment. The molecular weight of enalaprilat is 384.43.[6]

■ CASE MESSAGE

This example illustrates the importance of collecting pertinent background information, even for seemingly uncomplicated questions. Failure to understand exactly how the information that you provide will be used could result in an inaccurate or misleading response. In this case, providing the molecular weight without alerting the requestor that *in vitro* enalapril is pharmacologically inactive would have resulted in wasted time and money, and the results of the experiment would likely have been invalid.

Case Study 2–2

■ INITIAL QUESTION

What is the maximum dose of oprelvekin (Neumega)?

■ POTENTIAL RESPONSE IN THE ABSENCE OF RELEVANT BACKGROUND INFORMATION

The recommended dose of oprelvekin in adult patients is 50 µg/kg given once daily.[7] Larger doses of oprelvekin (75 to 100 µg/kg/day) have been studied in patients with breast cancer.[8] Constitutional symptoms associated with oprelvekin therapy, such as myalgias, arthralgias, and fatigue, were noted to increase in a dose-dependent fashion. One patient who received 100 µg/kg/day of oprelvekin experienced a cerebrovascular event after the third dose. Dose escalation greater than 75 µg/kg/day was discontinued in this study, and the maximum tolerated dose of oprelvekin was determined to be 75 µg/kg/day.[8]

■ PERTINENT BACKGROUND INFORMATION

The requestor is a physician who is managing a patient with human T-cell leukemia/lymphoma virus Type I (HTLV-1)-associated adult T-cell leukemia. The patient received myelosuppressive chemotherapy and subsequently developed prolonged and severe thrombocytopenia. Oprelvekin was prescribed in an attempt to improve the patient's platelet count and allow continuation of therapy. After 4 days of oprelvekin therapy at a dose of 50 µg/kg/day, the patient's platelet count did not increase substantially. The physician would like to know if doses greater than 50 µg/kg/day of oprelvekin have been studied. She is planning to increase the patient's dose to achieve a better response.

■ PERTINENT PATIENT FACTORS

R.R. is a 70-year-old man with HTLV-1–associated adult T-cell leukemia who has been treated with zidovudine plus interferon alfa-2b and four cycles of cyclophosphamide, hydroxydaunomycin (doxorubicin), vincristine (Oncovin), and prednisone, the combination of which is referred to as CHOP. After these treatments, R.R. developed severe and protracted thrombocytopenia, which has prevented further treatment.

Past Medical History

- HTLV-1 adult T-cell leukemia
- Cardiomegaly (ejection fraction 28%) secondary to zidovudine (AZT) and interferon alfa-2b treatment
- Peptic ulcer disease
- Hypertension
- Thrombocytopenia

Social History

- Ø alcohol
- Ø tobacco

Current Medications

- Oprelvekin 50 µg/kg/day subcutaneously
- Pantoprazole 40 mg orally daily
- Ramipril 5 mg orally daily
- Trimethoprim-sulfamethoxazole one double-strength tablet orally daily
- Dexamethasone 40 mg orally daily
- Loperamide 4 mg orally as needed for diarrhea
- Acetaminophen 325 mg orally as needed for headache
- Ø complementary/alternative or other over-the-counter (OTC) medications

Allergies/Intolerances

No known drug allergies.

Laboratory Results

Sodium 135 mmol/L, potassium 4.9 mmol/L, chloride 103 mmol/L, CO_2 22 mmol/L, creatinine 1.1 mg/dL, glucose 91 mg/dL, blood urea nitrogen (BUN) 25 mg/dL, albumin 3 g/dL, calcium (total) 2.49 mmol/L, magnesium 0.75 mmol/L, phosphorus 3.4 mg/dL, liver function tests (LFTs) within normal limits, white blood cells (WBCs) $28.3 \times 10^9/L$, hemoglobin (Hgb) 10.1 g/dL, hematocrit (Hct) 28.1%

Date	Platelet Count
7/13	25 K/mm^3
7/14[a]	21 K/mm^3
7/15	26 K/mm^3
7/16	29 K/mm^3
7/17	28 K/mm^3

[a]Day 1 of oprelvekin therapy.

■ PERTINENT DISEASE FACTORS

It is not known whether patients with adult T-cell leukemia respond differently to oprelvekin than those with other types of nonmyeloid malignancies.

■ PERTINENT MEDICATION FACTORS

Oprelvekin, or recombinant interleukin-11, is indicated for the prevention of severe thrombocytopenia and the reduction of the need for platelet transfusions following myelosuppressive chemotherapy in adult patients. The U.S. Food and Drug Administration (FDA)-approved dose of oprelvekin is 50 µg/kg once daily for up to 21 days.[7] Larger doses of oprelvekin (75 to 100 µg/kg/day) have been studied in patients with breast cancer.[7,8] Constitutional symptoms associated with oprelvekin therapy, such as myalgias, arthralgias, and fatigue, were noted to increase in a dose-dependent fashion. One patient who received 100 µg/kg/day of oprelvekin experienced a cerebrovascular event after the third dose. Dose escalation greater than 75 µg/kg/day was discontinued in this study, and the maximum tolerated dose of oprelvekin was determined to be 75 µg/kg/day.[8] However, the manufacturer warns that doses greater than 50 µg/kg/day may be associated with an increased incidence of fluid retention and cardiovascular events in adult patients.[4] After initiation of therapy, platelet counts usually begin to increase between 5 and 9 days, with peak counts occurring after about 14 to 19 days of therapy.[8]

■ ANALYSIS AND SYNTHESIS

Because R.R. has only received 4 days of oprelvekin treatment and platelet counts are expected to increase between 5 and 9 days after the initiation of therapy, adequate time for an optimal response to oprelvekin therapy has not been reached. In addition, oprelvekin doses greater than 75 µg/kg/day have been associated with serious adverse effects in adult patients. Therefore, increasing the dose of oprelvekin in this patient is probably not necessary, and may increase the risk of serious adverse effects without providing additional therapeutic benefits.

■ RESPONSE AND RECOMMENDATIONS

Oprelvekin, or recombinant human interleukin-11, is a thrombopoietic growth factor that stimulates the proliferation of hematopoietic stem cells and megakaryocyte progenitor cells, resulting in increased platelet production. Oprelvekin is indicated for the prevention of severe thrombocytopenia in patients with nonmyeloid malignancies who are at high risk for severe thrombocytopenia following chemotherapy.[7] Platelet counts usually begin to increase between 5 and 9 days after initiation of oprelvekin, with peak platelet counts occurring after 14 to 19 days of therapy.[7,8] R.R. has only received 4 days of oprelvekin treatment, which is insufficient for an optimal response. In addition, the adverse effects of oprelvekin therapy (e.g., myalgias, arthralgias, fatigue, fluid retention, and cardiovascular events) are dose dependent.[7,8] Therefore, increasing the oprelvekin dose at this time is not warranted. In fact, doing so may predispose the patient to an increased risk of adverse effects without the prospect of added therapeutic benefit.

■ CASE MESSAGE

This example demonstrates the importance of understanding the proper context of the query. In this case, the physician is asking the wrong question. The pharmacist must collect critical background information to determine the actual drug information needed. Had the pharmacist failed to collect pertinent patient information, the physician may have increased the dose of the medication after being told that doses of 75 µg/kg/day of oprelvekin have been used. This would have been inappropriate, given that this patient had not received the medication for a sufficient duration to achieve optimal response. Moreover, larger doses of this medication are associated with a higher incidence of adverse effects.

Case Study 2–3

■ INITIAL QUESTION

Are there any drug interactions between labetalol, clonidine, amlodipine, lorazepam, and minoxidil?

■ POTENTIAL RESPONSE IN THE ABSENCE OF RELEVANT BACKGROUND INFORMATION

An extensive search of tertiary[4,9-12] and secondary literature sources did not reveal any significant drug–drug interactions between labetalol, clonidine, amlodipine, lorazepam, and minoxidil. However, concomitant therapy with a β-adrenergic antagonist, an alpha-adrenergic antagonist, a calcium-channel antagonist, and a peripheral vasodilator may increase the potential for additive hypotension.

■ PERTINENT BACKGROUND INFORMATION

The requestor is a physician who is caring for a patient with severe hypertension. The physician plans to add minoxidil to the antihypertensive regimen because the patient's morning blood pressure is not optimally controlled. He would like to make sure that there are no drug interactions between minoxidil and the patient's other medications.

■ PERTINENT PATIENT FACTORS

S.L. is a 40-year-old human immunodeficiency virus (HIV)-infected man with severe hypertension and renal dysfunction.

Past Medical History

- HIV infection (2008)
- Hepatitis C (2006)
- Hypertension × 4 years
- Renal dysfunction

Social History

- 1 to 2 pints of vodka daily × 12 years
- 1 pack per day (PPD) of cigarettes × 25 years
- History of intravenous drug abuse

Current Medications

- Labetalol 400 mg orally daily (@9 AM)
- Clonidine transdermal patch 0.3 mg/day
- Amlodipine 10 mg orally daily (@9 AM)
- Lorazepam 1 mg orally as needed for anxiety
- Multiple vitamin tablet orally daily
- Ø complementary/alternative or other OTC medications

Allergies/Intolerances

- Lisinopril (angioedema)

Laboratory Results

- Sodium 136 mmol/L, potassium 4.7 mmol/L, chloride 102 mmol/L, CO_2 24 mmol/L, creatinine 2.9 mg/dL, glucose 98 mg/dL, BUN 14 mg/dL
- Viral DNA <100 copies/mL
- Cluster designation 4 (CD4) count 900 cells/mm^3

Blood Pressure Measurements

4/15		4/16		4/17	
@ 6 AM	172/116	@ 6 AM	168/110	@ 6 AM	178/114
@ noon	121/81	@ noon	116/86	@ noon	119/84
@ 8 PM	158/100	@ 8 PM	150/104	@ 8 PM	166/100

■ PERTINENT DISEASE FACTORS

It is not known whether patients with HIV infection respond differently to antihypertensive medications.

■ PERTINENT MEDICATION FACTORS

There are no primary or tertiary literature reports describing drug interactions between minoxidil and any of S.L.'s current medications.[4,9-12] A review of the patient's current antihypertensive medications suggests that the dose of each agent is appropriate for achieving adequate blood pressure control in the face of significant renal compromise.[13] However, the duration of action of labetalol is 8 to 12 hours, and this agent is typically dosed twice daily. S.L. is receiving 400 mg of labetalol daily at 9 AM.

■ ANALYSIS AND SYNTHESIS

S.L.'s blood pressure appears to be highest in the morning, just before the daily doses of labetalol and amlodipine are administered. He is receiving 400 mg of labetalol daily at 9 AM. Because the duration of action of labetalol is 8 to 12 hours, and the usual maintenance dose is 200 to 400 mg twice daily, the increase in blood pressure observed in the morning could be due, at least in part, to inappropriate dosing of labetalol. This medication should generally be administered twice daily to achieve maximal benefit. Adjustment of the labetalol dose should precede the addition of other antihypertensive agents to this patient's medication regimen. Although long-term cigarette smoking can increase the cardiovascular risk associated with hypertension, there is no indication that smoking or alcohol ingestion are contributing to this patient's present problem.

■ RESPONSE AND RECOMMENDATIONS

There do not appear to be any significant drug interactions between any of S.L.'s current medications and minoxidil.[4,9-12] Additionally, after considering the pharmacokinetics, pharmacodynamics, adverse effect profiles, and pharmaceutical properties of the patient's medications, the potential for a clinically significant drug interaction appears low. However, a review of the patient's current antihypertensive regimen suggests that the dosing of labetalol is inappropriate. The duration of action of labetalol is 8 to 12 hours, and the usual maintenance dose is 200 to 400 mg twice daily. Because S.L. is receiving 400 mg of labetalol once daily at 9 AM, the increase in blood pressure observed in the morning could be due to inappropriate labetalol dosing. The physician was directed to optimize labetalol therapy before the addition of another antihypertensive agent. If the patient's blood pressure is not controlled with proper dosing of labetalol and minoxidil therapy is required, the physician should be advised that minoxidil is usually administered with a diuretic to prevent fluid retention.

■ CASE MESSAGE

This is another example emphasizing the importance of the proper context of the question. In this case, the pharmacist was able to recommend appropriate drug therapy management, even though the initial question posed by the physician was not related to the dosage and administration of labetalol.

Case Study 2–4

■ INITIAL QUESTION

Can ranitidine cause thrombocytopenia?

■ POTENTIAL RESPONSE IN THE ABSENCE OF RELEVANT BACKGROUND INFORMATION

Ranitidine has been infrequently associated with thrombocytopenia.[4,14-16] This is a relatively rare but readily reversible complication of histamine-2 (H_2)-antagonist therapy.

■ PERTINENT BACKGROUND INFORMATION

The requestor is a physician who is evaluating a patient for suspected Cushing disease. The patient has been hospitalized for 8 days and has undergone extensive diagnostic tests, including serial blood sampling to establish the diagnosis. Over the last 4 days, the patient has experienced a rapid decline in her platelet count. The physician is aware that cimetidine can cause thrombocytopenia. Her patient is taking ranitidine, and she would like to know if the thrombocytopenia could be induced by this medication.

■ PERTINENT PATIENT FACTORS

L.B. is a 38-year-old obese woman with Type 2 diabetes who is being evaluated for Cushing disease.

Past Medical History

- Gastroesophageal reflux disease (GERD) × 6 years
- Type 2 diabetes × 1 year

Social History

- Ø alcohol
- Ø tobacco
- No occupational or environmental exposures

Current Medications

- Ranitidine 150 mg orally twice a day (intermittently for 6 years)
- Metformin 500 mg orally three times a day (for about 8 months)
- Heparin 100 USP units/mL (as needed for flushing heparin lock)
- Ø complementary/alternative or OTC medications

Allergies/Intolerances

- Penicillin (rash)

Laboratory Results

Sodium 137 mmol/L, potassium 4.9 mmol/L, chloride 102 mmol/L, CO_2 24 mmol/L, creatinine 0.9 mg/dL, glucose 133 mg/dL, BUN 12 mg/dL, albumin 3.4 g/dL, calcium 2.35 mmol/L, magnesium 0.81 mmol/L, phosphorus 3.8 mg/dL, liver function tests within normal limits, WBCs 5.6×10^9/L

Date	Platelet count
1/17	241 K/mm³
4/20[a]	230 K/mm³
4/24	212 K/mm³

4/25	159 K/mm^3
4/26	114 K/mm^3
4/27	97 K/mm^3
4/28	81 K/mm^3

[a]Day of admission.

■ PERTINENT DISEASE FACTORS

L.B.'s thrombocytopenia is of new onset and is characterized by a rapid decline in the platelet counts over a few days. This patient does not appear to have a readily identifiable medical condition as a likely cause of the thrombocytopenia. Furthermore, she does not have any clinical evidence of bleeding or thrombosis.

■ PERTINENT MEDICATION FACTORS

A review of the literature[4,14,17] indicates that metformin has not been reported as a cause of thrombocytopenia. Ranitidine, however, has been infrequently associated with thrombocytopenia.[4,14-16] This is a relatively rare but readily reversible complication of ranitidine therapy. Ranitidine-induced thrombocytopenia usually develops within the first 30 days of therapy, but its pathogenesis remains unclear. Most hematologic toxicities reported with the H$_2$-receptor antagonists appear to occur in patients with serious concomitant diseases or in those receiving other treatments more commonly associated with hematologic adverse effects.[14-16] Thrombocytopenia has been reported in about 5% of patients treated with porcine heparin.[4] Heparin-induced thrombocytopenia does not appear to be dose dependent and has been reported in patients receiving less than 500 units of heparin per day. This condition typically develops within 5 to 9 days after initiation of therapy and reverses readily after discontinuation of the drug.

■ ANALYSIS AND SYNTHESIS

Although both ranitidine and heparin have been reported to cause thrombocytopenia, heparin appears to be the most likely cause in this case. L.B. has been taking ranitidine intermittently for nearly 6 years. Thrombocytopenia induced by ranitidine usually develops within the first 30 days of therapy. Moreover, heparin-induced thrombocytopenia is a more common adverse effect and has been reported in patients receiving very small daily doses of heparin (including heparin lock flush solution). It usually develops within 5 to 9 days after initiation of therapy. Based on the presentation and temporal sequence of events, heparin-induced thrombocytopenia is the most likely explanation for L.B.'s acute drop in platelet count. Assessment of causality using the Naranjo algorithm (see Chapter 16 for more information on this algorithm) implicates heparin as a probable cause of thrombocytopenia in this case, with ranitidine and metformin as possible and unlikely causes, respectively.[18]

■ RESPONSE AND RECOMMENDATIONS

A review of L.B.'s current medications reveals two agents, ranitidine and heparin, that have been reported to cause thrombocytopenia.[4,9,14] Ranitidine-induced thrombocytopenia is most likely to occur within the first 30 days of therapy.[14-16] Because L.B. has been taking ranitidine intermittently for GERD for approximately 6 years, it is unlikely that ranitidine is responsible for the acute decrement in platelet count. Ranitidine, however, cannot be immediately ruled out as a possible cause. Heparin-induced thrombocytopenia is a more common adverse effect that has been reported even with very small daily doses of heparin (e.g., heparin lock flush solution).[4] The thrombocytopenia is acute and usually develops within 5 to 9 days after initiation of therapy. Based on the presentation and temporal relationship, heparin appears to be the most likely cause of thrombocytopenia in this patient. The physician was advised to discontinue the heparin lock flush solution, closely monitor the patient's platelet count, and test for heparin antibodies in order to establish the diagnosis and guide future therapy. If the platelet counts do not begin to normalize after discontinuation of heparin, other potential causes of thrombocytopenia should be considered.

■ CASE MESSAGE

This question highlights the importance of skillful problem solving. As always, collecting appropriate background information and patient data is critical. Analyzing this information before synthesizing a logical response is paramount for effective patient management. In this case, failure to recognize that the patient was receiving heparin lock flush solution could incorrectly have excluded heparin as a possible cause of the thrombocytopenia.

Conclusion

Formulating effective responses and recommendations requires the use of a structured, organized approach whereby critical factors are systematically considered and thoroughly evaluated. The steps in this process include organizing relevant patient information, gathering information about the disease states and affected body systems, collecting medication information, obtaining pertinent background information, and identifying other relevant factors or special circumstances. Once these data are collected and carefully assembled, they must be critically analyzed and evaluated in the proper context. Responses and recommendations are synthesized by integrating data from these diverse sources through the use of logic and deductive reasoning.

Self-Assessment Questions

1. Why is it necessary to gather background information and patient data? Why do pharmacists often fail to obtain this information?

2. What factors should be considered in making a recommendation regarding the dosage and administration of an antibiotic? Provide a justification for each factor you select.

3. Given the question, "Can naproxen cause nephrotoxicity?" list at least five related questions that should be considered.

4. List three patient-related factors that should be considered for a question pertaining to a potential drug interaction.

5. How would you handle a requester who may be difficult to understand, aggressive, or impatient.

6. How can you ensure that the information you provide is correctly applied? How will you know if you were successful?

7. Can patient-specific recommendations be made in the absence of adequate background information and patient data? Please elaborate.

8. What are your options in responding to patient-specific queries in cases where there is insufficient or inadequate clinical data? Please elaborate.

REFERENCES

1. Watanabe AS, Conner CS. Principles of Drug Information Services. Hamilton (IL): Drug Intelligence Publications Inc; 1978.
2. Galt KA, Calis KA, Turcasso NM. Clinical Skills Program: Module 3 Drug Information. Bethesda (MD): American Society of Health-System Pharmacists Inc; 1995.
3. Calis KA, Anderson DW, Auth DA, Mays DA, Turcasso NM, Meyer CC, Young LR. Quality of pharmacotherapy consultations provided by drug information centers in the United States. Pharmacotherapy. 2000;20(7):830-6.

4. McEvoy GK, ed. AHFS Drug Information 2010. Bethesda (MD): American Society of Health-System Pharmacists; 2010.

5. Vasotec [package insert]. Bridgewater (NJ): BTA Pharmaceuticals, Inc; 2010.

6. O'Neil MJ, Smith A, Heckelman PE, Obenchain JR Jr, eds. The Merck Index: An Encyclopedia of Chemicals, Drugs, and Biologicals. 14th ed. Whitehouse Station (NJ): Merck & Co; 2006.

7. Neumega [package insert]. Philadelphia (PA): Wyeth Pharmaceuticals; 2011.

8. Gordon MS, McCaskill-Stevens WJ, Battiato LA, et al. A phase I trial of recombinant human interleukin-11 (Neumega rhIL-11 growth factor) in women with breast cancer receiving chemotherapy. Blood. 1996;87(9):3615-24.

9. DRUG-REAX system. Greenwood Village, CO: Thomson MICROMEDEX [cited 2011 Apr 25]. Available from: http://thomsonhc.com.

10. Hansten PD, Horne JR. Drug Interactions: Analysis and Management. St. Louis (MO): Wolters Kluwer Health; 2009.

11. Tatro DS, ed. Drug Interaction Facts. St. Louis (MO): Wolters Kluwer Health; 2007.

12. Zucchero FJ, Hogan MJ, Sommer CD, eds. Evaluation of Drug Interactions. St. Louis (MO): First Databank; 2004.

13. Aronoff GR, Bennett WM, Berns JS, Bier ME, eds. Drug Prescribing in Renal Failure. 5th ed. Philadelphia (PA): American College of Physicians; 2007.

14. Aronson JK, Dukes MNG, Meyler L, eds. Meyler's Side Effects of Drugs. 15th ed. Amsterdam, The Netherlands: Elsevier Science; 2006.

15. Yim JM, Frazier JL. Ranitidine and thrombocytopenia. J Pharm Technol. 1995;11:263-6.

16. Wade EE, Rebuck JA, Healey MA, Rogers FB. H_2 antagonist-induced thrombocytopenia: is this a real phenomenon? Intensive Care Med. 2002;28(4):459-65.

17. Glucophage [package insert]. Princeton (NJ): Bristol-Myers Squibb; 2009.

18. Naranjo CA, Busto U, Sellers EM, et al. A method for estimating the probability of adverse drug reactions. Clin Pharmacol Ther. 1981;30:239-45.

3

Chapter Three

Drug Information Resources

Kelly M. Shields • Elaine Blythe

Learning Objectives

After completing this chapter, the reader will be able to

- Differentiate between primary, secondary, and tertiary sources of information.
- Identify resources relevant to different pharmacy practice areas.
- Select appropriate resources for a specific drug information request.
- Describe the role of Internet and personal digital assistant (PDA)/smartphone resources in the provision of drug information.
- Evaluate tertiary resources to determine appropriateness of information.
- Describe appropriate search strategy for use with computerized secondary databases.
- Recognize alternative resources for provision of drug information.
- Identify the most appropriate resource to verify a veterinary dose upon receiving a prescription for a companion animal in a community pharmacy setting.
- Select the best online resource to educate pharmacists on contemporary issues surrounding veterinary compounding.

Key Concepts

❶ Tertiary sources provide information that has been filtered and summarized by an author or editor to provide a quick easy summary of a topic.

❷ Community pharmacy settings are a unique environment to practice One Medicine, a blending of veterinary medicine and human medicine for the benefit of public health, and to better serve human and animal patients alike.

❸ Comprehensive searches for information will require the use of multiple databases and resources.

❹ Primary literature may be a variety of types of articles, not just clinical trials.

❺ At times even well-designed searches of standard medical literature will not yield sufficient information to make clinical decisions or recommendations, and alternative resources may be needed.

❻ Understanding where to access information is only the first step in the provision of quality drug information.

Introduction

The quantity of medical information and medical literature available is growing at an astounding rate. The technology by which this information can be accessed is also improving exponentially. The introduction of PDAs/smartphones and Internet resources has radically changed the methods and technology by which information is accessed, but not the process of providing drug information.

On a daily basis, pharmacists are being asked to provide responses to numerous drug information requests for a variety of people. It is tempting just to select the easiest, most familiar resources to find information; however, by doing that, there is the possibility of missing new resources or limiting the comprehensiveness of the information found. It is for these reasons that the systematic approach discussed in Chapter 2 is helpful in order to streamline the search process.

Generally the best method to find information includes a stepwise approach moving first through tertiary (e.g., textbooks, full-text databases, review articles), then secondary (e.g., indexing or abstracting service), and finally primary (e.g., clinical studies) literature. The tertiary sources will provide the practitioner with general information needed to familiarize the reader with the topic. This is also an opportunity for the practitioner to gain general information about the disease or drug in question, which will ultimately result in a more structured and productive search.

If the information obtained in the tertiary resources is not recent or comprehensive enough, a secondary database may be employed to direct the reader to review or primary literature articles that may provide more insight on the topic. Primary literature often provides the most recent and in-depth information about a topic, and allows the reader to analyze and critique the study methodology to determine if the conclusions are valid (see Chapters 4 and 5 for more information on critiquing the primary literature).

●   For some requests it may be necessary to consult news reports or other Internet sites to get background information before beginning the searching process. Also, other resources, including experts or specialists in particular areas of practice, may need to be consulted. More information will be provided about these resources later in the chapter.

●   Often a search for information will not employ all of these steps nor require the use of all three types of resources. For example, a question regarding commercial availability of a product formulation, or mechanism of action, could quickly be found in a tertiary resource. The information found there may be sufficient to conclude the search and provide a response. However, a question regarding the clinical trials supporting off-label use in a specific population will likely require a search of primary literature.

    The type of requestor may also substantially influence the resources used to respond to a question. Generally, a request from a consumer or patient could more appropriately be answered from available tertiary resources than from a stack of clinical trials. However, if the requestor is a prescriber requesting detailed information about the management of a specific disease state and role of investigational therapies, provision of primary literature may be appropriate.

    The provision of drug information is continually expanding into new areas and technologies that may impact selection of resources. For example, increased patient use of dietary supplements and alternative therapies has left medical professionals seeking information on these topics. Pharmacists are often expected to respond to questions about these topics and provide recommendations as to management of patients using these therapies. Also increasing interest in the practice of veterinary pharmacy underscores the need for pharmacists to be able to practically apply drug information resources for the benefit of animal patients, animal owners, and veterinary professionals. Additionally, the emergence of completely new fields of practice, like pharmacogenomics, offer opportunities for pharmacists to apply their training in nontraditional roles.

Tertiary Resources

● ❶ *Tertiary sources provide information that has been summarized and distilled by the author or editor to provide a quick easy summary of a topic.* Some examples of tertiary resources include textbooks, compendia, review articles in journals, and other general information, such as may be found on the Internet. These references may often serve as an initial place to identify information, since they provide a fairly complete and concise overview of information available on a specific topic. These resources are also convenient, easy to use, and familiar to most practitioners. Most of the information needed by a practitioner can be found in these sources, making these excellent first- line resources when dealing with a drug information question.

- The major drawback to tertiary resources, however, is the lag time associated with publication, resulting in less current information. Medical information changes so rapidly that it is possible that information may be out of date before a text is even published. Electronically available tertiary resources have to some extent helped this situation; however, the requirement for information to be reviewed and summarized requires an inherent
- delay in communicating new information. It is also possible that information in a tertiary text may be incomplete, due either to space limitations of the resource or incomplete literature searches by the author. Other problems that can be seen with tertiary information include errors in transcription, human bias, incorrect interpretation of information, or a lack of expertise by authors. For these reasons readers must judge the quality of tertiary references at often verify the information in multiple sources. Some questions that should be considered when evaluating tertiary literature are listed in Table 3–1.

It is impossible to compile a comprehensive list of tertiary resources that are useful in all areas of pharmacy practice. Differences in practice setting, available funding, patients seen, and types of information most commonly needed, all impact which tertiary resources should be available at a specific practice site. The legal requirements for information sources available at a practice setting vary from state to state, but rarely will the minimally required texts be sufficient to meet all information needs in a practice.

Another important factor in the selection of appropriate tertiary resources includes selecting a resource focused on the type of information needed for a specific request or situation. For example, a very well-written and comprehensive therapeutics text may have very limited use in providing information regarding pharmacokinetics of a specific drug. For this reason it is important to consider the categories of requests received in a particular practice setting to ensure that appropriate tertiary texts are available. Table 3–2 lists resources that may be useful for specific categories of drug information requests.

A brief summary of selected tertiary resources is listed to provide examples of some resources that may be useful in the general pharmacy practice. Information is provided about the features of the resource as well as the publisher and publisher Web site. While specific electronic resources may be hosted on a different Web site, the publisher site will direct users toward the appropriate link.

TABLE 3–1. EVALUATION OF TERTIARY LITERATURE

Does the author have appropriate experience/expertise to publish in this area?
Is the information likely to be timely based on publication date?
Is the information supported by appropriate citations?
Does the resource contain relevant information?
Does the resource appear free from bias or blatant errors?

TABLE 3–2. USEFUL RESOURCES FOR COMMON CATEGORIES OF DRUG INFORMATION

Type of Request	Useful Tertiary Sources	Secondary Resources
General Product Information	Major compendia*, Handbook of Nonprescription Drugs[1], product labeling,	MEDLINE, EMBASE, IPA, IDIS
Adverse Effects	Meyler's Side Effects of Drugs[2], Side Effects of Drugs Annual[3], product labeling, major compendia*	Reactions Weekly, MEDLINE, EMBASE, IPA, IDIS
Availability of Dosage Forms	Red Book[4], American Drug Index[5], major compendia*	
Compounding/Formulations	Remington: The Science and Practice of Pharmacy[6], Merck Index[7], A Practical Guide to Contemporary Pharmacy Practice[8], USP/NF[9], Trissel's Stability of Compounded Formulations[10], (Children's Hospital of Philadelphia) Extemporaneous Formulations[11], Ansel's Pharmaceutical Dosage Forms and Drug Delivery Systems[12], USP Pharmacists' Pharmacopeia[13]	IPA, IDIS, EMBASE, MEDLINE
Dietary Supplement	Natural Medicine Comprehensive Database[14], Review of Natural Products[15], Natural Standard[16], PDR for Herbal Medicine[17], Trease and Evans' Pharmacognosy[18], AltMedDex[19]	EMBASE, MEDLINE, IPA, IDIS
Dosage Recommendations (General and organ impairment)	Major compendia*, Drug Prescribing in Renal Failure[20]	MEDLINE, IPA, IDIS, EMBASE
Drug Interactions	Hansten and Horn's Drug Interaction Analysis and Management[21], Drug Interaction Facts[22], Stockley's Drug Interactions[23], Food-Medication Interactions[24], Drug Therapy Monitoring System[25], major compendia*	Reactions, IPA
Drug-Laboratory Interference	Basic Skills in Interpreting Laboratory Data[26], Laboratory Tests and Diagnostic Procedures[27]	———

continued

63

TABLE 3–2. USEFUL RESOURCES FOR COMMON CATEGORIES OF DRUG INFORMATION (CONTINUED)

Type of Request	Useful Tertiary Sources	Secondary Resources
Geriatric Dosage Recommendations	Geriatric Dosage Handbook[28], The Merck Manual of Geriatrics[29], major compendia*	MEDLINE, IPA, IDIS, EMBASE
Identification of Product	IDENTIDEX[30], Clinical Pharmacology[31], IDENT-A-DRUG[32], Clinical Reference Library[33], electronic Facts and Comparisons[34]	
Investigational Drug Information	FDA website[35], Clinicaltrials.gov[36], MedlinePlus[37], manufacturer websites	Current Contents, EMBASE, MEDLINE, Lexis-Nexis, IPA, IDIS
Incompatibility/Stability	Handbook of Injectable Drugs[38], King Guide to Parenteral Admixtures[39], Trissel's 2 Clinical Pharmaceutics Database[40], Extended Stability for Parenteral Drugs[41], Trissel's Stability of Compounded Formulations[10], Remington: the Science and Practice of Pharmacy[6]	IPA, IDIS, EMBASE, MEDLINE
International Drug Equivalency	Martindale: The complete drug reference[42], Index Nominum[43], Internet Search Engines, Specific country resources	
Method/Rate of Administration	Major compendia*	
Pediatric Dosage Recommendations	The Harriet Lane Handbook[44], Pediatric Dosage Handbook[45], Neofax[46], major compendia*	MEDLINE, IPA, IDIS, EMBASE
Pharmacokinetics	Applied Pharmacokinetics: Principles of Therapeutic Drug Monitoring[47], Basic Clinical Pharmacokinetics[48], Applied Biopharmaceutics and Pharmacokinetics[49], major compendia*	IPA, EMBASE, MEDLINE, IDIS
Pharmacology	Goodman & Gilman's: The Pharmacological Basis of Therapeutics[50], Basic & Clinical Pharmacology[51], Brody's Human Pharmacology: Molecular to Clinical[52], Modern Pharmacology with Clinical Applications[53], Principles of Pharmacology[54]	IDIS, IPA, EMBASE, MEDLINE

Pharmacy Law	Pharmacy Practice and the Law[55], Guide to Federal Pharmacy Law[56], State Board of Pharmacy web pages	Lexis Nexis
Teratogenicity/Lactation	Drugs in Pregnancy and Lactation[57], Medications and Mother's Milk[58], Catalog of Teratogenic Agents[59], Drugs during Pregnancy and Lactation[60], REPRORISK[61], major compendia*	Reactions, EMBASE, MEDLINE, IDIS, IPA
Therapy Evaluation/Drugs of Choice	Pharmacotherapy: a Pathophysiologic Approach[62], Applied Therapeutics: the clinical use of drugs[63], The Merck Manual of diagnosis and therapy[64], Harrison's Principles of Internal Medicine[65], Cecil Medicine[66], Textbook of Therapeutics[67], Conn's Current Therapy[68]	MEDLINE, EMBASE, IDIS, IPA
Toxicology Information	POISINDEX[69], Goldfrank's Toxicologic Emergencies[70], Casarett & Doull's Toxicology: The Basic Science of Poisons[71], Medical Toxicology[72], Poisoning & Toxicology Handbook[73], Haddad and Winchester's Clinical Management of Drug Overdose[74], TOXNET[75]	Reactions, EMBASE, MEDLINE, IPA, IDIS, BIOSIS
Veterinary Medicine	Textbook of Veterinary Internal Medicine[76], The Merck Veterinary Manual (MVM)[77], Pet Place[78], Pet education[79], Pets with Diabetes[80], Veterinary Drug Handbook[81], Compendium of Veterinary Products (CVP)[82], The Merck Veterinary Manual (MVM)[83], Exotic Animal Formulary[84], USP, Veterinary Medicine[85]	BIOSIS, EMBASE, MEDLINE

*Major compendia referred to in this table include: Facts and Comparisons[86], AHFS Drug Information, Physicians' Desk Reference, DRUGDEX, Clinical Reference Library[35], Clinical Pharmacology[33].

This list is not comprehensive and reflects only a limited number of resources available. The Basic Resources for Pharmacy Education listing distributed by the American Association of Colleges of Pharmacy (AACP)[87] was utilized in selecting the resources described in this chapter; additional commonly used resources in drug information[88] were also included. The complete document contains hundreds of other resources that may be useful depending on practice setting.

Veterinary pharmacy as a specialty practice is a growing area in the United States, and pharmacists are interested in obtaining veterinary-specific knowledge and skills. The growth in veterinary pharmacy has allowed pharmacists to apply their drug knowledge resources to veterinary situations.

Supporting the growth of veterinary pharmacy is the concept of "One Medicine," a blending of veterinary medicine and human medicine for the benefit of public health, and to better serve human and animal patients alike. From a clinical pharmacy perspective, veterinary medicine and human medicine complement each other, with the human-trained pharmacist being uniquely positioned to educate and serve veterinarians and animal owners.

❷ *Opportunities for the practical application of One Medicine can occur in community pharmacy settings as most pharmacists practicing in a community setting have been presented with prescriptions for animal patients at some time during the course of their careers. Veterinarians outsource more prescriptions to community pharmacists now than they did in the past; inventory control, high drug costs, and the need for compounded drug therapies have contributed to this shift.* The use of human-labeled pharmaceuticals prescribed in an off-label manner to treat companion animal disease states is a viable option for veterinary medicine. These factors contribute to a situation where pharmacists who receive veterinary prescriptions can be challenged in their knowledge of veterinary drugs, indications, dosages, disease states, and therapeutic monitoring parameters. Practice settings that provide care for animal patients may benefit from having access to the following resources. The resources used by someone who specializes in veterinary medicine are different from those found in a traditional pharmacy or drug information center. These resources are covered along with human references and are included below.

General Product Information

AHFS DRUG INFORMATION

American Society of Health-System Pharmacists (http://www.ashp.org). This drug information resource is organized by monographs containing information on both

FDA-approved and off-label uses of medications. It is designated by the U.S. Congress as an appropriate source of information for determining reimbursement of unlabeled uses of medications. Information about dosing in specific populations is also included, as is a wide variety of general information about medications. Some information is also available about compatibility and stability of injectable formulations. AHFS is available in paper format (updated annually). This resource has also partnered with Lexicomp (described below) and ePocrates Rx online to offer an electronic subscription combining multiple resources, both on the Internet and for PDA/smartphone devices.

CLINICAL PHARMACOLOGY

Gold Standard (http://www.clinicalpharmacology.com). This electronic database contains monographs of prescription and nonprescription products as well as some dietary supplements. Tools within the database allow users to screen for drug interactions, create comparison tables for drug products, determine intravenous (IV) compatibility (based on Trissel's 2 Clinical Pharmaceutics Database), and search for tablets by description or imprint codes. Patient education information is available in English and Spanish. It is available via the Internet, CD-ROM, as a PDA program, or as a smart phone application. This resource has partnered with Pharmacist's Letter and Natural Medicine Comprehensive Database to allow searching within all three resources with institutional subscriptions to all three.

MICROMEDEX HEALTH CARE EVIDENCE

Thomson MICROMEDEX (http:///www.micromedex.com). This electronic resource contains multiple databases that are searched simultaneously. One of the most commonly used sections is DRUGDEX, a database that contains information about FDA-approved indications, off-label uses, pharmacokinetic data, safety information, and pharmacology. DrugPoints provides a summary of the most critical information for a medication. Multiple interactive tools are available to assess drug-drug/food/supplement interactions, incompatibilities, and pharmacokinetic adjustments. A brief summary of common diagnostic tests and nonpharmacologic and drug therapy is available for common disease states. The IDENTIDEX database allows identification of drugs based on imprint codes. REPRO-RISK provides information on teratogenicity and lactation based on human or animal data. POISINDEX and ToxPoints describes the presentation and management of many toxicology scenarios. An additional section DRUGDEX Consults provides information regarding common questions for some medications (e.g., rate of cross-sensitivity between penicillin and cephalosporins). Patient education materials are also included in this database. The resource also contains information from the Physicians' Desk Reference (described below) and Index Nominum. This resource is available on CD-ROM, mobile devices, and the Internet.

DRUG FACTS AND COMPARISONS

Wolters Kluwer Health, Inc. (http://www.factsandcomparisons.com). This reference contains information about prescription and nonprescription drugs organized by drug class. Information is provided about specific agents, including inactive ingredients in commercial preparations. There are comparative monographs of drug classes to help discern differences between agents of the same class. This resource is available via hardcopy, CD-ROM, online, and for mobile devices. The electronic version of this resource allows for an integrated search across a variety of Facts and Comparison publications (depending on subscription purchased).

DRUG INFORMATION HANDBOOK

Lexicomp Inc. (http://www.lexi.com). This handbook is organized in brief product monographs, where information is presented regarding clinical use, safety, and monitoring for a variety of drugs. Data is presented about FDA-approved and off-label use of medications. There is a tablet identification section as part of the electronic format. The resource also has several helpful appendices providing treatment options and comparing agents in the same class. This resource is available in CD-ROM, PDA/smartphone, and online formats. The electronic versions allow for integrated searches of various Lexicomp Inc products (depending on subscription purchased) through the online Clinical Reference Library (http://www.crlonline.com). The online resource also includes medication pricing information provided by drugstore.com. This resource has also partnered with AHFS (described above) to offer an electronic subscription combining their two databases in a seamless search.

HANDBOOK OF NONPRESCRIPTION DRUGS: AN INTERACTIVE APPROACH TO SELF-CARE

American Pharmacists Association (http://www.pharmacist.com). This text is organized by body system, focusing on those disease states for which self-care may be appropriate. Information is provided about comparative efficacy of various over-the-counter (OTC) agents, as well as contraindications for self-treatment, drug interactions, and other safety information. Use of treatment algorithms and patient care cases make this resource especially helpful for students and new practitioners. The text is also available as an e-book.

PHYSICIANS' DESK REFERENCE (PDR)

Thomson Healthcare (http://www.thomsonreuters.com). This resource is a compilation of prescription product package inserts. Additional information includes contact information for manufacturers, a list of poison control centers, and very limited tablet identification. The company maintains a Web site, PDRhealth, which contains patient appropriate information. Information from the PDR is also available online at http://www.pdr.net or http://www.pdrhealth.com, via MICROMEDEX or in a PDA/smartphone format. In addition to the original PDR, there are a variety of specialty texts, including the PDR for Herbal Medicines, PDR for Nutritional Supplements, PDR for Ophthalmic Medicines, PDR for Nonprescription Drugs and Dietary Supplements.

USP DICTIONARY

U.S. Pharmacopeia (http://www.usp.org). This is the official resource for determining generic and chemical names of drugs, as well as the international nonproprietary name. Additionally, useful information such as chemical structure, molecular weight, Chemical Abstracts Services (CAS) registry number, and a pronunciation guide are provided. This resource is also available in an online format and in print.

Adverse Effects

MEYLER'S SIDE EFFECTS OF DRUGS

Elsevier Publishing (http://www.elsevier.com). This reference, published every four years, provides a critical review of international literature in the area of adverse events. Chapters are organized by drug classification; adverse events are organized by drug name and then by organ system within each drug. Information is provided about adverse events and management.

SIDE EFFECTS OF DRUGS ANNUAL: A WORLDWIDE YEARLY SURVEY OF NEW DATA AND TRENDS IN ADVERSE DRUG REACTIONS

Elsevier Publishing (http://www.elsevier.com). This reference which is updated annually serves as a companion to the text Meyler's Side Effects of Drugs. A team evaluates international literature published each year identifying new information and summarizing that information in this resource.

■ PERTINENT BACKGROUND INFORMATION

A 15-year-old patient has recently been started on atomoxetine for treatment of attention deficit/hyperactivity disorder. He is taking no other medications. He has noted recently that his hair is thinning and wants to know if this might be drug-related.

- *What are appropriate tertiary resources to consult for a response to this request?*

Availability of Dosage Forms

AMERICAN DRUG INDEX

Wolters Kluwer Health, Inc. (http://www.factsandcomparisons.com). Contains brief entries, indexed by product and generic name, with information about product use, available dosage forms and sizes, and manufacturer information. Several helpful charts are also available, including: look-alike/sound-alike medications, pregnancy categories, normal lab values, as well as common pharmacy calculations.

RED BOOK (RED BOOK DRUG TOPICS)

Thomson Healthcare (http://www.thomsonreuters.com). This resource primarily contains data regarding Rx and OTC product availability and pricing. There are also a number of tables listing information such as sugar-free, lactose-free, or alcohol-free preparations. Additionally information such as NDC numbers, routes of administration, dosage form, size, and strength are included. This resource is available in paper copy and CD-ROM.

Compounding Formulations

Some journals are especially useful for compounding formulations or "recipes," for example the International Journal of Pharmacy Compounding, U.S. Pharmacist, or American Druggist.

EXTEMPORANEOUS FORMULATIONS (CHILDREN'S HOSPITAL OF PHILADELPHIA)

American Society of Health-System Pharmacists (http://www.ashp.org). This resource is a compilation of published formulations with stability data. Most products are oral formulations to reflect the unique needs of some pediatric patients. Information is also provided about legal and technical issues in compounding practices.

MERCK INDEX

Merck & Co., Inc. (http://www.merck.com). This resource provides descriptions of chemical and pharmacological information about a variety of chemicals, drugs, and biologicals. Data includes Chemical Abstracts Service (CAS) number, chemical structure, molecular weight, and physical data, including solubility, which may be especially useful in compounding. This reference is available in print, online, and on CD-ROM.

REMINGTON: THE SCIENCE AND PRACTICE OF PHARMACY

Lippincott Williams & Wilkins (http://www.lww.com). This classic text contains information about all aspects of pharmacy practice. There is discussion of social issues impacting pharmacy as well as information about the basics of pharmaceutics, manufacturing, pharmacodynamics, and medicinal chemistry. Information is provided regarding common compounding techniques and ingredients. The paper text also includes a companion CD-ROM.

A PRACTICAL GUIDE TO CONTEMPORARY PHARMACY PRACTICE

Lippincott Williams & Wilkins (http://www.lww.com). This text resource with CD-ROM is organized in an outline format to easily find information. Discussion of compounding techniques and explanations of additives used in compounding are very useful. Students and young practitioners may find the sample cases especially helpful.

TRISSEL'S STABILITY OF COMPOUNDED FORMULATIONS

American Pharmacists Association (http://www.pharmacist.com). This text provides information about preparation of sterile and non-sterile dosage forms. The text is organized by drug and provides a summary of the properties of a drug, general stability considerations and stability reports of compounded preparations. There also is extensive information provided about beyond-use dating.

USP/NF

United States Pharmacopeial Convention (http://www.usp.org). This resource, available in both text and CD-ROM format, contains the official substance and product standards. Also, official preparation instructions are given for a limited number of commonly compounded products.

Dietary Supplements

NATURAL MEDICINE COMPREHENSIVE DATABASE

Therapeutic Research Faculty (http://www.naturaldatabase.com). This resource is available in a text form as well as online. It provides a summary of the information available for various dietary supplements and rates the relative safety and efficacy of those products. Searches can be performed by brand name of supplement or by a variety of common names. The electronic version includes an interaction checker and disease state/condition search. The electronic resource has also partnered with the USP Verified program to indicate which supplements have been certified to contain a quality product by USP Verified. This resource is also available for PDA.

NATURAL STANDARD

Natural Standard (http://www.naturalstandard.com). This resource is available in text and electronic forms. Extensive evidenced-based information regarding efficacy is provided. The monographs utilize tables to quickly summarize published literature and to grade the quality of that evidence. The monographs also provide detailed dosing information reflecting the doses used in clinical studies as well as those recommended by expert opinion. This resource is also available in a PDA/handheld version.

PDR FOR HERBAL MEDICINES

Thomson Healthcare (http://www.thomson.com). Products in this reference are indexed by common name, and information is provided regarding action, usage, dosage, and other clinically useful information. Citations to the primary literature are also provided at the conclusion of each monograph. The focus on strictly herbal products, rather than nonbotanical dietary supplements, may limit utility in some settings.

REVIEW OF NATURAL PRODUCTS

Wolters Kluwer Health, Inc. (http://www.factsandcomparisons.com). This resource provides information about the chemistry, pharmacology, and toxicology of a number of natural products, based on references to primary literature. A summary of relevant clinical trials is also available. There is also limited patient counseling information, but the strength of this resource is in the chemistry and pharmacology information. Recent revisions have dramatically increased the amount of information included in patient counseling sections. This is available in loose-leaf, bound, CD-ROM online, and mobile device formats.

TREASE AND EVANS' PHARMACOGNOSY

Saunders Ltd. (http://www.elsevier.com). This text offers a mixture of more classic pharmacognosy, crude plant-based drug classification and examination, and some of the more clinical applications, pharmacology, and phytochemistry. This is not a resource focused on patient-care issues.

Dosage Recommendations (Organ Impairment)

DRUG PRESCRIBING IN RENAL FAILURE

American College of Physicians (http://www.acponline.org). This resource addresses the changes in pharmacokinetics that occur as a result of renal impairment, and provides specific recommendations for dosing adjustment for medications. Information is provided in a variety of tables. Tables also include recommendations for dosage modifications for patients undergoing hemodialysis, chronic ambulatory peritoneal dialysis, and continuous renal replacement therapy. Citations to the primary literature are also provided.

Drug Interactions

HANSTEN AND HORN'S DRUG INTERACTIONS ANALYSIS AND MANAGEMENT

Wolters Kluwer Health, Inc. (http://www.hanstenandhorn.com). This resource provides summaries of, mechanism of, and management options for reported drug interactions. The authors also provide information regarding severity of interaction and any risk factors that may predispose patients to this event. The loose-leaf version of the reference is updated quarterly, while the bound is updated annually. Both provide rapid information regarding severity and likelihood of an interaction and actions needed to minimize this risk based on the case studies and primary literature available. Some of this content is integrated into other electronic Facts and Comparisons products.

DRUG INTERACTION FACTS

Wolters Kluwer Health, Inc. (http://www.factsandcomparisons.com). This resource provides information about drug-drug or drug-food interactions. Discussions of significance of the interaction as well as suggestions for management are included. This resource is available in both bound and loose-leaf texts. Electronically, it is available via CD-ROM and as integrated in other online Facts and Comparisons products.

EVALUATIONS OF DRUG INTERACTIONS

First DataBank (http://www.firstdatabank.com). This loose-leaf reference, updated six times per year, contains information, organized by drug class, about the management of various drug interactions. Information is provided regarding mechanism of drug interaction, recommendations for management, and clinical significance. This information is also available in an electronic database.

DRUG THERAPY MONITORING SYSTEM

Medi-Span (http://www.medi-span.com). This CD-ROM resource offers information about drug-drug, drug-food, and drug-alcohol interactions. Discussion regarding onset of interaction, severity, mechanism, and management are provided. Also summaries of primary literature are provided.

STOCKLEY'S DRUG INTERACTIONS

Pharmaceutical Press (http://www.pharmpress.com). This resource, available in CD-ROM, Internet, and print formats, contains concise summaries of drug interactions with supporting primary reference citations. The text uses of both British (BAN) and American (USAN) drug names.

FOOD-MEDICATION INTERACTIONS

Food-Medication Interactions (http://www.foodmedinteractions.com). This resource is available in print, PDA, and online formats. This focuses on the impact food may have on mediations and also highlights what foods should be avoided with specific medications.

Geriatric Dosage Recommendations

GERIATRIC DOSAGE HANDBOOK

Lexicomp Inc. (http://www.lexi.com). The monographs in this resource contain traditional sections of drug information, but focus on dosing recommendations for geriatric patients. There is a special section of each monograph addressing concerns specific to the geriatric population. Limited references to primary literature are provided. This reference is also available online, on CD-ROM, and in PDA/smartphone format.

THE MERCK MANUAL OF GERIATRICS

Merck & Co. Inc. (http://www.merck.com). This resource, available in print and online (http://www.merck.com/mkgr/mmg/home.jsp), focuses primarily on management of diseases and conditions common in geriatric patients. There is some discussion of appropriate dosing of medications in this population.

Identification of Product

IDENT-A-DRUG

Therapeutic Research Faculty (http://www.indentadrug.com). This resource is organized by imprint codes and provides identification of drugs based on those codes. Descriptions of medications as well as U.S. National Drug Code (NDC) and Canadian Drug Identification Number (DIN) are provided. Electronic and text versions of this reference are available.

Other resources, discussed elsewhere, also have some tablet identification features including Clinical Pharmacology, Lexicomp Online, MICROMEDEX, and Facts and Comparisons online.

Incompatibility and Stability

HANDBOOK ON INJECTABLE DRUGS

American Society of Health-System Pharmacists (http://www.ashp.org). This resource, commonly called Trissel's, includes information regarding the compatibility and stability of various parenteral medications. Information is primarily provided in the form of charts and tables, making finding information relatively quick. This resource also provides information about routes of administration and commercially available strengths. A pocket-sized handbook and a CD-ROM version are also available.

KING GUIDE TO PARENTERAL ADMIXTURES

King Guide Publications (http://www.kingguide.com). Over 450 intravenous drug monographs are provided, focused on compatibility information. Also limited information about stability is available. This resource is available in loose-leaf, bound copy, online, and for PDAs/smartphones.

TRISSEL'S 2 CLINICAL PHARMACEUTICS DATABASE

TriPharma (http://compoundingtoday.com/Trissels/). This electronic resource compiles data from other Trissel publications. Information about parenteral admixtures, compounded formulations, physical compatibility, and chemotherapy formulations is included. Extensive information is provided describing published information in advice in applying this information to specific clinical situations. This resource is available for the Intranet, as well as via CD-ROM and the Internet.

International Drug Equivalency

INDEX NOMINUM: INTERNATIONAL DRUG DIRECTORY

Medpharm Publishers (http://www.medpharm.de). This drug information source contains information on drugs available in over 130 countries. Information is included regarding structure, therapeutic class, and proprietary names for single entity medications. A CD-ROM is included containing contact information for pharmaceutical manufacturers worldwide. The information from this resource is also included in the MICROMEDEX Healthcare Series.

MARTINDALE: THE COMPLETE DRUG REFERENCE

Pharmaceutical Press (http://www.pharmpress.com). This resource includes information on a variety of domestic and international drugs. Proprietary names and manufacturer contact information are available for a variety of countries. Some information is provided about common herbal products as well as diagnostic agents, radioactive pharmaceuticals, and some veterinary products. This information is available in hardcopy, CD-ROM, via online subscription, and is also included in some MICROMEDEX Healthcare Series packages.

Additional resources are available that are specific to individual countries including Diccionario de Especialidases Farmaceuticas (Mexico), British Pharmacopoeia (United Kingdom), Rote Liste (Germany), Dictionary Vidal (France), Compendium of Pharmaceuticals and Specialties (Canada), and Repertorio Farmaceutico Italiano (Italy). Please note that each resource is in the native language of the country.

Pediatric Dosage Recommendations

THE HARRIET LANE HANDBOOK

Mosby (http://www.us.elsevierhealth.com). This resource, assembled by medical residents, contains a succinct discussion of common diseases and conditions of newborn to adolescent patients. A significant portion of the book is dedicated to medication dosing, specifically pediatrics. This section also contains information about common side effects and dosage forms available. This resource is also available for a PDA/smartphone.

NEOFAX

Thomson Reuters (http://www.neofax.com). This reference, available in print, mobile device, and online forms, contains brief drug monographs arranged by drug therapeutic class. Each monograph has information about dose, monitoring, adverse reactions, preparation of drugs, and limited references to primary literature.

PEDIATRIC DOSAGE HANDBOOK

Lexicomp Inc. (http://www.lexi.com). The monographs in this resource contain traditional sections of drug information, but focus on detailed dosing recommendations for pediatrics. There is also information about common extemporaneous preparations. Limited references to primary literature are provided. This reference is also available online, on CD-ROM, and for mobile devices.

Pharmacokinetics

APPLIED PHARMACOKINETICS: PRINCIPLES OF THERAPEUTIC DRUG MONITORING

Lippincott Williams & Wilkins (http://www.lww.com). The first section of this text includes general information about pharmacokinetics and pharmacodynamics as well as how these parameters may differ in specified patient populations. This text also addresses pharmacokinetics of specific drugs and drug classes. Case studies are included to allow experience applying the theory explained in the text. An appendix describes outcome studies with therapeutic drug monitoring.

BASIC CLINICAL PHARMACOKINETICS

Lippincott Williams & Wilkins (http://www.lww.com). This text discusses the basic principles of pharmacokinetics especially interpretation and implications of plasma concentrations. The second section of the book provides monographs and discussions focused on drugs most commonly assessed by blood concentration levels.

APPLIED BIOPHARMACEUTICS AND PHARMACOKINETICS

McGraw-Hill (http://www.mcgraw-hill.com). This text describes the role of pharmacokinetics as it relates to drug development and to patient care. This covers the clinical application of pharmacokinetics and also addresses the impact of pharmacogenetics on drug metabolism. This text is also included in the Access Pharmacy electronic subscription.

Pharmacology

GOODMAN & GILMAN'S: THE PHARMACOLOGICAL BASIS OF THERAPEUTICS

McGraw-Hill (http://www.mcgraw-hill.com). This classic pharmacology text also provides information about pharmacokinetics and pharmacodynamics of a number of drugs. The focus of the resource is to provide a correlation between principles of pharmacology and contemporary clinical practice. The text makes extensive use of charts and tables to convey information. This text is also included in the Access Pharmacy electronic subscription.

BASIC AND CLINICAL PHARMACOLOGY

McGraw-Hill (http://www.mcgraw-hill.com). This text, organized by therapeutic class of agents, provides general discussion of pharmacology principles as well as more detailed discussion of specific agents. Figures and tables are frequently used to illustrate difficult material. This text is also included in the Access Pharmacy electronic subscription.

BRODY'S HUMAN PHARMACOLOGY: MOLECULAR TO CLINICAL

Elsevier (http://www.elsevier.com). This text is designed with a student focus and emphasizes therapeutic impact of pharmacology. The text is organized by organ system impacted. The text also has accompanying PDA downloads and Internet updates.

MODERN PHARMACOLOGY WITH CLINICAL APPLICATIONS

Lippincott Williams & Wilkins (http://www.lww.com). This textbook is focused on the clinical application of drugs. The text has moved away from an emphasis on chemical structures to an emphasis on structure-activity relationships. This text also includes information on some common dietary supplements.

Pharmacy Law

Information about individual state pharmacy law is best obtained through the individual state boards of pharmacy. A listing of state board Web site URLs is available at http://www.nabp.net/boards-of-pharmacy/. Often the Board will have this information available in PDF format on the Web page. The Code of Federal Regulations containing aspects of federal law is available at http://www.gpoaccess.gov/cfr/index.html. General texts about federal law and the practice of pharmacy are listed below.

GUIDE TO FEDERAL PHARMACY LAW

Apothecary Press (http://www.apothecarypress.com). This text is geared toward students preparing to take the pharmacy licensure exam. Discussion is provided about major legislation and the impact of these laws on pharmacy practice. Practice exam questions and answers are also provided.

PHARMACY PRACTICE AND THE LAW

Jones and Bartlett Publishers (http://www.jblearning.com). This resource contains information about federal laws and regulations impacting pharmacy practice. Additional implications for pharmacy practice are provided for some legislation. Information is provided about federal and state regulation of product development, dispensing, and development. Various summaries of case law are provided. Additional information regarding Internet pharmacies and electronic transmission of prescriptions has been added.

Teratogenicity/Lactation

DRUGS IN PREGNANCY AND LACTATION

Lippincott Williams & Wilkins (http://www.lww.com). As the title implies, this text (often referred to as Briggs') focuses exclusively on information available about the use of medications in pregnant or lactating women. Summaries of the literature available regarding fetal exposure *in utero* or exposure through breast milk are provided. Animal literature is provided in cases where human literature is lacking. Additional information about recommendations by organizations such as the American Academy of Pediatrics is provided.

MEDICATIONS AND MOTHER'S MILK

Hale Publishing (http://www.ibreastfeeding.com). Information focused on safe use of medications, supplements, and vaccines in lactation is addressed in this text. Numerous case reports are cited and discussed; also some basic pharmacokinetic data of interest is provided. The text is organized by drug monograph, and for relevant sections alternative treatment options are provided.

CATALOG OF TERATOGENIC AGENTS

Johns Hopkins University Press (http://www.press.jhu.edu). This resource covers pharmaceuticals, chemicals, environmental pollutants, food additives, household products, and viruses and their possible teratogenicity. Special attention has been paid to international as well as domestic information.

■ PERTINENT BACKGROUND INFORMATION

A new mother has been breastfeeding her child for three months. The mother has recently been prescribed levofloxacin for treatment of an infection.

- *Is it safe for her to continue breastfeeding during this therapy?*
- *What sources could be consulted?*
- *What additional information is needed to answer this patient's question?*

Therapy Evaluation/Drug of Choice

APPLIED THERAPEUTICS: THE CLINICAL USE OF DRUGS

Lippincott Williams & Wilkins (http://www.lww.com). This text includes information about disease states and treatment options. Information is presented in the form of cases with follow-up discussion. Its focus is on clinical case-based presentation of information. There is also a pocket-sized handbook designed to accompany the text. This print resource is updated every 3-4 years and comes with a CD-ROM. A version is also available for use on a PDA/smartphone.

CECIL MEDICINE

Saunders (http://www.us.elsevierhealth.com). This text is available in print, CD-ROM, PDA/smartphone, and Internet (http://www.cecilmedicine.com) formats. Information is organized by disease state and color-coded to speed usage. Information about etiology, manifestations, diagnosis, treatment, and prognosis are provided.

HARRISON'S PRINCIPLES OF INTERNAL MEDICINE

McGraw-Hill (http://www.mcgraw-hill.com). This text serves as a fairly comprehensive introduction to clinical medicine. It is available in text, PDA/smartphone, and electronic formats. Comprehensive information is presented including pathophysiology, differential diagnosis, and disease management. This text is also included in the Access Pharmacy electronic subscription.

THE MERCK MANUAL OF DIAGNOSIS AND THERAPY

Merck & Co. Inc. (http://www.merck.com). This source provides a quick summary of disease state information, including pathology, symptoms, diagnosis, and treatment. This resource is also available online as a free resource at http://www.merck.com/mrkshared/mmanual/home.jsp, and as a CD-ROM and a PDA/smartphone version.

PHARMACOTHERAPY: A PATHOPHYSIOLOGICAL APPROACH

McGraw-Hill (http://www.mcgraw-hill.com). This text focuses on the management of a variety of disease states. Information provided about disorders includes epidemiology, etiology, presentation of disease, treatment, and treatment outcomes. This is available in text and electronic formats. This resource also has accompanying texts: *Pharmacotherapy Casebook: A Patient-Focused Approach* and *Pharmacotherapy Handbook*. These texts are also included in the Access Pharmacy electronic subscription.

PHARMACOTHERAPY PRINCIPLES AND PRACTICE

McGraw-Hill (http://www.mcgraw-hill.com). This winner of the Medical Book Award from the American Medical Writers Association focuses on the management of a variety of disease states. Information provided about disorders includes epidemiology, etiology, presentation of disease, treatment, and treatment outcomes. While similar to *Pharmacotherapy: A Pathophysiologic Approach*, it is condensed and contains additional features to assist students. This is available in text and electronic formats. This resource also has the accompanying text, *Pharmacotherapy Principles and Practice Study Guide*.

TEXTBOOK OF THERAPEUTICS

Lippincott Williams & Wilkins (http://www.lww.com). PDA/smartphone, CD-ROM, and print versions of this resource are available. While the resource focuses on treatment of disease states and development of a therapeutic plan, sections regarding pathophysiology and clinical presentation are also provided.

Toxicology

CASARETT & DOULL'S TOXICOLOGY: THE BASIC SCIENCE OF POISONS

McGraw-Hill Medical Publishing (http://www.mcgraw-hill.com). This resource is designed to serve as a textbook rather than a quick resource for toxicology information.

Extensive information is provided regarding organ- and non-organ-directed toxicity. This text is also included in the Access Pharmacy electronic subscription.

GOLDFRANK'S TOXICOLOGIC EMERGENCIES

McGraw-Hill Medical Publishing (http://www.mcgraw-hill.com). This text is designed to offer a case study approach to toxicology. Initial basic toxicology data is provided, but the majority of this text focuses on management of toxicologic emergencies with a variety of common drugs, botanicals, pesticides, and other occupational or environmental hazards.

MEDICAL TOXICOLOGY

Lippincott Williams & Wilkins (http://www.lww.com). This text outlines the diagnosis and treatment of poisonings or drug overdoses. Chapters are included focused on biological and chemical weapons. One section is focused on the diagnosis of patients with poisoning symptoms when the cause is unknown.

Case Study 3–3

■ PERTINENT BACKGROUND INFORMATION

A pharmacy student is working on a presentation involving illicit drugs. She knows that there have been recent news stories about adolescents using Coricidin HBR products for recreational use, and she is curious to know the doses at which these products are toxic.

- *Which resources would be useful for her project?*
- *What search terms might she utilize?*

Veterinary Medicine

VETERINARY MEDICINE: GENERAL

The first five resources listed are some of the most useful, practical, and easily accessed resources that any health care professional can use to augment the clinical care of veterinary patients.

Veterinary Drug Handbook

This sixth edition textbook is written by a pharmacist and is considered one of the most useful references for extra-label drug dosages, indications, and specific drug information on human and veterinary labeled pharmaceuticals. Blackwell Publishing (http://www. blackwellpublishing.com/vet). Monographs are listed in alphabetical order, and categorize the drugs' chemistry, pharmacology, indications, species dosing, contraindications, and interactions into an easily identifiable format. It is often referred to as "The Virus" in veterinary medicine because it is everywhere. A client information booklet is also available.

Textbook of Veterinary Internal Medicine

Saunders (http://www.us.elsevierhealth.com). This is a practical, valuable, and informative two-volume resource, focusing on internal medicine topics in canines and felines. The text provides extensive coverage of pathophysiology, diagnosis, and treatment of diseases affecting dogs and cats.

Compendium of Veterinary Products (CVP)

North American Compendiums (http://www.nacusastore.com). This online reference is similar to the human Physicians' Desk Reference (PDR) in terms of information provided and format. The resource contains the product monographs for over 5000 FDA-approved pharmaceuticals, USDA-approved biologicals, diagnostic, feed-additive, and EPA-approved pesticide products that are currently available. The reference contains indexes of manufacturers and distributors, brand name/ingredient indexes, and product category indexes. It can be accessed online at no cost, but users must register at https://www.bayerdvm.com/index.cfm.

FDA, Center for Veterinary Medicine (FDA/CVM) Homepage

http://fda.gov/cvm. This Web site provides information for pharmacists about the legal or regulatory issues that affect the practice of veterinary pharmacy or veterinary medicine. It is useful for regulatory issues pertaining to animal health. The compliance policy guide (CPG 608.400) "Compounding of Drugs for Use in Animals" and the Animal Medicinal Drug Use Clarification Act (AMDUCA) can be found at this site; these documents are considered essential reading for any pharmacist who practices veterinary pharmacy. CVM updates are available that detail the prohibited use of drugs in certain animal populations. Updates on the judicious use of antibiotics in food-producing animals are posted at this site. A listing of all FDA-approved animal drug products, also known as the "Green Book," is available and searchable at this site. Patent information, manufacturer lists, indications, approval numbers, general drug information, code of regulations, and trade/generic names are just a few pieces of information that can be gathered from this Web site. Practitioners can also access the FDA Veterinarian Newsletter from this site.

American Veterinary Medical Association (AVMA), Scientific Reference Material on Veterinary Compounding

The American Veterinary Medical Association has a wealth of information at its home page (http://www.avma.org). For pharmacists and veterinarians alike, there is a collection of valuable veterinary compounding guidelines, brochures, federal regulations, frequently asked questions, definitions of compounding, and the AVMA compounding position statements at http://www.avma.org/issues/drugs/compounding/veterinary_compounding_brochure.asp. This information is an excellent starting point for any health care professional wishing to prescribe, provide, or utilize compounded drug products for animal patients.

Case Study 3–4

■ PERTINENT BACKGROUND INFORMATION

You have an appointment to discuss new compounded drug services with a local veterinarian. Your pharmacy has just begun offering veterinary compounding, and you are letting the local veterinarians know about your services. The first veterinarian you speak to starts referencing "AMDUCA." You have never heard of this.

- *What would be your search strategy to find out the meaning and relevance of this term?*

VETERINARY DRUG DOSING AND PHARMACOLOGY

The following print and Internet resources are useful for obtaining information on veterinary pharmacology and toxicology subjects.

Animal Poison Control Center

This Web site (http://www.aspca.org/about-us/animal-poison-control-center.aspx) focuses on animal toxicology and safety and is the premier resource for pharmacists in a community setting who may receive poisoning questions about animals. The American Society for the Prevention of Cruelty to Animals (ASPCA), Animal Poison Control Center, is a nonprofit organization dedicated to helping animals exposed to potentially hazardous substances by providing 24-hour veterinary diagnostic and treatment recommendations. A toll-free number is available for immediate assistance when faced with a toxicology problem (888-426-4435), and a fee is required. The Center has extensive experience in assisting veterinarians in poison management by providing immediate and specific treatment recommendations. The site also provides useful information on poison prevention, human medications that are poisonous to pets, and guidance on what to do if a pet is poisoned. References to toxicology publications and general consultation are listed in this Web site.

Exotic Animal Formulary

Elsevier (http://www.elsevier.com). This pocket guide provides quick, convenient access to essential pharmacology information for exotic animals. Indications and dosages for fish, reptiles, birds, rodents, amphibians, primates, and other exotic species are provided. The text contains tables, appendices, and a formulary containing commonly needed information for each exotic group.

The Exotic Animal Drug Compendium: An International Formulary

Veterinary Learning Systems (http://www.exoticanimal.net/drugbook/). This text provides a formulary reference for numerous exotic animal species (wildlife, laboratory animals, zoo animals, and exotic pets). The formulary contains 28 drug sections, with each section constructed as tables according to species, drug, dosage, and additional comments. Each listed dosage is accompanied by a notation as to how the dose was developed: pharmacokinetics research, clinical trials, anecdotal, or manufacturer. The book is written for veterinarians who care for exotic animal species and veterinary pharmacists who dispense the drugs.

POISINDEX

Thomson MICROMEDEX, (http:///www.micromedex.com). This electronic resource is a database within the MICROMEDEX Healthcare Series, and provides some information on the toxicology parameters of human medications in animal patients. While the information presented is based on human case reports, animal data is extensively referenced.

Small Animal Clinical Pharmacology and Therapeutics

Saunders Ltd. (http://www.elseiver.com). A useful pharmacology reference textbook focusing on pharmaceuticals for the prevention and treatment of small animal diseases. The book is divided into three sections detailing principles of drug therapy with special attention to clinical relevancy, the use of drugs from a categorical basis, and pharmaceutical use from a body systems approach.

USP, Veterinary Medicine

The site (http://www.usp.org) provides drug information, quality reviews, and veterinary news. The USP veterinary drug information monographs on antibiotic use in animals are available online at no cost; however, you must register first (http://www.usp.org/audiences/veterinary/). The site also provides information on drug standards for veterinary products and vaccine associated feline sarcomas.

Veterinary Pharmacology and Therapeutics

Wiley-Blackwell (http://www.wiley.com). This textbook provides comprehensive information on the basic and applied principles of veterinary pharmacology and therapeutics. Information on mechanisms of action, pharmacodynamics, and pharmacokinetics is detailed.

_____ Case Study 3–5

■ PERTINENT BACKGROUND INFORMATION

A decimal error has been discovered in the dosing of a 4-pound Yorkshire terrier. The prescribing veterinarian is calling you for specific information on the toxicological parameters of metronidazole, specifically the mechanism of toxic action. You have access to the local university's health science library.

* _What is the best resource to utilize to answer the veterinarian's question?_

VETERINARY DISEASE STATE

The following print and Internet resources are useful for obtaining information regarding veterinary disease states. There are also animal health Web sites that contain educational information written for laypeople.

The Merck Veterinary Manual (MVM)

Merck & Co. Inc. (http://www.merck.com). The manual has served veterinarians and other health care professionals as a concise and reliable animal health reference for over 45 years. The full-text electronic version is available for free online at http://www.merckvetmanual.com. A guide to abbreviations used in veterinary medicine is also included.

Vet Med Center

VetMedCenter (http://www.vetmedcenter.com). Vet Med Center's mission is to address and satisfy the information needs of the animal health care community. This site serves as a point of access for veterinary professionals and pet owners to comprehensive animal health information, reference materials, clinical databases, and news. The site is searchable by specialty (e.g., cardiology, dermatology, ophthalmology), current news, or wellness topics. The drug formulary can also be searched. Most of the information focuses on canines and felines.

Pet Place

The site (http://www.petplace.com) has pet centers focusing on different species (e.g., dog, cat, bird, horses, fish, reptiles, and small mammals) and is written for laypersons. The database includes articles on veterinary disease states and preventative medicine. The drug library search tool allows the user to find drug information on a specific pharmaceutical. There are also text and graphics describing medication administration techniques for dogs and cats.

Pet Education

This Web site (http://www.peteducation.com) contains a variety of information on many species such as the dog, cat, birds, fish, reptiles, and small pets and is written for laypersons. The site features a category on drug information, with subcategories on antibiotics, eye medications, ear and skin medications, pain relievers, and wormers. The site offers information about the common veterinary prescription and OTC medications, supplements, and nutraceuticals used in dogs and cats.

Pets with Diabetes

This Web site (http://www.petdiabetes.com) contains information on diabetes in small animals particularly dogs and cats. The site offers general diabetes education, drug information, and is written for laypersons. The site also offers insight and information on home testing and complications. There are also resources to support owners of diabetic animals.

CURRENT VETERINARY PRACTICE

American Veterinarian Medical Association (AVMA)

From this site, pharmacists can read about the latest developments in One Medicine, public health issues affecting human and veterinary patients, peer-reviewed journal articles, and legal/regulatory issues and recent developments in veterinary medicine. The site provides numerous links organized by discipline for locating information. Under the scientific resources tab, there is a resource titled Veterinary Therapeutics that is valuable for educating veterinary pharmacists about current therapeutics issues in veterinary medicine (http://www.avma.org/products/scientific/therapeutics.asp).

DVM Newsmagazine

A very informative magazine, found at http://www.dvmnewsmagazine.com, that reports on current issues within the veterinary profession, disease state updates, breaking news, practice management, and new products and devices for small animal, food animal, and equine practitioners.

Selecting a Format for Tertiary Resources

Pharmacists should also be aware that more resources are becoming available in a variety of formats. Many resources that have been traditionally only available in a paper text are now accessible via CD-ROM, the Internet, or via PDA/smartphone. Selection of the appropriate format (e.g., hardcopy, online, PDA/smartphone) is now another factor that pharmacists should consider when selecting resources for a practice site. Electronic resources are often preferred because they may be easier to use, allow quicker access to information, allow multiple searches to be performed simultaneously, and often contain the most recent information available regarding a topic. Additionally, many electronic networked resources allow use of the same resource at more than one location. This lets many practitioners access information from a variety of physical locations rather than being restricted to only medical libraries or drug information centers. Also, the use of PDA/smartphone references allows easy accessibility to a considerable amount of information from a mobile device.

Many texts are now being combined into one electronic package, for example the McGraw-Hill product AccessPharmacy (http://www.accesspharmacy.com/index.aspx). The combination of multiple resources in one package may make selection of resources for a practice site much easier, but also more costly. As these combination packages increase in popularity with students and universities, the expectations practitioners have for access to resources in work settings will likely also continue to increase.

References for PDA/Mobile Devices

The increasing incorporation of mobile devices into clinical practice settings has prompted an expanding choice of drug information databases for that medium. As described earlier in the chapter many of the major compendia available electronically also offer a product for a mobile device. It is important to recognize that the information available in a PDA/smartphone version of a database may differ from that available in the online or hardcopy forms.[89] One study looking specifically at dietary supplements databases highlighted some of the variations that may exist between different forms of the same resource.[90] Due to factors such as cost and memory requirements, practitioners must be judicious in their selection of databases to purchase for a mobile device.

A limited number of critical evaluations of these databases have been performed to aid in the selection of the highest quality databases.[91-93] Based on the limited data available Lexicomp, ePocrates, and Clinical Pharmacology OnHand appear to be among the best-quality PDA drug information databases available at the time of these studies. One additional study[94] evaluating the efficacy of PDA databases specifically for addressing drug interaction information found slightly different results from previous studies but did find Lexi-Interact to be one of the top performers, in addition to iFacts (www.skyscape.com).

Secondary Literature

Secondary literature refers to references that either index or abstract the primary literature, with the goal of directing the user to relevant primary literature. This type of literature can be used for multiple purposes; one can be to help keep a practitioner keep abreast of recently published information[95] or to help find more recent or detailed information on a specified treatment or disease. When discussing secondary literature, there are two very commonly used terms, *indexing* and *abstracting*; the two terms differ slightly. Indexing consists of providing bibliographic citation information (e.g., title, author, and citation of the article), while abstracting also includes a brief description (or abstract) of the information provided by the article or resource cited. ❸ *Various systems will index or abstract literature from different journals, meetings, or publications; therefore, in order to perform a comprehensive search, multiple secondary databases must be used.*

The vast majority of secondary resources are available and used electronically, although some may still have a print form. Using a paper resource will often require more time than the electronic formats, due to the need to look at multiple editions and indexes (possibly an annual or quarterly listing).

Electronic versions offer multiple advantages over print listings: notably, for online listings, the more frequent updating of listings and information. In searching most electronic databases, a user will follow a similar search strategy, with small changes to reflect differences in database systems. There are several challenges in searching secondary database systems. Systems do not index all terms the same, and so it is necessary to determine what terms a database is using in order to conduct a successful search. For example, databases through the National Library of Medicine index terms by their Medical Subject Heading (MeSH term), while the Iowa Drug Information System uses the United States Adopted Name and the International Classification of Diseases. To give an example to show the importance of these indexing systems, consider a search of Acquired Immune Deficiency Syndrome. If the indexing/abstracting system files things under that term, a search of it should produce the largest number of citations on the topic. However, some systems may instead file the citations under Acquired Immunodeficiency Syndrome (i.e., Immunodeficiency instead of Immune Deficiency), and some might just use AIDS, the acronym. If the researcher uses the incorrect term, the number of citations found is likely to drop dramatically. Sometimes, just the addition of the letter *s* to the end of a term can have a dramatic effect on the number of citations found. Most computerized databases also include a free-text search option, which is very useful when the defined index terms are not identifying relevant data. This option may also be helpful when the term is newly emerging or before an official index term is defined, but it is still the best practice to use whatever officially defined term is used by the indexing/abstracting system that is being searched and to realize that term may be different when another system is searched.

The need to utilize a variety of terms for search strategy is illustrated in the following sample question "Is clonidine effective in the treatment of attention deficit hyperactivity disorder (ADHD) in adolescents?" It is first important to identify the key terms. These terms might include *clonidine, attention deficit hyperactivity disorder,* and *adolescents.* However some databases may not recognize the term *adolescent* and instead use the terms *pediatric* or *child.* Additionally the use of the term *pediatric* may just refer to the medical specialty caring for pediatric in some resources, rather than treatment of a pediatric patient population. Therefore it is important to recognize that different databases may require different search terms to be used. Also the name of the disease state, attention deficit/hyperactivity disorder, has changed over time and so it may be necessary to use other terms, such as attention deficit disorder.

Electronic searches generally use the Boolean operators AND, OR, and NOT (see Figure 3–1), although some systems (e.g., Google Scholar) use proprietary systems that allow the user to put in their search in manners that seem more like a natural language. The use of logical operators, however, may help the searcher to best center a search more precisely on the topic of interest. The operator AND will combine two terms, returning only citations containing both of those concepts or terms. Combining two terms with the operator OR will result in an equal or greater number of returns since it will include any citation where either term is used. Use of the term NOT should be used with caution as it will always decrease the number of returns; since it eliminates any references having that term it may eliminate articles that may be appropriate, simply because the term being eliminated happens to appear somewhere in the article.

For example, in the earlier clonidine for ADHD question, the appropriate search terms (clonidine AND attention deficit/hyperactivity disorder) may be used with the

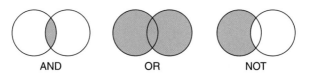

Figure 3–1. Boolean operators.

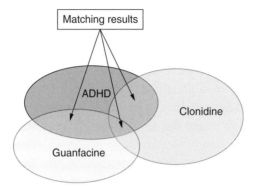

Figure 3–2. ADHD AND (clonidine OR guanfacine).

AND operator. However, if the requestor wanted information regarding use of either clonidine or guanfacine in this disease state, then the term OR might be used. See Figure 3–2 for a graphic presentation of this search. A search using OR will return a number of results equal to or larger than a search using the term AND. The term OR might also be useful when searching for a term with synonyms, for example, *attention deficit disorder* OR *attention deficit hyperactivity disorder*. The operator NOT would be helpful if a user wants to exclude certain topics, for example, a specific disease state. In this case a search might be performed for attention deficit hyperactivity disorder NOT Tourette disorder. Since the use of the term NOT will exclude any article mentioning Tourette disease, an article focused on treatment of ADHD with a small section about Tourette disease would also be excluded. It is for that reason that the use of the NOT logical operator is often avoided. Parentheses can also be used to further streamline a search. In this example, a search may be performed for clonidine AND (attention deficit disorder OR attention deficit hyperactivity disorder), this would retrieve articles that contain the drug of interest as well as either of the two disease states of interest. An additional example of search strategy using Boolean operators is provided in Appendix 3–1.

Some databases will also use the terms WITH or NEAR. These operators are similar to AND; however, they require the terms to be within a set number of words of each other. These terms may be useful when other searches are identifying a large number of articles where both terms are mentioned, but not in conjunction with each other.

Most databases allow results to be restricted via use of "limit" fields. For example, this may include language of publication, year of publication, type of article (e.g., human study, review, case report), or by type of journal where publication is found. This is most helpful when the initial search terms return a large number of possible matches. Using too many limits with the initial search may eliminate articles or citations that would be helpful.

Some databases have a surprising number of other terms that can be used. For example, the Medline system, even in the early 1980s, had methods to limit searches to authors in specific geographic areas or to search for a specific chemical structure.

One additional point to bear in mind when performing electronic searches is that the same search phrase could be indexed under a variety of search terms or spellings, and in order to provide a comprehensive search it is important to address all of those. For example, if looking for information regarding the herbal product ginkgo it may be helpful to search under the botanical name, common name(s), as well as common alternative spellings. So a possible search strategy may be to use the terms "ginkgo," "ginkgo biloba," the Latin name "Ginkgoaceae" as well as the misspelled word "gingko". This same principle holds true when considering disease states whose names may have changed over time.

Listed below are some examples of secondary databases and types of requests that are helpful in addressing.

BIOLOGICAL ABSTRACTS/BIOSIS PREVIEWS

Thompson Medical (http://www.scientific.thomson.com). This is a comprehensive database of biological information, covering biological and biomedical information. BIOSIS also covers abstracts from conferences relating to basic sciences. This is most helpful when seeking more basic science information about activity of compounds on a cellular level.

CANCERLIT

National Cancer Institute (http://www.cancer.gov/). This database is maintained by the National Cancer Institute and indexes literature from a variety of sources specific to cancer literature. This resource is most useful when looking for information about oncology therapies or quality-of-life issues. This resource is updated monthly and is available electronically at http://www.cancer.gov/search/cancer_literature/.

CINAHL

CINAHL Information Systems (http://www.cinahl.com). This is an indexing service that covers primarily literature in the fields of nursing and allied health. This database is useful when seeking information about patient care from the perspective of allied health professionals. It is updated monthly.

COCHRANE LIBRARY

Cochrane Library (http://www.cochrane.org). This database has three components including indexes of Cochrane reviews about a variety of medical treatments, conditions, and alternative therapies; abstracts of international systematic reviews, and a bibliography of systematic reviews in worldwide literature. These evidence-based medicine reviews are based on extensive analysis of current literature, and provide treatment recommendations (see Chapter 7 on Evidence-Based Medicine).

CURRENT CONTENTS SEARCH

Thompson Medical (http://scientific.thomsonreuters.com/index.html). This electronic service offers an overview of very recently published literature as it relates to scientific information. There are multiple subsets; the clinical medicine and life science subgroups are likely the most useful for practitioners and focus on useful information about recent drug research or developments.

EMBASE

Elsevier (http://www.embase.com). EMBASE is a comprehensive abstracting service covering biomedical literature worldwide. This database covers material similar to that covered by MEDLINE, but with greater coverage of international publications. Additionally there is less lag time between publication and inclusion in the database. This database is useful when seeking information about dietary supplements or medications that may be available in other countries.

GOOGLE SCHOLAR

Google (http://scholar.google.com). An Internet search engine that is designed to target scholarly materials available online, in a variety of professional areas including health care. Information from a variety of scholarly journals and publications is able to be searched; however, in some cases the searcher may not be able to access full-text versions of articles or works due to password restrictions.

INTERNATIONAL PHARMACEUTICAL ABSTRACTS (IPA)

American Society of Health-System Pharmacists (http://www.ashp.org). Coverage includes drug-related information, including drug use and development. This database also abstracts a variety of meeting presentations. The main focus of this database is pharmacy information, including pharmacy administration and clinical services, making it the most comprehensive database for pharmacy-specific information.

IOWA DRUG INFORMATION SYSTEM (IDIS)

Division of Drug Information Service, University of Iowa (http://itsnt14.its.uiowa.edu/). This is an indexing service that allows retrieval of complete articles from a variety of biomedical publications. Indexing is done by database-specific terms, which at times makes searching challenging. This database is useful for information about standard medications. It is unique in that it provides full articles, in either PDF form or, for older articles, microfiche. There are a limited number of journals covered, and not all articles from a specific journal issue are included (i.e., some articles may not be included if the editorial staff did not feel that they had sufficient focus on relevant drug or disease state information).

JOURNAL WATCH

Massachusetts Medical Society (http://www.jwatch.org). Journal Watch is an abstracting service including recent information, summarized by physicians, from a variety of medical literature. A general newsletter covering major medical stories of interest to generalists is published as well as additional newsletters in specific specialty areas. This is most helpful when monitoring for new clinical trials involving specific medications.

LEXISNEXIS

LexisNexis Academic & Library Solutions (http://www.lexisnexis.com). This indexing and abstracting service provides coverage of a variety of types of information, including medical, legal, and business news. Some publications are available full text through this service. This resource is helpful when attempting to locate information about recent medical news or research.

MEDLINE

National Library of Medicine (http://www.nlm.nih.gov). Coverage includes basic and clinical sciences as well as nursing, dentistry, veterinary medicine, and many other health care disciplines. Information comes from more than 5000 journals in 40 different languages. This database is available through a variety of publishers; free access to content is available via PubMed (http://www.ncbi.nlm.nih.gov/pubmed/). A sample search is provided in Appendix 3–1.

PHARMACOECONOMICS & OUTCOMES NEWS WEEKLY

Adis International (http://www.adis.com). This biweekly publication covers recent publications regarding economic use of health care resources, as well as information on prescribing trends, recent health care news and regulatory updates. The focus of this publication is the economic impact of disease states and medical interventions.

REACTIONS WEEKLY

Adis International (http://www.adis.com). A weekly indexing/abstracting service summarizing literature involving adverse events, drug interactions, drug dependence, and toxicology data. This resource is especially useful when seeking case reports of adverse reactions or other information on drug safety.

Case Study 3–6

■ PERTINENT BACKGROUND INFORMATION

A physician requests information about the use of sildenafil for treatment of female sexual arousal disorder. She also requests information about use of any of the other phosphodiesterase 5 inhibitors.

- *What resources might be good places to look for this information?*
- *What search terms should be used?*
- *Should limits/restrictors be used?*

In addition, there are a variety of publications targeting specific therapeutic areas that are available. For example, Adis (http://www.adisonline.com) compiles Anti-infectives Today, Cancer Today, CNS Disorders Today, and Pediatrics Today.

Also, it is worth mentioning that the various search engines may provide other services. For example, many of them allow practitioners to set up a search that they frequently want updated because of their practice situation. Once set up, the search can then be automatically run on that search engine, with the results being sent via e-mail to the requestor on a regular basis.

Primary Literature

Primary literature consists of clinical research studies and reports, both published and unpublished. Not all literature published in a journal is classified as primary literature, for example review articles or editorials are not primary literature. ❹ *There are several types of publications considered primary, including: controlled trials, cohort studies, case series, and case reports.* Additional information about study designs commonly found in medical literature and how to evaluate them is found in the two chapters on Drug Literature Evaluation.

Advantages to the use of primary literature include access to detailed information about a topic and the ability to personally assess the validity and applicability of study results. Additionally, primary literature tends to be more recent than tertiary or secondary literature. However, there are several disadvantages to the use of primary literature alone. These disadvantages include misleading conclusions based on only one trial without the context of other research, the need to have good skills in medical literature evaluation, and the time needed to evaluate the large volume of literature available.

Due to the rapidly increasing number of specialty journals being published it is difficult to determine which journals are really most essential in a pharmacy practice setting. A listing of core holdings for a college of pharmacy assembled by the American Association of Colleges of Pharmacy is available at http://www.aacp.org/governance/SECTIONS/libraryeducationalresources/Pages/LibraryEducationalResourcesSpecial ProjectsandInformation.aspx.[96] While this list may be more extensive than what is required in most practice settings, it does provide a core listing of journals. Each practice setting will require slightly different primary literature based on the specific areas that are of greatest importance to that facility and the patients cared for in that location.

In addition, the following reference is suggested for practitioners needing access to the veterinary literature.

JOURNAL OF THE AMERICAN VETERINARY MEDICAL ASSOCIATION

This periodical from the American Veterinary Medical Association is published twice a month, and abstracts can be found on a Medline search. The journal is peer reviewed and contains articles with a research or clinical focus. Full-text articles are available online with registration (http://avmajournals.avma.org/loi/javma). Regulatory issues and current topics in veterinary medicine are included in most issues.

OBTAINING THE PRIMARY LITERATURE

Once literature has been identified in a secondary searching system, the actual articles can be obtained in various ways. Many databases link users directly to the article of interest. For example, PubMed links users to open access journal publications and articles resulting from NIH-funded research through PubMed Central (http://www.pubmedcentral.nih.gov/).

However, many articles are not available via open access routes; in those cases alternative techniques may be needed. Once a citation is identified, then utilizing a local library catalog is a good next step. Often a local library may carry the journal needed, or may be affiliated with other facilities that can provide that article. Articles are often available for a fee via the publisher's Web site. If neither of these options is available, then the Loansome Doc ordering system may be used. This system is available through the National Library of Medicine and offered for a fee to any user. Articles identified in PubMed can be easily ordered from that database through this system. Additional information about this program is available at http://www.nlm.nih.gov/pubs/factsheets/loansome_doc.html.

Alternative Resources

INTERNET SEARCHES

❺ *At times even well-designed searches of standard medical literature will not yield sufficient information to make clinical decisions or recommendations. In these cases alternative resources may need to be employed.* One such method to identify relevant resources might be a general Internet search for information. This can be especially helpful to serve as a starting point for questions about uncommon diseases, new terms, drugs in development, or about marketed over-the-counter products and combination dietary supplements. For example, if a requester asked about use of a dietary supplement product called GABA Plus in ADHD, it would be difficult to search for information, unless the requester was able to provide a list of ingredients contained in the product. Often requesters may not have that information, and, therefore, it may be necessary to search for a manufacturer's Web site to identify the specific individual ingredients and then look for information on the individual components. This is also helpful in identifying information or specific product claims provided by the manufacturer. Additionally Internet searches may be useful for topics that have recently been in the news, where information is changing more rapidly than standard paper resources can be updated.

It is important to remember that different search engines use different techniques to identify Web pages, and that no search engines will identify all Web sites. Some search engines are geared toward scholarly content (such as Google Scholar, http://scholar.google.com) or toward scientific research (Scirus, http://www.scirus.com), rather than general information. These might be more useful for identifying recent research about a disease or disorder, rather than the ingredients in "GABA Plus." In order to efficiently perform a search, it is important to consider which search engine would most likely index the desired materials. Additional discussion of search engines is found elsewhere in this book.

There are however several caveats to finding information on the Internet. The first is to carefully evaluate the quality of all information provided. There are literally millions of

Web sites, and there are no true quality assurance measures in place to evaluate the reliability of information available. There are some general tenets to keep in mind when evaluating this type of literature. Generally sites maintained by educational institutions, not-for-profit medical organizations, or a division of the U.S. government are likely to contain high-quality information, whereas information maintained by a company selling a promoting a specific product may be more questionable.

In order to assess quality of online information several standards and programs now exist. These include organizations such as Health on the Net (HON code, http://www.hon.ch), which clearly define rules to evaluate the quality of information available via a Web site. These organizations do not evaluate every Web site available, but instead only those who request evaluation; since many Web sites do not request evaluation, the lack of an organization's quality seal does not necessarily indicate that the information is of low quality.

The following criteria may be some points to bear in mind when determining quality of online material.

- Is the source credible, without a vested interest in promoting one particular treatment or product?
- Is the information accurate and current?
- Does the site link to other nonaffiliated sites that provide consistently good information?
- Is the information appropriately detailed and referenced?
- Is it possible to identify the author of the site to contact with additional questions or comments?

Alternative Information Sources

Occasionally sufficient information to address a drug information request cannot be obtained from standard resources and may require the use of some alternative sources of information. If a question involves, for example, a recent news story reporting a removal of a medication from the market, a logical first place to find initial information would be to identify the original news story. This can be done by searching various newswire services like PR Newswire or even major news network Web sites such as CNN. LexisNexis (http://www.lexisnexis.com) indexes a variety of newswire stories as well as transcripts of news reports. While this news story may not provide all the information needed, it might at least serve as a point from which to search for additional information.

TABLE 3–3. **MAJOR NEWS SOURCES ONLINE**

News Source	URL
ABC	http://www.abcnews.go.com
AP (Associated Press)	http://www.ap.org
CBS	http://www.cbsnews.com
CNN	http://www.cnn.com
FDC Reports	http://www.healthnewsdaily.com/FDC/Daily/hnd/TOC.htm
MSNBC	http://www.msnbc.msn.com
Reuters Health News	http://www.reutershealth.com
PR Newswire	http://www.prnewswire.com

Case Study 3–7

■ PERTINENT BACKGROUND INFORMATION

A patient tells you she saw a news story on NBC that said all patients should stop taking Coumadin. She tells you she is not planning to take it anymore and wants the physician to find a different medication. She is indignant that you as a health care professional didn't know this was going on.

- *Where might you find a copy of the news story that this patient saw to help her better understand what the news reporter was trying to convey?*

In some cases there may be such limited information available that it would be wise to seek out an expert in the field, for example, a question about the use of heparin in a troche dosage form. In these cases it may be prudent to contact persons performing research in this area or practitioners who are currently using that therapy to identify information that might have been missed in an initial search or may not have been published. Some experts may be identified via medical organizations focusing on specific disease states, leadership of medical societies, or persons who have authored numerous papers on a specific medication or medical condition.

When looking for recent recommendations regarding treatment of a specific disease state, it may be helpful to identify an organization affiliated with that disease state. For example, when looking for treatment recommendations for management of irritable bowel syndrome it might be appropriate to contact the International Foundation for

Functional Gastrointestinal Disorders (http://www.iffgd.org/) to obtain information about current practice standards as well as possible emerging therapies.

Additionally when seeking information about a specific drug therapy it may be helpful to contact the product manufacturer via their medical information department to identify information that may be available in-house. This resource could be especially helpful for obtaining difficult-to-access literature if a product is newly approved, or identifying a possible rare adverse drug reaction.

Consumer Health Information

As consumers become more active and educated in their health care and disease management and more computer literate, the demand for health information sources designed for consumers has been increasing. Currently there are a variety of sources where consumers obtain their health information. Since many consumers find at least some of their information online, pharmacists should be prepared to help consumers evaluate the quality of information found on line as well as recommend sites where information might be found. Table 3–4 contains a listing of just a few of the sources that may be useful for consumers.

Consumers may also benefit from some text resources available at a local library. Some resources are published by organizations that produce references for health care professionals, while others are published by lay press companies. There is great variation in the quality of information provided from resource to resource. Some of the most popular resources may not be written at an appropriate level for a consumer to understand or may not provide helpful information for the patient. For this reason, it is important to discuss with patients what other resources they are using to find additional drug and medical information. Opening a dialogue with patients about this topic is fairly simple and can consist open-ended questions such as "Where else have you found information on your disease state?" or "What other material have you read about your medication/disease state?"

If being asked to recommend a source of online information for a patient, one confidently can recommend health care organizations or disease societies, both of which usually provide helpful, high-quality disease-specific information geared for the average consumer. The FDA and WebMD have now launched a joint online venture (http://www.webmd.com/fda) which directs consumers to reliable information. Also many drug companies offer Web pages with helpful disease or disease management information.

In addition to these resources aimed at consumers, there are consumer-specific sections of many tertiary resources discussed earlier. Electronic resources such as MICROMEDEX or Clinical Pharmacology have subsections dedicated to consumer-level information.

TABLE 3–4. **ONLINE CONSUMER INFORMATION SOURCES**

Website URL	Maintained By	Information
http://www.medlineplus.gov	National Library of Medicine	Contains information about various medications as well as disease states and conditions.
http://www.fda.gov/cder	Food and Drug Administration	Contains information about new drugs as well as dietary supplements. Also contains information about recalls of drug or food.
http://www.gettingwell.com	Thomson Health care	Contains information about a variety of prescription drugs.
http://www.merckhomeedition.com	Merck	This is a consumer-based version of the *Merck Manual*. It includes a variety of interactive features.
http://www.healthfinder.gov	Department of Health and Human Services	This site contains information about a variety of common medical conditions and diseases.
http://www.4women.gov	National Women's Health Information Center	This site contains information about the conditions and diseases of special interest to women.
http://www.cdc.gov	Centers for Disease Control and Prevention	This site has information about the treatment and prevention of infectious diseases. It also contains a listing of public health hoaxes.
dirline.nlm.nih.gov	National Library of Medicine and National Institute of Health	This contains a directory of health care organizations online.
ods.od.nih.gov	National Institute of Health	This site compiles some of the scientific information available about the efficacy and safety of dietary supplements.
nccam.nih.gov	National Center for Complementary and Alternative Medicine	This site is a government maintained in the area of dietary supplements, as well as detailing efficacy information currently available.
http://www.safemedication.com	American Society of Health-System Pharmacists	This site provides a patient version of AHFS Drug Information Resource, as well as tips about medication administration and resources to empower patients to better track/manage their own health care.

Conclusion

Given the rapid rate at which medical information is increasing and the amount of available technology to organize and locate this information, it is easy to become overwhelmed by the volume of data available. However, as pharmacists develop a better understanding of where to access information, provision of drug information will occur more quickly.

As technological advances continue, which may change the face of physical pharmacy dispensing and compounding, reliance on pharmacists for information retrieval and interpretation will continue to grow.

Practitioners must not, however, be satisfied with merely identifying sources for drug information. ❻ *Understanding where to access information is only the first step in the provision of quality drug information.* Information must be interpreted and evaluated to become knowledge, as is described in other chapters. It is this unique knowledge that will enable practitioners to optimize patient care.

The information in this chapter helps provide guidance as to where specific types of drug information might be found and how to begin a search for drug information. The next several chapters will provide additional guidance on how to interpret and apply the information that is gathered.

Case Study 3–8

■ PERTINENT BACKGROUND INFORMATION

A physician is seeking information about the use of chondroitin in the management of osteoarthritis. He sees a large number of patients in his practice and is seeking information about efficacy, safety, and appropriate dosing of this product.

- *What are the advantages and disadvantages of tertiary resources in responding to this request?*
- *What are the advantages and disadvantages of primary literature in this scenario?*
- *What might be appropriate key words to use to identify relevant information in a secondary database?*
- *Might information on the Internet be helpful in responding to this question?*

Self-Assessment Questions

1. If you were looking for information on an interaction between St. John's wort (an herb) and Prozac (a prescription drug), which source would likely provide this information?
   a. Review of Natural Products
   b. Drug in Pregnancy and Lactation
   c. American Drug Index

   d. Remington: The Science and Practice of Pharmacy

   e. The Harriet Lane Handbook

2. Which of the following would be the most useful resource when determining the U.S. equivalent of an international drug?

   a. Trissel's Handbook of Injectable Drugs

   b. Pharmacy Practice and the Law

   c. Index Nominum

   d. Merck Index

3. Which database would be best for finding information about a recent business merger of two large pharmaceutical manufacturers?

   a. International Pharmaceutical Abstracts (IPA)

   b. Iowa Drug Information System (IDIS)

   c. LexisNexis

   d. CINAHL

   e. Reactions

4. While searching for information on a specific medication, you find an electronic document describing a clinical experience of a practitioner with a patient who had an adverse reaction to a medication. What kind of literature is this?

   a. Primary

   b. Secondary

   c. Tertiary

   d. None of the above (electronic documents are not reliable)

   e. None of the above (electronic documents do not fulfil the criteria for any type of literature)

5. Which of the following references would contain information on the normal dose of a prescription medication?

   a. Red Book

   b. AHFS Drug Information

   c. American Drug Index

   d. Catalog of Teratogenic Agents

   e. Handbook of Nonprescription Drugs

6. A nurse calls you from the Intensive Care Unit, and she has a patient who is receiving an intravenous solution containing amoxicillin. The doctor has now ordered morphine to be injected into the Y site of the intravenous solution every 4 hours. The nurse wants to know if these drugs will be compatible at the Y site. Which reference would provide you with this information?

   a. Merck Manual

   b. Review of Natural Products

   c. Trissel's: Handbook on Injectable Drugs

   d. Index Nominum

   e. Red Book

7. A 75-year-old patient asks if docusate (an over-the-counter product) is safe for him to use with his other medications. Which resource would *not* be a good place to look for this information?

   a. Micromedex

   b. Drug Information Handbook

   c. Geriatric Dosage Handbook

   d. IDENTIDEX

   e. All of the above would be good sources for this information

8. Which of the following statements is true when considering drug information programs for PDAs?

   a. No major drug information database companies offer PDA programs.

   b. PDA versions of databases are identical to the online database.

   c. The quality of PDA programs have not yet been evaluated.

   d. The only PDA programs available are drug interaction checkers.

   e. None of the above are true.

9. A health care setting that wants to be able to perform comprehensive searches should make available which secondary resources to their practitioners?

   a. MEDLINE

   b. EMBASE

   c. Iowa Drug Information Service (IDIS)

   d. International Pharmaceutical Abstracts (IPA)

   e. All of the above

10. A physician calls you to compound an ointment called Whitfield's Ointment (which his father used to prescribe in the early 1950s). He wants you to start compounding this for his patients. Where might you look to find the formulation?

   a. Merck Manual

   b. Index Nominum

   c. Meyler's Side Effects of Drugs

   d. Remington: The Science and Practice of Pharmacy

   e. Natural Medicine Comprehensive Database

11. Which of the following would be classified as primary literature?
    a. Clinical trial
    b. Textbook
    c. Case report
    d. a and b
    e. a and c

REFERENCES

1. Berardi RR, Shimp LA, Tietze KJ, Kroon LA, McDermott JH, Newton GD, Oszko MA, Popovich NG, Remington TL, Rollins CJ. Handbook of nonprescription drugs. 16th ed. Washington, DC: American Pharmacists Association; 2009.

2. Aronson JK. Meyler's side effects of drugs: the international encyclopedia of adverse drug reactions and interactions. 15th ed. Amsterdam: Elsevier; 2006.

3. Aronson JK. Side effects of drugs annual: a worldwide yearly survey of new data and trends in adverse drug reactions. 31th ed. Amsterdam: Elsevier; 2009.

4. Red Book: Pharmacy's fundamental reference. 2010 edition. Montvale (NJ): Thomson Healthcare; 2010.

5. Billups NF, Billups SM. American Drug Index 2010. 54th ed. St Louis (MO): Wolters Kluwer Health; 2007.

6. Remington: The science and practice of pharmacy. 21st ed. Philadelphia (PA): Lippincott Williams & Wilkins; 2006.

7. O'Neil MJ. Merck Index: an encyclopedia of chemicals, drugs and biologicals. 14th ed. Whitehouse Station (NJ): Merck & Co. Inc; 2006.

8. Thompson JE. A practical guide to contemporary pharmacy practice. 3rd ed. Philadelphia (PA): Lippincott Williams & Wilkins; 2009.

9. USP 33/NF 28 2010: The official compendia of standards. Rockville (MD): United States Pharmacopeial Convention; 2010.

10. Trissel LA. Trissel's stability of compounded formulations. 4th ed. Washington, DC: American Pharmacists Association; 2009.

11. Jew RK, Mullen RJ, Soo-Hoo W. Extemporaneous formulations. Bethesda (MD): American Society of Health-System Pharmacists; 2003.

12. Allen LV, Popovich NG, Ansel HC. Ansel's pharmaceutical dosage forms and delivery systems. 9th ed. Philadelphia (PA): Lippincott Williams & Wilkins; 2010.

13. 2008-2009 USP pharmacists' pharmacopeia. Rockville (MD): United States Pharmacopeial Convention; 2008.

14. Natural Medicines Comprehensive Database [Internet]. Stockton (CA): Therapeutic Research Faculty. 1995 [cited 1 Jun 2010]. Available from: http://www.naturaldatabase.com

15. DerMarderosian A, Beutler JA. The review of natural products. 5th ed. St. Louis (MO): Wolters Kluwer; 2008.

16. Natural Standard [Internet]. St. Louis (MO): Mosby. 2001 [cited 1 Jun 2010]. Available from: http://www.naturalstandard.com

17. PDR for herbal medicine. 4th ed. Montvale (NJ): Thomson Healthcare Inc; 2007.

18. Evans WC. Trease and Evans' Pharmacognosy. 16th ed. Edinburg (TX): W. B. Saunders; 2009.

19. AltMedDex [Internet]. Montvale (NJ): Thomson Healthcare. 2002 [cited 1 Jun 2010]. Available from: www.thomsonhc.com

20. Aronoff GR, Bennett WM, Berns JS, Brier ME, Kasbekar N, Mueller BA, Pasko DA, Smoyer WE. Drug prescribing in renal failure. 5th ed. Philadelphia (PA): American College of Physicians; 2007.

21. Hansten PD, Horn JR. Drug interaction analysis and management 2009. 4th ed. St. Louis (MO): Wolters Kluwer; 2009.

22. Taro DS. Drug interaction facts. 2010 edition. St. Louis (MO): Facts and Comparisons; 2009.

23. Baxter K. Stockley's drug interactions. 9th ed. London: Pharmaceutical Press; 2010.

24. Pronsky ZM, Crowe JP, Elbe D, Young VSL, Epstein S, Roberts W, Ayoob TK. Food medication interactions. 16th ed. Birchrunville (MO): Food-Medication Interactions; 2010.

25. Drug therapy monitoring system v2.1 [Internet]. St. Louis (MO): Wolters Kluwer. [cited 1 Jun 2010]. Available from: http://www.medispan.com

26. Lee M. Basic skills in interpreting laboratory data. 4th ed. Bethesda (MD): American Society of Health-System Pharmacists; 2009.

27. Chernecky CC, Berger BJ. Laboratory Tests and Diagnostic Procedures. 5th ed. Philadelphia (PA): Saunders; 2007.

28. Semla TP, Beizer JL, Higbee MD. Geriatric Dosage Handbook. 15th ed. Hudson (OH): Lexicomp; 2010.

29. Beers MH, Berkow R. The merck manual of geriatrics. 3rd ed. Whitehouse Station (NJ): Merck Research Laboratories; 2000.

30. IDENTIDEX [Internet]. Montvale (NJ): Thomson Healthcare. 2002 [cited 1 Jun 2010]. Available from: http://www.thomsonhc.com

31. Clinical Pharmacology [Internet]. Tampa: Clinical Pharmacology. 2006 [cited 1 Jun 2010]. Available from: www.clinicalpharmacology.com

32. IDENT-A-DRUG Reference [Internet]. Stockton (MO): Therapeutic Research Center. 1995-2010 [cited 1 Jun 2010]. Available from: http://www.indentadrug.com

33. Clinical Reference Library [Internet]. Hudson (OH): Lexi-Comp. 1978- [cited 1 Jun 2010]. Available from: http://www.crlonline.com

34. Facts & Comparisons E Answers [Internet]. St. Louis (MO): Wolters Kluwer Health. 2003 [cited 1 Jun 2010]. Available from: http://online.factsandcomparisons.com

35. US Food and Drug Administration homepage [Internet]. Washington, DC: US Food and Drug Administration; [cited 1 Jun 2010]. Available from: http://www.fda.gov

36. ClinicalTrials.gov [Internet]. Washington, DC: US National Institutes of Health; [cited 1 Jun 2010]. Available from http://www.clinicaltrials.gov

37. MedlinePlus Health Information from the National Library of Medicine [Internet]. Washington, DC: National Library of Medicine; [cited 1 Jun 2010]. Available from: http//medlineplus.gov

38. Trissel LA. Handbook of injectable drugs. 15th ed. Bethesda (MD): American Society of Health-System Pharmacists; 2009.

39. King JC, Catania PN. King guide to parenteral admixtures. 35th ed. Napa (CA): King Guide Publications; 2006.

40. Trissel's 2 Clinical Pharmaceutics Database [Internet]. Cashier: TriPharma Communications [cited 1 Jun 2010]. Available from: http://trissels2.rcl.com/tsweb/

41. Bing CM, Chamallas SN. Extended stability for parenteral drugs. 4th ed. Bethesda (MD): American Society of Health-System Pharmacists; 2009.

42. Sweetman SC. Martindale: The complete drug reference. 36th ed. London: Pharmaceutical Press; 2009.

43. Index Nominum: International drug directory. 19th ed. Stuttgart: Medpharm Scientific Publishers; 2008.

44. Custer JW, Rau RE. The Harriet Lane Handbook. 18th ed. Philadelphia (PA): Mosby; 2009.

45. Taketomo CK, Hodding JH, Kraus DM. Pediatric Dosage Handbook. 16th ed. Hudson (OH): Lexi-Comp; 2009.

46. Young TE, Magnum B. Neofax 2009. 22nd ed. Montvale (NJ): Thomson Reuters Healthcare; 2009.

47. Burton ME, Shaw LM, Schentag JJ, Evans WE. Applied Pharmacokinetics: Principles of Therapeutic Drug Monitoring. 4th ed. Philadelphia (PA): Lippincott Williams & Wilkins; 2005.

48. Winter ME. Basic clinical pharmacokinetics. 5th ed. Philadelphia (PA): Lippincott Williams & Wilkins; 2009.

49. Shargel L, Wu-Pong S, Yu AB Applied Biopharmaceutics and Pharmacokinetics. 5th ed. New York (NY): McGraw-Hill; 2004.

50. Brunton LL. Goodman & Gilman's: The Pharmacological Basis of Therapeutics. 11th ed. New York (NY): McGraw Hill; 2006.

51. Katzung BG. Basic & Clinical Pharmacology. 11th ed. New York: McGraw Hill; 2009.

52. Wecker L, Crespo L, Dunaway G, Faingold C, Watts S. Brody's Human Pharmacology: Molecular to Clinical. 5th ed. Philadelphia (PA): Elsevier; 2009.

53. Craig CR, Stitzel RE. Modern Pharmacology with Clinical Applications. 6th ed. Philadelphia (PA): Lippincott Williams & Wilkins; 2004.

54. Golan DE. Principles of Pharmacology: the pathophysiologic basis of drug therapy. 2nd ed. Philadelphia (PA): Lippincott Williams & Wilkins; 2008.

55. Abood RR Pharmacy Practice and the Law. 5th ed. Sudbury (MA): Jones and Bartlett Publishers; 2008.

56. Reiss BS, Hall GD. Guide to Federal Pharmacy Law. 6th ed. Delmar (NY): Apothecary Press; 2009.

57. Briggs GG, Freeman RK, Yaffe YJ. Drugs in Pregnancy and Lactation: a reference guide to fetal and neonatal risk. 8th ed. Philadelphia (PA): Lippincott Williams & Wilkins; 2008.

58. Hale TW. Medications and Mother's Milk. 13th ed. Amarillo (TX): Hale Pub; 2008.

59. Shepard TH, Lemire RJ. Catalog of Teratogenic Agents. 12th ed. Baltimore (MD): Johns Hopkins University Press; 2007.

60. Schaefer C, Peters P, Miller RK. Drugs during Pregnancy and Lactation: treatment options and risk assessment. 2nd ed. Amsterdam: Elsevier Academic Press; 2007.

61. REPOTOX [Internet]. Montvale (NJ): Thomson Healthcare. 2002 [cited 1 Jun 2010]. Available from: http://www.thomsonhc.com

62. DiPiro JT. Pharmacotherapy: a Pathophysiologic Approach. 7th ed. New York (NY): McGraw Hill; 2008.

63. Koda-Kimble M, Young LY, Kradjan WA, Guglielmo BJ, Alldredge BK.. Applied Therapeutics: the clinical use of drugs. 9th ed. Philadelphia (PA): Lippincott Williams & Wilkins

64. Beers MH. The Merck Manual of diagnosis and therapy. 18th ed. Whitehouse Station (NJ): Merck Research Laboratories; 2006.

65. Fauci AS, Braunwald E, Kasper DL, Hauser SL, Longo DL, Jameson JL, Loscalzo J. Harrison's Principles of Internal Medicine. 17th ed. New York (NY): McGraw Hill; 2008.

66. Goldman L, Ausiello D. Cecil Medicine. 23rd ed. Philadelphia (PA): Saunders Elsevier; 2008.

67. Helms RA, Quan DJ. Textbook of therapeutics: drug and disease management. 8th ed. Philadelphia (PA): Lippincott Williams & Wilkins; 2006.

68. Bope ET, Rakel RE Kellerman RD. Conn's current therapy 2010. 2010 edition. Philadelphia (PA): Saunders Elsevier; 2009.

69. POISONDEX [Internet]. Montvale (NJ): Thomson Healthcare. 2002 [cited 1 Jun 2010]. Available from: http://www.thomsonhc.com

70. Flomenbaum N, Goldfrank L, Hoffman R, Howland MA, Lewin N, Nelson L. Goldfrank's toxicologic emergencies. 8th ed. New York (NY): McGraw Hill; 2006.

71. Klaassen C. Casarett & Doull's Toxicology: The Basic Science of Poisons. 7th ed. New York (NY): McGraw Hill; 2008.

72. Dart RC. Medical toxicology. 3rd ed. Philadelphia (PA): Lippincott Williams & Wilkins; 2003.

73. Leikin JB, Paloucek FP. Poisoning and toxicology handbook. 4th ed. Boca Raton: CRC; 2007.

74. Shannon MW. Borron SW, Burns MJ, Haddad LM, Winchester JF. Haddad and Winchester's Clinical Management of Drug Overdose. 4th ed. Philadelphia (PA): Saunders/Elsevier; 2007.

75. TOXNET [Internet] Washington, DC: US National Institutes of Health; [cited 1 Jun 2010]. Available from: http://toxnet.nlm.nih.gov/

76. Ettinger SJ, Feldman EL, editors. Textbook of veterinary internal medicine. 7th ed. Philadelphia (PA): W.B. Saunders; 2009.

77. Merck Veterinary Manual [homepage on the Internet]. Whitehouse Station (NJ): Merck & Co, Inc.; [cited 1 Jun 2010]. Available from: http://www.merckvetmanual.com.

78. PetPlace.com [homepage on the Internet]. Weston (FL): Intelligent Content Corp.; c1999-2010 [cited 1 Jun 2010]. Available from: http://www.petplace.com.

79. PetEducation.com [homepage on the Internet]. Drs. Foster & Smith Inc.; c1997-2010 [cited 1 Jun 2010]. Available from: http://www.petplace.com.

80. Pets with Diabetes [homepage on the Internet]. Petdiabetes.com c2000-2010 [cited 1 Jun 2010]. Available from http://www.petdiabetes.com.

81. Plumb DC. Plumb's veterinary drug handbook. 6th ed. Stockholm (WI): Wiley-Blackwell; 2008.

82. Compendium of Veterinary Products. 11th ed. Port Huron (MI): North American Compendiums; 2008.

83. Merck Veterinary Manual [homepage on the Internet]. Whitehouse Station (NJ): Merck & Co, Inc.; c2008 [cited 1 Jun 2010]. Available from: http://www.merckvetmanual.com.

84. Carpenter JW, Mashima TY, Rupier DJ, editors. Exotic animal formulary. 3rd ed. Philadelphia (PA): W.B, Saunders; 2005.

85. USP Veterinary Medicine [homepage on the Internet]. Rockville (MD): United States Pharmacopeia, c1997-2008. [cited 1 Jun 2010]. Available from: http://www.usp.org/veterinary.

86. Drug facts and comparisons 2010. 2010 edition. St. Louis (MO); Wolters Kluwer Health; 2009.

87. American Association of Colleges of Pharmacy [Internet]. Alexandria: American Association of Colleges of Pharmacy; c2008. Basic Resources for Pharmacy Education 2008; 2008 Dec [cited 2009 Jan 8]; [57 pages]. Available from: http://www.aacp.org/Docs/MainNavigation/Resources/9673_2008BasicResources.pdf.

88. Rosenberg JM, Kourmis T, Nathan JP, Cicero LA, McGuireH. Current status of pharmacist-operated drug information centers in the United States. Am J Health-Syst Pharm. 2004;61(19):2023-32.

89. Clauson KA, Polen HH, Marsh WA. Clinical decision support tools: performance of personal digital assistants versus online drug information databases. Pharmacother. 2007;27(12):1651-8.

90. Clauson KA, Polen HH, Peak AS, March WA, DiScala SL. Clinical decision support tools: personal digital assistant versus online dietary supplement databases. Ann Pharmacother. 2008;42:1592-9.

91. Enders SH, Enders JM, Holstad SG. Drug-information software for palm operating system personal digital assistants: breadth, clincical dependability and ease of use. Pharmacother. 2002;22:1036-40.

92. Lowry CM, Kostka-Rokosz MD, McClowskey WW. Evaluation of personal digital assistant drug information databases for the managed care pharmacist. J Manag Care Pharm. 2003;9(5):441-8.

93. Clauson KA, Seamon MJ, Clauson AS, Van TB. Evaluation of core and supplemental drug information databases for the Palm OS and Pocket PC. Am J Health-Syst Pharm. 2004;61:1015-24.

94. Barrons R. Evaluation of personal digital assistant software for drug interactions. Am J Health-Syst Pharm. 2004;61:1036-40.

95. Shaughnessy AF. Keeping up with the medical literature: how to set up a system. Am Fam Physician. 2009;79(1):25-26.

96. American Association of Colleges of Pharmacy [Internet]. Alexandria: American Association of Colleges of Pharmacy; c2008. AACP Core list of journals for libraries that serve schools and colleges of pharmacy 2009; 2009 Jan [cited 2009 Jan 8]; [4 pages]. Available from: http://www.aacp.org/site/page.asp?TRACKID=&VID=1&CID=380&DID=3619.

Chapter Four

Literature Evaluation I: Controlled Clinical Trial Evaluation

Michael Kendrach • Maisha Kelly Freeman
• Terri M. Wensel • Peter J. Hughes

Learning Objectives

● *After completing this chapter, the reader will be able to*

- List and explain the skills pharmacists need to locate and evaluate current information for pharmacy practice activities.
- Describe special characteristics of a controlled clinical trial that distinguish this research design as the prototype for clinical research.
- Differentiate between the types of data and measures of central tendency.
- Prepare a null hypothesis (H_0) based upon the clinical trial objective and endpoints.
- Differentiate between Type I and Type II errors; discuss methods to reduce the possibility of either of these errors occurring.
- Interpret p-values and 95% confidence interval (CI); discuss whether to reject or fail-to-reject the H_0 by using clinical trial results.
- Calculate and interpret relative risk (RR), relative risk reduction (RRR), absolute risk reduction (ARR), and number-needed-to-treat (NNT).
- State whether a statistical significance and clinical difference are present, using the clinical trial results.
- Explain the purpose and usage of editorials, letters to the editor, and secondary journals in critiquing clinical trials and in the decision-making process of applying the results into practice.

Key Concepts

❶ Pharmacists need to efficiently locate, critically analyze, and effectively communicate data from the primary literature in daily activities of patient care and the medication use process.

❷ A controlled clinical trial is the premier study design to measure and quantify differences in effect between the intervention versus control.

❸ Decision making should not rely solely on reading abstracts; the entire manuscript is to be read and thoroughly evaluated.

❹ The results of a controlled clinical trial should be extrapolated to the type of patient enrolled in the study, and readers should be aware of the limitations of surrogate endpoints and subgroup analysis results.

❺ Randomization is an essential component of controlled clinical trials and a significant differentiator from other study designs.

❻ The controlled clinical trial primary endpoint should be appropriate for the study purpose and measured using valid techniques and methods.

❼ An appropriate sample size in a controlled clinical trial is vital for the study results to have any significant meaning; conducting a power analysis is important to determine a suitable sample size.

❽ Correctly interpreting the p-values is crucial in evaluating a controlled clinical trial; not all statistically significant p-values are clinically important. The magnitude of difference in effect between the intervention and control cannot be determined solely with the p-value.

❾ The use of 95% confidence intervals can assist the reader in assessing the magnitude of difference in effect between the intervention and control.

❿ Calculating measures of association (RR, ARR, RRR, NNT) for nominal data provides further information to evaluate the meaning of controlled clinical trial results.

⓫ Non-statistically significant results do not equate to the intervention and control being the same or equal.

⓬ All controlled clinical trial results need to be assessed to determine the clinical relevance (i.e., meaningfulness) of the intervention versus control.

⓭ Controlled clinical trial investigators and authors should disclose any funding sources and potential conflicts of interest.

⓮ Editorials, letters to the editor, and commentary publications can assist in interpreting controlled clinical trial results.

Pharmacists continually rely upon the biomedical/pharmacy literature for many day-to-day activities. The practice of medicine and pharmacy are dynamic, and drug facts acquired during formal education cannot sustain a health care provider in future practice. Changes include new medications, dosage formulations, and uses approved by the Food and Drug Administration (FDA), revised drug safety information (i.e., adverse drug effects, drug interactions), and updated disease state therapeutic guidelines. During 2009, more than 20 new molecular entities/biological agents were approved by the FDA,[1] more than 80 drug safety alerts/notices for human medical products were issued by the FDA,[2] and over 500 published articles classified as human practice guidelines were added to the National Library of Medicine database.[3] Pharmacists must employ methods to keep current with these advances in order to remain competent, trustworthy health care professionals.[4] ❶ *Pharmacists need to efficiently locate, critically analyze, and effectively communicate data from the primary literature in daily activities of patient care and the medication use process.* Therefore, skills such as drug literature evaluation are necessary to prepare the health care provider for practice.

Multiple resources are available for pharmacists to provide answers to questions, care for patients, make decisions, and solve problems. But pharmacists need to recognize both the advantages and limitations of the information resources to meet the challenges encountered during their daily practice activities. Advantages include ready access and electronic formats. Potential disadvantages include biases, costs, and lag-time (i.e., lack of current content) that hinder the usefulness of some references. In addition, misinterpretation of the information can lead to improper patient care.

Although access to information for both health care professionals and laypersons has increased exponentially, not all information can be deemed accurate, and pharmacists are repeatedly relied upon to clarify, explain, defend, and/or refute information.[5] Thus, pharmacists must have skills in efficiently locating and critically analyzing drug information to appropriately formulate and effectively communicate a response. In addition, pharmacists are frequently consulted by other health care providers to assist in individual patient care regarding appropriate drug use.[5-7] Furthermore, pharmacists are in a position to select drugs for use in a multitude of patients (e.g., third-party health care plans, drug formulary decisions).[8,9] All these activities require pharmacists to carefully review and critique the literature instead of accepting the authors' conclusions. Many studies have very positive conclusions, but include study design errors that limit the clinical usefulness of the results. Also, medical/pharmacy continuing education presentations may contain biases and/or inaccuracies, while textbooks/review articles may contain misinterpreted, outdated, and/or noncomprehensive information. Due to the important contribution pharmacists have in patient care, pharmacists need to have skill in identifying the strengths and limitations of the biomedical literature. This chapter is devoted to explaining and discussing core concepts for critiquing one essential type of biomedical literature, controlled clinical trials.

Biomedical/Pharmacy Literature

Three types of literature serve as information resources for pharmacists: tertiary, secondary, and primary (Table 4–1).[10] Readers are referred to Chapter 3 in this text for more in-depth discussions of these three literature types.

Primary literature, specifically controlled clinical trials, serves as the foundation for clinical practice by providing the documentation for using therapy. Although vast numbers of primary literature articles are published each year, individuals can efficiently locate information specific and useful to their needs by incorporating appropriate search techniques.[11,12] Clinical trials are one particular type of primary literature that can be a reliable source of new information to change health care practices.[13-15] ❷ *A controlled clinical trial is the premier study design to measure and quantify differences in effect of the intervention versus control.* New information may either counter or serve as the root for altering existing practice regimens; thus, pharmacists need to critique clinical trials. The special features of clinical trial design allow investigators to determine which therapeutic interventions should be used in practice.[16,17] In fact, the FDA requires clinical trials to be conducted and the results submitted before a new molecular entity (i.e., medication) can be marketed and/or receive new indications for use.[18] Proper interpretation of clinical trials is vital to providing appropriate health care. Chapter 5 reviews evaluating publications using the other types of research designs.

In general, a controlled clinical trial consists of an investigational (intervention) group being directly compared to a control group (e.g., standard therapy, placebo).[16,17] The intervention under investigation may be a new medication, different medication dosing regimen, diet, surgery, behavioral process, exercise program, diagnostic procedure, or

TABLE 4–1. THREE TYPES OF LITERATURE

Literature Type	Description	Examples
Tertiary	Established knowledge	Textbooks, review articles, MD Consult, WebMD, Lexicomp
Secondary	Indexing/abstracting services (i.e., databases)	PubMed or MEDLINE (National Library of Medicine), Embase (Elsevier), International Pharmaceutical Abstracts (Thomson Scientific Inc.)
		CINHAL (Cumulative Index to Nursing and Allied Health),
		InfoTrac OneFile (Gale CENGAGE Learning), Academic Lexi-Nexis (Reed Elsevier Inc)
Primary	Original research	Controlled clinical trials, case-control studies, crossover trials, case reports

something else. The goal of the clinical trial is to measure and quantify the difference in effect between the investigational and control groups. The results then can allow decisions to be made regarding proper care for patients (i.e., to use or not use the investigational therapy).[16] Although the origins of the controlled trial date back to the eighteenth century,[19] a formalized process of conducting controlled clinical trials was not implemented until the late 1940s.[20] However, poorly designed clinical trials are still published, and the existence of a clinical trial may not translate into clinically useful information. Research has reported that results of well-designed clinical trials are considered to be of better quality and are usually more clinically relevant than clinical trials that are poorly designed.[21]

The published clinical trial is presented in a manner that explains the research process in an orderly format to improve the readers' comprehension of the study, results, and conclusions. Table 4–2 displays the style in which a clinical trial usually appears in printed resources.[22,23] This chapter discusses the information presented in these sections according to the CONSORT (Consolidated Standards of Reporting Trials) format. The CONSORT

TABLE 4–2. **FORMAT AND CONTENT OF CONTROLLED CLINICAL TRIALS**

Controlled Clinical Trial Section	Type of Information Presented
Abstract	Brief overview of the research project
Introduction	Research background
	Clinical trial objective
Methods	Study design
	Patient inclusion and exclusion criteria
	Intervention and control groups
	Randomization
	Blinding
	Endpoints
	Follow-up procedure
	Sample size calculations/power analysis
	Statistical analysis
Results	Subject characteristics
	Subject drop-outs/compliance
	Endpoints quantified
	Safety assessments
Discussion	Result interpretations
	Other study results compared
	Limitations
Acknowledgments	Other contributors
	Funding source
	Peer-review dates/manuscript acceptance date (not all trials)
References/Bibliography	Citations for information included from other resources (e.g., trials and reports)

format was formulated to improve the quality of reporting clinical trials in the published literature, since inadequate reporting methods hinder the interpretation of results produced by clinical trials. CONSORT has been supported by an increasing number of medical and health care journals, such as *Journal of the American Medical Association* (*JAMA*) and editorial groups, such as the International Committee of Medical Journal Editors.[23] Other research types (e.g., case-control studies) can report the investigation using the style of reporting a controlled clinical trial. Therefore, one should not assume all publications using this format are controlled clinical trials.

Evidence from clinical trials is used by health care providers to base their patient-care decisions.[13,14,24,25] A controlled clinical trial is the most robust method to measure and quantify differences in effects between a therapy under study and the control group.[16,17] Many clinical studies are published annually, but not every study initiated is reported in the published literature.[26-28] Primary reasons for not publishing trials are lack of time, funds, or other resources.[27] In order to treat patients most appropriately, all relevant information and data, both positive and negative, are needed in the decision-making process.[27,29,30]

Readers of the biomedical literature need to consider the issues of selective reporting (i.e., publishing positive study results but not negative studies). In addition, usually one clinical trial is not sufficient to adopt a therapy under investigation as the first choice to treat patients. Results of multiple trials are usually combined together to serve as the evidence for either incorporating a newly developed therapy into practice or changing the existing method of treating a disease (see Chapter 7 on Evidence-Based Clinical Guidelines).[31,32] Journal editors have an obligation and should publish negative studies. Results of these studies are important in formulating practice patterns based upon the available evidence. Failure by investigators and journal editors to publish negative studies contributes to publication bias.[29,33,34]

The intent of this chapter is for readers not to be misled by the literature, but to correctly critique the controlled clinical trial, then properly use the results and conclusions in health care practice settings. In addition to the discussions of critiquing clinical trials from this chapter, readers should use the principles of evidence-based medicine (Chapter 7) of this text in providing patient care.

Approach to Evaluating Research Studies (True Experiments)

Many different research designs are published, but the most common of these are prospective studies in which an intervention is directly compared to a control, and differences between these are measured. Examples of prospective studies include clinical trials (e.g., drug A versus drug B; drug versus exercise), stability of compounded drug formulation (e.g., suspension made from drug tablets), compatibility of intravenous drug mixtures, and drug pharmacokinetic interactions. Regardless of the study design and objective, fundamental elements should be present in all studies, including appropriate qualifications of the researchers conducting the research; valid investigational methods; proper research techniques; and appropriate analysis plus interpretation of the results. A similar process is used to evaluate prospective studies. A checklist for pertinent information to be included in a clinical trial is located in Appendix 4–1. Answering the questions contained in Appendix 4–1 can allow readers to determine the strengths and limitations of a clinical trial. The remainder of this chapter discusses the questions presented in the appendix plus techniques for critiquing a clinical trial.

Journal, Peer-Review, and Investigators

Numerous journals are published covering the professions of medicine and pharmacy. Health care practitioners need to regularly access professional journals (either print or electronic) to assist them in keeping current in their practice responsibilities.[35] Misleading information may be presented to health care providers by pharmaceutical industry representatives.[36] In addition, not all studies will be published in reliable journals[35] (i.e., in non-peer-reviewed journals[37,38]). One essential journal feature is the peer-review process. Simply defined, peer-reviewed articles are evaluated by someone other than the editorial staff (i.e., evaluation by one's peers).[33,39] Most journals incorporate the peer-review process in selecting articles for publication. Briefly, manuscripts submitted to the journal for publication consideration are screened by the editor; those deemed as potential publications are sent to individuals with expertise in the appropriate area. These individuals read the manuscript and comment upon the strengths and limitations, plus offer a recommendation to the journal editor regarding accepting or rejecting the manuscript for publication. The peer reviewers' comments are sent to the authors for the manuscript to be revised and, if necessary, resubmitted for publication consideration. In some cases, manuscripts may be rejected as being too flawed or inappropriate for the journal.

Although the peer-review process increases the time required before publication, the goal is to reduce the publication of manuscripts that have inappropriate methods/design, are poorly written, and/or do not meet the needs of the journal's audience.[39] However, the peer-review process does not always prevent publication of articles without deficiencies, and readers should assess the quality and critique each published article. Two journal sections can be checked for information addressing whether the peer-review process is used: instructions for authors and journal scope/purpose. Readers of the biomedical/pharmacy literature need to be aware of journals not incorporating a peer-review process and, therefore, not having this safeguard built in. Regardless of whether a clinical trial is published in a peer-reviewed or non-peer-reviewed journal, the article needs to be evaluated closely for biases and interpreted appropriately.[35]

As readers become more familiar with the professional literature, they will find certain journals have a reputation for good-quality publications, such as the *New England Journal of Medicine (N Engl J Med)* and *Annals of Pharmacotherapy*. This too can be considered in the evaluation of literature, although poor articles can still be found in well-respected journals, and excellent articles are published in other journals.

Research results can be published in other venues besides journals. A very common publication type is meeting abstracts. Research presented during a professional organization's meeting, whether as platform or poster, requires an abstract to be available for meeting attendees to review. These abstracts usually undergo the peer-review process to be selected, but readers should be cautious of the abstract content. The peer-review process may not be as thorough, and the entire study details are not available to the reader. Another common publication type for research is journal supplements. The purpose of such supplements is to publish a collection of articles related to a specific topic in a separate journal issue.[33] Many, but not all, supplements are sponsored by an outside entity (i.e., pharmaceutical company), which serves as another source of revenue for the journal. The articles may undergo peer review, but the process may not be as rigorous. Not all articles published in journal supplements should be automatically discarded or classified as inferior information. An example of a very informative journal supplement is the American College of Chest Physicians' supplement addressing antithrombotic therapy.[40] Many of the articles in this supplement are authored by recognized leaders and researchers in their field of practice.

Other factors to evaluate are the investigators' credentials and the practice site of these individuals. Investigators need to be properly trained and have active practice experience in the area of study. The site where the clinical trial was conducted should not immediately endorse or condemn the quality of the research, other than it should be a site that has the capability to perform the study (i.e., have the resources to properly and completely perform the necessary study methods). The quality of the research must be evaluated because even prestigious institutions can conduct poor clinical trials. Also, persons involved with the study need to be ethical and responsible to protect patients enrolled in the study.[41] Persons with specialized credentials in biostatistics need to contribute with statistical analysis of the data. Furthermore, all authors listed should have made substantial contributions to the research and/or publication. The "Uniform Requirements for Manuscripts Submitted to Biomedical Journals," prepared by journal editors, explicitly outlines the criteria for persons to be listed as authors for a published article. According to this publication, "An author is generally considered to be someone who has made a substantive intellectual contribution to a published study...."[33] The topics of authorship and publishing are discussed in detail in Chapter 9.

Articles with authors who are employees of a pharmaceutical company should be more selectively analyzed, since there may be concern about potential bias. The pharmaceutical industry must conduct research for new therapies to be introduced to the marketplace, and many companies are collaborating with academic researchers.[36,42] The concern regarding influence from the pharmaceutical industry on health care providers has not gone unnoticed, particularly involving practitioners conducting research for the pharmaceutical industry. In response, many journals now are requiring article authors to declare any conflict of interests with the research and outside interests.[33,41] A conflict of interest is possible even though investigators may not consider that their relationship affects their scientific judgement.[33] Authors need to state they have received honorariums and/or research grants or are members of the speaker's bureau for pharmaceutical companies. Readers should be informed of potential bias of the investigators. However, immediately discarding or discounting clinical trials in which investigators declare relationships with the pharmaceutical industry may be premature. Many investigators are required to obtain external funding for research projects and academic promotion. Clinical trials that have researchers with relationships with multiple pharmaceutical companies may not be considered to be overtly biased. Investigators have an ethical obligation to submit credible research results for publication.[33] Biases may be present, but readers having the skills of identifying study strengths and limitations can still use the clinical trial results appropriately.

Title

The clinical trial title is important and should be carefully evaluated by the reader. A title should be reflective of the work, unbiased, specific, and concise (i.e., usually ≤ 10 words), but not too general or detailed. Declarative sentences, which tend to overemphasize a conclusion, are not preferred for scientific articles.[43] In addition, the title should not be phrased as a question, and randomized clinical trials should be identified in the title.[23] Furthermore, the title should include terms both sensitive (easing the task of locating the appropriate articles) and specific (excluding those not being searched for) that allow electronic retrieval of the article.[33]

The following is an example of a biased study title: "Improved bronchodilation with levalbuterol compared with racemic albuterol in patients with asthma."[44] The title implies levalbuterol to be better than racemic albuterol. Although the average change in lung function parameters was slightly greater with levalbuterol, no significant differences were reported.[44] Thus, one could have been misled by reading only the title, believing levalbuterol to be a superior agent. A suggested unbiased title for this trial is: "Comparison of levalbuterol and racemic albuterol bronchodilation in patients with asthma: a randomized clinical trial."

Abstract

An abstract is considered to be a concise overview of the study or a synopsis of the major principles of the article. ❸ *Decision-making should not rely solely on reading abstracts; the entire manuscript is to be read and thoroughly evaluated.* Abstracts include information addressing the article objective, methods, results, and conclusions. A primary use of abstracts is for readers to obtain an immediate overview of the article to determine if the entire article should be read.[45,46] Another use is publishing the abstract in secondary resources (e.g., PubMed, International Pharmaceutical Abstracts [IPA]) for individuals conducting literature searches.

Although unique for each journal, authors are required to follow specific requirements while preparing an abstract. Many journals now require abstracts to be prepared in an organized format (i.e., structured abstract) and usually contain ≤ 500 words. The structured abstract includes the following sections: objective, research design, clinical setting, participants, interventions, main outcome measurements, results, and conclusions.[33,45] Structured abstracts, compared to non-structured abstracts, do have some advantages, including being more informative, easier to read, and generally preferred by readers.[47,48] However, structured abstracts usually require more journal space. Informative abstracts may entice some individuals to read the study; thus, abstracts should be thorough, complete, and unbiased in wording selection.[48]

Abstracts should be consistent with the manuscript and should not present biased and/or inaccurate information.[45,46,48] For further information regarding abstracts and preparation, please refer to the appendices in Chapter 9. Regardless of the abstract presentation style, readers should not make decisions based upon abstract information only. Results of three published studies illustrate the dangers of reading only the abstract.[49-51] These studies provided evidence of omissions and discrepancies between the abstract and the manuscript in medical, psychology, and pharmacy journals.

Introduction

The introduction section serves two specific purposes: discussing the study rationale and study purpose.[23,52] Usually, readers are first briefly educated on the issues that were the basis for conducting the study. The study investigators may state that the reason the research was conducted is due to the lack of data to answer a question or that available data are conflicting regarding an issue. Every clinical trial is designed to answer one or more primary questions. The investigators should explain how the clinical trial will overcome the shortcomings of the prior research, if applicable. The study objective is often stated within the last paragraph, if not the last sentence, of this section. Well-written studies present a clearly stated research purpose, and this statement should be understood by the reader before continuing with the remaining article content. Studies with a well-written purpose statement enable the reader to better comprehend and assess the research methods.

Once the clinical trial objective is determined, the investigators need to formulate a research and null hypothesis. A research hypothesis (also known as the alternative hypothesis) is a difference between the therapy under investigation and the control while the null hypothesis (H_0) is no difference between these two groups (see next paragraph for an example). After the study is completed, the researchers analyze the data and then the research hypothesis is either accepted (which also includes rejecting H_0) or rejected (which then means H_0 is accepted). Readers should recognize that not all clinical trials will include the specific research and null hypotheses in the introduction section. While this can be considered a deficiency in the paper, it does not necessarily indicate that the paper contains incorrect information.

An example to explain some of the material thus far included in this chapter is the "Ezetimibe and Simvastatin in Hypercholesterolemia Enhances Atherosclerosis Regression (ENHANCE)" trial, which assessed carotid artery thickness as a marker for progression of atherosclerosis in persons with familial hypercholesterolemia. The ENHANCE trial compared simvastatin 80 mg daily with ezetimibe 10 mg daily or placebo.[53] The investigators expressed in the introduction section that the rationale for conducting this clinical trial was that patients with familial hypercholesterolemia have an increased risk of early coronary artery disease, and artery thickness begins in childhood and progresses quickly. The actual ENHANCE trial study objective was stated as, "...to determine whether the daily administration of ezetimibe 10 mg in combination with simvastatin 80 mg could reduce the progression of atherosclerosis in patients with familial hypercholesterolemia, as assessed by measurement of arterial intima-media thickness."[53] The research hypothesis of the ENHANCE trial was: "There is a difference in the arterial intima-media thickness between simvastatin plus ezetimibe versus simvastatin plus placebo." The H_0 for this clinical trial was: "There is no difference in the arterial intima-media thickness between simvastatin plus ezetimibe versus simvastatin plus placebo." After reading the ENHANCE trial introduction, the reader has a clear understanding of the study rationale and purpose: Patients with familial hypercholesterolemia are at increased cardiovascular risk with progressive arterial thickening, and the results of this trial should provide health care providers with evidence to prescribe simvastatin with or without ezetimibe.

As with all sections of a clinical trial, this section needs to be carefully read. Authors may set the stage by presenting only selective (i.e., not comprehensive) information and/ or weak references (to be later discussed in the chapter) to support the rationale for conducting the study. Also, the information may be presented using biased wording, which predisposes the reader to believing the prior research was insignificant in providing evidence applicable to practice.

Methods

Following a well-designed plan is essential for the clinical trial results to be acceptable and useful to practitioners. The design of a study (i.e., methods) is important for the results to be valid, just as abiding by the blueprints is vital to building a house. The methods section of a clinical trial contains a large amount of information that includes the type of subjects enrolled, the comparative therapy description, outcome measures, and statistics. Flaws within the design of a clinical trial limit the application and significance of the results. Poor study design leads to reduced study internal validity, thus resulting in limited external study validity (Table 4–3).[19,54] The methods section needs to be thorough in describing to the reader the process in which the study was conducted. In fact, a reader should devote the majority of time used to assess the trial in this section.

Clinical trials follow a pattern in presenting the information within the methods section.[23] This standardized format allows study details to be in an orderly fashion and quickly located. Readers of the biomedical literature should have an understanding of the overall design to appropriately critique clinical trials and use the study results for patient care activities.

STUDY DESIGN

Several study designs are available for investigators to select from when conducting research. The study questions the researchers wish to answer dictate which study design

TABLE 4–3. **INTERNAL VS. EXTERNAL VALIDITY OF CLINICAL TRIALS**

Term	Meaning	Application
Internal validity	Quality of the study design	Strong design should translate into reliable results
External validity	Ability to apply results into practice	Study results meaningful to practitioners and can be used for patient care

is selected to conduct the research.[55,56] Both investigators and readers of the literature need to identify the strengths and limitations of the research designs. Although many study designs are available, this chapter only discusses controlled clinical trials. For additional information on other study designs the reader is referred to Chapter 5.

● A simple description of a controlled clinical trial is that it prospectively measures a difference in effect between two or more therapies. The groups are similar and treated identically with the exception of the therapies under study. The subjects in the study are assigned to one of the groups and monitored.[16,17,24,56] This study type, called parallel design, is the primary study design encountered in the literature.

● Controlled clinical trials offer investigators the most rigorous method of establishing a cause-and-effect relation between treatment and outcome.[17] Simply explained, the treatment under study is the cause, and the consequence of giving the treatment is measured as the effect. The effect of the treatment under study is compared to the effect of the other group(s). Thus, investigators can use a clinical trial to claim that a treatment has some effect that may be important in curing or relieving disease symptoms. In addition, the magnitude (i.e., size) of the difference in the effect between the groups can be estimated.[17]

An example of a controlled clinical trial measuring a cause-and-effect is a study that compared atorvastatin to a placebo. The study objective was to compare atorvastatin (cause) to placebo and measure the reduction in average LDL-cholesterol (LDL-C) levels (effect) between the two groups.[57] A clinical trial also quantifies the differences in the effect, such as atorvastatin compared to simvastatin in lowering LDL-C.[58] The results of these studies can be used to determine the magnitude of LDL-C lowering by atorvastatin and make the decision to use, or not use, this medication in practice.

PATIENT INCLUSION/EXCLUSION CRITERIA

❹ *The results of a controlled clinical trial should be extrapolated to the patient type enrolled in the study.* The inclusion criteria lists subject demographics that must be present to be enrolled into the trial, while exclusion criteria are characteristics that prevent enrollment into the trial or necessitate withdrawal from the study, if they are later determined to be present.[23] Diagnostic criteria for conditions under study and definitions of the inclusion/exclusion criteria must be included in an article reporting study results. For instance, if subjects with hypertension are the target group to be enrolled in a trial, hypertension needs to be defined in terms of the minimal and maximum systolic blood pressure (SBP) and diastolic blood pressure (DBP). The study participant features should reflect the disease under investigation, but the existence of complex and/or extensive comorbid conditions (e.g., terminal cancer, pregnancy, numerous other disease states) in the study patients may not allow the researchers to accurately measure the differences in effect between the groups. The presence of these complex and/or extensive comorbid conditions can make for difficult decisions regarding including subjects representative of real patients versus excluding typical persons whose complicating conditions will make it impossible to accurately assess a new treatment. Whenever possible and appropriate, typical individuals with the condition being assessed, who in all probability will receive the therapy in real practice, should be represented in the trial. This includes ensuring a realistic representation of the gender, race, and other demographics. Subjects with one or more (but not numerous) other disease states and taking a few other medications are usually entered into the clinical trial, so the typical patients in which the therapy under investigation is intended are represented.

The inclusion/exclusion criteria are pertinent to the extrapolation of the study results (i.e., applying the study results into practice [external validity]).[54] Trial results are only applicable to the type of subject included in the study. The investigators of the ENHANCE trial enrolled men and women with heterozygous familial hypercholesterolemia.[53] The combination therapy did not reduce or slow the progression of carotid artery buildup compared with simvastatin-alone therapy. However, this does not mean that this medication should not be prescribed to any patient with high cholesterol. The patients in the ENHANCE study were not typical patients with elevated cholesterol levels (only 1 in 500 patients [0.2%] have this type of hyperlipidemia [a LDL receptor disorder] leading to elevated serum cholesterol). Thus, the results of the ENHANCE trial cannot be extrapolated to typical patients with hypercholesterolemia.

Researchers are careful in deciding which subjects to include and exclude in the clinical trial. Standard types of subjects disqualified are pregnant and lactating females; also, most clinical trials will not enroll subjects with severe conditions that may alter the medication's pharmacokinetics and/or pharmacodynamics (e.g., renal and/or hepatic dysfunction). Generally, the inclusion criteria attempt to include subjects that are homogeneous and are similar to the common type of patients in practice.[52]

During the process of the investigators selecting subjects to be included into a study, readers of clinical trials need to be conscious of the potential for a selection bias that may be present. A selection bias can occur due to various reasons, but can seriously affect the study results in a negative fashion. In general, a selection bias occurs after subjects meet the inclusion and exclusion criteria, but are not enrolled into the study.[59] The investigators may prevent a subject from being enrolled since this person may either positively or negatively alter the results.[16,24,59,60]

Although it may be difficult for the reader to detect the above form of selection bias, the following paragraphs describe selection biases that can be more readily identified, but are not present in all clinical trials.[59] One common form of a selection bias is requiring the subjects to complete a run-in phase (also called lead-in phase) before being officially enrolled in the study. This phase is usually short in duration (usually 2 to 4 weeks) in which the subjects may take a placebo or the therapy being investigated. The investigators should inform the reader of the intent of the run-in phase. Typical reasons include identifying subjects that may or may not be compliant with the therapy regimen, experience side effects from the therapy, or not meet pre-specific criteria (e.g., blood pressure less than a set value). Afterwards, these identified subjects are excluded from participating in the study even though they meet the original inclusion criteria. The run-in phase produces a bias by selecting a group of subjects who do not completely represent the population, since a selected group of the subjects meeting the study inclusion criteria are not included in the study and their run-in phase results are not included in the final analysis.[61] In addition, a run-in phase can delay the time from identifying candidates to actually enrolling into the clinical trial, which can increase the chance of patients withdrawing from the study.[62]

The following examples explain a selection bias by a run-in phase. Subjects meeting the hypothetical trial inclusion criteria complete a 4-week run-in phase in which a new therapy under investigation is given to all these persons. Those persons experiencing side effects to the new therapy during the run-in phase are not allowed to be enrolled into the study. By excluding those persons eliminated after the run-in phase, the incidence and severity of the side effects of the therapy are not accurately measured during the actual study since subjects experiencing the side effects during the run-in phase were not enrolled in the study. A second example is where researchers may include a run-in phase in which only those persons achieving a pre-set goal are allowed to be included in the study. For instance, only subjects achieving at least a 25% reduction in LDL-C after a 4-week phase with a new therapy are enrolled in the 12-week study comparing the new therapy to placebo. By only including those with a favorable response, the final average reduction in LDL-C with the new therapy is falsely elevated since only selected subjects were allowed into the study. Those persons with less than a 25% reduction in LDL-C were excluded from the 12-week trial; if these individuals were included in the 12-week trial, the final average reduction in LDL-C most likely would have been significantly lower than actually measured.

Trials including a run-in phase are not always considered to be a study limitation.[61] The investigators may stop a therapy previously prescribed to the subjects and give a placebo during the run-in phase. This allows the effects of the prior therapy to diminish and not interfere with the effects of the therapy under study. Furthermore, a clinical trial may be designed in which the investigators enroll a very specific type of subject, which can be considered a selection bias in the inclusion criteria. The purpose of this type of selection bias is to evaluate a therapy in a very unique group of individuals, usually those who met some predetermined criteria. For instance, a trial was designed so that only subjects who experienced a gastrointestinal (GI) bleed with aspirin alone were enrolled.[63] The investigators were specifically selecting a unique group of subjects (having a GI bleed due to aspirin). The combination of aspirin plus esomeprazole was compared to clopidogrel to determine which therapy had a lower recurrence of GI bleeding. Even though the trial results indicated that the aspirin plus esomeprazole combination has a lower GI bleeding recurrence rate, this does not mean this drug combination should be used instead of aspirin alone in those people needing aspirin therapy. The results of this trial can only be used for selected patients, those who had a GI bleed while taking aspirin and need to continue antiplatelet therapy.

Investigators also should explain the process of recruiting subjects and define the time period of which the recruitment occurred.[23] Sponsors of clinical trials and investigators typically recruit subjects for clinical trials by four main strategies: sponsors may offer financial and other incentives to investigators to increase enrollment; investigators may target their own patients as potential subjects; investigators may seek additional subjects from other sources (e.g., physician referrals and disease registries); or sponsors and investigators may advertise and promote their studies. The most common means for advertising for recruitment to clinical trials is through newspapers, radio, Internet, television, or as posters on public transportation and in hospitals.[64] The methods in which investigators recruit subjects may have implications on the generalizability of the research results to the population (i.e., external validity). Newspaper and Internet advertisements are common; however, there are inherent problems with this form of advertisement. Surveys results indicate that the majority of persons who read the newspapers are older in age, Caucasian, wealthier, more educated, and own more upscale homes than the average American. Gender bias also can affect recruitment rates as it has been documented that female readers consider newspaper advertising to be more important than do male readers.[65]

Internet recruitment is not without similar problems. Typically, minority and elderly individuals are less familiar and have less access to the Internet. A study described the process of registering persons with cancer for clinical trials via the Internet and telephone call center. Most of the subjects registered via the Internet compared to the telephone call center (88% versus 12%). The majority of subjects who registered were female (73% versus 27% male), Caucasian (88.9%), and received colorectal cancer screening (59%); the median age was 49 years. No differences with respect to ethnicity or gender were observed for patients registering via the Internet compared to the call center; however, subjects registering via the Internet were significantly younger than those registering through the call center. Recruitment via newspapers and the Internet may offer some benefits in terms of recruitment, although the lack of uniformity with respect to access to newspapers and the Internet for elderly and minority subjects may increase the difficulty of applying the clinical trial results to these underrepresented populations because of the lack of this subject type included in the trials.[66]

Another important issue that affects the recruitment of patients is the increasing number of clinical studies that are outsourced to other countries due to decreased costs associated with conducting clinical trials abroad. Although outsourcing clinical trials to other countries may decrease the problems associated with insufficient recruitment of patients who enroll in clinical trials, other issues may occur as a result of including a large number of foreign patients in clinical trials.[67] More relaxed governmental standards of research and an increased numbers of scientists may be sacrificed for the inclusion of patients with who may serve as volunteers for the enticement that participation in clinical trials may offer.[68] In addition, potential ethnic differences may affect the way drugs are handled in the body (e.g., overall response, drug distribution, metabolism, excretion). Therefore, readers of clinical studies that have included foreign patients need to ensure that the results of the study are generalizable to the patient population in which they serve.

INTERVENTION AND CONTROL GROUPS

Once the subjects to be enrolled in the clinical trial have been selected, these persons will be assigned to either the intervention or control group. The intervention group consists of the new therapy under investigation (e.g., medication, procedure). The intervention is compared to a control so that the fundamental principle of a controlled clinical trial can be accomplished, measuring cause and effect. The control group can consist of no therapy (e.g., placebo), another therapy (a.k.a. active control) for instance, drug or exercise, or compared to existing data (i.e., historical data). Both the intervention and control groups are to be the same in all respects other than the treatment received. Afterwards, the investigators will measure and quantify a difference in effect between the group assigned to the intervention with those in the control group. Thus, any identified differences in the measured effect can be attributed to intervention rather than other factors.[16,69,70]

A key term in the phrase *controlled clinical trial is* the word *control,* indicating another therapy is serving as the measuring point for the effect of the intervention to be assessed. Reports have been published documenting placebo effects (i.e., measured change even though no therapy was given).[71] Without a control, the effects measured by the intervention may be by chance or falsely quantified. For example, investigators of a study reported that oxandrolone caused an average increase in body weight in patients with chronic obstructive pulmonary disease (COPD).[72] However, all the subjects were treated with oxandrolone, and no control group was included in the study. Although these patients gained weight, oxandrolone may not be the sole reason for this effect. Weight gain may have occurred naturally, even without the medication or by some unidentified reason. The results of this non-controlled clinical trial may be the rationale for a clinical trial being conducted to evaluate the weight-gaining effects of oxandrolone. However, they cannot be used as evidence that weight gain was solely attributed to this drug. The results of studies designed without a control can be useful, but since no control group was present, readers cannot be certain that the intervention caused the effect.

Researchers can select from a few different types of controls, including historical, placebo, or active. Historical controls are described as data that have been collected prior to the beginning of a clinical trial. Investigators conduct the study with only the intervention group and then compare the results to the existing data.[73] One advantage of using historical controls is only one group is needed to be enrolled, which may result in less time, expense, and so on. Another advantage is the usefulness of studying a disease with a low occurrence or a disease with high incidence of death or other serious sequelae in which some form of therapy should not be denied.[73] Disadvantages include usually overestimating the effect of the intervention,[21] lack of homogeneity between patients in the trial and historical controls, and differences in therapeutic procedures, or techniques from one study period to the next.[73]

Historical controls are not used very often in published clinical trials, but are acceptable in selected situations. For example, investigators of a clinical trial evaluated the efficacy and safety of the direct thrombin inhibitor, argatroban in patients with heparin-induced thrombocytopenia (HIT), or HIT with thrombosis syndrome (HITTS) and compared the results with a historical control. Historical controls consisted of patients who met the same inclusion/exclusion criteria who experienced HIT 4 years prior to the initiation of the trial. The use of a historical control was appropriate in this study because, at the time of the study, no approved alternative therapy was available, and a placebo control was deemed unethical.[74]

An intervention under investigation is compared to a placebo in many clinical trials to document and measure the pharmacological effect of the intervention. These studies are generally conducted as a requirement by the FDA to document that drug therapy is better than no therapy (placebo) for a given disease state.[71] Those trials reporting a significant difference in effect of the intervention compared to placebo could be used to support the use of the intervention in treating patients. Simvastatin was compared to placebo to determine if the incidence of a death would be lowered in subjects with a history of angina pectoris or MI.[75] Before this study was conducted, health care providers did not have any information indicating that simvastatin would benefit or harm this subject type. At the time this trial was designed and initiated, persons with angina pectoris or history of MI were not routinely treated with a HMG-CoA reductase inhibitor (i.e., statins); thus, a placebo was selected as the control. However, the place in therapy for the intervention may be difficult to determine when a placebo is the control, since other drugs may be found to be better than the drug in question, upon further research. For example, in this case, although simvastatin lowers LDL-C greater than placebo,[76] it is not directly known how simvastatin compares to other drugs that lower LDL-C based solely on these trial results.

Not all clinical trials will have a placebo as the control group for various valid reasons. For example, including a placebo as one of the groups in a trial may decrease the willingness of subjects to participate; some may not wish to be treated with a placebo.[77] But more importantly, denying therapy that has been documented to reduce morbidity and/or mortality to patients with selected diseases may be unethical. These studies would not include a placebo as the control, but instead may use active therapy (i.e., standard therapy).[71,78] Patients with cancer enrolled in a clinical trial are prime examples where trials will not include a placebo as the control.

Usually after the new therapy is compared to a placebo, a trial using an active therapy as the control is used to assess the difference in effect between the groups. Readers should be aware that clinical trials with a placebo as the control, particularly those funded by the pharmaceutical industry, yield a larger treatment effect than if an active therapy was selected as the control group.[79,80] For instance, the difference in the LDL-C lowering effect is expected to be significantly greater with a new statin versus placebo instead of another statin or other lipid-lowering agent. Thus, the treatment effect may appear to be substantial versus placebo, but could be minimally different from another active drug that was used as the control. Also, the possibility exists that the new treatment, in fact, may be inferior in efficacy and/or safety compared to an active drug, even though the new treatment appears better in comparison to a placebo.

An appropriate control needs to be included in the study for the results to be applicable for practice. The use of historical or placebo as the control is acceptable in some clinical trials (as described above). Some studies may be designed with a control that may no longer be the preferred treatment after the trial results are published. The study may have been designed and initiated based upon either recommendations of the FDA or before new therapy recommendations were available.

Also, investigators including a medication as the control need to use the dosing regimen (i.e., dose, frequency) deemed suitable.[79] Standard references should be consulted to ensure appropriate dosing regimens were included in the trial to reduce the chance of obtaining biased results. A trial concluding a new analgesic relieved pain better than morphine dosed 0.05 mg intravenously (IV) every 24 hours post-surgery in otherwise healthy adult subjects is biased because an appropriate morphine regimen was not used. However, at times investigators may not know the equivalent dosing regimen of the intervention relative to the control. Investigators directly comparing rosuvastatin to atorvastatin, both 10 mg once daily for 12 weeks, reported a greater lowering of mean LDL-C with rosuvastatin (43% versus 35%).[81] Other studies comparing these two medications have reported that average LDL-C levels are similar with atorvastatin doses two times that of the rosuvastatin dose.[82] Thus, concluding rosuvastatin is a superior LDL-C-lowering agent to atorvastatin based solely upon the results of a single trial evaluating both agents dosed 10 mg once daily is incorrect. A more appropriate conclusion is these two agents do not have an equivalent pharmacological effect at this dose.

INSTITUTIONAL REVIEW BOARD (IRB)/SUBJECT CONSENT

Research projects that use humans as study subjects must be approved before investigators begin enrolling subjects into the trial. The Institutional Review Board (IRB) is the committee charged with ensuring the subjects are protected and not exposed to unnecessary harm or unethical medical procedures,[83,84] in particular vulnerable populations (e.g., pediatrics, pregnant women, impaired persons[85]). The name of the actual committee may differ from place to place (e.g., local ethics committee), although the purpose of the committee remains to protect the study subjects. This committee consists of both health care and non-health care professionals; people specialized in ethics also need to be included.[86] The rules and regulations of human research require the study to be assessed prior to the initiation of the project.

Another primary responsibility of the IRB is to approve the informed consent form.[87,88] Before agreeing to participate in a trial, each subject is presented with an informed consent form that notifies the subjects of the study procedures, their rights and responsibilities of participating in the study, plus at least eight major points that include risks, benefits, compensation, voluntary participation, and right to withdraw from the study without any penalty. In addition to the content of the informed consent form, the IRB provides investigators with suggestions on how to write the form in language that laypersons can comprehend.[86-90] Additional information regarding clinical trial research can be obtained at http://www.cancer.gov/clinicaltrials/education/main/Page1. Also, the reader may refer to Chapter 17 (Investigational Drugs). According to the Uniform Requirements, articles describing clinical trials using humans as research subjects are required to include a statement that the research was approved by the IRB (or other committee that protects subjects) and consent was obtained from the subject to participate in the research project.[33] Over the past 10 years, more medical journals include IRB/ethics approval information within the published studies.[89] Trials not including the IRB/informed consent information should be questioned.

BLINDING

Since clinical trials measure differences in effect between groups, outside influences (i.e., biases) should be minimized. This is especially important in studies measuring subjective outcomes (e.g., pain, depression scores). Blinding is a technique in which subjects and/or the investigators are unaware of who is in the intervention or control group. Blinding techniques are incorporated to reduce possible bias (defined as "Differences between the true value and that actually obtained [are] due to all causes other than sampling variability").[24] Patients knowing they are taking a placebo to reduce depression symptoms are very likely to report no change or worsening of the disease. The results are biased

TABLE 4–4. **TYPES OF BLINDING**

Type of Blinding	Definition
No blinding (open-label)	Investigators and subjects are aware of the assignment of subjects to the intervention or control group
Single	Either investigators or subjects, but not both, are aware of the assignment of subjects to the intervention or control group
Double	Both investigators and subjects are not aware of the assignment of subjects to the intervention or control group
Triple	In addition to both investigators and subjects not being aware of the assignment of subjects to the intervention or control group, trial personnel involved with data interpretation are not aware of subject assignment

since subjects knowingly are taking a substance that does not reduce symptoms. Therefore, blinding techniques are important to reduce the influence of bias on measuring a difference in effect between the intervention and control. Four types of blinding can be used in a clinical trial (Table 4–4). The specific blinding type usually is dictated by the effect being measured during the trial.

Single- and no-blinding techniques are primarily incorporated in clinical trials that have study objectives not conducible to blinding (e.g., surgery versus medication). Some trials may include a procedure that is difficult to blind (e.g., surgery), and it may not be ideal to include a placebo procedure because sham surgery is not without risks as death or infection-related complications are possible.[91] The use of placebo procedures to ensure a trial remains blinded, which may increase the risk of adverse effects or other dangers, is controversial and possibly unethical if the investigators do not thoroughly discuss the rationale for including and/or not using other methods to blind the trial.[92] A clinical trial designed to compare surgery to a medication is an example of using no-blinding methods since both the investigators and subjects know which group the subjects have been assigned.

An example of single-blinding is when one group of subjects is administered a medication subcutaneously once daily versus the other group who took an oral anticoagulation medication. The subjects were not blinded since the risk of injecting a saline solution subcutaneously (i.e., bleeding complications may develop in persons taking an anticoagulant agent plus unnecessary injections) may outweigh the benefit. The investigators measured the occurrence of a blood clot, an objective outcome that cannot be biased or influenced by the subjects. Therefore, the subjects' knowledge of which therapy they were receiving cannot influence the incidence of the blood clots. Since the investigators do not know which therapy is administered, the potential for the results to be biased is minimized. There are also cases in which the subjects were blinded, but not the investigator.

Double-blinding, where neither the investigator nor patient know who is receiving which treatment, is considered the gold standard blinding technique and is most commonly used in clinical trials.[25] As a general rule, and regardless whether the outcome is a subjective or objective measure, the study should be double-blinded. A clinical trial measuring an objective outcome usually assesses other study outcome measures, such as the incidence and severity of side effects, which may be biased if double-blinding was not incorporated into the trial. For instance, double-blinding was used in the ENHANCE trial[53] to not only minimize biases in the objective measurements (carotid artery intima-media thickness) but also subjective assessments (side effects) in those patients assigned to intervention or control.

In order to ensure that blinding remains intact, the therapy each group receives should be exact in frequency of administration, appearance, size, taste, and smell and other variables. Studies that compare regimens taken once daily to twice daily will require the once daily group to take a placebo as the second dose (i.e., double-dummy).[16] Double-dummy methods are included in clinical trials when two therapies being compared are not the same (e.g., different routes of administration, different formulations). Patients receive two formulations, one active and one control, to ensure that blinding is maintained.[16] For example, investigators of a clinical trial evaluating the blood pressure–lowering effects of amlodipine (a tablet) and the combination product of amlodipine plus benazepril (a capsule) should administer amlodipine tablets plus placebo capsules to those subjects randomized to amlodipine therapy and amlodipine/benazepril capsules plus placebo tablets to the other subjects. A similar situation may present in clinical trials in which the formulations being compared are administered via different routes. Investigators evaluating the efficacy of a once daily oral contraceptive tablet to an intramuscular contraceptive agent administered every 3 months may allocate an intramuscular placebo to those patients randomized to once-daily oral contraceptives and a once-daily placebo tablet to those patients randomized to the intramuscular contraceptive. Each patient receives a formulation that represents each therapy, and both subjects and investigators would be less likely to determine which formulation is active.

Sometimes it is necessary to triple-blind a study. In addition to the trial investigators and subjects, other personnel involved with the trial (e.g., data collection, analysis, or monitoring; drug administration or dispensing) can have opinions regarding the outcome of the therapy being studied based on their interaction with the subjects involved in the trial or their experience with the intervention and/or control being assessed. These opinions may cause inappropriate data collection, measurement, analysis, and/or interpretation of the results by the study personnel. Also, data collection personnel having a bias for or against the intervention may not be as consistent in their data collection procedures if they know which group the subjects were assigned. This may result in an inappropriate interpretation (e.g., overestimation of the treatment effects) of the study results.[16,21,25] Therefore, it is often necessary to blind these other individuals (i.e., triple-blinding).

RANDOMIZATION

Randomization is a distinguishing study attribute that separates controlled clinical trials from other study designs (e.g., case-control, cohort). ❺ *Randomization is an essential component of all controlled clinical trials and a significant differentiator from other study designs.* "Randomization can be simply described as all persons in a clinical trial have an equal chance to be in the intervention or control group."[93] Research has indicated that the results obtained from randomized trials are more dependable than non-randomized trials. An analysis of randomized versus non-randomized trials reported that, on average, investigators of non-randomized trials overestimated the treatment effects of the intervention compared to the control primarily due to bias.[21] Even though including randomization in a clinical trial is important for more reliable results, it is necessary to remember not all randomized trials are without faults.

Subjects are eligible for randomization after meeting the trial inclusion criteria.[16] Subjects are randomized so the investigators cannot purposely assign selected persons to one group over another (i.e., sicker individuals in the control versus less sick in the intervention group). Randomization minimizes bias by lowering the potential for an imbalance of risk factors or prognostic variations between the intervention and control groups.[24] A difference in effect measured by a clinical trial may result from many causes, and treatment may be just one of these. Disparities between the groups at baseline may cause a false result instead of measuring differences in effect between the intervention and control.[94] Therefore to be assured that the difference is truly due to the intervention, the groups need to be as equal as possible, and other outside factors that may affect the overall results of the trial need to be equally distributed between the groups.[69] Besides reducing bias,[16,95] an additional reason to include randomization in a clinical trial is so statistical tests are valid. Most statistical tests require subjects to be randomized so that similar groups are being compared, and selected statistical tests can determine whether certain subject characteristics are equivalent between groups.[24]

Measuring differences in the effect between the intervention and control group requires the groups to be as similar in as many characteristics as possible (e.g., age, gender, severity of illness) so that outside factors (i.e., confounders) do not influence the results.[95] Baseline discrepancies between the groups do not allow the true difference in effect between the intervention and group to be measured and quantified. If unbalanced factors are present between the two groups, the outcome measure is biased, and the treatment effect may be either under- or overestimated.[94]

Many randomization techniques are available and range from very simple to complex processes. The nature of the study and outcomes measured influence the randomization procedure. Various methods are available that include random number tables and computer programs. The randomization procedures should be unbiased and unpredictable by not allowing the subjects or investigators to know in advance to which group the subject will be assigned.[16,95]

Specific randomization methods include from simple (i.e., coin toss) to more advanced techniques (i.e., stratification). Simple randomization is an easy technique to implement and includes assigning subjects according to some criteria (e.g., day of the week, subject birthday, or subject medical record number). But this method is not considered a proper randomization method since the number of subjects in the groups can be imbalanced due to the technique. If investigators assign all subjects with an office visit on a specific day of the week to one group (i.e., control), then these subjects did not have equal opportunity to be assigned to either group. These may lead to a reduction in the ability of the investigators to detect differences in effects between the two groups. Few trials use simple randomization techniques due to the limitations of this randomization method.[24]

The more sophisticated randomization procedure, stratification, is designed to achieve similarities in both known and unknown baseline patient characteristics between the groups. Selected factors are identified (e.g., age, smoking, presence of other disease states) and used in determining which group the subjects will be assigned so significant imbalances of these factors are not present among the groups, while all subjects with any specific factor have an equal chance of being in each group.[96]

The persons randomizing study participants should be at a distant location, so that they may not be able to obtain any information that could bias the randomization process. Unduly influencing the randomization sequence by randomizing subjects to either therapy based on some preference can occur with personal contact with the subject.[24] Thus, to minimize these issues, investigators may contact a central randomization center who randomizes the subject to either the intervention or control group.

ENDPOINTS

Clinical trials measure some effect caused by the intervention and control in order to compare these groups.[17,25,97] All trials specify one effect caused by the intervention and control as the primary endpoint, which can be referred to as what the investigators measured to achieve the study objective. Since significant time, money, and effort are devoted to conduct a clinical trial, researchers usually measure a primary endpoint plus secondary endpoints. These secondary endpoints are important, but not considered to be the primary purpose of the study. The selected primary endpoint should be a routine and useful measure.[25,97] For example, a trial evaluating the cholesterol-lowering effect of a statin compared to placebo selected a change in average LDL-C value, an appropriate measure, as the primary endpoint to satisfy the study objective. However measuring a change in serum creatinine between losartan and captopril to improve heart failure (HF) symptoms[98] is not ideal, since serum creatinine is not the predominate parameter used in practice to monitor the progression or improvement in HF status.

❻ *The controlled clinical trial primary endpoint should be appropriate for the study purpose and measured using valid techniques and methods.* Investigators may combine a group of endpoint measures into one primary endpoint, referred to as a composite endpoint. The group usually consists of clinical outcomes directly related to morbidity and mortality as opposed to a pharmacological action (e.g., reduction in any incidence of stroke/MI/CV-related death versus lowering cholesterol levels). The investigators select a group of endpoints that can occur during therapy that are considered clinically important. For example, after experiencing a MI, a therapy is prescribed to reduce the occurrence of multiple adverse outcomes (e.g., reinfarction, death, chest pain), not just one clinical outcome. The rationale for measuring composite endpoints is to measure an overall effect of therapy, since one specific outcome cannot be deemed to be most important for the study subjects.[79,99,100]

The use of composite endpoints is not without debate.[79,99-103] The results of the individual components of the composite should be reported separately and analyzed.[99,100,102] Investigators may claim the investigational therapy is better than the control based upon the overall result of the composite endpoint, even though the investigational therapy was shown to significantly affect only one or a few (but not all) of the composite endpoint components. Also, the most important component of the composite may not be affected by the intervention under study.

The following example explains composite endpoints and issues encountered with these. The investigators of the "Efficacy and Safety of Subcutaneous Enoxaparin in Non-Q-Wave Coronary Events (ESSENCE)" trial used a composite primary endpoint, which consisted of death, MI [or reinfarction], or recurrent angina after 14 days of follow-up.[104] The incidence of the primary endpoint was lower with enoxaparin (intervention) than unfractionated heparin (control) (16.6% versus 19.8%, respectively; p = 0.02) in patients with angina at rest or non-Q-wave MI. However, only one of the three components of the composite endpoint was significantly different with enoxaparin, recurrent angina (12.9% versus 15.5%, respectively; p = 0.03).[104] As seen by the percentages, the majority of primary endpoint composite (~78%) consisted of this single event, which is the least robust of the three outcomes.[105] Although lowering the incidence of recurrent angina is clinically important, this outcome is not as severe as death or reinfarction. The composite endpoint effect of enoxaparin appears to be superior to heparin, even though the incidence of two of the three components of the composite endpoint indicates no difference between these two drugs. Enoxaparin was considered to be a useful therapy in this patient type, but further research was recommended to determine if the therapy reduces the occurrence of death and MI in these patients.[106]

The primary and other endpoint definitions, plus valid measuring techniques, need to be determined prior to the start of the clinical trial and incorporated in the study design.[16,25] By doing so, the investigators can be consistent throughout the trial in measuring the endpoints, thereby reducing study variances or biases. To illustrate, the ENHANCE trial primary endpoint was change in ultrasonographic measurement of the mean carotid artery intima-media thickness, defined as "the average of the means of the far-wall intima-media thickness of the right and left common carotid arteries, carotid bulbs, and internal carotid arteries in the two study groups."[53] If readers are informed of the measurement types and methods under investigation, they can judge whether practical methods were used to measure the endpoints and can determine if the study can be replicated by future investigators or by individuals wanting to implement the trial results into practice to actual patients. Furthermore, the internal and external validity of the clinical trial can be assessed. Endpoints involving human judgment (e.g., need for coronary revascularization) also can contribute to the complexity of analyzing and interpreting the study results if strict criteria or a blinded clinical events committee designed to produce valid recommendations are not incorporated and utilized during the trial.[99]

A final type of endpoint that may be seen is a surrogate endpoint. This will be discussed later in the chapter.

FOLLOW-UP SCHEDULE/DATA COLLECTION/COMPLIANCE

A few important issues are considered here. First, a study should be conducted for an appropriate duration; second, data need to be consistently collected throughout the entire trial. A magical number of weeks or months has not been established as a rule for all clinical trials, but the length of the study (i.e., follow-up time) should be an ideal representation to answer the question being researched.[25] Statins usually exert the maximum cholesterol-lowering effect after approximately 6 weeks of stable dosing.[107] Thus, the results of a study directly comparing atorvastatin 10 mg once daily to simvastatin 20 mg once daily for 6 weeks to compare the LDL-C level lowering differences between these two agents would be considered acceptable.[58]

A number of trials do not have an extensive follow-up time, and the reader may have difficulty in interpreting the results for clinical practice. For example, in one study, the antipsychotic agent aripiprazole and placebo were administered to subjects for 4 weeks to determine the efficacy of aripiprazole in treating psychosis.[108] The investigators of the clinical trial detected a pharmacological effect of aripiprazole during this time period, but the clinical effects and tolerability of the medication beyond this time period could not be assessed due to the short duration of the trial. Considering the actual duration of aripiprazole and other antipsychotic therapy for patients with psychosis exceeds four weeks,[109,110] the trial should have been longer so investigators could determine the long-term clinical effects of this drug in practice.

Monitoring of the trial results at predetermined intervals is important throughout the duration of the trial. The Code of Federal Regulations and good clinical practice guidelines for clinical research state that subject monitoring is required during the clinical investigation.[25] Larger trials may have a clinical trial investigator subgroup who serve as the data and safety monitoring board members. These individuals are blinded to the subject groupings and are responsible for reviewing the results obtained while the trial is ongoing. Interim analyses of the study results may indicate the intervention produces either a favorable outcome or increased risk over the control before the established duration of the study has been completed. Typically, the protocol for discontinuing the clinical trial early is established prior to enrolling study subjects.[29,34]

By stopping the study early after finding the intervention results in significant harm compared to the control; subjects randomized to the intervention would not be at a greater risk for experiencing the harmful effects if a trial was allowed to continue. Conversely, if the intervention was shown to be more beneficial than the control, the investigators would be denying useful therapy to those subjects randomized to the control if the trial continued.[29]

Prior to the start of the study, data collection methods are established. These should be reasonable in that extensive time and/or procedures are not required, so that incomplete follow-up by trial personnel and subjects at each follow-up time can be minimized. In addition, investigators should ensure trial personnel are properly trained and have sufficient resources to complete data collection.[111]

Another data collection and follow-up issue is measuring the compliance of therapy in the study participants.[25] This includes medication pill counts, serum drug levels, or regular follow-up communications (e.g., telephone conversations). Subjects not complying with the therapy regimen may cause inaccuracies and less reliable data. Insufficient and/or inappropriate data collection methods and noncompliance usually lead to biased results that may make the extrapolation of results to clinical practice difficult.[16]

SAMPLE SIZE

❼ *An appropriate controlled clinical trial sample size is vital for the study results to have any significant meaning; conducting a power analysis is important to determine a suitable sample size.* Sample size (denoted by the letter n) refers to the number of subjects randomized into a study and is of considerable importance to the validity of the study results. Financial and logistical limitations prevent all subjects with the specific inclusion criteria from being enrolled into the study.[25,111] For example, investigators may want to evaluate a new drug to treat hypertension. It would be virtually impossible to enroll all people with hypertension into this clinical trial. In response, investigators will draw a representative group (i.e., sample) of individuals from all those with hypertension (i.e., population). Researchers do not wish to include too few nor too many subjects in the trial. Obviously having only one subject each in the intervention and control group is insufficient to determine differences in effect between groups since chance alone may be the reason for a difference found (if any) between the two groups. On the other hand, having too many subjects can be excessive, costly, and may expose some subjects to unnecessary treatment. The sample size should not be determined on the basis of convenience, arbitrarily, or by the number of easily recruited subjects.[112]

The number of subjects to enroll in a clinical trial is dependent upon the expected magnitude of difference in the endpoint effect between the intervention and control. The expected magnitude of difference in effect between groups is estimated based on the results of previously conducted trials or other research results assessing the intervention. In general, an inverse relationship exists between the sample size and the effect size. A large sample size is needed to detect a small difference in effect between the intervention and control outcome, while a smaller sample size is needed to detect large differences between the two groups.[20,112] A large sample size is needed to detect differences in blood pressure between two antihypertensive therapies (small difference in blood pressure reductions), while a smaller sample size is needed to measure the difference in relieving postoperative pain between morphine and placebo (large difference in pain relief).

Researchers use various procedures from table/charts to manual calculations in estimating the necessary sample size for a particular trial.[70,112] Regardless of the method selected to determine the appropriate sample size, it must be calculated prior to initiating the clinical trial. A study lacking a sample size calculation may be biased since the reader is not informed of the basis on which the investigators determined the number of subjects to enroll. Also, another important issue is that the sample size is calculated based upon the differences in the primary endpoint effect between the intervention and control groups. Investigators intending to measure differences in effect for other endpoints besides the primary endpoint need to include this in the process of calculating the sample size. Clinical trials consisting of larger sample sizes can be considered more reliable in measuring and detecting true difference in the effect (if it exists) between the intervention and control.[113] Consequences of a clinical trial not having a sufficient sample size (i.e., too small or too large) is discussed later in the Type I and Type II errors section of this chapter and in Chapter 8.

The importance of an appropriate study sample size is exemplified in the following example. Investigators conducted a small study (51 patients) to evaluate fenoldopam mesylate compared with 0.45% sodium chloride infusion in enhancing renal plasma flow in patients undergoing contrast angiography. Fewer subjects receiving the fenoldopam developed a specific adverse event (radiocontrast-induced nephropathy [RCN]) at 48 hours than those treated with 0.45% sodium chloride infusion (21% versus 41%, respectively).[114] One primary contributor to the large difference in the results was the small number of subjects enrolled; the incidence of RCN is increased by 4% for each subject developing this outcome. Even though the percent difference was 20% (41% minus 21%), this represents a difference of only five subjects developing RCN. After the results of this large difference in reducing RCN incidence were released, fenoldopam was frequently used in these patients.[115] However, the CONTRAST study (Evaluation of Corlopam in Patients at Risk for Renal Failure—A Safety and Efficacy Trial) was designed to determine if fenoldopam reduces RCN in patients after receiving iodine-based dye during cardiac angioplasty,[115] but this study had a much larger sample size (157 patients in the fenoldopam group and 158 in the placebo) compared to the previous study evaluating fenoldopam therapy. At 48 hours, RCN incidence was 19.9% versus 15.9% with fenoldopam and placebo, respectively. At 96 hours, incidence was 33.6% versus 30.1%, respectively. The investigators recruited slightly more than 300 subjects to accommodate potential subject discontinuations. Based upon the results of this clinical trial, the incidence of RCN was actually higher with fenoldopam than placebo. By conducting a study with a larger sample size, the treatment effect of fenoldopam was more accurately measured compared to the study of only 51 subjects.

STATISTICAL ANALYSIS

Within controlled clinical trials, the use of statistics is a means to analyze sample data and apply to the population. Many statistical tests are available, and readers should be familiar with and have a basic understanding of the most common tests used in clinical trials. Some statistical analysis can be easily conducted using simple computer programs, while others require specialized training and extensive skill. Typically, a biostatistician is consulted as one of the trial investigators to perform the statistical analysis of the trial results.[116,117] However, even with biostatisticians evaluating the data, study results may be biased by using incorrect statistical analyses.[118]

The purpose of statistical analysis of the study data is to collect sufficient evidence to reject the null hypothesis (H_0) in favor of accepting the research hypothesis (H_1) (new terminology may refer to this as failure to accept the null hypothesis).[118,119] Prior to the start of the study, the appropriate tests are selected based upon the type of data that will be collected and analyzed. Since the selection of statistical tests is dependent upon the type of data,[93] an overview of the types of data is presented here. There are four types of data (Table 4–5)[120]: nominal, ordinal, interval, and ratio (the latter two are usually referred collectively as continuous). Nominal data are categorical without any sense of order; these data only can be categorized into one of the possible groups (e.g., either dead or alive, but not both). Nominal data are mutually exclusive, meaning that the data can be in only one group. Ordinal data (i.e., ranking) are categorical data with an intrinsic order, but do not have equal intervals between units. Pain severity (or other type of subjective data) measured by a scale is a typical example of ordinal data. For example, a 5-point pain scale with a score of zero indicating no pain, while a score of five indicates severe pain. A 1-point change in pain intensity on this 5-point pain scale is not necessarily the same from one-to-two as from four-to-five on the scale. Interval and ratio data both have measurable

TABLE 4–5. **TYPES OF DATA**

Type of Data	Definition	Examples
Nominal	Categorical data; Data placed in one category, but not more than one category	Yes/No; alive/dead; colors of cars in a parking lot into five categories of either red, white, blue, black, or other
Ordinal	Ranking, ordered	Likert scale; visual analog scale
Interval	Data with measurable equal distances between points, but no absolute zero	Temperature in degrees Fahrenheit
Ratio	Data with measurable equal distances between points and an absolute zero	Temperature in degrees Kelvin, blood pressure, cholesterol levels, white blood count

equal intervals between data points, but interval data have no absolute zero (e.g., Fahrenheit temperature) while an absolute zero point (e.g., white blood cell count) is a characteristic for ratio data. Readers need to differentiate between the types of data to ensure correct statistical tests were selected in addition to the study being designed appropriately with correct data collection methods.

The type of data collected also dictates the use of inferential or descriptive statistical methods. Inferential statistics (e.g., Student t-test, Chi Square test) are used to draw conclusions, based upon the sample, for the application of the trial results to the population.[121,122] In other words, data are analyzed to make a conclusion of the study results from the sample that is then inferred to the population. Descriptive statistics describe the characteristics of the sample (e.g., average subject age, baseline endpoint values, number of subjects with another disease present), and the results in some studies (e.g., X% had an adverse effect). Descriptive data are typically presented as measures of central tendency (e.g., mean [average], median, mode) and/or measure of variability (e.g., range, standard deviation) (Table 4–6).[123] Refer to Chapter 8 for further information on descriptive and inferential statistics.

TABLE 4–6. **DATA PRESENTATION METHODS**

Type of Data	Mode	Median	Mean	Range	Interquartile Range	Standard Deviation
Nominal	X					
Ordinal	X	X		X	X	
Interval and Ratio	X	X	X	X	X	X

NOTE: Mode: most frequently occurring data point; Median: midpoint of the data (point at which the data lie 50% above and below); Mean: average of the data points; Range: officially the difference between the smallest and largest data point in the data set, although usually described by listing the smallest and largest data points (e.g., "The range is from 5 to 9"); interquartile range: difference between the scores at the 75th and 25th percentile; Standard Deviation: degree in which individual data points deviate from the mean value of the data set.

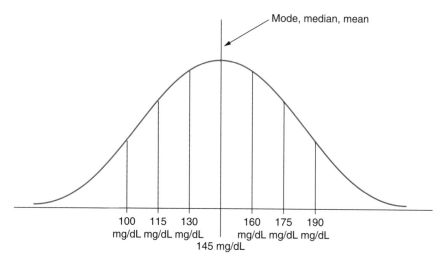

Figure 4-1. Histogram of LDL-C with standard deviation ± 15 mg/dL.

Explaining the terms in Table 4–6 can be done best via an example of a trial in which the change in LDL-C was measured. A total of 200 subjects were enrolled in a clinical study designed to measure the reduction in LDL-C with a statin versus placebo. The LDL-C is measured in all subjects at the beginning of the trial. The values are then plotted using a histogram (Figure 4–1). For each subject with a specific LDL-C value, a mark is placed on the graph for that value. As each subject with the same LDL-C value is plotted on the graph, an upward column for that LDL-C value forms. If the sample of subjects was randomly taken from the population, all the plotted LDL-C values would form a bell-shaped curve (also known as a normally distributed data set). After all LDL-C values are obtained, the values for the terms in Table 4–6 can be calculated. As seen from the graph, the mode (most commonly occurring LDL-C value), median (point at which 50% of the LDL-C values lie above and below) and the mean (average) LDL-C are the same. In this data set, a LDL-C of 145 mg/dL represents these three measures of central tendencies. In addition, the range for the LDL-C values can be determined by identifying the lowest and highest LDL-C value. The data also can be organized into quartiles, four groups containing 25% of the data points. The data are arranged from the lowest to highest value; afterwards, the data points are divided into four groups: 25th, 50th, 75th, and 100th percentile. Therefore, a LDL-C value that corresponds to the 75th percentile would be in the upper limit of this third quartile of the distribution. In addition, the upper limit of the 50th quartile would equal the median value for the data set. The interquartile range is the difference between the scores at the 75th and the 25th percentile.[123]

Since many trials present the results as an average (mean), a more detailed discussion of this measure of central tendency is warranted. Using the LDL-C example, an average

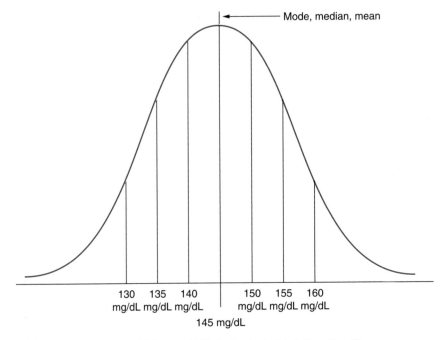

Figure 4–2. Histogram of LDL-C with standard deviation ± 5 mg/dL.

LDL-C value is calculated using all the measured values. However, presenting only the sample average does not inform the reader of the diversity in the set of values. Thus, a standard deviation (SD) is calculated using all of the LDL-C values. The SD is presented with the mean value of the sample (e.g., 145 mg/dL ± 15, where the former number is the mean and the latter number is the SD). The SD is important since the average LDL-C from two distinct samples may be the same, but the dispersion of the LDL-C values may be considerably different. Figure 4–2 displays another set of LDL-C values taken from a different sample of subjects. The average LDL-C value is the same as Figure 4–1, but the spread of the values are not very dispersed away from the average.

The presentation of the average ± SD allows the readers to calculate the percentage of LDL-C values within portions of the graph. Figure 4–3 illustrates the distribution of LDL-C within one, two, and three SDs from the average in a data set that has normal distribution of the values. As a rule, ~68% of the LDL-C values would be in ± 1 SD, ~95% in ±2 SDs, and ~99% in ± 3 SDs. Using Figure 4–1, the average LDL-C is 145 ± 15 mg/dL. Based upon these numbers, 68% of the LDL-C values are in the range of 130 to 160 mg/dL, 95% between 115 to 175 mg/dL, and 99% between 100 to 190 mg/dL. In Figure 4–2, the mean ± SD is 145 ± 5 mg/dL with corresponding values of: 140 to 150 mg/dL, 135 to 155 mg/ dL, and 130 to 160 mg/dL, respectively. Notice that even though the average of both

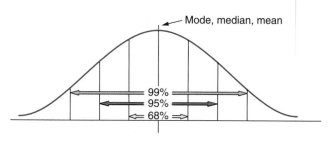

Figure 4–3. Histogram of normal distribution with standard deviations.

LDL-C data sets is the same, 95% of the LDL-C values are in the range of 115 to 175 mg/dL in Figure 4–1, but 135 to 155 mg/dL in Figure 4–2. The SD allows for the readers to assess more than just the mean for a set of data.

Although SD is commonly used, some investigators may present the standard error of the mean (SEM), which is calculated as the SD divided by the square root of the sample size (SD/$\sqrt{n}$).[122,124,125] As seen by this formula, the SEM is smaller than the SD, which implies a smaller dispersion of the data points away from the average. Presenting SEM instead of SD may occur when the investigators want the reader to interpret a small dispersion of the data from the mean value instead of a large variance from the mean if the SD was presented. While standard deviation measures the deviation of the individual values from the mean of the sample, SEM measures the deviation of the individual sample means from the mean of the population.[122] The SEM identifies the variability in the population; 95% of the time, the true mean of the population lies within two SEM of the sample mean.[125] At times SEM is used appropriately (more than one clinical trial) while at most times SEM is incorrectly presented.[125] Readers should be aware of these distinctions and interpret the data accordingly.

Inferential statistics are used to determine if a statistical difference is present between the intervention and control groups. A p-value is calculated based upon trial results and statistical tests; afterwards, the p-value is compared to the alpha (α) value established prior to the beginning of the trial[121,124] (see Statistical Significance versus Clinical Difference later in this chapter for further discussion). The selection of the statistical test depends upon the data being parametric (i.e., normal distribution) versus nonparametric. Typically, continuous data are assessed via parametric statistics; common tests are Student's t-test, analysis of variance (ANOVA), and analysis of covariance (ANCOVA). Nonparametric tests are used for nominal and ordinal data; examples are Chi square (χ^2) and Mann-Whitney U test.[93,121] A multitude of other statistical analytical procedures are available. An analysis of all research articles in six common pharmacy journals published during 2001 identified Chi square (χ^2), Student's t-test, and analysis of variance (ANOVA) as the three most common statistical tests used.[126] Chapter 8 in this textbook is devoted to a more in-depth discussion of statistical analyses.

Other statistical terms encountered while reading clinical trials are unpaired versus paired and one-tailed versus two-tailed statistical analysis. Comparing results between independent groups is referred to as unpaired analysis, while a paired analysis involves the same subject compared to themselves or to a similar matched subject.[120,127] For example, measuring the mean change in LDL-C from baseline to 12 weeks within the same subject receiving simvastatin would be a paired analysis. Analyzing the mean difference in the LDL-C reduction after 12 weeks between two independent groups, one being treated with simvastatin and the other with atorvastatin, would be considered an unpaired test. Two two-tailed (also known as two-sided) statistical tests are used for trials in which investigators are not sure in which direction the primary endpoint will be affected by the intervention. These tests analyze the results in both directions, for positive or negative effects in comparison to the control.[113] Two-tailed tests are more common because the direction of change (and the degree) is not known.[29,113] For example, a two-tailed test is used for an investigational drug compared to placebo to treat elevated LDL-C. The investigators do not know the effect of the intervention on the LDL-C levels (i.e., the levels can increase or decrease relative to the placebo). A one-tailed test is primarily used in a study in which the direction of the effect of the intervention and active control (e.g., another medication, but not placebo, such as a non-inferiority study) are known or can only go in one direction. The intent of this study type is to measure more precisely the difference in effect between the two groups. Some investigators have used a one-tailed test to determine differences in LDL-C changes in patients receiving statins. Prior research has documented the LDL-C lowering effects of atorvastatin and simvastatin being compared to other medications or placebo. Since these research results are available, a one-tailed test could be used to increase the statistical accuracy of detecting a difference in effect between the two statins in lowering LDL-C.

TYPE I AND II ERRORS/POWER ANALYSIS

A clinical trial is conducted to test a research hypothesis that a difference in effect exists between the intervention and control treatments. Before the trial begins, the investigators develop a null hypothesis (H_0; no difference between the groups) and research hypothesis (H_1; a difference is present between the groups). The trial is conducted and the investigators measure the difference in effect between the groups (if any). If a difference is present, this could actually be due to the intervention or happen by random chance (error).[118,119] Hypothesis testing is conducted to examine how likely any observed difference between the intervention and control would be due to chance if the H_0 were true. As the trial results diverge farther and farther from the finding of no difference, the H_0 is rejected (i.e., failure to accept the H_0) between the intervention and control group.[119]

TABLE 4–7. **TYPE I AND TYPE II ERRORS POSSIBILITIES**

Error Type	Action Decision	Interpretation
Type I	Statistical difference calculated, even though it is not really present; reject H_0	H_0 is really true, but was rejected, which leads to a false-positive result. The probability equals the α-error rate. There is one reason for a Type I error: chance.
Type II	No statistical difference calculated, even though there is one. Fail-to-reject ("accept") H_0.	H_0 is really false, but was accepted, which leads to a false-negative result. The probability equals the β-error rate. There are two reasons for a Type II error: chance or small sample size.

Two types of errors are possible in hypothesis testing (Table 4–7). A Type I error can occur when the H_0 is falsely rejected and the H_1 is falsely accepted. Thus, the investigators are stating a difference in effect was measured even though there really is no difference between the intervention and control groups (also known as a false-positive finding).[95,111,113,124] On the other hand, a Type II error can occur when H_0 is falsely accepted and the H_1 is falsely rejected. In this case, the investigators are stating no difference in effect is present between the intervention and control even though there really is a difference between the groups (also known as a false-negative finding).[70,113,124,128]

Investigators attempt to control for Type I and II error occurrence by setting limits on the probability of these occurring. The only reason that a Type I error can occur is by chance. Since no research is error-proof, methods usually are developed to allow up to a 5% probability that chance was the reason a difference in effect was measured between the intervention and control. The process of setting the probability of a Type I error (false-positive result) to occur no greater than 5% is termed as establishing the alpha (α) value.[111,113,124] This is also referred to setting the statistical significance to 0.05, but can also be phrased significance level of 0.05 or setting the alpha rate at 0.05. Another phrase commonly used to establish the α value is p-values < 0.05 are statistically significant. This rate is the norm for most studies, but a few trials may have $\alpha = 0.01$. This latter rate indicates the investigators are more stringent by reducing the possibility of a Type I error to 1%. However, setting $\alpha = 0.1$ is too relaxed and permits the Type I error possibility to be very high (at 10%). The alpha rate is a measure of how willing the researchers are to accept the chance of making a Type I error.[118] With the alpha rate at 0.05, this is indicating that in 1 of 20 trials, a difference in effect being measured between the groups can be due to chance.[70,111] An alpha rate of 0.002 indicates that in 2 out of 1000 trials, a difference in the measured effect between groups can be due to chance. Thus, the smaller the p-values, the less likely that chance (error) was the reason for finding the differences. Also, the p-value can be expressed as the probability of rejecting a true Ho.[121] This last statement will be explained in the statistical significance section later.

The probability of making a Type II error is referred to as beta (β).[70,113,128] Although investigators want to avoid a Type II error, appropriately designed clinical trials allow this error (false-negative) to occur no greater than 20% of the time.[70,128] Even though investigators want to avoid making both a Type I and Type II error, they are more willing to make a Type II error than Type I error because a Type II error may be easier to determine than a Type I error.[118] Also, Type I errors are more dangerous in terms of the possible direct effects on patients (see next paragraph). Therefore, this is why the alpha rate is set lower than the beta rate. Investigators, in designing the clinical trial, aim to balance the possibility of a Type I and Type II error knowing that decreasing the probability of one error may increase the probability of the other error occurring.

Making a Type I error means a difference in effect was measured by chance but really no difference in effect exists between the two groups. The danger of using a therapy no different from the control is more serious when the control is a placebo versus an active therapy. A Type II error indicates no difference was measured between the two groups. If the control group is another therapy, then the intervention is shown to be no different. If the control is a placebo, then the intervention may not be considered as a therapy to treat patients. Although the false-negative result is a concern (i.e., a useful therapy may be not used), this is less severe than a false-positive results (i.e., using a therapy that really is no different in effect from the control but was found to be by chance).

A Type II error can occur by either chance or small sample size in which the later is usually the reason if the error occurs.[113] The ultimate goal of each clinical trial is to ensure that the difference in effect size is properly measured between the intervention and control groups, which requires a sufficient sample size.[70] One method for the investigators to ensure that a sufficient number of subjects are enrolled in the trial is by conducting a power analysis. The power of a study is defined as the ability to detect a difference in the outcome between the intervention and control if a difference truly exists. Power is calculated from the β-error rate (power = 1-β).[112,128] As seen from this formula, the lower the β-error rate, the higher the power. Increasing the sample size then reduces the β-error rate, increases study power, and reduces the chance of a false-negative result.[112] In addition, the magnitude of difference in the effect that can be detected between the intervention and control group is related to the sample size; smaller differences in the effect between the intervention and control can be detected with larger sample sizes.[20,112]

Another factor important to ensure a clinical trial has the power to detect differences in effect is estimating the absolute difference in the effect (δ) between intervention and control groups.[24] This value is not as easily determined as the two other rates; the δ is usually based upon prior preliminary research results or even consensus discussion among the researchers (i.e., educated guess).[112]

The sample size needed is influence by the α-, β-, and δ-values. The purpose of the sample size calculation is to provide sufficient power to be able to reject the H_0 established for the clinical trial primary endpoint if it is false and should be rejected.[70] Hopefully, a clinical trial with an appropriate sample size will not lead to erroneously detecting a difference in effect when there is no real difference (Type I error), but also have a degree of certainty that the true difference in effects was not missed (Type II error).[111] A trial having an appropriate sample size increases the precision of estimating the difference in effect (effect size) of the intervention compared to the control.[16] The total number of subjects completing the trial should be similar to the actual sample size calculation for the study to have appropriate power.[112] Normally, the investigators will increase the sample size by some factor above the number calculated to be necessary (i.e., 10%) to account for subject attrition and therapy noncompliance.

Results

After the methods section, the results of the clinical trial are presented. This section contains primary and secondary endpoint results and other useful information, which includes patient demographics, dropout information, and side effect incidence. This section is to be critically appraised to verify if the study objective was met, based upon the data, but also to evaluate the other types of outcomes that may have occurred. Normally tables, charts, figures, or other illustrative forms present many of the results, which can expedite the understanding and analysis process.

SUBJECT DEMOGRAPHICS

The first type of information provided in the results section describes the subjects actually enrolled and randomized in the clinical trial.[23] A general overview of the average subject is described, and is usually presented in a table of demographic information.[129] Typical information in the table includes average age, male-to-female ratio, disease states, and/or drug therapy among the study participants at the time of enrollment. In addition, any complicating factors that can affect the endpoint(s) or trial outcome(s) may be described, such as the number of subjects who smoke, amount of caffeine intake, and so forth.

The patient baseline demographic data need to be compared between treatment groups to ensure the groups are as similar as possible. The groups should not have any significant differences if proper randomization techniques are incorporated by the study investigators; but a few differences can still occur due to chance.[16] Significant dissimilarities between the groups that could contribute to differences in the outcome between the groups need to be closely scrutinized. If the patient baseline differences are substantial, a confounding variable is present, and the study investigators must analyze the results to determine if these differences have affected the outcome of the study. Otherwise, the results may not be applicable to practice.[113]

An example of baseline subject demographics is illustrated by select patient information from the ENHANCE trial: 46.1 years average age; 53.5% male; 80% previously took statins; and 18% had hypertension as a risk factor. Only 10 baseline subject demographics were listed in the trial and only one was significantly different between the patients randomized to simvastatin plus ezetimibe versus simvastatin alone: body mass index (BMI), 26.7 versus 27.4, respectively.[53] Although a statistical difference is present, clinical judgment suggests the magnitude is not great and this would not significantly alter the study results in favor of one group.

SUBJECT DROPOUTS/COMPLIANCE

After the baseline subject information, data regarding the follow-up (i.e., subject dropout) and compliance should be presented. Not all subjects randomized in a clinical trial will complete the entire duration, at which time they are then termed a study dropout or lost to follow-up.[69] Reasons vary for discontinuing study participation and include lack of desire to continue, subject relocation (e.g., moving to another city), subject violating study protocol, side effects, and death. Also, not all subjects will be compliant with the therapy. Not accounting for the number of dropouts and noncompliance can have an effect on the trial results.[69,130,131] Thus, the investigators need to report the number of subjects and major reasons for discontinuing the study, compliance rates, and the techniques of assessing the data for the readers to draw appropriate conclusions about the intervention under study and subsequent trial results.

The impact of dropouts on the overall study results is dependent on the magnitude of subject discontinuations. A few subjects dropping out of the study may not cause a substantial difference in the results, whereas a sizable percentage may alter the study results significantly. No threshold of dropout rates have been established that deems the trial results to be of no clinical value. The overall effect of the dropouts on the significance of the trial results is dependent upon the trial endpoints and readers' interpretation. For example, a hypothetical clinical trial had 100 patients each in the intervention and control group, all who had an infection. At study end, patients in the intervention group experienced greater infection cure rates (75% versus 40%). However, 60 patients discontinued the intervention compared to only 10 patients from the control due to side effects, and these data were not included in the overall study results. If all subjects were included in the analysis (counting the dropouts as therapy failures), the cure rate would be lower in the intervention than control group (30% versus 36%). This illustrates the importance of reporting results for all subjects enrolled, not just those completing the clinical trial.

Frequently, the study results will be analyzed using data collected from all randomized subjects, regardless of whether they completed the entire study duration (i.e., results from dropouts are not discarded, but are considered to be treatment failures). This technique is referred to as the intention-to-treat (ITT) principle (see Chapter 5 for more on ITT and per-protocol [PP]). Even in cases where the subject may have only taken one dose of the medication under investigation, these results are still included in the ITT analysis. The advantage of the ITT analysis is this analysis better mimics real-life application of an intervention into practice because, similar to real-life, all subjects in a clinical trial may not complete therapy as prescribed.[130,131] However, a concern with the ITT analysis is that data from subjects discontinuing a trial early may bias the analysis. This is of considerable importance for an endpoint measurement that worsens over time (e.g., cognitive function in subjects with dementia). The last score obtained in a subject discontinuing the trial early may suggest a better response than the last score obtained if this subject discontinued later in the trial.[132]

At times, the study results are analyzed via ITT and the per-protocol (PP) procedure. The latter term refers to analyzing data only from subjects completing the trial. The advantage of this technique is for determining the effects of the intervention in subjects that followed the study protocol and completed the entire course of therapy.

An example of analyzing study data according to ITT and PP methods follows. The West of Scotland Coronary Prevention Study (WOSCOPS) reported the ITT results of pravastatin lowering mean LDL-C by –15.8% compared to –26.3% via the PP analysis (from a baseline of 190 mg/dL to 160 mg/dL and 140 mg/dL, respectively). The change for the control group was virtually unchanged, as expected.[133] Both the ITT and PP results can be useful to apply into practice; a subject meeting the inclusion criteria of this trial who is compliant and correctly taking pravastatin may achieve on average LDL-C lowering of 26%, while as a whole this value would decrease by an average of 16% in the group of patients treated with this medication.

Clinical trials including only the PP results are to be scrutinized more because results from all subjects are not assessed. Reasons for the subjects discontinuing should be evaluated to interpret the PP analysis. Assessing the results only via PP in a trial that had the majority of subjects discontinuing due to adverse drug effects leads to overestimation of the results. If the subjects discontinued the trial due to relocating to another city, then analyzing the trial results via PP is not affected as significantly as in the prior case. Investigators not accounting for discontinuations directly caused by the therapies leads to biased results since these subjects can be counted as treatment failures but are not.

ENDPOINTS/SAFETY

A critical component of the results section is the primary endpoint results. These results can be displayed as tables, graphs, or other illustrations. The information should be presented clearly and completely, using clear and unbiased methods. In addition, the investigators need to explain the results and present p-values. Results of secondary endpoints follow and are presented in a fashion similar to the primary endpoints; however, endpoints other than the primary endpoint may not be adequately powered to detect differences in effect between the intervention and control. Therefore, if statistically significant results occur with these other endpoints, the results may be due to chance. Other endpoints should be adequately powered to draw meaningful conclusions regarding use in practice.[23]

One issue to consider in evaluating the results in some clinical trials is whether medication dosing titration is allowed in the methods. The final medication dose of one group may be maximized while the other group did not require maximum doses. The investigators may make a conclusion based upon misleading information. An example is a hypothetical trial beginning with losartan 50 mg once daily. The dose is increased to 100 mg once daily and hydrochlorothiazide (HCTZ) 25 mg once daily can be added so that goal DBP of < 90 mm Hg is achieved. The control group received amlodipine 5 mg once daily; the dose also could be increased to 10 mg once daily and HCTZ 25 mg once daily could be added. Approximately 85% of patients randomized to losartan also received HCTZ while only 45% randomized to amlodipine received HCTZ. The investigators concluded that losartan was as effective as amlodipine in achieving goal DBP even though a disproportionate number of subjects received the maximum losartan dose plus HCTZ compared to amlodipine and only 15% of the losartan-treated subjects received monotherapy versus 55% of the amlodipine-treated subjects. The final losartan and amlodipine doses need to be assessed in regard to the number of subjects receiving the higher medication dose and those with HCTZ. The number of patients who received HCTZ should also be assessed to determine if clinically meaningful results can be drawn between losartan and amlodipine despite differences in doses and HCTZ therapy. Readers should be cautious in accepting investigators' conclusion that two drugs are equal in effect in a trial with methods that allow dose titrations and/or additional medications added to therapy without analyzing the final doses.

Safety assessments or tolerability of all therapies should be included in the results section.[23] Investigators need to implement valid methods of defining, collecting, and analyzing these results. As with the secondary endpoints, the study may not be powered sufficiently to definitively quantify the safety/tolerability of the intervention. In addition, the frequency and severity of these results may be dissimilar to those observed in clinical practice. Investigators need to monitor the subjects closely and collect these data.[41] Other factors need to be considered that include the clinical trial duration, limited sample size, and exclusion of selected subjects from being enrolled into the trial.

Surrogate Endpoints

Investigators of some clinical trials select a primary endpoint that can be classified as a surrogate endpoint,[134] which is described as "a measure of the efficacy of a treatment [that] can be defined as laboratory values (e.g., HDL-C/LDL-C), symptoms (e.g., pain), or clinical parameters (e.g., blood pressure) which are employed as a substitute for a clinical endpoint (e.g., morbidity, mortality). Here it is assumed that changes in the surrogate endpoint can be directly translated into changes in the definitive clinical endpoint."[135] The primary reason surrogate endpoints are selected for clinical trials is to quickly measure an effect at a lower cost.[135] Also, surrogate endpoints are measured instead of clinical endpoints due to a lower clinical trial financial burden and shorter time commitment. The established efficacy and other data collected from trials measuring surrogate endpoint provide the rationale for larger trials with clinical endpoints (i.e., MI, stroke, death).[25] The following conditions should be fulfilled before a surrogate endpoint is considered as a valid substitute for a clinical endpoint: convenience (easily and readily assessable); well-established relationship between the surrogate and clinical outcomes (e.g., LDL-C and risk of MI); and determination of clinical benefit as a result of changes in the surrogate endpoint.[135]

The ENHANCE trial was designed to utilize a surrogate endpoint (arterial thickness) in order to determine the progression of atherosclerosis. As previously described, this study compared simvastatin 80 mg plus ezetimibe 10 mg to simvastatin 80 mg and measured arterial thickness at baseline and 24 months.[53] Arterial thickness is a surrogate endpoint because the investigators hypothesized this would correlate to disease progression. However, many researchers disagree with this assessment. They do not believe this to be a validated measure as a surrogate endpoint that correlates with a decrease in morbidity and mortality.

The primary limitation of surrogate endpoints is illustrated by an excellent example. Investigators of the ILLUMINATE trial reported a significant increase in mean HDL-C with adding torcetrapib to atorvastatin versus atorvastatin alone (+72% versus +2%, respectively) along with change in LDL-C (−25% versus +3%, respectively) after 12 months of therapy. One would expect these two changes in cholesterol levels to reduce the risk of cardiovascular events (e.g., nonfatal MI, stroke). However, the incidence of a major cardiovascular event was significantly higher in patients treated with the drug combination than atorvastatin alone (6.2% versus 5%, respectively).[136] As can be seen, the use of surrogate endpoints to support benefit in clinical outcomes is not always guaranteed.

SUBGROUP ANALYSIS

Investigators often analyze the results of subsets of the study subjects, as divided into various groups that often include gender, age, and presence of diseases or other complicating factors (i.e., diabetes versus no diabetes).[137] Reasons to analyze the results in these subgroups vary, but usually relate to providing additional information in these specific patient types as opposed to just the overall trial results from all the randomized subjects. For example, trial investigators may analyze the results according to various demographics that included age (i.e. ≤ 65 years and > 65 years), race/ethnicity, or gender.[53]

Although the investigators may be able to obtain more information from a trial by using subgroup analysis, limitations and other issues need to be recognized.[23,79,102,137,138] A few prerequisites should be present before subgroup analyses are conducted. First, the clinical trial should be well-designed with sound study methods. A subgroup analysis should be defined prior to the initiation of the trial and have documented justification (e.g., past studies suggest a benefit in that patient group). Subgroup analyses should come from trials with well-defined study methods (e.g., ITT, randomization, blinding). If results from studies are sufficiently flawed, there is no reason to perform subgroup analysis. Additionally, data analysis should only be conducted from those studies in which the primary endpoint was statistically significant; otherwise, investigators may be searching for statistically significant results.[138] Second, the investigator may have conducted a multitude of subgroup analyses and only reported the statistically significant results. As the number of statistical evaluations increases, the likelihood of finding a statistical difference by chance alone increases.[137] Therefore, multiple subgroup analyses should be avoided, unless authors can show they have powered the endpoint for the analysis *a priori* and/or have adjusted error rates statistically to control for multiple comparisons. Third, the power of the assessment is reduced, since results from a smaller number of subjects are analyzed as compared to the entire trial sample. Reduced power may lead to false-positive results.[137,138] Fourth, the subgroup analyses should be defined prior to the initiation of the trial and have documented justification to be conducted (e.g., past studies results suggest an effect in this group). Also, the ITT data are preferred for these evaluations since subject discontinuations may not be balanced between the two groups. Sixth, outcomes that can be influenced by either the intervention or control (i.e., compliance) should not be selected for a subgroup analysis. Last, the reader needs to review the appropriate subgroup analysis, but keep the primary endpoint as their focus.[137] Subgroup analysis can be helpful in determining future research questions, but unless powered appropriately should not be used to base changes in clinical practice.

The reader should recognize both positive and negative features of subgroup analyses. Further details of the trial results in a specific patient type are provided and may be justification to conduct clinical trials with a larger sample with just this subject type. For instance, the PROSPER study was the first study to evaluate a statin (pravastatin) specifically in the elderly to reduce adverse events (primary endpoint measured as a combination of definite or suspected death from CHD, nonfatal MI, and fatal or nonfatal stroke). Prior clinical trials evaluating reduction of clinical events (e.g., MI, death) with a statin enrolled few elderly subjects. Analysis of the results in only the elderly subjects of these trials suggested statins were clinically useful for this patient type. Thus, investigators conducted a specific clinical trial in which elderly men and women between 70 and 82 years of age with a history of, or risk factors for, vascular disease (e.g., coronary, cerebral, or peripheral) or at risk (e.g., hypertension, diabetes, and smoking) were enrolled. The incidence of the primary endpoint was lower with pravastatin than placebo (16.2% versus 14.1%; p = 0.014).[139] The results of this study provided the evidence to prescribe a statin (specifically pravastatin) in this patient type, instead of extrapolating this decision upon subgroup analysis of previous statin studies that included elderly individuals (but not as the primary subject type).

However, subgroup analysis limitations need to be recognized. Overinterpretation of subgroup results can occur, usually because the overall study results did not demonstrate the desired difference in effect as expected by the investigators.[134] The sample size included in a clinical trial is based upon the primary endpoint for all enrolled subjects. Reducing the sample size via a subgroup analysis can lead to a positive result that may have occurred by chance.[79,130,137,138] An illustration of this effect was documented by the African-American Antiplatelet Stroke Prevention Study (AAASPS),[140] which was conducted in response to the subgroup analysis of Ticlopidine Aspirin Stroke Study (TASS).[141] The TASS investigators documented a lower incidence of nonfatal stroke or death from any cause in subjects with recent transient or mild persistent focal cerebral or retinal ischemia taking ticlopidine compared to aspirin (17% versus 19%; p = 0.048). In addition to this overall study result, the investigators reported fewer cases of stroke and death with ticlopidine compared to aspirin in a subgroup analysis of African-Americans enrolled in this trial. The AAASPS results documented a slightly higher incidence of the composite endpoint (recurrent stroke, MI, or vascular death) in patients taking ticlopidine compared to aspirin (14.8% versus 12.4%; p = 0.12). Although the study designs of these two studies were not identical, the AAASPS results serves as an example to the limitations of selecting therapy based upon subgroup analysis. Thus, practitioners should be aware that although subgroup analysis may document greater benefits in selected individuals, the differences in effect may be due to chance or other factors.

ANCILLARY VERSUS ADJUNCTIVE THERAPIES

Clinical trials are designed to have identical groups with the only difference between the groups being the assignment to the intervention or control. At times, the study design may allow ancillary therapy to be included, in which subjects can take another therapy that can distort or interfere with the results.[69] The effect of the ancillary therapy on the study results needs to be assessed and included in the study evaluation. However, readers should not confuse ancillary therapy with adjunctive therapy. Some studies may include in the methods an adjunctive therapy, which all participants receive as treatment, while ancillary therapy is not equally distributed between the intervention and control groups. Thus, any significant difference in effect between the outcomes measured between the groups should be due to the therapies under investigation, not the adjunctive therapy. An example is a study comparing atorvastatin with simvastatin to lower LDL-C, where each patient has to follow a specified diet.[58] Although this diet can lower LDL-C, all patients are receiving the diet, and any effects of the diet on the LDL-C change should be similar between the groups. However, ancillary therapy with antacids (amount not regulated, patient takes as many as they wish) in a study comparing heartburn relief between esome-prazole as needed versus lansoprazole taken every day can lead to biased results.[142] At the end of the study, esomeprazole relieved heartburn symptoms better between the two groups, but the investigators did not report the antacid amount consumed by patients in either group (i.e., the average daily intake could have been 8.2 versus 1.2 tablets for the esomeprazole versus lansoprazole group, respectively). Antacids can reduce heartburn symptoms, but a significant imbalance may have been present between the two groups which could be the reason esomeprazole was reported to relieve symptoms better.

Discussion/Conclusion

The primary purpose of discussion/conclusion is to evaluate and/or interpret the results of the clinical trial. Investigators should begin with a summary of the key findings of the study. Potential explanations of the study results should be addressed, in addition to discussing internal and external validity of outcomes.[23] The investigators should also interpret the trial results in comparison with results of other similarly designed studies. Also, the trial may be discussed in comparison to other trials assessing the intervention or the disease state under investigation. This is also where clinical trial limitations are identified and discussed.[23] Even though all clinical trials have limitations, these may vary from minor to those that seriously hinder the usefulness of the results, including completely invalidating the study. The discussion section should also address the clinical importance of the clinical trial results and how these results should be used in practice. All of this information should allow the reader to understand the application of the clinical trial results in practice. However, this section needs to be read just as carefully as the other sections, because it can contain biased wording. In addition, only selected items may be discussed in relationship to the clinical trial.[79]

The investigators should ensure that strategies are included within the study design to minimize biases that may occur. Some of the strategies can include blinding, randomization, and appropriate inclusion/exclusion criteria. In addition, investigators should not be biased in interpreting the results of the trial. Readers should determine the degree that the study results compare with patients encountered in practice. One of the most commonly cited criticisms of clinical trials by clinicians is the lack of external validity of the trials, which may be one explanation for the underuse of reportedly favorable treatment options in clinical trials by clinicians.[143] Although some investigators may report beneficial results of an intervention under investigation, the patient population in the clinical trial may be so dissimilar to patients encountered in practice that clinicians are not convinced that the favorable results may be beneficial in their patient population. Several issues may potentially affect the external validity of the clinical trial and should be evaluated to assess the effects of the results in practice. These include the setting of the trial, selection of patients, characteristics of randomized patients, differences between the trial protocol and routine practice, outcome measures, follow-up, and adverse effects of treatment.[143] If the characteristics of the patients and setting are very different from those encountered in practice, the clinical usefulness of the reported information may be questionable.

Study strengths and limitations should be addressed in the discussion section. Potential limitations may include small sample size, short duration of the study, endpoint assessment techniques, or other factors that hinder the clinical usefulness of the study. The investigators should also address methods to circumvent trial limitations in subsequent clinical studies. Although there is no minimum or maximum limitation number that investigators should address, a thorough discussion of the limitations should be provided so that readers can determine the applicability of the trial results to their patient population.

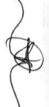

Comparison of the current study to previous studies should be conducted. According to the results of one study, discussion sections of trial reports were lacking complete analysis of previous clinical trial results.[144] A total of 33 randomized trials were identified in 19 issues of leading medical journals (e.g., *Annals of Internal Medicine, JAMA)* in May 2001. The authors of four reports claimed that their study was a first-of-a-kind study; however, reports of similar trials were located for one of these studies. In three of the reports, systematic reviews of earlier trials were mentioned; however, no attempts to incorporate the results of the new trial with the existing results were identified in the remaining 27 reports. The results of other trials should be included to allow the reader to assess the results of the current trial in context to previous trial results. The readers can determine if the study is a first-of-a-kind study that adds substantial information to a topic or is a me-too study that adds no new information to existing knowledge. The discussion section should also address future concerns and unanswered questions.

The conclusion section should provide an overall research recommendation to the readers. The investigators' conclusion should focus on the primary endpoint results, especially if no statistically significant differences between the intervention and control group were observed, rather than favorable, secondary endpoint results. Conclusions should be limited to only that information discussed in previous sections of the trial; no new information should be discussed in this section. Also, the conclusions should be aligned with the results of the trial. Investigators should not make erroneous conclusions that are not supported by the results of the trial.

Clinical Trial Result Interpretation

STATISTICAL SIGNIFICANCE VERSUS CLINICAL DIFFERENCE

❽ *Correctly interpreting the p-values is crucial in evaluating a controlled clinical trial; not all statistically significant p-values are clinically important. The magnitude of difference in effect between the intervention and control cannot be determined solely with the p-value.* Once the clinical trial is completed, the investigators calculate a p-value for the endpoints using the collected study results and statistical tests. The p-value is an abbreviation for probability-value and is compared to the alpha (α) value established prior to the beginning of the clinical trial (*a priori*) that serves as the benchmark to which p-values are compared to determine if statistical significance is present. Also, since the entire population is not included, the investigators have to estimate the difference in effect from the sample.[118,119,145] Without statistical analysis, the likelihood of chance being the reason for any measured difference in effect is not known.[113] A p-value for the primary endpoint that is less than the alpha value indicates the H_0 is rejected and a statistically significant difference is declared between the intervention and control groups. This also indicates chance alone was not likely the reason that a difference in effect was measured. The H_0 is accepted (failed to be rejected) with a p-value equal to or greater than the alpha value and no statistically significant difference is declared.[119,145]

Statistical significance does not automatically mean a clinical difference in the effect between the intervention and control groups.[146] (See next section regarding the assessment of clinical difference.) The reader needs to make a decision in determining if the intervention is worth using instead of the control therapy, which can be dependent upon the judgment and experiences of the reader (i.e., assessing both internal and external validity). Not all statistically significant studies have clinically different results (Figure 4–4). A p-value less than the alpha value only represents the probability that a true H_0 has been rejected. In other words, the p-value can be translated into "what is the probability of the difference in the effect between the intervention and control due to chance?"[118] Lower p-values indicate a lower probability that chance alone could be the reason a difference in effect was measured between the intervention and control. Alternatively stated, "what is the chance of observing this difference if there really was no difference between the two groups?"[113] Recall that a Type I error is possible after rejecting the H_0; the results may be statistically significant due to chance alone.

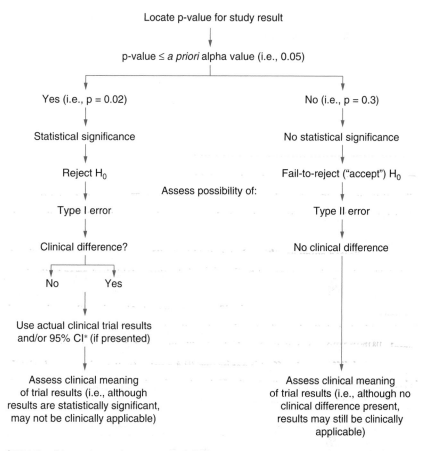

Locate p-value for study result

p-value ≤ *a priori* alpha value (i.e., 0.05)

| Yes (i.e., p = 0.02) | | No (i.e., p = 0.3) |

| Statistical significance | | No statistical significance |

| Reject H_0 | Assess possibility of: | Fail-to-reject ("accept") H_0 |

| Type I error | | Type II error |

| Clinical difference? | | No clinical difference |

No   Yes

Use actual clinical trial results
and/or 95% CI* (if presented)

| Assess clinical meaning of trial results (i.e., although results are statistically significant, may not be clinically applicable) | | Assess clinical meaning of trial results (i.e., although no clinical difference present, results may still be clinically applicable) |

*95% Confidence interval.

Figure 4–4. Determining statistical significance, clinical difference, and clinical meaningfulness.

Another paramount issue in understanding clinical trials is that the p-value does not express the magnitude of difference in the effect between the intervention and control.[119] Statistically significant results simply signify that the alternative hypothesis (H_1) is accepted. The H_1 states a difference in the effect is present between the intervention and control. From this information, the reader cannot determine complex quantitative differences in effect (i.e., clinical difference between intervention and control groups).[113,121]

In addition, specific p-values should be stated in the text of the article (i.e., p = 0.0012 instead of p < 0.05) to be more informative and helpful to the reader.[113,119] Also, all p-values should be presented in conjunction with associated endpoint results (e.g., *the clinical trial concluded that drug A lowered mean DBP more than placebo, –12 versus –3 mm Hg, respectively [p = 0.001]* as opposed to *the clinical trial concluded that drug A lowered mean*

DBP more than placebo [p = 0.001]). Readers should scrutinize study data that presents p-values without endpoint results (naked p-values). Such a situation should prompt the reader to ask, "Were the endpoint results not presented with the p-value because the actual difference in the effect was minimal?" Without the endpoint results being presented, statistical significance alone can be concluded with the p-value; clinical differences cannot be assessed without accompanying endpoint results. See next sections for further discussion of this issue.

ASSESSING CLINICAL DIFFERENCE

Two critical items needed to assess clinical difference between the intervention and control groups of a clinical trial are the p-value and actual study results used to calculate the p-value. A fundamental first step of determining clinical difference in a given trial begins with determining if statistical significance exists (i.e., p < *a priori* alpha value) (see Figure 4–4). The reader must keep in mind that clinical difference is predicated on statistical significance. Put another way, clinical difference between the intervention and control cannot exist with study outcome data if the results are not statistically significant. The second step in assessing clinical differences is evaluating the results used to calculate the p-value. The reader must analyze the magnitude of endpoint difference between the intervention and control results.[113,146] Once a reader determines statistical significance is present with given study data, no magical formula is available to conclude whether clinical difference exists between the intervention and control.[119] The remainder of the process is based upon clinical knowledge and experience and may be relative in the reader's opinion to whether clinical difference is present or not. For example, an antihypertensive therapy lowers mean DBP by 14 mm Hg versus 3 mm Hg with placebo in subjects with a mean baseline DBP of 98 mm Hg. In this case, the results are clinically different due to 11 mm Hg average difference and subjects are achieving goal DBP values from baseline (< 85 mm Hg). However, atorvastatin lowering mean LDL-C by 1.7% greater than simvastatin (37.1% versus 35.4%; p = 0.0097[71]) can be considered not clinically different in subjects with a mean baseline LDL-C of 181 mg/dL. The mean LDL-C was reduced by < 2% with atorvastatin than simvastatin, a difference that most likely is not associated with producing clinical differences in effect. In addition, the actual mean LDL-C lowering was almost identical (66 mg/dL), and the mean LDL-C level at study end was < 116 mg/dL in both groups.

Some readers may consider the trial results to be clinically different while others may not. In fact, two people may have different conclusions after reading the same clinical trial. This situation is very common when interpreting clinical trials in health care practice. In response, readers must justify their own conclusion regarding their decision of clinical difference. A few suggestions and examples are provided to assist in determining clinical difference.

Understanding the instrument that was used in measuring the endpoint is important in assessing clinically significant differences in trials. For example, ordinal data typically use scales or ranking (e.g., pain, depression scales).[120] Thus, the definitions of the minimum and maximum numbers of these scales need to be known. As an example, investigators of a hypothetical clinical trial concluded that glucosamine (500 mg three times a day) reduced pain greater than placebo in men with osteoarthritis (OA) of the knee. Pain intensity difference at rest was assessed by a 10-point visual analog scale (0 = no pain; 10 = severe pain). The median scores were 3.6 with placebo versus 3.3 with glucosamine (p = 0.03) at the end of the trial. Although results are statistically significant between glucosamine and placebo, the difference in scores between these two groups is minimal, only 0.3 points on a 10-point scale. Stating a clinical difference between glucosamine and placebo would be considered incorrect.

Another issue to consider is that clinical trials with too large a sample size (i.e., overpowered) lead to smaller p-values versus those with smaller sample sizes.[112,119] The magnitude of the p-value is dependent upon sample size; small differences in effect can be statistically significant with large sample size.[113] Thus, statistically significant results can occur even though a small absolute difference in effect is present. An example of this issue is a clinical trial that compared esomeprazole (n = 2624) versus lansoprazole (n = 2617). The primary endpoint, incidence of erosive esophagitis healing, was statistically significant in favor of esomeprazole (92.6% versus 88.8%; p = 0.0001).[147] The investigators (and marketing advertisements) concluded esomeprazole to be superior to lansoprazole, although the absolute difference in healing was only 4% between these two drugs. In addition, a significant number of subjects in each group (> 88%) experienced erosive esophagitis healing. Readers can debate whether the difference in effect is clinically different.

A data assessment technique that can be misleading is converting a continuous endpoint measure into a dichotomous value. For instance, blood pressure (continuous value) is measured after an intervention (rofecoxib) and control (celecoxib) are administered. Those subjects with a blood pressure above a predefined cut-off point are classified as being hypertensive (nominal data because subject has a blood pressure value below or above this cut-off point). Significantly more subjects taking rofecoxib versus celecoxib were diagnosed with systolic hypertension (17% versus 11%, respectively; p = 0.032). However, the change in the mean for SBP values was +2.6 versus –0.5 mm Hg, respectively (p = 0.007).[148] These two data sets assessed together indicate that rofecoxib may not negatively affect SBP compared to celecoxib. The actual SBP in the subjects taking rofecoxib may have just exceeded the cut-off hypertensive value (increase > 20 mm Hg with absolute value > 140 mm Hg) while just below this value for the celecoxib (i.e., 141 versus 139 mm Hg, respectively). The absolute difference between these two blood pressure values is minimal (3 mm Hg), but the number of subjects counted as hypertensive is different (6%).

The change in SBP between these two medications does not appear to be clinically different. Even though the measured endpoints between subjects randomized to the intervention are numerically close to the control, the subjects were categorized differently based upon cut-off blood pressure values. This example illustrates the potential biases of this form of data analysis and presentation.

The foundation in determining clinical difference between an intervention and control is the p-value and actual study results. Other items can assist the reader in this endeavor and include 95% confidence intervals and calculating measures of association; both of these are described below. However, readers must remember that not all clinical trials may have these latter two items. Thus, the importance of analyzing and interpreting p-values and the magnitude of difference between the intervention and control cannot be over emphasized.

CONFIDENCE INTERVALS

More clinical trials are including 95% confidence intervals (CI) with the study results, which can assist in assessing clinical difference between the intervention and control. ❾ *The use of 95% confidence intervals can assist the reader in assessing the magnitude of difference in effect between the intervention and control to apply to the population.* Confidence intervals provide data that address the size of effect (e.g., mean reduction in DBP) of the intervention under investigation in a clinical trial by presenting a range that likely covers the true but unknown value.[149,150] Although the basis of accepting or rejecting the H_0 is based upon the p-value, a limitation of the p-value is that the magnitude of difference in effect between the intervention and control groups of a clinical trial is not known, since it is not able to be determined based upon a statistical calculation.[119,146] Because of this, the use of a CI can assist in judging the clinical usefulness of the study result.[113] Clinical trials report the effect of an intervention as a point estimate, a single value that can be considered to represent the true effect (e.g., mean reduction in DBP; incidence of MI). For instance, an angiotensin-converting enzyme (ACE) inhibitor lowered mean DBP by 8 mm Hg; this value would be termed the point estimate. If the study was repeated, a similar, but not exact, reduction in mean DBP may occur (e.g., –10 mm Hg, –12 mm Hg). The presentation of the results only as a point estimate provides the reader with limited information. Clinical trials presenting 95% CI in conjunction with the point estimate enables the readers to further critique the study results and determine the usefulness for practice.

 A confidence interval provides an indication of the outcome within the population and is interpreted as a range of values in which the true value is included. The 95% CI for an average is calculated using the standard error of the mean (SEM) from the trial sample. Recalling the formula for SEM, the standard deviation is divided by the square root of the sample size ($SD/\sqrt{n}$). A 95% CI is equivalent to approximately two SEM from the sample mean, with an exact formula of: CI = mean ±1.96 ∗ SEM. The SEM is used as opposed to the SD since SEM is more reflective of the population variance, while SD is indicative of the dispersion within the sample.[119,150] A 95% CI is not the only CI reported in the literature, and readers of clinical trials need to recognize the changes in the interpretation. A 99% CI indicates more confidence that the true, but unknown, endpoint value is in this range than does a 95% CI. Thus, the 99% CI range is wider in value than a 95% CI, where as a 90% CI range is more narrow (i.e., less confident).[150,151]

A 95% CI for a point estimate is a common method of data presentation. Investigators of a clinical trial reported the mean reduction in DBP with an ACE inhibitor was –11.3 mm Hg (95% CI, –8.2 to –14.4 mm Hg) in subjects with a mean baseline DBP of 99 mm Hg. This indicates that the investigators are 95% confident that the mean DBP reduction in the population is between –8.2 to –14.4 mm Hg. An important issue to recognize in interpreting a 95% CI is that there is a lower probability for the mean reduction in DBP at the upper and lower end of the 95% CI range compared to numbers near the point estimate value.[122] The further away a value lies from the point estimate within the 95% CI range, the lower the probability that this value is representative of the given population. A low probability exists that the ACE inhibitor lowers mean DBP in the population by only –8.2 mm Hg compared to a higher probability that mean DBP reduction is closer to the point estimate of 11.3 mm Hg (the same is true with the upper end of the 95% CI).

Within this trial, the ACE inhibitor was compared to hydrochlorothiazide (HCTZ) and the mean DBP reduction with HCTZ was –9.9 mm Hg (95% CI, –7.5 to –13.3 mm Hg). The same principles are used to interpret this 95% CI as with the ACE inhibitor 95% CI; the investigators are 95% confident that the mean reduction of DBP in the population with HCTZ is between 7.5 and 13.3 mm Hg. In addition, these two 95% CI ranges can be compared to determine any difference in effect between these two agents. Since both 95% CI ranges overlap considerably, no difference in effect is concluded.[113,119,151] However, if no overlap of the 95% CI for the two groups is present, a clinical difference can be concluded.

Another common method of data presentation is calculating a 95% CI for the difference of the point estimates between two groups. In the above trial example, the point estimate of mean DBP lowering with the ACE inhibitor was –11.3 mm Hg while –9.9 mm Hg for HCTZ. The difference in mean DBP between these two equals –1.4 mm Hg (–11.3 minus –9.9 = –1.4). The 95% CI for the difference in the point estimates is calculated to be –3.9 to +1.1 mm Hg. This is interpreted as being 95% confident that the difference in mean DBP reduction can be 1.1 mm Hg greater with HCTZ (e.g., –13.1 mm Hg for HCTZ versus –12 mm Hg for ACE inhibitor) or 3.9 mm Hg greater with the ACE inhibitor (e.g., –16.9 mm Hg for ACE inhibitor versus –13 mm Hg for HCTZ). Notice the upper end of the 95% CI of the difference in point estimates is a positive number (+1.1 mm Hg). This does not indicate the mean DBP was increased, only that the difference in mean DBP lowering was 1.1 mm Hg greater with HCTZ compared to ACE inhibitor (e.g., –12 minus

–13.1 mm Hg for ACE inhibitor and HCTZ, respectively). Also, in this 95% CI is the number zero (value of equality); this indicates with 95% confidence that no difference in mean DBP between these two groups (e.g., –13.2 minus –13.2 mm Hg for both agents equals zero). If no zero is in the 95% CI of the difference between the two point estimates, then a clinical difference in effect between the intervention and control could be concluded.

The interpretation of clinical difference using 95% CI is dependent upon clinical experience and appropriate assessment. A 95% CI without a zero in the range does not always indicate a clinical difference between the intervention and control. For example, a 95% CI for mean DBP lowering in a trial comparing an ACE inhibitor and HCTZ was –1.9 to –0.5 mm Hg. Even though this 95% CI range does not contain a zero, a mean difference of only 0.5 to 1.9 mm Hg greater DBP lowering effect with one agent would not be considered clinically different.

INTERPRETING RISKS AND NUMBERS-NEEDED-TO-TREAT

Another technique to critique and interpret clinical trial results is to calculate the measures of association: relative risk (RR), relative risk reduction (RRR), absolute risk reduction (ARR), and number-needed-to-treat (NNT). ⑩ *Calculating measures-of-association (RR, ARR, RRR, NNT) for nominal data provides further information to evaluate the meaning of controlled clinical trial results.* However, these calculations only can be performed with clinical trials designed to determine if there is a reduction in an outcome that occurs with modification of a risk factor when comparing the intervention to the control. Examples of outcomes could include the incidence of MI, stroke, hospitalization, or death. Since the endpoint is dichotomous (i.e., occurred or did not occur), the results can be set up in a table, as illustrated in Table 4–8. As seen from Table 4–8, the subjects randomized to the intervention are represented by either A (number of subjects experiencing the outcome) or B (those without the outcome). Subjects assigned to the control group and experiencing the outcome are designated by C while those without the outcome by D.[151,152]

Table 4–9 displays the formulas to calculate the four measure of association values plus provides a description of these measures;[151,152] a description of interpreting these values follows. The RR is calculated as the proportion of the intervention group

TABLE 4–8. PRESENTING NOMINAL DATA STUDY RESULTS

Group	Adverse Event	
	Yes	No
Intervention	A	B
Control	C	D

TABLE 4–9. **MEASURES OF ASSOCIATION DESCRIPTION AND FORMULAS**

Measure of Association	Description	Formula
RR	Amount of risk removed by the intervention compared to the control	[A/(A + B)]/[C/(C + D)]
RRR	Percent of baseline risk removed	1-RR
ARR	Percentage of subjects treated with the intervention spared the adverse outcome compared with the control	[C/(C + D)] – [A/(A + B)]
NNT	Number of subjects needed to be treated to prevent one adverse event. A time course is included that represents the average (or median) duration of follow-up during the trial	1/(ARR)

experiencing the outcome divided by the proportion of the control group with the event. The RR equaled to 1 indicates no difference between the intervention and control (i.e., the incidence of the outcome was not increased nor decreased with the intervention compared to control). Anytime a numerator divided by a denominator calculates to 1, these two variables are equal. The RR < 1 signifies the intervention lowered the risk of the outcome compared to the control (i.e., protective effect); a lower proportion of the intervention group compared to the control experienced the outcome. The RR > 1 indicates the intervention increased the risk of the outcome; a greater proportion of the intervention group had the outcome compared to control. As an example, a RR of death equal to 0.70 was reported in a clinical trial in which subjects were randomized to either simvastatin (n = 2221) or placebo (n = 2223).[75] The RR was calculated by dividing the proportion of the subjects who died taking simvastatin (n = 182) by the proportion of those who died taking placebo (n = 256). The calculation of RR for this trial is: (182/2221)/(256/2223). The RR is < 1, which indicates simvastatin lowered the risk of death by almost one-third of the baseline risk compared to placebo. Relative risk reduction (RRR) indicates the relative change in the outcome rate between the intervention and control groups. The RRR was calculated as 30% (1–0.70). Thus, the risk of experiencing death was 30% lower by treating these subjects with simvastatin instead of placebo. Absolute risk reduction (ARR) refers to the difference in the outcome rate between the intervention and control groups. A higher proportion of subjects taking placebo died (n = 256 of 2223 or 11.5%) compared to those taking simvastatin (182 of 2221 or 8.2%). The ARR for death associated with simvastatin in this trial equals 3.3% (ARR = 11.5% – 8.2%). Thus, 3.3% of the subjects receiving simvastatin were spared death compared to placebo. The NNT of this study equals 30 (NNT = 1/0.033), meaning 30 subjects need to be treated for a median of 5.4 years with simvastatin instead of placebo to prevent one case of death. The trial had a median follow-up time period of 5.4 years.

Many clinical trials present an endpoint as a relative change, which can be a misleading value. For instance, the RRR of stroke associated with atorvastatin was 48% compared to placebo. Although this value appears very beneficial to subjects at risk for stroke, the absolute risk needs to be evaluated besides just the RRR value. The actual incidence of stroke was 1.5% (21 of 1428 subjects treated with atorvastatin) versus 2.8% (39 of 1409 subjects treated with placebo), which calculates to an absolute difference of 1.3% (ARR). Even though almost 50% fewer subjects (a relative difference) experienced a stroke with atorvastatin, this represents only a difference of 18 of just over 2800 subjects.[153]

All four measures of association can be calculated for clinical trials measuring nominal data and assessed together for the reader to determine the clinical difference in effect between the intervention and control. As seen by the simvastatin example above (plus Table 4–9), the same study result (e.g., death) can be presented using four different methods with different meanings. However, readers should not be misled by clinical trials that only present and discuss one of these values, which usually is the most appealing value (i.e., the one that seems to show the greatest difference). In fact, studies have documented that practitioners are more inclined to select a therapy presented as RRR more often if the same study result was presented as all four values (i.e., ARR, RR, RRR, NNT).[154] Thus, investigators may be biased and selectively present the most appealing of these four values to mislead the reader in concluding a greater difference in effect among the intervention and control, even though the difference may be minimal.

Confidence intervals also can be calculated for nominal endpoints presented as relative risk (RR) or hazard ratio (HR). The latter is used to describe risks associated with adverse events and/or mortality data. The same formula for RR is used to calculate HR, which refers to whether the hazard of the adverse event (i.e., MI, hospitalization) is lowered or increased with the intervention compared to the control.[155] According to the formula for RR (and HR), a calculated value of 1 signifies that the incidence of the adverse event is equal between the intervention and control (i.e., numerator and denominator are equal and therefore no difference).[113,151] As previously mentioned, a RR < 1 signifies the intervention lowered the risk, and a RR > 1 is interpreted as the intervention increasing the risk of the adverse event compared to the control. Therefore investigators of a clinical trial presenting a RR (or HR) with a 95% CI that lies entirely on one side of 1 (i.e., up to 0.99 or 1.01 and upwards) indicates a difference in effect between the intervention and control. The 95% CI range for death in the simvastatin study was entirely below 1 (0.58 to 0.85),[75] which is interpreted as the investigators are 95% confident that the RR associated with simvastatin is between 0.58 and 0.85 for the population. Also since 1 is not in this range, the investigators are 95% confident that the RR of experiencing the adverse event is reduced with simvastatin (i.e., difference in effect). Using another example, the calculated

HR for the primary endpoint of CHD was 1.82 with a 95% CI of 1.49 to 2.01. This information indicates the investigators are 95% confident that the risk of CHD is increased with the intervention versus placebo in the population since the HR is > 1. Also, the investigators were 95% confident that the intervention increased CHD risk in the population since the 95% CI for this endpoint did not go below 1. However, a 95% CI containing the value of 1 indicates the intervention may have neither lowered nor increased the risk (or hazard) of the adverse event. For instance, a HR for death due to other causes was calculated as 0.92 (95% CI, 0.74 – 1.14). The 95% CI range lies on both sides of 1 and indicates the risk of death could be lowered to 0.74 or increased to 1.14 with the intervention. Thus, the investigator (or reader) would conclude that the intervention is no different from placebo in decreasing or increasing the risk of death.

NO DIFFERENCE DOES NOT INDICATE EQUIVALENCY

Clinical studies reporting p-values greater than the alpha value translate into no statistical significance; thus, no clinical difference in effect is declared between the intervention and control group. The H_0 is accepted (fail to be rejected) and the H_1 is rejected; in response, the statement of *no difference* is accepted.[118,145] The H_0 is not written to state the intervention and control are the same, but stated as no difference in the effect (i.e., endpoint measurement) between the intervention and control. ⓫ *Non-statistically significant results do not equate to the intervention and control being the same or equal.* Studies accepting the H_0 have the possibility of a Type II error. A difference in effect between the intervention and control group may be present, but either by chance or a small trial sample size the difference in effect was not detected. In this latter instance, the clinical trial may not have been powered sufficiently to detect the difference. Usually (but not all of the time) clinical trials in which the H_0 is accepted have too small a sample size.[113] In fact, some studies may even be designed with an insufficient sample size so the investigators may claim equivalence between the intervention and active control after rejecting the H_0 even though a trial with an appropriate sample size could detect a difference. Unfortunately, the trial results may be incorrectly interpreted as though the intervention and control were the same. This situation can occur in biased articles and/or presentations. However, the correct interpretation should be no difference detected. As one author stated, "absence of evidence is not evidence of absence."[112]

ASSESSING THE CLINICAL RELEVANCE OF THE RESULTS

⓬ *All controlled clinical trial results need to be assessed to determine the clinical relevance (i.e., meaningfulness) of the intervention versus control.*[31,121,146] In other words, what do these results mean to practice? Small treatment effects and/or differences may be statistically different, but really not mean much clinically.[60,79,113] For example, an antihypertensive medication lowered mean DBP by 5 mm Hg versus 2 mm Hg for placebo (p = 0.04). The H_0 was rejected due to statistical difference. However, mean baseline DBP was 98 mm Hg, and this antihypertensive medication only lowered mean DBP to 93 mm Hg, which is still classified as hypertensive.[156] Thus, practitioners would consider these results to be not clinically meaningful. In other words, these results are not useful in treating patients with hypertension.

On the other hand, a small difference in effect that is statistically different may be of clinical importance, depending upon the perspective of the reader. A long-term care pharmacist who specializes in geriatrics may consider a trial reporting a reduced number of incontinence episodes, on average, by two in a 24-hour period with a new anticholinergic agent compared to placebo to be clinically meaningful compared to an infectious disease pharmacist. The new drug may reduce nursing time and improve the overall quality of life in patients with incontinence.

Not all clinical trials reporting non-statistically significant results are completely devoid of clinical importance. The overall effect of the intervention and control need to be assessed. A study compared lansoprazole (30 mg; n = 421) to omeprazole (20 mg; n = 431); each group received once-daily therapy for a duration of 8 weeks. The healing rates of erosive reflux esophagitis was 87.2% versus 87%, respectively, via ITT analysis (p = NS).[157] No clinical difference is concluded from this study, but these results would be considered to be clinically meaningful (i.e., clinically relevant) since > 85% of patients were healed with either therapy.

As previously mentioned, clinical trial results of the intervention may be statistically significant and clinically different from the control, but may be not clinically practical. The clinical trial methods need to be reviewed for the ability to replicate these into everyday patient care. A clinical trial may be designed that consists of technologies and/or include personnel that may not be readily accessible in patient care areas. In addition, patients may not be able to afford the new intervention. Another issue to consider is the demands on the actual patient. At times investigators offer incentives (e.g., monetary compensation, free medical care) for the subjects to strictly follow the study protocol (i.e., more motivated to be compliant). But in practice, real patients may not be as eager to follow an intricate schedule. For example, bismuth subsalicylate can be taken as a prophylaxis against traveler's diarrhea.[158] Although a clinical trial reported the suspension of subsalicylate bismuth 60 mL four times daily reduced the incidence of this unfortunate experience during travel,[159] some individuals may not be willing to adhere to this dosing schedule. Another issue to consider before applying the clinical trial results into practice is the normal care for patients with the disease/condition under study. Endpoint results of an intervention may be statistically significant and clinically different from the active control, but the control is not normally prescribed for patients with the disease/condition.[79]

Bibliography

References are a very important part of the manuscript. The reference or bibliography section is at the end of the manuscript and provides documentation to support the information provided in the manuscript or acknowledgement for the work of other authors.[43] Any material that the author uses in the manuscript should be appropriately cited. References included in the manuscript should be recent (e.g., outdated articles should not be used unless the results of the article are pertinent to the manuscript) and complete. Readers should scan the references listed in the bibliography to determine if the authors used material from reputable sources. In addition, authors should refrain from extensively citing only their own work.[160] References typically should be listed in numerical order (e.g., Arabic numerals) in which these appear in the manuscript; however, several referencing styles exist and are journal dependent (refer to Appendix 9–3 for further information about referencing). At minimum, the information in the reference section should be sufficient to lead the reader to locating the same article. Some readers may wish to verify the cited information, while others search for articles in the reference section to gather additional information regarding a topic.[43]

Acknowledgments

Individuals contributing to the clinical trial, but who do not meet the requirements for authorship, can be recognized in this section (see Chapter 9 for more information). Examples of persons identified are those providing manuscript preparation, technical assistance, or donors of equipment or supplies. Medical writers or editors also may be listed if their contributions were significant. A collaboration or group may receive recognition in the acknowledgement section; however, many journals have a pre-specified amount of space for the acknowledgement section that must be adhered to by authors. Authors must obtain written permission from persons acknowledged before listing in this section, so the readers do not infer endorsements of the data and conclusions from these contributors.[33,43]

Other types of information may be included in this section. Such items are financial support (see below for further information) and an indication that the manuscript underwent peer-review, signified by a series of dates and titled received/revised/accepted.

Typically, at least 4 to 8 weeks are between these dates since it is necessary to allow time for the reviewers to comment, the authors to revise, and then for another review of the manuscript. Some journals only present the manuscript acceptance date, which allows readers to determine the lag time between the article being accepted in final form to publication. Hopefully, a minimal time period exists between acceptance and the publication date, which increases content currency.

Funding

⑬ *Controlled clinical trial investigators and authors should disclose any funding sources and potential conflicts of interest.* Due to the enormous expense required to conduct a clinical trial, investigators seek financial assistance to conduct the research. Various funding sources are available that include pharmaceutical companies, government agencies (e.g., National Institutes of Health [NIH]), national organizations (e.g., American Cancer Society), university grants (e.g., faculty development grants), and private donations. According to an assessment of 500 randomly selected clinical trials published in five highly recognized medical journals from 1981 to 2000 (e.g., *N Engl J Med, JAMA*), the primary funding source (36% of the studies) was the pharmaceutical industry, either independently or jointly. In addition, a trend was observed toward a greater percentage increase of trials with pharmaceutical industry support over this time period. Furthermore, the study results documented a significant increase in the number of authors being affiliated with a pharmaceutical company.[161]

During 2008, an estimated $65 billion was spent by the pharmaceutical companies for research and development (which includes clinical drug trials); approximately 75% of this figure consisted of domestic research and development.[162] The pharmaceutical industry is responsible for a significant amount of the clinical research conducted worldwide. Thus, readers of industry-sponsored research should be cognizant of possible conflicts of interest, defined as "a set of conditions in which professional judgment concerning a primary interest (such as a patient's welfare or the validity of research) tends to be unduly influenced by a secondary interest (such as financial gain)"[163] that may result in potential bias. Conflicts of interest arise because the industry may be prompted to publish articles as a means of making their product appear better for a disease state in relation to the standard of care. This research may result in methods bias, premature termination of trials for nonscientific/non-ethical reasons, or reporting/publication bias.[164] The International Committee of Medical Journal Editors (ICMJE) has adopted a disclosure form for all their member journals to obtain financial associations of the authors submitting manuscripts. The form is posted on the ICMJE Web site (http://www.icmje.org/oi_disclosure.pdf).[165]

The study design, result presentation style, data interpretations, and study conclusions should be assessed appropriately to determine if the funding source had any influences on the overall clinical trial. A clinical trial should not be automatically rejected by the reader due to the funding agency. Pharmaceutical companies need to determine the clinical usefulness of newly developed medications. These companies are expecting to profit from the new medication being approved by the FDA and marketed to prescribers. Many organizations (e.g., government, nonprofit) are not prime candidates to offer funding for these studies, which leaves the pharmaceutical company to sponsor the study.

Not all investigator-pharmaceutical industry relationships have the potential to cause a conflict of interest, but readers should decide if a publication is biased. In fact, many well-designed, clinically important studies documenting a reduction in morbidity and mortality have been sponsored by the pharmaceutical industry, and these have changed the standards of practice in treating patients.

However, there have been reports in the literature of selected pharmaceutical companies: terminating studies for various reasons unrelated to efficacy and safety;[166] employing inappropriate comparators;[167] using inappropriate study samples;[168] and suppressing the results of negative studies.[169] Also, it can be assumed that a pharmaceutical company would design studies that are most likely to show superiority of their drug in some aspect or another. Furthermore, reports have been published that indicate a favorable conclusion of studies financially supported by the pharmaceutical industry, which can be referred to as publication bias. This type of sponsored research usually yields larger treatment effects than not-for-profit-funded studies.[79]

Research has documented that the conclusions of some trials funded by for-profit organizations significantly were in favor of the experimental drug as the treatment of choice. But not all pharmaceutical industry-sponsored research is biased; many study results are clinically meaningful. Readers need to be aware that the pharmaceutical company has a lot at stake for an investigational drug to be approved by the FDA. In response, the pharmaceutical company attempts to design a clinical trial to meet the FDA-approval standards. However, the methods of presenting (i.e., Results section), interpreting (i.e., Introduction and/or Discussion sections), and summarizing the data and results (i.e., Conclusion) can be biased and are not governed by the regulations of the FDA. Consequently, readers need to evaluate the trial data critically to assess the appropriateness and validity of the reported conclusions based upon the trial results.[170]

Furthermore, trial registration with an official governmental entity is another method for the reader to discern if publication bias exists in favor of a particular interventional therapy. Specifically, the national clinical trials registry (http://www.clinicaltrials.gov),[171] which is hosted by the National Institutes of Health is a very useful resource for the reader of biomedical literature to determine if potentially negative study results are being excluded from discussion in clinical trials or promotional materials. The Food and Drug

Administration Amendments Act of 2007, passed on September 27, 2007, mandates registration and results reporting certain clinical trials utilizing certain drugs, biologics, and devices, regardless of study outcome.[172]

ClinicalTrials.gov indexes > 90,000 federally and privately funded clinical trials conducted in the United States and abroad. Furthermore, this resource provides the user with details about a trial's purpose, guidelines for participation, study locations, and contact information for more details. The information contained within the national trial registry should be strictly viewed as supplementary to competent care from a health care professional. This Web site can be searched by a variety of functions, including investigational agent or disease state. With this in mind, the national clinical trials registry is also a very useful tool for the practicing pharmacist who may need to identify treatment options for a patient who cannot afford conventional intervention or who has a rare or terminal disease state and is seeking additional treatment options.[171]

Commentaries/Clinical Trial Critiques

All journals should provide its readership the opportunity for correspondence to exchange ideas about a topic or relay new information about articles published in the journal.[33,43] ⑭ *Editorials, letters to the editor, and commentary publications can assist in interpreting controlled clinical trial results.* Commentaries can be essential in assisting readers in interpreting and/or critiquing articles published within the journals by providing strengths and limitations of the original research, an update to published information, or questions to the authors of the original research manuscript.

Editorials, defined as, "a written expression of opinion that may reflect the official position of the publication"[43] are short essays from the editor or other experts in a particular field that are written to convey additional opinions about an article, typically, in the same issue of a journal. Not all editorials reflect the ideas/thoughts of the journal because these are opinions of the editorial author. Although editorials may contain some bias, this literature should always be considered when evaluating a clinical trial by providing additional insight of the results and aiding in the comprehension of the clinical application of the trial results. For instance, an editorial in response to the ENHANCE trial[53] was published in the same journal issue. The editorial authors discussed many issues ranging from the dangers of surrogate endpoints (specifically the paradox of improved cholesterol markers with worsened intimal thickness) to the premature disclosure of interim data by study investigators. The authors concluded that documented therapies should be employed in high-risk patients until the clinical effects of ezetimibe using clinical markers are published in other trials in the near future.[173]

Several issues should be considered during the preparation or evaluation of editorials. Quality editorials are original; those editorials with non-original ideas need to include a clear justification of repeating these ideas. The editorial objective should be clearly presented and reflect a complete message. The content should be significant to merit publication. The editorial points should be timely with respect to the publication in which the author is responding. Finally, the editorial author should mention the facts clearly, and the material should be applicable to the readership of the publication.[174]

Not all original research reports are accompanied by an editorial. Persons seeking an editorial associated with a clinical trial can use a few methods to locate the publication. First, the journal issue that contains the clinical trial will list the editorial title in the journal issue table of contents. Another, but not always present in all clinical trials, is a notation printed on the first page of the clinical trial referring the reader to another page (e.g., "For comment, see page..."; Commentary, page ..."). Readers not having access to the actual clinical trial or journal issue table of contents can locate the trial citation in PubMed (using the Single Citation Matcher at http://www.pubmed.gov). Those clinical trials with an accompanying editorial will contain a notation of Comment in and an abbreviated journal citation (i.e., journal name, date, plus volume, issue, and page numbers). Another method is to search the clinical trial topic (i.e., via Medical Subject Heading term in PubMed) and limit the search to the publication type of editorial.

Some journals/Web sites are published for the primary purpose of providing editorials/commentaries addressing a clinical trial. These resources are known as secondary journals and are independent of the journals that directly publish the clinical trials.[35,79,175] Secondary journals are publications that assist the busy practitioners in a few vital methods: keeping them current regarding important and relevant studies, plus presenting key study information in a concise format. Clinical trials are presented, usually in a structured abstract style, but not just copying and pasting the exact abstract prepared by the trial investigators. These prepared abstracts may present additional and/or more precise information. In addition, a commentary addressing the study strengths, limitations, and application into practice is authored by a leading practitioner in the field of study. Readers should use these resources while critiquing the biomedical/pharmacy literature.

Examples of secondary journal Web sites include http://www.theheart.org, and http://www.medscape.com. Typically, these publications provide an overview of the study followed by a commentary. Medscape is particularly useful for pharmacists since pharmacy-specific topics are addressed in a section of this Web site. *ACP Journal Club* is an online and print resource in which biomedical literature (i.e., original research, systematic reviews) is selected based on predefined criteria and summarized by an expert in the field in the form of structured abstracts followed by a commentary. More than 100 journals are reviewed and are selected due to their potential impact on clinical practice.[176]

Another example is *Journal Watch,* a print and online resource that is published at least monthly in print[177] and daily on the Internet.[178] Updated information for 13 specialty areas of medical practice along with 20 topic areas (e.g., diabetes) is provided by physicians along with a commentary to help clinicians determine the impact or the research results on their practice.[176] Several specialty editions of *Journal Watch* are available including *Journal Watch Dermatology, Journal Watch Emergency Medicine, Journal Watch Gastroenterology,* and *Journal Watch Infectious Diseases.*[175]

LETTERS TO THE EDITOR

Letters to the editor can provide valuable insight into original research and can include various types of contributions. These may be in the form of comments, addenda, or updates from previously published articles, alerts regarding potential problems in practice, observations/comments on trends in medication use, opinions on trends or controversies in therapy or research, or original research. Authors of letters to the editor must adhere to strict guidelines from the journals regarding the length, number of tables, and format of the publication.[179] The primary content of letters to the editor is feedback from the journal readers regarding the published materials in the journal. Typically, these letters are published within three to six months of the original publication. The letters may disagree with the design, result interpretation, and/or conclusions of the publication. Also, the letters may ask for additional information that can be used to interpret/clarify, comprehend, and/or critique the information within the publication. Afterwards, the authors of the original publication may provide a response to these published letters. The letters to the editor serve as another source of valuable information for those using and critiquing the biomedical literature.

Conclusion

Pharmacists are characterized by having the skills to problem-solve, critically think, and formulate recommendations based upon the literature. All pharmacists need the skill of efficiently locating, critically evaluating, plus effectively formulating and communicating an evidence-based recommendation, regardless of the practice setting. As the role of the pharmacist in direct patient care continues to increase, incorporating these skills on a daily basis is essential. A multitude of literature is published each year and the quality varies significantly. Readers of the literature should not immediately accept the authors' conclusions but assess the strengths and limitations of the source. The information within this chapter identifies and discusses many issues to consider while reading and analyzing controlled clinical trials. Although every clinical trial has limitations, those trials with appropriate design and well-presented results are still important to apply into clinical practice. Using the proper techniques in evaluating clinical trials can allow pharmacists to contribute as key stakeholders in an ever increasing interdisciplinary health care arena.

Case Study 4-1

■ RELEVANT BACKGROUND INFORMATION

A patient of yours visits you with an advertisement and coupon for a nonprescription product consisting of plant sterols (a.k.a., encapsulated phytosterol esters [EPE]). Your patient was very impressed with the advertisement, which claims people taking this product had their cholesterol levels lowered. Certain advertisement statements were: "REMOVE CHOLESTEROL"; "... natural plant sterols are clinically proven to help remove cholesterol from your body"; "In a national survey of 310 cardiologists, four out of five cardiologists endorse this product." Your patient wants to lower his cholesterol naturally and is interested in purchasing the EPE product. But he wanted to obtain your opinion of how useful the EPE would be in lowering cholesterol. You conduct a literature search and located only one published study evaluating EPE. Below is a summary of this study.

A randomized, double-blind, placebo-controlled study was conducted to evaluate the cholesterol-lowering effects of encapsulated phytosterol esters (EPE) over a 12-week period. The study, which was the first to evaluate EPE, enrolled 54 patients between the ages of 20 and 70 years with low-density lipoprotein cholesterol (LDL-C) levels at or above 130 mg/dL. Patients who smoked, received lipid-lowering agents in the previous 6 months, consumed more than three alcoholic beverages a day, or had elevated blood pressure were excluded from the study. Patients were randomized to EPE 2.6 g per day (n = 25) or placebo (n = 29). All patients in the study were required to follow a low cholesterol diet. The primary endpoint of the study was mean change in LDL-C. Secondary endpoints included mean changes in high-density lipoprotein cholesterol (HDL-C), triglycerides (TG), and total cholesterol (TC).

Data were presented as mean ± standard deviation; statistical significance was set at p < 0.05. Patient demographics were similar for both groups. Baseline lipid values were as follows (EPE and placebo, respectively): LDL-C, 164 mg/dL versus 154 mg/dL; TC, 241 mg/dL versus 231 mg/dL. After 12 weeks, LDL-C values for EPE and placebo were 156 mg/dL and 160 mg/dL, respectively (p < 0.045). Mean changes in HDL-C and TG were not significant. The TC levels at study end were 233 mg/dL and 236 mg/dL, respectively (p < 0.05). No adverse reactions were reported during the study. The investigators concluded EPE is an effective and safe agent to lower LDL-C and TC.

1. Does this study need IRB approval?
2. Is the use of a placebo as the control group appropriate, considering many FDA-approved agents are available that can lower LDL-C?
3. Interpret the standard deviation of "± 28 mg/dL" associated with the end-of-study mean LDL-C value for patients taking EPE.
4. Is the low-cholesterol diet followed by all subjects in this study considered adjunctive or ancillary therapy?
5. Interpret the primary endpoint p-value in terms of probability.
6. Please formulate a recommendation regarding the use of this EPE product for your patient.

_____ Case Study 4–2

■ RELEVANT BACKGROUND INFORMATION

A pharmaceutical company representative visits you to promote an analgesic agent. She claims her company's analgesic product (tapentadol) is a very effective agent to reduce pain for all types of patients in need of an analgesic agent and should be selected instead of other agents. She presents a study to support her claim. Below is a summary of this study.

> A randomized, active- and placebo-controlled clinical trial compared the efficacy and tolerability of tapentadol-IR, oxycodone-IR, and placebo over a 10-day period in patients with uncontrolled osteoarthritis (OA) pain. These patients were candidates for total hip replacement (THR) or knee replacement (TKR) secondary to end-stage degenerative joint disease. The study consisted of a screening period (20 days), a run-in phase (6 days), a treatment period (10 days), and a follow-up period (10–15 days). During the treatment phase, subjects were randomized to therapy with tapentadol-IR 50 mg (n = 161), tapentadol-IR 75 mg (n = 169), oxycodone-IR 10 mg (n = 172), or placebo (n = 169) every 4 to 6 hours during waking hours. The primary endpoint was the sum of pain-intensity difference (SPID) over 5 days, calculated as the sum of all pain intensity measurements (measured twice daily) from the evening of day one to the morning of day 6. The mean age of participants was 61 years, and gender was equally distributed within and between groups.

Five-day SPID was significantly reduced in subjects treated with active therapies versus placebo (tapentadol-IR 50 mg: least squares mean difference from placebo [LSMD] = 101.2 [95% CI: 51.81–143.89]; tapentadol-IR 75 mg: LSMD = 97.5 [95% CI: 51.81–143.26]) or oxycodone-IR 10 mg (LSMD = 111.9 [95% CI, 66.49–157.38]), ($p < 0.0001$ for all active therapies versus placebo; $p > 0.05$ for active therapy compared to each other). The incidence of select gastrointestinal side effects (nausea, vomiting, constipation) were less in subjects receiving both doses of tapentadol-IR compared to oxycodone-IR ($p < 0.001$). The investigators concluded that tapentadol-IR is an effective agent to reduce pain.

1. Which blinding type is the most appropriate for this study?
2. What type of data is being evaluated for the primary endpoint?
3. Which measures of central tendency is/are appropriate to present the primary endpoint?
4. Can the run-in phase of this study be considered a study design bias?
5. Is the pharmaceutical representative correct in her statement that tapentadol is a very effective agent to reduce pain for all types of patients in need of an analgesic agent and should be selected instead of other agents?

Case Study 4–3

■ RELEVANT BACKGROUND INFORMATION

One of your female friends (19 years old) who plays university soccer and is a non-health care major asks for your advice. She read on the Internet that taking calcium and vitamin D supplements prevents stress fractures in young female athletes. She wants to know if she should start taking these supplements. She knows that not all information from the Internet can be trusted, so she is seeking your recommendation. Plus, she does not want to take anything that can cause side effects. You conduct a literature search and locate only one study addressing this issue. You read this study (below) to formulate an evidence-based response for her.

A double-blinded clinical trial was designed to determine whether the combination of calcium plus vitamin D (CaVitD) reduces the incidence of stress fractures (Sfx) in female Navy recruits during basic training. Prior research indicated that intense training increases calcium demands for bone formation and increases cutaneous calcium losses. Females at least 17 years of age recruited into the Navy and considered to be healthy were enrolled in this study; no exclusion criteria were listed in the study. The primary endpoint was the incidence of Sfx measured by patients reporting to the clinic with symptoms. All Sfx were confirmed with radiography or technetium scan. The females were randomized to either the combination of calcium 2000 mg plus vitamin D 800 IU per day (n = 2626) or identical placebo tablets (n = 2575). All the females underwent the same training programs/conditions during the 8 weeks of study. The CaVitD or placebo tablets were distributed to the patients during breakfast and dinner. The results were analyzed via ITT and a level of significance of 0.05 was set for the analyses. The median age was 19 years (range, 17–35 years), and most females were Caucasian (54%). Fewer patients taking CaVitD than placebo had a Sfx (5.3% versus 6.6%, respectively; p = 0.026). Median time to Sfx was 37 versus 34 days, respectively. A total of 3700 patients completed the study. Reasons for not finishing were (similar between groups): Navy discharge (7%), just quit (16%), adverse effects (4%). The CaVitD was well tolerated. No specific adverse effect incidences were reported other than 4% of the patients discontinued due to adverse effects (constipation, upset stomach, diarrhea). The investigators concluded that CaVitD reduces the incidence of Sfx.

1. Calculate the RRR for the primary endpoint and interpret this value.
2. Calculate the ARR for the primary endpoint and interpret this value.
3. Interpret the primary endpoint 95% CI: RR = 0.80 (95% CI, 0.64 to 0.97).
4. The investigators also analyzed the study results with only the patients who completed the entire 8-week study (n = 3700). Fewer patients treated with the intervention had the primary endpoint than the control group (6.8% vs. 8.6%, respectively; p = 0.02). State this type of result analysis and compare to the ITT (intention-to-treat) analysis method.
5. What would your evidence-based recommendation be to this female?

Self-Assessment Questions

Read the excerpt of the following clinical trial summary and answer the questions that follow.

A randomized, controlled clinical trial was conducted to assess rosuvastatin as primary prevention to decrease the risk of first major cardiovascular (CV) adverse events in subjects with baseline LDL-cholesterol (LDL-C) levels <130 mg/dL. The primary end-point was the composite endpoint: occurrence of first major CV event, defined as a nonfatal myocardial infarction (MI), nonfatal stroke, hospitalization for unstable angina, an arterial revascularization procedure, or confirmed death from CV causes.

Investigators also assessed secondary endpoints, which were the components of the primary endpoint considered individually (arterial revascularization, or hospitalization for unstable angina, MI, stroke, or death from cardiovascular causes; another secondary end-point was death from any cause).

Subjects included in the trial were men (≥ 50 years of age) and women (≥ 60 years of age) with no history of CV disease. Other baseline values to be included were high-sensitivity C-reactive protein (CRP) level ≥ 2 mg/L and triglycerides (TG) < 500 mg/dL. Patients had to have medication compliance of at least 80% during the 4-week placebo run-in phase. This trial had many exclusion criteria, which included diagnosis of diabetes or inflammatory conditions (e.g., severe arthritis or lupus) or taking immunosuppressant agents (e.g., azathioprine, long-term oral glucocorticoids).

Subjects were randomized to rosuvastatin 20 mg once daily or placebo (n = 8901 in each group). Neither investigators nor subjects knew which treatment they were receiving. A sample size was estimated for a 5-year follow-up time period to detect at least a 25% greater reduction in the primary endpoint with rosuvastatin. The investigators esti-mated that a 10% beta-error was possible. All results were analyzed using the intention-to-treat analysis. P-values < 0.05 were considered statistically significant. The trial was concluded earlier (median 1.9 years) than originally planned.

Majority of the clinical trial participants were white (71%) and male (62%); the average age was 66 years. The median baseline values were: LDL-C, 108 mg/dL; high-sensitivity CRP, 4.2 mg/L; and TG was 118 mg/dL. Approximately 75% of the randomized subjects were taking their assigned therapy at the closure of the clinical trial. After 12 months, the median LDL-C and high-sensitivity CRP levels were reduced to 55 mg/dL and 2.2 mg/L with rosu-vastatin therapy; these values were 110 mg/L and 3.5 mg/dL, respectively, with placebo.

The incidence of the primary endpoint was lower in the rosuvastatin group versus placebo group (1.6% versus 2.8%, respectively; HR = 0.56, 95% CI, 0.46 to 0.69; $p < 0.00001$). Rates of the primary endpoint were 0.77 and 1.36 per 100 person-years of follow-up, respectively. Secondary endpoints were statistically reduced with rosuvastatin therapy versus placebo and included MI ($p = 0.0002$), stroke ($p = 0.002$), arterial revascularization or unstable angina ($p < 0.0001$), and death from any cause ($p = 0.02$). All subgroup analy-ses indicated a statistically significant reduction in the primary endpoint with rosuvasta-tin. These included patients at least 65 years of age, males and females, those with hypertension, and current smokers. The adverse effect profile was similar between the two groups. No differences in the incidence of myopathy, rhabdomyolysis, hepatic disor-der, or cancer were reported ($p > 0.05$).

The investigators concluded that rosuvastatin reduces the incidence of major CV events in persons with elevated high-sensitivity CRP but normal LDL levels. This agent can be considered for primary prevention of CV adverse events.

1. Which of the following is the *best* rationale for selecting a controlled clinical trial as the study design for this study?
   a. Controlled clinical trials are the best study design to determine cause and effect and quantify the difference between the intervention and control.
   b. Controlled clinical trials are retrospective in nature and provide a means of looking backward in time to determine the cause of an effect between the intervention and control.
   c. Controlled clinical trials are the only study design that allows for calculation of measures of association.
   d. Controlled clinical trials allow for randomization that can improve the validity of statistical tests.
   e. Controlled clinical trials allow for the evaluation of multiple endpoints during the trial.

2. Neither the investigators nor the subjects knew which treatment they were receiving. Which type of blinding is included in this study?
   a. No blinding
   b. Single-blinding
   c. Double-blinding
   d. Triple-blinding
   e. Endpoint-assessment blinding

3. Subjects in the study were randomized to rosuvastatin 20 mg once daily or placebo. Which of the following is a characteristic of randomization?
   a. Included in all study design types.
   b. Allows for each subject to have an equal opportunity to be assigned to either the intervention or control group.
   c. Appropriate techniques increase the chance of selection bias that can measure the difference in effect between the intervention and control.
   d. Invalidates statistical tests.
   e. Assures that treatment effects are due to confounders.

4. Which of the following statements is the correct null hypothesis (H$_0$) for this study? The composite endpoint is the occurrence of first major CV event, defined as a nonfatal myocardial infarction, nonfatal stroke, hospitalization for unstable angina, an arterial revascularization procedure, or confirmed death from CV causes.

a. There is a difference in the composite endpoint incidence between rosuvastatin and placebo.
b. The composite endpoint efficacy and safety are different between rosuvastatin and placebo.
c. Rosuvastatin decreases the risk of the composite endpoint versus placebo.
d. There is no difference in the composite endpoint incidence between rosuvastatin and placebo.
e. There is no difference in the composite efficacy and safety between rosuvastatin and placebo.

5. Which of the following represents the type of data being collected and evaluated for the primary endpoint in this study?
   a. Nominal
   b. Ordinal
   c. Interval
   d. Ratio
   e. Continuous

6. Which of the following endpoints measured in the study represents a surrogate endpoint?
   a. Unstable angina
   b. Occurrence of first major CV event
   c. Death from CV causes
   d. Myocardial infarction
   e. LDL-cholesterol level

7. Which of the following is correct regarding the power of this study?
   a. Since at least 70% of the patients completed the trial, the power is at least 70%.
   b. Included to estimate a sample size to reduce a Type II error.
   c. Set at 95% to reduce a Type I error.
   d. Calculated to be equivalent to 80%.
   e. No evidence of a power analysis was calculated for this study.

8. Which of the following statements should be selected based upon the primary endpoint p-value ($p < 0.00001$) of this study?
   a. Accept the H_0 since the p-value is less than the study alpha.
   b. Accept the H_0 since the p-value is greater than the study alpha.
   c. Reject the H_0 since the p-value is less than the study alpha.
   d. Reject the H_0 since the p-value is greater than the study alpha.
   e. Since no study alpha value was stated in the study summary, cannot accept or reject the H_0.

9. Which of the following statements should be selected based upon the primary endpoint p-value (p < 0.00001) of this study?
   a. Statistical significance is not present, and a Type I error is possible.
   b. Statistical significance is present, and a Type II error is possible.
   c. Statistical significance is not present, and a Type II error is possible.
   d. Statistical significance is present, and a Type I error is possible.
   e. Since no study alpha value was stated in the study summary, statistical difference cannot be determined.

10. What is the *best* interpretation of the primary endpoint p-value (p < 0.00001) for this study?
   a. The probability of accepting a false H_0 is < 0.00001%.
   b. The probability of a Type I error is < 0.00001%.
   c. The probability of a Type II error is < 0.001%.
   d. The probability of accepting a true H_0 is < 0.0001%.
   e. The probability of rejecting a true H_0 is < 0.001%.

11. The incidence of the primary endpoint in the rosuvastatin group versus placebo group was 1.6% and 2.8%, respectively. Which of the following measures of association calculation and interpretation of the primary endpoint is correct?
   a. A HR (RR) = 0.56 represents the percentage of baseline risk removed as a result of therapy with rosuvastatin.
   b. The ARR = 1.2% and means 1.2% of subjects treated with the intervention was spared the primary endpoint compared with the control.
   c. NNT = 8.3 indicating that 8.3 patients need to be treated over the course of 1 year to prevent one case of the primary outcome.
   d. RRR = 44% and refers to the amount of risk removed by rosuvastatin therapy compared to the control.
   e. Measures of association cannot be calculated based on the endpoint type of data.

12. Which of the following is the most appropriate interpretation of the primary endpoint 95% CI (HR = 0.56; 95% CI, 0.46 to 0.69)?
   a. A clinical difference is present because the value of equality (zero) is not included in the 95% confidence interval range.
   b. The investigators are confident that 5% of the patients will not experience the primary endpoint with rosuvastatin therapy.
   c. A clinician may expect that 46% to 69% of the patients will achieve a reduction in the primary endpoint with rosuvastatin therapy.

d. If the study were repeated, 95% confident that the calculated HR associated with the primary endpoint would be between 0.46 and 0.69.

e. Indicates that the 10% β-rate that was established *a priori* was achieved, as evidenced by the difference between the HR and the lower bounds of the 95% CI (0.56 − 0.46 = 10%).

13. Which statement is the *best* in regard to whether a clinical difference between rosuvastatin and placebo exists (primary endpoints: 1.6% versus 2.8%, respectively; HR = 0.56, 95% CI, 0.46 to 0.69; p < 0.00001)?

a. Clinical difference may exist due to the p-value and HR calculation.

b. Clinical difference does not exist because the study was not appropriately powered to detect differences in the intervention and control groups.

c. Clinical difference does not exist because the results are not statistically significant.

d. Clinical difference exists because the results are statistically significant.

e. Clinical differences between the intervention and control cannot be determined based on the information provided.

14. A subgroup analysis revealed that patients who were at least 65 years of age, those with hypertension, and those who were currently smoking experienced a significant reduction in the primary endpoint with rosuvastatin. Which of the following is the *best* interpretation of this subgroup analysis?

a. All patients who are at least 65 years of age, those with hypertension, and current smokers should receive rosuvastatin therapy for the prevention of the primary endpoint.

b. Subgroup analysis reduces limitations associated with clinical trials and provides a means of evaluating the effects of therapy in several different patient populations.

c. Subgroup analysis increases the power of the study.

d. The likelihood of finding a statistical significance in a subgroup analysis decreases according to the number of analyses that are conducted.

e. Interpret with caution since this analysis may not be appropriately powered to detect differences between the intervention and control.

15. Which of the following is the *best* place for a letter to the editor to be published in response to this study? The study was published in the November 20, 2008, issue of the *New England Journal of Medicine* (*N Engl J Med*).

a. November 20, 2008, issue of *N Engl J Med*.

b. A secondary journal (e.g., *Journal Watch*).

c. March 5, 2009 issue of *N Engl J Med*.

d. A secondary Web site (e.g., theheart.org).

e. Readers are not provided an opportunity to comment on published studies.

REFERENCES

1. Drugs @ FDA [homepage on the Internet]. FDA approved drug products. [cited 2010 Jan 7]. Drug Approval Reports. Available from: http://www.accessdata.fda.gov/scripts/cder/drugsatfda/index.cfm?fuseaction= Reports.ReportsMenu.

2. 2009 Safety Alerts for Human Medical Products [database on the Internet]. [cited 2010 Jan 7]. Available from: http://www.fda.gov/Safety/MedWatch/SafetyInformation/SafetyAlertsforHumanMedicalProducts/ucm091428.htm.

3. PubMed [database on the Internet] [cited 2010 Jan 7]. National Library of Medicine. Available from: http://www.ncbi.nlm.nih.gov/sites/entrez.

4. Pharmacists rank among "most trusted" for 27th straight year [cited 2009 Sept 7]. Available from: http://www.pharmacytimes.com/issue/pharmacy/2007/2007-02/2007-02-6250.

5. Calis KA, Hutchison LC, Elliott ME, Ives TJ, Zillich AJ, Poirier T, et al. Healthy People 2010: challenges, opportunities, and a call to action for America's pharmacists. Pharmacotherapy. 2004 Sept;24(9):1241-94.

6. Bohenek WS, Grossbart SR. Pharmacists' role in improving quality of care. Am J Health-Syst Pharm. 2008 Aug 15;65(16):1566-70.

7. Zellmer WA. . Pharmacy vision and leadership: revisiting the fundamentals. Pharmacotherapy. 2008 Dec;28(12):1437-42.

8. Elliott GR, Brien JA, Aslani P, Chen TF. Quality patient care and pharmacists' role in its continuity–a systematic review. Ann Pharmacother. 2009 Apr;43(4):677-91.

9. American Society of Health-System Pharmacists. ASHP statement on the role of health-system pharmacists in public health. Am J Health-Syst Pharm. 2008 Mar 1;65(5):462-7.

10. Wright SG, LeCroy RL, Kendrach MG. The three types of biomedical literature and systematic approach to handle a drug information request. J Pharm Pract. 1998 June;11(3): 148-62.

11. Schrimsher RS, Kendrach MG. Searching PubMed. Hosp Pharm. 2006 Sept;41(9):855-67.

12. Lowe HJ, Barnett GO. Understanding and using the medical subject headings (MeSH) vocabulary to perform literature searches. JAMA. 1994 Apr 13;271(14):1103-8.

13. Bhandari M, Giannoudis PV. Evidence-based medicine: what it is and what it is not. Injury. 2006 Apr;37(4):302-6.

14. Sackett DL, Straus SE, Richardson WS, Rosenberg W, Haynes RB. Evidence-based medicine: how to practice and teach EBM. 2nd ed. London (UK) Churchill Livingstone; 2000.

15. Whitcomb ME. Why we must teach evidence-based medicine. Acad Med. 2005 Jan;80(1):1-2.

16. Green SB. Design of randomized trials. Epidemiol Rev. 2002;24(1):4-11.

17. Sibbald B, Roland M. Understanding controlled trials. Why are randomised controlled trials important? BMJ. 1998 Jan 17;316(7126):201.

18. New drug application (nda) process (CBER). [cited 2010 Jan 7]. Available from: http://www.fda.gov/BiologicsBloodVaccines/DevelopmentApprovalProcess/NewDrugApplicationNDAProcess/default.htm.

19. Gehlbach S. Interpreting the medical literature. 5th ed. New York (NY): McGraw-Hill Company; 2006.

20. Doll R. Controlled trials: the 1948 watershed. BMJ. 1998 Oct 31;317(7167):1217-20.

21. Kunz R, Oxman AD. The unpredictability paradox: review of empirical comparisons of randomised and non-randomised clinical trials. BMJ. 1998 Oct 31;317(7167):1185-90.

22. Kendrach MG, Anderson HG. Fundamentals of controlled clinical trials. J Pharm Pract. 1998 June;11(3):163-80.

23. Schulz KF, Altman DG, Moher D, for the CONSORT Group. CONSORT 2010 Statement: updated guidelines for reporting parallel group randomised trials. BMJ 2010;340:c332. doi: 10.1136/bmj.c332. [cited 2010 June 9]. Available from: http://www.bmj.com/cgi/section_pdf/340/mar23_1/c332.pdf.

24. Friedman L, Furberg C, DeMets D. Fundamentals of clinical trials. 3rd ed. New York (NY): Springer; 1998.

25. Lader EW, Cannon CP, Ohman EM, Newby LK, Sulmasy DP, Barst RJ, et al. The clinician as investigator: participating in clinical trials in the practice setting: Appendix 1: fundamentals of study design. Circulation. 2004;109:e302-4.

26. Mathieu S, Boutron I, Moher D, Altman DG, Ravaud P. Comparison of registered and published primary outcomes in randomized controlled trials. JAMA. 2009 Sep 2;302(9): 977-84.

27. Krzyzanowska MK, Pintilie M, Tannock IF. Factors associated with failure to publish large randomized trials presented at an oncology meeting. JAMA. 2003 Jul 24;290(3):495-501.

28. Irwin RS. The role of conflict of interest in reporting of scientific information. Chest. 2009 Jul;136(1):253-9.

29. DeMets DL, Pocock SJ, Julian DG. The agonising negative trend in monitoring of clinical trials. Lancet. 1999 Dec 4;354(9194):1983-8.

30. Sridharan L, Greenland P. Editorial policies and publication bias: the importance of negative studies. Arch Intern Med. 2009 Jun 8;169(11):1022-3.

31. Stone GW, Pocock SJ. Randomized trials, statistics, and clinical inference. J Am Coll Cardiol. 2010 Feb 2;55(5):428-31.

32. Kaptchuk TJ. Effect of interpretive bias on research evidence. BMJ. 2003 Jun 28;326(7404):1453-5.

33. Uniform requirements for manuscripts submitted to biomedical journals: writing and editing for biomedical publication. [cited 2010 Jan 7]. Available from: http://www.icmje.org/urm_main.html.

34. Armstrong PW, Newby LK, Granger CB, Lee KL, Simes RJ, Van de Werf F, et al. Lessons learned from a clinical trial. Circulation. 2004 Dec 7;110(23):3610-4.

35. Cook DJ, Meade MO, Fink MP. How to keep up with the critical care literature and avoid being buried alive. Crit Care Med. 1996 Oct;24(10):1757-68.

36. Blumenthal D. Doctors and drug companies. N Engl J Med. 2004 Oct 28;351(18):1885-90.

37. Campbell B. "Throw-away journals": tactics for dealing with office waste. CMAJ. 1990 Jan 15;142(2):100.

38. Hasso AN. How to review and retrieve information from the AJNR; or, how to read the AJNR and still have time to ski. AJNR Am J Neuroradiol. 1997 Aug;18(7):1323-4.

39. Weller A. Editorial peer review: Its strengths and weaknesses. Medford (NJ): American Society for Information Science and Technology; 2001.

40. Hirsh J,. Guyatt G, Albers GW, Harrington R, Schünemann HJ; American College of Chest Physicians. Executive summary: American College of Chest Physicians evidence-based clinical practice guidelines (8th Edition). Chest. 2008 Jun;133(6 Suppl):71S-109S.

41. Lader EW, Cannon CP, Ohman EM, Newby LK, Sulmasy DP, Barst RJ, et al. The clinician as investigator: participating in clinical trials in the practice setting. Circulation. 2004 Jun 1;109(21):2672-9.

42. Studdert DM, Mello MM, Brennan TA. Financial conflicts of interest in physicians' relationships with the pharmaceutical industry—self-regulation in the shadow of federal prosecution. N Engl J Med. 2004 Oct 28;351(18):1891-900.

43. Iverson C, Flanagin A, Fontanarosa P, Glass R, Glitman P, Lantz J, et al., editors. American Medical Association manual of style: A guide for authors and editors. 10th ed. Baltimore (MD): Williams & Wilkins; 2007.

44. Nelson HS, Bensch G, Pleskow WW, DiSantostefano R, DeGraw S, Reasner DS, et al. Improved bronchodilation with levalbuterol compared with racemic albuterol in patients with asthma. J Allergy Clin Immunol. 1998 Dec;102(6 Pt 1):943-52.

45. Peat J, Elliott E, Baur L, Keena V. Scientific writing: easy when you know how. London (England): BMJ Books; 2002.

46. Widerquist JG. Abstract writing. Hosp Mater Manage Q. 2000 Nov;22(2):58-63.

47. Guimarães CA. Structured abstracts: narrative review. Acta Cir Bras. 2006 Jul-Aug;21(4):263-8.

48. Hartley J. Current findings from research on structured abstracts. J Med Libr Assoc. 2004 Jul;92(3):368-71.

49. Harris AH, Standard S, Brunning JL, Casey SL, Goldberg JH, Oliver L, et al. The accuracy of abstracts in psychology journals. J Psychol. 2002 Mar;136(2):141-8.

50. Pitkin RM, Branagan MA, Burmeister LF. Accuracy of data in abstracts of published research articles. JAMA. 1999 Mar 24-31;281(12):1110-1.

51. Ward LG, Kendrach MG, Price SO. Accuracy of abstracts for original research articles in pharmacy journals. Ann Pharmacother. 2004 Jul-Aug;38(7-8):1173-7.

52. Cuddy PG, Elenbaas RM, Elenbaas JK. Evaluating the medical literature. Part I: Abstract, introduction, methods. Ann Emerg Med. 1983 Sept;12(9):549-55.

53. Kastelein JJ, Akdim F, Stroes ES, et al for the ENHANCE Investigators. Simvastatin with or without ezetimibe in familial hypercholesterolemia. N Engl J Med. 2008 Apr 3;358(14):1431-43.

54. Motheral B. Research methodology: Hypotheses, measurement, reliability, and validity. J Manage Care Pharm. 1998 Jul/Aug;4(4):382-8.

55. Hulley SB, Cummings SR, Browner WS, Grady DG, Newman TB. Designing clinical research. 3rd ed. Philadelphia (PA): Lippincott Williams & Wilkins; 2006.

56. Mednick D, Day D. Method is everything: evaluating results by study design. J Manage Care Pharm. 1997 Jan/Feb;3(1):66-8,71-2,75-6.

57. Bakker-Arkema RG, Davidson MH, Goldstein RJ, Davignon J, Isaacsohn JL, Weiss SR, et al. Efficacy and safety of a new HMG-CoA reductase inhibitor, atorvastatin, in patients with hypertriglyceridemia. JAMA. 1996 Jan 10;275(2):128-33.

58. Karalis DG, Ross AM, Vacari RM, Zarren H, Scott R. Comparison of efficacy and safety of atorvastatin and simvastatin in patients with dyslipidemia with and without coronary heart disease. Am J Cardiol. 2002 Mar 15;89(6):667-71.

59. Berger VW, Exner DV. Detecting selection bias in randomized clinical trials. Control Clin Trials. 1999 Aug;20(4):319-27.

60. Naylor CD, Guyatt GH. Users' guides to the medical literature. X. How to use an article reporting variations in the outcomes of health services. The Evidence-Based Medicine Working Group. JAMA. 1996 Feb 21;275(7):554-8.

61. Berger VW, Rezvani A, Makarewicz VA. Direct effect on validity of response run-in selection in clinical trials. Control Clin Trials. 2003 Apr;24(2):156-66.

62. Siddiqi AE, Sikorskii A, Given CW, Given B. Early participant attrition from clinical trials: role of trial design and logistics. Clin Trials. 2008;5(4):328-35.

63. Chan FK, Ching JY, Hung LC, Wong VW, Leung VK, Kung NN, et al. Clopidogrel versus aspirin and esomeprazole to prevent recurrent ulcer bleeding. N Engl J Med. 2005 Jan 20;352(3):238-44.

64. Department of Health and Human Services. Recruiting human subjects: pressures in industry-sponsored clinical research. Available from: http://oig.hhs.gov/oei/reports/oei-01-97-00195.pdf. Accessed October 14, 2009.

65. Hebert R. Newspaper advertising could distort research results. Nicotine Tob Res. 2000;2(4):317-8.

66. Wei SJ, Metz JM, Coyle C, Hampshire M, Jones HA, Markowitz S, et al. Recruitment of patients into an internet-based clinical trials database: the experience of OncoLink and the National Colorectal Cancer Research Alliance J Clin Oncol. 2004 Dec 1;22(23):4730-6.

67. Maiti R, M R. Clinical trials in India. Pharmacol Res. 2007 Jul;56(1):1-10.

68. Acharya S. Ethical issues in research outsourcing. J Dent Educ. 2007 Apr;71(4):447-8.

69. Guyatt GH, Sackett DL, Cook DJ. Users' guides to the medical literature. II. How to use an article about therapy or prevention. A. Are the results of the study valid? Evidence-Based Medicine Working Group. JAMA. 1993 Dec 1;270(21):2598-601.

70. Julious SA. Sample sizes for clinical trials with normal data. Stat Med. 2004 Jun 30;23(12):1921-86.

71. Vickers AJ, de Craen AJ. Why use placebos in clinical trials? A narrative review of the methodological literature. J Clin Epidemiol. 2000 Feb;53(2):157-61.

72. Yeh SS, DeGuzman B, Kramer T. Reversal of COPD-associated weight loss using the anabolic agent oxandrolone. Chest. 2002 Aug;122(2):421-8.

73. Baker SG, Lindeman KS. Rethinking historical controls. Biostatistics. 2001 Dec;2(4):383-96.

74. Lewis BE, Wallis DE, Berkowitz SD, Matthai WH, Fareed J, Walenga JM, et al. Argatroban anticoagulant therapy in patients with heparin-induced thrombocytopenia. Circulation. 2001 Apr 10;103(14):1838-43.

75. Randomised trial of cholesterol lowering in 4444 patients with coronary heart disease: the Scandinavian Simvastatin Survival Study (4S). Lancet. 1994 Nov 19;344(8934):1383-9.

76. Simons LA, Nestel PJ, Calvert GD, Jennings GL. Effects of MK-733 on plasma lipid and lipoprotein levels in subjects with hypercholesterolaemia. Med J Aust. 1987 Jul 20;147(2):65-8.

77. Avenell A, Grant AM, McGee M, McPherson G, Campbell MK, McGee MA, et al. The effects of an open design on trial participant recruitment, compliance, and retention: a randomized controlled trial comparison with a blinded, placebo-controlled design. Clin Trials. 2004;1(6):490-98.

78. Tramer MR, Reynolds DJ, Moore RA, McQuay HJ. When placebo controlled trials are essential and equivalence trials are inadequate. BMJ. 1998 Sep 26;317(7162):875-80.

79. Montori VM, Jaeschke R, Schunemann HJ, Bhandari M, Brozek JL, Devereaux PJ, et al. Users' guide to detecting misleading claims in clinical research reports. BMJ. 2004 Nov 6;329(7474):1093-6.

80. Gluud LL. Bias in clinical intervention research. Am J Epidemiol. 2006 Mar 15;163(6):493-501.

81. Davidson M, Ma P, Stein EA, Gotto AM, Jr., Raza A, Chitra R, et al. Comparison of effects on low-density lipoprotein cholesterol and high-density lipoprotein cholesterol with rosuvastatin versus atorvastatin in patients with Type IIa or IIb hypercholesterolemia. Am J Cardiol. 2002 Feb 1;89(3):268-75.

82. Kendrach MG, Kelly-Freeman M. Approximate equivalent rosuvastatin doses for temporary statin interchange programs. Ann Pharmacother. 2004 Jul-Aug;38(7-8):1286-92.

83. Schwenzer KJ. Practical tips for working effectively with your institutional review board. Respir Care. 2008 Oct;53(10):1354-61.

84. Enfield KB, Truwit JD. The purpose, composition, and function of an institutional review board: balancing priorities. Respir Care. 2008 Oct;53(10):1330-6.

85. Schwenzer KJ. Protecting vulnerable subjects in clinical research: children, pregnant women, prisoners, and employees. Respir Care. 2008 Oct;53(10):1342-9.

86. Montori A, Onorato M. Why there is a need of an ethics committee in scientific medical societies. Dig Dis. 2008;26(1):32-5.

87. Lema VM, Mbondo M, Kamau EM. Informed consent for clinical trials: a review. East Afr Med J. 2009 Mar;86(3):133-42.

88. Freeman SR, Lundahl K, Schilling LM, Jensen JD, Dellavalle RP. Human research review committee requirements in medical journals. Clin Invest Med. 2008;31(1):E49-54.

89. Byerly WG. Working with the institutional review board. Am J Health-Syst Pharm. 2009 Jan 15;66(2):176-84.

90. Mertl SL. The fundamentals of Institutional Review Board operations. J Pharm Pract. 1996;IX:437-43.

91. Macklin R. The ethical problems with sham surgery in clinical research. N Engl J Med. 1999 Sep 23;341(13):992-6.

92. Horng S, Miller FG. Is placebo surgery unethical? N Engl J Med. 2002 Jul 11;347(2):137-9.

93. Riegelman RK. Studying a study and testing a test: How to read the medical literature. 5th ed. Philadelphia (PA): Lippincott William & Wilkins; 2004.

94. Guyatt G, Rennie D. User's guide to the medical literature: essentials of evidence-based clinical practice. Chicago (IL): AMA Press; 2002.

95. Collins R, MacMahon S. Reliable assessment of the effects of treatment on mortality and major morbidity, I: clinical trials. Lancet. 2001 Feb 3;357(9253):373-80.

96. Roberts C, Torgerson D. Randomisation methods in controlled trials. BMJ. 1998 Nov 7;317(7168):1301.

97. Roland M, Torgerson D. Understanding controlled trials: what outcomes should be measured? BMJ. 1998 Oct 17;317(7165):1075.

98. Pitt B, Segal R, Martinez FA, Meurers G, Cowley AJ, Thomas I, et al. Randomised trial of losartan versus captopril in patients over 65 with heart failure (Evaluation of Losartan in the Elderly Study, ELITE). Lancet. 1997 Mar 15;349(9054):747-52.

99. Freemantle N, Calvert M, Wood J, Eastaugh J, Griffin C. Composite outcomes in randomized trials: greater precision but with greater uncertainty? JAMA. 2003 May 21;289(19):2554-9.

100. Lubsen J, Kirwan BA. Combined endpoints: can we use them? Stat Med. 2002 Oct 15;21919):2959-70.

101. Buzney EA, Kimball AB. A critical assessment of composite and coprimary endpoints: a complex problem. J Am Acad Dermatol. 2008 Nov;59(5):890-6.

102. Kaul S, Diamond GA. Trial and error: how to avoid commonly encountered limitations of published clinical trials. J Am Coll Cardiol. 2010;55(5):415-27.

103. Montori VM, Busse JW, Permanyer-Miralda G, Ferreira I, Guyatt GH. How should clinicians interpret results reflecting the effect of an intervention on composite endpoints: should I dump this lump? ACP J Club. 2005 Nov-Dec;143(3):A8.

104. Cohen M, Demers C, Gurfinkel EP, Turpie AG, Fromell GJ, Goodman S, et al. A comparison of low-molecular-weight heparin with unfractionated heparin for unstable coronary artery disease. Efficacy and Safety of Subcutaneous Enoxaparin in Non-Q-Wave Coronary Events Study Group. N Engl J Med. 1997 Aug 14;337(7):447-52.

105. Armstrong PW. Heparin in acute coronary disease: requiem for a heavyweight? N Engl J Med. 1997 Aug 14;337(7):492-4.

106. Ohman EM. Enoxaparin reduced combined coronary events in unstable angina and non-Q-wave MI at 14 and 30 days [Comment]. ACP J Club. 1998;128:34.

107. Executive Summary of the Third Report of the National Cholesterol Education Program (NCEP) Expert Panel on Detection, Evaluation, and Treatment of High Blood Cholesterol in Adults (Adult Treatment Panel III). JAMA. 2001 May 16;285(19):2486-97.

108. Potkin SG, Saha AR, Kujawa MJ, Carson WH, Ali M, Stock E, et al. Aripiprazole, an antipsychotic with a novel mechanism of action, and risperidone vs. placebo in patients with schizophrenia and schizoaffective disorder. Arch Gen Psychiatry. 2003 Jul;60(7):681-90.

109. American Psychiatric Association. Practice guidelines for the treatment of psychiatric disorders. Arlington (VA): American Psychiatric Association; 2006.

110. Woo TUW, Canuso CM, Wojcik JD, Brunette MF, Green AI. Treatment of schizophrenia. In: Schatzberg AF, Nemeroff CB, eds. Textbook of psychopharmacology. 4th ed. Washington, DC: American Psychiatric Publishing, Inc: 2009:1135-69.

111. Lader EW, Cannon CP, Ohman EM, Newby LK, Sulmasy DP, Barst RJ, et al. The clinician as investigator: participating in clinical trials in the practice setting: Appendix 2: statistical concepts in study design and analysis. Circulation. 2004;109:e305-7.

112. Whitley E, Ball J. Statistics review 4: sample size calculations. Crit Care. 2002 Aug;6(4):335-41.

113. Guller U, DeLong ER. Interpreting statistics in medical literature: a vade mecum for surgeons. J Am Coll Surg. 2004 Mar;198(3):441-58.

114. Tumlin JA, Wang A, Murray PT, Mathur VS. Fenoldopam mesylate blocks reductions in renal plasma flow after radiocontrast dye infusion: a pilot trial in the prevention of contrast nephropathy. Am Heart J. 2002 May;143(5):894-903.

115. Stone GW, McCullough PA, Tumlin JA, Lepor NE, Madyoon H, Murray P, et al. Fenoldopam mesylate for the prevention of contrast-induced nephropathy: a randomized controlled trial. JAMA. 2003 Nov 5;290(17):2284-91.

116. Altman DG, Goodman SN, Schroter S. How statistical expertise is used in medical research. JAMA. 2002 Jun 5;287(21):2817-20.

117. Delgado-Rodriguez M, Ruiz-Canela M, De Irala-Estevez J, Llorca J, Martinez-Gonzalez A. Participation of epidemiologists and/or biostatisticians and methodological quality of published controlled clinical trials. J Epidemiol Community Health. 2001 Aug;55(8): 569-72.

118. Guyatt G, Jaeschke R, Heddle N, Cook D, Shannon H, Walter S. Basic statistics for clinicians: 1. Hypothesis testing. CMAJ. 1995 Jan 1;152(1):27-32.

119. Whitley E, Ball J. Statistics review 3: hypothesis testing and P values. Crit Care. 2002 Jun;6(3):222-5.

120. DeMuth JE. Overview of biostatistics used in clinical research. Am J Health-Syst Pharm. 2009 Jan 1;66(1):70-81.

121. Salkind NJ. Statistics for people who (think they) hate statistics. Thousand Oaks (CA): Sage Publications, Inc; 2000.

122. Whitley E, Ball J. Statistics review 2: samples and populations. Crit Care. 2002 Apr;6(2):143-8.

123. Whitley E, Ball J. Statistics review 1: presenting and summarising data. Crit Care. 2002 Feb;6(1):66-71.

124. Evans RB, O'Connor A. Statistics and evidence-based veterinary medicine: answers to 21 common statistical questions that arise from reading scientific manuscripts. Vet Clin North Am Small Anim Pract. 2007 May;37(3):477-86.

125. Glantz SA. Primer of biostatistics. 5th ed. New York (NY): McGraw-Hill; 2002.

126. Lee CM, Soin HK, Einarson TR. Statistics in the pharmacy literature. Ann Pharmacother. 2004 Sep;38(9):1412-8.

127. Swinscow TDV. Statistics at square one. London (England): British Medical Association; 1983.

128. Kirby A, Gebski V, Keech AC. Determining the sample size in a clinical trial. Med J Aust. 2002 Sep 2;177(5):256-7.

129. Elenbaas JK, Cuddy PG, Elenbaas RM. Evaluating the medical literature, Part III: Results and discussion. Ann Emerg Med. 1983 Nov;12(11):679-86.

130. DeMets DL. Statistical issues in interpreting clinical trials. J Intern Med. 2004 May;255(5):529-37.

131. Hardin JM. Principle of intention to treat analysis in clinical studies: its use and controversies. J Pharm Pract. 1998 Jun;11(3):231-8.

132. Le Bars PL, Katz MM, Berman N, Itil TM, Freedman AM, Schatzberg AF. A placebo-controlled, double-blind, randomized trial of an extract of Ginkgo biloba for dementia. North American EGb Study Group. JAMA. 1997 Oct 22-29;278(16):1327-32.

133. Shepherd J, Cobbe SM, Ford I, Isles CG, Lorimer AR, MacFarlane PW, et al. Prevention of coronary heart disease with pravastatin in men with hypercholesterolemia. West of Scotland Coronary Prevention Study Group. N Engl J Med. 1995 Nov 16;333(20): 1301-7.

134. Bucher HC, Guyatt GH, Cook DJ, Holbrook A, McAlister FA. Users' guides to the medical literature: XIX. Applying clinical trial results. A. How to use an article measuring the effect of an intervention on surrogate end points. Evidence-Based Medicine Working Group. JAMA. 1999 Aug 25;282(8):771-8.

135. Weihrauch TR, Demol P. Value of surrogate endpoints for evaluation of therapeutic efficacy. Drug Inf J. 1998;32:737-43.

136. Barter PJ, Caulfield M, Eriksson M, Grundy SM, Kastelein JJ, Komajda M, et al for the ILLUMINATE Investigators. Effects of torcetrapib in patients at high risk for coronary events. N Engl J Med. 2007 Nov 22;357(21):2109-22.

137. Cook DI, Gebski VJ, Keech AC. Subgroup analysis in clinical trials. Med J Aust. 2004 Mar 15;180(6):289-91.

138. Oxman AD, Guyatt GH. A consumer's guide to subgroup analyses. Ann Intern Med. 1992 Jan 1;116(1):78-84.

139. Shepherd J, Blauw GJ, Murphy MB, Bollen EL, Buckley BM, Cobbe SM, et al. Pravastatin in elderly individuals at risk of vascular disease (PROSPER): a randomised controlled trial. Lancet. 2002 Nov 23;360(9346):1623-30.

140. Gorelick PB, Richardson D, Kelly M, Ruland S, Hung E, Harris Y, et al. Aspirin and ticlopidine for prevention of recurrent stroke in black patients: a randomized trial. JAMA. 2003 Jun 11;289(22):2947-57.

141. Hass WK, Easton JD, Adams HP, Jr., Pryse-Phillips W, Molony BA, Anderson S, et al. A randomized trial comparing ticlopidine hydrochloride with aspirin for the prevention of stroke in high-risk patients. Ticlopidine Aspirin Stroke Study Group. N Engl J Med. 1989 Aug 24;321(8):501-7.

142. Tsai HH, Chapman R, Shepherd A, McKeith D, Anderson M, Vearer D, et al. Esomeprazole 20 mg on-demand is more acceptable to patients than continuous lansoprazole 15 mg in the long-term maintenance of endoscopy-negative gastro-oesophageal reflux patients: the COMMAND Study. Aliment Pharmacol Ther. 2004 Sep 15;20(6):657-65.

143. Rothwell PM. External validity of randomised controlled trials: "to whom do the results of this trial apply?" Lancet. 2005 Jan 1-7;365(9453):82-93.

144. Clarke M, Alderson P, Chalmers I. Discussion sections in reports of controlled trials published in general medical journals. JAMA. 2002 Jun 5;287(21):2799-801.

145. Anderson G, Kendrach MG, Trice S. Basic biostatistics and hypothesis testing. J Pharm Pract. 1998 Jun;11(3):181-95.

146. Pocock SJ, Ware JH. Translating statistical findings into plain English. Lancet. 2009 Jun 6;373(9679):1926-8.

147. Castell DO, Kahrilas PJ, Richter JE, Vakil NB, Johnson DA, Zuckerman S, et al. Esomeprazole (40 mg) compared with lansoprazole (30 mg) in the treatment of erosive esophagitis. Am J Gastroenterol. 2002 Mar;97(3):575-83.

148. Whelton A, Fort JG, Puma JA, Normandin D, Bello AE, Verburg KM. Cyclooxygenase-2-specific inhibitors and cardiorenal function: a randomized, controlled trial of celecoxib and rofecoxib in older hypertensive osteoarthritis patients. Am J Ther. 2001 Mar-Apr;8(2):85-95.

149. Borenstein M. The case for confidence intervals in controlled clinical trials. Control Clin Trials. 1994 Oct;15(5):411-28.

150. Guyatt G, Jaeschke R, Heddle N, Cook D, Shannon H, Walter S. Basic statistics for clinicians: 2. Interpreting study results: confidence intervals. CMAJ. 1995 Jan 15;152(2): 169-73.

151. Guyatt GH, Sackett DL, Cook DJ. Users' guides to the medical literature. II. How to use an article about therapy or prevention. B. What were the results and will they help me in caring for my patients? Evidence-Based Medicine Working Group. JAMA. 1994 Jan 5;271(1):59-63.

152. Jaeschke R, Guyatt G, Shannon H, Walter S, Cook D, Heddle N. Basic statistics for clinicians: 3. Assessing the effects of treatment: measures of association. CMAJ. 1995 Feb 1;152(3):351-7.

153. Colhoun HM, Betteridge DJ, Durrington PN, Hitman GA, Neil HA, Livingstone SJ, et al for the CARDS investigators. Primary prevention of cardiovascular disease with atorvastatin in type 2 diabetes in the Collaborative Atorvastatin Diabetes Study (CARDS): multicentre randomised placebo-controlled trial. Lancet. 2004 Aug 21-27;364(9435):685-96.

154. Kendrach MG, Covington TR, McCarthy MW, Harris CM. Calculating risks and number-needed-to-treat: a method of data interpretation. J Managed Care Pharm. 1997 Mar/Apr;3(2):179-83.

155. Feinstein AR. Principles of medical statistics. Boca Raton (FL): Chapman & Hall/CRC Press Co; 2002.

156. Chobanian AV, Bakris GL, Black HR, Cushman WC, Green LA, Izzo JL, Jr., et al. The Seventh Report of the Joint National Committee on Prevention, Detection, Evaluation, and Treatment of High Blood Pressure: the JNC 7 report. JAMA. 2003 May 21;289(19):2560-72.

157. Castell DO, Richter JE, Robinson M, Sontag SJ, Haber MM. Efficacy and safety of lansoprazole in the treatment of erosive reflux esophagitis. The Lansoprazole Group. Am J Gastroenterol. 1996 Sep;91(9):1749-57.

158. Advice for travelers. Treat Guidel Med Lett. 2009 Nov;87:83-94.

159. DuPont HL, Sullivan P, Evans DG, Pickering LK, Evans DJ, Jr., Vollet JJ, et al. Prevention of traveler's diarrhea (emporiatric enteritis). Prophylactic administration of subsalicylate bismuth). JAMA. 1980 Jan 18;243(3):237-41.

160. Mosdell KW. Literature evaluation I: controlled clinical trials. In: Malone PM, Mosdell KW, Kier KL, Stanovich JE, editors. Drug information: a guide for pharmacists. 2nd ed. New York (NY): McGraw-Hill; 2001. p. 160.

161. Buchkowsky SS, Jewesson PJ. Industry sponsorship and authorship of clinical trials over 20 years. Ann Pharmacother. 2004 Apr;38(4):579-85.

162. Pharmaceutical Research and Manufacturers of America. Pharmaceutical Industry Profile 2009. [cited 2009 July 27]. Available from: http://www.phrma.org/files/PhRMA%202009%20Profile%20FINAL.pdf.

163. Thompson DF. Understanding financial conflicts of interest. N Engl J Med. 1993 Aug 19;329(8):573-6.

164. Wynia M, Boren D. Better regulation of industry-sponsored clinical trials is long overdue. J Law Med Ethics. 2009;37(3):395, 410-9.

165. Drazen JM, Van Der Weyden MB, Sahni P, Rosenberg J, Marusic A, Laine C, et al. Uniform format for disclosure of competing interests in ICMJE journals. Ann Intern Med. 2010 Jan 19;152(2):125-6.

166. Lievre M, Menard J, Bruckert E, Cogneau J, Delahaye F, Giral P, et al. Premature discontinuation of clinical trial for reasons not related to efficacy, safety, or feasibility. BMJ. 2001 Mar 10;322(7286):603-5.

167. Gotzsche PC, Johansen HK. Meta-analysis of prophylactic or empirical antifungal treatment versus placebo or no treatment in patients with cancer complicated by neutropenia. BMJ. 1997 Apr 26;314(7089):1238-44.

168. Rochon PA, Berger PB, Gordon M. The evolution of clinical trials: inclusion and representation. CMAJ. 1998 Dec 1;159(11):1373-4.

169. Blumenthal D, Campbell EG, Anderson MS, Causino N, Louis KS. Withholding research results in academic life science: evidence from a national survey of faculty. JAMA. 1997 Apr 16;277(15):1224-8.

170. Als-Nielsen B, Chen W, Gluud C, Kjaergard LL. Association of funding and conclusions in randomized drug trials: a reflection of treatment effect or adverse events? JAMA. 2003 Aug 20;290(7):921-8.

171. ClinicalTrials.gov Web site. [cited 2010 June 21]. Available from: http://www.clinicaltrials.gov/.

172. ClinicalTrials.gov investigator instructions Web site. [cited 2010 June 21]. Available from: http://prsinfo.clinicaltrials.gov/fdaaa.html.

173. Drazen JM, Jarcho JA, Morrissey S, Curfman GD. Cholesterol lowering and ezetimibe [editorial]. N Engl J Med. 2008 Apr 3;358(14):1507-8.

174. Annals of Pharmcotherapy journal Web site. [cited 2009 Sept 7]. Available from: http://www.hwbooks.com/annals/guides.html#eo.

175. Devereaux PJ, Manns BJ, Ghali WA, Quan H, Guyatt GH. Reviewing the reviewers: the quality of reporting in three secondary journals. CMAJ. 2001 May 29;164(11):1573-6.

176. ACP Journal Club Purpose and Procedure. [cited 2009 Sept 7]. Available from: http://www.acpjc.org/shared/purpose_and_procedure.htm.

177. Subscribe to Journal Watch Newsletters. [cited 2009 Sept 7]. Available from: https://secure.jwatch.org/ecom/subscribe/sub_product.aspx.

178. About Journal Watch Online. [cited 2009 Sept 7]. Available from: http://www.jwatch.org/misc/about.dtl.

179. Columns of AJHP. American Journal of Health-System Pharmacy Web site. [cited 2009 Sept 7]. Available from: http://www.ajhp.org/misc/about.dtl.

SUGGESTED READINGS

1. Schulz KF, Altman DG, Moher D, for the CONSORT Group. CONSORT 2010 Statement: updated guidelines for reporting parallel group randomised trials. BMJ. 2010;340:c332. doi: 10.1136/bmj.c332.

2. Stone GW, Pocock SJ. Randomized trials, statistics, and clinical inference. J Am Coll Cardiol. 2010 Feb 2;55(5):428-31.

3. Guyatt G, Rennie D. User's Guide to the Medical Literature: Essentials of Evidence-Based Clinical Practice. Chicago (IL): AMA Press; 2002.

4. Kaul S, Diamond GA. Trial and error: how to avoid commonly encountered limitations of published clinical trials. J Am Coll Cardiol. 2010 Feb 2;55(5):415-27.

5. Pocock SJ, Ware JH. Translating statistical findings into plain English. Lancet. 2009 Jun 6;373(9679):1926-8.

6. Guller U, DeLong ER. Interpreting statistics in medical literature: a *vade mecum* for surgeons. J Am Coll Surg. 2004 Mar;198(3):441-58.

7. Green SB. Design of randomized trials. Epidemiol Rev. 2002;24(1):4-11.

8. DeMuth JE. Overview of biostatistics used in clinical research. Am J Health-Syst Pharm. 2009 Jan 1;66(1):70-81.

9. Whitley E, Ball J. Statistics review 3: hypothesis testing and P values. Crit Care. 2002 Jun;6(3):222-5.

10. Kendrach MG, Covington TR, McCarthy MW, Harris CM. Calculating risks and number-needed-to-treat: a method of data interpretation. J Managed Care Pharm. 1997 Mar/Apr;3(2):179-83.

5

Chapter Five

Literature Evaluation II: Beyond the Basics

Patrick J. Bryant • Karen P. Norris • Cydney E. McQueen • Elizabeth A. Poole

Learning Objectives

After completing this chapter, the reader will be able to

- Describe examples of other study designs besides the basic controlled clinical trial.
- Discuss the potential utility, limitations, and questions to ask when evaluating other study designs.
- Describe the characteristics of various observational trial designs.
- Differentiate between the three types of literature reviews: narrative (nonsystematic) review, systematic review, and meta-analysis.
- Describe common quality of life (QOL) measures used in health outcomes research and discuss the appropriate use of these measures in the medical literature.
- Discuss common issues encountered in dietary supplement (botanical and nonbotanical) medical literature.
- Describe how to efficiently and effectively evaluate the available evidence associated with a clinical question and categorize the quality of that evidence to develop a recommendation/clinical decision.

Key Concepts

1 Although the randomized, controlled trial is the most frequently used study design for clinical research, several other designs are used in specific situations, such as investigating rare outcome incidences, studying equivalency/non-inferiority between drugs, or minimizing patient exposure to new drugs with inadequate efficacy.

2 Observational study designs offer an alternative to interventional trials. These designs are used in specific situations such as when large populations of patients must be followed over extended periods of time. They can be prospective, retrospective, or a single snapshot (or slice) in time. Interpretation of results from these trials only allows associations to be formed rather than true cause-and-effect relationships.

3 Reports describing observations made regarding a patient or patient group exposure to a drug or technology can be valuable to record preliminary findings that will lead to further study. A key characteristic to these reports is the lack of a control or comparison group. These observational or interventional reports are referred to as case studies, case reports, or case series.

4 Survey research is commonly used and represents information gathered from an identified group from which conclusions are drawn and applied to a larger population. This gathered information is considered either descriptive (such as opinions and attitudes) or explanatory (such as explaining a cause and effect) in nature. Validity of the results depends on the quality of the study's internal rigor.

5 Reviews provide support for clinical decisions when large, well-conducted trials are lacking. Meta-analyses are the only type of review that provides new quantitative data. This new data is derived from combining the results of each study included in the meta-analysis and performing a statistical analysis on that data set. The overall reliability of conclusions stemming from a meta-analysis is ultimately dependent upon the quality of the individual studies and the homogeneity between these studies involved in the analysis.

6 Multiple health outcome measurements have been developed to address a patient's quality of life (QOL). Physical and social environment, in addition to the emotional and existential reactions to this environment, all affect QOL. The value assigned to quality and quantity of life affected by many different variables including disease, injury, treatment, or policy is termed health-related quality of life (HR-QOL). This HR-QOL value is used to assist in decision-making regarding interventions such as procedures and pharmacotherapy.

7 The same principles and criteria used to analyze the quality of drug literature are used to analyze dietary supplement literature; however, there are some unique additional points such as standardization and purity that must be considered.

❽ Given the numerous novel study designs being used by investigators to create new knowledge and medical evidence today, an understanding of strengths and limitations inherent with each design is essential to determine the overall quality of the evidence produced. Those trial designs with a high level of quality provide the most reliable evidence, and that translates into the strongest recommendation/clinical decision.

Introduction

Question: Why is it important to understand principles of study design and evaluation beyond the prospective, randomized, controlled, clinical trial?

Answer: Principles that apply to well-designed randomized, controlled trials (see Chapter 4) also apply to other types of study designs; however, there are situations where other research designs are more effective in answering specific questions or provide the only data available to answer the questions. For example, only a handful of small, randomized, controlled trials may be available to address a particular clinical situation. This is apparent in the many small trials of gabapentin for treatment of neuropathic pain. In this case, a meta-analysis may be more effective at answering the question because data from these small trials is pooled to achieve statistical power needed to answer the question. As another example, it may not be feasible to study the toxicity of certain agents (e.g., cardiovascular risks associated with cyclooxygenase inhibitors) in prospective, randomized, controlled, clinical trials; therefore, observational cohort trials and/or retrospective case-control studies must be employed. To effectively determine the quality of these trials, the practitioner must first evaluate the major considerations that apply. One approach uses a list of essential study components referred to as the Ten Major Considerations Checklist.[1] The Ten Major Considerations include:

1. Power of the study set and met (to estimate adequate sample size that will identify a difference between groups if one truly exists)?
2. Dosage/treatment regimen appropriate?
3. Length of study appropriate to show effect?
4. Inclusion criteria adequate to identify target study population?
5. Exclusion criteria adequate to exclude patients who may be harmed in study?
6. Blinding present?
7. Randomization resulted in similar groups?

8. Biostatistical tests appropriate for type of data analyzed?
9. Measurement(s) standard/validated/accepted?
10. Author's conclusions are supported by the results?

Once this is completed, additional considerations unique to study designs discussed in this chapter must be evaluated. The purpose of this chapter is to familiarize the practitioner with these unique study designs. In addition, specific considerations unique to each design and in addition to the Ten Major Considerations are identified for the practitioner to evaluate (see Appendix 5–1). Finally, a process is provided to bring all the results of trials focused on a particular clinical question together and develop a recommendation/clinical decision based on this evidence.

This chapter covers the variations on randomized clinical trial design (non-inferiority, N-of-1, adaptive clinical trials), observational trial design (cohort, case-control, cross-sectional), and uncontrolled study designs (case studies, case series, case reports). Specific types of studies such as bioequivalency, postmarketing surveillance, and programmatic research are discussed. Differences between narrative (qualitative), systematic (qualitative), and meta-analysis (quantitative) reviews are addressed. A discussion of the specialized area of health outcomes research is included to introduce concepts directly related to patient quality of life trials. A section on evaluation of dietary supplement medical literature, including issues specific to these trials and common methodological flaws, is provided.

Good literature evaluation skills and application of a systematic evidence-based medicine process provide the foundation that allows clinicians to make the best recommendations and decisions. In light of rapidly emerging evidence and busy practitioner schedules, an understanding of inherent strengths and limitations of various types of clinical trial design provides a powerful clinical tool. Those trials with a greater number of strengths than limitations provide a higher level of reliability and thus, a stronger recommendation/clinical decision. This in turn ensures the highest level of patient care, whether for one specific patient or large patient populations.

Beyond the Basic Controlled Trial

❶ *Although the randomized, controlled trial is the most frequently used study design for clinical research, several other designs are used in specific situations, such as investigating rare outcome incidences, studying equivalency/non-inferiority between drugs, or minimizing patient exposure to new drugs with inadequate efficacy.* The randomized, controlled, clinical trial is sometimes referred to as an "interventional trial." The intervention provided could be in the form of a treatment, an educational program, a medical procedure, or something else. Students often ask why the strongest experimental designs are not used exclusively by all individuals performing research. "Doing the best with what one has" may be the best answer. Study designs are developed in an effort to reasonably achieve three key research objectives: (1) to have equivalent sampling groups; (2) to isolate and control the intervention; and (3) to obtain reliable measurements of the response. Attainment of these objectives requires significant resource allocation including time, materials, subjects, and money. Interventional designs require large quantities of each resource. These studies may be impractical or inefficient when investigating rare outcome incidences, when finances are limited, or when concerns arise regarding the ethical feasibility of allocating patients to potentially hazardous interventions. Table 5–1 lists commonly encountered biomedical literature.

TABLE 5–1. COMMONLY ENCOUNTERED BIOMEDICAL LITERATURE

Study Design	Study Purpose
Clinical study (true experiment)	Determine cause and effect relationships
N-of-1 study	Compare effects of drug to control during multiple observation periods in a single patient
Stability study	Evaluate stability of drugs in various preparations (e.g., ophthalmologic, intravenous, topical, and oral)
Bioequivalence study	Assess the bioequivalency of two or more products
Programmatic research	Determine the impact and/or economic value of clinical services
Cohort (follow-up) study	Determine association between various factors and disease state development
Case-control (trohoc) study	Determine association between disease states and exposure to various risk factors
Cross-sectional study	Identify prevalence of characteristics of diseases in populations
Case study, case report, or case series	Report observations in a single patient or series of patients
Survey research	Study the incidence, distribution, and relationships of sociologic and psychologic variables through use of questionnaires applied to various populations
Postmarketing surveillance study	Evaluate use and adverse effects associated with newly approved drug therapies
Narrative review	Nonsystematic, subjective summary of data from multiple studies
Systematic review	Systematic, qualitative, and objective summary of data from multiple studies
Meta-analysis	Combine, statistically evaluate, and summarize data from multiple studies
Outcomes studies (pharmacoeconomic and health related-QOL measures)	Compare outcomes (QOL) and costs (pharmacoeconomics) of drug therapies or services

ABBREVIATION: QOL = quality of life.

NON-INFERIORITY TRIALS

Randomized, controlled, clinical trials are utilized to determine one of three different outcomes between comparative drugs: superiority, equivalency, or non-inferiority (NI).[2] All three trial designs involve a new test drug compared to the accepted active control or standard drug. With superiority trials, the aim is to determine that one drug is superior to the other.[3] In contrast, equivalency trials are designed to determine if the new drug is therapeutically similar to the control drug. This trial design is used primarily to determine bioequivalence between two drugs. Non-inferiority trials seek to show that any difference between two treatments is small enough to conclude the test drug has "an effect not too much smaller than the active control" or reference drug.[4] This section will focus on description, interpretation, and evaluation of NI trials.

A NI study design is often considered when superiority of a test drug over a reference drug (for instance standard of care) is not anticipated.[5] In this case, the objective is showing the test drug to be statistically and clinically not inferior to the reference drug. Non-inferiority trials are also considered when the use of a superiority trial would be considered unethical.[3] For example, it is unethical to use a placebo when there is available effective treatment that possesses an important benefit such as preventing death or irreversible injury to the patient. For this reason, non-inferiority trials can provide an alternative method to using superiority trials for meeting Food and Drug Administration (FDA) marketing approval requirements.[3] Rather than going through the process of showing a new drug is therapeutically superior to the standard of therapy or a placebo, pharmaceutical companies are choosing NI trial design. This is a relatively new developmental strategy to confirm the new drug has a valid therapeutic effect and that its effect is not, at minimum, worse than a reference drug, which is generally considered standard of therapy. Often the anticipated key differentiating factor for the test drug in this situation is improved safety profile. For example, a new drug for cardiac arrhythmias is anticipated to have similar efficacy but less serious side effects than standard of care therapy.

The NI trial design focuses on the mean difference in efficacy measures between the test drug versus reference drug (Figure 5–1). A NI margin is how much better the reference drug's effect can be and still allow the test drug to be considered non-inferior. Confidence intervals (95% CI) around the mean difference in efficacy between the test drug and reference drug are compared against this NI margin. If the 95% CI around the mean difference in treatment effect includes (or crosses) the NI margin, then the possibility of the test drug being inferior to the reference drug cannot be ruled out, and thus, non-inferiority is not demonstrated (see Figure 5–1A). However, if the 95% CI around the mean difference in treatments does not include or cross the NI margin, then one can conclude that the test drug is non-inferior to the reference drug (see Figure 5–1B and C).

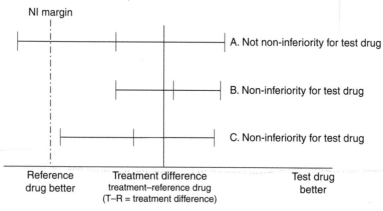

Figure 5–1. Non-inferiority trial design concept.

For instance, a NI study of a new antihypertensive agent (test drug) compared to standard of therapy (reference drug) is published in the literature. The NI margin is established based on the reference drug's performance confirmed in previous published studies. That margin of a clinically significant difference between the two drugs is set at 6 mmHg sitting diastolic pressure (Figure 5–2). The test drug's lower bound of the 95% CI will need to not include (or cross) this NI margin to confirm non-inferiority for the test drug. If the test drug's lower bound 95% CI includes (or crosses) the margin of NI, this would suggest that the test drug did not demonstrate non-inferiority. In other words, the test drug could be inferior to the reference drug (see Figure 5–2A). Upon completion of the antihypertensive NI study, the actual results confirm non-inferiority of the new

*SUPERIORITY CAN BE DECLARED IN A NON-INFERIORITY STUDY IF THE LOWER BOUND OF THE INTERVAL WERE ABOVE ZERO (NOT SIMPLY ABOVE THE MARGIN)

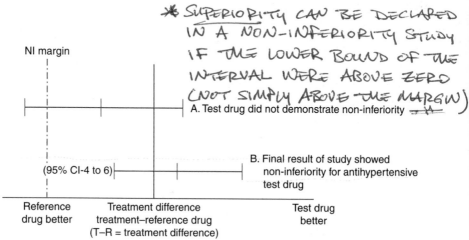

Figure 5–2. Non-inferiority trial design example.

antihypertensive agent based on the lower bound of the 95% CI for the test drug not including (or crossing) the NI margin (see Figure 5–2B). This whole concept of NI is based on the mean difference between the test and reference drug, the 95% CI around that mean, and whether the CI crosses the NI margin of clinical significance.

The statistical rationale for NI trials differs from that used with superiority trials.[6,7] Specifically, the defining parameters for the null and alternative hypotheses differ from those used with superiority trials. The null hypothesis for a superiority trial postulates there is no significant difference between treatment groups, and the alternative hypothesis states there is a significant difference between the treatment groups. With NI trials, the opposite approach is taken: the null hypothesis states the reference drug is significantly different from the test drug by at least the established NI margin.[5] The alternative hypothesis states that the reference drug is not significantly different from the test drug by not exceeding the established NI margin. Even though the reference drug may have slightly better efficacy compared to the test drug, as long as the 95% CI around the mean difference does not cross the NI margin, the difference in drug effect would not be considered clinically significant. With NI trials, the null hypothesis must be rejected to conclude non-inferiority for the test drug.

Some controversy exists whether a NI trial alone can show superiority of the test drug over the reference drug.[2,5,8] According to guidance from the FDA, a NI study can be designed to first test for non-inferiority with a predetermined NI margin, and if successful proving non-inferiority, then analyze the study for potential superiority of the test drug. Note the importance of the sequential process of first proving non-inferiority, then analyzing for superiority. For instance, if the new antihypertensive NI trial discussed earlier provided results that showed the test drug to be non-inferior, then an analysis of superiority would be appropriate and acceptable. In contrast, seeking the conclusion of NI from a failed superiority trial is almost never acceptable because of the obvious bias introduced when specifying a NI margin after the data has already been analyzed.[3] Rather, if a non-inferiority conclusion is anticipated, a NI study design should be the initial choice.

Several study design characteristics must be considered when evaluating the quality of a NI trial.[2] The Ten Major Considerations Checklist discussed earlier in the Introduction is used to identify specific major strengths and limitations.

Of significant importance is how the NI margin used to determine non-inferiority is defined.[5] Correctly determining this margin is considered the greatest challenge in the design and interpretation of NI trials.[3] If non-inferiority is established for the test drug, further concluding the test drug is effective can only be made if the reference drug's efficacy has been confirmed against placebo. This is referred to as assay sensitivity. The NI margin is set using historical studies to determine the actual effect of the reference drug. Historical evidence of sensitivity to drug effects (HESDE) is a term used to describe appropriately designed and conducted past trials using the reference drug and regularly exhibiting the reference drug to be superior to placebo. Meta-analytic methods can be used to develop more precise estimates of reference drug effect when several studies are available. When multiple studies exist, all studies should be considered to avoid overestimating the reference drug's effect.[3] Only after a determination is made that these past studies are similar in design and conduct compared to the NI trial regarding features that could alter the effect size can the HESDE be used to select the NI margin. In other words, the historical and new NI study should be as identical as possible regarding important characteristics. This is called the "constancy assumption."[4]

Case Study 5-1

■ PERTINENT BACKGROUND INFORMATION

A non-inferiority (NI) trial was conducted to determine if dronedarone, a new antiarrythmic drug, is therapeutically non-inferior to the standard of care amiodarone for maintaining sinus rhythm after cardioversion. In addition, safety was compared between the two drugs throughout the study. The primary outcome measure was reoccurrence of atrial fibrillation/flutter after initiation of either study drug. The NI margin was set based on previous placebo-controlled trials with amiodarone. An intention-to-treat analysis was used. Safety was assessed by the number of reported adverse drug reactions for each drug.

1. Identify the null hypothesis and alternative hypothesis for this non-inferiority study.
2. When setting the NI margin, what specific things did the investigators need to take into consideration?
3. Did the investigators use the appropriate analysis type for a NI study?
4. What is your conclusion if the 95% CI around the mean difference in reoccurrence rate of atrial fibrillation/flutter between dronedarone and amiodarone does not include or cross over the established NI margin?
5. If the 95% CI around the mean difference in reoccurrence rate of atrial fibrillation/flutter between dronedarone and amiodarone includes or crosses over the established NI margin, what is your conclusion?
6. After showing non-inferiority for the two drugs, the investigators performed a superiority analysis on the data. What is your reaction to this second analysis?

Setting the NI margin post hoc can be interpreted as potential manipulation by investigators to show desired results. For this reason, it is critical that the NI margin be set prospectively before the beginning of the trial. This is considered acceptable practice. A practical consideration associated with choice of the NI margin involves the sample size requirement. A small margin requires a smaller lower bound of the 95% CI, which in turn requires a larger sample size due to the higher level of precision required. Conversely, selecting a NI margin that represents a value greater than the actual effect of the reference drug can lead to an incorrect conclusion that the test drug is non-inferior. For all of these reasons, the investigators should provide a detailed description of how the NI margin was determined.

The type of analysis used should also be determined prospectively. For the purposes of NI study analysis, a per protocol analysis where only the patients that completed the study are included is preferred over an intention-to-treat analysis (ITT).[2,5] The ITT analysis includes all patients that were randomized to treatment regardless of whether they completed the study duration. With the ITT analysis, smaller observed treatment effects can result, since patients did not necessarily complete the duration of the trial. Using an ITT analysis with a NI trail can significantly increase the risk of falsely claiming non-inferiority due to the potential of smaller observed treatment effects. For this reason, a per-protocol analysis is preferred over an ITT analysis. However, the FDA suggests conducting both, a per protocol and ITT analysis. Any differences in results between these two separate analyses should be examined closely.[3]

Determining adequate sample size to ensure the trial will have the statistical power to show NI if the test drug is truly non-inferior is important.[3] Unfortunately, this task is not always easy to perform prior to study initiation. Both variance of the estimated treatment effect and event rate are unknown for the test drug at this point. This problem is similar to sample size determination in a superiority trial. In superiority trials, the blinded information is examined during the trial by an independent data-monitoring committee. This committee is looking for an unexpectedly low event rate, so an upward adjustment in sample size can be proposed. This same approach is applied to NI trials. For this reason, a clear explanation of how the blinded information was handled and how the independent data-monitoring committee was conducted is necessary.

As mentioned previously, an attempt to rescue a failed superiority study that concludes the results really demonstrate NI should not be accepted.[5] Unfortunately, this situation is more common than would be expected.[9] The plan to determine NI of a test drug compared to the reference drug must be established prospectively utilizing the proper study design to test for NI. In other words, lack of superiority in a superiority trial design does not equal NI.

Appendix 5–1 contains a list of additional questions specific to NI studies. These specific questions are in addition to the standard questions used to evaluate other randomized clinical trials noted in Chapter 4 and using basic tools like the Ten Major Considerations Checklist discussed in the Introduction section.

N-OF-1 TRIALS

The N-of-1 trial attempts to apply the principles of clinical trials, such as randomization and blinding, to individual patients.[10] These trials are useful when the beneficial effects of a particular treatment in an individual patient are in doubt. It is advantageous if the treatment has a short half-life (allowing multiple crossover periods without carryover effects) and is being used for symptomatic relief of a chronic condition.[11] An N-of-1 trial can be used to determine whether a drug is effective in an individual patient. Taken as a whole, a group of N-of-1 trials can help to identify characteristics that differentiate responders from nonresponders. Trials of multiple doses can identify the most effective dose and the clinical endpoints most influenced by the drug.[12]

An N-of-1 trial is similar to a crossover study conducted in a single patient who receives treatments in pairs (one period of the experimental therapy and one period of either alternative treatment or placebo) in random order. [12] As described below, the study usually consists of several treatment periods that are continued until effectiveness is proven or refuted. Randomization to active drug or placebo and blinding of the physician and patient to the treatment being administered reduce treatment order effects (the order in which patients receive the treatments in the trial affects the results), placebo effects (therapeutic activity provided by administering a placebo), and observer bias (person collecting the data from the trial knows or has some idea what study drug each patient is receiving, and therefore this may have some affect on the results reported). Desired outcomes are identified prior to initiation of the study to ensure that objective criteria that are meaningful to both the physician and patient are used to assess treatment efficacy.[11]

N-of-1 trials may improve appropriate prescribing of drugs in individual patients. For example, carbamazepine may be an option for relief of pain in a patient with diabetic neuropathy, but definitive information on the efficacy of such treatment is limited. Therefore, investigators may conduct an N-of-1 trial to determine whether such therapy is useful in a particular patient. N-of-1 trials are especially useful when long-term treatment with a specific drug may result in toxicity and the physician wishes to determine whether benefits outweigh potential risks.[11]

The effectiveness of N-of-1 trials has been evaluated.[12,13] Of 57 N-of-1 trials completed, 50 (88%) provided a definite clinical or statistical answer to a clinical question leading to the conclusion by the authors that N-of-1 trials were useful and feasible in clinical practice.[13] Simply stated, the goal of an N-of-1 trial is to clarify a management decision.[13] Of 34 completed N-of-1 trials evaluated over a 2-year period, 17 (50%) were judged to provide definitive results (10 showed treatment to be effective, five showed treatment no better than no treatment, and two demonstrated harmful effects to the patients).[14] The remaining 17 completed N-of-1 trials showed trends toward equivalence to control or actually favored placebo. Overall, physician confidence in the therapy was found to increase or decrease depending on the direction of trial results.[14]

General requirements have been recommended for N-of-1 trials.[14] Readers should determine whether the treatment target (or measure of effectiveness) was evaluated during each treatment period.[15] This target should be a symptom or diagnostic test result, but must be directly relevant to the patient's well-being (e.g., the visual analog scale for pain in the example of carbamazepine). Two other critical characteristics of an N-of-1 study are that the symptom under investigation shows a rapid improvement when effective treatment is begun and that this improvement regresses quickly (but not permanently) when effective treatment is discontinued.[15] The longer it takes to see a therapeutic effect provided by a drug, the longer the testing period of the trial. This also holds true for how long it takes for the therapeutic effect to disappear after stopping the drug, the longer the washout period must be, which translates into an overall increase in trial duration. The length of the treatment period is important to know. For those diseases that remain constant, this treatment period is easy to establish. When dealing with a disease that is not constant such as multiple sclerosis, the treatment period must be long enough to observe an exacerbation of the condition. A general rule is that if an event occurs an average of once every X days, then a clinician needs to observe 3 times X days to be 95% confident of observing at least one event. One should ask if a clinically relevant treatment target is used and can it be accurately measured? It is advisable to measure symptoms or the patient's quality of life (QOL) directly, with patients rating each symptom at least twice during each study period.

It is important to determine if sensible criteria for stopping the trial are established. Specification of the number of treatment pairs in advance strengthens the statistical analysis of the results, and it has been advised that at least two pairs of treatment periods be conducted before the study is unblinded.[12]

N-of-1 trials provide more objective information than case reports or case studies, and are useful for providing definitive information for drug prescribing in individual patients. See Table 5–2 for a comparison of N-of-1 trials and case studies.

Appendix 5–1 contains a list of additional questions specific to N-of-1 studies. These specific questions are in addition to the standard questions used to evaluate other randomized clinical trials noted in Chapter 4 and using basic tools like the Ten Major Considerations Checklist discussed in the Introduction section.

ADAPTIVE CLINICAL TRIALS

Adaptive clinical trial (ACT) design has become a topic of great interest recently by both the pharmaceutical industry and the United States FDA.[15] Classical clinical trial design is rigidly structured to investigate a set number of variables and prevent additional variables from being introduced that will confound the results. For instance, a traditional, randomized, controlled trial stipulates inclusion and exclusion criteria to allow only a specific population of patients entrance into the trial. The benefit of these strict criteria is a

TABLE 5–2. COMPARISON OF N-OF-1 TRIALS AND CASE STUDIES

	N-of-1 Trial	Case Study
Design	Prospective	Retrospective (most often)
Predefined methods	Yes	No
Clearly defined outcome measures	Yes	No
Randomization	Yes	No
Blinding	Yes	No
Multiple treatment periods	Yes	Not usually

Data from reference 51.

well-defined population to be studied that excludes patients predicted to be potentially harmed if entered into the trial. However, the disadvantage of such rigidity is the inability to make adjustments to the inclusion and exclusion criteria as the study progresses and new information comes from those patients that have completed the trial. If the investigators discover there is a specific patient group that responds to the treatment during the trial, adjustments to include only that patient population are not allowed. For that reason, a significant number of patients that are not going to respond are exposed to a treatment that may cause severe side effects. ACT design provides enough flexibility to incorporate continuously emerging knowledge generated as a trial is carried out. In essence, the ACT design provides the researcher an opportunity to change some study methodology when they identify things that may need to be done differently, such as using a different dose, different patients, or measuring different outcomes over a different period of time. Ideas from industry, academia, and regulatory agencies, such as the FDA Critical Path Initiative (http://www.fda.gov/ScienceResearch/SpecialTopics/CriticalPathInitiative/default. htm), are leading a movement towards ACT design as a potential alternative method to gather data for use in the FDA approval of a drug.

In simplest form, the ACT is known as a staged protocol or group sequential trial.[16] One example of this group sequential design is called a 3+3 trial used in Phase I to identify the maximum-tolerated dose (MTD). Three patients start at a specific dose, and if no toxicity is noted, a second group of three patients are given a higher dose. If one patient experiences a limiting toxicity, then a third group of three patients are given that same dose. From this third group, two or maybe all three patients experience toxicity which leads to claiming that the previous lower dose is the MTD. This is the basic framework of the design that can have many different variations.

Key to this study design is that ACT provides the ability to use more adaptive sampling strategies. These strategies include response-adaptive designs for clinical trials where the emerging data or observations from the trial are used to make adjustments in the ongoing study.[17] As illustrated in this example where an ACT design is incorporated into a dose-response study, emerging patient outcomes are utilized to adjust allocation of future enrolled patients or some other study design component.

The primary benefit of ACT design is that fewer patients are allocated to a less-effective therapy, a greater number of responding patients can be monitored for safety of the effective therapy, and fewer patients overall may be required to determine statistical and clinical significance of the drug.[18] Other potential benefits include a more efficient developmental pathway for the drug, patients benefit from effective therapies earlier, and physicians have more information on patients most likely to benefit from the drug.

The majority of studies utilizing the ACT design have been dose-response trials used to identify the range of effective doses to be used in future efficacy confirmatory studies.[18] A much smaller number of pivotal efficacy-confirming studies have used this design due to company concerns about FDA's skepticism of ACT design, including potential bias and increase in false-positive rates. With time, the ACT design is becoming more common in agreements made between the FDA and sponsors (also known as Special Protocol Assessments) for later stages of clinical development.

Higher-level, more powerful, and complex ACTs require the use of Bayesian statistics that allow for much more flexibility than traditional statistical approaches can provide.[17] The more familiar statistical approach determines the likelihood that the efficacy of a specific drug could have happened by chance. On the other hand, the Bayesian approach provides a probability (or relative likelihood) that the drug is effective. This approach estimates the relative likelihood by using new data as it is created from the ongoing study. The Bayesian approach continuously updates the relative likelihood of the subject being investigated.

Pfizer's ASTIN trial (Acute Stroke Therapy by Inhibition of Neutrophils) is an example of how ACT methodology can be incorporated into a randomized, double-blind, placebo-controlled dose-response study.[19] This trial represents the first time that computer-assisted, real-time learning was successfully implemented in a large international study to look at dose-response effects. In this study, ACT design methodology was used to help determine the maximum-effective dose and ensure the study drug's best chance of showing efficacy. At the same time, the use of the ACT design decreased the exposure of patients to a drug that was found not efficacious in this particular disease state. The ACT study design is computationally and logistically complex, but today's rapid data collection methods and computing power are adequate to meet the requirements. Software programs developed in-house by pharmaceutical industry statisticians are used to handle these complexities.

Studies based on the ACT design are evaluated similarly to other randomized clinical trials; however, there are some questions that are specific for assessing the ACT component. These questions are best understood using the ASTIN trial as an example.

The specific methodologies used to make adaptive changes in the trial are important. In the ASTIN trial, allocation of treatment was carried out centrally at baseline, days 7, 21, and 90 using a computer-generated Bayesian design algorithm. This algorithm determined the current real-time optimal dose and provided information regarding the need to vary the number of patients required, distribute the patients differently between placebo and the study drug, and correct the optimal dose of the study drug. An automated fax system from other patients on the study drug provided information that was used to adjust and optimize the dose. In addition, an independent data-monitoring committee was established to utilize a termination rule for recommending discontinuation of the study after futility or efficacy was established. Termination for futility could be recommended only after a minimum of 500 evaluable patients had completed the study. A minimum of 250 evaluable patients were required before a recommendation could be made to terminate the study for efficacy reasons. Those patients with confirmed ischemic stroke by Computerized Axial Tomography (CAT) scan that were still alive at study day 90 were termed evaluable patients.

Existing logistical issues and how they are being handled are important to know when evaluating an ACT study. In the ASTIN study, patient-response information was transferred to a central location using an automated fax system. The adjusted-dosing information was then sent back to the study site using this same fax system.

In ACTs, all proposed adaptive changes should be based on evidence and good clinical judgment. In the ASTIN study, the proposed adaptive changes were based on the dose-response information from other patients active and/or completed in the trial. The computer-generated specific adaptations that determined the current real-time optimal dose were provided by the Bayesian design algorithm. As mentioned earlier, information regarding the need to vary the number of patients required, distribute the patients differently between placebo and the study drug, and correct the optimal dose of the study drug was provided by this algorithm. A termination rule was established with specific criteria to be applied to the actual patient response information. This was developed to assist the independent data-monitoring committee in making a recommendation to discontinue the study after futility or efficacy was established.

It is important to know if extensive adaptation to the protocol occurred during the ACT. When adaptation is extensive in efficacy confirming trials, the key hypothesis can become unclear and protection of the study's integrity is at risk. The ASTIN study was a dose-response trial, not an efficacy-confirming trial. Adaptations of the dosing strength did occur, and these were associated primarily with lack of efficacy or safety issues. The study's integrity was not jeopardized.

As with other study designs, obvious indications of bias entering the study and having effects on the results should be identified. *Bias* is a term used to describe a preference toward a particular result, when this preference interferes with the ability to be impartial or objective. Several types of bias have been identified that can have major effects on the results of a study. See Table 5–3 for a list of biases from different causes that should be

TABLE 5-3. TYPES OF BIAS THAT MAY OCCUR WITHIN OBSERVATIONAL STUDY DESIGNS AND METHODS OF CONTROL

Category of Bias	Name of Bias	Description	Methods of Control	Cohort	Case-Control	Cross-Sectional
Selection bias	Admission rate (Berkson) bias	Admission rates of exposed and unexposed cases and controls differ, resulting in a distortion of odds of exposure in hospital-based studies	A priori define inclusion and exclusion criteria. All groups of subjects should have undergone identical diagnostic testing and there should be no difference in how exposure or disease status is determined		X	
	Nonresponse bias	Nonrespondents may exhibit exposures or outcomes that differ from respondents, resulting in over or under estimation of odds or risk	Match or adjust for confounding variables. Use more than one control group	X	X	X
	Prevalence-incidence (Neyman) bias	Timing of exposure identification causes some cases to be missed		X	X	
	Unmasking bias	An innocent exposure causes a sign or symptom that precipitates search for a disease, but does not itself cause the disease		X	X	±
Information bias	Family history bias	Family members tend to share more information with family members who have similar diseases or exposures. Those family members without the disease or exposure may be unaware. Family historical information may vary widely depending on whether the person is a case or a control	Establish a priori explicit criteria for data collection methods on exposures and outcomes. Blinded interviewer and subject to the hypotheses investigated. Standardize data collection procedure, i.e., train observers, develop and refine survey questions and methods of recording answers	X	N/A	X

	Bias	Definition	Methods to minimize			
	Recall bias	Difference in how data collection occurs exists between cases and controls, or the exposed and unexposed, resulting in an abnormally high rate of recall of exposure or outcome in one group	Maintain aggressive contact with subjects to limit attrition (cohort designs) For surveys, obtain response rates $\geq 80\%$ Assess for effects of potential confounders	X	N/A	X
	Exposure suspicion bias	Knowledge of a subject's disease status may influence both intensity and outcome of a search for exposure		X	N/A	±
Data-analysis bias	Post hoc significance bias	When decisions regarding level of significance are selected a posteriori, conclusion may be biased	Establish a priori the statistical methods to be used to evaluate data Report how missing data are handled	X	X	X
	Data-dredging bias	When data are reviewed for all possible associations without prior hypotheses, results are only suitable for hypothesis-forming activities	Assess associations between confounders and exposures and outcomes	X	X	X
	Significance bias	Confusing statistical significance with clinical significance		X	X	X
	Correlation bias	Correlations do not equate with causation; concluding that correlation equates with causation can lead to serious errors		X	X	X

Data from reference 38.

ruled out as having significant effects on the results of an ACT. Possible ways that bias could have entered the study should be identified and confirm the effect of that bias on the results determined. In the ASTIN study, several measures were instituted to minimize the chance of bias. An independent data-monitoring committee consisting of three stroke clinicians and a statistician was established prospectively. This group worked independently of the study investigators and would make recommendations based on the patient information to the steering committee. For instance, changing doses based on patient safety and determining if the trial should be terminated according to predetermined criteria for efficacy or futility are two types of recommendations made by this committee. The executive steering committee also worked independently of the study investigators. In addition, the study was double-blinded so neither the patient nor the study investigators were aware of what treatment the patient was receiving.

- If an interim analysis was conducted, exactly who had access to the information created from the interim analysis and how could this have affected any of the results is crucial to know. As mentioned previously, the ASTIN study had an independent data-monitoring committee formed to conduct interim analyses on the patient information received from the ongoing study. It would appear members of that committee had little if any interactions with Pfizer, the company sponsoring the trial.

- Sometimes the ACT is stopped early based on an interim analysis. A determination should be made if stopping the trial early had any effect on the results that would prevent development of strong conclusions. If the discontinuation significantly shortens the period of treatment, evidence may be lacking for any conclusions to be made. The ASTIN study was stopped early. The effect on the evidence was minimal since the specific numbers of patients that needed to be enrolled before discontinuation could even be considered were predetermined before the study was initiated. A minimum of 500 evaluable patients were required before termination for futility could be recommended. In addition, a minimum of 250 evaluable patients were necessary before a recommendation to terminate for efficacy could be made. Actually, 551 evaluable patients had been enrolled, received some dose of the study drug within the allotted range, and completed the study to day 90 before the trial was discontinued. An adequate sample size appeared to be obtained to meet the set power.

The benefits of ACT design are obvious, and this encourages further exploration for appropriate application to clinical programs. Adaptations to number of patients, eligibility criteria, drug dose, and randomization allocation can significantly improve the efficiency of drug development and overall patient care. This is an emerging area of study design research that deserves further consideration for specific uses.

Appendix 5–1 contains a list of additional questions specific to adaptive clinical trials. These specific questions are in addition to the standard questions used to evaluate other randomized clinical trials noted in Chapter 4 and using basic tools like the Ten Major Considerations Checklist discussed in the Introduction section.

STABILITY STUDIES/*IN VITRO* STUDIES

Stability studies determine the stability of drugs in various preparations (e.g., ophthalmologic, intravenous, topical, and oral) under various conditions (e.g., heat, freezing, refrigeration, and room temperature). These trials are very similar to a traditional clinical trial design in many ways. There are some minor changes to what one considers while evaluating the trial, which are mentioned in this section. Stability studies are extremely important to the practice of pharmacy. For example, pharmacists who prepare intravenous solutions for use by patients at home often want to know how long a drug admixed in a particular solution is stable. Another stability question associated with this admixture would be whether freezing increases the length of time the admixture is stable. This information helps to determine how many intravenous admixtures may be dispensed at a time. It is also important for pharmacists involved with extemporaneous compounding to know the length of time a particular preparation is stable.

The quality of stability studies conducted 20 plus years ago were poor, and this prompted Trissel and associates to prepare study guidelines.[20] These guidelines state that investigators conducting stability studies should provide a complete description of study methodology and test conditions. Appropriate, validated assays should be used. Samples should include a baseline time zero measurement and an appropriate number of samples to assess stability over the time period. For example, if the goal of the study is to determine the stability of an antibiotic at room temperature, then taking measurements at time zero and 30 days may not be adequate. Planning the study so that testing is done at multiple time points (e.g., time zero, 6 hours, 12 hours, 18 hours, and 24 hours) would yield more information about the degradation timeline of the product. As with all studies, conclusions should be consistent with the results.

Appendix 5–1 contains a list of additional questions specific to stability studies. These specific questions are in addition to the standard questions used to evaluate other randomized clinical trials noted in Chapter 4 and using basic tools like the Ten Major Considerations Checklist discussed in the Introduction section.

BIOEQUIVALENCE TRIALS

An ever-increasing number of generic products are becoming available in the marketplace, and there is a need to establish that the quality, safety, and efficacy of these generic drugs are the same as the brand name product, which is the purpose of this type of trial.[21] The health care practitioner is often placed in the position of having to select one from among several apparently equivalent products for individual patients or for use on formularies of health care organizations. The more skilled the health care practitioner is at interpreting the data, the more comfortable he or she will be in selecting the appropriate product for the specific patient or organization.

Current FDA regulations require that bioequivalence between the generic product and the brand name product be demonstrated, but do not require that bioequivalence among generic copies of the same brand name drug be demonstrated. As a result, it is a common concern whether these generic drugs can be used interchangeably.

Bioequivalent products are products that are equivalent in rate and extent of absorption (by definition, the rate and extent of absorption differ by –20%/+ 25% or less).[22] These criteria are based on an arbitrary medical decision that, for most products, a –20%/+ 25% difference in the concentration of the active ingredient in blood will not be clinically significant.[23] For some drugs with a narrow therapeutic index (NTI) such as certain anticonvulsants and antipsychotics, there is concern this large of margin may be unsafe. The area under the blood concentration time curve (AUC), the peak height concentration (C_{max}), and the time of the peak concentration (T_{max}) are the primary pharmacokinetic parameters used to assess the rate and extent of drug absorption. Additionally, for approval of a generic product, a manufacturer must show that a 90% confidence interval for the ratio of the mean response of its product compared to that of the innovator product is within the limits of 0.8 to 1.25 (80%-125%).[23]

Bioequivalence trials are often conducted under standardized conditions in normal healthy adult volunteers unless safety considerations prohibit administering the drug to healthy individuals. Standardized conditions and normal healthy adult volunteers are preferred because of availability and lack of confounding factors in this population.[23] This procedure has been questioned in situations where the disease state along with comorbid diseases may have an effect on absorption. In these cases, studying the bioequivalence in patients with this clinical picture would probably yield more accurate results.

Single doses of the test and control drugs are administered, and blood or plasma levels of the drug are measured over time. Multidose studies are also conducted on occasion to establish bioequivalence at steady state. A crossover study design is used so that the subject serves as his own control, thus improving precision of results.[24]

When examining the results of bioequivalence studies, lack of statistical significance does not equate to bioequivalence.[24] This is a commonly encountered problem. The standards for a bioequivalency trial are completely different from a superiority trial. In a bioequivalence trial, a 10% difference between products would be equivalent, whereas, a 10% difference between the products in a superiority trial could easily be deemed as meaning that there is a difference. Even the null hypothesis is different, which reflects on the complexity of the bioequivalency study design. Practitioners should also note whether the acceptable age and weight range for the subjects are defined in the methods, and clinical parameters used to characterize a normal, healthy adult (e.g., physical examination observations, hematological evaluations) are described.[25] Subjects should be free of all drugs, including caffeine, nicotine, alcohol, and other recreational drugs, for at least 2 weeks prior to testing, because these factors can affect pharmacokinetic parameters. All subjects should receive the drug under the same conditions, and all blood levels should be taken at the same intervals, which should be based on the half-life of the drug. Bioequivalency testing may be performed in both fasting and fed states to assess the impact of food on bioavailability; however, food intake should be closely monitored and controlled. An important exclusion criteria frequently not specified is use of dietary supplements. Subjects should be free of all dietary supplements (botanical and nonbotanical), because many of these products can interact with products under bioequivalence review.

One of the most common errors in the use of bioavailability data is comparing two products based on data obtained from separate studies.[25] Different subject populations, study conditions, and assay methodologies are all reasons why comparisons of data from different studies are dangerous and can lead to false conclusions.[25] For example, a pharmacy and therapeutics committee may locate two generic products that each have individually shown bioequivalence to the brand product in two separate studies. A false conclusion can be made that both generic products are bioequivalent to each other. As another example, for some products, multiple assays are available for measuring serum levels. Using the same assay, results for the two drugs may demonstrate equivalence; however, if one assay type is used for the reference drug and another assay type is used for the test drug, the results may not demonstrate equivalence because the sensitivity and specificity of assays may be different. Finally, it is important to remember that data from healthy volunteers may not reflect the population for whom the medication is prescribed. This should be a consideration when evaluating bioequivalence studies in making formulary decisions.

For additional information, scientific and medical evaluations by the FDA are published in the FDA's Orange Book *Approved Drug Products with Therapeutic Equivalence Evaluations* and are also available on the FDA Web site at: http://www.accessdata.fda.gov/scripts/cder/ob/default.cfm.[23]

Bioequivalence studies represent an increasingly important part of the medical literature. When evaluating such trials for application in clinical practice, it is important to focus on the methods of the study. Specifically, the reader must determine if a crossover study design was used, if the assay was validated, and if consistent conditions were maintained to minimize subject variability (e.g., food intake, timing of blood levels, and nicotine use).

Appendix 5–1 contains a list of additional questions specific to bioequivalence studies. These specific questions are in addition to the standard questions used to evaluate other randomized clinical trials noted in Chapter 4 and using basic tools like the Ten Major Considerations Checklist discussed in the Introduction section.

PROGRAMMATIC RESEARCH

Another type of research important to the practice of pharmacy is focused on the impact and economic value of programs and services provided by pharmacists in community and institutional settings. Programmatic research is particularly important because limited resources and budget constraints demand that only those services that improve patient care in a cost-effective manner should be implemented. A diverse body of evidence in support of the economic benefit of pharmacists providing clinical pharmacy services has grown over the past decade.[26] The evidence includes contemporary practice sites and services. The study design and methodology has improved, in addition to economic, clinical, and humanistic outcomes assessed in many practice environments. Pharmacists, working in interdisciplinary settings with physicians and other health care providers, have demonstrated that they can improve drug therapy effectiveness and safety.[27] This study also showed that pharmacists enhanced the efficient delivery of health care as physician enhancers, applying their specific drug therapy knowledge, skills, and abilities to complement the other types of care provided by the collaborating professionals. The American College of Clinical Pharmacy (ACCP) has published a succession of position statements that review published literature regarding the value of clinical pharmacy services.[27,28] These position papers discuss strengths and limitations of existing literature, and include recommendations for further studies in order to facilitate continued documentation of value provided by pharmacists in progressive roles and settings, while utilizing methodology that ensures a high level of evidence-based rigor.

Appendix 5–1 contains a list of additional questions specific to programmatic research studies. These specific questions are in addition to the standard questions used to evaluate other randomized clinical trials noted in Chapter 4 and using basic tools like the Ten Major Considerations Checklist discussed in the Introduction section.

Observational Study Design

❷ *Observational study designs are used in specific situations such as when large populations of patients must be followed over extended periods of time. They can be prospective, retrospective, or a single snapshot (or slice) in time. Interpretation of results from these types of trials only allows associations to be formed, rather than true cause-and-effect relationships.* Observational study designs involve subject groups that are based on presence or absence of a disease or exposure with observations being made and recorded regarding patient characteristics. The observational study design seeks to evaluate questions based on less rigidly controlled practice conditions than those used in experimental study designs. Research questions are addressed by comparing outcomes or experiences of patients arising from naturally occurring assignment to different treatments, subject characteristics, or exposures.[28,29] For instance, if an agent is particularly toxic and of no therapeutic value, it would be unethical to ask subjects to voluntarily expose themselves to the agent;

thus an observational study design would be used.[30] An example of this type of situation is the evaluation of risk factors for diseases such as cancer. An investigator wishing to evaluate the toxicity of environmental or industrial hazards or the teratogenicity of drugs administered during pregnancy would have to employ epidemiologic research techniques such as cohort or case-control studies to study these problems. These research techniques allow associations rather than cause and effect relationships to be determined. Thus, when evaluating overall results of any observational study (cohort, case-control, cross-sectional, or case study), it is important to remember that a correlation or an association between exposure and outcome does not prove causation.[31] Other factors possibly related to both the exposure and outcome must be considered.

The following discussion will present observational study designs commonly encountered within health literature: the cohort, case-control, and cross-sectional designs. Differences between these study designs will be discussed and specific uses identified for each design. In addition, evaluation techniques for each will be discussed.

See Table 5–4 for differentiating factors between observational trial designs: cohort, case-control, and cross-sectional. In addition, see Table 5–3 for specific types of bias associated especially with observational studies. Note the suggested methods to control for bias and which types of observational studies are at highest risk for each bias discussed.

COHORT STUDIES

The term *cohort* is derived from the Latin word *cohors*, which means a group of soldiers.[32] In ancient Roman times, soldiers were assigned into one of 10 divisions of a legion where they remained over the duration of their service. This term is used today to describe a group of individuals with a common characteristic or experience.[33] That experience is often a specific exposure to a particular agent such as a vaccine, medication, procedure, or environmental toxin.[33] Participants in a cohort study are grouped by their exposure and followed over time to determine the incidence of symptoms, disease, or death.[33] Two

TABLE 5–4. CHARACTERISTICS OF OBSERVATIONAL STUDY DESIGNS

Observational Study Design	Prospective Data Collection	Retrospective Data Collection	Exposure Known at Beginning of Study	Outcome Known at Beginning of Study	Study Determines Exposure Status	Study Determines Outcome Occurrence
Cohort	X		X			X
Case-control (trohoc)		X		X	X	
Cross-sectional	X				X	X

groups are usually compared. Generally, these two groups are made up of those participants exposed and those non-exposed. Other terms for cohort are *follow-up*, *incidence*, and *longitudinal studies*. See Figure 5–3 for a schematic representation of this study design.

• There are three basic categories of cohort studies used based on timing of the events: prospective (looking forward in time), retrospective (looking back in time), and ambidirectional (looking both forward and backward in time).[33] The prospective cohort study, also known as concurrent because participants are monitored over time, groups the participants based on current or past exposure and then follows these groups over time, observing the various predetermined outcomes. In the prospective cohort design, outcomes have yet to develop and investigators are required to wait for their occurrence. For example, observing the long-term effects of lead exposure on cognitive function as children grow to be adults.

• Retrospective or historical cohort studies, also referred to as nonconcurrent since both the exposure and the outcome are already recorded in a database, uses computerized

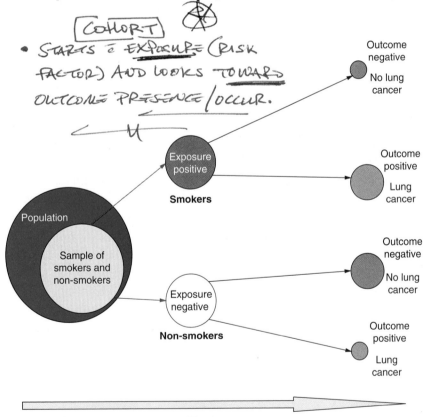

> COHORT
> • STARTS c̄ EXPOSURE (RISK
>   FACTOR) AND LOOKS TOWARD
>   OUTCOME PRESENCE/OCCUR.
>   ← H

Figure 5–3. Schematic diagram of a cohort study.

data on patients that has been recorded over the natural course of their health care.[34,35] For instance, information regarding the treatment received by individuals in 2000 is obtained from a database in 2010. In addition, the assessment of outcomes due to this treatment is known and recorded in this database by 2010. A computer database is searched for all patients that received medication or surgical treatment for a disease in 2000. Once identified, the investigators observe the assignment to study or control groups. The database is then searched to determine the outcomes occurring for each group from 2000 to 2010.

Finally, the ambidirectional cohort study involves both prospective and retrospective components.[33] An example of this type of cohort is the Air Force Health Study looking at pilots involved in aerial spraying of herbicides including Agent Orange during the Vietnam War. The retrospective portion of the study observed the incidence of cancer and mortality from time of exposure in the war through the 1980s while the prospective component involves observing these men well into the future.

Other terms describing cohort studies are based on the characteristics of the population that makes up the cohort, changes or no changes in the exposure over time, and existence of losses to follow-up.[33] Cohort studies where the participants may enter or leave based on changing characteristics, such as smoking, alcohol consumption, occupation, specific geographical location, are referred to as open or dynamic. For instance, participants are members of an open cohort group of Kansas City residents as long as they continue to live in Kansas City. A fixed cohort is identified by an unchangeable event such as having undergone a surgical procedure or been exposed to a potential toxin like Agent Orange at a specific time like the 1960s and place such as Vietnam. For this reason, exposures do not change or are considered fixed in this type of cohort. A third type of cohort is referred to as "closed." Similar to the fixed cohort, a closed cohort involves an unchangeable event. A closed cohort also has a specific starting and ending point that involves follow-up. For example, a closed cohort may be conducted with participants attending a high school football game to determine if the nachos and spicy cheese consumed at the game provided them discomfort such as gastritis throughout the remainder of the evening until morning.

Cohort study designs are primarily used to investigate the cause of a disease or the benefits and safety risks of both medication and procedures.[35] For instance, important information on the risks of cancer in individuals undergoing radiation therapy for noncancerous disease states has been identified. The cohort study is the simplest approach for studying disease incidence.[36] Key characteristics of each participant are determined prior to the study initiation and monitored during the follow-up period. From this information, important risk factors relating to the disease incidence are identified. In this way, risk factors are measured prospectively before the disease occurs. For example, cohort studies have been responsible for identifying the risk factors associated with cardiovascular disease such as high blood pressure, high blood cholesterol, physical inactivity, obesity, and smoking.

Primary disadvantages of cohort studies are expense and time consumption.[37] For example, a prospective study investigating the occurrence of rare outcomes such as the occurrence of aplastic anemia with clonazapine use is conducted. This type of study may require extremely large numbers of patients, take decades of data collection, and accrue large project costs to obtain answers. It takes many years for adequate assessment of disease development or to establish disease-free status.[32] Such research questions are investigated more efficiently with the retrospective case-control design.

The study hypothesis for a cohort study attempts to establish a relationship between an exposure or risk factor and a subsequent outcome.[35] A measurement such as relative risk is frequently used to determine the extent of this relationship. Relative risk is the risk of developing a disease or adverse event in those participants exposed to a specific variable compared to those not exposed to that variable[1,36]

$$\text{Relative Risk} = \frac{\text{Outcome or Adverse Event (treatment group)}}{\text{Outcome or Adverse Event (control group)}}$$

The relative risk values can be greater than, less than, or equal to one. For instance, if the relative risk calculated for a relationship between a specific drug exposure and cervical cancer is 5, this means that participants are five times more likely to contract cervical cancer when given the drug compared to those not being exposed to the drug. Other measurements such as attributable risk, number needed to treat, and life-table methods can be used to analyze the data from cohort studies.[35]

Relative risk gives an idea of the magnitude of an effect, but does not provide information about precision or statistical significance of the result.[38] Alternatively, calculation of confidence intervals (usually at a level of 95%) is utilized for evaluation of statistical significance of results. The confidence interval provides a range in which the true value for the population lies. The concept is that the wider the confidence interval, the greater the variability and therefore range that contains the true value. Because a relative risk of 1 indicates no difference exists between groups, the confidence interval cannot include 1 and still maintain statistical significance.

When critically evaluating a cohort study, the practitioner should be concerned with several points.[86] With a cohort study, there is no randomization process that occurs to ensure that each participant has an equal opportunity to be in either the exposed or non-exposed group. The investigator selects the group to which each participant is assigned for the duration of the study. Certainly, those who have been, are, or will be exposed are assigned to that group, as are those who never have or never will be exposed assigned to the non-exposed group. Unlike a randomized controlled trial where patients are anticipated to be similar in their demographic characteristics between groups due to the randomization schedule, a cohort study has no assurance of this similarity. For this reason, two concerns arise: selection bias and confounders.[8,39,40] Selection bias is a potential whenever the investigator is allowed to decide who is brought into the study and who is not selected to participate. This can result in differences within and/or between the groups that can have an impact on the final study results. For instance, an investigator either knowingly or unknowingly selects from the general population only the healthiest individuals to be assigned to the non-exposure group while at the same time a mixture of healthy and unhealthy participants are selected for the exposure group. With this scenario, there is an imbalance between groups that could set the exposed group up for an exaggerated negative effect to the exposure. When compared to the non-exposed group who were extremely healthy from the start of the study, this selection bias can produce an amplified difference that would not have been observed if both groups were balanced in regard to the initial healthiness of the participants. Simply stated, when a study starts out with dissimilar groups, the observed results at the study completion may be due to the exposure or due to the fact that the groups were different from the start. An example of selection bias would be a cohort study that shows dark chocolate increases participants' life span. Upon further examination of each group's characteristics, one can see that the participants exposed to dark chocolate were considerably healthier than the non-exposed group at the time of assignment to their respective groups.

A confounding factor or confounder is a variable related to one or more variables defined in the study.[41] These confounding factors can be known or unknown depending whether they have been discovered. Confounding factors are common in cohort studies since they are the product of not using a randomization schedule that evenly distributes the confounding factors between the exposure and non-exposure groups. For instance, in a cohort trial that is studying the effects of sleep deprivation on pharmacy students during their schooling, sleep deprivation is a defined variable (exposure), and various outcomes associated with sleep deprivation such as grades, interaction during lectures, and volunteer time provided to student organizations are other defined variables. An example of a confounder would be age. If there were a greater number of older students in the exposure group, the outcomes could be poorer since older students have established lives with families and possibly other activities competing for their time. These confounding factors could certainly have an effect on the outcome measures, but have nothing to do with sleep deprivation. Confounding factors can mask actual associations or falsely demonstrate an apparent association that actually does not exist between variables in a study.[39] In the example of sleep-deprived pharmacy students, time taken away from studying and volunteer work that results in a negative effect on grades and volunteer time for organizations could be due to other competing activities related with older age (confounding factor) of participants. With age as a confounding factor in this example, it is possible to see how this confounder falsely demonstrates an apparent association between sleep deprivation and negative outcomes. In other words, an association between sleep deprivation and poorer grades or less volunteer time can be made when in reality the difference in age between groups is the real cause of the negative outcomes. Whether the investigators have used a systematic process to identify known confounders should be identified. In addition, careful consideration can sometimes identify confounders not mentioned by the authors. This would be considered a limitation and should raise caution with regard to reliability of the results.

There are methods and techniques that can be used to assess, correct, control, or adjust for confounding variables.[40,41] One method is putting restrictions on the selection criteria.[40] If the investigators had recognized age as a potential confounding factor prior to initiating the pharmacy student sleep deprivation study described earlier, an age range restriction such as 20 to 25 years of age could have been incorporated into the selection criteria. By restricting the age to no greater than 25 years, the confounding factor of older age and the potential effects on the results are removed from the scenario. Other analytical strategies can be used on the data to increase confidence that confounding factors had no or minimal effects on the results.[42] One analytical technique is regression that uses the data to determine if confounders are related to the outcomes. If regression analysis determines confounders have affected the results, an adjusted estimate of the actual exposure effect of interest on the outcomes is provided. For example, if age was shown by regression analysis to have affected the outcomes in the pharmacy student study, an adjusted estimate of actual sleep deprivation without the confounder effect on the outcomes would be provided. Stratification is another analytical technique that creates subgroups which are more balanced regarding baseline participant characteristics than the entire study population. Confounders such as age are balanced between subgroups. For example, applying a stratification analysis to the sleep deprivation study would result in age being more balanced between subgroups. The overall effect of sleep deprivation is calculated from the difference in average outcomes between the exposure and non-exposure groups within each stratum. The result of stratification is less confounder effect on the results of the association between sleep deprivation and measured outcomes of pharmacy student grades, lecture interaction, and volunteer time. Whether the investigators have used any of these techniques should be identified. Use of the technique can determine if confounding factors played a significant role in the final results based on what these analysis strategies reveal.

Accurate measurement of the outcome is essential.[8] Surveillance bias is a potential problem when one group, generally the exposed group is more intensely monitored for changes in the outcome measure than the comparison group. Blinding the investigator responsible for performing the outcome measurement is one potential way of minimizing the chances for surveillance bias. Sources for acquiring the outcome data can vary. When this happens, the different sources can affect the results since one source can be more sensitive than others. For example, the details provided regarding follow-up can be significantly different when looking at medical chart versus nursing notes versus the actual interpretation of the radiology report by an expert. Making sure that the same source is used to obtain all measurements for both groups is crucial. Furthermore, information bias can occur if the same efforts to measure outcomes are not made for both the exposed and non-exposed groups.[32,39]

Adequate follow-up is important.[8,33] The practitioner must ensure that the length of follow-up was adequate for the outcome being measured. For instance, a three-month cohort study to determine risk factors associated with long-term cardiovascular events such as myocardial infarction is inadequate. Also, dropouts should be accounted for by the authors and assessed to determine if there were factors that caused a greater number in one group compared to the other. For instance, participants who are sicker in one group might drop out of the study due to death that is not associated with the risk factor being studied, but rather because they were more prone to death due to some other cause. Studies where loss to follow-up exceeds 20% in either the exposed or non-exposed cohort should be interpreted with caution.[32]

Appendix 5–1 contains a list of additional questions specific to cohort studies. These specific questions are in addition to the standard questions used to evaluate other randomized clinical trials noted in Chapter 4 and using basic tools like the Ten Major Considerations Checklist discussed in the Introduction section.

Case Study 5–2

■ PERTINENT BACKGROUND INFORMATION

A cohort study is published in *New England Journal of Medicine*. The study compares two similar groups of subjects in New York City, one exposed to drinking water from the tap and the other drinking water that has been purified and bottled. Subjects for the study were picked by the investigator based on a private interview. The results of the study showed that there was a greater incidence of illness associated with those patients receiving water directly from the tap. The investigator concluded that the tap water was causing these illnesses.

1. What would indicate that there is some potential for selection bias in this study?
2. What would be some of the potential confounding factors associated with this study?

3. What are some of the other characteristics of a cohort study that should be evaluated?

4. What cause-effect relationship can be established with this study?

CASE-CONTROLLED STUDIES

Case-control studies (also termed "case-referent," "case history," or "retrospective studies") are a type of observational study that offers an epidemiologic research alternative to cohort studies. The latter requires a large number of subjects, and is often expensive and time-consuming.[31] Case-control studies seek to retrospectively identify potential risk factors of diseases or outcomes. In a case-control study, subjects (cases) with a particular characteristic or outcome of interest (e.g., disease) are recruited, matched with, and compared to a similar group of subjects (controls) who have not experienced the characteristic or outcome.[31,42,43] Data regarding exposures are collected retrospectively via patient interviews or by reviewing subject data records, and the two groups are compared to identify possible risk factors or contributors for development of the disease or outcome of interest. Of note, not only is the outcome of interest known at the beginning of the study, but also which subjects (cases) the outcome occurs in are also known. This is a key differentiating factor for case-control versus cohort study design. See Figure 5–4 for a schematic of the case-control study design.

Case-control studies can be more useful than cohort studies when diseases have a rare prevalence or when many years of exposure to the risk factor is required.[27,32,43] Case-control studies are always conducted in a retrospective design compared to randomized clinical trials and cohort studies, which are usually performed in a prospective manner and that is why case-control studies are sometimes called trohoc studies (i.e., cohort spelled backward).[43]

Exposure of study subjects to the risk factor should reflect what occurs in the general population. If subjects with higher or lower exposure rates to the risk factor are excluded from the study, determination of possible associations between the exposure and a particular disease may be biased and inaccurate.[43] For example, case-controls often use subjects drawn from hospitalized populations, whose risk factor exposure may differ from individuals in the community, a problem termed Berkson bias.[43] See Table 5–3, which presents this and other types of bias that may be found within observational study designs, along with methods that provide control of potential biasing factors.

Predisposition to the disease of interest should be similar in both cases and controls, except for exposure to the risk factor under investigation; however, this is extremely

[handwritten: CASE CONTROL]

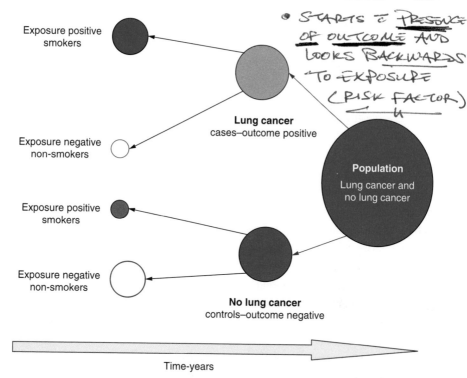

[handwritten annotations to the right of figure:]
- STARTS c̄ PRESENCE OF OUTCOME AND LOOKS BACKWARDS TO EXPOSURE (RISK FACTOR)

Figure 5–4. Schematic diagram of a case-control study.

difficult to ensure.[39,44,45] Matching is often used to ensure that cases and controls are similar. With matching, each case has a comparable control or controls in terms of demographic and exposure characteristics. At the beginning of the study in Figure 5–4, patients with lung cancer and those without have matching demographics and exposure characteristics. Often it is difficult to determine which variables should be used to match cases to controls (e.g., sex, age, and date of admission). Matching allows assessment of only the risk factor under investigation such as smoking. No other variables that may have contributed to the disease such as indirect sampling are taken into consideration.[43,44,46] Matching may even result in a negative impact on the interpretation of study results if cases and controls are matched for a factor that is itself related to exposure.[32] Using the example, this type of situation could exist if the patients were required to have a family background of smokers. The result is both groups being exposed to indirect smoking in the past that may contribute to the development of lung cancer.

Cases and controls should undergo the same diagnostic evaluation to determine presence or absence of the disease under investigation (e.g., chest x-ray and bronchoscopy for definitive diagnosis of lung cancer), because detection of a disease is more likely to be found in individuals who undergo extensive diagnostic testing.[45] In addition, individuals administering the tests should be blinded to the presence or absence of the risk factor to eliminate diagnostic-review bias.[43,45] This blinding can be achieved if the x-rays and bronchoscopies are reviewed and interpreted by an independent, non-investigator who is unaware of the study protocol details. A problem is that many diagnostic tests can only be performed in individuals suspected of having a particular disease state due to risks associated with their use. This would be the situation with bronchoscopies due to the invasiveness of the test, therefore leaving only chest x-ray and trust in the physician that made the final diagnosis in the medical records.

Case-control study designs have both benefits and disadvantages. These studies are relatively inexpensive and can be completed in a shorter timeframe than cohorts.[47] Both of these advantages are related to how subjects are recruited and data are acquired. When rare events are studied prospectively in a cohort design, recruitment of large numbers of patients is required due to the uncertainty of events occurring during the study period and the resulting need to ensure study power. In contrast, case-control studies reduce the need for large sample sizes, as subjects are recruited based on *a priori* knowledge of occurrence of outcomes as stated in the medical records.

Several points should be considered when evaluating these types of trials. Most limitations inherent to case-control studies are due to the retrospective design.[44] Overall, the two major methodological issues include appropriate selection of controls and accurate determination of the level of exposure.[39] Historical data used in case-control studies that is obtained from medical records may be inaccurate or incomplete.[43,44,46] When patients are interviewed regarding historical events, equal distribution of patients' ability to recall events that have happened in the past between the two groups may not be ensured.[45] For example, patients with lung cancer may be more likely to recall events preceding development of the disease than patients who are healthy. Patients with disease have probably contemplated factors they believe may have contributed to disease development (recall bias). For this reason, there should be some explanation in the study addressing the issue of recall bias. Unblinded investigators who collect data also may question individuals exposed to the disease more intensely than control subjects. To reduce variation in data obtained from cases and controls, data collectors should be blinded to the status of the subjects as cases or controls (lung cancer or no lung cancer).[43]

Another prominent disadvantage is that information about the exposure and outcome is collected simultaneously, so it is difficult to sort out the temporal relationship between the two.[39] For instance, it is often difficult to determine if the outcome preceded the exposure, a situation termed "protopathic bias," where the disease may lead to risk factor exposure rather than vice versa.[39,45] Consider the following illustration. Abnormal vaginal bleeding may be an early sign of uterine cancer. Vaginal bleeding, however, may lead to prescribing hormonal therapies such as progesterone. An investigator may later erroneously

TABLE 5–5. CASE-CONTROL STUDY—DETERMINATION OF ODDS RATIOS IN INDUSTRIAL FORMALDEHYDE EXPOSURE IN PATIENTS WITH RESPIRATORY ILLNESS

Risk Factor	Respiratory Illness	No Respiratory Illness	Total
Formaldehyde exposure	20	5	25
No industrial exposure to formaldehyde	180	195	375
Total	200	200	400

conclude that use of progesterone was associated with development of uterine cancer, when in fact the cancer preceded use of the progesterone in this case.[45]

Some experts have suggested use of several control groups selected on the basis of different criteria in an attempt to reduce some of the biases discussed above.[43] A well-designed case-control study may have multiple controls for each case. If results of comparing cases to the various control groups are in agreement with one another, bias in the control groups is less likely to be present.[43]

Odds ratios are used to help interpret the results from case-control studies. Odds ratio is an estimate of relative risk.[31] Although relative risk is preferred for prospective trials, the odds ratio is the measure of choice for retrospective studies.[8] Consider the situation presented in Table 5–5, where industrial exposure to formaldehyde in patients with and without respiratory illness is assessed. Odds of exposure to formaldehyde is 20/180 (0.11) in the cases with respiratory illness and 2/195 (0.01) in the controls. The odds ratio is calculated as 0.11/0.01 (11), which approximates the relative risk determined in the cohort study example. Interpretation is the same; greater than one denotes increased risk, equal to one indicates no effect, and less than one indicates a protective effect. As with cohort studies, 95% confidence intervals should be calculated.[48] Confidence intervals are preferred because they provide some indication of precision and variability of the individual participant's outcome. A narrow confidence interval suggests precision and less variability of the individual outcome measures. The wider the confidence interval, the more variability observed between outcome measurements that make up the mean.

Appendix 5–1 contains a list of additional questions specific to case-control studies. These specific questions are in addition to the standard questions used to evaluate other randomized clinical trials noted in Chapter 4 and using basic tools like the Ten Major Considerations Checklist discussed in the Introduction section.

CROSS-SECTIONAL STUDIES

Cross-sectional studies or prevalence surveys can be thought of as a snapshot (or slice) of time because data are collected and evaluated at a single point in time.[49] This type of study design is hypothesis generating as opposed to hypothesis testing, and is not suited for testing the effectiveness of interventions.[39] Only an association can be drawn from the results, not a cause-effect relationship. Typical examples of cross-sectional studies are surveys that evaluate opinions or situations at a fixed point in time. For a hypothetical situation concerning a drug, a cross-sectional study design could be developed to look into a large insurance database and determine how many people died suddenly within five years of receiving that drug. Cross-sectional studies are relatively quick and easy to perform and may be useful for measuring current health status or setting priorities for disease control.[39]

A study is classified as cross-sectional because measurements are taken at a single point in time, even though observations may cover a period of several months or years. For example, a survey of smokers is cross-sectional when the questionnaire is administered once, even though the questions contained in the survey may focus on smoking habits over the past 10 years.

As in other observational trial designs, the research question and the relevant inclusion and exclusion criteria must be clearly and unambiguously stated.[39] Also, selection of cases must be clearly described.[32]

Problems that may occur during cross-sectional studies include errors in data collection and transient effects that may influence observations. Because measurements occur at only one point in time, inaccuracies in data collection may go unnoticed because there are no prior data for comparison. In studies where multiple observations occur, data collection errors, seen as outlier data, may be more easily recognized. For instance, the prevalence of a disease state may be recorded in 2007 as 15% of the United States population. However, if looking at the same statistics for 2006, 2008, and 2009 it is possible to see the prevalence was 2.1%, 2.2%, and 2.0%, respectively. Obviously, the 2007 prevalence of 15% is quite different from the prevalence 1 year before and the next 2 years after this observation. The 2007 observation would be considered a data outlier that probably represents a data collection error. The problem is, taken as a single observation without the other years, the 2007 prevalence would appear accurate and not recognized as an error in data collection. Transient effects are temporary occurrences that are found at the time a cross-sectional study is conducted, but are not identified if the study were repeated. A good example of transient effects is student evaluations of university professors. If a professor chooses to have students evaluate a course after a particularly grueling examination, chances are the evaluations would be poor based on students' response to the examination just taken. However, if the evaluations were administered after a curve had been applied for final grades, students may reflect on the course positively based on the overall knowledge they received from the instructor, rather than a single negative experience. Transient effects are difficult to identify by a study evaluator. They may only be uncovered through retrospective evaluation of the study by the investigator. The investigator must perform a thorough assessment of all factors that may have impacted the results of the trial.

Appendix 5-1 contains a list of additional questions specific to cross-sectional studies. These specific questions are in addition to the standard questions used to evaluate other randomized clinical trials noted in Chapter 4 and using basic tools like the Ten Major Considerations Checklist discussed in the Introduction section.

Reports Without Control Group

CASE STUDIES, CASE REPORTS, AND CASE SERIES

● ❸ *Reports describing observations made regarding a patient or patient group exposure to a drug or technology can be valuable to record preliminary findings that will lead to further study. A key characteristic to these reports is the lack of a control or comparison group. These observational or interventional reports are referred to as "case studies," "case reports," or "case series."* Because these reports lack comparison to a control group, they do not take into consideration other influencing factors that may also have played a role in observed outcomes. In contrast to N-of-1 trials, a case study (either interventional or observational) does not apply clinical trial principles such as randomization and blinding to individual patients. The case study can be prospective or retrospective whereas the N-of-1 trial design is prospective. The case study usually does not involve multiple treatment periods like that seen with N-of-1 trials. Comparisons of single-patient clinical trials (N-of-1) and case studies are presented in Table 5-2.[50]

● Interpretation of case studies can be difficult.[51] Design and methods describing conduct of a case study are not well defined.[52] For example, beneficial effects attributed to a drug or treatment under investigation may actually be a function of spontaneous regression of signs and symptoms of the disease, a placebo effect, and/or related to physicians' attitudes that may influence patient outcome.[52]

● Case studies, however, are an integral part of the biomedical literature. They have played an important role in identifying treatments for rare disorders where large subject pools cannot be identified.[52] Case studies, reports, or series may also be useful for early recognition of drug toxicities and teratogenicity. A newly recognized value of case reports is utilization for understanding potential toxicities of dietary supplement products (botanical and nonbotanical). Because the FDA does not regulate these products and adverse event reporting is scarce, often safety information is not well-defined for these products. Thus, published case reports may play a somewhat larger role for dietary supplements in suggesting potential safety problems than for traditional drug products.

When possible, results of case studies, reports, or series should be confirmed with randomized controlled clinical trials. Case studies, reports, and series serve as an important initial step in the formulation of hypotheses.[53] When case studies, reports, or series show a beneficial effect of a drug or treatment in diseases whose outcomes are consistently grim, or when all other treatments have failed, the results can be applied to patients in clinical practice.[53]

Appendix 5–1 contains a list of additional questions specific to case studies, reports, and series. These specific questions are in addition to the standard questions used to evaluate other randomized clinical trials noted in Chapter 4 and using basic tools like the Ten Major Considerations Checklist discussed in the Introduction section.

Survey Research

❹ *Survey research is commonly used and represents information gathered from an identified group from which conclusions are drawn and applied to a larger population. This gathered information is considered either descriptive (such as opinions and attitudes) or explanatory (such as explaining a cause and effect) in nature. Validity of the results depends on the quality of the study's internal rigor.* Survey research is used to study the incidence, distribution, and relationships of sociologic and psychological variables.[53] It is used to collect information from a sample and generalize the findings to a larger, target population.[54] Data obtained from survey research have been used for many purposes including helping investigators identify, assess, and compare respondents' ideas, feelings, plans, beliefs, and demographics.[55] In pharmacy practice, surveys may be used to determine how programs should be implemented by utilizing the opinions of experts with experience in a particular area, to study effectiveness of a program by questioning individuals who have used its services, or to understand attitudes and behaviors of patients or members of the profession. For example, directors of pharmacy may survey other hospitals to determine salary ranges in order to decide whether salary increases are needed to remain competitive in the job market. The ability to critically evaluate such literature has become a necessity for the practicing pharmacist due to an increased emphasis on this type of research in the medical literature.[55]

There are two basic types of surveys published in the biomedical literature. Descriptive surveys attempt to identify psychosocial variables such as attitudes, opinions, knowledge, and behaviors in a population, while explanatory surveys attempt to explain causal relationships between variables.[55] These dependent variables such as knowledge and behavior are often compared to independent variables such as age, sex, or education.[56]

Several types of data are collected in survey research and include incidence, attitudinal, knowledge, and behavior measurements. Incidence data try to determine the occurrence of events without drawing any relationships between variables.[57] An example of incidence data is the morbidity or mortality data reported weekly in the Centers for Disease Control and Prevention's Morbidity and Mortality Weekly Report (http://www.cdc.gov/mmwr). Manpower data are also incidence data frequently reported in pharmacy literature.[57] The number of residency-trained specialists in drug information centers is an example of data that might be collected in a nationwide manpower survey. Attitudinal data such as job satisfaction surveys often try to compare this dependent variable with independent variables such as age, education, or salary. Knowledge data attempt to document a person's knowledge or level of understanding about a specific topic. Examples include surveys asking physicians' knowledge of retail prices of medications or pharmacists' knowledge of state pharmacy laws.[57] Behavior data documents what a person actually does in a particular situation rather than asking him or her in a survey, which may reflect an attitude rather than the actual observed behavior. Observing the number of specific points that a pharmacist addresses during patient education sessions is an example of behavior data.[57]

Data collection for surveys may involve questionnaires, examination of historical records, telephone interviews, face-to-face interviews, Web-based questionnaires, or panel interviews.[57] Well-conducted surveys have several important characteristics—they are objective and carefully planned, data are quantifiable, and subjects surveyed are representative of the target population.[58] In evaluating survey research, just like any other research, one must ask if the results are reliable and valid, and if they can be generalized.[55]

Four sources of error have been described that can threaten the precision and accuracy (i.e., reliability) of survey results, and must be evaluated by readers.[55] The first type of error, coverage error (sampling bias), occurs when there is a discrepancy between the target population and the population from which the sample was derived. This type of error can compromise the ability to generalize study results.[55] For example, people without telephones or those with unlisted numbers would be excluded from a sample frame of names from a telephone directory. In the case of a Web-based survey of a target population that includes urban and rural areas, those persons without a computer or e-mail address would be excluded from the list of e-mail addresses provided for the survey.

Sampling error (or random error) occurs when the researcher surveys only a subset (sample) of all possible subjects within the population of interest.[55] The use of random sampling procedures and larger sample sizes can be used to minimize sampling error. *Sampling error* is a statistical term that describes the rate of random error in sample selection. This error describes variation around the true value of the population mean seen when multiple samples are pulled from the same population.[58] Sample error is reported usually as the mean ±1 standard error from the mean, which is known as standard error of the mean (SEM).

• Measurement error (response bias) occurs when the collection of data is influenced by the interviewer or when the survey item itself is unclear from the respondent's point of view. When measurement error occurs, a subject's response cannot be compared to other responses.[55] The survey method used to collect the data may be one source of measurement error. Face-to-face interviewers may influence the responses of the person being surveyed. The survey instrument itself may be ambiguous and open to interpretation. Bias can be introduced into a survey by the cover letter or sponsoring body; either may lead the respondent to one desired response rather than measuring the true response.

• A fourth type of measurement error occurs when a respondent replies with a preferred or more socially acceptable answer rather than the real answer. A well-designed survey instrument can minimize the chances of this type of error occurring. The well-designed survey instrument takes into account the abilities and motivation of the respondent to respond correctly (i.e., written at an appropriate educational level). Parallel forms (usually consisting of alternatively worded items placed throughout the survey) of either specific survey items or the entire survey instrument have been used to increase reliability of survey research. The use of such forms requires the calculation of correlation coefficients between the parallel items and survey instruments.

Accurate assessment of measurement error relies on the availability of the questionnaire or tool used to collect data so that readers may analyze wording. Unfortunately, many articles relating results of survey research do not include the actual questionnaire used in the survey due to space and ownership issues. Lengthy questionnaires take up valuable journal space, and the publisher may decide not to include them. Some authors do not want to give away the intellectual work that they invested in developing a good questionnaire and decide not to publish it. These factors make it impossible for the reader to evaluate the wording and, thus, the objectivity of questions or quality of the survey instrument.

Finally, nonresponse error (nonresponse bias) occurs when a significant number of subjects in a sample do not respond to the survey. If the responder's demographics, characteristics, or responses differ significantly from the nonresponders in a way that influences the results, then nonresponse error would be suspect.[55] Unfortunately, this error is difficult to assess since the nonresponder's answers are never known. One way researchers attempt to minimize the chances of this error is to strive for response rates in the 80% to 90% range. This level of response rate provides some assurance that the small number of nonresponders will not alter results and therefore, the author's conclusions.[57] Other authors argue that response rates of 80% for face-to-face interviews, 70% for telephone interviews, and 50% for mailed questionnaires are acceptable.[56]

In order to accurately assess the survey's validity (i.e., robustness) and evaluate these potential sources of error and bias, the Methods section, which must be explicit, should be heavily scrutinized. Foremost, a description of study methodology with enough detail to replicate the study should be provided. Additionally, the Methods section should relate each type of error associated with survey research and state how investigators attempted to control those errors.[59]

Attempts to assess validity and reliability of the survey and efforts made to validate factual data should be described. For example, demographics of individual hospitals can be verified using American Hospital Association data. Asking more than one question about a concept can increase the internal validity of a survey.[55] For example, a respondent who answers yes to a positively worded statement would be expected to answer no to the same concept when worded in a negative fashion. A coefficient alpha (or similar statistical test) that measures correlation between items should be calculated and reported in the article if this technique is used.[55] The coefficient alpha is interpreted in the same fashion that coefficients of reliability are interpreted, (i.e., 0 indicates no consistency between responses while increasing consistency is seen as you approach 1).

The Methods section should report sample size, along with a description of how it was determined. The validity of both survey research and clinical trials relies on sample size. In order to have sufficient statistical power to demonstrate a difference between two groups, studies must have an adequate sample size. In designing survey research, the population of interest is first determined, and then subdivided into smaller groups around a variable of interest. For example, the population of interest may be all patients who attend a pharmacist-managed asthma clinic. This population could be subdivided into smaller groups based on the severity of asthma and then surveyed as to level of customer satisfaction. In establishing sample size for survey research, investigators must then determine the minimum number of subjects that must be sampled for the sample to be representative of the entire population.[59] This determination is made by consulting references that describe variability in sampling.

Additionally, the reader should evaluate the comprehensiveness, probability of selection, and efficiency of the sample frame. A sample frame describes the population that will actually be drawn from to make up the survey sample. A sample is comprehensive if all members of a population had a chance to be chosen and no one was systematically excluded.[59] Determining efficiency of a sample relates to how well the sample frame excluded individuals who are not the subject of the survey. For example, to survey elderly people, it is appropriate to survey all households to determine if elderly individuals live there.[59] In addition to providing information about the sampling frame, the Methods section should provide a description of interviewers (age, sex, ethnicity, and so forth) and the effect interviewers may have had on the data.

Sampling strategy and response rates should also be stated. The Methods section should supply the reader with enough information to ensure that nonresponse error was assessed and measures were taken to control the error.[55] Repeated attempts to obtain completed questionnaires from initial nonrespondents will yield higher response rates and more accurate results than if no follow-ups are performed.[59] For example, attempts at other times of the day should be made for phone surveys and a second reminder postcard should be sent for mailed surveys. For Web-based surveys, e-mail reminders serve as follow-ups. Additionally, one way to minimize the problem of poor response rates is to sample (by phone) a small group of non-responders to determine if their responses differ substantially from responders, although this may not be possible.[58] If results do not differ, the survey remains valid. Furthermore, authors should relate as much information about nonrespondents as possible. Although survey result information has not been gathered, authors may have demographic and geographic data based on addresses and other information originally obtained.

The Methods section should also describe techniques used to assess the reliability (i.e., can the results of the survey be repeated by another investigator?) of the survey instrument and present the results of reliability estimates.[55] In general, the higher the reliability estimate, the more confidence the reader may place in the results published. A more complete review of reliability coefficients is presented later (see Chapter 8). Additionally, any relevant elements of the survey research administration process (i.e., whether a pretest or pilot test was used) should be described. A pretest or pilot test is an assessment of a questionnaire made before full-scale implementation to identify and correct problems such as faulty questions, flawed response options, or interviewer training deficiencies.[60] Subjects administered the pretest not only answer the survey questions, but also answer questions about the clarity, length, and ease of understanding the actual instrument and may contribute other questions that should be included.[56]

Of note, informed consent is generally not required in survey research as the risk is minimal and the respondent has the opportunity to withdraw from participating every time a new question is asked.[59] However, it is wise to check with the institution's investigational review board (IRB) before initiating a survey study to confirm the need for informed consent. If the respondent does withdraw partway through the survey or interview, the data should not be included in the final analysis. In situations where sensitive information might potentially harm the subject, asking for an informed consent document to be signed allows the researchers the opportunity to reassure their commitment to confidentiality and reinforce the limits of how the data can be used.

Surveys are a commonly used research tool and are capable of providing a wealth of information on many aspects of a given target population. Ensuring validity of information gained through survey research, however, relies on critical evaluation of results through a thorough assessment of the study's internal rigor.[55] The ability to evaluate such research results is highly dependent on the amount and quality of information presented in the Methods section.

Appendix 5–1 contains a list of additional questions specific to survey research studies. These specific questions are in addition to the standard questions used to evaluate other randomized clinical trials noted in Chapter 4 and using basic tools like the Ten Major Considerations Checklist discussed in the Introduction section.

Postmarketing Surveillance Studies

Prior to approval by the FDA, drugs undergo testing in a limited number of patients. Once approved, experience in patients escalates, and previously unrecognized rare adverse events may be identified. The drug also may be found to be useful for conditions not described in the product labeling.

Postmarketing surveillance studies are phase IV studies that follow drug use after market approval and are sometimes referred to as pharmacoepidemiologic studies. They are useful in identifying new, potentially serious effects of drugs. A number of drugs have been removed from the market after approval following identification of such problems (e.g., fenfluramine, rofecoxib [Vioxx], valdecoxib [Bextra], and more recently, hydromorphone hydrochloride extended-release capsules [Palladone Extended-Release]). Postmarketing surveillance studies also allow assessment of drug use outside of product labeling and may identify areas for further research.

Many types of study designs are used in phase IV studies, including cross-sectional, case-control, cohort, and randomized, controlled clinical trials. These studies can answer questions about drug interactions, identify potential new indications for the product, and gather information about the consequences of overdose. In addition, the studies can provide efficacy in a larger and broader population (patients with different disease states and demographics that may not have been fully evaluated in the original clinical trials).[60]

Perhaps one of the most important functions of postmarketing surveillance is in the area of adverse-event reporting. Currently, most of the information on postmarketing safety of the product comes from spontaneous adverse-reaction reports. Reports of events associated with a product by the health care practitioner to a regulatory agency or the pharmaceutical company that markets the product are the primary means for gathering this information. Each pharmaceutical company is required to maintain a database of these spontaneous reports. This database is monitored for increases in frequency of certain events or the appearance of serious unexpected events. If it is determined that there is a causal relationship between the drug and event, the product labeling may be changed to reflect either new events or events with increasing frequency. For more information about this topic see Chapter 15.

There are several limitations to this type of data collection. The information is taken from the reporter, who must make a diagnosis and assessment of causality. Data may be underreported because it is a voluntary system, and this may bias the estimation of incidence. Reports may vary in quality or thoroughness, and the database may not be suitable for detecting adverse reactions with high background rates in the population.[61] See Chapter 15 for additional information.

The principles of literature evaluation described in previous sections are also applicable to these studies. The method used to evaluate the study is dependent upon the type of information collected. The reader is directed to the specific section of this chapter or book for the exact method to evaluate the study.

Appendix 5–1 contains a list of additional questions specific to postmarketing surveillance studies. These specific questions are in addition to the standard questions used to evaluate other randomized clinical trials noted in Chapter 4 and using basic tools like the Ten Major Considerations Checklist discussed in the Introduction section.

Review Articles

⑤ *Reviews provide support for clinical decisions when large, well-conducted trials are lacking. Meta-analyses are the only type of review that provides new quantitative data. This new data is derived from combining the results of each study included in the meta-analysis and performing a statistical analysis on that data set. The overall reliability of conclusions stemming from a meta-analysis is ultimately dependent upon the quality of the individual studies and homogeneity between these studies involved in the analysis.* Once a reader understands differences between individual study designs and characteristics for evaluating strengths and weaknesses within individual studies, it will become easier to analyze differences between publications that attempt to combine results from multiple studies.

Review articles consist of three very different entities—the narrative or nonsystematic review (qualitative review), the systematic review (qualitative review), and the meta-analysis (quantitative review). Reviews are becoming more common in the literature and are relied on as an efficient method for keeping up with the large amount of information presented to the health care professional each day.

Review articles, with the exception of meta-analyses, that essentially consist of analysis and interpretation of previously conducted research studies, are classified as tertiary literature, although they are often used as secondary sources because they can lead readers to primary literature references. Meta-analyses are classified as primary literature since they create new data. Review articles discussing treatment of disease states or clinical aspects of drug therapy enable practitioners to gain insight into a topic or question of interest and may provide more current information than textbooks.

Although the purpose of review articles is to present the truth found among conflicting and variable primary literature, this does not always occur. Reviews may be subject to author biases or inaccuracies in the literature search.[61] Narrative (nonsystematic) literature reviews generally do not apply systematic methods, such as formal criteria for selection of studies, and they address broad rather than focused clinical questions. In addition, they provide qualitative rather than quantitative information. They often educate readers about the author's interpretations of selected evidence, rather than using a systematic approach to evidence evaluation. Frequently, authors are experts on the topic and know the conclusions prior to conducting the review.

In contrast, systematic reviews do use formal criteria for trial selection and interpretation of study results, and authors determine the conclusions based on the data reviewed. These reviews provide qualitative information that is of a higher quality than narrative reviews because a systematic approach was utilized. Meta-analyses (sometimes referred to as quantitative systematic reviews) differ from both narrative and systematic reviews in that they provide new data that is quantitative in nature. Due to increased emphasis on evidence-based practice, narrative reviews have largely been replaced by both systematic reviews and meta-analyses as a source of authoritative, summative information.

It is important to note that it is not uncommon to find conclusions of general overviews, systematic reviews, or meta-analyses conflict with one another.[62,63] Differences in research methodology may explain conflicting conclusions noted in selected published studies. Other explanations for conflicting conclusions include differences in study populations, type of intervention, or study endpoint, as well as chance or confounding issues.[64] In some cases, the amount of high-quality data may not be sufficient to come to a valid conclusion; in others, clinical judgment of authors may place more weight on certain findings over other results. Readers of review articles need to determine whether studies included in the review are broad enough to apply to their clinical situation.

NARRATIVE (NONSYSTEMATIC) REVIEW: QUALITATIVE

A narrative (nonsystematic) review is a summary of research that lacks a description of systematic methods. Narrative reviews are considered tertiary literature because they provide information in much the same manner as found in textbooks, but are sometimes used like secondary references because they also contain extensive and up-to-date bibliographies. Narrative reviews may pertain to one specific clinical question or disease state, or to topics related to pharmacy administration (e.g., pharmacy and therapeutics committees).

Appendix 5–1 contains a list questions specific to narrative reviews that can be used to evaluate the quality of these reviews. These specific questions are in addition to the standard questions used to evaluate other randomized clinical trials noted in Chapter 4 and using basic tools like the Ten Major Considerations Checklist discussed in the Introduction section. Such evaluative questions are necessary, considering the poor quality of many published narrative reviews.[62] As a specific example of shortcomings of narrative reviews, Joyce and associates[64] found that citation of the literature is influenced by the review authors' discipline and nationality. For example, infectious disease specialists reviewing a disease state were more likely to cite laboratory literature than psychiatrists reviewing the same disease state. The reverse was true for neuropsychiatry literature; a review author in the United Kingdom was more likely to cite articles that originate in the United Kingdom than in other countries. This study also found that, of 89 reviews, only three (3.4%) described the methods used in the literature search. Legitimate differences in authors' clinical judgment can also affect results. For example, if a treatment has been shown to be effective and has a 7% incidence of a fairly severe adverse event, some authors will feel this is an acceptable risk compared to risks of the disease state, while others will deem that level of risk unacceptable.

SYSTEMATIC REVIEW: QUALITATIVE

If the purpose of nonsystematic reviews is to find the truth, then the purpose of the systematic review is finding the whole truth.[65] Cook and associates describe systematic reviews as scientific investigations with predefined methods and original studies as their subjects.[66] Two general types of systematic reviews exist. The term *systematic review* has been applied to a summary of results of primary studies where the results are not statistically combined.[67] In contrast, a quantitative systematic review, or meta-analysis, has been described as a systematic review that uses statistical methods to combine the results of two or more studies. Perhaps, more appropriately, meta-analyses can be thought of as a specific methodological and statistical technique (or tool) for combining quantitative data that generates new data. Table 5–6 illustrates the primary differences between narrative reviews—qualitative, systematic reviews—qualitative, and meta-analyses—quantitative reviews.[67]

Systematic overviews that summarize scientific evidence (in contrast to nonsystematic narrative reviews that mix opinions and evidence) are becoming increasingly prevalent. These overviews address questions of treatment, causation, diagnosis, or prognosis and are considered superior to nonsystematic (narrative) reviews of any given topic.[63]

Systematic reviews should concentrate on a clearly defined issue that is of importance to practice.[63,64] Specific criteria should be used to select articles from the primary literature to be included in the review.[63] For valid conclusions to be derived from systematic reviews, authors must clearly define the study population or topic of interest and include only those studies using valid research methods.[63] For example, authors would have the choice of assessing patients who are either pre- or postmenopausal in a systematic review focused on the utility of chemotherapy in improving survival following mastectomy in breast cancer patients. Conclusions of this systematic review are likely to be very different depending on which subsets of breast cancer patients are selected. In addition, the authors' initial literature search would probably reveal a collection of studies that use a wide variety of research techniques. Only those studies meeting strict criteria for validity as discussed in Chapter 4 should be included in the review. To produce the most reliable results, poorly controlled, nonrandomized, unblinded studies should be excluded.

TABLE 5–6.   **COMPARISON OF DIFFERENT TYPES OF REVIEWS**

Feature	Nonsystematic Review	Qualitative Systematic Review	Quantitative Systematic Review
Clinical question	Often broadly defined	Clearly defined and focused	Clearly defined and focused
Literature search	Methods of literature search usually not explicitly described	Explicit description of predefined and comprehensive search strategy	Explicit description of predefined and comprehensive search strategy
Studies included	Methods for determining which studies to include not usually described	Predefined inclusion and exclusion criteria	Predefined inclusion and exclusion criteria
Includes unpublished literature	Not usually	Possibly	Possibly
Blinding of reviewers	No	Yes	Yes
Analysis of data	Variable and subjective	Rigorous and objective	Rigorous and objective
Results statistically evaluated	No	No	Yes
Types of results	Qualitative	Qualitative	Quantitative

Source: Adapted from Cook DJ et al.[65] and Bryant PJ et al.[1] Copyright 2009, American Society of Health-System Pharmacists. Used with permission.

Authors should use a variety of resources to identify studies for the systematic review. Use of a single database is not likely to capture all relevant studies and results in reference bias. A combination of databases (such as MEDLINE, PubMed, Iowa Drug Information Service, International Pharmaceutical Abstracts, and EMBASE for literature published outside the United States), study bibliographies, and experts in the field should be used to identify studies for evaluation.[63,64]

Consideration should be given to inclusion of unpublished data (e.g., data on file at the manufacturer or personal communication with investigators) in addition to published studies, because it has been determined that published studies are more often of a positive nature than unpublished studies, a situation termed publication bias.[63] Researchers are now required to register their studies and provide data to an FDA Web site (http://www.clinicaltrials.gov): this is a good site to find unpublished studies ongoing or completed. Unfortunately, this Web site only provides summative information, so the quality of the evidence often cannot be determined. The benefit of using unpublished studies is to include more data from which to draw a conclusion. A drawback is that unpublished studies have likely not undergone a peer-review and revision process; errors and unclearly stated conclusions may be present. Language bias, in which only articles published in the author's primary language are used, may also affect results. In order to reduce selection bias, review authors choosing articles should be blinded to (1) names of the study authors (to avoid political or personal issues), (2) institution of publication, and (3) results of the studies. For the initial choice of study inclusion, only the Methods section should be reviewed.[67,68] In addition, because of the subjective nature of some aspects of analysis, two or more authors should critique each study under consideration, and all evaluators should concur on which studies will be included in the systematic review.[63]

A systematic review article should provide a table that summarizes the results from each study included in the review.[63] Outcomes described in the systematic review article should be meaningful, and, if the trial is a clinical trial, clinically relevant.[63] For example, improved survival rate is a more desirable endpoint than reduction in total cholesterol for the hydroxymethylglutaryl-CoA (HMG-CoA) reductase inhibitors literature. Authors should also assess benefits versus risks associated with the therapy under review.[63]

Systematic reviews are retrospective observational trials and for this reason are subject to systematic and random error.[67] Just as for nonsystematic reviews, techniques can be applied to evaluate the quality of systematic reviews.[69]

Appendix 5–1 contains a list of additional questions specific to systematic reviews. These specific questions are in addition to the standard questions used to evaluate other randomized clinical trials noted in Chapter 4 and using basic tools like the Ten Major Considerations Checklist discussed in the Introduction section.

META-ANALYSIS: QUANTITATIVE

Meta-analysis is a technique that has been developed to provide a quantitative and objective assessment.[70] These analyses are widely used to provide supporting evidence for clinical decision-making. In a meta-analysis, results of previously conducted clinical trials are combined and statistically analyzed.[68,71] Meta-analyses are designed to provide greater insight into clinical dilemmas than individual clinical trials. They are especially useful when previous studies have been inconclusive or contradictory, or in situations where sample size may have been too small to detect a statistically significant difference between treatment and control groups (i.e., power not met with required sample size). Meta-analyses assist in (1) supporting or refuting lesser-quality evidence, (2) overcoming reduced statistical power of small studies, (3) assessing occurrence of rare events, (4) providing guidance with limited/conflicting data, (5) displaying sample sizes and treatment effects graphically, (6) assessing heterogeneity between studies and publication bias, (7) evaluating the natural history of disease, (8) improving estimates of effect size , and (9) answering new questions not posed at the start of individual trials.[68,71] Meta-analyses can be used to look at both clinical trials and epidemiologic research, such as cohort and case-control studies, and are particularly useful when definitive trials cannot be conducted, results of available trials are inconclusive, or while awaiting the results of definitive trials.[68,69,71] The meta-analysis study design has been used to address important clinical questions, such as whether aspirin reduces the risk of pregnancy-induced hypertension, cholesterol lowering decreases mortality, fluoxetine increases suicidal ideations, or estrogen replacement therapy increases the risk of breast cancer.[71] The thought process involved in identifying the need for this type of analysis can be presented with a hypothetical situation regarding a drug used for the treatment of myocardial infarction. Suppose this drug is shown to be related to increases in sudden death through proarrhythmic effects based on results from a number of small trials. A meta-analysis could be performed to statistically combine the results of these small trials increasing the total sample size, and thus increasing the power of the finding that there is an association or lack of association with increased sudden death for this drug.

Methodological problems with meta-analyses have lead to controversy surrounding their use in clinical decision-making. Potential errors and biases to watch out for are associated with specific vulnerable steps in the meta-analysis process.[72] These vulnerable steps include study identification, study selection for inclusion, availability of information, data extraction, data analysis and synthesis, and data interpretation and reporting. When results from multiple trials are combined, biases of the individual studies are incorporated and new sources of bias arise.

The quality of the meta-analysis depends on the quality of the individual studies used to develop the meta-analysis.[73] Indeed, LeLorier and coworkers have compared the results of a series of large randomized controlled trials with those of previously published meta-analyses examining the same questions. They found that outcomes of 12 large randomized controlled trials studied were predicted inaccurately by previously published meta-analyses 35% of the time.[74] The randomized controlled clinical trials corresponded to meta-analyses in terms of population studied, therapeutic intervention, and at least one outcome. In this study, 46% of divergences in results involved a positive meta-analysis being followed by a negative randomized controlled trial while the remaining 54% of identified divergences involved a negative meta-analysis followed by a positive randomized controlled trial. Reasons for divergences, as cited by the authors, included the heterogeneity of the trials included in the meta-analyses and publication bias (tendency of investigators to preferentially submit studies with positive results for publication).[74]

Several points should be considered when evaluating meta-analyses. A good-quality meta-analysis must clearly define the clinical question addressed by the analysis.[68,69] Prior to conducting a meta-analysis, the hypothesis should be stated and a detailed protocol developed.[73] As with systematic reviews, details of literature searches that were conducted to locate primary research articles must be given, and criteria for inclusion of studies in the meta-analysis must be determined prior to conducting the analysis.[68,69,71] Because computerized searches may not locate all of the relevant articles, other resources such as textbooks, experts in the field, and reference lists from clinical studies should also be consulted.[68] Whether to include trials from gray literature (i.e., documents provided in limited numbers outside the formal channels of publication and distribution) is controversial.[75] There are risks in using data from gray literature including inaccurate information (not completely correct information), misinformation (incorrect information), and disinformation (false information deliberately provided in order to influence opinions) that can confound the meta-analysis results.

A major problem of meta-analyses is the issue of publication bias found by LeLorier and associates described above.[68,70,71] Publication bias is a form of selection bias where publication of studies is based on the magnitude, direction, or statistical significance of the results.[76] It has been documented that researchers are more likely to publish studies that demonstrate positive effects of drugs. Therefore, studies that show lack of efficacy are less likely to be located than those that demonstrate beneficial effects of a drug. Funnel plots are used to identify the potential existence of publication bias. A funnel plot is a scatter plot of treatment effect versus sample size of the studies included in the meta-analysis.[77] The treatment effect estimates should cluster around a constant value with variability in this treatment effect decreasing as size of the trial increases with a resultant funnel shape.[77] If the funnel plot shows an inverted symmetrical funnel shape, publication bias is probably not present (Figure 5–5). However, if an asymmetrical funnel is noted, this suggests a relationship between treatment effect and study size. An asymmetrical funnel plot indicates the possibility that publication bias is present.

Trials included in and excluded from the meta-analysis should be listed, along with explanation of reasons for exclusion. Authors of meta-analyses should be blinded and choose trials to include in the meta-analysis that match prespecified criteria based solely on the Methods section of studies. Strict standards should be established prior to the initiation of the meta-analysis to ensure that criteria used for inclusion of participants, administration

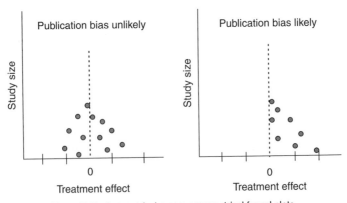

Figure 5–5. Symmetrical versus asymmetrical funnel plots.

of the principal treatment, and measurement of outcome events are similar in all trials studied.[75] Types of patients, their diagnosis, treatments, and therapeutic endpoints used in the original clinical studies should be given. The source of financial support for the original articles should be identified; however, as with analysis of individual trials, this becomes a major source of concern only when evidence of possible bias is present (e.g., strong positive conclusions, when results are inconclusive or only weakly positive).[68,69] Interpretation of meta-analyses results are limited by what studies were included or were excluded, how homogeneous (or heterogeneous) the studies were, and the methodological quality of the studies.[32]

Authors should address the validity of articles used in the meta-analysis (see Chapter 4) such as randomization techniques, compliance, blinding, appropriate dosing and length of studies, and intention-to-treat analyses.[68,71] Some experts believe that studies should receive higher weight in the analysis if they are deemed to be of higher quality, but this practice is controversial because it is felt such assessments are too subjective.[71]

The studies should be similar enough to allow pooling of data.[68,69] Statistical tests that evaluate homogeneity should be used to assess similarity of studies.[69] The more statistically significant the results of these tests, the more likely differences in study results are due to chance alone. If results of the tests of homogeneity are not significant, the studies are heterogeneous and differences in study results may be due to research design, rather than chance alone. Caution should be used when pooling results of heterogeneous studies. Factors that preclude pooling of results include discrepancies and poor quality of studies in general, inconsistencies in methods, improper conduct of the trial and reporting of data, and widely disparate findings.[73]

Appropriate statistical analyses should be undertaken (usually the Mantel-Haenszel test or mixed effects modeling). In addition, the probability of false-positive (e.g., Type I error) and false-negative (e.g., Type II error) results should be discussed. The 95% confidence intervals for each study included should be calculated.[68] These confidence intervals provide the range of values where the true value of the mean lies 95% of the time.

The preferred method to present results obtained from meta-analyses is the forest plot.[75] The forest plot illustrated in Figure 5–6 describes the results of a meta-analysis conducted to determine the 1-year effectiveness of transdermal nicotine versus placebo patches for smoking cessation.[78] A closer look reveals the mean odds ratio (including the confidence interval for nicotine patch) compared to placebo patch is plotted for each study. The odds ratio represents a ratio between two values, for instance, abstinence rates from smoking between two interventions such as nicotine patch and placebo patch. Odds ratio is the preferred measurement over relative risk to be calculated for retrospective analyses. The null hypothesis value defined as no difference between treatment groups for the odds ratio (nicotine patch versus placebo patch) is one. Because of this, a statistically significant difference in favor of the nicotine patch would be illustrated as a mean

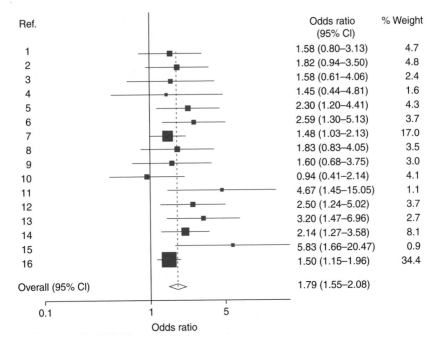

Ref.		Odds ratio (95% CI)	% Weight
1		1.58 (0.80–3.13)	4.7
2		1.82 (0.94–3.50)	4.8
3		1.58 (0.61–4.06)	2.4
4		1.45 (0.44–4.81)	1.6
5		2.30 (1.20–4.41)	4.3
6		2.59 (1.30–5.13)	3.7
7		1.48 (1.03–2.13)	17.0
8		1.83 (0.83–4.05)	3.5
9		1.60 (0.68–3.75)	3.0
10		0.94 (0.41–2.14)	4.1
11		4.67 (1.45–15.05)	1.1
12		2.50 (1.24–5.02)	3.7
13		3.20 (1.47–6.96)	2.7
14		2.14 (1.27–3.58)	8.1
15		5.83 (1.66–20.47)	0.9
16		1.50 (1.15–1.96)	34.4
Overall (95% CI)		1.79 (1.55–2.08)	

0.1   1   5
Odds ratio

Heterogeneity chi-square statistic $Q = 16.59$ (d.f. = 15), $p = 0.344$
Test of OR = 1: $z = 7.74$, $p = 0.000$

Figure 5–6. Forest plot.
Source: Myung SK et al.[77]

odds ratio and confidence interval greater than 1 (e.g., mean=2.30 with 95% CI, 1.20-4.41) as noted by D'Agostino and associates in the Forest plot. A statistically significant difference in favor of placebo over the nicotine patch would be represented as a mean odds ratio less than 1 (0.40 with 95% CI, 0.23-0.80). Note there were no studies in this meta-analysis, that favored placebo over nicotine patch. At the bottom of the forest plot is the pooled odds ratio from all the individually plotted studies included in the meta-analysis. For this meta-analysis, the overall mean odds ratio was 1.79 with a 95% CI of 1.55-2.08. These values represent a statistically significant difference in odds ratios favoring nicotine patch compared to placebo. The advantage of illustrating the meta-analysis results using a forest plot is that each study's results are presented in a visual display. With this visual display, the practitioner can quickly interpret the overall results of the meta-analysis while at the same time being able to see the contributions made to the overall result by each included study.

Sensitivity testing is an integral part of the analysis and should be conducted to determine how the results of the meta-analysis vary depending on use of different variables such as assumptions, tests, and criteria.[68,69] This allows a better understanding of how these different variables affect the results of the meta-analysis. Sensitivity testing is essential to confirm the accuracy of the results produced by the meta-analysis. For example, in the meta-analysis for smoking cessation discussed earlier, the investigators only included studies with a follow-up of 1 year. The question that sensitivity testing will answer is whether limiting the follow-up criteria to 6 months changes the overall results of the meta-analysis. In addition, the economic implications of the meta-analysis should be considered.

Overall, meta-analyses should be interpreted with caution, remembering that conclusions depend on the quality of the studies included. Findings of subsequent randomized controlled trials may differ from those of the meta-analysis.[32] This point was recently illustrated when the results of subsequent randomized controlled trials did not support previously published meta-analyses on the same subject.[74] Meta-analyses, on the surface, appear to be an extremely valuable tool allowing the practitioner to efficiently stay abreast of new information; however, oversimplification may lead to inappropriate conclusions.[74] Like all types of research evidence, meta-analyses require careful evaluation to determine their validity and applicability in practice.[76]

Appendix 5–1 contains a list of additional questions specific to meta-analyses.[79] These specific questions are in addition to the standard questions used to evaluate other randomized clinical trials noted in Chapter 4 and using basic tools like the Ten Major Considerations Checklist discussed in the Introduction section.

Case Study 5–3

■ PERTINENT BACKGROUND INFORMATION

A meta-analysis was performed to combine five smaller studies that individually do not meet power. This was done to obtain enough pooled patients to meet a set power of 0.80. All five of the smaller studies show no statistically significant difference between the two antidepressants being compared. You perform a funnel plot analysis that reveals a symmetrical inverted funnel. A closer look at these individual studies reveals low quality of study design in two trials and inconsistencies in methods between all five studies. Finally, the results of this meta-analysis are provided in the text of the article.

1. The quality of the meta-analysis depends on the quality of what?
2. One concern with meta-analyses is publication bias. What is publication bias, and what does the inverted symmetrical funnel plot suggest about publication bias as it relates to this meta-analysis?

3. The studies included in a meta-analysis should be similar enough to allow pooling of the data. What factors associated with these five studies suggest there may be a problem pooling the results?
4. The results of this meta-analysis are provided in the text of the article. What method should the authors of this meta-analysis have used to provide the results, and why is this method preferred?

Practice Guidelines

Three types of practice guidelines are published at the present time: evidence-based medicine (EBM), formal consensus-based, and a mixture of EBM and consensus-based. These various types are differentiated by the source of information used to develop the practice guideline as well as the rigor of the process for evaluating that information. EBM practice guidelines utilize a rigorous systematic process involving review and critical evaluation of the medical literature to develop final recommendations. Formal consensus-based practice guidelines utilize experience of experts in their practice area to draw conclusions and develop recommendations. This is useful for those instances where the evidence does not exist, is not complete, or not conclusive enough to allow the development of a final recommendation. In these situations, experts are used to assist completion of practice guidelines using their expertise in those deficient areas. The mixed EBM and consensus-based practice guideline uses evidence to construct the guideline and supplements those steps without evidence with experience of the experts.

Practice guidelines are created primarily for facilitating clinical decision-making, improving the quality of health care, providing consistent treatment across environments, decreasing costs, diminishing professional liability, and identifying individualized alternative treatment.[80,81] Key questions to be considered when evaluating a practice guideline are proposed.[82,83] Appendix 5–1 contains a list of these questions in addition to information presented in Chapter 7.

Useful guidelines provide information regarding therapeutic options and most appropriate choices for a specific disease and patient.[84] Important attributes for useful guidelines include validity, reproducibility/reliability, clinical applicability, clinical flexibility, accessibility, clarity, multidisciplinary development process, scheduled review, and documentation.[85] To be applicable, practice guidelines must be regularly maintained. Research has shown that within 2 years of development, a practice guideline may become outdated.[84]

Practice guidelines are becoming a common tool to use for patient population decisions. Factors are identified that influence the impact of a particular practice guideline.[86] One of the most important factors is strength of the evidence used to develop guidelines. Other factors include intensity of dissemination, follow-through of dissemination, type of problem addressed, source of guidelines, physician participation in development and adoption, format and specificity of the guideline recommendation, legal considerations, and financial/administrative issues.

Health Outcomes Research

Health outcomes research encompasses literature pertaining to discussion of pharmacoeconomic, therapeutic, and nontherapeutic outcomes (such as number of visits to the emergency room and number of hospital admissions), along with quality of life (QOL) outcomes. Readers are referred to Chapter 6 for information on evaluating pharmacoeconomic outcome studies. Therapeutic and nontherapeutic outcomes are covered in previous sections. This section will focus on evaluating literature that includes QOL outcome measures.

QUALITY-OF-LIFE MEASURES

Clinical trials have traditionally focused on health outcomes related to physical or laboratory measurements of response.[87] How the patient feels and functions relative to daily activities is not always captured by these measurements. A patient's perception of well-being can be the most important outcome in specific disease states. Investigators make assumptions that changes in therapy improve the patient's QOL. These assumptions require testing. For this reason, additional health outcome measurements have been developed to address a patient's QOL.

QOL is a term that has acquired several different definitions. General agreement exists that QOL is a multidimensional concept focusing on impact of a disease and treatment relative to the well-being of a patient.[88] Physical and social environment affects QOL. Emotional and existential reactions to this physical and social environment also have an influence. *Health-related quality of life (HR-QOL)* is an accepted term used to represent the value assigned to quality and quantity of life "as modified by impairments, functional states, perceptions, and social opportunities that are influenced by disease, injury, treatment, or policy."[88] Direct measure of HR-QOL is impossible. Only inferences from patient symptoms and reported perceptions provide measurement of HR-QOL.

Two types of HR-QOL measurements exist: health-status assessment and patient-preference assessment.[80] Heath-status assessment is a self-assessment that measures multiple aspects of a patient's perceived well-being. This assessment is primarily designed to either compare groups of patients receiving different treatments or effect of a treatment for a single group over time. Thus, health-status assessments are most often used in clinical trials comparing treatment regimens. Context of questions used range from perceived impact of disease and treatments to disease frequency and severity. Examples of health-status assessments include Functional Living Index-Cancer (FLIC), European Organization for Research and Treatment of Cancer (EORTC QLQ-C30), and the Functional Assessment of Cancer Therapy (FACT).[89-91] Health-status assessments take approximately 5 to 10 minutes to complete.

● Patient-preference assessments reflect an individual's decision-making process at a time when the eventual outcome is unknown.[88] These assessments measure the patient's tradeoff between quality and quantity of life. For example, a patient with a terminal illness may be assisted with decision-making of treatment options based on a time tradeoff instrument. This instrument is designed to assess a patient's preference with respect to their wishes regarding QOL versus quantity of life. Specifics of patient-preference assessments are beyond the scope of this discussion because they are seldom used in clinical trials.

● Two types of instruments are used to measure HR-QOL: generic and disease-specific.[92] Generic instruments assess HR-QOL in patients with and without active disease. An example of a generic instrument is Sickness Impact Profile, a health profile instrument that attempts to measure multiple aspects of HR-QOL. Generic instruments are useful for comparing completely different groups or following groups after treatment is discontinued. Disease-specific instruments are narrower in scope, more sensitive, and focus on specific treatment or disease impact. A battery of several disease-specific instruments can be used to obtain a comprehensive understanding of impact associated with different interventions. For example, a variety of disease-specific instruments, including sleep, sexual dysfunction, and physical activity, can be used to demonstrate differing effects of antihypertensive therapy on HR-QOL. HR-QOL trials should use validated HR-QOL instruments.[93] Reviewers can confirm validation of HR-QOL instruments from statements, backed by citations, indicating the questionnaires have been validated. Lack of these references or some other description of a validation process should cause concern and skepticism. Similarly, use of a combination or a series of valid HR-QOL measurements as described above should also document validity for the resultant HR-QOL battery. In practice, this integrative approach may reduce validity of HR-QOL measurements due to interactions of the various instruments on one another. Investigators must document the validity of each test used in a series as well as validity of the series as a whole. Reviewers should be aware of potential bias or problems resulting from this.

When reviewing a study containing HR-QOL measurements, the reader should consider several study characteristics,[94] and list suggested questions to ask when reviewing these trials. Appendix 5–1 contains a list of these questions. These specific questions are in addition to the standard questions used to evaluate other randomized clinical trials noted in Chapter 4 and using basic tools like the Ten Major Considerations Checklist discussed in the Introduction section.

Because there is no commonly accepted method to determine clinical significance of changes in most HR-QOL measurements, interpretation of HR-QOL results from clinical trials can be difficult.[95] A standardized method to indicate appropriate interpretation of clinically important changes and/or differences between groups in HR-QOL measurements is needed.

Trials measuring HR-QOL should be powered to detect a statistically significant difference.[88] Adequate sample size is calculated by the investigator to meet a designated level of power with a resultant number of subjects required to detect a statistically significant difference, if a difference truly exists. For example, if a study required 400 patients in each group to meet power but only 270 patients in each group were included in the final statistical analysis, power would not have been met. This is particularly important if no difference is noted between groups, in which case a difference may actually exist, but due to inadequate sample size that difference was not detected. Inadequate enrollment to allow for attrition, large patient dropout rates, and numerous protocol violators all contribute to a reduced sample size. Often HR-QOL is designated as a secondary endpoint with study power calculated to detect differences in only primary outcome measurements. Note that if subgroups are analyzed, sample size of those subgroups must also be determined prior to analysis and whether those sample sizes are adequate to meet power. Additional information regarding power can be found in Figure 5–7 and in Chapter 8.

Authors should document inclusion and applicability of relevant HR-QOL measurements in the assessment instrument.[96,97] For instance, if the study is evaluating a drug for

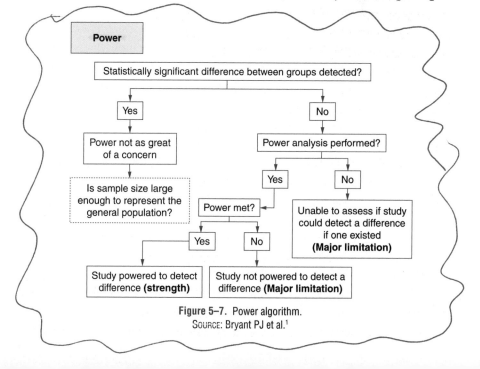

Figure 5–7. Power algorithm.
SOURCE: Bryant PJ et al.[1]

treatment of a particular disease state, rheumatoid arthritis, outcome measurements should be specific to this disease (e.g., outcome measures for rheumatoid arthritis would include mobility, hand activities, personal care, home chores, and interpersonal activities). The HR-QOL measurements represent unique personal perceptions that reflect how individual patients feel about their health status and/or nonmedical aspects of their lives. These perceptions can be difficult to capture, resulting in HR-QOL measurements that inadequately reflect patient's values and preferences.[98] The reviewer should evaluate the HR-QOL measurements to determine if individual patients are given opportunities to express opinions and reactions rather than just an assessment of disease progression. For example, the HR-QOL measurement instrument for hand activities associated with rheumatoid arthritis should capture patients' perception of how well they can move their hand, not just a determination of range of hand motion. In addition, the HR-QOL instrument should be sensitive to changes in patients' status throughout the clinical trial and should measure aspects of their lives considered important by the patients.[99] Benchmarking these measures with those used in similar published studies helps identify standard or accepted measurements for a specific disease state.

These can be difficult parameters to isolate, and thus, many measurements of HR-QOL fall short of capturing this important concept.[77] Trials overlooking important issues related to patients' health status and/or nonmedical aspects of their lives can provide misleading results.

Timing of HR-QOL measurements should be appropriate to answer research questions.[88] This timing of test administration should be related to the anticipated timing of clinical effects. In some cases, outcomes may lag behind clinical effects, and in other situations they could precede clinical effects. For instance, when evaluating a subject's perception of mood improvement following initiation of a course of antidepressant drug therapy, the measurement should not occur for several weeks to allow the medication adequate time to demonstrate efficacy. Alternatively, a HR-QOL measurement of overall QOL related to cancer therapy may include pretreatment anxiety and anticipatory nausea and vomiting preceding a chemotherapy session.

HR-QOL measurements should occupy the same timing within test sequences. For example, it is recommended that HR-QOL measurements be obtained at the beginning of clinic visits, unless there are substantial reasons provided by the authors to perform these tests at a different time. This is due to cognitively-demanding assessment instruments and the fact that most subjects are fresh at the beginning of the visit. Additionally, if several measurements are obtained for each subject throughout the course of a trial, care should be taken to ensure similar timing between subjects occurs for sequential testing.

The mode of data collection is important because self-reporting is sufficient with some types of questions, while other specific types of questions are better asked by an interviewer.[88] When a trained interviewer is used, interview location is important to obtaining unbiased answers. In a case regarding a treatment for a terminal illness, the patient may be more interested in QOL, while the family member is prioritizing quantity of life. An interview conducted in the presence of that family member could affect that patient's QOL response. Thus, HR-QOL measurements are best obtained in a private setting to reduce risk of biased responses.

Results are usually reported as a composite; however, individual patient data are often reported in smaller studies; for instance, when a rare disease limits sample size. When individual patient data are reported, the reviewer should attempt to determine if patients' answers were potentially biased due to their awareness of this public disclosure.

Assessment instrument response rates are critical since nonresponse can introduce significant bias into the results.[100] In addition, data should be reasonably complete throughout the study since missing data can suggest investigator's bias.[88] The reviewer should determine if data appear to be randomly missing. If a pattern of missing data is recognized (e.g., if a specific question or group has been excluded), the omission should be explained by authors. In this situation, the reviewer should determine if missing data have the potential to counter the author's hypothesis, thus identifying one explanation for incomplete data reporting. Reviewers must determine if HR-QOL measurements in a multicenter trial were performed at all sites. If HR-QOL measurements are not performed at all sites, authors should provide the reason for this methodology deviation.

Repeated use of HR-QOL measurements can lead to a training effect on the patient and/or interviewer, resulting in misleading conclusions.[99] The reviewer should determine if this effect is present and how that affects results. Showing test subjects their prior responses to HR-QOL measurement questions in an attempt to decrease variability should generally not be done unless acceptable supportive rationale for this procedure is given by the authors.

For the HR-QOL analysis, appropriate statistical tests should be used for the type of data analyzed such as use of categorical tests like the Mann-Whitney U test for nonparametric data. For example, data regarding attitudes about patient satisfaction with use of inhaled insulin may be measured by a Likert scale (ordinal data), and should be analyzed using nonparametric tests. All specific analytical features should be described at the time of trial design (i.e., *a priori*). A reviewer should look for an author explanation of which specific tests are used on QOL data and should not assume that the same statistical tests are used on the QOL data as are discussed for the other trial outcomes (i.e., efficacy or safety outcome data) if not directly discussed. Selective reporting of favorable or statistically significant results is also a problem. Both positive and negative findings, in addition to neutral or insignificant results, should be reported for completeness.

Several other items are worth consideration when evaluating trials with HR-QOL outcome measurements. Use of HR-QOL measurements for reporting of adverse drug events is not appropriate.[95] Trials should evaluate efficacy, safety, and HR-QOL separately and as distinctly different outcomes. An assumption that adverse events determine HR-QOL (or vice versa) can lead to erroneous results. For instance, consider a trial with breast cancer patients in whom surgery and chemotherapy are expected to eradicate all cancer cells. An appropriate assessment of HR-QOL outcomes for some patients may be positive despite troublesome adverse reactions such as low blood counts, decreased energy, and increased susceptibility to infection, based on the perception that treatment will ultimately result in a complete cure. Alternatively, other patients' HR-QOL outcomes may reflect poor QOL, even in the absence of treatment-related adverse events but instead, due to an overall situational depression. Without separate assessments of adverse events experienced and HR-QOL outcomes, linking adverse events with QOL can result in inaccurate interpretations.

Finally, culturally defined factors may impact patient's QOL and assessment of HR-QOL measurements. Validity of HR-QOL measurements across different cultures or subcultures should be considered by the reviewer. For instance, a HR-QOL instrument may effectively measure outcomes for HIV-infected men living in the United States, but may be completely inadequate for measuring outcomes in HIV-infected women living in Africa. Assessment instruments must account for and reflect the variability between outcomes perceived as important to patients, considering that perceptions may be quite diverse between cultures, and must be assessed accordingly.

Dietary Supplement Medical Literature

❼ *The same principles and criteria used to analyze the quality of drug literature are used to analyze dietary supplement literature; however, there are some unique additional points such as standardization and purity that must be considered.* Dietary supplement (botanical and nonbotanical) information is a rapidly growing body of medical literature that many health practitioners delve into more frequently as patients continue to use herbal and non-herbal supplements. As with standard drug literature, the ability to discern solid clinical evidence from weak clinical evidence is an important skill to aid practitioners in making recommendations to patients and to other health care professionals.

The provision of dietary supplement information is not dissimilar to that of standard drug information. Evidence is described and ranked according to the quality of the literature supporting or refuting dietary supplement product claims. The same evidence-based criteria utilized for drug literature analysis apply to the dietary supplement literature for determining study strengths and weaknesses. Thus, large, well-designed, randomized, controlled clinical trials or well-done meta-analyses lend stronger support versus uncontrolled or retrospective data, case series or reports, observational data, and experiential testimonials. Unfortunately, however, it is not unusual to only have poorly designed published trial data supporting or refuting a dietary supplement product's claims. This means that, for some products, the only data available concerning theoretical actions, interactions, and side effects are animal and/or *in vitro* data. To further compound misinformation, often trials touted as supporting claims for efficacy or actions of a dietary supplement have instead been conducted using chemical extracts or single chemical agents, and the results inappropriately extrapolated to apply to the supplement. For example, a trial of a concentrated, specially prepared echinacea extract showing positive results for shortening duration and severity of cold symptoms cannot be used to support a claim of similar efficacy for an echinacea product consisting of ground whole root capsules.

Unlike standard medications, dietary supplements are not legally required to be proven safe and effective in humans prior to marketing. In situations where the only safety and efficacy data for a product are theoretical, from case reports or flawed trials, or from animal and/or *in vitro* studies, practitioners must weigh risks of occurrence of the interaction or side effect against possible benefits when counseling or recommending a product to the patient.

While many EBM principles are easily applied to dietary supplement literature, what follows are some issues unique to dietary supplement trials as well as the most commonly encountered methodological flaws. Chemical entity standardization, inclusion of international literature, adequate trial duration and sample size, limited availability of high-quality evidence-based literature, and quality and purity of product formulations are specifics to consider in addition to standard literature evaluation criteria.

STANDARDIZATION

One important characteristic to look for in a botanical dietary supplement study is standardization of the chemical components of the product. Plant-derived products often contain many different chemical entities that fluctuate depending upon growing and harvesting conditions of the plant, the plant's age, and which part of the plant is used. There may be one or more chemical entities that are considered active constituents, that is, responsible for desired pharmacologic action, which may or may not be accurately identified. Others may be marker compounds that allow scientists to estimate levels of other, less-easily assayed chemicals. Standardization of one chemical entity, either an active constituent (if known) or a marker compound, is used to calibrate the product. Using a standardized chemical concentration allows for uniformity between study product and marketed product as well as between various brands of one product. When evaluating dietary supplement product trials, it is important to assess standardization methods used by investigators. Investigators should discuss and document the plant or chemical substance as well as the strength or salt form utilized in the trial.

Plant parts are also important to consider. If a trial evaluated the use of an herb's root, but the product about which a practitioner is searching for information contains the herb's leaves and flowers, the results cannot be extrapolated. This simple concept of comparing apples-to-apples also applies to nonbotanical products. However, in these cases, it refers to differences in salt forms. For example, glucosamine sulfate has a great deal of evidence documenting benefit in osteoarthritis patients, while other salt forms of glucosamine have little supportive evidence.

Because chemical constituents of botanicals, or products derived from them, can be volatile, possible degradation must be considered in interpreting results of a trial.[101] Researchers should verify that products used in studies have appropriate stability throughout the duration of a clinical trial.

INTERNATIONAL TRIALS AND INFORMATION RETRIEVAL

The majority of dietary supplement trials are conducted in Europe and Asia. Appropriateness of generalizability of results to a practitioner's own patient population must always be considered, just as with standard drug trials. This may even be of greater concern for supplement trials, as many supplements are often used as food products as well.

Studies of supplements published in foreign-language journals may be overlooked when doing a literature search that only uses the MEDLINE database, with which most health professionals are familiar. EMBASE (http://www.embase.com) is another large, commonly used database that indexes abstracts from additional international journals. It must be remembered that while abstracts can be used to get an idea of the volume of potential supportive data, they do not contain enough information to properly analyze a trial's quality. Therefore, the original studies must be reviewed.

Whatever databases are searched, use of adequate keywords or indexing terms is important. This is especially true for botanical supplements—plants have multiple common names and different spellings, different plants share common names, and official taxonomy can change frequently. A database search should include multiple search terms in order to ensure thoroughness. Additionally, searching the references of obtained articles (i.e., bibliographic searches) is useful to identify citations of trials.

DURATION

As with drug clinical trials, duration of therapy is important. Inadequate duration for appropriate assessment is a common flaw in dietary supplement trials. Because of the mechanism of action, some supplements may take several weeks to several months before patients experience benefit. Dietary supplements may appear less efficacious than they actually are if study duration is too short. If benefits are only small to moderate, a short trial may tend to overestimate responses as patients will often exhibit greater responses in the beginning of clinical trials, perhaps because of contributing placebo effect that may attenuate somewhat as the trial proceeds. As with drug clinical trials, shorter study periods cannot always predict outcomes or safety issues associated with long-term use.

TRIAL SIZE

● Small subject population is another common flaw with dietary supplement trials. Small-sized groups may not have adequate statistical power to detect a potential difference between a dietary supplement and a placebo. Adverse reactions or drug interactions can be overlooked in smaller groups versus a larger one. In addition, a small subject population can decrease trial generalizability to broader patient populations.

LACK OF EVIDENCE

● Few large controlled methodologically-sound clinical trials exist for most dietary supplements. Many products have only animal, *in vitro*, or theoretical data to support their claims. However, more sound studies are underway as dietary supplement use becomes more prevalent, acceptable, and recognized by health practitioners. All dietary supplement clinical trials should be evaluated for quality with the same criteria as those used for FDA-approved medications. However, there are additional questions that become important when considering both internal and external validity of the trial:

- Which plant part was utilized?
- Was a standardized botanical extract utilized?
- Was the study product standardization appropriate?
- Was a specific plant species or specific salt form utilized?

Appendix 5–1 contains a list of additional questions to evaluate natural product studies. These specific questions are in addition to the standard questions used to evaluate other randomized clinical trials noted in Chapter 4 and using basic tools like the Ten Major Considerations Checklist discussed in the Introduction section.

OTHER CONSIDERATIONS

● Unlike prescription drugs, dietary supplements are not reviewed or regulated by the FDA for labeling or purity prior to marketing; action can be taken if problems are discovered with either once a product is available to consumers. The bottle a consumer purchases in the health store or supermarket is not guaranteed to be labeled or dosed appropriately. Therefore, even when clinical evidence clearly supports use of an herb or supplement, the

patient may not experience a benefit because the product is mislabeled, dosed subthera-
peutically, or incorrectly standardized.

Dietary supplements can be adulterated with heavy metals or prescription medications. ConsumerLab (http://www.consumerlab.com) is an example of an organization
that independently evaluates specific brands of dietary supplements for accurate labeling
and purity. Approved or validated products receive a seal of approval, which companies
may place on product labels. Manufacturers may also voluntarily agree to have manufacturing plants and products inspected to earn approval from agencies such as the USP-
Dietary Supplement Verification Program (USP-DSVP, http://www.uspverified.org/).
Approved manufacturers are permitted to display a seal of approval on product labels and
are listed on the USP-DSVP Web site.

Dietary supplement use continues to be prevalent despite fluctuations in age groups
choosing to use supplements and changes in the popularity of specific products.[102] Health
practitioners must serve as reliable and approachable information resources for dietary
supplement information just as they do for other medications. In the retail setting, dietary
supplements are often placed with over-the-counter products near the pharmacy, making
pharmacists easily accessible for consumer questions and counseling. The ability to effectively evaluate dietary supplement literature is essential to making informed recommendations and appropriately counseling patients with dietary supplement questions.

Case Study 5–4

■ PERTINENT BACKGROUND INFORMATION

You are evaluating a trial comparing a natural product called echinacea to placebo for stim-
ulating the immune system as an adjunct to 10-day postsurgical prophylactic antibiotics.
The trial utilized capsules containing echinacea plant roots. In addition, the trial was conducted in Germany. Forty patients were randomized to receive either echinacea or identical placebo capsules for 4 days postoperatively. The results of the study showed there was
no difference in the incidence of postoperative infections between the two groups (p =
0.43). Power was set at 0.80 with an alpha of 0.05 and required 30 patients per group to
meet that power. The investigators used an intention-to-treat analysis.

1. You are evaluating this trial because a physician has asked if there is any evidence to
   support the use of echinacea extract to enhance the effect of postoperative antibiotic
   prophylaxis. How could standardization be a problem regarding extrapolating the
   results of this trial to the present situation?

2. Like this trial, many natural product trials are conducted outside the United States. Why should you take this into consideration?
3. Is there any concern with the duration of echinacea therapy?
4. Do you see any issues with the relatively small number of patients entered into the trial?

Conclusion

❽ *Given the numerous novel study designs being used by investigators to create new knowledge and medical evidence today, an understanding of strengths and limitations inherent with each design is essential to determine the overall quality of the evidence produced. Those trial designs with a high level of quality provide the most reliable evidence and that translates into the strongest recommendation/clinical decision.* Research is accomplished with the use of various types of study designs. The design is chosen based on the specific clinical questions needing to be answered. In some cases, a design is used because it represents the only way a particular data set can be obtained ethically. There are general questions that should be answered when evaluating any study design type. This chapter provides additional questions/points to consider that are unique for each specific design.

Once the study is evaluated, the overall quality of that trial must be determined. Categorizing the quality of the trial is the bridge from literature evaluation to developing a defensible conclusion/recommendation/clinical decision. In general, trial designs can be categorized by quality. This categorization ranks each study design from very low to high in quality. These categories of different quality are referred to as levels of evidence.[1]

Several different scales that rank the quality of evidence have been developed.[103] Although many of these levels-of-evidence scales follow a similar continuum of quality, labeling of each level is highly variable. For instance, one scale may use an alphabetical system (A = highest quality and D = lowest quality of evidence) while another scale uses a numerical system (1 to 5). There are even scales that combine the two systems (e.g., 1a, 1b, 1c, 2a, 2b) to rank the study design from highest to lowest quality within each level. In addition, several of these levels of evidence scales use ambiguous descriptors such as "poorly designed" or "high-quality study." This complicates the use of the scale and adds

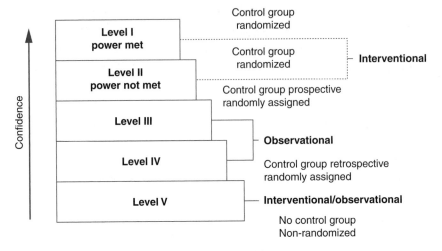

Figure 5–8. Levels of evidence.
SOURCE: Bryant PJ et al.[1] Copyright 2009, American Society of Health-System Pharmacists. Used with permission[1]

subjectivity, which leads to variability between scales. In other words, reproducing the same ratings between scales is difficult.

A standard level-of-evidence scale developed by combining the best attributes from several individual scales that are currently available has been proposed.[104] Figure 5–8 illustrates this proposed level of evidence scale. Using the level of evidence scale illustrated, the level of quality can be assigned to a trial based on the specific study design characteristics. For example, a randomized double-blind controlled N-of-1 trial used to test the efficacy and safety of a new antihypertensive would be assigned either a Level 1 or Level 2 ranking. Upon further examination of the study's methodology section, the practitioner identifies that power was set; however, an inadequate number of patients were entered into the trial to meet the set power. In this case there is a high risk of a Type II error being present or in other words, no difference is noted when in fact a true difference actually exists. It is unknown whether adding the additional patients needed to meet power would have resulted in actually observing the true difference between treatment groups. Using the diagram, the practitioner can identify that this study design is categorized as a Level 2 ranking of quality. Note the one difference between the Level 1 and Level 2 categories is power being set and met. See Figure 5–7 for a better understanding of how power can affect the quality of a study design. As mentioned in the Introduction of this chapter, additional study characteristics are also considered to further evaluate the strengths and limitations and how these attributes impact the results of the trial. The greater the number of individual strengths identified, the greater the quality and reliability of the evidence produced by that trial. From the assigned level of evidence based on the study design and attributes, the practitioner has an understanding of the overall quality of the trial. This understanding allows the practitioner to develop a clinical decision that can be easily defended based on the evidence. Three inputs have been identified that are involved with developing an EBM recommendation/clinical decision.[1] These three inputs include quality of evidence, logical reasoning, and clinical judgment. Organizing the trials by highest level of evidence, outcome of the trial, and associated limitations allows the practitioner to formulate an initial recommendation/clinical decision statement. Identifying key points associated with efficacy, safety, cost, and special considerations/special populations can help practitioners justify and defend their recommendation/clinical decision. Note that a conservative approach is taken with population-based decisions such as drug additions to a hospital formulary. These types of decisions require a more conservative approach, since a whole population is affected and little detail exists about each patient in that group. This is in contrast to an individual patient therapeutic decision where a great amount of detail from the medical chart is known about that single patient, and for this reason the decision requires a less conservative approach. Putting it all together, in an EBM manner is critically important to clinical decision-making. No matter what study design is used, a thorough evaluation and categorization of the quality of that evidence is necessary. Practitioners need high-quality and reliable evidence to make firm clinical recommendations/decisions. Caution should be exhibited making these decisions when lower quality or no evidence is available. In this situation, the practitioner must rely on the other two components mentioned: logical reasoning and clinical judgment. Unfortunately, clinical decisions made in this manner tend to overestimate the efficacy of the intervention and underestimate the safety risk to patients.[104] For this reason, clinical decisions and recommendations should be made using the highest quality of evidence available to ensure the best patient care.

Acknowledgments

Authors wish to gratefully acknowledge Denise Woolf at the University of Missouri—Kansas City School of Pharmacy Drug Information Center for her editing, macro-formatting, and proofreading of the text and Kerry Cain for her assistance with citations. Also, the authors wish to thank and acknowledge N. Seth Berry, Pharm.D., Associate Director, Clinical PK/PD Modeling & Simulation at Quintiles for his assistance with the non-inferiority trial and adaptive clinical trial sections, in addition to consultation on appropriate statistical methodologies. Many thanks to Timothy A. Candy, Pharm.D., M.S., BCPS, Senior Manager, Global Regulatory Affairs and Pharmacovigilance at Baxter Health Care

Corporation for his assistance with the non-inferiority trial section. Additional thanks to Eve C. Elias, Pharm.D., Director, UMKC Columbia Satellite Drug Information Center for her help with the non-inferiority trial section.

Self-Assessment Questions

For each of the following questions, please select the *best* answer regarding which study design is presented.

1. A physician designs a crossover study to prospectively evaluate the use of an anticonvulsant drug for treatment of chronic fatigue syndrome in an individual patient.
   a. N-of-1 study
   b. Case report
   c. Postmarketing

2. A clinician notes that a patient develops erythema multiforme after administration of phenytoin. In what form does the clinician write and publish her observations regarding this patient.
   a. N-of-1study
   b. Case report
   c. Postmarketing

3. An investigator must determine if three different levothyroxine products can be used interchangeably.
   a. Case series
   b. Stability
   c. Bioequivalence
   d. Postmarketing

4. Non-inferiority trials are designed to determine if the new drug is therapeutically:
   a. Worse than the control drug
   b. Superior to the control drug
   c. No worse than the control drug
   d. Similar to the control drug

5. Adaptive clinical trial (ACT) design provides the ability to use:
   a. Less-adaptive sampling designs for reallocation of patients
   b. Emerging data to make adjustments in the study
   c. Less flexible non-interim analysis strategies
   d. All of the above

6. After reading the following three cases, identify the study design for each trial in the correct order.

   Trial #1: It is hypothesized that hormone replacement therapy (HRT) in postmenopausal women may play a beneficial role in preventing osteoporosis. A group of patients receiving HRT and a group of patients not receiving HRT are followed over a 20-year period. The development of osteoporosis as assessed by bone mineral density in each group is compared, and the relative risk associated with the use of HRT and the development of osteoporosis is calculated.

   Trial #2: There is a concern that the use of hormone replacement therapy (HRT) in postmenopausal women may cause an increased risk of breast cancer. A study is conducted to test this hypothesis. Medical charts from a group of patients previously admitted to the hospital with the diagnosis of breast cancer are compared to medical charts from a group of patients previously admitted to the hospital without breast cancer. The groups are matched by age, sex, date of admission, and other confounding factors such as alcohol use. Use of HRT in each group is assessed and compared. An odds ratio for the risk of breast cancer related to use of HRT is calculated.

   Trial #3: An investigator identifies a study sample of women aged 20 to 45 years. During a single office visit, the investigator measures bone mass in the women. He also questions them about their past and present exercise habits. The investigator determines that women involved with rigorous exercise before the onset of menses have a greater bone mass.

   a. Cohort, cross sectional, case control
   b. Cross sectional, case control, cohort
   c. Case control, cohort, case series
   d. Cohort, case control, cross sectional
   e. Cohort, case control, case series

7. Indicate which selection ranks trial designs in order of decreasing rigor.

   a. Cohort → Case series → Case control
   b. Non-powered randomized controlled trial → Powered randomized controlled trial.
   c. Case control → → Case report → Cohort
   d. Cohort → Case control → Case series

8. Match the correct example for a retrospective observational study design with control group.

   a. N-of-1 study
   b. Case control
   c. Cohort
   d. Case series

9. Match the correct example for an uncontrolled study design.
   a. N-of-1 study
   b. Case control
   c. Cohort
   d. Case series

10. Conflicting reports exist about the effect of combining heparin with thrombolytic therapy on mortality in acute myocardial infarction. An investigator systematically identifies both published and unpublished studies in this area, combines the results, and performs a statistical analysis to create new data. Which of the following best describes this resulting document?
    a. Narrative (nonsystematic) review—Qualitative
    b. Systematic review—Qualitative
    c. Meta-analysis—Quantitative

11. Key points to note regarding the appropriate use of quality of life measures in a study are:
    a. Has the measure been validated?
    b. Does there appear to be investigator's bias present?
    c. Are the instruments used culturally relevant?
    d. All of the above.

12. One important characteristic to look for in a dietary supplement study is:
    a. Standardization since plant-derived products often contain many different chemical entities
    b. FDA approval since plant-derived products are regulated by the FDA
    c. Trial duration because studies with plant-derived products are often long and drawn out
    d. All of the above

13. All reputable EBM processes:
    a. Use a universal standardized method for ranking quality of the evidence.
    b. Avoid ranking quality of evidence.
    c. Use very complex and time-intensive methods when ranking quality of evidence.
    d. Use different methods for ranking quality of the evidence.

14. Key components to an EBM process include a:
    a. Systematic method to evaluate the evidence
    b. Method to determine the quality of evidence

    c. Method to determine a defensible recommendation/clinical decision

    d. All of the above

15. The quality-of-evidence equation includes:

    a. Key study attributes and study design characteristics

    b. Only these trials of highest quality

    c. Every unpublished study and clinical research report

    d. Risk to patients that is greater than what should be accepted

REFERENCES

1. Bryant PJ, Pace HA, editors. The pharmacist's guide to evidence based medicine for clinical decision making. Bethesda (MD): American Society of Health-system Pharmacists; 2009. p. 198.

2. De Muth JE. Basic statistics and pharmaceutical statistical applications. 2nd ed. Boca Raton (FL): Chapman & Hall/CRC; 2006. p. 714.

3. Piaggio G, Elbourne DR, Altman DG, Pocock SJ, Evans SJ. Reporting of non-inferiority and equivalence randomized trials: an extension of the CONSORT statement. JAMA. 2006;295: 1152-60.

4. U.S. Department of Health and Human Services, Food and Drug Administration, Center for Drug Evaluation and Research, and Center for Biologics Evaluation and Research. Guidance for industry non-inferiority clinical trials. [Internet]. Silver Springs (MD); 2010 Mar [cited 2010 June 11]. Available from: http://www.fda.gov/Drugs/GuidanceComplianceRegulatoryInformation/Guidances/default.htm.

5. D'Agostino RB Sr, Massaro JM, Sullivan LM. Non-inferiority trials: design concepts and issues—the encounters of academic consultants in statistics. Statist Med. 2003;22:169-86.

6. Norman GR, Streiner DL, editors. Biostatistics: the bare essentials. Shelton (CT): People's Medical Publishing House; 2008. p. 393.

7. Chiquette E, Posey LM, editors. Evidence-based pharmacotherapy. Washington DC: American Pharmaceutical Association; 2007. p. 211.

8. Pater C. Equivalence and noninferiority trials—are they viable alternatives for registration of new drugs? (III). Current Controlled Trials in Cardiovascular Medicine [Internet]. 2004 Aug 17 [cited 2010 Feb 4];5(8): Available from: http://trialsjournal.com/content/5/1/8.

9. Green WL, Concato J, Feinstein AR. Claims of equivalence in medical research: are they supported by the evidence? Ann Int Med. 2000;132:715-22.

10. Larson EB, Ellsworth AJ. N-of-1 trials: increasing precision in therapeutics [editorial]. ACP J Club. 1993 July/Aug:A16-7.

11. Cook DJ. Randomized trials in single subjects: the N of 1 study. Psychopharmacol Bull. 1996;32:363-77.

12. Guyatt GH, Keller JL, Jaeschke R, Rosenbloom D, Adachi JD, Newhouse MT. The n-of-1 randomized controlled trial: clinical usefulness. Our three year experience. Ann Intern Med. 1990;112:293-9.

13. Larson EB, Ellsworth AJ, Oas J. Randomized clinical trials in single patients during a 2-year period. JAMA. 1993;270:2708-12.

14. Guyatt G, Sackett D, Taylor DW, Chong J, Roberts R, Puosley S. Determining optimal therapy-randomized trials in individual patients. N Engl J Med. 1986;314:889-92.

15. Durham TA, Turner JR, editors. Introduction to statistics in pharmaceutical clinical trials. London: Pharmaceutical Press; 2008. p. 226.

16. Lowe D. What you need to know about adaptive trials. Pharm Exec [Internet]. 2006 July 1 [cited 2008 Dec 18]. Available from: http://pharmexec.findpharma.com/pharmexec/article/articleDetail. jsp?id=352793&pageID=1&sk=&date=.

17. Gottlieb S. Adaptive trial design. Paper presented at: Conference on Adaptive Trial Design. 2006 Jul 10; Washington DC.

18. Adaptive designs in the real world by Deborah Borfitz [Internet]. WHERE: BioIT World. com. Despite potential advantages, pharma is taking a cautious approach to adaptive designs, resulting in a slow but sure restyling of the research enterprise; 2008 Jun 10 [cited 2008 Dec 18]. Available from: http://www.bio-itworld.com/issues/2008/june/cover-story-adaptive-trial-designs.html?terms=tessella.

19. Krams M, Lees KR, Hacke W, Grieve AP, Orgogozo J, Ford GA. Acute stroke therapy by inhibition of neutrophils (ASTIN): an adaptive dose-response study of UK-279,276 in acute ischemic stroke. Stroke. 2003;34:2543-8.

20. Trissel LA, Flora KP. Stability studies: five years later. Am J Hosp Pharm. 1988;45:1569-71.

21. Chow SC. Individual bioequivalence—a review of the FDA draft guidance. Drug Inf J. 1999;33:435-44.

22. The United States Pharmacopeial Convention, Inc. Food and Drug Administration Center for Drug Evaluation and Research approved drug products with therapeutic equivalence evaluations. USPDI, 27th ed. Vol. 3, Approved drug products and legal requirements. Massachusetts; 2007:I/5-I/17.

23. The United States Pharmacopeial Convention, Inc. Food and Drug Administration Center for Drug Evaluation and Research approved drug products with therapeutic equivalence evaluations. USPDI, 27th ed. Vol. 3, Approved drug products and legal requirements. Greenwood Village (CO): Thompson Healthcare; c2007. p. 1700.

24. DiSanto AR. Bioavailability and bioequivalency testing. In: Gennaro AR, Chase GD, Marderostan AD, Harvey SC, Hussar DA, Medwick T, et al., editors. Remington's pharmaceutical sciences. 18th ed. Easton (PA): Mack Publishing; 1990. p. 1451-8.

25. Malinowski HJ. Bioavailability and bioequivalency testing. In: Hendrickson R (Chair), Beringer P, DerMarderosian A, Felton L, Gelone S, Gennaro AR, Gupta PK, Hoover JE, Popovick NG, Reilly WJ Jr. Gennaro AR, Chase GD, Marderosian AD, Hanson GR, Medwick T, Popovich NG, Reilly WJ Jr, editors. Remington: the science and practice of pharmacy. 21st ed. Philadelphia (PA): Lippincott Williams & Williams; 2000. p. 1037-46.

26. Willett MS, Bertch KE, Rich DS, Eveshehefsky L. Prospectus on the economic value of clinical pharmacy services. A position statement of the American College of Clinical Pharmacy. Pharmacother. 1989;9:45-56.

27. Collaborative drug therapy management by pharmacists: Pharmacother. 2003;23(9): 1210-25.

28. Mann CJ. Observational research methods. Research design II: cohort, cross sectional, and case-control studies. Emerg Med J. 2003;20:54-60.

29. Gottlieb M, Anderson G, Lepor H. Basic epidemiologic and statistical methods in clinical research. Urol Clin North Am. 1992;19:641-53.

30. Feinstein AR, Horwitz RI. Double standards, scientific methods, and epidemiologic research. N Engl J Med. 1982;307:1611-7.

31. Dolan MS. Interpretation of the literature. Clin Obstet Gynecol. 1998;41:307-14.

32. Aschengran A, Seage GR III, editors. Essentials of epidemiology in public health. 2nd ed. Sudbury (MA): Jones and Bartlett Publishers; 2008. p. 516.

33. Greenhalgh T. How to read a paper. 3rd ed. Malden (MA): Blackwell Publishing Ltd.; 2006. p. 229.

34. Riegelman R. Studying a study and testing a test. 5th ed. Philadelphia (PA): Lippincott Williams & Wilkins; 2005. p. 356.

35. Slaughter RL, Edwards DJ, editors. Evaluating drug literature: a statistical approach. New York: McGraw-Hill; 2001. p. 369.

36. Matthews DE, Farewll VT, editors. Using and understanding medical statistics. 4th ed. Basel (Switzerland): Karger; 2007. p. 322.

37. Fletcher RH, Fletcher SW, Wagner EH, editors. Risk. In: Clinical epidemiology: the essentials. 3rd ed. Baltimore (MD): Williams & Wilkins; 1996. p. 94-110.

38. Peipert JF, Glennon Phipps M. Observational studies. Clin Obstet Gynecol. 1998; 41:235-44.

39. Rochon PA, Gurwitz JH, Sykora K, Mamdani M, Streiner DL, Gafinkel S, et al. Reader's guide to critical appraisal of cohort studies: 1. role and design. BMJ. 2005;330:895-7.

40. Mamdani M, Sykora K, Li P, Normand ST, Austin PC, Rochon PA, et al. Reader's guide to critical appraisal of cohort studies: 2. assessing potential for confounding. BMJ. 2005;330: 960-2.

41. Normand ST, Sykora K, Li P, Mamdani M, Rochon PA, Anderson GM. Reader's guide to critical appraisal of cohort studies: 3. analytical strategies to reduce confounding. BMJ. 330:1021-3.

42. Hayden GF, Kramer MS, Horwitz RI. The case-control study. A practical review for the clinician. JAMA. 1982;247:326-31.

43. Niemcryk SJ, Kraus TJ, Mallory TH. Empirical considerations in orthopaedic research design and data analysis. Part I: strategies in research design. J Arthroplasty. 1990;5: 97-103.

44. Horwitz RI, Feinstein AR. Methodologic standards and contradictory results in case-control research. Am J Med. 1979;66:556-64.

45. Study design: The case-control approach. In: Gehlbach SH, editor. Interpreting the medical literature. 4th ed. New York: McGraw-Hill; 2002:31-54.

46. Gullen WH. A danger in matched-control studies. JAMA. 1980;244:2279-80.

47. Kleinbaum DG, Kupper LL, Morganstern H, editors. Typology of observational study designs. In: Epidemiologic research: principles and quantitative methods. New York: John Wiley & Sons; 1982:62-95.

48. Hartzema AG. Guide to interpreting and evaluating the pharmacoepidemiologic literature. Ann Pharmacother. 1992;26:96-8.

49. Grimes DA, Schulz KF. Cohort studies: marching towards outcomes. Lancet. 2002;359: 341-5.

50. Spilker B. Single patient clinical trials. Guide to clinical trials. New York: Lippincott-Raven; 1996:277-82.

51. Jaeschke R, Sackett DL. Research methods for obtaining primary evidence. Int J Technol Assess Health Care. 1989;5:503-19.

52. Lukoff D, Edwards D, Miller M. The case study as a scientific method for researching alternative therapies. Altern Ther Health Med. 1998;4:44-52.

53. Kerlinger FN. Foundations of behavioral research. 2nd ed. New York: Holt, Rinehart & Winston; 1973. p. 401.

54. Harrison DL, Draugalis JR. Evaluating the results of mail survey research. J Am Pharm Assoc. 1997;NS37:662-6.

55. Shi L. Health services research methods. In: Williams S, editors. Delmar series in health services administration. Albany (NY): International Thomson Publishing; 1997.

56. Manasse H, Lambert R. Types of research: a synopsis of the major categories and data collection methods. Am J Hosp Pharm. 1980;37:694-701.

57. Segal R. Designing a pharmacy survey. Top Hosp Pharm Manage. 1985:37-45.

58. Fowler F. Survey research methods. In: Bickman L, Rog D, editors. Applied social research methods series, vol. 1. Newbury Park (CA): Sage; 1993.

59. Fairman K. Going to the source: a guide to using surveys in health care research. J Manag Care Pharm. 1999;5:150-9.

60. Spilker B. Classification and description of phase IV postmarketing study designs. Guide to clinical trials. New York (NY): Lippincott-Raven; 1996. p. 44-58.

61. Mulrow CD. The medical review article. State of the science. Ann Intern Med. 1987;106:485-8.

62. Oxman AD, Cook DJ, Guyatt GH. Users' guides to the medical literature. VI. How to use an overview. JAMA. 1994;272:1367-71.

63. Oxman AD, Guyatt GH. Guidelines for reading literature reviews. CMAJ. 1988;138: 697-703.

64. Joyce J, Rabe-Hesketh S, Wessely S. Reviewing the reviews. The example of chronic fatigue syndrome. JAMA. 1998;280:264-6.

65. Mulrow CD, Cook DJ, Davidoff F. Systematic reviews: critical links in the great chain of evidence [editorial]. Ann Intern Med. 1997;126:389-91.

66. Cook DJ, Mulrow CD, Haynes RB. Systematic reviews: synthesis of best evidence for clinical decisions. Ann Intern Med. 1997;126:376-80.

67. Sacks HS, Berrier J, Reitman D, Pagano D, Chalmers TC. Meta-analyses of randomized control trials. An update of the quality and methodology. In: Bailar JC, Mosteller F, editors. Medical uses of statistics. 2nd ed. Boston (MA): NEJM Books; 1992:427-42.

68. Einarson TR, Leeder JS, Koren G. A method for meta-analysis of epidemiological studies. Drug Intell Clin Pharm. 1988;22:813-24.

69. Greenhalgh T. Papers that summarize other papers (systematic reviews and meta-analyses). BMJ. 1997;315:672-5.

70. Gibaldi M. Meta-analysis. A review of its place in therapeutic decision-making. Drugs. 1993;46:805-18.

71. Pucino F. Use of meta-analysis to support clinical decision making. Paper presented at: Meta-analysis: Principles and Practice Session. Proceedings of the 43rd American Society of Health-System Pharmacists Midyear Clinical Meeting; 2008 Dec 7-11; Orlando, Florida.

72. Calis KA. Pitfall and limitations of meta-analysis. Paper presented at: Meta-Analysis: Principles and Practice Session. Proceedings of the 43rd American Society of Health-System Pharmacists Midyear Clinical Meeting; 2008 Dec 7-11; Orlando, Florida.

73. LeLorier J, Gregoire G, Benhaddad A, Lapierre J, Derderian F. Discrepancies between meta-analyses and subsequent large randomized, controlled trials. N Engl J Med. 1997;337:536-42.

74. Moores KG. Meta-Analysis: principles and practice. Paper presented at: Meta-Analysis. Principles and Practice Session. Proceedings of the 43rd American Society of Health-System Pharmacists Midyear Clinical Meeting; 2008 Dec 7-11; Orlando, Florida.

75. Cook DJ, Guyatt GH, Ryan G, Clifton J, Buckinham L, Willan A, et al. Should unpublished data be included in meta-analyses? Current convictions and controversies. JAMA. 1993;269(21):2749-53.

76. Guyatt G, Rennie D, editors. User's guides to the medical literature: a manual for evidence-based clinical practice. Chicago (IL): AMA Press; 2002.

77. Armitage P, Berry G, Matthews JN, editors. Statistical methods in medical research, 4th ed. Malden (MA): Blackwell Science, Inc.; 2005. p. 817.

78. Myung SK, Yoo KY, Oh SW, Park SH, Seo HG, Hwang SS, et al. Meta-analysis of studies investigating one-year effectiveness of transdermal nicotine patches for smoking cessation. Am J Health-Syst Pharm. 2007;64:2471-6.

79. Thacker SB, Stroup DF, Peterson HB. Meta-analysis for the practicing obstetrician gynecologist. Clin Obstet Gynecol. 1998;41:275-81.

80. Zinberg S. Practice guidelines—a continuing debate. Clin Obstet Gynecol. 1998;41:343-7.

81. Rush AJ, Crismon ML, Toprac MG, Trivedi MH, Rago WV. Consensus guidelines in the treatment of major depressive disorder. J Clin Psychiatry. 1998;59(Suppl 20):73-84.

82. Hayward RS, Wilson MC, Tunis SR, Bass EB, Guyatt G. Users' guide to the medical literature. VIII. How to use clinical practice guidelines. A. Are the recommendations valid? JAMA. 1995; 274:570-4.

83. Shekelle PG, Ortiz E, Rhodes S, Morton SC, Eccles MP, Grimshaw JM, et al. Validity of the agency for health care research and quality clinical practice guidelines: how quickly do guidelines become outdated? JAMA. 2001;286(12):1461-7.

84. Wilson MC, Hayward RS, Tunis SR, Bass EB, Guyatt G. User's guide to the medical literature. VII. How to use clinical practice guidelines. B. What are the recommendations and will they help you in caring for your patients? JAMA. 1995;274:1630-2.

85. Field MJ, Lohr KN. Clinical practice guidelines: directions for a new program. US Dept. of Health and Human Services. US Institute of Medicine Committee to advise the public health service on clinical practice guidelines, Washington (DC): National Academy Press; 1990.

86. Katz DA. Barriers between guidelines and improved patient care: an analysis of AHCPR's unstable angina clinical practice guideline. Health Serv Res. 1999;34(1):377-89.

87. Fairclough DL. Design and analysis of quality of life studies in clinical trials. Boca Raton (FL): Chapman & Hall; 2002.

88. Patrick D, Erickson P. Health status and health policy: allocating resources to health care. New York (NY): Oxford University Press; 1993.

89. Aaronson NK, Cull AM, Kaasa S, Spranger MA. The European Organization for Research and Treatment of Cancer (EORTC) modular approach to quality of life assessment in oncology: an update. In: Spilker B, editor. Quality of life and pharmacoeconomics in clinical trials. 2nd ed. Philadelphia (PA): Lippincott-Raven; 1996. p. 179-89.

90. Cella DF, Bonomi AE. The functional assessment of cancer therapy (FACT) and functional assessment of HIV infection (FAHI) quality of life measurement system. In: Spilker B, editor. Quality of life and pharmacoeconomics in clinical trials. 2nd ed. Philadelphia (PA): Lippincott-Raven; 1996. p 203-10.

91. Clinch JJ. The functional living index-cancer: ten years later. In: Spilker B, editor. Quality of life and pharmacoeconomics in clinical trials. 2nd ed. Philadelphia (PA): Lippincott-Raven; 1996. p. 215-25.

92. Guyatt GH, Jaeschke R, Feeny DH, Patrick DL. Measurements in clinical trials: choosing the right approach. In: Spilker B, editor. Quality of life and pharmacoeconomics in clinical trials. 2nd ed. Philadelphia (PA): Lippincott-Raven; 1996. p. 44-5.

93. Juniper EF, Guyatt GH, Jaeschke R. How to develop and validate a new health-related quality of life instrument. In: Spilker B, editor. Quality of life and pharmacoeconomics in clinical trials, 2nd ed. Philadelphia (PA): Lippincott-Raven; 1996. p. 49-56.

94. International Society for Pharmacoeconomics & Outcomes Research Consensus Group. ISPOR quality of life regulatory guidance issues. ISPOR Website 1999 [cited 2010 Apr 8]. 26 screens. Available from: http://www.ispor.org/workpaper/consensus/index.asp.

95. Samsa G, Edelman D, Rothman ML, Williams GR, Lipscomb J, Matchar D. Determining clinically important difference in health status measures. A general approach with illustration to the Health Utilities Index Mark II. Pharmacoeconom. 1999;15:141-55.

96. Bowling A. Measuring health: a review of quality of life measurement scales. 2nd ed. Philadelphia (PA): Open University Press; 1997.

97. Spilker B. Quality of life and pharmacoeconomics in clinical trials. New York: Lippincott-Raven; 1996. p. 1259.

98. Gill TM, Feinstein AR. A critical appraisal of the quality of quality of life measurements. JAMA. 1994;272:619-26.

99. Guyatt GH, Naylor CD, Juniper E, Heyland DK, Jaeschke R, Cook DJ. User's guides to the medical literature. XII. How to use articles about health-related quality of life. JAMA. 1997;277:1232-7.

100. Sanders C, Egger M, Donovan J, Tallon D, Frankel S. Reporting on quality of life in randomized controlled trials: bibliographic study. BMJ. 1998;317:1191-4.

101. Stoney CM, Coates P, Briggs JP. Integrity of active components of botanical products used in complementary and alternative medicine. JAMA. 2008;300(17):1995.

102. Kelly JP, Kaufman DW, Kelley K, Rosenberg L, Anderson TE, Mitchell AA. Recent trends in use of herbal and other natural products. Arch Intern Med. 2005;165:281-6.

103. Croom M, Bryant PJ, Pace HA, Schnabel L. A comparative analysis of identified hierarchical categorizations of evidence. Paper presented at: Innovations in Drug Information Session. Proceedings of the 42nd American Society of Health-System Pharmacists Midyear Clinical Meeting; 2007 Dec 3; Las Vegas, Nevada.

104. Cook DJ, Guyatt GH, Laupacis A, Sackett DL. Rules of evidence and clinical recommendations on the use of antithrombotic agents. Chest. 1992;102(4 suppl):305S-311S.

6

Chapter Six

Pharmacoeconomics

James P. Wilson • Karen L. Rascati

Learning Objectives

After completing this chapter, the reader will be able to

- Describe the four types of pharmacoeconomic analysis: cost-minimization analysis (CMA), cost-benefit analysis (CBA), cost-effectiveness analysis (CEA), and cost-utility analysis (CUA).
- Describe the advantages and disadvantages of the different types of pharmacoeconomic analyses.
- List and explain the 10 steps that should be found in a well-conducted pharmacoeconomic study.
- List the six steps in a decision analysis.
- Give examples of the application of the pharmacoeconomic evaluation techniques to the formulary decision process, including decision analysis.
- Apply a systematic approach to the evaluation of the pharmacoeconomic literature.

Key Concepts

❶ Pharmacoeconomics has been defined as the description and analysis of the costs of drug therapy to health care systems and society—it identifies, measures, and compares the costs and consequences of pharmaceutical products and services.

❷ Pharmacoeconomic studies categorize costs into four types: direct medical, direct nonmedical, indirect, and intangible.

❸ *Perspective* is a pharmacoeconomic term that describes whose costs are relevant based on the purpose of the study.

❹ There are four ways to measure outcomes, and each type of outcome measurement is associated with a different type of pharmacoeconomic analysis: cost-minimization analysis (CMA), cost-benefit analysis (CBA), cost-effectiveness analysis (CEA), and cost-utility analysis (CUA).

❺ There are two common methods that economists use to estimate a value for health-related consequences, the human capital approach and the willingness-to-pay approach.

❻ A CUA takes patient preferences, also referred to as utilities, into account when measuring health consequences.

❼ All four types of analyses described (CMA, CBA, CEA, and CUA) should follow 10 general steps.

❽ A sensitivity analysis allows one to determine how the results of an analysis would change when these best guesses or assumptions are varied over a relevant range of values.

❾ Decision analysis is the application of an analytical method for systematically comparing different decision options. Decision analysis graphically displays choices and performs the calculations needed to compare these options.

Introduction

Many changes have recently taken place in health care. The continued introduction of new technologies, including many new drugs, has been among these changes. From 2006 to 2008, 138 new drugs were approved by the Food and Drug Administration (FDA).[1] New biotechnology drugs can cost over $10,000 per course of therapy. The increase in the number of new drugs combined with the increase in costs of drugs provides a great challenge for managed care organizations (MCOs) as they struggle to deliver quality care while minimizing costs.[2]

Pharmacy and therapeutics (P&T) committees are responsible for evaluating these new drugs and determining their potential value to organizations. Evaluating drugs for formulary inclusion can often be an overwhelming task. The application of pharmacoeconomic methods to the evaluation process may help streamline formulary decisions.

This chapter presents an overview of the practical application of pharmacoeconomic principles as they apply to the formulary decision process. Students and health professionals are often asked to gather and evaluate literature to support the decision process.

Pharmacoeconomics: What Is It and Why Do It?

❶ *Pharmacoeconomics has been defined as the description and analysis of the costs of drug therapy to health care systems and society—it identifies, measures, and compares the costs and consequences of pharmaceutical products and services.*[3] Decision-makers can use these methods to evaluate and compare the total costs of treatment options and the outcomes associated with these options. To show this graphically, think of two sides of an equation: (1) the inputs (costs) used to obtain and use the drug and (2) the health-related outcomes (Figure 6–1).

The center of the equation, the drug product, is symbolized by R_x. If only the left-hand side of the equation is measured without regard for outcomes, this is a cost analysis (or a partial economic analysis). If only the right-hand side of the equation is measured without regard to costs, this is a clinical or outcome study (not an economic analysis). In order to be a true pharmacoeconomic analysis, both sides of the equation must be considered and compared.

Relationship of Pharmacoeconomics to Outcomes Research

Outcomes research is defined as an attempt to identify, measure, and evaluate the end results of health care services. It may include not only clinical and economic consequences, but also outcomes, such as patient health status and satisfaction with their health care. Pharmacoeconomics is a type of outcomes research, but not all outcomes research is pharmacoeconomic research.[4]

Models of Pharmacoeconomic Analysis

The four types of pharmacoeconomic analyses all follow the diagram shown in Figure 6–1; they measure costs or inputs in dollars and assess the outcomes associated with these

$$\text{Costs(\$)} \longrightarrow \boxed{R_x} \longrightarrow \text{Outcomes}$$

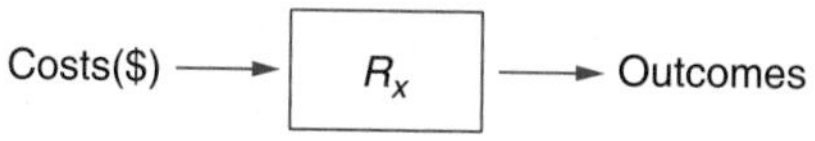

Figure 6–1. The pharmacoeconomic equation.

TABLE 6–1.   FOUR TYPES OF PHARMACOECONOMIC ANALYSIS

Methodology	Cost Measurement Unit	Outcome Measurement Unit
Cost-minimization analysis (CMA)	Dollars	Assumed to be equivalent in comparable groups analysis
Cost-benefit analysis (CBA)	Dollars	Dollars
Cost-effectiveness analysis (CEA)	Dollars	Natural units (life years gained, mm Hg blood analysis (CEA) pressure, mmol/L blood glucose)
Cost-utility analysis (CUA)	Dollars	Quality-adjusted life year (QALY) or other utilities

costs.   Pharmacoeconomic analyses are categorized by the method used to assess outcomes. If the outcomes are assumed to be equivalent, the study is called a cost-minimization analysis (CMA); if the outcomes are measured in dollars, the study is called a cost-benefit analysis (CBA); if the costs are measured in natural units (e.g., cures, years of life, blood pressure), the study is called a cost-effectiveness analysis (CEA); if the outcomes take into account patient preferences (or utilities), the study is called a cost-utility analysis (CUA) (Table 6–1). Each type of analysis includes a measurement of costs in dollars. Measurement of these costs is discussed first, followed by further examples of how outcomes are measured for these four types of studies.

Assessment of Costs

First, the assessment of costs (the left-hand side of the equation) will be discussed. A discussion of the four types of costs and timing adjustments for costs follows.

TYPES OF COSTS

Costs are calculated to estimate the resources (or inputs) that are used in the production of an outcome. ❷ *Pharmacoeconomic studies categorize costs into four types.* Direct medical costs are the most obvious costs to measure. These are the medically-related inputs used directly in providing the treatment. Examples of direct medical costs would include costs associated with pharmaceutical products, physician visits, emergency room visits, and hospitalizations. Direct nonmedical costs are costs directly associated with treatment, but are not medical in nature. Examples include the cost of traveling to and from the physician's office or hospital, babysitting for the children of a patient, and food and lodging required for patients and their families during out-of-town treatment. Indirect costs involve costs that result from the loss of productivity due to illness or death. Please note that the accounting term *indirect costs*, which is used to assign overhead, is different from the economic term, which refers to a loss of productivity of the patient or the patient's family due to illness. Intangible costs include the costs of pain, suffering, anxiety, or fatigue that occur because of an illness or the treatment of an illness. It is difficult to measure or assign values to intangible costs.

Treatment of an illness may include all four types of costs. For example, the cost of surgery would include the direct medical costs of the surgery (medication, room charges, laboratory tests, and physician services), direct nonmedical costs (travel and lodging for the preoperative day), indirect costs (cost due to the patient missing work during the surgery and recuperative period), and intangible costs (due to pain and anxiety). Most studies only report the direct medical costs. This may be appropriate depending on the objective of the study or the perspective of the study. For example, if the objective is to measure the costs to the hospital for two surgical procedures that differ in direct medical costs (e.g., using high-dose versus low-dose aprotinin in cardiac bypass surgery), but that are expected to have similar nonmedical, indirect, and intangible costs, measuring all four types of costs may not be warranted.

In order to determine what costs are important to measure, the perspective of the study must be determined. ❸ *Perspective is a pharmacoeconomic term that describes whose costs are relevant based on the purpose of the study.* Economic theory suggests that the most appropriate perspective is that of society. Societal costs would include costs to the insurance company, costs to the patient, and indirect costs due to the loss of productivity. Although this may be the most appropriate perspective according to economic theory, it is rarely seen in the pharmacoeconomic literature. The most common perspectives used in pharmacoeconomic studies are the perspective of the institution or the perspective of the payer. The payer perspective may include the costs to the third-party plan, the patient, or a combination of the patient copay and the third-party plan costs.

TIMING ADJUSTMENTS FOR COSTS

When costs are estimated from information collected for more than a year before the study or for more than a year into the future, adjustment of costs is needed. If retrospective data are used to assess resources used over a number of years, these costs should be adjusted to the present year. For example, if the objective of the study is to estimate the difference in the costs of antibiotic A versus B in the treatment of a specific type of infection, information on the past utilization of these two antibiotics might be collected from a review of medical records. If the retrospective review of these medical records dates back for more than a year, it may be necessary to adjust the cost of both medications by calculating the number of units (doses) used per case and multiplying this number by the current unit cost for each medication.

If costs are estimated based on dollars spent or saved in future years, another type of adjustment, called discounting, is needed. There is a time value associated with money. Most people (and businesses) prefer to receive money today, rather than at a later time. Therefore, a dollar received today is worth more than a dollar received next year—the time value of money. Discount rate, a term from finance, approximates the cost of capital by taking into account the projected inflation rate and the interest rates of borrowed money and then estimates the time value of money. From this parameter, the present value (PV) of future expenditures and savings can be calculated. The discount factor is equal to $1/(1 + r)^n$, where r is the discount rate and n is the year in which the cost or savings occur. For example, if the costs of a new pharmaceutical care program are $5000 per year for the next 3 years, and the discount rate is 5%, the PV of these costs is $14,297 ($5000 year one + $5000/1.05 year two + $5000/$[1.05]^2$ year three) (note that discounting does not start until year two). The most common discount rates currently seen in the literature are 3% to 5%, the approximate cost of borrowing money today.

Assessment of Outcomes

The methods associated with measuring outcomes (the right-hand side of the equation) will be discussed in this section. ❹ *As shown in Table 6–1, there are four ways to measure outcomes: CMA, CBA, CEA, and CUA.* Each type of outcome measurement is associated with a different type of pharmacoeconomic analysis. The advantages and disadvantages of each type of analysis will be discussed in this section.

COST-MINIMIZATION ANALYSIS

For a CMA, costs are measured in dollars, and outcomes are assumed to be equivalent. One example of a CMA is the measurement and comparison of costs for two therapeutically equivalent products, like glipizide and glyburide.[5] Another example is the measurement and comparison of using prostaglandin E2 on an inpatient versus an outpatient basis.[6] In both cases, all the outcomes (e.g., efficacy, incidence of adverse drug interactions) are expected to be equal, but the costs are not. Some researchers contend that a CMA is not a true pharmacoeconomic study, because costs are measured, but outcomes are not. Others say that the strength of a CMA depends on the evidence that the outcomes are the same. This evidence can be based on previous studies, publications, FDA data, or expert opinion. The advantage of this type of study is that it is relatively simple compared to the other types of analyses because outcomes need not be measured. The disadvantage of this type of analysis is that it can only be used when outcomes are assumed to be identical.

Examples

A hospital needs to decide if it should add a new intravenous antibiotic to the formulary, which is therapeutically equivalent to the current antibiotic used in the institution and has the same side effect profile. The advantage of the new antibiotic is that it only has to be administered once per day versus three times a day for the comparison antibiotic. Because the outcomes are expected to be nearly identical, and the objective is to assess the costs to the hospital (e.g., the hospital perspective), only direct medical costs need to be estimated and compared. The direct medical costs include the daily costs of each medication, the pharmacy personnel time used in the preparation of each dose, and the nursing personnel time used in the administration of each dose. Even if the cost of the new medication is a little higher than the cost of the current antibiotic, the lower cost of preparing and administering the new drug (once a day vs. three times per day) may off-set this difference. Direct nonmedical, indirect, and intangible costs are not expected to differ between these two alternatives and they need not be included if the perspective is that of the hospital, so these costs are not included in the comparison.

Mithani and Brown[7] examined once-daily intravenous administration of an aminoglycoside versus the conventional every 8-hour administration (Table 6-2). The drug acquisition cost was in Canadian dollars ($Can) 43.70 for every 8 hours dosing, and $Can 55.39 for the single dose administration. Not including laboratory drug level measurements, the costs of minibags ($Can 29.32), preparation ($Can 13.81), and administration ($Can 67.63) were $Can 110.76 for the three-times daily administration versus $Can 42.23 (minibags $Can 10.90, preparation $Can 6.20, and administration $Can 25.13) for the single daily dose. With essentially equivalent clinical outcomes, the once-daily administration of the aminoglycoside minimized hospital costs ($Can 97.62 versus $Can 154.46).

TABLE 6-2. **EXAMPLE OF COST MINIMIZATION**

Type of Cost	Every 8 Hours	Once Daily
Drug acquisition cost	$43.70	$55.39
Minibag cost	$29.32	$10.90
Preparation cost	$13.81	$6.20
Administration costs	$67.63	$25.13
Total cost	$154.46	$97.62

NOTE: Costs are presented in Canadian dollars.

COST-BENEFIT ANALYSIS

A CBA measures both inputs and outcomes in monetary terms. One advantage to using a CBA is that alternatives with different outcomes can be compared, because each outcome is converted to the same unit (dollars). For example, the costs (inputs) of providing a pharmacokinetic service versus a diabetes clinic can be compared with the cost savings (outcomes) associated with each service, even though different types of outcomes are expected for each alternative. Many CBAs are performed to determine how institutions can best spend their resources to produce monetary benefits. For example, a study conducted at Walter Reed Army Medical Center looked at costs and savings associated with the addition of a pharmacist to its medical teams.[8] Discounting of both the costs of the treatment or services and the benefits or cost savings is needed if they extend for more than a year. Comparing costs and benefits (outcomes in monetary terms) is accomplished by either of the two methods. One method divides the estimated benefits by the estimated costs to produce a benefit-to-cost ratio. If this ratio is more than 1.0, the choice is cost beneficial. The other method is to subtract the costs from the benefits to produce a net benefit calculation. If this difference is positive, the choice is cost beneficial. The example at the end of this section will use both methods for illustrative purposes.

Another more complex use of CBA consists of measuring clinical outcomes (e.g., avoidance of death, reduction of blood pressure, and reduction of pain) and placing a dollar value on these clinical outcomes. This type of CBA is not often seen in the pharmacy literature, but will be discussed here briefly. This use of the method still offers the advantage that alternatives with different types of outcomes can be assessed, but a disadvantage is that it is difficult to put a monetary value on pain, suffering, and human life. ❺ *There are two common methods that economists use to estimate a value for these types of consequences, the human capital (HC) approach and the willingness-to-pay (WTP) approach.* The human capital approach assumes that the values of health benefits are equal to the economic productivity that they permit. The cost of disease is the cost of the lost productivity due to the disease. A person's expected income before taxes and/or an inputted value for nonmarket activities (e.g., housework and child care) is used as an estimate of the value of any health benefits for that person. The human capital approach was used when calculating the costs and benefits of administering a meningococcal vaccine to college students. The value of the future productivity of a college student was estimated at $1 million in this study.[9] There are disadvantages to using this method. People's earnings may not reflect their true value to society, and this method lacks a solid literature of research to back this notion. The willingness-to-pay method estimates the value of health benefits by estimating how much people would pay to reduce their chance of an adverse health outcome. For example, if a group of people is willing to pay, on average, $100 to reduce their chance of dying from 1:1000 to 1:2000, theoretically a life would be worth $200,000 [$100/(0.001–0.0005)]. Problems with this method include the issue that what people say they are willing to pay may not correspond to what they actually would pay, and it is debatable if people can meaningfully answer questions about a 0.0005 reduction in outcomes.

Example

An independent pharmacy owner is considering the provision of a new clinical pharmacy service. The objective of the analysis is to estimate the costs and monetary benefits of two possible services over the next 3 years (Table 6–3). Clinical Service A would cost $50,000 in start-up and operating costs during the first year, and $20,000 in years two and three. Clinical Service A would provide an added revenue of $40,000 each of the three years, Clinical Service B would cost $40,000 in start-up and operating costs the first year and $30,000 for years two and three. Clinical Service B would provide added revenue of $45,000 for each of the three years. Table 6–3 illustrates the comparison of both options using the perspective of the independent pharmacy with no discounting and when a discount rate of 5% is used. Although both services are estimated to be cost beneficial, Clinical Service B has both a higher benefit-to-cost ratio and a higher net benefit when compared to Clinical Service A.

COST-EFFECTIVENESS ANALYSIS

This is the most common type of pharmacoeconomic analysis found in the pharmacy literature. A CEA measures costs in dollars and outcomes in natural health units such as cures, lives saved, or blood pressure. An advantage of using a CEA is that health units are common outcomes practitioners can readily understand and these outcomes do not need to be converted to monetary values. On the other hand, the alternatives used in the comparison must have outcomes that are measured in the same units, such as lives saved with each of two treatments. If more than one natural unit outcome is important when conducting the comparison, a cost-effectiveness ratio should be calculated for each type of outcome. Outcomes cannot be collapsed into one unit measure in CEAs as they can with CBAs (outcome = dollars) or CUAs (outcome = quality-adjusted life years [QALYs]). Because CEA is the most common type of pharmacoeconomic study in the pharmacy literature, many examples are available. Bloom and others[10] compared two medical treatments for gastroesophageal reflux disease (GERD), using both healed ulcers confirmed by endoscopy and symptom-free days as the outcomes measured. Law and others[11] assessed two antidiabetic medications by comparing the percentage of patients who achieved good glycemic control as the outcome measure.

A cost-effectiveness grid (Table 6–4) can be used to illustrate the definition of cost-effectiveness. In order to determine if a therapy or service is cost-effective, both the

TABLE 6–3. CBA EXAMPLE CALCULATIONS

	Year 1 Dollars (No Discounting in Year 1)	Year 2 Dollars (Discounted Dollars)	Year 3 Dollars (Discounted Dollars)	Total Dollars (Discounted Dollars)	Benefit-to-Cost Ratio Dollars (Discounted Dollars)	Net Benefit Dollars (Discounted Dollars)
Costs of A	$50,000 ($50,000)	$20,000 ($19,048)	$20,000 ($18,140)	$90,000 ($87,188)	$120,000/$90,000 = 1.33:1 ($114,376/87,188 = 1.31:1)	$120,000 − $90,000 = $30,000 ($114,376 − 87,188 = 27,188)
Benefits of A	$40,000 ($40,000)	$40,000 ($38,095)	$40,000 ($36,281)	$120,000 ($114,376)		
Costs of B	$40,000 ($40,000)	$30,000 ($28,571)	$30,000 ($27,211)	$100,000 ($95,782)	$135,000/100,000 = 1.35:1 ($128,673/95,782 = 1.34:1)	$135,000 − 100,000 = 35,000 ($128,673 − 95,782 = 32,891)
Benefits of B	$45,000 ($45,000)	$45,000 ($42,857)	$45,000 ($40,816)	$135,000 ($128,673)		

278

TABLE 6–4. **COST-EFFECTIVENESS GRID**

Cost-Effectiveness	Lower Cost	Same Cost	Higher Cost
Lower effectiveness	A	B	C
Same effectiveness	D	E	F
Higher effectiveness	G	H	I

costs and effectiveness must be considered. Think of comparing a new drug with the current standard treatment. If the new treatment is (1) both more effective and less costly (cell G), (2) more effective at the same price (cell H), or (3) has the same effectiveness at a lower price (cell D) , the new therapy is considered cost-effective. On the other hand, if the new drug is (1) less effective and more costly (cell C), (2) has the same effectiveness but costs more (cell F), or (3) has lower effectiveness for the same costs (cell B), then the new product is *not* cost-effective. There are three other possibilities: (1) that the new drug is more expensive and more effective (cell I)—a very common finding—(2) less expensive but less effective (cell A), or (3) has the same price and the same effectiveness as the standard product (cell E). For the middle cell E, other factors may be considered to determine which medication might be best. For the other two cells, an incremental cost-effectiveness ratio (ICER) is calculated to determine the extra cost for each extra unit of outcome. It is left up to the readers to determine if they think the new product is cost-effective, based on a value judgment. The underlying subjectivity as to whether the added benefit is worth the added cost is a disadvantage of CEA.

Example

A MCO is trying to decide whether to add a new cholesterol-lowering agent to its preferred formulary. The new product has a greater effect on lowering cholesterol than the current preferred agent, but a daily dose of the new medication is also more expensive. Using the perspective of the MCO (e.g., direct medical costs of the product to the MCO), the results will be presented in three ways in Tables 6–5 to 6–7 to illustrate the various ways that costs and effectiveness are presented in the literature. Table 6–5 presents the

TABLE 6–5. **LISTING OF COSTS AND OUTCOMES**

Alternative	Costs for 12 Months of Medication	Lowering of LDL in 12 Months (mg/dL)
Current preferred medication	$1,000	25
New medication	$1,500	30

NOTE: LDL = low-density lipoprotein.

TABLE 6–6. **COST-EFFECTIVENESS RATIOS**

Alternative	Costs for 12 Months of Medication	Lowering of LDL in 12 Months	Average Cost per Reduction in LDL
Current preferred medication	$1,000	25 mg/dL	$40 per mg/dL
New medication	$1,500	30 mg/dL	$50 per mg/dL

NOTE: LDL = low-density lipoprotein.

simple listing of the costs and benefits of the two alternatives. Sometimes for each alternative, the costs and various outcomes are listed but no ratios are conducted—this is termed a cost-consequence analysis (CCA).

The second method of presenting results includes calculating the average cost-effectiveness ratio (CER) for each alternative. Table 6–6 shows the cost-effectiveness ratio for the two alternatives. The CER is the ratio of resources used per unit of clinical benefit, and implies that this calculation has been made in relation to doing nothing or no treatment. In this case, the current medication costs $40 for every 1 mg/dL decrease in LDL while the new medication under consideration costs $50 for the same decrease. In clinical practice, the question is infrequently "Should we treat the patient or not?" or "What are the costs and outcomes of this intervention versus no intervention?" More often the question is "How does one treatment compare with another treatment in costs and outcomes?" To answer this more common question, an incremental cost-effectiveness ratio (ICER) is calculated. The ICER is the ratio of the *difference* in costs divided by the *difference* in outcomes. Most economists agree that an ICER (the extra cost for each added unit of benefit) is the more appropriate way to present CEA results. Table 6–7 shows the incremental cost-effectiveness (the extra cost of producing one extra unit) of the new medication compared to the current medication. For the new medication, it costs an *additional* $100 for every *additional* decrease in LDL of 1 mg/dL. The formulary committee would need to decide if this increase in cost is worth the increase in benefit (improved clinical outcome). In this example, the costs and benefits of the medications are estimated for

TABLE 6–7. **INCREMENTAL COST-EFFECTIVENESS RATIO**

Alternative	Costs for 12 Months of Medication	Lowering of LDL in 12 Months	Incremental Cost per Marginal Reduction in LDL
Current preferred medication	$1,000	25 mg/dL	($1,500 – $1,000)/ (30 mg/dL – 25 mg/dL)= $100 per mg/dL
New medication	$1,500	30 mg/dL	

NOTE: LDL = low-density lipoprotein.

only 1 year; discounting is not needed. If incremental calculations produce negative numbers, this indicates that one treatment is both more effective and less expensive, or dominant, compared to the other option. The magnitude of the negative ratio is difficult to interpret, so it is suggested that authors instead indicate which treatment is the dominant one. As mentioned before, when one of the alternatives is both more expensive and more effective than another, the ICER is used to determine the magnitude of added cost for each unit in health improvement (see CEA grid, cell I, Table 6–4).

Clinicians must then wrestle with this type of information—it becomes a clinical call. Many economists will argue that this uncertainty is why cost-effectiveness may not be the preferred method of pharmacoeconomic analysis.

COST-UTILITY ANALYSIS

❻ *A CUA takes patient preferences, also referred to as utilities, into account when measuring health consequences.*[12] The most common unit used in conducting CUAs is QALYs (Quality Adjusted Life Year[s]). A QALY is a health-utility measure combining quality and quantity of life, as determined by some valuations process. The advantage of using this method is that different types of health outcomes can be compared using one common unit (QALYs) without placing a monetary value on these health outcomes (like CBA). The disadvantage of this method is that it is difficult to determine an accurate QALY value. This is a relatively new type of outcome measure and is not understood or embraced by all providers and decision-makers. Therefore, this method is not commonly seen in the pharmacy literature. One reason researchers are working to establish methods for measuring QALYs is the belief that 1 year of life (a natural unit outcome that can be used in CEAs) in one health state should not be given the same weight as 1 year of life in another health state. For example, if two treatments both add 10 years of life, but one provides an added 10 years of being in a healthy state and the other adds 10 years of being in a disabled health state, the outcomes of the two treatments should not be considered equal. Adjusting for the quality of those extra years is warranted. When calculating QALYs, 1 year of life in perfect health has a score of 1.0 QALY. If health-related quality of life (HR-QOL) is diminished by disease or treatment, 1 year of life in this state is less than 1.0 QALY. This unit allows comparisons of morbidity and mortality. By convention, perfect health is assigned 1.0 per year and death is assigned 0.0 per year, but how are scores between these two determined? Different techniques for determining scales of measurement for QALY are discussed below.

There are three common methods for determining QALY scores: rating scales (RS), standard gamble (SG), and time trade-off (TTO). A rating scale consists of a line on a page, somewhat like a thermometer, with perfect health at the top (100) and death at bottom (0). Different disease states are described to subjects, and they are asked to place the different disease states somewhere on the scale indicating preferences relative to all diseases described. As an example, if they place a disease state at 70 on the scale, the disease state is given a score of 0.7 QALYs.

The second method for determining patient preference (or utility) scores is the standard gamble method. For this method, each subject is offered two alternatives. Alternative one is treatment with two possible outcomes: either the return to normal health or immediate death. Alternative two is the certain outcome of a chronic disease state for life. The probability (p) of dying is varied until the subject is indifferent between alternative one and alternative two. As an example, a person considers two options: a kidney transplant with a 20% probability of dying during the operation (alternative one) or dialysis for the rest of his life (alternative two). If this percent is his point of indifference (he would not have the operation if the chances of dying during the operation were any higher than 20%), the QALY is calculated as 1-p or 0.8 QALY.

The third technique for measuring health preferences is the TTO method. Again, the subject is offered two alternatives. Alternative one is a certain disease state for a specific length of time t, the life expectancy for a person with the disease, then death. Alternative two is being healthy for time x, which is less than t. Time x is varied until the respondent is indifferent between the two alternatives. The proportion of the number of years of life a person is willing to give up $(t - x)$ to have her remaining years (x) of life in a healthy state is used to assess her QALY estimate. For example, a person with a life expectancy of 50 years is given two options: being blind for 50 years or being completely healthy (including being able to see) for 25 years. If the person is indifferent between these two options (she would rather be blind than give up any more years of life), the QALY for this disease state (blindness) would be 0.5. Table 6–8 contains examples of disease states and QALY estimates for each disease state listed.

As one might surmise, QALY measurement is not regarded as being as precise or scientific as natural health unit measurements (like blood pressure and cholesterol levels) used in CEAs. Some issues in the measurement of QALYs are debated in the literature. One issue concerns whose viewpoint is the most valid. An advantage of having patients with the disease of interest determine health state scores is that these patients

TABLE 6–8. **SELECTED QALY ESTIMATES**

Disease State	QALY Estimate
Complete health	1.00
Moderate angina	0.83
Breast cancer: removed breast, unconcerned	0.80
Severe angina	0.53
Cancer spread, constant pain, tired, not expected to live long	0.16
Death	0.00

may understand the effects of the disease better than the general population, whereas, some believe these patients would provide a biased view of their disease compared with other diseases they have not experienced. Some contend that health care professionals could provide good estimates because they understand various diseases and others argue that these professionals may not rate discomfort and disability as seriously as patients or the general population.

Another issue that has been addressed regarding patient preference or utility-score measures is the debate over which is the best measure. Utility scores calculated using one method may differ from those using another. Finally, utility measures have been criticized for not being sensitive to small, but clinically meaningful, changes in health status.

Example

An article by Kennedy and associates[13] assessed the costs and utilities associated with two common chemotherapy regimens (vindesine and cisplatin [VP], and cyclophosphamide, doxorubicin, and cisplatin [CAP]) and compared the results with the costs and utilities of using best supportive care (BSC) in patients with non–small cell lung cancer. The perspective was that of the health care system or the payer. Using the TTO method, treatment utility scores were estimated by personnel of the oncology ward. Although the chemotherapy regimens provide a longer survival (VP = 214 days, CAP = 165 days) than BSC (112 days), the quality of life TTO score was higher for BSC (0.61) compared with the chemotherapy regimens (0.34). When survival time is multiplied by the TTO scores, the use of BSC results in an estimated 0.19 QALYs, which is similar to VP (0.19 QALYs), but higher than CAP (0.15 QALY). The costs to the health care system for the three options are about $5000 for BSC, $10,000 for VP, and $7000 for CAP (the authors reported median costs instead of average costs due to the abnormality of the cost data). Cost-utility ratios are calculated similarly to cost-effectiveness ratios, except that the outcome unit is QALYs. Therefore the cost-utility ratio is about $26,000/QALY for BSC and about $44,000 to $52,000/QALY for the chemotherapy regimens. Because BSC is at least as effective, as measured by QALYs, and is less expensive than the other two options, a marginal (or incremental) cost-utility ratio does not need to be calculated. Marginal cost-utility ratios only need to be calculated to estimate the added cost for an added benefit, not when the added benefit comes at a lower cost.

Performing an Economic Analysis

Conducting a pharmacoeconomic analysis can be challenging. Resources (time, expertise, data, and money) are limited. Data used to construct a model may be impossible to obtain due to lack of computer automation. Comparative studies of drug treatments may

TABLE 6–9. **STEPS IN PERFORMING AN ECONOMIC ANALYSIS**

Step 1	Define the problem
Step 2	Determine the study's perspective
Step 3	Determine specific treatment alternatives and outcomes
Step 4	Select the appropriate pharmacoeconomic method or model
Step 5	Measure inputs and outcomes
Step 6	Identify the resources necessary to conduct the analysis
Step 7	Establish the probabilities for the outcomes of the treatment alternatives
Step 8	Construct a decision tree
Step 9	Conduct a sensitivity analysis
Step 10	Present the results

not be available or poorly designed. Results of clinical trials may not apply at the institution performing the analysis due to lack of resources.

❼ *Methods for conducting a pharmacoeconomic analysis have been described. All four types of analyses described (CMA, CBA, CEA, and CUA) should follow 10 general steps.* See Table 6–9. A modified practical approach to these steps based on the work developed by Jolicoeur and others.[14] will be reviewed.

STEP 1: DEFINE THE PROBLEM

This step is self-explanatory. What is the question or objective that is the focus of the analysis? An example might be, "The objective of the analysis is to determine what medications for the treatment of urinary tract infections (UTIs) should be included on our formulary." Perhaps one of the drugs being evaluated is a new drug recently approved by the FDA. Should the new drug be added to the drug formulary? The important thing to remember with this step is to be specific.

STEP 2: DETERMINE THE STUDY'S PERSPECTIVE

It is important to identify from whose perspective the analysis will be conducted. As mentioned in the Assessment of Costs section, this will determine the costs to be evaluated. Is the analysis being conducted from the perspective of the patient or from that of the hospital, clinic, insurance company, or society? Depending on the perspective assigned to the analysis, different results and recommendations based on those results may be identified. If deciding on whether to add a new antibiotic to a formulary for treating UTIs, the perspective of the institution or payer would probably be used.

STEP 3: DETERMINE SPECIFIC TREATMENT ALTERNATIVES AND OUTCOMES

In this step, all treatment alternatives to be compared in the analysis should be identified. This selection should include the best clinical options and/or the options that are used most often in that setting at the time of the study. If a new treatment option is being considered, comparing it with an outdated treatment or a treatment with low efficacy rates is a waste of time and money. This new treatment should be compared with the next-best alternative or the alternative it may replace. Keep in mind that alternatives may include drug treatments and nondrug treatments. For the UTI example, a new antibiotic would probably be compared with fluoroquinolones or sulfa drugs, or even the use of cranberry juice—old or gold standard therapy—but still the usual and most commonly used therapy. Today's expensive new chemical entities are very unlikely to cost less than standard therapy, and because of this, newer drugs are sometimes compared to the most recent, more expensive drugs used as alternative therapy.

The outcomes of those alternatives should include all anticipated positive and negative consequences or events that can be measured. Remember, outcomes may be measured in a variety of ways: lives saved, emergency room visits, hospitalizations, adverse drug reactions, dollars saved, QALYs, and so forth. For the UTI example, cure rates would be the most important outcome.

STEP 4: SELECT THE APPROPRIATE PHARMACOECONOMIC METHOD OR MODEL

The pharmacoeconomic method selected will depend on how the outcomes are measured (see Table 6–1). Costs (inputs) for all four types of analyses are measured in dollars. When all outcomes for each alternative are expected to be the same, a CMA is used. If all outcomes for each alternative considered are measured in monetary units, a CBA is used. When outcomes of each treatment alternative are measured in the same nonmonetary units, a CEA is used. When patient preferences for alternative treatments are being considered, a CUA is used. For the UTI example, cure rates are a natural clinical unit measure, so a CEA would be conducted.

STEP 5: MEASURE INPUTS AND OUTCOMES

All resources consumed by each alternative should be identified and measured in monetary value. The cost for each alternative should be listed and estimated (see Assessment of Costs section). The types of costs that will be measured will depend on the perspective chosen in Step 2. When evaluating alternatives over a long period of time (e.g., greater than 1 year), the concept of discounting should be applied. For the UTI example, if the perspective is an acute care hospital, only inpatient costs of treatment are measured. If the perspective is that of the third-party payer, all direct medical costs for the treatment are included whether they are provided on an inpatient or outpatient basis.

Measuring outcomes can be relatively simple (e.g., cure rates) or relatively difficult (e.g., QALYs). Outcomes may be measured prospectively or retrospectively. Prospective measurements tend to be more accurate and complete, but may take considerably more time and resources than retrospective data retrieval. Prospectively it is possible to define exactly what data to capture, but because it is necessary to wait for the patients to complete therapy, these types of studies may take months to years to complete. A data set on the shelf (computer) can be available now, and may have all the data fields of interest. For the UTI example, cure rates attributed to the new product may be estimated from previous clinical trials, expert opinion, or measured prospectively in the population of interest.

STEP 6: IDENTIFY THE RESOURCES NECESSARY TO CONDUCT THE ANALYSIS

The availability of resources to conduct the study is an important consideration. Lack of access to important data can severely limit the validity of an analysis, as can the accuracy of the data itself. Data may be obtained from a variety of sources, including clinical trials, medical literature, medical records, prescription profiles, or computer databases. Before proceeding with the project, evaluate whether reliable sources of data are accessible or the data can be collected within the timeframe and budget allocated for the project.

STEP 7: ESTABLISH THE PROBABILITIES FOR THE OUTCOMES OF THE TREATMENT ALTERNATIVES

Probabilities for the outcomes identified in Step 3 should be determined. This may include the probability of treatment failures or success, or adverse reactions to a given treatment or alternative. Data for these can be obtained from the medical literature, clinical trials, medical records, expert opinion, prescription databases, as well as institutional databases. For the UTI example, probabilities of a cure rate for the new medication can be found in clinical trials or obtained from the FDA-approved labeling information. See Figure 6–2. Probabilities of cure rates for the previous treatments (e.g., sulfas) can also be found in clinical trials or by accessing medical records. If prospective data collection is conducted, the probabilities of all alternatives will be directly measured instead of estimated.

STEP 8: CONSTRUCT A DECISION TREE

Decision analysis can be a very useful tool when conducting a pharmacoeconomic analysis (see the section on Decision Analysis for a step-by-step review). Constructing a

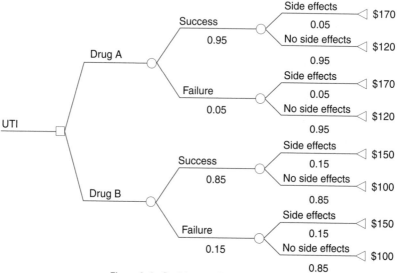

Figure 6–2. Decision tree for UTI example.

decision tree creates a graphic display of the outcomes of each treatment alternative and the probability of their occurrence. Costs associated with each treatment alternative can be determined and the respective cost ratios derived. An example using a decision tree is provided in Figure 6–2.

STEP 9: CONDUCT A SENSITIVITY ANALYSIS

Whenever estimates are used, there is a possibility that these estimates are not precise. These estimates may be referred to as assumptions. For example, if the researcher assumes the discount rate is 5%, or assumes the efficacy rate found in clinical trials will be the same as the effectiveness rate in the general population, this is a best guess used to conduct the calculations. ❽ *A sensitivity analysis allows one to determine how the results of an analysis would change when these best guesses or assumptions are varied over a relevant range of values.* For example, if the researcher makes the assumption that the appropriate discount rate is 5%, this estimate should be varied from 0 to 10% to determine if the same alternative would still be chosen within this range. In order to vary many assumptions at one time, a probabilistic sensitivity analysis can be conducted that simulates many patients randomly being processed through the decision model using a range of estimates chosen for the analysis.[15]

This method will help determine the robustness of the analysis. Do small changes in probabilities produce significant differences in the outcomes of the treatment alternatives? Another example of a sensitivity analysis will be provided in the Decision Analysis section.

STEP 10: PRESENT THE RESULTS

The results of the analysis should be presented to the appropriate audience, such as P&T committees, medical staff, or third-party payers. The steps outlined in this section should be employed when presenting the results. State the problem, identify the perspective, and so on. It is imperative to acknowledge or clarify any assumptions.

Although none of the models presented above are perfect, their utility may lead to better decision-making when faced with the difficult task of evaluating new drugs or technology for health care systems.

What Is Decision Analysis?

❾ *Decision analysis is a tool that can help visualize a pharmacoeconomic analysis. It is the application of an analytical method for systematically comparing different decision options. Decision analysis graphically displays choices and performs the calculations needed to compare these options.* It assists with selecting the best or most cost-effective alternative. Decision analysis is a tool that has been utilized for years in many fields, but has been applied to medical decision-making more frequently in the last 10 years. This method of analysis assists in making decisions when the decision is complex and there is uncertainty about some of the information.

Discussions of the medical uses of decision analysis have been included in collections of pharmacoeconomic bibliographies,[16-20] and in such specific topic areas as CEAs,[21] CUAs,[22] CBAs,[23] CMAs,[24] policies,[25] formulary processes,[26] pharmacy practices,[27] and drug product development.[28]

STEPS IN DECISION ANALYSIS

The steps in the decision process are enumerated in greater detail in several articles,[29-33] and are relatively straightforward, especially with the availability of computer programs that greatly simplify the calculations.[33] Articles reporting a decision analysis should include a picture of the decision tree, including the costs and probabilities utilized. The steps in a decision analysis will be outlined using the UTI example. The six steps involved in performing a decision analysis are provided below, and in Table 6–10.

TABLE 6–10. **STEPS IN DECISION ANALYSIS**

Step 1	Identify the specific decision (therapeutic or medical problem)
Step 2	Specify alternatives
Step 3	Specify possible outcomes and probabilities
Step 4	Draw the decision analysis structure
Step 5	Perform calculations
Step 6	Conduct a sensitivity analysis (vary cost estimates)

Step 1: Identify the Specific Decision

- Clearly define the specific decision to be evaluated (what is the objective of the study?). Over what period of time will the analysis be conducted (e.g., the episode of care, a year)? Will the perspective be that of the ill patient, the medical care plan, an institution/ organization, or society? Specifying who will be responsible for the costs of the treatment will determine how costs are measured. For the UTI example, the decision was whether to add a new antibiotic to the formulary to treat UTIs. The perspective was that of the institution and the time period is 2 weeks.

Step 2: Specify Alternatives

- Ideally, the two most effective treatments or alternatives should be compared. In pharmacotherapy evaluations, makers of innovative new products may compare or measure themselves against a standard (older or well-established) therapy. This is most often the case with new chemical entities. For pharmaceutical products, dosage and duration of therapy should be included. When analyzing costs and outcomes of pharmaceutical services, these services should be described in detail. For the UTI example, the use of the new medication (drug A) will be compared with that of a sulfa drug (drug B).

Step 3: Specify Possible Outcomes and Probabilities

- Consequences and outcomes calculated in dollars yield a cost per outcome in natural medical units, such as mg/dL, which is a CEA. For each potential outcome, an estimated probability must be determined (e.g., 95% probability of a cure or a 7% incidence of side effects).

  Table 6–11 shows the outcomes and probabilities for the UTI example. The probabilities represent the chances or likelihood of treatment success or side effects, and the costs associated with them.

Step 4: Draw the Decision Analysis Structure

- Lines are drawn to joint decision points (branches or arms of a decision tree), represented either as choice nodes, chance nodes, or final outcomes. Nodes are places in the decision tree where decisions are allowed; a branching becomes possible at this point. There are

TABLE 6–11. OUTCOMES AND PROBABILITIES, UTI EXAMPLE

	Drug A	Drug B
Effectiveness probability	0.95	0.85
Side effect probability	0.05	0.15
Cost of medication	$120	$100
Cost of side effects	$50	$50

three types of nodes: (1) a choice node is where a choice is allowed (as between two drugs or two treatments), (2) a chance node is a place where chance (natural occurrence) may influence the decision or outcome expressed as a probability, and (3) a terminal node is the final outcome of interest for that decision. Probabilities are assigned for each possible outcome, and the sum of the probabilities must add up to one. Most computer-aided software programs utilize a square box to represent a choice node, a circle to represent a chance node, and a triangle for a terminal branch or final outcome. Figure 6–2 illustrates the decision tree for the UTI example.

Step 5: Perform Calculations

The first consideration should be the present value, or cost, of money. If the study is over a period of less than 1 year, actual costs are utilized in the calculations. If the study period is greater than 1 year, then costs should be discounted (converted to PV). For each branch of the tree, costs are totaled and multiplied by the probability of that arm of the tree. These numbers (costs × probabilities) calculated for each arm of the option are added for each alternative. Example calculations are given in Tables 6–12, 6–13, and 6–14. The UTI example would be a cost-effectiveness type of study, so the difference in the cost for each arm would be divided by the difference in effectiveness for each arm to produce a marginal cost-effectiveness ratio (see Table 6–14).

Step 6: Conduct a Sensitivity Analysis (Vary Cost Estimates)

Because these decision trees or models are constructed with best guesses, a sensitivity analysis is conducted. The highest and lowest estimates of costs and probabilities are

TABLE 6–12. DECISION ANALYSIS CALCULATIONS FOR DRUG A

	Cost	Probability	Probability × Cost ($)
Outcome 1	$120 + $50 = $170	0.95 × 0.05 = 0.0475	8.08
Outcome 2	$120	0.95 × 0.95 = 0.9025	108.30
Outcome 3	$120 + $50 = $170	0.05 × 0.05 = 0.0025	0.42
Outcome 4	$120	0.05 × 0.95 = 0.0475	5.70
Total		1	122.5

TABLE 6–13. **DECISION ANALYSIS CALCULATIONS FOR DRUG B**

	Cost	Probability	Probability × Cost ($)
Outcome 1	$100 + $50 = $150	0.85 × 0.15 = 0.1275	19.12
Outcome 2	$100	0.85 × 0.85 = 0.7225	72.25
Outcome 3	$100 + $50 = $150	0.15 × 0.15 = 0.0225	3.38
Outcome 4	$100	0.15 × 0.85 = 0.1275	12.75
Total		1	107.50

inserted into the equations, to determine the best case and worse case answers. These estimates should be sufficiently varied to reflect all possible true variations in values. For the UTI example, the new drug (drug A) would be added to the formulary if the committee thought the added cost ($150) was worth the added benefit (one more successful treatment) (see Table 6–12). Some might not agree with the probability of the side effects of drug A; because the therapy is new, they may believe 5% may be an underestimate. If the estimate is increased to a 10% side effect rate for the new drug and the marginal cost-effectiveness ratio is recalculated, the recalculated ratio would be $175 per added treatment success. Again, the committee would have to decide if the added cost is worth the added benefit.

Decision analysis is being used more commonly in pharmacoeconomic evaluations. The use and availability of computer programs[32] to assist with the multiple calculations makes it fairly easy for someone to automate their evaluations. Examples of software available for this purpose include TreeAge Pro (http://www.treeage.com), DPL (http://www.syncopation.com), and DecisionPro (http://www.decisionpro.biz). The prices for these software packages range from less than $100 for student versions to almost $1000 for professional versions. Decision analyses can also be conducted using Microsoft Excel (http://office.microsoft.com/en-us/excel).

Example

An article by Botteman and others[34] used a decision tree analysis to model the cost-effectiveness of enoxaparin compared to warfarin for the prevention of complications

TABLE 6–14. **INCREMENTAL COST-EFFECTIVENESS RATIO**

	Alternative Costs of Drug and Treating Side Effects ($)	Effectiveness in Treating UTI (%)	Incremental Cost per Treatment Success
Drug A	$122.50	95	($122.50 − $107.50)/ (0.95 − 0.85) = $150
Drug B	$107.50	85	

(deep vein thrombosis, venous thromboembolisms, and postthrombotic syndromes) due to hip replacement surgery. Data for this model were obtained through published literature and expert opinion. The model was created to assess both short-term (immediately after surgery) and long-term (followed until death or 100 years old) costs and consequences. The perspective was that of the payer, and a discount rate of 3% was used for the long-term analysis. For the short-term model, therapy with enoxaparin was more expensive (+ $133 per patient), but had a better outcome (+ 0.04 QALY per patient). For the long-term model, therapy with enoxaparin saved money (– $89 per patient) and had a better outcome (+ 0.16 QALY per patient), and was therefore the dominant choice. Both univariate and probabilistic sensitivity analyses were conducted and indicated that the results were robust.

Steps in Reviewing Published Literature

It is more likely that a practicing pharmacist will be asked to evaluate published literature on the topic of pharmacoeconomics, rather than actually conduct a study. When evaluating the pharmacoeconomics literature for making a formulary decision, or selecting a best product for an institution, a systematic approach to evaluating the pharmacoeconomics literature can make the task easier.

Several authors[14, 35-40] cite methodology to assist in systematically reviewing the pharmacoeconomic literature. If a study is carefully reviewed to ensure that the author(s) included all meaningful components of an economic evaluation, the likelihood of finding valid and useful results is high. The steps for evaluating studies are similar to the steps for conducting studies, because the readers are determining if the proper steps were followed when the researcher conducted the study. When evaluating a pharmacoeconomic study, at least the following 10 questions should be considered.

1. Was a well-defined question posed in an answerable form? The specific questions and hypotheses should be clearly stated at the beginning of the article.
2. Is the perspective of the study addressed? The perspective should be explicitly stated, not implied.
3. Were the appropriate alternatives considered? Head-to-head comparisons of the best alternatives provide more information than comparing a new product or service with an outdated or ineffective alternative.
4. Was a comprehensive description of the competing alternatives given? If products are compared, dosage and length of therapy should be included. If services are compared, explicit details of the services make the paper more useful. Could another researcher replicate the study based on the information given?

5. What type of analysis was conducted? The paper should address if a CMA, CEA, CBA, or CUA was conducted. Some studies may conduct more than one type of analysis (i.e., a combination of a CEA and a CUA). Some studies, especially older published studies, incorrectly placed the terms *benefit* or *effectiveness analysis* in the title of the article, when many were actually CMA studies.

6. Were all the important and relevant costs and outcomes included? Check to see that all pertinent costs and consequences were mentioned. The clinician needs to evaluate his or her situation and compare it to his or her practice situation.

7. Was there justification for any important costs or consequences that were not included? Sometimes, the authors will admit that although certain costs or consequences are important, they were impractical (or impossible) to measure in their study. It is better that the authors state these limitations, than to ignore them.

8. Was discounting appropriate? If so, was it conducted? If the treatment cost or outcomes are extrapolated for more than 1 year, the time value of money must be incorporated into the cost estimates.

9. Are all assumptions stated? Were sensitivity analyses conducted for these assumptions? Many of the values used in pharmacoeconomic studies are based on assumptions. For example, authors may assume the side effect rate is 5%, or that compliance with a regimen will be 80%. These types of assumptions should be stated explicitly. For important assumptions, was the estimate varied within a reasonable range of values?

10. Was an unbiased summary of the results presented? Sometimes, the conclusions seem to overstate or exaggerate the data presented in the results section. Did the authors use unbiased reasonable estimates when determining the results? In general, are the study results believable?

Case Study 6–1

An example of an evaluation is given below. Due to space limitations, a manuscript abstract rather than a full article will be evaluated. The names and details of the products are fictional.

Title: Pharmacoeconomic Analysis of Ultraceph and Megaceph

Background: Two new antibiotics were recently approved by the FDA—Ultraceph and Megaceph. Both have similar spectrums of activity. Ultraceph is dosed orally 50 mg once per day. Ultraceph affects liver function, so monitoring is needed. Megaceph is also dosed orally 25 mg twice per day and is associated with a 1% chance of hearing loss, which is reversible if caught within the first 2 days of treatment.

Methods: The purpose of this study was to calculate the net benefit/cost when comparing Ultraceph and Megaceph. Costs paid by third-party payers were assessed. Costs of the medications, administration time, and lab monitoring were included as input costs. The average number of hospital days was assessed for patients on each medication. An estimated cost of $1500 per hospital-day was used to calculate the outcome costs.

Results: The net savings of using Ultraceph compared to Megaceph were $700 per patient. The average cost estimates of hospitalization varied from $500 to $2000 per day and results still favored Ultraceph (range of $200 to $950 net savings).

Conclusion: Although the costs associated with administering Ultraceph are higher than Megaceph, Ultraceph may allow patients to leave the hospital sooner, thus third-party payers may realize a net benefit.

■ EVALUATION

1. Was a well-defined question posed in an answerable form?
2. Is the perspective of the study addressed?
3. Were appropriate alternatives considered?
4. Was a comprehensive description of competing alternatives given?
5. What type of analysis was conducted?
6. Were appropriate costs and consequences measured?
7. Was there justification for any important costs or consequences that were not included?
8. Was discounting appropriate? Conducted?
9. Were assumptions stated—were they reasonable?
10. Was an unbiased summary of the results presented?

Many articles, several journals, and numerous texts have been devoted to pharmacoeconomics. Research and further development and refinement of the analysis tools are ongoing. It can be expected that the literature on pharmacoeconomics will continue to expand rapidly, not only for use in proving the value of new therapies, but for invalidating the worth of standard therapies. Draugalis,[35] Baskin,[36] Greenhalgh,[37] and Mullins and Flowers[40] among others, cite references to assist readers in understanding and assessing

TABLE 6–15. SELECTED WEB SITE REFERENCES

Canadian Coordinating Office of Health Technology Assessment	http://www.cadth.ca/en
Cochrane Collaboration Home Page	http://www.cochrane.org
Department of Defense Pharmacoeconomic Center	http://www.pec.ha.osd.mil/
Institute of Health Economics	http://www.ihe.ca
International Society for Pharmacoeconomics and Outcomes Research	http://www.ispor.org/links_index.asp

economic analyses of health care as well as providing checklists (with examples and explanations) to evaluate published articles.

Selected Pharmacoeconomics Web Sites

Articles that provide an overview of the field of pharmacoeconomics, its changing methodologies, and recent advances can often be found readily at Internet sites devoted to this area of specialization. These sites usually highlight articles that are not necessarily drug or therapy specific, but many present an overview or validation of methodologies. Several pharmacoeconomic Web sites are included as references. They were selected because they all have multiple links to other pharmacoeconomic-related sites; see Table 6–15.

Educational opportunities in pharmacoeconomics have grown tremendously over the past 10 years, especially in United States Colleges of Pharmacy.[41] A Web site that lists links to over 60 other Web sites that offer pharmacoeconomic education can be found at http://www.healtheconomics.com/education.cfm.[42]

Conclusion

Many health care organizations continue to be challenged with managing costs of pharmacotherapy. Pharmacoeconomic models can be useful tools for evaluating the costs of pharmaceuticals. The ability to objectively measure and compare costs may also produce better decisions about the choice of pharmaceuticals for a formulary. Decision analysis is one of the many tools finding increased utilization in the field of medicine, and pharmacoeconomics specifically. As the science of pharmacoeconomics becomes more standardized, rigorous comparisons among several papers on the same topic will be possible (and necessary). For a more in-depth review of the principles and concepts of pharmacoeconomics, please see textbooks devoted to the topic, such as *Essentials of Pharmacoeconomics*[43] or *Methods for the Economic Evaluation of Health Care Programmes.*[44]

Study Questions

1. Describe the differences in CEA, CBA, CMA, and CUA.

2. What are the steps in the decision analysis process?

3. Why is a sensitivity analysis performed as part of the decision analysis?

4. Would all articles presenting pharmacoeconomic studies contain essentially the same steps? Why?

Self-Assessment Questions

1. A patient is anxious about waiting 2 weeks for a test result—this can be categorized as what type of cost?
   a. Direct medical cost
   b. Direct nonmedical cost
   c. Indirect cost
   d. Intangible cost

2. A home health care visit by a pharmacist is categorized as what type of cost?
   a. Direct medical cost
   b. Direct nonmedical cost
   c. Indirect cost
   d. Intangible cost

3. For which of the following would Alternative A be considered cost-effective when compared to the standard Alternative B.
   a. Alternative A costs less than Alternative B.
   b. Alternative A is more effective than Alternative B.
   c. Alternative A is more effective than Alternative B, and Alternative A costs less than Alternative B.
   d. Alternative A is less effective than Alternative B, but Alternative A costs more than Alternative B.

4. When an article states that the results of an analysis are sensitive to a particular variable, this means:
   a. The results vary depending on the range of that variable, thereby strengthening your confidence in the study results.
   b. The results vary depending on the range of that variable, thereby weakening your confidence in the study results.
   c. The results do not vary depending on the range of that variable, thereby strengthening your confidence in the study results.
   d. The results do not vary depending on the range of that variable, thereby weakening your confidence in the study results.

5. If Project A costs $20,000 this year, $30,000 in year 2, and $30,000 in year 3, what are the total 3 years costs in present value (PV) terms using a 5% discount rate. Do not begin discounting until year 2. Round to the nearest $1000.
   a. $76,000
   b. $80,000
   c. $85,000
   d. $88,000

6. If a researcher evaluates cost per quality-adjusted life year saved, what type of study is being conducted?
   a. CEA
   b. CBA
   c. CMA
   d. CUA

7. Most economists agree that the most appropriate way to present cost-effectiveness data is using:
   a. An incremental cost-effectiveness ratio
   b. A simple cost-effectiveness ratio
   c. A net benefit ratio
   d. A benefit-to-cost ratio

8. In order to estimate utilities, researchers use:
   a. Rating scale methods.
   b. Time trade-off methods.
   c. Standard gamble methods.
   d. Any of the above methods may be used.

9. In order to estimate the monetary value of health, researchers use:
   a. Human capital methods
   b. Willingness-to-pay methods

c. Both of the above methods

d. Neither of the above methods

10. Drug A costs $3000 and saves $5000. What is the benefit-to-cost ratio for Drug A?

a. 0.60:1

b. 0.80:1

c. 1.67:1

d. 2.50:1

11. Drug B costs $3000 and saves $4000. What is the benefit-to-cost ratio for Drug B?

a. 0.75:1

b. 0.80:1

c. 1.67:1

d. 1.33:1

12. Based on these results from questions 10 and 11, which option would you choose?

a. Drug A is the most cost-beneficial option.

b. Drug B is the most cost-beneficial option.

c. They are equally cost-beneficial.

d. Not able to calculate based on information given.

For questions 13-15 use the following abstract:

TITLE: Cost-utility of asthmazolimide (fictitious drug) in the treatment of severe persistent asthma. BACKGOUND: Some patients with severe persistent asthma are not controlled with standard treatment (defined in this study as a combination of long-acting beta agonists (LABAs) and inhaled corticosteroids (ICS). Clinical trials have shown improved outcomes for these patients if asthmazolimide is added to their regimen.

OBJECTIVE: The objective of this study was to estimate the cost per quality-adjusted life year (QALY) of the addition of asthmazolimide to standard treatment for patients enrolled in a randomized controlled trial. The perspective of the study was the third-party payer.

METHODS: Patients with severe persistent asthma in a health plan were enrolled in the study using a pre-post study design. The index date for each patient was their date of enrollment. Two years of pre-index utilization and costs of medical services were recorded using retrospective data collection, and patients were followed prospectively for 1 year after their index date. For the first 12 months after enrollment, patients recorded their use of any asthma-related medical services and prescriptions and kept a daily symptom diary. Then patients had asthmazolimide added to their regimen for the next 12-month period and again kept tract of their asthma-related medical services and prescriptions and a diary of daily symptoms. Costs of pre-index services were adjusted to 2008 costs to the health plan. QALYs were calculated using utility weights for various asthma-related symptoms that were estimated from a previous study using the time trade-off (TTO) method.

RESULTS: A total of 216 patients were enrolled in and completed the study. Asthma-related health plan costs increased after the addition of asthmazolimide (mostly from an increase in prescription costs) by an average of $800 per year. Fewer symptoms and less-severe symptoms were reported after the addition of the new drug, resulting in an average increase of 0.1 QALY, for an incremental cost per QALY ratio of [for calculating the answer, see question 13, below]

CONCLUSION: For these 216 patients, the addition of asthmazolimide to their medication regimen resulted in a reduction of symptoms at a reasonable cost to the health plan.

13. What number should be included in the blank in the above abstract?
    a. $800
    b. $8,000
    c. $80
    d. $80,000

14. In the above abstract, was discounting needed? Was it conducted?
    a. Not needed, not conducted
    b. Needed, not conducted
    c. Needed, conducted
    d. Not needed, conducted

15. In the above abstract, was adjustment needed? Was it conducted?
    a. Not needed, not conducted
    b. Needed, not conducted
    c. Needed, conducted
    d. Not needed, conducted

REFERENCES

1. Centerwatch: Clinical trials listing service. [cited 2011 June 26]. Available from: http://www.centerwatch.com/drug-information/fda-approvals/default.aspx?DrugYear=2008.
2. Wang Z, Salmon JW, Walton SM. Cost-effectiveness analysis and the formulary decision-making process. J Manag Care Pharm. 2004;10(10):48-59.

3. Bootman JL, Townsend RJ, McGhan WF. Introduction to pharmacoeconomics. In: Bootman JL, Townsend RJ, McGhan WF, editors. Principles of pharmacoeconomics. 2nd ed. Cincinnati (OH): Harvey Whitney Books; 1996. p. 5-11.

4. Rascati KL. Essentials of Pharmacoeconomics. Philadelphia (PA): WoltersKluwer/ Lippincott Williams & Wilkins; 2009. p. 3.

5. Nadel HL. Formulary conversion from glipizide to glyburide: a cost-minimization analysis. Hosp Pharm. 1995;30(6):467-9, 472-4.

6. Farmer KC, Schwartz WJ, Rayburn WF, Turnball G. A cost-minimization analysis of intra-cervical Prostaglandin E2 for cervical ripening in an outpatient versus inpatient setting. Clin Ther. 1996;18(4):747–56.

7. Mithani H, Brown G. The economic impact of once-daily versus conventional administration of gentamicin and tobramycin. PharmacoEconom. 1996;10(5):494-503.

8. Bjornson DC, Hiner WO, Potyk RP, Nelson BA, Lombardo FA, Morton TA, et al. Effects of pharmacists on health care outcomes in hospitalized patients. Am J Hosp Pharm. 1993; 50:1875–84.

9. Jackson LA, Schuchat A, Gorsky RD, Wenger JD. Should college students be vaccinated against meningococcal disease? A cost-benefit analysis. Am J Public Health. 1995; 85(6): 843-5.

10. Bloom BS, Hillman AL, LaMont B, Liss C, Schwartz JS, Stever GJ. Omeprazole or ranitidine plus metoclopramide for patients with severe erosive oesophagitis. PharmacoEconom. 1995;8(4):343-9.

11. Law AV, Pathak DS, Segraves AM, Weinstein CR, Arneson WH. Cost-effectiveness analysis of the conversion of patients with non-insulin-dependent diabetes mellitus from glipizide to glyburide and of the accompanying pharmacy follow-up clinic. Clin Ther. 1995;17(5):977-87.

12. Kaplan RM. Utility assessment for estimating quality-adjusted life years. In: Sloan FA, editor. Valuing health care: costs, benefits, and effectiveness of pharmaceuticals and other medical technologies. Cambridge (NY): Cambridge University Press; 1995.

13. Kennedy W, Reinharz D, Tessier G, Contandriopoulos AP, Trabut I, Champagne F, et al. Cost-utility analysis of chemotherapy and best supportive care in non-small cell lung cancer. PharmacoEconom. 1995;8(4):316-23.

14. Jolicoeur LM, Jones-Grizzle AJ, Boyer JG. Guidelines for performing a pharmacoeconomic analysis. Am J Hosp Pharm. 1992;49:1741-7.

15. Shaw JW, Zachry WM. Application of probabilistic sensitivity analysis in decision analytic modeling. Formulary (USA). 2002;37:32–4, 37-40.

16. McGhan WF, Lewis NJW. Basic bibliographies: pharmacoeconomics. Hosp Pharm. 1992;27:547-8.

17. Wanke LA, Huber SL. Basic bibliographies: cancer therapy pharmacoeconomics. Hosp Pharm.1994;29:402.

18. Skaer TL, Williams LM. Basic bibliographies: biotechnology pharmacoeconomics I. Hosp Pharm.1994;29:1053-4.

19. Skaer TL, Williams LM. Basic bibliographies: biotechnology pharmacoeconomics II. Hosp Pharm.1994;29:1136.

20. McGhan WF. Basic bibliographies: pharmacoeconomics. Hosp Pharm. 1998;33:1270, 1273.

21. Duggan AE, Tolley K, Hawkey CJ, Logan RF. Varying efficacy of Helicobacter pylori eradication regimens: cost effectiveness study using a decision analysis model. BMJ. 1998;316:1648–54.

22. Messori A, Trippoli S, Becagli P, Cincotta M, Labbate MG, Zaccara G. Adjunctive lamotrigine therapy in patients with refractory seizures: a lifetime cost-utility analysis. Eur J Clin Pharmacol. 1998;53(6):421-7.

23. Ginsberg G, Shani S, Lev B. Cost benefit analysis of risperidone and clozapine in the treatment of schizophrenia in Israel. PharmacoEconom. 1998 Feb 13;231-41.

24. Sesti AM, Armitstead JA, Hall KN, Jang R, Milne S. Cost-minimization analysis of hand held nebulizer vs. metered dose inhaler protocol for management of acute asthma exacerbations in the emergency department. ASHP Midyear Clinical Meeting; 32: MCS-7: 1997; 1996 Dec 8–12; New Orleans, Louisiana.

25. Hinman AR, Koplan JP, Orenstein WA, Brink EW. Decision analysis and polio immunization policy. Am J Pub Health. 1988;78:301-3.

26. Kessler JM. Decision analysis in the formulary process. Am J Health Syst Pharm. 1997;54:S5-S8.

27. Einarson TR, McGhan WF, Bootman JL. Decision analysis applied to pharmacy practice. Am J Hosp Pharm. 1985;42:364-71.

28. Walking D, Appino JP. Decision analysis in drug product development. Drug Cosmet Ind. 1973;112:39-41.

29. Rascati KL. Decision analysis techniques practical aspects of using personal computers for decision analytic modeling. Drug Benefit Trends. 1998; July:33-36.

30. Richardson WS, Detsky AS. Users' guides to the medical literature. Part 7. How to use a clinical decision analysis. Part A. Are the results of the study valid? JAMA. 1995;273:1292-5.

31. Richardson WS, Detsky AS. Users' guides to the medical literature. Part 7. How to use a clinical decision analysis. Part B. What are the results and will they help me in caring for my patients? JAMA. 1995;273:1610-3.

32. Baskin LE. Practical pharmacoeconomics. Cleveland (OH): Advanstar Communications; 1998.

33. Sacristán JA, Soto J, Galende I. Evaluation of pharmacoeconomic studies: utilization of a checklist. Ann Pharmacother. 1993;27:1126-32.

34. Botteman MF, Caprini J, Stephens JM, Nadipelli V, Bell CF, Pashos CL, et al. Results of an economic model to assess cost-effectiveness of enoxaparin, a low-molecular-weight heparin, versus warfarin for the prophylaxis of DVT and associated long-term complications in total hip replacement surgery in the United States. Clin Ther. 2002:24(11):1960-86.

35. Draugalis JR. Assessing pharmacoeconomic studies. In: Bootman JL, Townsend RJ, McGhan WF, editors. Principles of pharmacoeconomics. Cincinnati (OH): Harvey Whitney Books; 1996. p. 278-9.

36. Baskin LE. How to evaluate the validity and usefulness of pharmacoeconomic literature. In: Practical pharmacoeconomics. Cleveland (OH): Advanstar Communications; 1998. p. 95-102.

37. Greenhalgh T. How to read a paper: papers that tell you what things cost (economic analyses). BMJ. 1997;315:596-9.

38. Drummond MF, Richardson WS, O'Brien BJ, Levine M, Heyland D. Users' guides to the medical literature. XIII. How to use an article on economic analysis of clinical practice. A. Are the results of the study valid? Evidence-Based Medicine Working Group. JAMA. 1997;277(19):1552-7.
39. O'Brien BJ, Heyland D, Richardson WS, Levine M, Drummond MF. Users' guides to the medical literature. XIII. How to use an article on economic analysis of clinical practice. B. What are the results and will they help me in caring for my patients? Evidence-Based Medicine Working Group [erratum JAMA. 1997;278(13):1064]. JAMA. 1997;277(22):1802-6.
40. Mullins CD, Flowers LR. Evaluating economic outcomes literature. In: Grauer DW et al., editors. Pharmacoeconomics and outcomes: applications for patient care. 2nd ed. Kansas City (MO): American College of Clinical Pharmacy; 2003.
41. Rascati KL, Drummond MF, Annemans L, Davey PG. Education in pharmacoeconomics: an international multidisciplinary view. PharmacoEconom. 2004;22(3):139-47.
42. HealthEconomics.com. [cited 2011 June 26]. Available from: http://www.healtheconomics.com/education.cfm.
43. Rascati KL. Essentials of Pharmacoeconomics. Philadelphia (PA): WoltersKluwer/Lippincott Williams & Wilkins. 2009.
44. Drummond MF, Sculpher MJ, Torrance GW, O'Brien BJ, and Stoddart GL. Methods for the economic evaluation of health care programmes. 3rd ed. Oxford (NY): Oxford University Press; 2005.

SUGGESTED READINGS

1. Bingefors K, Pashos CL, Smith MD, Berger ML, Hedbloom EC, Torrance GW. Health care costs, quality, and outcomes ISPOR book of terms. Lawrenceville (NJ): International Society for Pharmacoeconomics and Outcomes Research; 2003.
2. Drummond M and McGuire A. Economic evaluation in health care: merging theory with practice. New York: Oxford University Press; 2002. Drummond MF, Sculpher MJ, Torrance GW, O'Brien BJ, Stoddart GL. Methods for the economic evaluation of health care programmes. New York: Oxford University Press; 2005.
3. Rascati KL. Essentials of pharmacoeconomics. Philadelphia (PA): Wolters Kluwer/Lippincott Williams & Wilkins; 2009.

7

Chapter Seven

Evidence-Based Clinical Practice Guidelines

Kevin G. Moores

Learning Objectives

● *After completing this chapter, the reader will be able to*

- Define clinical practice guideline.
- Describe the role of clinical practice guidelines in pharmacy practice and the pharmacist's role in development and use of these guidelines.
- Identify sources of published guidelines and organizations currently involved in guideline activities.
- Describe intended purposes for the development and implementation of clinical practice guidelines.
- Explain the methodology for development of clinical practice guidelines.
- Describe the process of the systematic review of scientific evidence as part of the early steps involved in drafting clinical practice guidelines to assess benefits and harms of therapeutic interventions.
- Apply structured criteria to evaluate the validity of clinical practice guidelines.
- Identify the key issues in interpreting clinical practice guidelines and issues involved in their implementation.

Key Concepts

1 Properly developed, valid practice guidelines provide a concise summary of current best evidence on what works and what does not when considering specific health care interventions. Recommended methods for development of valid practice guidelines emphasize evidence-based approaches, formal quantitative techniques to calculate risks and benefits, and incorporation of the patient's preference.

2 The practice of evidence-based medicine (EBM) involves integrating individual clinical expertise with the best available external clinical evidence from systematic research. Development and application of clinical practice guidelines are two of the tools used in EBM.

3 Practitioners should have a thorough understanding of practice guideline methodology for involvement in appropriate evaluation and implementation of these guidelines. Although several methodologies exist, those incorporating EBM are considered most valid. Specifically, the Agency for Healthcare Research and Quality (AHRQ) developed methodology that has influenced major guideline development programs.

4 Once a topic for guideline development has been selected, a multidisciplinary panel of health care practitioners associated with the topic should be formed to develop the practice guideline. Steps involving guideline development include defining the clinical questions to be addressed, determining criteria for evidence to be included, conducting systematic search for the evidence, performing systematic evaluation and grading of the evidence, and preparing a synthesis of the evidence.

5 Synthesis of the evidence from selected studies is most useful to the practitioner when summarized in a format that facilitates consideration of individual study characteristics and quality, consistency of results between studies, size of the evidence database, and treatment effect size regarding benefits and harm. When high-quality evidence is unavailable, a summary of identified evidence is often provided with no specific recommendation, or, in some cases, a consensus method is considered to derive a recommendation.

6 Once synthesis is completed, recommendations are developed based on benefits, harms, costs, and quality of evidence. A draft guideline document is then prepared from these recommendations, tested by pilot peer-review, revised based on feedback, and implementation strategies devised with follow-up and guideline updating plans established.

7 Substantial inconsistencies exist between the many methods used to evaluate the quality of evidence. This can affect the interpretation of the evidence and hence, the quality of recommendations based on this evidence made in various practice guidelines. The practitioner must understand the particular method used with a given guideline to correctly interpret the strength of a guideline recommendation, quality of evidence used to form the recommendation, and balance between benefits and harms of interventions considered.

8 Determination of the quality of published practice guidelines is crucial before selecting and implementing one in a health care system. A guideline evaluation tool can be extremely helpful in this situation. The AGREE collaboration produced a structured, reliable, and reasonably easy-to-use instrument for critical appraisal of clinical practice guidelines. This evaluative instrument looks at how biases associated with development, presentation, and applicability of a guideline have been minimized. In addition, each step of development is required to be clearly reported.

9 Although the most effective methods for implementing new practice guidelines have not been confirmed, things to consider when developing an implementation strategy include local factors, potential facilitators, and barriers to implementation. Any factor that limits or restricts physician adherence to a guideline is considered a barrier to implementation. These factors include lack of physician awareness, familiarity, agreement, self-efficacy, and outcome expectancy. In addition, inertia of previous practice and external barriers such as patient nonadherence are noted.

10 Complete clinical practice guidelines can be found on Web sites such as the National Guideline Clearinghouse and in the peer-reviewed medical literature located in MEDLINE and other secondary databases. Systematic reviews that can be helpful in developing or assessing specific practice guidelines are available from organizations such as the Cochrane Library, in addition to other Web sites that collect and provide health care–related information designed to support evidence-based medicine such as the Agency for Healthcare Research and Quality (AHRQ), Health Information Research Unit at McMaster University, and the Centre for Evidence-Based Medicine at Oxford.

Introduction

Evidence-based clinical practice guidelines are "systematically developed statements to assist practitioner and patient decisions about health care for specific circumstances."[1] Clinical practice guidelines are developed by a variety of groups and organizations including federal and state government, professional societies and associations, managed care organizations, third-party payers, quality assurance organizations, and utilization review groups. ❶ *Properly developed, valid practice guidelines provide a concise summary of current best evidence on what works and what does not when considering specific health care interventions. Recommended methods for development of valid practice guidelines emphasize evidence-based approach, formal quantitative techniques to calculate risks and benefits, and incorporation of the patient's preference.* The purpose of the guidelines, development methods used, format of the documents, and the strategies for implementation vary widely. Considering the potential for clinical practice guidelines to influence thousands to millions of decisions on medical interventions, it is incumbent on all health care practitioners to be thoroughly familiar with criteria to judge the validity of guidelines, and be skilled in determining their appropriate application.

Development and implementation of clinical practice guidelines have many characteristics in common with traditional activities performed by drug information practitioners, such as evaluation of new drugs for formulary consideration, medication use evaluation, and quality improvement. Many of the skills required for guideline development are required of drug information practitioners, including clear, specific definition of clinical questions, literature search and evaluation, epidemiology, biostatistics, clinical expertise, writing, editing, formatting, and education. Drug information practitioners benefit from the use of clinical practice guidelines as information resources for their work, and based on their skills are logical professionals to participate in guideline development and implementation. Other pharmacists also find clinical practice guidelines to be useful in their practices.

The primary attraction for all health care practitioners in properly developed, valid practice guidelines is that they provide a concise summary of current best evidence on what works and what does not when considering specific health care interventions. New information and new technology in health care are developed at a rapid pace. It is very difficult for individual practitioners to systematically evaluate the benefits and risks of all new technology, including new medications. By presenting a summary of best evidence, guidelines assist the practitioner in decision-making for specific patients and also facilitate discussion of care options most consistent with individual patient needs and preferences. Guidelines may also enhance provider communication and continuity of care, especially when decisions are made by multiple providers in different care settings.[2]

There is a growing awareness in health care that a significant time lag occurs in getting research information into practice. There are several examples of treatments that have been well studied and proven effective that are substantially underutilized, and interventions that have been proven ineffective or harmful that continue to be provided.[3] One of the goals of development and implementation of evidence-based clinical practice guidelines is to help speed up the process of getting evidence into practice.

Clinical practice guidelines to assist with health care decision-making, and to identify indicators for monitoring quality of care, are frequently mentioned in connection with efforts to improve quality and efficiency of services. The key issues in reorganizing the

U.S. health care system are access to care, cost, and quality. Quality and safety are a major focus as evidenced by legislative proposals for specific requirements of health insurance coverage, critical recommendations in the report from the President's Advisory Commission on Consumer Protection and Quality in the Health Care Industry,[3] and the conclusions of The Institute of Medicine National Roundtable on Health Care Quality.[4] In addition, The Institute of Medicine (IOM) has published landmark reports in the past few years regarding quality of care problems in the United States,[5] recommendations to improve the health care system,[6] and specific recommendations to focus on improvements in patient safety.[7] A central concept in these reports and recommendations relates to utilizing the best available evidence, providing decision support tools, use of informatics, and participation of patients in health care decisions and responsibilities. These concepts are also central to clinical practice guidelines.

Methods currently recommended as the most valid for development of clinical practice guidelines emphasize an evidence-based approach, formal quantitative techniques to calculate risks and benefits, and incorporation of the patient's preferences. The concepts of an evidence-based approach and use of methods to grade the quality of evidence and strength of recommendations are critical elements that will be reviewed in more detail in this chapter in the sections on methodology for clinical practice guideline development and interpretation of guideline recommendations. The evidence-based health care movement and the implementation of continuous quality improvement (CQI) programs have stimulated growth in guideline development. There have also been advancements in methods of evaluation and summarizing the best available evidence (e.g., systematic reviews, meta-analyses, and decision analyses). Development of new information databases of systematic reviews and new informatics resources facilitate the production of clinical practice guidelines and improve access to this information.

This chapter will present a review of the background to explain why clinical practice guidelines have become a common element in health care; describe the activities of selected major organizations involved with guidelines; review evidence-based methods for guideline development, evaluation, and implementation; describe interpretation skills for guideline recommendations; and provide directions to locate sources of guidelines and further information.

Evidence-Based Practice and Clinical Practice Guidelines

❷ *The practice of evidence-based medicine (EBM) involves integrating individual clinical expertise with the best available external clinical evidence from systematic research. Development and application of clinical practice guidelines are tools used in EBM.*

Evidence-based medicine (EBM) is a philosophy of practice and an approach to decision-making in the clinical care of patients. Sackett and colleagues have defined EBM as the "conscientious, explicit, and judicious use of current best evidence in making decisions about the care of individual patients."[8] The practice of EBM refers to integrating individual clinical expertise with the best available external clinical evidence from systematic research. EBM is often mistaken for, or reduced to, just one of its several components, critical appraisal of the literature. However, to be useful EBM requires both clinical expertise and an intimate knowledge of the individual patient's situation, beliefs, priorities, and values. External evidence must be used to inform, but not replace, individual clinical expertise. It is clinical expertise that determines if the external evidence may be applied to the individual patient and, if so, how it should be used in decision-making by the patient and the health care provider. The development and application of clinical practice guidelines are among the tools used in EBM. In fact, David Eddy, who remains one of the most recognized individuals for development of EBM, writes that the first published use of the term *evidence-based* was in fact in the context of clinical guidelines.[9] An understanding of EBM is necessary to understand recommended methods for production and implementation of guidelines.

Physicians working at McMaster University in Hamilton, Ontario, first used the terminology evidence-based medicine. This group, called The Evidence-Based Medicine Working Group, published a description of what they considered a new paradigm for medical practice and teaching.[10] In that article they presented their views on changes that were occurring in medical practice relating to the use of medical literature to more effectively guide decision-making. They state that the foundation for the paradigm shift rests in the significant developments in clinical research over the past 30 years, particularly the randomized-controlled trial. Also considered important is meta-analysis as a method of summarizing the results of a number of randomized trials that may have profound effects on setting treatment policy.

The Evidence-Based Medicine Working Group cites the following changes that document the development of the new philosophy: (1) proposals to apply the principles of clinical epidemiology to day-to-day clinical practice; (2) numerous articles published instructing clinicians on how to access, evaluate, and interpret the medical literature; (3) growing demand for courses that instruct physicians on how to use the medical literature; (4) improvements in the format of journal articles; (5) textbooks with more rigorous review of available evidence; (6) new information resources like the American College of Physicians (ACP) Journal Club; and (7) the development of practice guidelines based on rigorous methodological review.

The practice of EBM has been described as focusing on five linked activities[11]: (1) express information needs in clearly defined answerable clinical questions, (2) conduct a systematic search for the best available evidence for the problem, (3) evaluate the validity and applicability of the evidence, (4) prepare a synthesis or summary of the evidence for decision-making and implement the decision in practice, and (5) evaluate performance and follow-up on any areas for improvement. Those who are familiar with the literature in drug information practice will recognize that these activities are remarkably similar to the systematic approach to drug information requests as outlined by Watanabe and colleagues over 30 years ago.[12] This process is still very similar to the approach to drug information questions today (see Chapter 2).

In 2000, the lead individuals in the Evidence-Based Medicine Working Group published a slightly modified description for what the practice of evidence-based care represents.[13] This description recognizes that not all practitioners will be "interested in gaining a high level of sophistication in using the original literature, and secondly, those who do will often be short of time in applying these skills." The modified description notes that sources of appropriately pre-appraised evidence can be used by "highly competent, up-to-date practitioners who deliver evidence-based care." Examples of pre-appraised evidence would include clinical practice guidelines and systematic reviews that have been produced with evidence-based methods. These authors note that skill in interpreting the medical literature is still necessary to judge the quality of the pre-appraised resources, to know when the recommendations in the pre-appraised resources are not applicable to selected patients, and to use the original literature when pre-appraised resources are unavailable.[13]

In his most recent review of the philosophy of EBM, Eddy describes an approach that is similar to the Evidence-Based Medicine Working Group.[9] Eddy refers to the Evidence-Based Medicine Working Group's original description of the practice as "evidence-based individual decision-making." He refers to a second approach to EBM as being "evidence-based guidelines." In this second approach he describes four important features: "first, the work of analyzing the evidence and developing a guideline, or other type of policy is done by small groups of specially trained people, usually sponsored by an organization. Second, they all use an explicit, rigorous process. Third, for all of them the 'product'—whether it is an evidence review, a guideline, or another type of policy—is generic. It is intended to apply to a class or group of patients defined by some clinical criteria, rather than to an individual patient. Fourth, their effects are indirect. That is, they are intended to enable, guide, motivate, or sometimes force physicians and other types of providers to deliver certain types of care to people; they do not directly determine the care provided to a particular patient."[9] Eddy goes on to explain that the most appropriate definition of EBM is a combination of these two approaches. The combination provides for medical practice that will achieve the most efficient and effective use of evidence.

Medical education has also taken on philosophies related to EBM and guidelines. International trends in continuing medical education were described in a series of seven articles published in the *British Medical Journal*.[14-20] The major themes of these articles include the following:

- Individual responsibility for health professionals to direct their own learning.
- Self-assessment and specific needs–directed education.
- Wider aspects of continuing professional development including computer literacy, literature appraisal, information management, problem solving skills, and EBM.
- Improved working and collaboration among different health professionals to achieve gains in quality and savings in cost.
- Innovative portfolio-based programs to capture learning issues and achievements that occur in everyday practice.
- Programs for better communications with patients and with other health care providers.
- Programs based on skill development rather than the traditional lecture format.
- Distance learning and use of technology to support learning.
- Focus on education that will affect behaviors and improve outcomes of care.
- Problem-based learning and small-group activities.
- Quality improvement tools.
- Programs based on the theories of adult learning.

The U.S. IOM made recommendations for reform of health professions education in 2003.[21] In this report it was stated, "The committee believes that the following should serve as an overarching vision for all programs and institutions engaged in the clinical education of health professionals, and further that such organizations should develop operating principals that will allow this vision to be achieved. All health care professionals should be educated to deliver patient-centered care as members of an interdisciplinary team, emphasizing evidence-based practice, quality improvement approaches, and informatics."[21] This statement has been referred to as the five core competencies for health professionals. The recommendations provided in this report were a follow-up to the influential IOM report *Crossing the Quality Chasm* from 2001.[6] Examination of these five core competencies and the goals of evidence-based clinical practice guidelines demonstrate significant overlap.

Health care professionals face the complicated reality of constantly changing and increasing medical knowledge. What is required to practice effective, high-quality medicine is not an encyclopedic memory, but the skills to acquire and critically assess the specific information that is necessary to make clinical decisions. The philosophy of EBM is consistent with the philosophy of clinical practice guidelines. The decision-making process of EBM is supported by access and use of clinical practice guidelines.

Guideline Development Methods

❸ *Practitioners should have a thorough understanding of practice guideline methodology for involvement in appropriate evaluation and implementation of these guidelines. Although several methodologies exist, those incorporating EBM are considered most valid. Specifically, the Agency for Healthcare Research and Quality (AHRQ) developed methodology that has influenced major guideline development programs.*

A thorough understanding of the methodology used for clinical practice guideline development is critical for pharmacists. Although relatively few pharmacists actually participate in guideline development, this understanding will prepare practitioners for involvement in appropriate evaluation and implementation of these guidelines. Evaluation of the quality of a guideline, and the appropriateness of its use in a given setting, depends primarily on an ability to distinguish methods that minimize potential biases in development. A strong indication of the quality of guideline development methods can be obtained by a quick scan to determine if the recommendations are based on focused clinical questions, the recommendations are specifically linked to evidence, the quality of the evidence and strength of recommendations have been graded, and evidence tables and a balance sheet are available. A lack of understanding of the requirements for guideline development could lead to inappropriate interpretation, or acceptance of inappropriate levels of enforcement of biased guideline recommendations. Application of biased guidelines may result in provision of ineffective or harmful therapy. Because of the central importance of guideline development methods, a significant portion of this chapter is devoted to this topic.

Several methods for developing practice guidelines have been described, including informal consensus development, formal consensus development, evidence-based guideline development, and explicit guideline development.[22] For decades, informal consensus methods have been used as the basis of guideline development. These guidelines were produced following a meeting of an expert panel in which agreement was reached through open discussion—sometimes producing recommendations in a single meeting. The actual guideline document would often provide only the recommendation, with little background on the evidence that was used or information on the methodology of the group. This practice made it difficult or impossible for readers to verify the accuracy of the recommendation or that bias did not significantly influence the results. Informal consensus development remains a common approach to developing practice guidelines because it is a relatively fast, easy, and inexpensive process. However, this approach generally results in guidelines of questionable quality. The fact that explicit methods for how the decisions were made are often not provided leaves doubt about how consensus was reached. Treatment recommendations are notoriously fallible when they are the result of efficacy evaluations based primarily on opinion. In addition, the ability to implement such guidelines will be seriously hampered based on the inability of the user to verify the accuracy and a resultant lack of confidence.[22]

The formal consensus development process was once used by the National Institutes of Health Consensus Development Program.[23] The National Institutes of Health (NIH) uses a structured 2.5-day conference in which guidelines are developed in closed session after a plenary session and open discussion, and are presented to an audience and press conference on the third day.[22] In some instances, the usual 2.5-day format of the conference is not sufficient, and alternative formats are used.[24] It should also be noted that substantial planning occurs for presentations of up-to-date reviews of available evidence by experts. This process provides more structure than informal consensus; however, it has been criticized for its requirement to produce recommendations in a relatively short period, the absence of explicit criteria, the variability in the type and degree of referencing of the recommendations to the literature, and the inconsistent degree of labeling recommendations as to the level of certainty provided by empirical evidence.

Most recently the NIH has been using evidence-based methods for guideline development, for example, the Third Report of the National Cholesterol Education Program (NCEP) Expert Panel on Detection Evaluation, and Treatment of High Blood Cholesterol in Adults (Adult Treatment Panel III [ATP III]).[25] In keeping with evidence-based methodology, an update to this guideline was published in July 2004 based on the results of five major studies that were completed after the ATP III guidelines were released. These clinical trials provided evidence regarding several significant issues pertaining to the benefits of cholesterol lowering. The purpose of the update was to "translate the scientific evidence into guidance that helps professionals and the public take appropriate action to reduce the risk for coronary heart disease (CHD) and cardiovascular disease."[26] Another example guideline produced with evidence-based methods by the NIH is the Seventh Report of the Joint National Committee on Prevention, Detection, Evaluation, and Treatment of High Blood Pressure (JNC 7).[27]

Guideline development procedures that can be considered evidence-based were first used in the late 1970s by the Canadian Task Force on Preventive Health Care (formerly known as the Canadian Task Force on the Periodic Health Examination).[28] The U.S. Preventive Services Task Force (USPSTF), which was first convened by the U.S. Public Health Service in 1984, adapted the Canadian Task Force methodology and also uses a systematic evidence-based methodology to review the evidence of effectiveness of clinical preventive services.[29] The USPSTF efforts culminated in the 1989 *Guide to Clinical Preventive Services*. A second edition of the *Guide* was published in 1996. For the third edition of the *Guide*, recommendations are being released incrementally as they become available as periodic updates at the following Web site: http://www.uspreventiveservicestaskforce. org/recommendations.htm

The most influential early publications on evidence-based guideline development methods were the writings of Eddy,[30-33] and the *Manual for Clinical Practice Guideline Development* prepared by the Agency for Healthcare Research and Quality (AHRQ) (the agency was known as the Agency for Healthcare Policy and Research [AHCPR] at that time).[34] Even though the AHRQ no longer produces guidelines directly, the methodology has been adopted, and in some cases slightly modified, by other groups. The AHCPR evidence-based guideline methodology is still recognized as a rigorous valid method. Most major guideline development programs in the United States, as well as those internationally, use an evidence-based process.[35] Examples of some of these organizations in the United States include the American College of Cardiology (ACC) / American Heart Association (AHA),[36] the American College of Rheumatology,[37] the American College of Chest Physicians (ACCP),[38] the American Academy of Pediatrics,[39] and the Infectious Diseases Society of America (IDSA).[40] Prominent international guideline development groups have published methodologies that focus on evidence-based principles. These programs include the National Institute for Clinical Excellence (NICE) in the United Kingdom,[41] the New Zealand Guidelines Group (NZGG),[42] and the Scottish Intercollegiate Guidelines Network (SIGN).[43]

Considering that the AHRQ had a large role in the development of evidence-based guideline methods, additional information about this agency is helpful for understanding current issues regarding guidelines. This agency was created in November 1989, when Congress amended the Public Health Service Act. Under the terms of Public Law 101-239 (also known as Omnibus Budget Reconciliation Act of 1989, OBRA'89) this agency was given responsibility for supporting research, data development, and other activities to "enhance the quality, appropriateness, and effectiveness of health care services." The AHCPR was also charged with the responsibility to "arrange for" the development and periodic review and updating of (1) clinically relevant guidelines that may be used by physicians, educators, and health care practitioners to assist in determining how diseases, disorders, and other health conditions can most effectively and appropriately be prevented, diagnosed, treated, and managed clinically; and (2) standards of quality, performance measures, and medical review criteria through which health care providers and other appropriate entities may assess or review the provision of health care and assure the quality of such care.[44] That legislation also reflected the increased importance of quality, safety, and access issues in national health policy and elevated the activities of the AHCPR to the level of a full Public Health Service (PHS) agency; on the same level as the Centers for Disease Control (CDC) and Prevention, the National Institutes of Health (NIH), and the Food and Drug Administration (FDA).

Between 1990 and 1996, the AHCPR-supported panels produced 19 clinical practice guidelines. However, the agency discontinued the guideline development program in the fall of 1996 after political conflicts developed based on recommendations in some of these guidelines. It was also recognized that convening separate national panels to develop each guideline was expensive and time-consuming. The demand for evidence-based information far exceeded the resources that could be devoted to the guideline development program. Furthermore, the agency recognized that many professional organizations, health plans, and commercial firms were producing thousands of guidelines. Therefore, the agency initiated the *Evidence-Based Practice Program*, and now serves as a science partner with private- and public-sector organizations to develop evidence reports. Evidence reports are based on comprehensive reviews and rigorous analysis of relevant scientific evidence. These reports are intended for use as the scientific foundation for public and private organizations to develop tools (including guidelines, technology assessments, and quality indicators) for improving quality of care.

The methodology developed by the AHRQ has influenced all major guideline development programs. The description of guideline development methods provided in this chapter are based primarily on the early publications of guideline methods that were mentioned above, and the publications on guideline development methods from the ACCP,[38-47] the NICE in the United Kingdom,[41] the NZGG,[42] and the SIGN.[43] Each publication dealing with methods for evidence-based guideline development describes a multistep process (see Appendices 7–1 and 7–2 for examples of the steps described for different programs). Major steps common in the evidence-based guideline development process used by these major organizations include the following:

- Select an appropriate topic for creation of a guideline.
- Recruit appropriate multidisciplinary membership for a panel to be involved in development of the guideline.
- Define the clinical questions to be addressed.
- Determine the criteria for evidence that will be considered.
- Conduct a systematic search for the qualifying evidence.
- Perform a systematic evaluation and grading of the evidence.
- Prepare a synthesis of the evidence.
- Agree on procedures for a consensus process, or other procedures for making recommendations, in the absence of higher levels of evidence for decision-making.
- Formulate and grade recommendations based on the grade of evidence and balance of benefits, harms, and costs of treatment options.
- Draft the guideline document.
- Conduct peer-review and pilot testing of the guideline.
- Revise the guideline as appropriate.
- Create tools for implementation of the guideline.
- Establish a plan for follow-up and periodic updating of the guideline.

Additional details for each of these steps are described below. The description provided for evidence-based guideline development provided in this chapter incorporates the recommendations from several groups. Not all groups describe all procedures or methods included in this chapter. If the reader wishes to review the specific details of a single organization's procedures for guideline development, the references provided should be consulted. Readers who wish to examine other details of guideline development that are not addressed in this chapter, such as organizational details for coordination of the guideline development, group work planning, a development timeline, and other administrative steps, which are beyond the methodology issues discussed in this chapter, should consult the references provided. A systematic review of evidence represents a substantial amount of the work that goes into development of a clinical practice guideline; therefore, guides for creating a systematic review are also valuable for anyone involved in performing this work. Two such excellent guides are the *Cochrane Handbook for Systematic Reviews of Interventions,*[48] and the *Centre for Reviews and Dissemination Guidance for those Carrying Out or Commissioning Reviews.*[49]

SELECT A TOPIC FOR GUIDELINE DEVELOPMENT

Selection of a topic for guideline development has aspects in common with selection of topics for a medication use evaluation program or in a broader sense for any quality improvement program. Considering that guidelines are intended to improve the quality of care process and outcomes of care, it is important to consider the potential to achieve this improvement when a topic is chosen. As with a clinical management decision, the potential benefits of development and implementation of a guideline should be assessed. Disease conditions with the maximum potential for benefit from guideline development and implementation share common characteristics, including the following:

- High prevalence
- High frequency and/or severity of associated morbidity or mortality
- Availability of high-quality evidence for the efficacy of treatments that reduce morbidity or mortality
- Feasibility of implementation of the treatment based on expertise and other resources required
- Potential cost-effectiveness
- Evidence that current practice is not optimal
- Evidence of practice variation
- Availability of personnel, expertise, and resources to develop and implement the practice guideline

As an example, the AHA/ACC identified the following reasons for developing evidence-based guidelines for cardiovascular disease prevention in women:[50]

- Cardiovascular disease remains the leading killer of women in the United States.
- Because coronary heart disease (CHD) is often fatal, and two-thirds of women who die suddenly have no previously recognized symptoms, it is essential to prevent CHD.
- In the wake of the reports of the Women's Health Initiative (WHI) and the Heart and Estrogen/Progestin Replacement Study (HERS), there is a heightened need to critically review and document strategies to prevent CHD in women.
- There has been an increase in the number and proportion of women who have participated in clinical trials, which provides more evidence of efficacy of different treatment strategies.
- Because patients seen in clinical practice may have characteristics that are not similar to those of clinical trial participants, it is necessary to evaluate the ability to apply these data in practice.

Individual guideline development programs will also use criteria for selecting a topic for guideline development that will maximize the potential benefit for the stakeholders that program serves. For an example of these criteria, see Appendix 7–3, criteria for selecting topics used by the NICE in the United Kingdom.[51] In addition to the characteristics mentioned above, the potential to achieve improvements in care by implementing a guideline in a practice depends on characteristics related to the individual practice. For example, has a recognized leader been identified to promote implementation of the guideline within the organization and to make sure it will proceed in a timely fashion? Also, achievement of improvement in care is more likely to be realized if there are systems in place to allow the change to be measured, and to provide feedback to individuals and to the implementation team.

RECRUIT APPROPRIATE MULTIDISCIPLINARY MEMBERSHIP FOR A PANEL TO BE INVOLVED IN DEVELOPMENT OF THE GUIDELINE

❹ *Once a topic for guideline development has been selected, a multidisciplinary panel of health care practitioners associated with the topic should be formed to develop the practice guideline. Steps involving guideline development include defining the clinical questions to be addressed, determine criteria for evidence to be included, conduct systematic search for the evidence, perform systematic evaluation and grading of the evidence, and prepare a synthesis of the evidence.*

The development of a clinical practice guideline should be a multidisciplinary process. Ideally, all groups that have a stake in the development and implementation of a guideline are represented in the process. Participants should include physicians with special expertise in the condition being considered; primary care practitioners involved in treatment of patients with the identified condition; representatives of other health disciplines involved in providing care for the identified condition (e.g., pharmacy, physical therapy, respiratory therapy, nursing, occupational therapy, social work, dentistry); experts in research methods applicable to the topic; individuals, such as drug information specialists, with expertise in conducting a systematic search for evidence; individuals with administrative, health services, economics, and other health care systems expertise; and patient representatives or caregivers. Organizational skills, project management, and editorial ability are also key to the success of a guideline program. As an example, the AHA/ACC selected the following panel membership to produce evidence-based guidelines for cardiovascular disease prevention in women[50]:

> the leaders of each of the 13 AHA Scientific Councils were asked to nominate a recognized expert in cardiovascular disease (CVD) prevention with particular knowledge about women; the president of the AHA appointed at large members to fill gaps in specific areas of expertise; the AHA Manuscript Oversight Committee approved the chair of the expert panel; major professional or government organizations with a mission consistent with CVD prevention were solicited to serve as cosponsors and were asked to nominate one representative to serve on the expert panel; diverse professionals and community organizations were also suggested to endorse the final document after its approval by the AHA Scientific Advisory Coordinating Committee and cosponsoring organizations.[50]

Individuals being considered for membership on a guideline development panel should also be asked to declare potential conflicts of interest. Individuals with a potential conflict of interest may still be considered for participation on a panel depending on the type and degree of conflict, along with appropriate levels of management and disclosure.[52] Rigid, complete exclusion of any possible conflict could result in guideline panels excluding the majority of individuals with the critical expertise needed. Surveys have shown the need for attention to this issue as guideline authors frequently have some relationship with pharmaceutical manufacturers.[53] The controversy that may occur has been manifest with challenges voiced regarding the sponsorship of guideline development and publication,[54] and potential conflicts of interest by panel members.[55] Public criticism of potential conflicts of interest by panel members involved in the NCEP Expert Panel on Detection, Evaluation, and Treatment of High Blood Cholesterol in Adults (ATP III) prompted a response from Barbara Alving, MD, Acting Director, National Heart, Lung, and Blood Institute (NHLBI). She issued a statement on July 29, 2004,[56] another on September 24, 2004,[57] and an 11-page letter on October 22, 2004,[58] to explain the development and review methodology used by the panel, defend the integrity of the process, and the scientific basis for the recommendations.

Expertise in guideline development methods that facilitate implementation of practice guidelines would also be valuable to the panel. Substantial research has been conducted in the past 10 years to identify methods of guideline implementation and guideline characteristics that facilitate adherence.[59] Recognized characteristics of guidelines that facilitate implementation include aspects of format, provision of clear unambiguous recommendations, and ability to incorporate the guideline recommendations into a decision support tool. These characteristics should be considered during the production process when possible. For example, significant progress has been made in translating document-based knowledge into systems or tools that can be conveniently integrated in the normal clinical workflow.[60] In order to accomplish this, Shiffman and colleagues (http://gem.med.yale.edu/default.htm) have developed a Guideline Elements Model (GEM II) for translation of the typical document-based clinical practice guideline into a format that can be integrated into clinical workflow with computerized decision support systems.[60] This method attempts to deal with guidelines that lack explicit definitions, contain excessive ambiguity, do not consider sequencing or timing of interventions, do not account for important patient-specific variables, lack prioritization of key recommendations, and otherwise do not include all parameters that must be considered for decision-making. Attention to these details is needed for computer decision support systems because they work best when clear dichotomous responses can be made one at a time to reach the desired endpoint. Ambiguity, lack of prioritization, and lack of required variables present significant obstacles to computerized decision support systems. It is also worth considering that the process of decision-making in health care is not always well understood, and in some instances it may not be possible to create the explicit linear process just described. If that is the case, it may be necessary for the guideline panel to recommend reconsideration of the specific questions to be addressed by the guideline. Or it may be necessary for the panel to make other specific recommendations about how best to implement the guideline in a way to facilitate adoption.

However, even with the advantages offered by information technology, there are potential barriers created by the technology itself that should be considered in guideline implementation plans.[61] Lyons and colleagues identified that physicians, nurses, and administrators perceive some aspects of the use of information technology for guideline implementation as facilitators and others as barriers. Information technology can facilitate guideline implementation because computerization may improve accessibility of some information, may facilitate documentation, assist with guideline updating, and provide useful decision support tools. However, there may be barriers to guideline implementation when there are problems with computer literacy, availability of equipment, and computer glitches or downtime. Lyons also identified that the different disciplines had opposing opinions on the overall importance and reality in the work place for some of these elements.[61] Consideration of these facilitators and barriers during the development process can ultimately improve the success of implementation.

Finally, techniques as simple as writing guidelines with concrete, precise behavioral terms (what, who, when, where, and how) may be effective to achieve guideline adherence.[62] Ensuring that the guideline development panel includes members with expertise to address each of these issues is important to maximize the desired endpoint, a well-constructed guideline that will be followed by practitioners and patients.

DEFINE THE CLINICAL QUESTIONS TO BE ADDRESSED

After the disease or condition is selected and the panel with applicable expertise is formed, the panel will accomplish the next step; further definition of the specific issues for which recommendations will ultimately be provided. The panel will consider what specific decision-making or action steps related to surveillance or screening for the disease, diagnosis, or treatment can be improved with specific recommendations. The decision-making points can be expressed as clinical questions. The definition of the clinical questions to be addressed by a guideline is a key step that provides direction for the activities to follow. The questions are important to provide direction to the systematic review of the literature, and also provide the outline for the recommendations that the guideline will provide. The importance of this phase cannot be overemphasized. Just as in the systematic approach to a drug information question, it is critical to first clearly define the question to be successful in searching for the necessary evidence, and subsequently be able to provide useful valid conclusions.

A clear description of the questions to be addressed by the guideline is also a good starting point for practitioners to determine if a guideline could be useful in their practice. Depending on the overall goals of a guideline, questions may be about prognosis, the best diagnostic test, methods of screening, what forms of treatment or prevention are most effective, quantification of the potential harms of treatment, what comorbidities change recommendations, or what costs are associated with different management strategies. Many of the guideline development groups use the PICO format for framing the questions, which includes the following parts:

- Patients: Which patients are being considered for the question, how can they be described, and are there any subgroups that require special consideration? (Similar to inclusion and exclusion criteria in a clinical study, however, usually not as restrictive.)
- Interventions: Which intervention or treatment should be considered?
- Comparison: What are the main alternatives that should be compared with the intervention?
- Outcome: What is most important to the patient (e.g., mortality, morbidity, treatment complications, rates of relapse, physical function, quality of life, and costs)?

Another format for question framework used by some groups is PECOT. The additional part added for this question format is Time, (i.e., over what timeframe are the benefits or the outcomes of care expected to occur?) In this format the E represents Exposure: which may be treatment, a risk factor, or management approach of interest.

The clinical questions should define the relevant patient population, the management strategies that will and will not be considered, and the outcomes of care that the guideline intends to achieve. In addition, the guideline development panel should describe the care setting for use of the guideline, for example, primary care, secondary care, or tertiary referral centers. All the questions that are necessary for consideration of patient management in a given clinical scenario are delineated to make sure that the recommendations provided by the guideline will be of sufficient scope to avoid important gaps in decision-making. There is no specific standard for the number of questions required for each guideline; however, most guideline development groups state that if the number exceeds 30, or in some cases 40 questions, it may be necessary to break the guideline into subtopics.

In some instances, a preliminary review of the literature may be necessary to assist with delineation of the focused clinical questions to be considered in the guideline. Clinical experts in the field as well as patients provide critical input in formulating the clinical questions. The SIGN places particular emphasis on obtaining input from patients. They obtain published studies, both qualitative and quantitative, that reflect patients' and caregivers' experiences and preferences in relation to the clinical topic. The program manager presents a summarized report of these findings to the panel at their first meeting to underline the significance of patient needs and preferences in the guideline development.

DETERMINE THE CRITERIA FOR EVIDENCE

It is necessary to define the admissible evidence; that is, the types of published or unpublished research to be considered so that an appropriate literature search may be performed. Key words from the focused clinical questions define the types of patients, interventions, comparators, and outcomes of studies that are considered to provide useful evidence. The guideline panel may decide that it will consider evidence from previous guidelines, meta-analyses or systematic reviews, and randomized-controlled trials. The panel may also decide to consider evidence from observational studies, diagnostic studies, economic studies, and qualitative studies. This direction is necessary for the information specialists that will conduct the search for evidence. Detailed criteria are also important in this step so that evidence will be retrieved and selected for inclusion in the review with a minimum of bias, so that the search is reproducible, and so that the entire process is as transparent as possible. In most cases, more than one person is involved in searching for evidence and selecting evidence for consideration in the review. Clear criteria must be used so that there is consistency among all individuals involved in this process. Inconsistency in the retrieval of evidence between evaluators would add a significant potential for bias in the review.

The process to define admissible evidence may also be revisited at a later stage of guideline development depending on the results of the initial search. It is conceivable, and in fact not uncommon, that based on the initial review of evidence, the questions may be modified or new questions formed, and a decision may be made to expand the scope of admissible evidence. Documentation of these decisions, and the reasons for any changes, is another indicator of a guideline that has been developed with rigorous methods. The Cochrane Collaboration recommends the following considerations when a change in the review questions or criteria for admissible evidence is made:

- What is the motivation for the refinement?
- Was it made after you had seen and been influenced by results from a particular study or was it simply that you had not initially considered alternate but acceptable ways of defining the participants, interventions, or outcomes of interest?
- Are your search strategies appropriate for the refined question (especially any that have already been undertaken)?
- Is your data collection tailored to the refined question?[48]

Case Study 7–1

You have been selected to lead the formation of a panel to be involved in the development of clinical practice guidelines in your institution. No additional information or guidance has been provided to you. As you sit in your office thinking about the many different activities that are going to be required of this panel, what are the first four steps that should be performed and what do they entail?

CONDUCT A SYSTEMATIC SEARCH FOR THE QUALIFYING EVIDENCE

Evidence-based guidelines require that all relevant evidence be located and appraised; therefore, a thorough literature search must be conducted. Many of the guideline development groups will first conduct a search to identify previously completed guidelines or systematic reviews of the same or closely related questions. The literature retrieval process should include a search of the available bibliographic resources such as MEDLINE, Current Contents, Embase, Science Citation Index, Cochrane Library, and Cummulative Index to Nursing and Allied Health Literature (CINAHL). A number of specialized databases exist and should be considered depending on the subject of the search. Also evidence may be obtained from citations listed in published bibliographies, textbooks, and any literature that may be identified by researchers and other individuals on the expert list that the panel may create. Specific keywords and other search constraints, for example MeSH (Medical Subject Headings from MEDLINE) terms, limits by publication year, language, randomized-controlled trials or other study types, and so forth should be recorded to allow verification of the process. Each retrieved article should then be judged for its relevance and compliance to criteria for inclusion as predetermined by the panel. When possible, it is helpful to have more than one reviewer judge the inclusion of studies. A log should be kept of excluded studies and the rationale for their rejection. The Centre for Reviews and Dissemination (CRD) has created a flow diagram to illustrate steps involved in selecting studies for inclusion in a systematic review (see Appendix 7–4). The CRD has also identified key points for consideration in this process (see Appendix 7–5).

A review of all the details regarding search strategies, such as controlled vocabulary searching, text word searching, truncation of terms, use of the vocabulary tree structures to explore select terms, and adjacency of terms are beyond the scope of this chapter. Most guideline development groups use highly trained methodologists and librarians to perform this critical search for evidence. Drug information specialists are also well qualified to complete these tasks. A carefully planned and executed search is necessary to obtain a result that is very sensitive to avoid missing important evidence and at the same time as specific as possible to avoid the requirement to manually screen many irrelevant citations. The Cochrane Collaboration has developed detailed search strategies and filters for use in conducting searches for literature.[48] The Cochrane Collaboration has also made specific recommendations for guideline developers for documentation of the search process; for example, for the search of an electronic data set the following should be documented:

- Title of database searched (e.g., MEDLINE).
- Name of the host (e.g., EBSCO Host).
- Date search was run (month, day, year).
- Years covered by the search.
- Complete search strategy used, including all search terms (preferably electronically cut and pasted rather than retyped).

- One or two sentence summary of the search strategy indicating which lines of the search strategy were used to identify records related to the health condition and intervention, and which lines were used to identify studies of the appropriate design.
- The absence of any language restrictions.[48]

Other details that should be documented include search methods for obtaining conference proceedings, hand searching of selected resources, whether the guideline developers contacted other methodologists or researchers to ask for references or to obtain information about unpublished studies, whether contact is made with product manufacturers for additional data, and any other efforts made to obtain published or unpublished evidence.

PERFORM A SYSTEMATIC EVALUATION AND GRADING OF THE EVIDENCE

There are a variety of methods for evaluating individual studies, many of which are discussed in other sections of this text. The purpose of this process is to identify issues with the trial design or any biases that would affect internal or external validity. Issues to consider include the basic trial design (i.e., randomized, controlled, clinical trial, cohort study, and case-control study), sample size, statistical power, selection bias, inclusion/exclusion criteria, choice of control group, randomization methods, comparability of groups, definition of exposure or intervention, definition of outcome measures, accuracy and appropriateness of outcome measures, attrition rates, data collection methods, methods of statistical analysis, confounding variables, unique characteristics of the study population, and adequacy of blinding. Formal methods may also be used to assign a quality score to each trial. Other factors considered in the overall body of evidence, for example, are the results of different trials consistent with each other or is there significant heterogeneity. The amount of evidence is also an important consideration—how many individuals have been evaluated over what length of time. The amount of available evidence is particularly important in consideration of the safety of treatments. Potentially serious adverse events that occur infrequently will not be identified in a database that does not contain a sufficient sample size or in a sample population that is too narrowly defined.

Many additional issues of evaluation of evidence are provided in other chapters in this text and will not be repeated here. There are other resources available to provide assistance with methods for this critical process. Each of the guideline development manuals that have been described in this chapter include significant sections on evaluation of the evidence.[1,41-43] The *Cochrane Handbook for Systematic Reviews of Interventions*[48] (available to download at http://www.cochrane.org/training/cochrane-handbook), and the Centre for Reviews and Dissemination Guidance for those Carrying Out or Commissioning

Reviews, are particularly useful for this purpose.[49] In addition, the AHRQ commissioned the Research Triangle Institute–University of North Carolina Evidenced-Based Practice Center to "prepare a report on methods or systems to assess health care research results, particularly methods or systems to rate the strength of the scientific evidence underlying health care practice, recommendations in the research literature, and technology assessments."[63] The overarching goals of this project were to "describe systems to rate the strength of scientific evidence, including evaluating the quality of individual articles that make up a body of evidence on a specific scientific question in health care, and to provide some guidance as to 'best practices' in this field today."[63] This report can be obtained at http://www.ahrq.gov/clinic/epcindex.htm, for a downloadable zip file, or http://www.ncbi.nlm.nih.gov/books/bv.fcgi?rid=hstat1.chapter.70996 for online access via the Health Services Technology/ Assessment Texts (HSTAT). HSTAT is a free, Web-based resource of full-text documents that provide health information and support health care decision-making.

Evaluation of the evidence, and grading of the recommendations, are critical aspects for users of guidelines to understand in order to appropriately interpret the recommendations. Because these aspects are critical to users of guidelines, a separate expanded section on the topic of Interpretation of Guideline Recommendations is provided in another section of this chapter.

PREPARE A SYNTHESIS OF THE EVIDENCE

❺ *Synthesis of the evidence from selected studies is most useful to the practitioner when summarized in format that facilitates consideration of individual study characteristics and quality, consistency of results between studies, size of the evidence database, and treatment effect size regarding benefits and harm. When high quality of evidence is unavailable, a summary of identified evidence is often provided with no specific recommendation or in some cases a consensus method is considered to derive a recommendation.*

The evidence from the selected studies should be summarized in a format that facilitates consideration of the characteristics and quality of individual studies, the consistency of the results between studies, the overall size of the evidence database, and the size of the treatment effects for benefits and harms. These key concepts for consideration in synthesis of evidence have been described by the CRD (see Appendix 7–6). The NICE has a standard format that they recommend for evidence tables (see Appendix 7–7). Most guideline development groups use a similar format. If the necessary evidence is available, it may be appropriate to perform a meta-analysis to present the summary estimate of the size of a treatment effect. Readers interested in a detailed description of meta-analysis may wish to consult the *Cochrane Handbook for Systematic Reviews of Interventions.*[48]

Formal methods for grading the quality of the evidence should be used as described above. The level of evidence assigned to each study is included in the evidence table. A detailed description of a consensus recommendation for methods to grade the quality of evidence and strength of guideline recommendations is provided in the section on Interpretation of Guideline Recommendations in this chapter.

The SIGN group and the NZGG use a form to document how the evidence synthesis was used to reach guideline recommendations. This process is called considered judgment. See Appendix 7–8 for a representation of the considered judgment form.

Methods for incorporation of economic evidence in practice guidelines are not well developed. In some instances, the ability to employ economic evaluations from one setting to another is very limited. The SIGN stated in their March 2004 guideline developers' handbook that none of the approaches to incorporation of resource use were regarded as sufficiently well proven or appropriate for SIGN methodology.[43] The SIGN does, however, include published economic studies in evidence tables, and uses a structured method to evaluate this evidence. They also have a form similar to the considered judgment form mentioned above that can be used to present information relating to economic issues associated with guideline implementation. In addition, they may include a commentary on economic issues in the published guideline.

The NICE includes a six-page chapter on incorporating health economics in their guidelines development manual.[41] The NICE utilizes a health economist as a core member of their guideline development team. They use the process of cost-effectiveness analysis to maximize the health gain by incorporating both costs and health benefits in the analysis. NICE may utilize published economic evidence, or may carry out or commission a cost-effectiveness or cost-utility analysis (see Chapter 6 for further information on these analyses). Formal quality appraisal and synthesis of the economic evidence is also performed, just as it is with epidemiologic or clinical study data, using study-type specific checklists. In regard to economic analysis, NICE employs the following general principles:

- An economic analysis should be underpinned by the best-quality clinical evidence.
- There should be the highest level of transparency in the reporting of methods.
- Uncertainty (around both internal and external validity) should be discussed fully and explored by sensitivity analysis (and, where data allow, statistical analysis).
- Limitations of the approach and methods taken should be fully discussed.
- Conventions on reporting economic evaluations should be followed (see Drummond and Jefferson[64]).
- Analysis should be carried out in collaboration between the health economist and the rest of the guideline development group.[41]

Users of practice guidelines should examine the document for inclusion of economic information. The primary concern should be to identify the methods used for obtaining and evaluating the economic information, and in what way, if any, the economic information was used in formulating recommendations for patient care.

AGREE ON PROCEDURES FOR A CONSENSUS PROCESS, OR OTHER PROCEDURES FOR MAKING RECOMMENDATIONS, IN THE ABSENCE OF HIGHER LEVELS OF EVIDENCE FOR DECISION-MAKING

In the absence of high levels of evidence, some guideline development groups will elect to state that the evidence for making a recommendation is inconclusive and will simply provide a summary of that evidence with no specific recommendation. Other guideline groups will consider a variety of consensus methods, to derive a recommendation. There is no one method for consensus that is considered the standard for this process. For more information about consensus methods, the reader may wish to review material in the guideline development references,[41-43] or the NIH Consensus Development Program Web site at http://consensus.nih.gov.

The key aspect for users of a guideline is to note the description of consensus methods, and to be certain to distinguish guideline recommendations that are made on the basis of high levels of evidence as opposed to those based on consensus only. A variety of designations are used by different guideline development groups to make this distinction. See Appendix 7–9 for a table from the Ontario Guidelines Advisory Committee (GAC), which shows a variety of designations used by nine guideline development groups. Guideline recommendations that are based on consensus opinion are generally considered the least reliable recommendations. They are suggestions for consideration and not standards for care.

Case Study 7–2

Building on the previous case, you have formed a practice guideline panel consisting of members from your institution with a vested interest. The first practice guideline for the panel to create has been identified along with clinical questions and criteria for the evidence to be used in creating this guideline. As the panel moves forward, what are the next three steps that should be performed and what does each step entail?

FORMULATE AND GRADE RECOMMENDATIONS BASED ON THE GRADE OF EVIDENCE AND BALANCE OF BENEFITS, HARMS, AND COSTS OF TREATMENT OPTIONS

❻ *Once synthesis is completed, recommendations are developed based on quality of evidence, benefits, harms, and costs. A draft guideline document is then prepared from these recommendations, tested by pilot peer-review, revised based on feedback, and implementation strategies devised with follow-up and guideline updating plans established.*

The details of this process are provided below in the section titled Interpretation of Guideline Recommendations. The specific recommendations in a guideline must be worded carefully, and must clearly communicate the confidence that the guideline panel has that the expected outcomes will be achieved if the recommendations are followed. Because many guideline users do not read the full guideline document, the recommendations should be written to stand alone as much as possible. NICE provides the following guidance regarding the wording of the recommendations (with slight modifications):

- Recommendations should stand alone.
- Recommendations should be action oriented.
- All recommendations should be assigned a grade (though these are not shown for the key priorities).
- Recommendations referring to drug use should use the generic drug name, avoid stating dosages, and indicate where the recommendation refers to off-label use.
- Tables can be used to present recommendations but only where this substantially improves clarity.
- Recommendations should take the patient into consideration and should try to avoid the use of words such as subjects rather than people or patients.[41]

DRAFT THE GUIDELINE DOCUMENT

The basis of the draft document is provided by the evidence tables and the graded recommendations. A formal narrative summary should also be provided with all relevant details of decisions made in the development of the guideline. It is highly desirable for the finished guideline to include details of the scope of the guideline including target patient population, restrictions on the population, interventions considered, specific outcomes or performance measures, who are the intended users of the guideline (e.g., specialty and care setting), and the overall objective of the guideline. A clear description of authorship, sponsorship, and any potential conflicts of interest should be provided. A detailed description of all production methods used (as detailed in this chapter), decision-making methods, recommendations for consideration in applying the guideline in practice (e.g., patient variables, setting, provider, and estimates of how the effects of these factors will alter outcomes are helpful for users to apply the guidelines locally), comments about ongoing studies which may affect recommendations, and any plans for updating the guideline. A detailed structure for a guideline as recommended by NICE is provided in Appendix 7–10.

Considering publication length limitations, some guideline producers are using Internet Web sites to provide some of the details recommended for finished guidelines. For example, the AHA/ACC Evidence-Based Guidelines for Cardiovascular Disease Prevention in Women uses the following Web site to provide access to the evidence tables: http://www.cardiosource.org/Science-And-Quality/Practice-Guidelines-and-Quality-Standards.aspx.

It is also desirable for a guideline to be written in different formats and levels of detail for different audiences and purposes. Many guideline developers produce quick reference guides, which give the essentials of the recommendations without the detailed background. These documents are more convenient to use as quick reminders and decision aids in a patient-care setting than a full guideline document. It is important, however, for users of the quick reference guides to review the full document before deciding that the guideline is one that is valid for their use, and to recognize any specific limitations in how they may wish to use that particular guideline. Another format that is useful is a guideline summary that may be used for a patient education purposes. As an example of the different formats, the Seventh Report of the Joint National Committee on Prevention, Detection, Evaluation, and Treatment of High Blood Pressure (JNC VII) was produced with a quick reference card (available at http://www.nhlbi.nih.gov/guidelines/hypertension/jnc7card.htm). There are also two different versions of the guideline document: an express version[65] and the complete version.[27] These two versions of the guideline, as well as patient education materials, media and press materials, and files for use on a PDA, are also available for download at the NHLBI Web site http://www.nhlbi.nih.gov/guidelines/hypertension/index.htm.

In preparation of the Seventh ACCP Conference on Antithrombotic and Thrombolytic Therapy, four editors (two methodologists and two content experts) worked with several authors for each chapter.[38] A number of drafts were prepared for each chapter with revisions recommended by each of the authors using a Web site to post recommendations to each other. At the conference, authors worked together to finalize and harmonize potentially controversial recommendations. Plenary meetings were also held to obtain feedback from other chapter authors for consideration of the guideline recommendations. "Authors continued this process after the conference until they reached agreement within their groups and with other group authors who provided critical feedback."[38]

Reaching clear decisions on recommendations for clinical practices is often difficult because the data are not adequate to clearly label the practice appropriate or inappropriate. Unfortunately, many practices fall into this gray zone category because of uncertainties about the benefits and harms, variability in patients and in their responses to treatment, and differences in patient preferences about the desirability of outcomes and aversion to risk. The use of rigid language in an effort to produce clear-cut recommendations can be dangerous, particularly when presented as simplistic algorithms that fail to recognize the complexity of medical decision-making and the need for individual clinical judgment. This danger can be avoided by describing uncertainty and providing broad boundaries for appropriate practice that allows for legitimate differences of opinion. Attempts to develop rigid guidelines, when the data are not conclusive, is clearly worse than having no written guidelines.

It is important to consider the information needs of the guideline's user. Practitioners will want specific, quantitative estimates of the relevant health outcomes if a recommendation is followed, a statement of the strength of the evidence and expert judgment supporting the guidelines, information on patient preferences, projections of cost, details of the reasoning behind the recommendations, and the ability to review the data independently if they so choose. Guidelines should be written such that they may be perceived as an explanation of the thinking process that is used in evaluating and applying the information. If guidelines are perceived as information only, they may be rejected as the cookbooks that practitioners fear guidelines will become. Such guidelines would also not achieve the educational goals to focus further research efforts (outcomes research or other) on gaps in the current evidence. The Manual for ACC/AHA Guideline Writing Committees Methodologies and Policies from the ACC/AHA Task Force on Practice Guidelines includes the following checklist for guideline authors to review the draft recommendations:

- Are the recommendations within the stated purpose and scope of the guideline?
- Are all recommendations cited and referenced (either in the text or in the evidence table)?
- Are all recommendations assigned a Classification of Recommendation and a Level of Evidence?
- Are clinically important and feasible recommendations made?
- Are areas of uncertainty and exceptions to the rule clearly identified?
- Are evidence tables and appropriate text provided to support recommendations, where applicable?
- Are recommendations and key clinical points displayed visually, when possible?[36]

Depending on the subject of the clinical practice guideline, more or less emphasis may be placed on the various sections of the guideline document. In addition, recommendations for future research may be included with the document. The process of developing practice guidelines often calls attention to the gaps in scientific information. The direction provided for future research is one of the important results of the practice guideline development process. Practice guidelines that fail to address research priorities may discourage innovation and negatively influence funding decisions for needed research in the involved area. For the few examples that exist in which clear answers are already provided by high-quality scientific evidence, waste of research resources may be avoided by stopping generation of data that would not increase understanding of a disease process or its treatment.

CONDUCT PEER-REVIEW AND PILOT TESTING OF THE GUIDELINE

Each guideline development group has its own methods for obtaining peer-review and feedback on the draft guidelines. In some cases, the peer-review is confined within that organization, in other groups specific requests will be made for review from targeted organizations, and in some guideline development groups open input from any interested party is sought by public notice. For example, SIGN holds a national open meeting that is widely publicized. This meeting is usually attended by 150 to 300 health care professionals and others interested in the guideline topic. The draft guideline is also available on the SIGN Web site for a limited time period to permit contributions to be submitted. Participation in the draft of the guideline can give a sense of ownership to the broader audience and may be a positive factor in the implementation of the guideline. SIGN also utilizes independent expert referees who are asked to comment on specific aspects of the guideline. In addition, they send the guideline for review by a non-health care professional to get comments from the patients' perspective. See Appendix 7–11 for a figure representing the consultation and peer-review steps used by SIGN.

The next step may be pretesting the guideline in practice settings. The pretesting panel should be given clear instructions on the observations that would be considered most useful and be asked to keep written notes of their experiences, observations, and suggestions. A summary report of these observations is provided to the development panel. In the final revision steps, the panel should examine all review comments and pretesting results in an unbiased fashion. A disposition record that documents how each recommendation was handled and the rationale for inclusion or exclusion in the final document should be kept. However, not all groups conduct pilot testing. For example, SIGN considers that pilot testing is more appropriate at a local level and leaves this to be done by local groups as part of their implementation process.

The guideline development process may be viewed in the philosophy of CQI from several aspects. The methodology emphasizes building quality in the production process, use of scientific principles and data, and plans to conduct follow-up studies on the outcomes of the use of the guideline, which are then used to update and improve the guideline.

REVISE THE GUIDELINE AS APPROPRIATE

Based on feedback from the peer-review process and any pilot testing of the application of the guideline, revisions may be required for the guideline to meet its intended goals. As with many steps in the guideline development process, one of the keys in this step is documentation. The decisions and actions taken in response to the recommendations from external review should be carefully documented. It is particularly important, if there are critical recommendations that the guideline panel decides to reject, that the reason for that decision be documented.

CREATE TOOLS FOR IMPLEMENTATION OF THE GUIDELINE

It is helpful if the guideline developers create tools that will assist target groups in the implementation step. A variety of tools may be used, including preparing various formats of the guideline for convenient use in the practice setting, creating guidelines that facilitate automated implementation, algorithms or flow charts that facilitate understanding of the use of the guideline, or educational programs. Many of the activities that the guideline development committee has performed in creating the guideline, careful wording of the recommendations and the documentation of all procedures, are done with this end in mind, that is, implementation. One of the simplest forms of implementation is to make the guideline accessible as freely and as widely as possible. Many of the development groups make the guidelines available as electronic documents and post them for free access on a Web site.

ESTABLISH A PLAN FOR FOLLOW-UP AND PERIODIC UPDATING OF THE GUIDELINE

In most cases, the guideline development group will determine a review interval for consideration to update the guideline. Depending on the topic and knowledge of ongoing studies, it may be reasonable to review the guideline after a period of between 2 and 5 years. However, if it is a topic in which rapid change may occur, more frequent review is necessary. In some instances, the guideline development group will designate a subgroup to monitor the literature and alert the entire group if new evidence becomes available that might necessitate revisions of the guideline recommendations. When it is time to consider updating a guideline, the careful records kept during the production of the previous edition are invaluable.

Interpretation of Guideline Recommendations

❼ *Substantial inconsistencies exist between the many methods used to evaluate the quality of evidence. This can affect the interpretation of the evidence and hence, the quality of recommendations based on this evidence made in various practice guidelines. The practitioner must understand the particular method used with a given guideline to correctly interpret the strength of a guideline recommendation, quality of evidence used to form the recommendation, and balance between benefits and harms of interventions considered.*

As mentioned previously, proper evaluation of a guideline and interpretation of the recommendations requires knowledge of methods for development. Interpretation of the recommendations in a guideline requires detailed understanding of the methods used for grading the quality of the evidence, the balance between the benefits and harms, and the strength of the recommendation. This can be difficult because a variety of grading systems are currently in use by different organizations producing guidelines—which creates confusion. If the grading system for the recommendations in a practice guideline is not interpreted correctly, a significant amount of information is lost. In addition, if guideline developers use methods that do not account for all the important decision-making factors, the recommendations cannot be presented with the necessary details. The Grades of Recommendation Assessment Development and Evaluation (GRADE) working group has provided a proposal to standardize the grading methods for the quality of the evidence and the strength of recommendations in practice guidelines.[66] The working group believes that consistent judgments about the quality of evidence and strength of recommendations combined with better communication about those judgments will be achieved by use of the GRADE system. Ultimately, it is believed that this will support better informed choices in health care.[66]

The quality of the evidence that forms the basis for recommendations is a key aspect for interpretation and use of a practice guideline. However, before deciding to implement a guideline recommendation it is also necessary for the user to have information for consideration of the balance between benefits and harms, and the ability to translate the evidence to specific circumstances (i.e., external validity). A system to communicate the strength of a recommendation should consider all of these factors. The designated strength of a recommendation should convey the amount of confidence one can have that adherence to that recommendation will do more good than harm.[66]

Substantial inconsistencies exist in the systems used by different guideline development groups to rate the quality or strength of evidence, and how that information is communicated within the guideline. Different systems may designate the same evidence and recommendation as II-a, B, C+, 1, Level III, or 2++ (see Appendix 7–9 for a comparison of the levels of evidence and grades of recommendation assembled by the Ontario GAC).

Since most health care professionals will encounter guidelines from many different groups, these various grading systems are confusing and reduce their effectiveness in communicating the amount of confidence one should have in a given recommendation.[66]

The GRADE working group began as an informal collaboration of people who recognized the shortcomings of the present grading systems and wished to offer recommendations for improvement.[66] The GRADE working group has conducted an analysis of six prominent grading systems that are used by ACCP, Australian National Health and Medical Research Council (ANHMRC), Oxford Centre for Evidence-based Medicine (OCEBM), SIGN, USPSTF, and U.S. Task Force on Community Preventive Services (USTFCPS).[67] Based on this evaluation, there was general agreement that none of these six systems addressed all of the important concepts and dimensions considered necessary for guideline recommendations. See Appendix 7–12 for a description of the GRADE working group's comparison of the proposed system to the other systems evaluated, including comments about the advantages of the GRADE system.

The system proposed by GRADE starts with explicit definitions of what is meant by quality of evidence and strength of recommendation. "Quality of evidence indicates the extent to which one can be confident that an estimate of effect is correct. The strength of a recommendation indicates the extent to which one can be confident that adherence to the recommendation will do more good than harm."[66] Using the GRADE system requires sequential judgments about the following:

- The validity of the results of individual studies for important outcomes.
- The quality of evidence across studies for each important outcome.
- Which outcomes are critical to a decision?
- The overall quality of evidence across these critical outcomes.
- The balance between benefits and harms.
- The strength of recommendations.

The GRADE system starts with clearly defined clinical questions and considers all outcomes that are important to patients. Each outcome is rated on a scale from low to high importance for a treatment decision as not critical, important, or critical. Critical outcomes are given more weight in the final recommendation than outcomes that are considered important. Outcomes that are considered not critical get little consideration.[66]

The quality of evidence for each outcome should be made on the basis of a systematic review using explicit criteria. The GRADE system recommends four key elements for consideration: (1) study design, (2) quality of study methods and execution, (3) consistency of results across studies, and (4) the directness of application of the results to the patients, interventions, and outcomes of interest. In terms of study design, randomized controlled trials have been considered to provide the highest level of evidence since the first efforts at grading evidence in health care were made by the Canadian Task Force on the Periodic Health Examination.[28] Over the years since that first hierarchy for evidence was described, there have been some refinements in designation of the quality of evidence. Basic study design does not tell the whole story of the quality of evidence. Randomization, when it is used correctly, has tremendous power to reduce the potential bias in the results. However, there are randomized controlled trials in which other aspects of the study design are seriously flawed, and there are observational studies (e.g., follow-up, case-control, interrupted time-series, and controlled before and after) with very strong methods that may produce high-quality evidence. Consideration of the quality of study methods must include criteria such as adequacy of allocation concealment, blinding, and follow-up. The consistency of results between different studies can also add to the confidence that the results are valid. The directness of the results refers to the extent to which the subjects, interventions, and outcomes of a study are similar to the ones of interest for a given treatment recommendation. If study subjects differ from your patients in ways that may predict a different level of response based on factors such as age, gender, race, other comorbidities, or severity of illness, the quality of evidence for your decision-making is not as great. In addition, studies using surrogate treatment outcomes, or intermediate outcomes, are not as reliable for estimation of ultimate treatment benefits. Surrogate outcomes include measurements like changes in bone mineral density rather than incidence of fractures, effects of a medication on the electrocardiogram (ECG) rather than mortality, changes in lipids rather than incidence of coronary artery disease events or mortality. Another example in which indirect evidence must be used is when there are no studies comparing different interventions directly and the evaluation must be made across different studies. This is a common problem with new drugs that have been studied only in comparison to placebo and not to other effective treatments. With this type of evidence comparison, it is difficult to determine which treatment is more effective, and it is even more difficult to estimate the size of a potential treatment difference.[66]

Based on consideration of the four components described above, the GRADE system arrives at a grade of evidence in one of the following categories:

- High: Further research is very unlikely to change the confidence in the estimate of effect.
- Moderate: Further research is likely to have an important impact on the confidence in the estimate of effect and may change the estimate.
- Low: Further research is very likely to have an important impact on the confidence in the estimate of effect and is likely to change the estimate.
- Very low: Any estimate of effect is very uncertain.[66]

Beginning with basic study design, a randomized trial would start with a grade of high, a quasi-randomized trial would start as moderate, an observational study would be low, and any other form of evidence would be graded very low. From that starting level, the grade of evidence could be decreased based on the other components as follows: serious limitations to study quality (subtract one level), very serious limitations to study quality (subtract two levels), important inconsistency between results of different studies (subtract one level), some uncertainty about directness of the evidence (subtract one level), major uncertainty about directness of the evidence (subtract two levels), imprecise or sparse data (subtract one level), and high probability of reporting bias (subtract one level).[66] The working group suggested that data be considered sparse if "the results include just a few events or observations and they are uninformative." In the GRADE system, the data are considered imprecise "if the confidence intervals are so wide that an estimate is consistent with either important harms or important benefits." Reporting bias (also referred to as publication bias) is a common concern in a systematic review as it is well known that small negative trials are less likely to be published than positive trials. This results in a bias in favor of an intervention on the basis of just the evidence that has been reported. Factors that can result in an increase in the grade of the evidence are "a strong measure of association, i.e., a significant relative risk of >2 or <0.5, based on consistent evidence from two or more observational studies with no plausible confounders (add one level); very strong evidence of association, i.e., a significant relative risk of >5 or <0.2, based on direct evidence with no major threats to validity (add two levels); evidence of a dose-response relationship (add one level); all plausible confounders would have reduced the size of the effect (add one level)."[66] All of these adjustments are cumulative, so that if more than one modifier exists for the quality of evidence, each modifier is applied.

The evidence for harms should be graded using the same system as the evidence for benefits. This creates somewhat of a challenge when making judgments about the balance of benefits and harms because the quality of evidence for harms is rarely on the same level as the evidence for benefits. One only has to look at the evidence for harms for rofecoxib (Vioxx) to note that obtaining high-quality evidence about harm is a more difficult process. The magnitude of the balance of the benefits compared to the harms, as well as value judgments of the desirability of the benefits and harms, must also be considered for treatment recommendations. In addition, information should be provided to demonstrate how the evidence translates into specific circumstances, and what adjustments may be necessary for individuals with different baseline risks, or who are receiving treatment in different settings. The GRADE working group recommends the following definitions to categorize the tradeoff between benefits and harms:

- Net benefits: The intervention clearly does more good than harm.
- Tradeoffs: There are important tradeoffs between the benefits and harms.

- Uncertain tradeoffs: It is not clear whether the intervention does more good than harm.
- No net benefits: The intervention clearly does not do more good than harm.[66]

Factors that should be considering in arriving at one of these designations include the estimated size and confidence intervals of the effect for the main outcomes, the quality of the evidence, ability to extrapolate the evidence to different patients or care settings, and uncertainty of the baseline risk of disease events in the population of interest.

Finally, the GRADE system assigns one of the following categories for a recommendation for an intervention:

- Do it (90% to 100% of people are likely to do it).
- Probably do it (60% to 90% of people are likely to do it).
- Maybe do it (40% to 60% of people are likely to do it).
- Probably do not do it (10% to 40% of people are likely to do it).
- Do not do it (0% to 10% of people are likely to do it).[65]

High grades of evidence, combined with net benefits and strong measures of association, would produce a recommendation of do it. High grades of evidence for no net benefits or possibly net harm would produce a recommendation of do not do it. Different grades of evidence and different categorization for the tradeoff of benefits and harms will produce recommendations between these extremes. For the intermediate strength of recommendation, individual patient values, different patient risk factors or circumstances, or different care settings will assume a more prominent role in the decision-making by the patient and the health care practitioner. The advantage of the GRADE system is that all of the evidence that is most important for making the decision has been judged with explicit criteria, the judgments are made transparent, evidence summary tables and balance sheets have been created, consequently facilitating the use of best evidence.

Although the system recommended by the GRADE working group may appear complex, with the number of steps involved, it provides a balance of the need for simplicity with a need for full explicit consideration of important issues in clinical decision-making, as well as transparency for the judgments made in arriving at recommendations. A pilot study on the use of this system identified some issues that warrant further improvements in the system, but on balance it was considered to be clear, understandable, sensible, and met the criteria for providing the communication necessary for guideline recommendations.[68]

Examples of evidence profiles using the GRADE system and additional information about the GRADE working group are available on their Web site http://www.gradeworkinggroup.org/.

The majority of published guidelines do not currently use the GRADE system, or any other system, for recommendations. Therefore for each guideline that is used, practitioners must carefully read the description of the grading scheme used by that particular guideline so that they will correctly interpret the strength of the recommendations, the quality of the evidence, and the balance between benefits and harms of the interventions considered.

Case Study 7–3

The practice guideline panel now has a series of conclusions derived from the summary tables of evidence they have evaluated. It is time to start moving toward the development of the specific practice guideline. What are the steps needed to develop the guideline, and what does each step entail?

Guideline Evaluation Tools

❽ *Determination of the quality of published practice guidelines is crucial before selecting and implementing one in a health care system. A guideline evaluation tool can be extremely helpful in this situation. The Appraisal of Guidelines for Research and Evaluation (AGREE) collaboration produced a structured, reliable, and reasonably easy to use instrument for critical appraisal of clinical practice guidelines. This evaluative instrument looks at how biases associated with development, presentation, and applicability of a guideline has been minimized. In addition, each step of development is required to be clearly reported.*

Prior to selecting a clinical practice guideline for implementation in a health care system, or for personal use by a health care professional, it is important that the quality of published guidelines be evaluated. Perhaps the most useful tool available for evaluation of a practice guideline is the one created by the AGREE collaboration. The purpose of AGREE is to improve the quality and effectiveness of clinical practice guidelines by establishing a shared framework for their development, reporting, and assessment.[69] The AGREE collaboration involves an international group of researchers and policy makers from 13 countries. This collaboration has produced a structured instrument that can be used for critical appraisal of clinical practice guidelines. The AGREE instrument is designed to assess the methodology used for guideline development and how completely and clearly the process is reported.[69] For groups or individuals who wish to perform an assessment of a guideline, the AGREE instrument provides a tool that is structured, reliable, and reasonable to use.

In development of the AGREE instrument, quality was defined as "the confidence that the biases linked to the rigor of development, presentation, and applicability of a clinical practice guideline have been minimized and that each step of the development process is clearly reported."[69] It should be noted the AGREE instrument does not assess clinical content, or the quality of evidence, it assesses the quality of the process of guideline development methods and the reporting quality. Individual items for consideration in developing the instrument were grouped into the following five quality domains: (1) scope and purpose, (2) stakeholder involvement, (3) rigor of development, (4) clarity and presentation, and (5) applicability. An initial set of 82 items was generated from previously validated appraisal instruments and other published literature. Based on coverage, overlap, and content validity, a working group within the collaboration reduced the list to 34 items. Further refinements were made after these items and a user's guide were pretested on two Dutch and two English guidelines. The AGREE partners and 15 international experts were then asked to comment on the clarity, comprehensiveness, relevance, and ease of use of the draft items and user's guide. In addition, each of the AGREE partners were asked to apply the instrument to two more guidelines. Following removal of overlapping items and revision of ambiguous items, there were 24 remaining items grouped into the five quality domains mentioned above. As part of the user's guide, a four-point scale was to be used to score each item: 1—strongly disagree; 2—disagree; 3—agree; and 4—strongly agree. An overall recommendation on whether the guideline should be used was also evaluated using the following three-point scale: 1—not recommended; 2—recommended with provisos or modifications; 3—strongly recommended.[69]

During development, the AGREE instrument was field tested twice; first by 194 appraisers using a structured protocol on a sample of 100 guidelines from 11 countries. At an AGREE workshop in spring 2000, the instrument was revised in response to the first field test. The second field test was based on a random sample of three guidelines per country (33 total) from the original 100 guidelines. In the second field test, 74 newly recruited appraisers used the instrument. Following field testing, a sixth quality domain was added to the instrument, editorial independence. The final form of the AGREE instrument includes 23 items grouped into six quality domains (see Appendix 7–13). A copy of the AGREE instrument, instructions for use, a training manual, and other details are available from the Web site http://www.agreecollaboration.org. Guideline users may benefit from using this instrument to evaluate the quality of guidelines before choosing to adopt them.

Although the AGREE instrument was developed with the primary intent of providing a tool for evaluation of a guideline by users, guideline developers may also use the AGREE instrument to ensure that the methods used to develop a guideline and the documentation provided with the guideline will meet minimum standards. In addition, if AGREE is adapted by editors of peer-reviewed journals it should provide a framework to improve the quality of reporting of published guidelines. This intent is similar to the Consolidated Standards of Reporting Trials (CONSORT) statement, which is well established for the reporting of randomized, controlled trials.[70] The full-text of the article describing revisions to the CONSORT statement, a detailed explanation of the statement, the CONSORT checklist, flow diagram, and a glossary are available at the Web site http://www.consort-statement.org. The quality of reporting of randomized trials has been proven to increase with use of the CONSORT statement.[71]

Another collaborative effort to improve guideline quality and reporting standards is the Conference on Guideline Standardization (COGS). The purpose of COGS is to "define a standard for guideline reporting that will promote guideline quality and facilitate implementation."[72] Problems arise in guideline implementation if the guideline is developed with inadequate methods, or if there is inadequate documentation of the methods used. It is the intent of COGS to improve the quality of guideline development methods, and the quality of reporting as well. The COGS panel developed a checklist to be used prospectively by guideline developers to improve documentation.[72] As opposed to the AGREE instrument, the COGS checklist is intended more for use by guideline developers or publication editors, but it is still a useful checklist for practitioners when considering quality issues of a published guideline.

The COGS panel included representatives from medical specialty societies, government agencies, private groups that develop guidelines, journal editors, the National Guideline Clearinghouse (NGC), managed care representatives, informatics experts, and academicians. With this broad representation, the panel included input from the perspectives involved in guideline development, dissemination, and implementation. Items considered for inclusion on the checklist were rated for their importance for establishing validity and practical application of the guideline. Using a formal consensus process in the development of the checklist, 44 items were considered necessary for reporting in a guideline; 36 items were considered necessary for establishing guideline validity, 24 items were considered necessary for practical implementation, and some were considered necessary for both. After consolidating closely related items, the checklist contained 18 topics. The titles for these topics are overview of material, focus, goal, users/setting, target population, developer, funding source/sponsor, evidence collection, recommendation grading criteria, method for synthesizing evidence, prerelease review, update plan, definitions, recommendations and rationale, potential benefits and harms, patient preferences, algorithm, and implementation considerations.[72] For a more detailed description of each of these topics, please see Appendix 7–14.

Twenty-two organizations that produce guidelines were sent the COGS checklist to survey their opinions. Sixteen of the organizations (73%) responded that the checklist would be helpful for creating more comprehensive guidelines; 19 (86%) responded that documenting the items on the checklist would fit within their guideline development methods; 15 (68%) stated that they would use the proposed checklist, and four indicated that they might use it. One comment from organizations that expressed possible reluctance for using the checklist was regarding the need to produce guidelines that are succinct and brief in order to increase health professional acceptance. Guidelines that are brief may conflict with the need for comprehensiveness required by the checklist.[72]

Authors of the COGS checklist have also commented that it can have an impact similar to the CONSORT statement as mentioned above for the AGREE instrument. The COGS checklist authors caution that although this checklist can help improve guideline development, documentation, and reporting, it should not be used alone to judge the quality or adequacy of a guideline. Updates for the COGS checklist are planned to be published on their Web site at http://gem.med.yale.edu/cogs/.

Implementation of Clinical Practice Guidelines

● **❾** *Although the most effective methods for implementing new practice guidelines have not been confirmed, things to consider when developing an implementation strategy include local factors, potential facilitators, and barriers to implementation. Any factor that limits or restricts physician adherence to a guideline is considered a barrier to implementation. These factors include lack of physician awareness, familiarity, agreement, self-efficacy, and outcome expectancy. In addition, inertia of previous practice and external barriers such as patient nonadherence are noted.*

David Eddy stated in a lecture to the IOM, "All the science in the world has no effect until it is implemented properly, and measuring performance is one of the most powerful tools for implementation."[73]

The most effective methods for implementing guidelines to achieve the desired effects of improved quality of care have not been determined. Institutional, organizational, local practice, political characteristics, and even individual practitioner characteristics should be considered when planning an implementation strategy for a practice guideline. It was previously believed that implementation strategies using multiple methods would be the most likely to succeed. In a systematic review of the adoption of clinical practice guidelines, variables that affected the success of implementation included qualities specific to the guidelines, characteristics of the health professional, characteristics of the practice setting, incentives, regulation, and patient factors.[74] The implementation methods shown to be weak were traditional continuing medical education (CME) and mailings. Audit and feedback were moderately effective, especially if it was concurrent, targeted to specific providers, and delivered by peers or opinion leaders. Strong methods were reminder systems, academic detailing (process by which a health care educator visits a physician to provide a 15–20 minute educational intervention on a specific topic. Information provided is based on the physician's prescribing patterns and evidence-based medicine), and the use of multiple intervention systems.[74]

However, the most current and extensive review of guideline dissemination and implementation strategies does not support the conclusion that multiple intervention methods are more effective.[59] Grimshaw and colleagues conducted a systematic review of 235 studies that reported 309 comparisons of strategies for guideline dissemination and implementation.[59] Overall, multifaceted interventions were involved in 73% of the comparisons. Eighty-four of the 309 comparisons (27%) were performed on a single intervention compared to no intervention or usual care. One hundred thirty-six (44%) of the comparisons were of multifaceted interventions compared to no intervention or a usual care group. Multifaceted interventions were compared to a control intervention, which was either a single intervention or an alternative multifaceted intervention, for 85 (27%) of the comparisons in the identified studies. Of the single interventions compared to no intervention, the most common strategies used and the percentage of all comparisons in the systematic review were reminders (13%), educational materials (6%), audit and feedback (4%), and patient-directed interventions (3%). The most frequent strategies used in multifaceted interventions and corresponding percentage of all comparisons were educational materials (48%), educational meetings (41%), reminders (31%), audit and feedback (24%), and patient-directed interventions (18%). For a more detailed description of these implementation strategies, please see Appendix 7–15.[59]

The effect size of the interventions was described in one of four categories on the basis of the absolute difference in the postintervention measures, which were generally process measures of care. The four categories of effect size were: small (an effect size ≤5%); modest (an effect size >5% and ≤10%); moderate (an effect size >10% and ≤20%); and large (an effect size >20%). Examples of the process measure of care included the frequency of prescribing a specific therapy, providing patient education, or test ordering that was in accordance with the guideline. Overall, 86% of interventions tested achieved positive improvements in process of care measures. There was considerable variation in the effect size of the interventions in different studies and in some studies between different interventions. The majority of interventions produced modest-to-moderate improvements in care. The lack of consistency of the differences between and within interventions did not permit any conclusion regarding the most effective strategy for guideline implementation.

Multifaceted interventions were not found to be consistently more effective than single intervention strategies, and the number of components in the multifaceted interventions did not appear to be associated with effect size. The authors of this systematic review also noted that the overall quality of the methodology and reporting of the included studies was poor.[59]

This systematic review provides the best evidence available and concludes that further research is required to develop and validate systems for estimation of the efficacy and efficiency of different strategies to implement patient, health professional, and organizational behavior change. Decision-makers will have to evaluate the choice for implementation strategies carefully. Local factors, potential facilitators and barriers to implementation are recommended for prominent consideration in this decision.[59]

The report of the systematic review by Grimshaw and colleagues is available at The National Coordinating Centre for Health Technology Assessment (NCCHTA) Web site at http://www.hta.ac.uk/fullmono/mon806.pdf. The NCCHTA programme is part of the United Kingdom National Health Service. Individuals involved in planning an implementation strategy for a practice guideline would benefit from review of this report.

As noted above, barriers to guideline implementation should be considered when making plans for this effort. Cabana and colleagues conducted a systematic review of the literature regarding barriers to physician adherence to clinical practice guidelines.[75] For this review, the authors conducted a search for articles published between January 1966 and January 1998 that focused on clinical practice guidelines, practice parameters, clinical policies, national recommendations or consensus statements, and that examined at least one barrier to adherence. A barrier was defined as any factor that limits or restricts complete physician adherence to a guideline. The full text of 423 articles was examined, and 76 met the criteria for inclusion in the review. After classifying possible barriers into common themes, the authors identified seven general categories of barriers. Table 7–1 lists the seven categories of barriers and provides examples or a description of each barrier. The relative importance of different barriers will vary depending on the characteristics of the specific guideline, and on many local health care system characteristics. However, this review provides a "differential diagnosis for why physicians do not follow practice guidelines."[75] Appropriate attention to these potential barriers in the planning and development of guidelines will facilitate successful implementation.

An observational study of general practice in the Netherlands identified the following characteristics that influenced the use of guidelines: (1) specific attributes of the guidelines determine whether they are used in practice, (2) evidence-based recommendations are better followed in practice than those not based on scientific evidence, (3) precise definitions of recommended performance improve use, (4) testing the feasibility and acceptance of clinical guidelines among target groups is important, and (5) the people setting the guidelines need to understand the attributes of effective evidence-based guidelines.[76]

TABLE 7–1. **SEVEN CATEGORIES OF BARRIERS**

Barrier Category	Examples of Barriers Identified or Description of Barrier
Lack of awareness	Did not know the guideline existed
Lack of familiarity	Could not correctly answer questions about guideline content or self-reported lack of familiarity
Lack of agreement	Difference in interpretation of the evidence Benefits not worth patient risk, discomfort, or cost Not applicable to patient population in their practice Credibility of authors questioned Oversimplified cookbook Reduces autonomy Decreases flexibility Decreases physician self-respect Not practical Makes patient-physician relationship impersonal
Lack of self-efficacy	Did not believe that they could actually perform the behavior or activity recommended by the guideline, e.g., nutrition or exercise counseling
Lack of outcome expectancy	Did not believe intended outcome would occur even if the practice was followed, e.g., counseling to stop smoking
Inertia of previous practice	This barrier relates primarily to motivation to change practice, whether the motivation is professional, personal, or social. It was also noted that guidelines that recommend eliminating a behavior are more difficult to implement than guidelines that recommend adding a new behavior
External barriers	Patient resistance/nonadherence Patient does not perceive need Perceived to be offensive to patient Causes patient embarrassment Lack of reminder system Not easy to use, inconvenient, cumbersome, confusing Lack of educational materials Cost to patient Insufficient staff, consultant support or other resources Lack of time Lack of reimbursement Increased malpractice liability Not compatible with practice setting

Computer-based clinical decision support (CDSS) is one method thought to facilitate guideline implementation. In 1998, a systematic review was published of controlled trials assessing the effects of CDSS systems. This systematic review indicated that CDSS can enhance clinical performance for drug dosing, preventive care, and other aspects of medical care, but was not convincing for effects on diagnosis.[77] The same research group published an updated systematic review of CDSS that produced only slightly different results.[78] One hundred studies published between 1998 and September 2004 met inclusion criteria for this updated review. Of the included trials, 88% were randomized; 49% of these were cluster randomized; and 40% used a cluster as the unit of analysis or adjusted for clustering. The methodological quality of the trials was noted to improve over time.

In the updated systematic review, there were 29 trials involving drug dosing or prescribing. Of 24 studies involving systems for single-drug dosing, 15 (62%) demonstrated improved practitioner performance with guidelines, and 2 of the 18 studies assessing patient outcomes showed positive improvement. Of the five systems using computer order entry for multidrug prescribing, four improved practitioner performance, but none improved patient outcomes. There were 40 studies of systems for disease management of conditions such as diabetes, cardiovascular disease prevention, urinary incontinence, human immunodeficiency virus infection, and acute respiratory distress. Thirty-seven of these studies evaluated practitioner performance with 23 (62%) demonstrating improvement. Only five (18%) of the 27 disease management trials evaluating patient outcomes demonstrated improvement. Of 21 trials of reminder systems for preventive care, 16 (72%) found improvements in practitioner performance according to practice guidelines. Of 10 trials that evaluated CDSS for diagnostic systems, only 4 (40%) found improvements in practitioner performance. Of the five trials of diagnostic systems that evaluated patient outcomes, none found improvement.[78]

Garg and colleagues also reported that improved practitioner performance was associated with CDSS systems that automatically prompted the practitioner to use the system compared to systems that required the practitioner to initiate system use. Improved performance was noted in 73% of trials of automated systems compared to 47% of user initiated systems ($p = 0.02$). It was also interesting to note that the best predictor of success of a CDSS was a study in which the authors were also the developers of the system. Studies conducted by the developer of the system were more likely to find success (74%), compared to 28% when the authors were not the developers ($p = 0.001$).[78] It is clear that as with other methods for implementation of guidelines and achieving performance or behavior change, further research is needed on use of CDSS to provide clear guidance on predictable success rates. Many individual factors will need to be considered in the decision-making for implementation of these systems.[79]

A randomized, controlled trial of CQI and academic detailing to implement clinical guidelines for the primary care of hypertension and depression produced mixed results.[80] The authors concluded that both academic detailing and CQI interventions involve complex social interactions that produce varied implementation across the different organizations.

One of the first systematic literature reviews and evaluations of the effect of practice guidelines was published in 1993.[81] The authors of this study conducted an extensive literature search and identified 59 studies that they considered to have appropriate methods to evaluate the effect of guidelines on either physician behavior or patient outcomes. All but four of the studies showed some benefit from the guidelines; however, the magnitude of the benefit and the patient care significance was not impressive in all cases.

• Guidelines represent an early application of decision support systems to facilitate providing quality clinical care. When done well, practice guidelines should contain all the necessary elements of routine care for most individuals with a specific condition. They should prompt consideration of what specific characteristics of an individual patient might warrant departures from the guideline. When effectively implemented, such systems save clinicians' time. They should be assisted by computerized systems that, among other functions, can catalogue past histories, check orders for medications against measures of hepatic and renal function, and schedule reminders for screening tests or preventive services. They should be part of the continuous improvement of systems of care. Guidelines will not be perfect at the outset; systems that use them must be constructed so that experience can be applied to improve the guidelines, just as the guidelines indicate where care delivery can be improved.[82]

Case Study 7–4

The practice guideline panel finally has a new practice guideline ready to be implemented. As you already know, the most effective methods for implementing guidelines have not been determined. You are also aware that barriers have been identified to guideline implementation that should be considered when developing the implementation plan. Since the most effective methods for implementing guidelines have not been determined, the successful implementation plan may very well include those methods that address these barriers. With this in mind, what are the seven categories of barriers to guideline implementation that have been identified to limit or restrict complete physician adherence to a practice guideline?

Sources of Clinical Practice Guidelines

• ⑩ Complete clinical practice guidelines can be found on Web sites such as the National Guideline Clearinghouse and in the peer-reviewed medical literature located in MEDLINE and other secondary databases. Systematic reviews that can be helpful in developing or assessing specific practice guidelines are available from organizations such as the Cochrane Library, in addition to other Web sites that collect and provide health care–related information designed to support evidence-based medicine such as the Agency for Healthcare Research and Quality (AHRQ), Health Information Research Unit at McMaster University, and the Centre for Evidence-Based Medicine at Oxford.

There are several mechanisms to locate completed clinical practice guidelines or systematic reviews. The Web-based NGC (http://www.guideline.gov) is an initiative of AHRQ, created in cooperation with the American Medical Association and the American Association of Health Plans. The mission of the NGC is to provide an accessible mechanism for obtaining objective, detailed information on clinical practice guidelines and to further their dissemination, implementation, and use. Components of the NGC include structured abstracts about the guideline and its development; a utility for comparing attributes of two or more guidelines in a side-by-side comparison; synthesis of guidelines covering similar topics, highlighting areas of similarity and difference; links to full-text guidelines where available and/or ordering information for print copies; an electronic forum for exchanging information on clinical practice guidelines, their development, implementation and use; and annotated bibliographies on guideline development methodology implementation and use. In order to be included in the NGC, the following criteria must be met:

1. The clinical practice guideline contains systematically developed statements that include recommendations, strategies, or information that assists health care practitioners and patients in making decisions about appropriate health care for specific clinical circumstances.

2. The clinical practice guideline was produced under the auspices of medical specialty associations; relevant professional societies, public or private organizations, government agencies at the federal, state, or local level; or health care organizations or plans. A clinical practice guideline developed and issued by an individual not officially sponsored or supported by one of the above types of organizations does not meet the inclusion criteria for NGC.

3. Corroborating documentation can be produced and verified that a systematic literature search and review of existing scientific evidence published in peer-reviewed journals was performed during the guideline development. A guideline is not excluded from NGC if corroborating documentation can be produced and verified detailing specific gaps in scientific evidence for some of the guideline's recommendations.

4. The full-text guideline is available on request in print or electronic format (for free or for a fee) in the English language. The guideline is current and the most recent version produced. Documented evidence can be produced or verified that the guideline was developed, reviewed, or revised within the last 5 years.[83]

The NGC provides a search function for identifying guidelines by disease, producer, bibliographic source, characteristics of the guideline, date, clinical specialty, objective, target population, and many other factors. The search engine allows the use of Boolean operators, truncation, automatic concept mapping, textword searching, and multiple sort and display options. The NGC premiered in January 1999 with 286 guidelines and as of September 2010, it contained 2371 disease guideline summaries.

Many guidelines have been published in the peer-reviewed medical literature and can therefore be located in MEDLINE. A variety of search techniques may be used, but the most efficient may be to search for *practice guideline* in the publication type field of the record, or use the MeSH term *practice guidelines* in conjunction with other terms for the specific disease or therapy of interest. Additional publication types in the NLM record that may be searched include the terms consensus development conference; consensus development conference, NIH; guideline; meta-analysis; and review, academic. Systematic review articles are also useful in preparation of clinical practice guidelines. The key differences with systematic reviews compared to the old forms of narrative review articles are that the systematic review begins with a focused clinical question, involves a comprehensive search for evidence, uses criterion-based selection that is uniformly applied to include evidence in the review, performs rigorous critical appraisal of the studies chosen, and provides a quantitative summary of the evidence.[84] Literature search strategies have been published for locating systematic reviews.[85,86]

The NIH Consensus Statements, NIH Technology Assessments, the USPSTF Guide to Clinical Preventive Services, AHRQ evidence reports, and other resources are available on Health Services Technology Assessment Texts (HSTAT). HSTAT was developed by the NLM Information Technology Branch and can be accessed at http://www.ncbi.nlm.nih.gov/books/bv.fcgi?rid=hstat.

The Guidelines International Network (GIN) is an international not-for-profit association of organizations and individuals involved in clinical practice guidelines. Founded in November 2002, GIN has now grown to 52 member organizations including World Health Organization (WHO) from 26 countries. According to the GIN Web site "GIN seeks to improve the quality of health care by promoting systematic development of clinical practice guidelines and their application into practice, through supporting international collaboration." GIN's Guideline Library contains updated information about guidelines for specific health topics, tools and resources for guideline development, training materials, and patient or consumer resources. In September 2010, over 7000 programs were available at http://www.g-i-n.net/. Some of the resources from this Web site require membership for access.

The Ontario GAC, a joint body of the Ontario Medical Association and the Ontario Ministry of Health and Long-Term Care with *ex officio* representation from the Institute for Clinical Evaluative Sciences, was formed in 1997. According to their Web site, "The Committee mandate is to develop and recommend appropriate strategies for the implementation and monitoring of practice and referral guidelines, make recommendations for assisting in the implementation of prescribing guidelines, consult widely with the profession in the development of its recommendations." The GAC assess the methodological quality and clinical relevance of existing practice guidelines and recommends one for use by practicing physicians. The GAC also develops and recommends strategies for implementation and evaluation of guidelines. The GAC has established a network of key stakeholders to assist in the development, implementation, and evaluation of these strategies (http://www.gacguidelines.ca/). Also, on their Web site is a group of links to guideline collections, guideline developers, research and education groups related to guidelines, and Canadian and International specialty societies.

The Turning Research Into Practice (TRIP) Database started in 1997 as a small search engine with a focus on medical articles considered evidence-based. The aims of the TRIP Database have remained the same since 1997—to allow health professionals to easily find the highest-quality material available on the Web. Content areas in this database include evidence-based, clinical guidelines, and others. TRIP is a subscription-based product (http://www.tripdatabase.com/).

As previously mentioned in this chapter, multiple professional organizations, academic centers, independent research centers, and government agencies are involved in development of clinical practice guideline activities. Updated information may be obtained by contacting these organizations directly and many have provided access to their guidelines on the Internet.

The Cochrane Library is based on the work of an international collaboration of health care providers and scientists who engage in preparing, maintaining, and disseminating systematic reviews of relevant randomized, controlled trials of health care.[87] This collaboration is named in honor of Archie Cochrane who in 1979 wrote that "it is surely a great criticism of our profession that we have not organized a critical summary, by specialty, adapted periodically, of all relevant, randomized, controlled trials." The Cochrane Library provides a collection of several databases: The Cochrane Database of Systematic Reviews (Cochrane Reviews), Database of Abstracts of Reviews of Effects (DARE), The Cochrane Central Register of Controlled Trials (CENTRAL), The Cochrane Database of Methodology Reviews (Methodology Reviews), The Cochrane Methodology Register (Methodology Register), Health Technology Assessment Database (HTA), NHS Economic Evaluation Database (NHS EED), About The Cochrane Collaboration, and the Cochrane Collaborative Review Groups (About). Full access to the Cochrane Library requires a subscription; however, abstracts of the systematic reviews are available at http://www.cochrane.org/reviews/index.htm.

The Cochrane Database of Systematic Reviews is a collection of highly structured and systematic reviews of research evidence in specific areas of health care. Data are often combined statistically (with meta-analysis) to increase the power of the findings from multiple studies. As of 2009, this database includes over 4000 complete reviews and is growing.

The CENTRAL is a bibliography of controlled trials identified by contributors to the Cochrane Collaboration as part of an international effort to create an unbiased source of data for systematic reviews of the medical literature. Additional information about the Cochrane Collaboration is available at their Web site (http://www.cochrane.org). Links to Cochrane training resources (including the previously mentioned Reviewers' Handbook), and training resources from other organizations are available at these sites, http://www.cochrane.org/resources/training.htm and http://www.cochrane.org/resources/revpro.htm.

The Internet has rapidly become a useful tool for access to health care–related information. Many sites are potentially useful. Three excellent sites that are specifically designed to support EBM are the AHRQ Web site http://www.ahrq.gov/, the Health Information Research Unit at McMaster University (http://hiru.mcmaster.ca/), and the Centre for Evidence-Based Medicine at Oxford (http://www.cebm.net/). These sites contain extensive information about systematic appraisal and use of evidence, worldwide projects for development of EBM including clinical practice guidelines, and links to many other quality sites.

Many activities conducted by professional organizations in pharmacy have principles in common with EBM and clinical practice guidelines. The American Society of Health-System Pharmacists (ASHP), in 1990 created a policy-recommending body called the Commission on Therapeutics. This commission develops therapeutic guidelines defined as "systematically developed documents that assist health care professionals on appropriate use of drugs for specific clinical circumstances."[88] With the publication of the ASHP Therapeutic Guidelines on Angiotensin-Converting-Enzyme Inhibitors in Patients with Left Ventricular Dysfunction,[89] the ASHP initiated an evidence-based style for its therapeutic guidelines.[90] The ASHP uses a process for preparation of the therapeutic guidelines similar to the one developed by the Agency for Healthcare Policy and Research.

Another example of a therapeutic guideline from ASHP is on stress ulcer prophylaxis.[91] This extensive review used the most current methods for guideline preparation including decision algorithms and a decision tree for pharmacoeconomic analysis. The authors employed methods for assessing the literature by using evidence tables and categorized the recommendations according to the strength of evidence using a system based on recommendations from the Evidence-Based Working Group at McMaster. This system for defining levels of evidence takes into consideration the information provided in meta-analyses, the consistency of results across trials, and the bounds of the 95% confidence interval compared to the numerical threshold for clinically important benefit. In keeping with EBM ideals, an update representing the implications of recent studies in this area has been published. In addition to therapeutic guidelines, ASHP produces Therapeutic Position Statements which are "concise statements that respond to specific therapeutic issues of concern to health care consumers and pharmacists, as approved by the board of directors" (http://www.ashp.org/Import/PRACTICEANDPOLICY/PolicyPositionsGuidelines BestPractices/BrowsebyDocumentType/TherapeuticPositionStatements.aspx).

More information about therapeutic guidelines and therapeutic position statements, and access to these documents is available at the ASHP Web site (http://www.ashp.org/).

Conclusion

Clinical practice guidelines have become a significant tool in health care with the focus on evidence-based practice. These guidelines fit well with the emphasis on CQI techniques. Guidelines have the potential to assist medical decision-making and ultimately improve the quality of care, improve patient outcomes, and make more efficient use of resources. Significant advances have been made in the methodology to produce valid guidelines. Information technology and greater understanding of optimal methods for implementation of guidelines will maximize their effect to improve quality of care. Pharmacists' active involvement in preparation and implementation of evidence-based clinical practice guidelines is vital. A thorough understanding of evidence-based methodology will prepare the pharmacist to participate in this process. A drug information–trained pharmacist is an ideal person to help prepare and/or implement evidence-based clinical practice guidelines.

Acknowledgment

The assistance of Patrick J. Bryant, Pharm.D. is acknowledged in preparing this chapter for publication.

Self-Assessment Questions

1. Which of the following groups or types of organizations have been involved in development of clinical practice guidelines?
   a. Federal and state government
   b. Professional societies and associations
   c. Managed care organizations
   d. Third-party payers
   e. All of the above

2. Which of the following is a common characteristic of practice guid‹ ment and traditional drug information practice activities?
   a. Decision-making and recommendations based on individual experience
   b. Assurance of cost savings
   c. Clear specific definition of clinical questions
   d. Lack of interdisciplinary participation
   e. All of the above

3. Clinical practice guidelines are important to getting research information into practice because:
   a. Research information is not readily available for implementation into practice.
   b. Well-studied new treatments proven effective are substantially underutilized.
   c. Interventions proven ineffective or harmful continue to be provided.
   d. a and b only.
   e. b and c only.

4. Which of the following methods of guideline development is currently recommended as the most valid?
   a. Evidence-based
   b. Informal consensus
   c. Formal consensus
   d. a and b
   e. a and c

5. Which of the following are included in the five core competencies for health professionals as recommended in the Institute of Medicine report Health Professions Education: A Bridge to Quality?
   a. Deliver patient-centered care.
   b. Participate in interdisciplinary teams.
   c. Emphasize evidence-based practice.
   d. Utilize informatics.
   e. All of the above.

6. The quality of guideline development methods can be estimated by a quick scan to determine if:
   a. Recommendations are based on focused clinical questions.
   b. Recommendations are specifically linked to evidence.
   c. Quality of evidence and strength of recommendations have been graded.
   d. Evidence tables and a balance sheet are available.
   e. All of the above.

7. Which of the following characteristics associated with a disease would suggest that it would be a good topic for development and implementation of a practice guideline?
   a. Low prevalence
   b. Evidence that current practice is optimal
   c. Evidence of little variation in current practiced
   d. Availability of high quality evidence for the efficacy of interventions
   e. Low frequency and severity of morbidity

8. Development of a clinical practice guideline should:
   a. Include a hospital administrator
   b. Be a multidisciplinary process
   c. Be made up of panel members without any conflicts of interest
   d. Have a pharmacist leading the effort
   e. All of the above

9. In the absence of high levels of evidence, guideline development groups would:
   a. Provide a statement that evidence for making a recommendation is inconclusive.
   b. Provide a summary of the evidence without specific recommendation.
   c. Use a consensus method to develop a recommendation.
   d. a and b only.
   e. a, b, and c.

10. Based on the GRADE working group, which of the following information should be incorporated with guideline recommendations?
    a. Quality of evidence from studies
    b. Balance of benefits and harms of interventions
    c. The strength of the recommendation
    d. a and c only
    e. a, b, and c

11. The GRADE working group includes all of the following elements in designating the quality of evidence *except*:
    a. Safety evaluation resulting from the study
    b. Basic trial design, e.g., randomized, controlled trial
    c. Quality of study methods and execution
    d. Consistency of results across studies
    e. Directness of application of results

12. All of the following are true regarding the AGREE instrument for guideline evaluation *except*:
    a. Created by an international panel of researchers and policy makers
    b. Assesses the quality of the guideline development methods and reporting

    c. Assesses the quality of the clinical content

    d. Intended for use by organizations and individuals

    e. Field tested twice

13. The purpose of the Conference on Guideline Standardization (COGS) include the following *except*:

    a. Define a standard for guideline reporting.

    b. Promote guideline quality.

    c. Facilitate guideline implementation.

    d. Provide support to guideline auditing.

    e. c and d.

14. Barriers that limit or restrict complete physician adherence to a practice guideline include all of the following *except* the lack of:

    a. Physician awareness that the guideline exists

    b. Physician familiarity with guideline content

    c. Patient desire to get better

    d. Patient adherence to guideline

    e. Physician agreement with interpretation of the evidence

15. Which of the following is true regarding studies of the effect of computer-based clinical decision support (CDSS) systems on patient care?

    a. The best predictor of success of the system is that the study to evaluate success is conducted by the system developer.

    b. Systematic reviews of these systems have shown enhanced clinical performance for drug dosing, preventive care, and diagnosis.

    c. Very few studies of these systems used randomization procedures.

    d. Most of the studies evaluate specific patient outcomes.

    e. The success of the system is not dependent on automatic prompting or practitioner-initiated use.

REFERENCES

1. Field JM, Lohr KN, editors. Guidelines for clinical practice: from development to use. Washington (DC): National Academy Press; 1992.

2. Jones RH, Ritchie JL, Fleming BB, Hammermeister KE, Leape LL. 28th Bethesda Conference. Task force 1: clinical practice guideline development, dissemination and computerization. J Am Coll Cardiol. 1997;29:1133-41.

3. President's Advisory Commission on Consumer Protection and Quality in the Health Care Industry. Quality first better health care for all Americans, 1998 [cited 1999 Jan 18]: [1 screen]. Available from: http://www.hcqualitycommission.gov/final/execsum.html.

4. Chassin MR, Galvin RW. The urgent need to improve health care quality. Institute of Medicine National Roundtable on Health Care Quality. JAMA. 1998;280:1000-5.

5. Kohn LT, Corrigan JM, Donaldson MS, editors. To err is human: building a safer health system. Institute of Medicine. Washington (DC): National Academy Press; 1999.

6. Corrigan JM, Donaldson MS, Kohn LT, editors. Crossing the quality chasm: a new health system for the 21st century. Washington (DC): National Academy Press; 2001.

7. Aspden P, Corrigan JM, Wolcott J, editors. Patient safety: achieving a new standard for care. Washington (DC): National Academy Press; 2004.

8. Sackett DL, Rosenberg WM, Gray JA, Haynes RB, Richardson WS. Evidence-based medicine: what it is and what it isn't. BMJ. 1996;312:71-2.

9. Eddy DM. Evidence-based medicine: a unified approach. Health Aff. 2005;24:9-17.

10. Evidence Based Medicine Working Group. Evidence based medicine: a new approach to teaching the practice of medicine. JAMA. 1992;268:2420-5.

11. Sackett DL, Straus SE, Richardson WS, Rosenberg W, Haynes RB. Evidence-based medicine: how to practice & teach EBM. 2nd ed. New York: Churchill-Livingstone; 2000.

12. Watanabe AS, McCart G, Shimomura S, Kayser S. Systematic approach to drug information requests. Am J Hosp Pharm. 1975;32:1282-5.

13. Guyatt GH, O Meade M, Jaeschke RZ, Cook DJ, Haynes RB. Practice of evidence based care. Not all clinicians need to appraise evidence from scratch but all need some skills. BMJ. 2000;320:954-5.

14. Towle A. Changes in health care and continuing medical education for the 21st century. BMJ. 1998;316:301-4.

15. Davis D. Continuing medical education. Global health, global learning. BMJ. 1998;316:385-9.

16. Fox RD, Bennett NL. Learning and change: implications for continuing medical education. BMJ. 1998;316:466-8.

17. Bashook PG, Parboosingh J. Recertification and the maintenance of competence. BMJ. 1998;316:545-8.

18. Holm HA. Quality issues in continuing medical education. BMJ. 1998;316:621-4.

19. Southgate L, Dauphinee D. Maintaining standards in British and Canadian medicine: the developing role of the regulatory body. BMJ. 1998;316:697-700.

20. Headrick LA, Wilcock PM, Batalden PB. Interprofessional working and continuing medical education. BMJ. 1998;316:771-4.

21. Greiner AC, Knebel E, eds. Health professions education: a bridge to quality. Washington (DC): National Academy Press; 2003.

22. Woolf SH. Practice guidelines: a new reality in medicine. II. Methods of developing guidelines. Arch Intern Med. 1992;152:946-52.

23. Perry S. The NIH consensus development program. A decade later. N Engl J Med. 1987;317:485-8.

24. Guidelines for the planning and management of NIH consensus development conferences, 1995 [cited 1999 Feb 22]: [1 screen]. Available from: http://odp.od.nih.gov/consensus/about/process.htm.

25. National Cholesterol Education Program (NCEP) Expert Panel on Detection, Evaluation, and Treatment of High Blood Cholesterol in Adults (Adult Treatment Panel III). Third Report of the National Cholesterol Education Program (NCEP) Expert Panel on Detection, Evaluation, and Treatment of High Blood Cholesterol in Adults (Adult Treatment Panel III) final report. Circulation. 2002;106:3143-21.

26. Gundy SM, Cleeman JI, Merz CNB, Brewer HB, Clark LT, Hunninghake DB, et al. Implications of recent clinical trials for the national cholesterol education program adult treatment panel III guidelines. Circulation. 2004;110:227-39.

27. Chobanian AV, Bakris GL, Black HR, Cushman WC, Green LA, Izzo JL, et al. Seventh report of the Joint National Committee on Prevention, Detection, Evaluation, and Treatment of High Blood Pressure. Hypertension. 2003;42:1206-52.

28. Canadian task force on the periodic health examination: the periodic health examination. Can Med Assoc J. 1979;121:1193-254.

29. About USPSTF. U.S. Preventive Services Task Force. AHRQ Publication No. 00-P046,2003. Rockville (MD): Agency for Healthcare Research and Quality. [cited 2004 Nov 17]. Available from: http://www.ahrq.gov/clinic/uspstfab.htm.

30. Eddy DM. Clinical decision-making: from theory to practice. Guidelines for policy statements: the explicit approach. JAMA. 1990;263:2239-40, 2243.

31. Eddy DM. Clinical decision-making: from theory to practice. Anatomy of a decision. JAMA. 1990;263:441-3.

32. Eddy DM. Clinical decision-making: from theory to practice. Practice policies: guidelines for methods. JAMA. 1990;263:1839-41.

33. Eddy DM. Designing a practice policy. Standards, guidelines, and options. JAMA. 1990;263:3077-81, 3084.

34. Woolf SH. Manual for clinical practice guideline development. AHCPR Publication No. 91-0007. Rockville, MD: Agency for Healthcare Policy and Research, Public Health Service, U.S. Department of Health and Human Services; 1991.

35. Burgers JS, Grol R, Klazinga NS, Makela M, Zaat J for the AGREE Collaboration. Towards evidence-based clinical practice: an international survey of 18 clinical guideline programs. Int J Qual Health Care. 2003;15:31-45.

36. Manual for ACC/AHA guideline writing committees: methodologies and policies from the ACC/AHA task for on practice guidelines [cited 2004 Nov 19]. Available from: http://circ.ahajournals.org/manual/index.shtml.

37. American College of Rheumatology. Guidelines for the development of practice guidelines, 1998. [cited 2004 Nov 19]. Available from: http://www.rheumatology.org/publications/guidelines/ guidesonguides.asp?aud=mem.

38. Schunemann HJ, Munger H, Brower S, O'Donnell M, Crowther M, Cook D, et al. Methodology for guideline development for the seventh American college of chest physicians conference on antithrombotic and thrombolytic therapy. Chest. 2004;126(suppl 3):174S-8S.

39. American Academy of Pediatrics and American Academy of Family Physicians. Clinical practice guideline: diagnosis and management of acute otitis media. Pediatrics. 2004;113:1451-65.

40. Mandell LA, Bartlett JG, Dowell SF, File TM, Musher DM, Whitney C. Update of practice guidelines for the management of community-acquired pneumonia in immunocompetent adults. Clin Infect Dis. 2003;37:1405-33.
41. National Institute for Clinical Excellence. Guideline development methods: information for national collaborating centres and guideline developers, 2004. London: National Institute for Clinical Excellence [accessed 2004 Nov 21]. Available from: http://www.nice.org.
42. New Zealand Guidelines Group. Handbook for the preparation of explicit evidence-based clinical practice guidelines, 2001. Available from: http://www.nzgg.org.nz/development/documents/nzgg_guideline_handbook.pdf.
43. Scottish Intercollegiate Guidelines Network. SIGN 50: a guideline developers' handbook. SIGN Publication No. 50 [cited 2004 Nov 21]. Available from: http://www.sign.ac.uk/guidelines/fulltext/50/index.html.
44. Field JM, Lohr KN, eds. Clinical practice guidelines: directions for a new program. Washington (DC): National Academy Press; 1990.
45. Hirsh J, Guyatt G, Albers GW, Schunemann HJ. The seventh ACCP conference on antithrombotic and thrombolytic therapy. Evidence-based guidelines. Chest. 2004;126 (suppl 3): 172S-3S.
46. Guyatt G, Schunemann HJ, Cook D, Jaeschke R, Pauker S. Applying the grades of recommendation for antithrombotic and thrombolytic therapy. The seventh ACCP conference on antithrombotic and thrombolytic therapy. Chest. 2004;126(suppl 3):179S-87S.
47. Schunemann HJ, Cook D, Grimshaw J, Liberati A, Heffner J, Tapson V, et al. Antithrombotic and thrombolytic therapy: from evidence to application. The seventh ACCP conference on antithrombotic and thrombolytic therapy. Chest. 2004;126(suppl 3):688S-96S.
48. Higgins JPT, Green S, eds. Cochrane Handbook for Systematic Reviews 5.0.2 [updated 2009 Sept; cited 2010 Sept 29]. Available from: http://www.cochrane.org/training/cochrane-handbook.
49. Khan KS, ter Riet G, Glanville J, eds. Undertaking systematic reviews of research on effectiveness CRD's guidance for those carrying out or commissioning reviews, 2nd ed. CRD Report No 4. Centre for Reviews and Dissemination, University of York, York, UK, 2001 [cited 2005 Feb 5]. Available from: http://www.york.ac.uk/inst/crd/report4.htm.
50. Mosca L, Appel LJ, Benjamin EJ, Berra K, Chandra-Strobos N, Fabunmi RP, et al. Evidence-based guidelines for cardiovascular disease prevention in women. J Am Coll Cardiol. 2004;43:900-21.
51. National Institute for Clinical Excellence. Topic suggestion and selection. criteria for selecting topics for the advisory committee on topic selection [cited 2005 Jan 29]. Available from: http://www. nice.org.uk/pdf/topicsuggestionselectiocriteria.pdf.
52. Fye WB. The power of clinical trials and guidelines, and the challenge of conflicts of interest. J Am Coll Cardiol. 2003;41:1237-42.
53. Choudhry NK, Stelfox HT, Detsky AS. Relationships between authors of clinical practice guidelines and the pharmaceutical industry. JAMA. 2002;287:612-7.
54. Curtiss FR. Consensus panel, national guidelines, and other potentially misleading terms. J Manag Care Pharm. 2003;9:574-5.

55. Van Der Weyden MB. Clinical practice guidelines: time to move the debate from the how to the who. Med J Aust. 2002;176:304-5.

56. Alving B. NHLBI clinical guidelines development. Statement from Barbara Alving, MD, Acting Director of the National Heart, Lung and Blood Institute [cited 2005 Jan 30]. Available from: http://www.nhlbi.nih.gov/new/press/04-07-29.htm.

57. Alving B. Cholesterol guidelines: the strength of the science base and the integrity of the development process. Statement from Barbara Alving, MD, Acting Director of the National Heart, Lung and Blood Institute [cited 2005 Jan 30]. Available from: http://www.nhlbi.nih.gov/new/press/04-09-24.htm.

58. Alving B. Letter to Mr. Merrill Goozner, Director, Integrity in Science Center for Science in the Public Interest. 2004 Oct 22. [cited 2005 Jan 30]. Available from: http://www.nhlbi.nih.gov/guidelines/ cholesterol/response.pdf.

59. Grimshaw JM, Thomas RE, MacLennan G, Fraser C, Ramsay CR, Vale L, et al. Effectiveness and efficiency of guideline dissemination and implementation strategies. Health Technol Assess. 2004;8(6) [cited 2005 Jan 29]. Available from: http://www.hta.ac.uk/fullmono/mon806.pdf.

60. Shiffman RN, Michel G, Essaihi A, Thornquist E. Bridging the guideline implementation gap: a systematic document-centered approach to guideline implementation. JAMIA. 2004; 11: 418-26.

61. Lyons SS, Tripp-Reimer T, Sorofman BA, DeWitt JE, Boots-Miller BJ, Vaughn T, et al. VA QUERI Informatics paper. Information technology for clinical guideline implementation: perceptions of multidisciplinary stakeholders. JAMIA. 2005;12:64-71.

62. Michie S, Johnston M. Changing clinical behaviour by making guidelines specific. BMJ. 2004;328:343-5.

63. West S, King V, Carey TS, Lohr KN, McKoy N, Sutton S, et al. Systems to rate the strength of scientific evidence. Evidence Report/Technology Assessment No. 47 (Prepared by the Research Triangle Institute-University of North Carolina Evidence-based Practice Center under Contract No. 290-97-0011). AHRQ Publication No. 02-E016. Rockville (MD): Agency for Healthcare Research and Quality; 2002.

64. Drummond MF, Jefferson TO. Guidelines for authors and peer reviewers of economic submissions to the BMJ. BMJ. 1996;313:275-83.

65. Chobanian AV, Bakris GL, Black HR, Cushman WC, Green LA, Izzo JL, et al. The seventh report of the Joint National Committee on Prevention, Detection, Evaluation, and Treatment of High Blood Pressure: the JNC 7 report. JAMA. 2003;289:2560-72.

66. Atkins D, Best D, Briss PA, Eccles M, Falck-Ytter Y, Flottorp S, et al. for the GRADE working group. Grading quality of evidence and strength of recommendations. BMJ. 2004; 328:1490.

67. Atkins D, Eccles M, Flottorp S, Guyatt GH, Henry D, Hill S, et al. Systems for grading the quality of evidence and the strength of recommendations I: critical appraisal of existing approaches. BMC Health Serv Res. 2004;4:38 [Epub ahead of print]. Available from: http://www.biomedcentral. com/1472-6963/4/38.

68. Atkins D, Briss PA, Eccles M, Flottorp S, Guyatt GH, Harbour RT, et al. The GRADE* working group. A pilot study of a new system for grading the quality of evidence and the strength of recommendations [cited 2005 Jan 31]. Available from: http://www.gradeworkinggroup.org/publications/ Grade_pilot_study_2004_01_20.pdf.

69. Cluzeau F, Burgers J, Brouwers M, Grol R, Makela M, Littlejohns P, et al. Development and validation of an international appraisal instrument for assessing the quality of clinical practice guidelines: the AGREE project. Qual Saf Health Care. 2003;12:18-23.

70. Moher D, Schulz KF, Altman DG, for the CONSORT Group. The CONSORT statement: revised recommendations for improving the quality of reports of parallel-group randomized trials. Ann Intern Med. 2001;134:657-62.

71. Moher D, Jones A, Lepage L. Use of the CONSORT statement and quality of reports of randomized trials: a comparative before-and-after study. JAMA. 2001;285:1992-5.

72. Shiffman RN, Shekelle P, Overhage M, Slutsky J, Grimshaw J, Deshpandey AM, et al. Standardized reporting of clinical practice guidelines: a proposal from the conference on guideline standardization. Ann Intern Med. 2003;139:493-8.

73. Eddy DM. Performance measurement: problems and solutions. Health Aff (Millwood). 1998;17(4):7-25.

74. Davis DA, Taylor-Vaisey A. Translating guidelines into practice. A systematic review of theoretic concepts, practical experience and research evidence in the adoption of clinical practice guidelines. CMAJ. 1997;157:408-16.

75. Cabana MD, Rand CS, Powe NR, Wu AW, Wilson MH, Abboud PAC, et al. Why don't physicians follow clinical practice guidelines? A framework for improvement. JAMA. 1999;282:1458-65.

76. Grol R, Dalhuijsen J, Thomas S, Veld C, Rutten G, Mokkink H. Attributes of clinical guidelines that influence use of guidelines in general practice: observational study. BMJ. 1998;317:858-61.

77. Hunt DL, Haynes RB, Hanna SE, Smith K. Effects of computer-based clinical decision support systems on physician performance and patient outcomes: a systematic review. JAMA. 1998;280:1339-46.

78. Garg AX, Adhikari NK, McDonald H, Rosas-Arellano MP, Devereaux PJ, Beyene J, et al. Effects of computerized clinical decision support systems on practitioner performance and patient outcomes. A systematic review. JAMA. 2005;293:1223-38.

79. Wears RL, Berg M. Computer technology and clinical work. Still waiting for Godot. JAMA. 2005;293:1261-3.

80. Horowitz CR, Goldberg HI, Martin DP, Wagner EH, Fihn SD, Chirstensen DB, et al. Conducting a randomized controlled trial of CQI and academic detailing to implement clinical guidelines. Jt Comm J Qual Improv. 1996;22:734-50.

81. Grimshaw JM, Russell IT. Effect of clinical guidelines on medical practice: a systematic review of rigorous evaluations. Lancet. 1993;342:1317-22.

82. Chassin MR. Is health care ready for six sigma quality? Milbank Q. 1998;76(4):565-91, 510.

83. Inclusion Criteria. Washington, DC: National Guideline Clearinghouse [updated 2005 May 23; cited 2005 May 23]. Available from: http://www.guideline.gov/about/inclusion.aspx.

84. Cook DJ, Mulrow CD, Haynes RB. Systematic review: synthesis of best evidence for clinical decisions. Ann Intern Med. 1997;126:376-80.

85. Hunt DL, McKibbon KA. Locating and appraising systematic reviews. Ann Intern Med. 1997;126:532-8.

86. Montori VM, Wilczynski NL, Morgan D, Haynes RB; for the Hedges Team. Optimal search strategies for retrieving systematic reviews from MEDLINE: analytical survey. BMJ. 2005;330(7482):68. Epub Dec 24, 2004.

87. Sackett DL. The Cochrane Collaboration [editorial]. ACP J Club. 1994;120(suppl 3):A11.

88. Practice Standards of ASHP 1993-1994. Bethesda (MD): American Society of Hospital Pharmacists; 1993.

89. American Society of Health-System Pharmacists. ASHP therapeutic guidelines on angiotensin-converting-enzyme inhibitors in patients with left ventricular dysfunction. This official ASHP practice standard was developed through the ASHP Commission on Therapeutics and approved by the ASHP Board of Directors on Nov 16, 1996. Am J Health-Syst Pharm. 1997;54:299-313.

90. Cooke-Ariel H. Promoting use of angiotensin-converting-enzyme inhibitors. Am J Health-Syst Pharm. 1997;54:264.

91. American Society of Health-System Pharmacists. ASHP therapeutic guidelines on stress ulcer prophylaxis. Am J Health-Syst Pharm. 1999;56:347-79.

Chapter Eight

The Application of Statistical Analysis in the Biomedical Sciences

Ryan W. Walters • Karen L. Kier

Learning Objectives

After completing this chapter, the reader will be able to

- Describe the importance of statistical analysis in completing and evaluating empirical studies.
- Identify and define the four scales of variable measurement.
- Define descriptive and inferential statistics.
- Describe several common epidemiological measures.
- Describe the properties of several commonly used probability distributions.
- Identify and describe the difference between parametric and nonparametric statistical tests.
- Discuss the assumptions of commonly used parametric and nonparametric statistical tests.
- Determine whether the appropriate statistical test has been performed when evaluating a study.
- Determine whether the statistical test was interpreted appropriately when evaluating a study.

Key Concepts

❶ There are four scales of measurement—nominal, ordinal, interval, and ratio.

❷ The mean is the most appropriate measure of central tendency for normally distributed interval or ratio variables, while the median is the most appropriate measure for ordinal variables or skewed distributions.

❸ The variance and standard deviation are the appropriate measures of variability for normally distributed variables measured on an interval or ratio scale.

❹ The central limit theorem states that when equally sized samples are drawn from a non-normal distribution, the plotted mean values for each sample will approximate a normal distribution.

❺ Clinical significance is far more important than statistical significance.

❻ Adaptive designs have strengths, but the limitations are substantial. Thus, researchers have to consider the limitations *a priori*.

❼ The decision of which statistical test to employ is based on several factors—research question, study design, dependent variable and independent variable considerations, and assumption violations—most of which are interconnected.

Knowledge of statistics is essential to understanding empirical literature within the biomedical sciences. This chapter will provide a basic understanding, and applied application, of descriptive and inferential statistics for the reader who has little or no statistical background. The focus of this chapter is to describe concepts as they relate to evaluating medical literature, as opposed to discussing the mathematical underpinnings, calculation, and programming of any specific statistical test. This chapter will enhance the ability of the student or evidence-based practitioner to interpret results of empirical literature within the biomedical sciences by evaluating the appropriateness of statistical tests employed, the conclusions drawn by the authors, and the overall quality of the study.

Before discussing the types of statistics used in biomedical literature, it may be helpful to review information regarding study design, dependent variable (DV) and independent variable (IV), and the four scales of measurement. The first section of this chapter will discuss basic concepts about populations, samples, data, and variables while the second section will discuss specific descriptive and inferential statistics.

Basic Concepts

POPULATIONS AND SAMPLES

When investigating a particular research question or hypothesis, researchers must first define the population to be studied. A population refers to all objects of a similar type in the universe, while a sample is a fraction of the population chosen to be representative of the specific population of interest. Thus, samples are chosen to make specific generalizations about the population of interest. Researchers typically do not attempt to study the entire population as most often data cannot be collected for everyone within a population. This emphasizes why the sample must be chosen at random; that is, each member of the population must have an equal chance of being included in the sample. For example, consider a study to evaluate the effect a calcium channel blocker (CCB) has on blood glucose levels in insulin-dependent diabetes mellitus (IDDM) patients. In this case, all IDDM patients would constitute the study population; however, because data could never be collected from all IDDM patients, a random sample that is representative of the IDDM population is selected. There are numerous random sampling methods, many beyond the scope of this text. Although only a few are discussed here, interested readers are urged to consult the list of recommended readings at the end of the chapter.

A random sample does not imply that the sample is drawn haphazardly or in an unplanned fashion. There are several approaches to selecting a random sample, with the most common method employing a random number table. A random number table theoretically contains all integers between one and infinity that have been selected without any trends or patterns (i.e., completely random). Thus, consider a random sample of IDDM patients; each patient in the population is assigned a number; say 1 to 1000 (ridiculously low, but as an example) from which a sample of 200 patients is requested. The random number table would randomly identify 200 patients from the population of 1000. There are numerous free random number tables and generators available online; simply search for random number table or random number generator in any search engine.

Depending on the type of study design, a simple random sample may not be the best method for selecting a representative sample. On occasion, it may be necessary to separate the population into mutually exclusive groups called strata, where a specific factor (e.g., patient race, gender) will be contained in separate strata to aid in analysis. In this case, the random sample is drawn within each stratum individually, termed a stratified random sample. For example, consider a situation where the race of the patient was an important variable in the IDDM study. To ensure each race is represented properly, the researcher stratifies by race and randomly selects patients within each stratum to achieve a study sample representative of the population of interest.

Another method of randomly sampling a population is known as cluster sampling. Cluster sampling is appropriate when there are natural groupings within the population of interest. For example, consider a researcher interested in the patient counseling practices of pharmacists across the United States. It would be difficult, if not impossible, to collect data from all pharmacists across the United States. However, the researcher has read literature suggesting regional differences within various pharmacy practices, not necessarily including counseling practices. Thus, he or she may decide to randomly sample within the four regions of the United States (U.S.) defined by the U.S. Census Bureau (i.e., West, Midwest, South, and Northeast) to assess for differences in patient counseling practices across regions.[1]

Another sampling method is known as systematic sampling. This method is used when information about the population is provided in list format, such as in the telephone book, election records, class lists, licensure records, and so forth. A form of systematic sampling is the equal-probability method where one individual is selected at random and every nth individual is then selected thereafter. For example, the researchers may decide to take every 10th individual listed after the first individual is chosen.

Finally, it should be noted that researchers often use convenience sampling. A convenience sample selects participants based on the convenience of the researcher. That is, no attempt is made to select a random sample representative of the population. However, within the convenience sample, participants may be selected randomly. For example, consider a researcher evaluating a new educational method to increase exam scores. Often, this type of research will use the convenience sample available to them; that is, a random sample of the students in their own classes or university. Obviously, there are significant weaknesses to this type of sampling, primarily, limited generalization (i.e., external validity).

VARIABLES AND DATA

A variable is a characteristic that is being observed or measured. Data are the measured values assigned to the variable for each individual member of the population. For example, a variable would be patient gender, while the data is whether the patient is male or female. There are three types of variables: dependent (DV), independent (IV), and confounding.

The DV is the response or outcome variable for a study, while an IV is a variable that is manipulated. A confounding variable is any variable that has an effect on the DV over and above the effect of the IV, but is not of specific research interest. For example, consider a study to evaluate the effect a new oral hypoglycemic medication has on glycosylated hemoglobin (HbA1c). Here, the DV consists of the HbA1c data for each patient, while the IV divides the sample into two groups: treatment (those who receive the medication) and placebo (those receiving an identical looking placebo or other innocuous solution). Initially, results may suggest the medication is very effective across the entire sample; however, previous literature has suggested patient race may affect the effectiveness of this type of medication. Thus, patient race is a confounding variable and would need to be controlled in the statistical analysis (discussed later). After statistically controlling for patient race, the results now suggest the medication is more effective in one race compared to all others which is an important finding.

Scales of Measurement

❶ *There are four levels of measurement: nominal, ordinal, interval, and ratio scales.*[2] Think of these four scales as relatively fluid; that is, as the data progress from nominal to ratio, the information about each variable is increased (this will become clearer below). The scale of measurement of the DV, IV(s), and confounding variable(s) is an important consideration when determining whether the appropriate statistical test was used to answer the research question and hypothesis. Further, when conducting analyses, it is important to recognize the relationship between the individual data points and the outcome or event they represent for each variable.

A nominal scale consists of categories that have no implied rank or order. Examples of nominal variables include patient gender (male versus female), patient race (Caucasian versus African American versus Hispanic), or disease state (absence versus presence). It is important to note that with nominal data, the patient can fit into only one category; that is, the data points are mutually exclusive.

An ordinal scale has all of the characteristics of a nominal variable; however, the data are placed into rank-ordered categories. It is important to note the distance between ordinal categories cannot be considered equal; that is, the data points can be ranked, but the distance between them may differ greatly. For example, in medicine a commonly used pain scale is the Wong-Baker Faces Pain Rating Scale.[3] Here, the patient ranks pain on a 0 to 10 scale; however, while it is known that a rating of 8 indicates the patient is in more pain than rating 4, there is no indication an 8 hurts twice as much as a 4.

Interval scales consist of ordered data points on a constant scale without a natural zero. That is, interval scales increase the information provided by an ordinal scale by allowing researchers to quantify a meaningful distance between two units. For example, temperature on a Celsius scale is measured on an interval scale (i.e., $10°C - 5°C = 20°C - 15°C$). However, $20°C/10°C$ cannot be quantified as twice as hot because there is no absolute zero (the selection of $0°C$ was arbitrary).

Finally, *ratio scales* differ from interval scales in that they have an absolute zero. The classic example of a ratio scale is temperature measured on the Kelvin scale, which has an absolute zero representing the absence of molecular motion. Although researchers should not confuse absolute and arbitrary zero points, this difference is nonessential as interval and ratio scales are analyzed by identical statistical procedures.

Continuous and Discrete Variables

Continuous variables typically consist of data measured on interval or ratio scales. However, if the number of ordinal categories is high (e.g., seven or more) and the assumptions of the statistical test are met, they may be considered continuous in the literature.[4] In the biomedical literature, continuous variables may also be referred to as interval or quantitative. Examples of continuous variables include age, body mass index (BMI), uncategorized lab values (e.g., 120/60 as opposed to high versus low blood pressure).

Discrete variables usually consist of data measured on nominal or ordinal scales; however, a discrete variable can be created from any continuous variable via categorization, with the important caveat that information will be lost. For example, consider the role of patient age when studying cardiac events. Although age is a continuous variable, younger patients typically will not experience the same number of cardiac events as older patients. In addition, a 1-year increase in age may not significantly affect the number of cardiac events until the patient is very old. Thus, age can be classified into categories (i.e., < 30, 31–49, 50–69, etc.) and used in analysis. Here, information is lost by using categorized age in analysis because the exact age of the patients is not considered, only their age category. Creating categories also allows the researcher to identify a reference category to compare to all other categories. For example, if 90+ is selected as the reference category, the analysis would then compare < 30 to 90+, 31–49 to 90+, 50–69 to 90+, and so on. Finally, in the literature, discrete variables are often termed nominal or categorical, or, if a variable is measured on a nominal scale with only two levels (e.g., male versus female), it may be termed dichotomous.

DESCRIPTIVE STATISTICS

● There are two types of statistics: descriptive and inferential. Descriptive statistics present, organize, and summarize data in a very basic sense, while providing information regarding the appearance of the data and distributional assumptions. Inferential statistics (discussed later) test for differences or relationships, against random variation, within the study sample, allowing reliable findings to be generalized to the population of interest.

Descriptive statistics are often used to summarize study data numerically and/or graphically. Measures of central tendency, variability, and shape are types of numerical representation, while histograms, boxplots, and scatterplots are common graphical representations.

Measures of Central Tendency

● Measures of central tendency are helpful in identifying the distribution of the data numerically. The most common measures of central tendency are the arithmetic mean (or simply, the mean), median, and mode. The most appropriate measure of central tendency depends on the scale of measurement for the variable being studied.

❷ *The mean is the most common and appropriate measure of central tendency for normally distributed data (discussed below) measured on an interval or ratio scale.* It is best described as the average numerical value for data within a variable. The mean is calculated by summing all data for a variable and dividing by the total number of patients with data on that specific variable (if data is complete, this number will be the total sample size, or simply n).

❷ *The median is most appropriate for data measured on an ordinal scale;* however, it can also be presented for continuous variables to assist in describing the variable distribution, as discussed below. The median is the absolute middle value in the data (exactly at the 50th percentile); that is, half of the data points fall above and half below the median. It is important to note that outliers (i.e., data points that are disconnected from the other data points) can significantly affect the mean, but not the median. Therefore, a comparison of the mean and median can give insight into whether outliers influenced the mean and overall distribution of the data points within a variable.

The mode is the most appropriate measure of central tendency for nominal data. The mode is the most frequently occurring value or category within a variable. Further, a variable could have two, three, or more modes; thus, a variable with two modes is referred to as bimodal, with three modes, trimodal, and so on.

Measures of Variability

The most common measures of variability (or dispersion) are the range, interquartile range, variance, and standard deviation. Measures of variability are useful in indicating the spread of data for a variable. These measures are also useful in association with measures of central tendency to assess how scattered the data are around the mean or median. For example, consider two nearly identical mean HbA1c values for the treatment and placebo groups in a study of IDDM patients. Taken at face value, the patients in these two groups may be considered similar; however, assessing the variability of the data within these two groups individually may illustrate a completely different picture. For instance, the treatment group may have considerably more variability (i.e., spread of HbA1c values) compared to the placebo group, which can affect results of statistical tests as well as affecting clinical significance. A clinician may find that the treatment group with more consistent HbA1c values is preferential. Considering measures of variability are vitally important when evaluating the biomedical literature, which will allow decisions to be made regarding the accuracy of the interpreted results.

The range can be used appropriately to describe data measured on an ordinal, interval, or ratio scale. The range is found by subtracting the minimum data point from the maximum data point. In the CCB example, say the maximum blood glucose was 357 mg/dL and the minimum was 54 mg/dL, the range would be equal to 303 mg/dL. In the medical literature, authors often provide the range simply by presenting the minimum and maximum values in the data. Although the range is easy to calculate, the measure is not very useful in describing or comparing data.

The interquartile range (IQR) is another measure of dispersion used to describe data measured on ordinal, interval, or ratio scales. The IQR is a measure of variability directly related to the median. The interquartile range is the difference between the 75th and 25th percentile. Remember, the median is located at exactly the 50th percentile; therefore, the interquartile range presents the middle 50% of the data and always includes the median. This value is a stable measure of spread and is not as affected by extreme values (i.e., outliers) in the data.

The final two measures of variability described are the variance and standard deviation. ❸ *These measures are appropriate for normally distributed continuous variables measured on interval or ratio scales.* Briefly, the variance for a variable is the average squared deviation from the mean for all data points within a specific variable. For example, say the mean value for HbA1c within the treatment group is 6.5%, and a specific patient had an HbA1c value of 6.0%. The squared deviation from the mean for this patient would be equal to 0.25% (i.e., 6.0% − 6.5% = −0.5%; $(−0.5\%)^2 = 0.25\%$). This calculation would continue for all patients in the study sample. When all squared deviations values are calculated, the squared deviations are summed and divided by the total sample size (assuming complete data) to obtain the variance. The reason deviations from the mean are squared is that otherwise, when summed, the unsquared deviations would equal zero. The variance is useful when calculating many of the inferential statistics discussed below; however, the standard deviation is typically used to describe the spread within continuous variables.

The standard deviation and variance are directly related, as the standard deviation is the square root of the variance. Thus, if one value is known, the other can be calculated. Standard deviation is often preferred over variance because it indicates the average deviation from the mean presented on the same scale as the original variable, unlike the variance, which is in square units. In comparing two groups with equal means, the standard deviation can provide insight into the dispersion of scores around the mean, with larger values indicating greater variability. For example, consider two variables with identical means. However, variable A has a standard deviation of 5.0, while variable B has a standard deviation of 15.1. Thus, variable B has greater variability in the data compared to variable A.

Finally, the coefficient of variation is a less commonly used measure that evaluates the dispersion of two or more variables measured on different scales. The coefficient of variation is typically expressed as a percentage, with higher percentages indicating greater variation. It is calculated by dividing the standard deviation by the mean and multiplying by 100. For example, it would not make sense to compare the standard deviations of blood glucose and HbA1c because they are measured on different scales. However, calculating the coefficient of variation for both blood glucose and HbA1c, say 67% and 33%, respectively, indicates there is less variability within the HbA1c values. It is important to note that extreme caution must be taken when interpreting the coefficient of variation, as a number of methodological issues can bias this value. It is advised to report and interpret the standard deviations of each continuous variable individually.

Measures of Shape

Skewness and kurtosis are appropriate for variables measured on interval or ratio scales, and indicate asymmetry and peakedness, respectively. They are typically used by researchers to evaluate the distributional assumptions of a variable, but both measures are usually omitted in the biomedical literature. The distribution of the DV is incredibly important when determining the most appropriate statistical test to employ, as most parametric statistical tests require a normal distribution (discussed in detail below).

The mean, median, and mode of a normal distribution (discussed below) are identical; thus, skewness can be indicated when the mean is not directly in the middle of the distribution. As stated above, skewness measures asymmetry within the distribution, and can be either positive or negative. Positive (or right) skewness occurs when the mode and median are less than the mean while negative (or left) skewness occurs when mode and median are greater than the mean. As stated previously, the mean is extremely sensitive to outlying values; thus, a researcher must identify true skewness as opposed to skewness due to outliers. True skewness is indicated by a steady decrease in data points toward the tails (i.e., ends) of the distribution. Skewness due to outliers in indicated when the mean is heavily influenced by data points that are extremely disconnected from the rest of the distribution.

Kurtosis refers to the peakedness of the distribution of data points. A curve with a wide, flat top is referred to as platykurtic, while a narrow, peaked distribution is termed leptokurtic. A platykurtic curve often is an indicator of greater variability; that is, the data is spread over a larger range. In contrast, a leptokurtic distribution has less variability with a large percentage of data points close to the mean.

It is often easier to visualize skewness and kurtosis with graphical representations as opposed to a numerical value. Significant skewness and kurtosis identified numerically may actually be spurious, especially for large sample sizes, as the denominator of the standard error calculation (used to identify significance) for skewness and kurtosis is sample size. Therefore, as sample size increases, standard error decreases, which may falsely indicate significant skewness or kurtosis. As a result, graphical representations of the data are presented in the next section, which provide researchers with a visual depiction of variable distributions.

Graphical Representations

Graphical representations of data are incredibly useful, especially when sample sizes are large. They allow researchers to inspect visually the distribution of individual variables. There are typically three graphical representations presented in the literature—histograms, boxplots, and scatterplots. Note that graphical representations are typically used for continuous variables measured on ordinal, interval, or ratio scales. By contrast, nominal, dichotomous, or categorical variables are best presented as count data, typically as frequency and percentage.

A histogram presents data as frequency counts over some interval; that is, the x-axis presents the values of the data points, whether individual data points or intervals, while the y-axis presents the number of times the data point or interval occurs in the variable

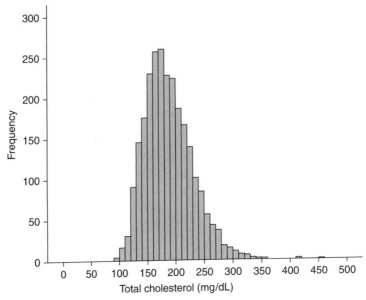

Figure 8–1. Histogram of total cholesterol with outliers.

(i.e., frequency). When data are plotted, it is easy to superimpose or visualize the normal distribution or bell curve to assess overall normality for the variable (i.e., skewness and kurtosis) as well as outliers. For example, consider the distribution of total cholesterol presented in Figure 8–1. Each vertical bar in the histogram represents a 20-unit interval. Further, the distribution has slight positive skewness and a few outliers (the disconnected scores between 420 mg/dL and 440 mg/dL in Figure 8–1).

A *boxplot*, also known as a box-and-whisker plot, provides the reader with five descriptive statistics.[5] Consider Figure 8–2, which presents identical data to the histogram in Figure 8–1. The box in a boxplot is the IQR, which identifies the 25th to 75th percentiles of data. Within the box is a broad line depicting the median, or 50th percentile. From both ends of the box extends a tail, or whisker, depicting the minimum and maximum data points. Further, a boxplot identifies and presents outliers (1.5 to 3.0 IQRs beyond the median) and extreme outliers (greater than 3.0 IQRs beyond the median) typically with circles and asterisks, respectively, as in Figure 8–2, or other symbols depending on the statistical software used.

A scatterplot presents bivariate (i.e., two variable) data for variables measured, typically, on continuous scales. That is, the *x*-axis contains the range of data for one variable, while the *y*-axis contains the range of data for the second variable. Figure 8–3 presents a scatterplot of total hospital cost (natural log transformed, discussed later) by the age of the patient. The individual circles in the scatterplot are participants' hospital cost

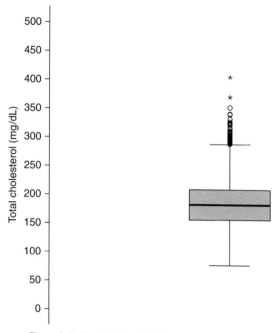

Figure 8–2. Boxplot of total cholesterol with outliers.

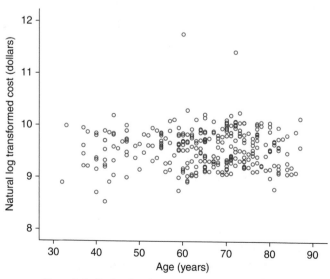

Figure 8–3. Scatterplot of natural log hospital cost and age.

in relation to their age. Therefore, participants are required to have data for both variables in order to be plotted. Scatterplots are useful in assessing association, or correlation (discussed below), between two variables as well as assessing other assumptions of various statistical tests (e.g., linearity, absence of outliers).

COMMON PROBABILITY DISTRIBUTIONS

• The distribution of the DV is of primary importance when determining which statistical test to employ. In the biomedical literature, a number of probability distributions are typically used to make inferences about the data and determine statistical significance. In the social, behavioral, and nursing sciences, the DV will often be continuous, requiring a normal distribution. In the biomedical literature, the DV could also be continuous, as well as categorical (e.g., dead versus alive, disease present versus disease absent), which requires binomial or Poisson distributions.

The Normal Distribution

• The normal distribution, also called Gaussian distribution, is one of the most important density curves. This distribution is the most commonly used distribution in statistics and one that occurs frequently in nature. It is very important to know whether a variable is distributed normally in the population, or whether the variable distribution approaches normal. As stated above, the statistical test employed often assumes variables are normal or approximately normal. This is vitally important when reading biomedical literature, as
• authors rarely state how variables are distributed. A normal curve has several easily identifiable properties uncovered by analyzing the numerical measures of central tendency, variability, and shape. Specifically, this includes the following characteristics:

1. The primary shape is a bell-curve.
2. The mean, median, and mode are identical.
3. The curve is symmetric around the mean; that is, the distribution is symmetrical and reflects itself perfectly when folded in half.
4. Skewness and kurtosis are zero.
5. The area under a normal distribution is, by definition, 1.

• It should be noted the five properties above are considered the gold standard. In practice, however, each of these properties may be approximated; namely, the curve will be roughly bell-shaped, the mean, median, and mode will be roughly equal, skewness and kurtosis may be evident but not significant, and so on.
• Finally, there are several additional aspects of a normal curve that are important. First, the curve is completely defined by the mean and standard deviation, meaning there are an infinite number of normal distributions as there are an infinite number of mean and

standard deviation combinations. Further, the standard deviation will always control the spread of the distribution (i.e., as the standard deviation increases, the distribution becomes wider). Third, the mean can always be identified as the topmost point of the curve. Finally, roughly 68% of the data will fall within one standard deviation (both positive and negative) of the mean, roughly 95% within two standard deviations, and roughly 99% within three standard deviations as shown in Figure 8–4.

The Standard Normal Distribution

Among the infinite number of possible normal distributions, only one can be compared to all other normal distributions—the standard normal distribution. When converting a normal distribution to a standard normal distribution, the variables are converted into standardized scores referred to as z-scores. A z-score is a means of expressing the original data in terms of the standard deviation; that is, how many standard deviations the score is from the mean. When converted to z-scores, the standard normal distribution has the same shape and characteristics as the normal distribution from which it originated, but with a mean of zero and a standard deviation and variance of one as seen in Figure 8–4. It should be noted that if the original distribution were skewed, z-score standardization would not normalize this distribution. That is, a skewed distribution will become a standardized skewed distribution.

Converting the original data to z-scores allows researchers to compare different variables as they are converted to the same scale (i.e., mean of zero; standard deviation of one). Therefore, differences between variables may be more easily detected and understood. For example, it is possible to compare similar standardized variables from different studies. The only assumption in this process is theoretical, and it requires that both

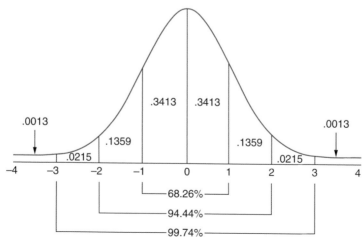

Figure 8–4. Area under the Normal Curve.

variables measure the same facet. For example, after z-score standardization, a study using low-density lipoprotein (LDL) cholesterol could be compared to another study using total cholesterol.[6]

The Binomial Distribution

Many discrete outcomes or events can be dichotomized into one of two mutually exclusive groups. The binomial distribution, also termed the Bernoulli distribution, is appropriate for this type of event or outcome (i.e., DV), and calculates the exact probability of the event or outcome. Note the binomial distribution approximates the normal distribution when n is large and the probability of the outcome is 0.50 (i.e., 50/50). The binomial distribution can only be used when an experiment assumes the four characteristics listed below:

1. The trial occurs a specified number of times (analogous to sample size, n).
2. Each trial has only two mutually exclusive outcomes (success or failure in a generic sense, x).
3. Each trial is independent, meaning that one outcome has no effect on the other.
4. The probability of success remains constant throughout the trial.

The binomial distribution counts the number of successes and failures during the study period. When all trials have been run, the probability of achieving exactly x successes (or failures) in n trials can be calculated. A classic example using the binomial distribution is flipping a coin. When the coin is flipped for a set number of trials, there are only two possible outcomes (i.e., heads or tails), each trial is not affected by the last, and the probability of flipping heads or tails remains constant (i.e., 0.50) throughout the trial. Say a coin is flipped ten times, of which it landed on heads six times. The binomial distribution allows for the calculation of the exact probability of achieving six heads in ten flips, which is 0.205. As mentioned above, if the coin was flipped 10,000 times, the binomial distribution would approximate the normal distribution.

In reality, however, the probability of an outcome is rarely 0.50. For example, often biomedical studies use all-cause mortality as the outcome variable. Most likely, the probability of suffering the event (i.e., death) is much lower than staying alive. Regardless, at the end of the trial, patients experience only one mutually exclusive outcome—dead or alive. In this example, say the sample consists of 1,000 patients, of which 154 die. The binomial distribution allows for the calculation of the exact probability of having 154 patients dying in a total sample of 1000 patients.

The Poisson Distribution

Similar to the binomial distribution, the Poisson distribution is a discrete probability distribution. However, the Poisson distribution typically involves count data or rates, allowing calculation of the mean probability of an event across time. The Poisson distribution can only be used when an experiment assumes the four characteristics listed below:

1. The probability of experiencing the event during a time interval is proportional to the length of the interval.
2. The probability of two events occurring during the time interval is low (i.e., rare events).
3. The probability of experiencing the event across time intervals remains constant.
4. The probability of experiencing the event in one time interval is independent of all other intervals.

For example, consider a study monitoring weekly drug-related hospital admissions over a 5-year study period. At the conclusion of the study, drug-related admissions occur on average 0.59 times per week. Assuming the four characteristics listed above, the Poisson distribution would allow for the calculation of the probability of experiencing anywhere from zero to an infinite number of drug-related hospital admissions per week. For example, based on a constant rate of 0.59 admissions per week, the probability of having one admission per week is 0.327.

DATA TRANSFORMATIONS

Various data transformations can be employed to remedy significant skewness, whether true skewness or skewness due to outliers. Significant kurtosis, on the other hand, is a much more difficult problem to remedy, but reasonable methods have been proposed for identifying and working with kurtotic distributions; however, these are outside the scope of this text.[7]

The transformations suggested for positive skewness differ from those suggested for negative skewness. Mild positive skewness is typically remedied by a square root transformation. Here, the square root of all data points for the variable is calculated and used in analysis. When positive skewness is severe, a natural log transformation is used, where the natural log is taken for all data points. For example, consider Figure 8–5. Here, the weight of approximately 10,000 participants was measured and the distribution is clearly skewed positively with several outliers. Because skewness did not appear severe, a square root transformation was used, as seen in Figure 8–6. However, very slight positive skewness is still evident along with several outliers; thus, the stronger natural log transformation is employed on the original data and presented in Figure 8–7.

When data are skewed negatively, power transformations are employed with higher powers being required for more severe skewness. For example, mild negative skewness may be remedied by squaring the data points, while severe skewness may require cubing

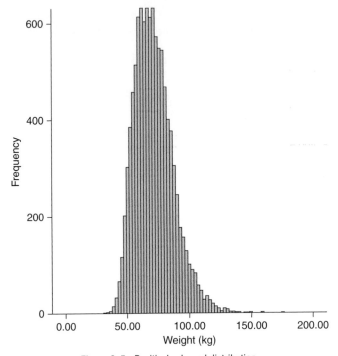

Figure 8–5. Positively skewed distribution.

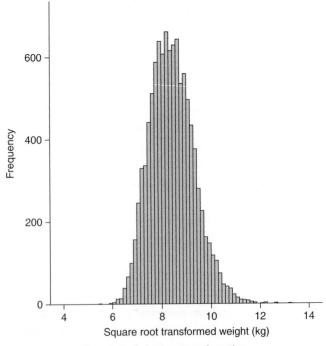

Figure 8–6. Square root transformation.

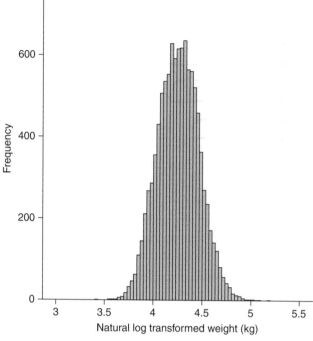

Figure 8–7. Natural log transformation.

or greater. The transformation process is identical to the example above. Depending on the severity of the skewness, several power transformations may be employed to identify which transformation better normalizes the distribution.

It should be noted while data transformation will not affect the rank order of the data; that is, participants with higher values prior to transformation will still have higher values following transformation, it will often cloud interpretation of inferential statistics significantly. That is, all results must be interpreted in transformed terminology, which can become convoluted quickly. Thus, when reading a journal article where the authors employed transformation, ensure the authors' interpretations were consistent with the transformed scale.

Epidemiological Statistics

The field of epidemiology investigates how diseases are distributed in the population and the various factors (or exposures) influencing this distribution.[8] Epidemiological statistics are not unique to the field of epidemiology, as much of the literature in the biomedical sciences incorporates some form of these statistics (e.g., odds ratios). Thus, it is important to have at least a basic understanding of these statistics. In this section, the most commonly used epidemiological statistics are discussed including ratios, proportions, rates, incidence and prevalence, relative risk and odds ratios as well as sensitivity, specificity, and predictive values.

RATIO, PROPORTIONS, AND RATES

Ratios, proportions, and *rates* are frequent terms used interchangeably in the medical literature without regard for the actual mathematical definitions. Further, there are a considerable number of proportions and rates available to researchers (some of which are discussed below), each providing unique information. Thus, researchers must be aware of how each of these measures was defined and calculated.[9]

A ratio expresses the relationship between two numbers. For example, consider the ratio of men to women diagnosed with multiple sclerosis (MS). If, in a sample consisting of only MS patients, 103 men and 57 women are diagnosed, the ratio of men to women is 103 to 57, or 103:57. Remember, that the order in which the ratio is presented is vitally important; that is, 103:57 is not the same as 57:103.

A proportion is a specific type of ratio indicating the probability or percentage of the total sample that experience an outcome or event without respect to time. Here, the numerator of the proportion (i.e., patients with the disease) is included in the denominator (i.e., all individuals at risk). For example, say 840 non-MS patients are added to the sample above for a total sample of 1000; thus, the proportion of patients with MS is 0.160 or 16.0% (i.e., 160/1,000). Note that the probability of a specific proportion is assessed by the binomial distribution.

A rate is a special form of proportion that includes a specific study period, typically used to assess the speed at which the event or outcome is developing.[10] A rate is equal to the number events, in a specified time period, divided by the length of the time period. For example, say over a 1-year period, 50 cases of MS were diagnosed. Thus, the rate of new cases of MS within this sample is 50 per year.

INCIDENCE AND PREVALENCE

Incidence quantifies the occurrence of an event or outcome, for a specific study period, within a specific population. The incidence rate is calculated by dividing the number of new events by the total number of people capable of experiencing the event (i.e., the population at risk). For example, consider the 50 new cases of MS that developed from the example above. The incidence rate is approximately 0.06 (i.e., 50/840). Note the denominator did not include the 160 patients already diagnosed (i.e., 1000 – 160 = 840) with MS because they were no longer considered at risk.

Prevalence quantifies the number of patients who have already experienced or outcome at a specific time point. Prevalence is calculated by dividing the total number of patients experiencing the event by the total number of individuals in the population. For example, including all MS cases above (i.e., $50 + 160 = 210$), the prevalence of MS in this sample is 0.21.

Finally, it is important to consider both incidence and prevalence when describing events or outcomes. Prevalence varies directly with incidence and the duration of the disease. For example, consider influenza. Here, the duration of the disease is relatively short; thus, while incidence (i.e., number of new cases) may be high, the overall prevalence may be low because most individuals recover or die quickly. By contrast, consider individuals diagnosed with asthma. Because asthma is incurable, the prevalence of the disease may be high because prevalence is an aggregate index, while incidence may be low depending on the total number of new cases diagnosed throughout the year. A good research article will describe both incidence and prevalence, as well as specify the specific study period.

RELATIVE RISK AND ODDS RATIO

Relative risk is defined as the ratio (or probability) of the incidence of an event occurring in individuals exposed to a risk compared to the incidence of the event in those not exposed to the risk. Relative risk can be calculated directly from the cohort study design (discussed previously in Chapter 5). Briefly, this design is typically a prospective observational design comparing the incidence of experiencing an event in exposed and unexposed individuals (i.e., the cohort) over time. For example, consider the risk of developing lung cancer in those who are exposed and unexposed to second-hand smoke over a 10-year study period. Upon study conclusion, the 2×2 contingency table, shown in Table 8–1, is created containing frequency counts of events for the exposed and unexposed groups. This table provides all data necessary to calculate the incidence of the event for both exposed and unexposed individuals. Relative risk is calculated by dividing the proportion of individuals who suffered the event in the exposed group (i.e., A/A+B) by the proportion of individuals who suffered the event in the unexposed group (i.e., C/C+D). When

TABLE 8–1. EXAMPLE OF A 2 × 2 CONTINGENCY TABLE

	Event	No Event	
Exposed	A	B	A+B
Unexposed	C	D	C+D
	A+C	B+D	A+B+C+D

calculated, relative risk provides a single number ranging from zero to infinity, and there are three interpretations resulting from this calculation.[8]

1. If relative risk equals 1, the exposed and unexposed have equal risk, indicating no association between the event and exposure.
2. If relative risk is greater than 1, the exposed group has greater risk than the unexposed group indicating a positive association with the risk factor.
3. If relative risk is less than 1, the exposed group has a lower risk than the unexposed group indicating a negative association or protective effect.

When relative risk cannot be calculated, researchers will present an odds ratio, which estimates relative risk. Odds are calculated by dividing the probability of experiencing an event by the probability of not experiencing an event. Thus, an odds ratio is a ratio of two odds; one for those exposed to the risk and the other for those not exposed to the risk. Odds ratios can be calculated for both cohort and case-control designs. A case-control study compares those who have experienced the event (i.e., cases) and those who have not (i.e., controls), and then assesses whether each individual was exposed to a risk. Thus, a case-control study is retrospective. For example, consider comparing a group of individuals who developed measles to those who did not and then determine whether they received all recommended vaccinations. The odds ratio is calculated differently depending on the design, but both calculations use a similar contingency table in Table 8–1. In a cohort study, the odds ratio is calculated by dividing the odds of experiencing the event in the exposed group (i.e., A/B) by the odds the unexposed group experienced the event (i.e., C/D). In a case-control study, the odds ratio is calculated by dividing the odds that cases were exposed to the risk (i.e., A/C) by the odds that the controls were exposed (i.e., B/D).

SENSITIVITY, SPECIFICITY, AND PREDICTIVE VALUES

Sensitivity, specificity, and predictive values (both positive and negative) measure the ability of a test to identify correctly those experiencing the event and those who did not. For example, consider the ability of a blood glucose screening test to correctly identify those with diabetes. Four outcomes result from this test, and are required for the calculation of sensitivity, specificity, and the predictive values:

1. True positives (TP) have the disease and have a positive test result.
2. False positives (FP) do not have the disease, but have a positive test result.
3. True negatives (TN) do not have the disease and have a negative test result.
4. False negatives (FN) have the disease, but have a negative test result.

Sensitivity is the probability a diseased individual will have a positive test result. It is the true positive rate of the test. It is calculated by dividing true positives by all individuals who actually have the disease (i.e., TP/TP + FN). Specificity is the probability a disease-free individual will have a negative test result, and is the true negative rate of the screening test. It is calculated by dividing true negatives by all disease-free individuals (i.e., TN/TN + FP).

Positive and negative predictive values are calculated to measure the accuracy of the screening test. Both predictive values are directly related to disease prevalence; that is, the higher the prevalence, the higher the predictive value.[8] Positive predictive value provides the proportion of individuals who test positive for the disease that actually have the disease. It is calculated by dividing true positives by all individuals with a positive test result (i.e., TP/TP + FP). Negative predictive value provides the proportion of individuals who test negative who are actually disease-free. It is calculated by dividing true negatives by all individuals with a negative test result (i.e., TN/TN + FN).

It is important to identify the implications all four values have to new and existing research. When designing a study involving a screening test, researchers must indicate a standard cutoff score for their screening. That is, qualify who is to be considered diseased and who will be considered disease-free. This decision clearly reflects the repercussions of classifying individuals as false negatives or false positives. For example, consider a screening tool for early stage breast cancer. There are considerable consequences for both false positives and false negatives. On one hand, a patient with a false positive may be referred for unnecessary testing that is painful and expensive, as well as emotionally taxing. On the other hand, a false negative also has serious implications, since the patient may not receive any treatment until the disease has progressed much farther.

Case Study 8–1

A researcher is considering a study to evaluate the effect of a new comprehensive intervention on reducing 30-day hospital readmissions for heart failure over a 1-year study period. The new intervention involves many levels of care, including hospitalists providing patient education; pharmacists ensuring medications are being taken, tolerated, and refilled accurately; and nurse practitioners checking on at home patient status. At the end of the study, patients receiving the intervention will be compared to a control group.

It is obvious the study will be costly; thus, the most important consideration is study design, allowing the researchers to evaluate the effectiveness of the intervention with few wasted resources. Please consider the items below:

1. Describe the population of interest.
2. What type of sampling strategy is most appropriate? Why?

3. What is the DV for this study? How many levels does the DV have? What is the scale of measurement?
4. What is the appropriate measure of central tendency for this DV? Why? How should this data be presented in an article?
5. What is the IV for this study? How many levels does the IV have? What is the scale of measurement?
6. What confounding variables should be considered? Why?
7. Describe the characteristics of an adequate control group.
8. What distribution will be used in data analysis? Why?
9. What epidemiological statistic(s) is most appropriate? Why?

Statistical Inference

Statistical analysis allows researchers to make rational decisions in the presence of random processes and variation. Inferential statistics provide the probability a conclusion is true in the population, based on the analysis of sample data. This section presents several considerations prior to conducting and evaluating the result of a statistical test. First, the sampling distribution and application of the central limit theorem is discussed, followed by hypothesis testing, as well as Type I and Type II errors and statistical power. Then, the difference between statistical and clinical significance is discussed. Next, the appropriate uses of parametric and nonparametric statistical tests are discussed. Finally, a brief discussion of experimental, nonexperimental, and quasi-experimental design, as well as the design and analysis of clinical trials, are presented.

SAMPLING DISTRIBUTIONS AND THE CENTRAL LIMIT THEOREM

As stated above, statistical inference employs sample data to make conclusion about populations. Because good samples are chosen randomly, the means produced from these samples are also random.[11] Thus, the mean may not be exactly representative of the population and varies from sample to sample. However, the law of large numbers states that as the size of the sample increases, the sample mean will move closer to the population mean. Further, as the number of samples increases, the mean of the sample means will begin to approximate the population mean. ❹ *The central limit theorem states when equally sized samples are drawn from a non-normal distribution, the plotted mean values from each sample will approximate a normal distribution as long as the non-normality was not due to outliers.* This distribution is termed the distribution of sampling means. For example, consider a study to analyze the mean value of blood urea nitrogen (BUN) in the general, healthy population, where the researcher selects 100 random samples of 10 healthy participants. Each sample of 10 will provide a mean BUN value, and although mean BUN will vary from sample to sample, when the 100 sample means are plotted in a histogram the distribution will begin to approximate the population distribution.

The central limit theorem states sufficiently large samples should produce an approximately normal distribution of sampling means as long as the data do not contain outliers. A sufficiently large sample is one that contains 30 or more participants or a situation where the degrees of freedom (discussed below) for the statistical test are greater than 20.[12] In addition, researchers must be careful not to confuse the issue of having a large enough sample to achieve statistical significance if it exists (i.e., statistical power; consult Chapter 4) and a large enough sample to be representative of the population.

As with any normal distribution, the standard deviation of the distribution of sampling means can be calculated, termed the standard error of the mean (SEM). The SEM is equal to the standard deviation divided by the square root of the sample size, and reflects variability within the sample means. It is important when evaluating the literature to distinguish between the standard deviation and the SEM. Researchers often use the SEM to show variability or noise in their data instead of using the standard deviation because the SEM will always be smaller. This incorrect use of SEM will show their data as less variable and more appealing.

HYPOTHESIS TESTING

A hypothesis indicates a theory about the population regarding an outcome the researcher is interested in studying. Statistical analyses test two types of hypotheses, the null and alternative. The null hypothesis assumes no difference or association between the different study groups or variables, while the alternative hypothesis states there is a difference or association. A representative, ideally random, sample is then drawn from the population of interest to estimate the population parameter (e.g., mean, odds ratio) and test whether a difference or association exists.

When testing hypotheses, researchers often need to determine whether their hypothesis is directional; that is, using a one-sided (directional) or two-sided (nondirectional) hypothesis test. For example, consider a hypothesis that states that initiating statin therapy will lower (i.e., directional) low-density lipoproteins (LDL). However, if the researchers were looking for any effect of statin therapy, whether lowering or raising LDL (i.e., nondirectional), they would have used a two-sided test. In the literature, it is generally more acceptable to use a two-sided test, even if the hypothesis is directional, as a two-sided test is considered stronger statistically and reduces the probability of committing a Type I error.

ERROR AND STATISTICAL POWER

It is essential that researchers establish how much error they are willing to accept before the initiation of the study. Type I and Type II have been discussed at length in Chapter 4. Briefly, a Type I error occurs when the researcher indicates a statistically significant difference exists when, in fact, one actually does not (i.e., false positive). Thus, a Type I error can only occur when the null hypothesis is true. A Type II error occurs when the researcher fails to indicate a statistically significant difference when one actually exists (i.e., false negative). Type I and Type II errors are interconnected; that is, as one type increases the other decreases. Researchers must consider these two errors carefully when designing studies, similar to the breast cancer example from above, weighing whether a false positive is more or less concerning than a false negative.

Statistical power was developed as a method allowing researchers to calculate the probability of finding a statistically significant result, when, in fact, one actually exists. This topic has been discussed in Chapter 4. Essentially, increasing statistical power reduces the probability of committing a Type II error; however, it can also increase the probability of committing a Type I error. Statistical power is influenced by four factors: alpha (the probability value at which the null hypothesis is rejected), effect size (the size of the treatment effect), error variance (the precision of the measurement instrument), and the sample size. Statistical power can be increased by increasing alpha (not advised), effect size, or sample size as well as deceasing error variance. Statistical power of at least 0.80 has been recommended.[13] However, some researchers use 0.90 or higher in the biomedical sciences, indicating that a false negative is more detrimental than a false positive.

Statistical Versus Clinical Significance

The next step in the research process is to employ a statistical test to assess whether a difference or relationship exists in the study sample. Primarily, the researcher is interested in determining whether to retain the null hypothesis or reject it in favor of the alternative hypothesis. Statistical tests produce probability values (i.e., p values) which range from 0 to 1. The p value produced from a statistical test is the probability of committing a Type I error based on the assumption that the null hypothesis is true (i.e., there is in reality no difference or relationship in the population and the actual observed difference or relationship is due to sampling error or random variation). If the p value is less than alpha, the difference or relationship is considered statistically significant.

Similar to p values, alpha ranges from 0 to 1; however, in most studies in the biomedical sciences use alpha set at 0.05. There may be occasions when alpha is set at 0.01 producing a more stringent statistical test (i.e., less likely to find statistical significance); however, this is rare. Statistical significance can never prove a hypothesis, only support it. A more stringent statistical test (i.e., alpha = 0.01 or 0.001) does not indicate in any way that a real treatment effect occurred. The set alpha level is a key contributor to the theoretical calculation of the true Type I error rate; that is, the level the researcher is willing to tolerate where a true null hypothesis may be falsely rejected. Again, most studies typically set alpha equal to 0.05; however, this value is technically an arbitrary value set by the researcher. A more lenient or stringent alpha may be used instead to attempt to better support the null hypothesis or make a stronger case for rejecting the null hypothesis, respectively. For all statistical tests, the alpha level has an associated critical value (i.e., the value the respective test statistic must exceed for the null hypothesis to be rejected) based on specific degrees of freedom (discussed below). Finally, alpha (and a p value) is directly indicative of the area under the distribution curve of interest (e.g., the standard normal distribution). Thus, an alpha (or p value) of 0.05 indicates 5% of the distribution's area is to the left or right of the associated critical value depending on whether the test statistic is positive or negative (e.g., a z-score of approximately 1.645 or –1.645 in Figure 8–4 leaves 5% of the distribution to the right and left, respectively, for a one-tailed test depending on the hypothesized direction). For a two-tailed test, the z-score for an alpha of 0.05 is 1.96 or –1.96, which leaves 2.5% of the distribution to the right or left of the z-score. When summed (2.5% + 2.5%) it equals 5% or 0.05 of the entire distribution. This highlights how a p value less than 0.05 indicates that less than 5% of the values (or area) lies beyond the critical value for the specific test statistic. Note, there is difficulty when interpreting p values, even among statisticians.[14] However, in general, if a p value is less than the set alpha value, the researcher rejects the null hypothesis in favor of the alternative hypothesis, and the difference or relationship is considered statistically significant. If the p value is equal to or greater than alpha, the null hypothesis is retained, and the difference or relationship is not considered statistically significant.

Statistical significance can also be established by calculating a confidence interval around the estimated population parameters (e.g., sample means) or test statistics. Confidence intervals account for sample size and variation; thus, a tighter confidence interval indicates less variability in the data. A confidence interval provides a range of scores likely to contain the unknown population parameter, and generally, a confidence interval is reported using a 95% confidence level. However, similar to alpha, the confidence level is arbitrary, with some researchers using 99% (note that as the confidence level increases, so does the width of the interval). A 95% confidence interval indicates that if repeated random sampling occurs within the population of interest under consistent conditions (e.g., sample size), the true population parameter would be included in the interval 95% of the time. Thus, every value within the interval is considered a possible value of the population parameter. Remember from above that roughly 95% of scores in a normal distribution fall within two standard deviations of the mean (actually, within approximately 1.96 standard deviations), and, according to the central limit theorem, this same value is applicable to 95% of means in the sampling distribution of means. A 95% confidence interval is calculated by multiplying 1.96 by the SEM and adding or subtracting this value from the estimated parameter to find the upper and lower confidence limits, respectively.

Using a confidence interval to indicate statistical significance varies according to whether the researcher is examining population parameters or test statistics. For example, consider Figures 8–8, 8–9, and 8–10. In each Figure, HbA1c values are being compared for a treatment and placebo group. Further, mean HbA1c for each group is presented as the circle, while the 95% confidence intervals are the whiskers extending above and below the means. The overlap of the confidence intervals between groups is directly related to p values; that is, less overlap (i.e., a larger difference) indicates smaller p values. Therefore, in Figure 8–8, the confidence intervals do not overlap; thus, this difference can be assumed statistically significant at least at $p < 0.05$. With that said, statistical significance can also be indicated when the confidence intervals overlap as long as the overlap is less than approximately 50% of a whisker, as in Figure 8–9.[15] Finally, as shown in Figure 8–10, substantial overlap in confidence intervals indicates a nonsignificant difference.

Determining statistical significance using confidence intervals around test statistics uses a different procedure, and varies based on the statistical test. For most parametric tests of group differences and correlation (discussed below), a 95% confidence interval around the test statistic containing zero is not considered statistically significant at an

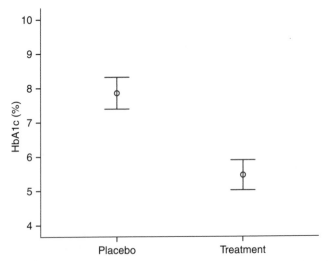

Figure 8–8. Statistically significant result indicated by non-overlapping 95% confidence intervals.

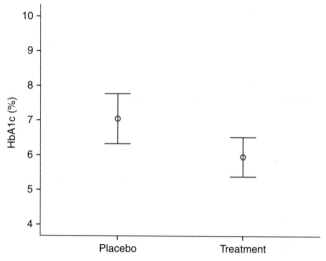

Figure 8–9. Statistically significant result indicated by overlapping 95% confidence intervals.

alpha of 0.05. That is, statistical significance for these types of analyses are essentially testing that the differences or relationship are different from zero. Thus, a 95% confidence interval containing zero essentially indicates that it is plausible that the true population difference or relationship could be zero.[16] For example, consider the commonly used independent samples *t* test (discussed below) testing for a difference between two group means. Say the test statistic produced as 2.0, but the confidence interval ranged from

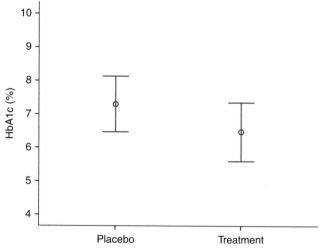

Figure 8–10. Overlapping 95% confidence interval indicating nonsignificance.

–0.50 to 4.50. Based on this sample, the difference would not be considered statistically significant because it is plausible that the true population parameter could in fact be zero.

Alternatively, the 95% confidence interval for test statistics based on ratios (e.g., logistic and Cox regression, discussed below) that contain 1 are not considered statistically significant at alpha equal to 0.05. Although this may seem different from above, it is actually very similar, and interpretation is identical. Statistical tests based on ratios produce odds or risks calculated by exponentiating the test statistic to create odds ratios (similar to above). A 95% confidence interval is calculated based on the exponentiated value. Because these values are exponentiated, converting these ratios back into the original unexponentiated metric requires calculating the natural log. Further, the natural log of 1 is zero. Thus, a 95% confidence interval containing 1 for an odds ratio produced by logistic regression indicates that it is plausible that the true population parameter could in fact be zero (i.e., the natural log of 1).

❺ *When evaluating the significance of the finding, keep in mind that statistical significance does not always indicate clinical significance.* Statistical significance can be manipulated in several ways, most easily by increasing sample size drastically. This sample size increase may artificially reduce error variance, which in turn reduces the standard error on which the test statistic is based thereby increasing the probability of statistical significance and the probability of committing a Type I error. As an example, with a sufficiently large sample, researchers may find a CCB reduced blood glucose significantly in IDDM patients. However, on examining the estimated parameters, the statistically significant difference in blood glucose was only 5 mg/dL, a decrease often considered clinically insignificant.

This example highlights the importance of identifying and interpreting the clinical significance (i.e., effect size) of all studies. While a complete discussion of effect size is beyond the scope of this chapter, in general, larger values are considered better (an interested reader should consult the recommended reading at the end of the chapter). However, it is important to remember that the definition of clinical significance varies by substantive area; thus, the definition of clinically significant to a researcher may be qualitatively different from an evidence-based practitioner. Finally, not all studies will provide an effect size estimate, especially in the biomedical sciences. Thus, research must be viewed with warranted skepticism until it can be determined whether the statistically significant difference or relationship is clinically meaningful.

PARAMETRIC AND NONPARAMETRIC TESTING

Regardless of whether a researcher is assessing for a statistically significant relationship or group difference, if the DV is continuous, the decision of which statistical test to employ typically begins with parametric options. All parametric tests have several conservative and easily violated assumptions, with the most critical requiring a defined probability distributions. That is, the estimated population parameters are evaluated against a defined distribution (several common distributions have been discussed above; e.g., normal, binomial, Poisson). Employing a parametric test in the presence of a non-defined distribution (e.g., skewed) will often lead to inaccurate and unreliable parameter estimates, because of violations to the assumptions necessary for parametric testing.

Some assumption violations challenge the robustness (i.e., correctness of the parameter estimate in the presence of assumption violations) of parametric tests greater than others. In most situations, any assumption violation requires the researcher to employ a nonparametric test, and most parametric tests have a widely used nonparametric alternative. Nonparametric statistical tests are distribution free, meaning that they do not make inferences based on a defined probability distribution. Further, the nonparametric tests can be employed for any scale of measurement (i.e., from nominal to ratio) and make few assumptions. Additional strengths of nonparametric tests include the ability to assess small sample sizes and the ability to assess data from several different populations.[17] However, it must be noted if the assumptions of a parametric test are assured these tests have greater statistical power than their nonparametric alternative(s).[18]

Although researchers rarely present information regarding assumption violations for parametric tests, it can be determined whether the test(s) was used appropriately based on the descriptive statistics authors typically present. In most cases, however, it will require some detective work. For example, consider an article where the author presents the mean, median, and standard deviation of the DV in a table. It is known that the parametric statistical test used requires a normally distributed DV and calculates the probability values of parameter estimates (i.e., statistical significance) of group means and standard deviations. From the descriptive statistics provided in the table, the spread of the distribution, indicated by the standard deviation, and presence of outliers as well as possible skewness, indicated by large discrepancies between the mean and median, can be determined. It is of benefit for readers to calculate these measures, whenever possible, since they should be skeptical of the statistics produced. However, if they do not have this particular expertise, they should find someone to help with the statistics.

EXPERIMENTAL, NONEXPERIMENTAL, AND QUASI-EXPERIMENTAL DESIGNS

The distinction between experimental, quasi-experimental, and nonexperimental research is important, both from a study design perspective and when evaluating literature. Although experimental designs are considered the gold standard by many, do not discount research conducted using quasi-experimental and nonexperimental designs, as long as the limitations are considered. Each of these types of designs will be discussed below.

Experimental Designs

In the biomedical sciences, experimental designs are typically referred to as a randomized control trial (RCT). Although a full treatment of experimental design is well beyond the scope of this chapter (refer to Chapter 4 for additional information on RCTs), it is important to note the key aspects of a quality experimental study. First, experimental designs always allow the researcher to manipulate levels of the IV(s). For example, consider a drug trial assessing the effectiveness of a new cancer medication. For this trial, four groups of participants are randomly assigned to a different dose of the medication (i.e., four levels of the IV). The researcher, within ethical and theoretical constraints, can manipulate the size of the dose, and, if the participants are measured multiple times, the length of the study period. Second, participants are randomly assigned to levels of the IV; thus, any participant has a chance of being placed into any single group. There are many different methods and theories of randomization, and the chance of being in one group versus another does not necessarily have to be equal. Third, causality can be determined with proper experimental control of error. For example, the effectiveness of a cancer drug can be better explained by reducing sources of error due to the participant (e.g., age, health status), setting (e.g., doctor), diagnostic tests (e.g., measurement accuracy), and so forth. However, it should be noted that an RCT has limitations. The primary limitation is cost. RCTs are extremely costly, requiring many considerations, such as space, personnel, and participants. RCTs also may have limited external validity and generalizability due to extreme control over experimental conditions, which do not necessarily translate to the real world. Third, it is difficult, if not impossible, to study rare events with an RCT due to the requirement of a considerable sample size. This discussion has only touched the tip of the iceberg on experimental designs; however, interested readers should consult the recommended readings referenced at the end of this chapter.

Nonexperimental Designs

Nonexperimental designs have several advantages over RCTs, primarily, low cost, quicker timeline to publication, and a broader range of patients.[19] The advantages of nonexperimental studies over RCTs have prompted their widespread use in the biomedical sciences. Overall, these studies tend to be nonrandomized, retrospective, and correlational in nature and are distinct because the researcher cannot manipulate the IV(s). For example, consider a 5-year retrospective study assessing the effectiveness of statin therapy on preventing cardiac events. The researcher has knowledge of which patients initiated statin therapy, but has no control over the drug, dose, adherence, and so on. Although the researcher may assign patients to groups based on the size of the dose, the researcher cannot randomly assign patients to drug or dose nor manipulate the dose the patients ingest. In addition, nonexperimental research often fails to indicate causality, which often is due to lack of experimental control and randomization as well as inability to identify all confounding variables. Finally, it is important to note that while nonexperimental designs are ubiquitous in the biomedical sciences, treatment effects may be different when compared to RCTs.[20]

Quasi-Experimental Designs

Quasi-experimental designs are seldom used in biomedical studies, and are much more common in the social sciences. On the surface, these types of designs appear to be experimental designs; however, they lack one key aspect, random assignment. For example, consider examining the effectiveness of a new dialysis treatment. Most dialysis patients are already in the care of a nephrologist at a specific clinic, and because nephrologists typically see numerous patients daily, randomizing patients to specific levels of treatment (i.e., the IV) may be unfeasible logistically. Thus, there is no choice, but to randomize entire clinics, where all patients in a specific clinic receive one treatment. Advantages to this type of design are similar to nonexperimental designs (e.g., cost, time) with the addition of possible increases in external validity due to conditions being more consistent with the real world. The disadvantages are considerable, primarily lack of random assignment. As with nonexperimental designs, nonrandom assignment may create dissimilar groups based on any number of characteristics related to the success of the treatment (e.g., patient demographics). Further, causation can rarely be implied and statistical analysis may be rendered useless.[21]

The Design and Analysis of Clinical Trials

The U.S. National Institutes of Health (NIH) defines five different types of clinical trials—treatment, prevention, diagnostic, screening, quality of life.[22] In this chapter, two specific types of treatment clinical trials are discussed—the randomized controlled trial (RCT) and adaptive clinical trial (ACT). The experimental design of RCTs and ACTs are discussed at length in Chapters 4 and 5. Briefly, both RCTs and ACTs are protocol-based (i.e., every step of the study from design to analysis is identified *a priori*), prospective studies (i.e., participants are followed over time) using strict experimental control to indicate reliably the causality between the manipulated IV (e.g., groups, dose) and DV (i.e., the outcome of interest).

THE DESIGN OF CLINICAL TRIALS

Parallel-Groups Design

The most common RCT is a parallel-groups design where the IV typically involves participants randomized into fixed levels of treatment (or arms), with each arm indicating a different treatment or comparison (e.g., placebo, active control).[23-26] That is, patients are randomly assigned to one, and only one, treatment or placebo group, and the sample size within each group is typically equal (however, sampling strategies vary). There are two parallel-groups designs frequently used in the biomedical sciences—group comparison and matched pairs.[25] Briefly, a group comparison design compares simultaneously at least two groups of participants, each group randomized to a different level of the IV. In a matched pairs design, participants are matched based on one or more characteristics (e.g., age, race) and then randomized to levels of the IV. This type of design closely resembles the within-subjects designs discussed later.

Crossover Design

The second most common RCT employs a crossover design, which has the primary purpose of having a participant serve as his or her own control.[23,25] The primary advantage of this type of design is that it typically requires fewer participants in comparison to a parallel-groups design. This happens because, at the end of the study, participants will have received all treatment arms. A disadvantage is that this type of trial cannot be used in a study where the first drug may have cured the patient (e.g., antibiotic), since there would be no reason to cross over to the other agent. For example, consider a 1-month study which includes two treatment arms. For a parallel-groups design, say 20 participants are required; that is, 10 participants are randomized to each treatment arm. By contrast, in a crossover design, only 10 subjects are required because each participant receives both treatments—10 participants receive the first arm, and the same 10 participants receive the second arm. While both designs have two total measurements, in the parallel-groups design, two individual groups of participants provide one measurement each, while in the crossover design, the same group of participants provides both measurements.

As another example, consider a 2×2 crossover design requiring one group of patients to receive treatment A followed by treatment B, while another group of patients receives treatment B followed by treatment A. Researchers will typically use a washout period between treatments to prevent the effects of the first treatment from carrying over to the second treatment. Note the length of the washout period varies depending on the treatment. For example, drugs with longer half-lives will require longer washout periods.

Adaptive Design

Finally, a more recent advancement to the RCT is the adaptive design or ACT. Although an adaptive trial is possibly cheaper and more ethical than an RCT, this design is much more complex to both implement and analyze; these considerations are discussed below. Briefly, adaptive designs implement changes (or adaptations) in the design or endpoint analyses based on the results of a predetermined (i.e., prior to initiation of the study) set of interim analyses. Interim analyses can be based on blinded or unblinded data, with the resulting adaptation(s) aimed at establishing a more efficient, safer, and informative trial that is more likely to demonstrate treatment effects.[27] For example, consider study examining the effect of three different doses of vitamin D on calcium absorption. Because this is a controversial area, ethical considerations require this study to be adaptive, as interim analyses provide important information regarding the effectiveness and safety of the doses. Thus, this ACT is scheduled to have interim analyses occurring quarterly. At the end of quarter two of the first year, the interim analyses indicated the group receiving the highest dose of vitamin D had twice the risk of developing kidney stones compared to the other two groups. Thus, this group was dropped from the study, and the study continues with the remaining two groups.

THE ANALYSIS OF CLINICAL TRIALS

The analysis of clinical trials typically involves studying longitudinal data (i.e., repeated measures); that is, participants are followed over time. This allows researchers to study the treatment effects over time in a smaller sample of participants due to the increased statistical power. Briefly, a repeated measures or longitudinal design increases statistical power by removing the error variance due to the participant, and thus reducing the overall error variance producing a larger test statistic. However, a repeated measures design has limitations relevant to clinical trials, primarily participant attrition and nonadherence. Attrition and nonadherence can assume many forms in a clinical trial. For example, participants may drop out of the study, fail to complete all required measurements, receive incorrect treatment or dose, or any other possible protocol violations. Thus, the first part of this section will discuss how the analysis of clinical trials typically handles missing data due to attrition and nonadherence. The subsequent sections discuss the analysis of parallel-group and crossover designs. Finally, the analysis of adaptive trials is discussed.

Intent-to-Treat and Per-Protocol Approaches

Two analytical approaches exist for clinical trials—intent-to-treat (ITT) and per-protocol (PP). The ITT approach is often employed in the presence of violations to protocol and patients being lost to follow-up, and is the approach most often used in the literature. ITT requires the analysis to include all participants in the arm to which they were randomized originally. That is, treatment effects are best evaluated by the planned treatment protocol rather than the actual treatment given.[28] For example, consider a participant randomized to receive Treatment A but instead receives Treatment B. For analysis, this participant would be considered as receiving Treatment A. It should be noted that if a large number of protocol violations of this nature occur, the study would be discontinued; thus, these occurrences are relatively rare. It is important to note that for ITT to be unbiased, attrition and nonadherence are considered to occur completely at random.[24] Further, the ITT approach may dilute treatment effects simply by including nonadherent participants by employing the last observation carried forward (LOCF) technique discussed below. By comparison, the PP approach evaluates only compliant participants with complete data. Although this analysis is straightforward analytically and allows researchers to evaluate a more accurate treatment effect, it has substantial limitations, primarily, reduced statistical power compared to an ITT approach, because participants with incomplete data are not considered in the analysis, and results in an inflated Type I error rate.[28]

Because the ITT approach considers all participants with at least one measurement, an imputation (i.e., replacement) method is employed for missing measurements, when necessary. The LOCF approach is one of the most commonly used imputation methods. This method uses the last recorded measurement (i.e., observation) for all missing values. For example, consider a study measuring HbA1c measured on six occasions over a 1-year study period. If a participant has only the first three measurements, the third (i.e., last) measurement would be imputed for measurements four through six. From this example, it is clear the ITT approach may dilute treatment effects. Other imputation approaches have been suggested including mean replacement, multiple imputation, and maximum likelihood estimation. However, these techniques only produce unbiased estimates if data are considered missing at random.[29,30]

Analyzing Parallel-Groups Designs

When analyzing a parallel-groups design, the traditional approach is to conduct an endpoint analysis, which typically involves employing an independent samples t test (for two groups), one-way analysis of variance (ANOVA) (for more than two groups), or analysis of covariance (ANCOVA) (two or more groups, statistically controlling for a baseline measurement) using only the final measurement (i.e., endpoint analysis). Note that these analyses are discussed in detail below.

For example, consider a study designed to assess the effect of lubiprostone compared to placebo (i.e., two arms) in treating chronic constipation associated with Parkinson disease. Following randomization, this 1-month study will assess constipation symptoms twice—at the end of weeks 2 and 4. An endpoint analysis will only consider the treatment effect at the week 4 measurement, ignoring the measurement at the end of week 2. Thus, this type of analysis does not consider the repeated measures and, as a result, does not consider the changes occurring over time, nor does it take full advantage of statistical power increases from a repeated measures design (as discussed above in the section titled Analysis of Clinical Trials).

By contrast, to assess for change over time, researchers often employ a two-way mixed ANOVA. Briefly, this analysis assesses between-subject factors (i.e., treatment versus placebo) and within-subject factors (i.e., participants measured two times). The major benefit of this analysis is provided by the interaction effect, which evaluates the change in repeated measurements over time between treatment arms. For example, consider the

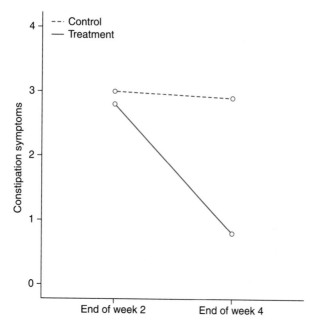

Figure 8–11. Statistically significant interaction effect.

lubiprostone example above. Results are presented graphically in Figure 8–11, where an apparent interaction is presented (indicated by the drastically different slopes between the two groups). Because a lower number of symptoms are indicative of treatment success, Figure 8–11 shows that the effect of lubiprostone is more effective compared to placebo over the study period. Following a statistically significant interaction effect, researchers can conduct follow-up (or *post hoc*) tests to determine where the significant difference occurred. Because this design used in the example was a 2×2 (i.e., group at 2 levels × the 2 repeated measures), no specific *post hoc* tests are necessarily required. However, if the design was larger, *post hoc* tests can assist researchers in identifying the shortest treatment time and minimum effective dose. That is, indicating where treatment effects diminish by assessing for plateaus or significant slope changes over the repeated measurements, or indicating when differences between doses converge and are no longer statistically significant. Finally, there are significant weakness in this type of analysis; however, it requires more statistical power to detect an interaction effect. That is, a larger sample size is required to detect this effect, which equates to a more costly study.

Analyzing Crossover Designs

The purpose of the crossover design is to study treatment effects using the participant as his or her own control. As discussed above, each participant receives all treatment arms, with an adequate washout period occurring between arms to eliminate carryover treatment effects. For example, consider the lubiprostone example above. Instead of having two treatment arms, all subjects are randomized into two groups, each receiving a different treatment order. Group A receives lubiprostone for the first 2 weeks, while Group B receives placebo. At the end of the 2-week study period, constipation symptoms are assessed. Next, all participants are required to have a 3-week washout period where no treatment or placebo are given, purported to effectively eliminate any carryover effects of the lubiprostone or placebo. After the washout period, Group A receives placebo for 2 weeks, while Group B receives lubiprostone. At the end of this second 2-week study period, constipations symptoms are assessed again.

A crossover design requires an initial test-for-order effect by assessing the interaction between order and the DV (i.e., constipation symptoms) by means of a two-way mixed ANOVA. When testing for order effects, a statistically significant interaction indicates that the order in which the treatments were received influenced the treatment effect. That is, receiving lubiprostone prior to placebo has a different treatment effect from receiving placebo prior to lubiprostone. A clear order effect is presented in Figure 8–12. Notice that the effect of placebo differs depending on the order in which it was received. The presence of a statistically significant order effect can have multiple explanations. Considering the example and Figure 8–12, it is clear that the washout period may not have been long enough, as the effectiveness of lubiprostone carried over to measurement of the placebo.

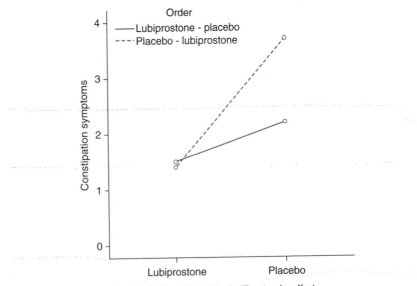

Figure 8–12. Statistically significant order effect.

In addition, the groups may have been initially different following randomization, a situation described in the randomization section above. Whenever a statistically significant order effect is identified, no further analysis is conducted as any subsequent analyses are biased by this order effect. However, if the interaction is nonsignificant (i.e., no order effect) an endpoint analysis is typically evaluated via paired samples t test. That is, treatment differences (i.e., lubiprostone versus placebo) are assessed without respect to the order in which the treatments were received.

Analyzing Adaptive Designs

The statistical analyses and considerations used when analyzing adaptive designs are similar to parallel-groups and crossover designs. The statistical tests used on the study endpoint typically include an independent samples t test (i.e., for comparing two groups), ANOVA (i.e., for comparing more than two groups), or ANCOVA (i.e., for statistically controlling baseline measurement). Further, Bayesian methods may be used as described briefly in Chapter 5. However, the endpoint for the interim analyses characteristic of adaptive designs will be the last recorded (i.e., most recent) measurement.

❻ *Several important considerations are required when analyzing and interpreting the results from adaptive designs.*[27] First, all interim and endpoint analyses suffer the risk of severely inflated Type I error rates; that is, as the number of interim analyses increases, the probability of finding spurious statistical significance increases. Thus, alpha has to be adjusted (i.e., reduced) appropriately, typically by dividing the experiment-wise alpha (i.e., 0.05 or the alpha the researcher decided is appropriate) by the number of interim analyses. This type of adjustment is known as a Bonferroni correction (discussed in detail in the Pearson's chi square section). Further, statistical power may be reduced by adjusting for Type I errors as alpha is being reduced drastically. This is a primary concern as inadequate statistical power increases the probability of Type II error, a situation that may lead to discontinuing an effective treatment. Remember, as the probability of Type I error decreases (e.g., by using a Bonferroni correction to reduce alpha), the probability of Type II error increases (e.g., by lowering statistical power). Second, estimates of population parameters may be biased. That is, any adaptation can reduce the generalizability to the original population sampled, produce underestimated or overestimated parameter estimates, and, thus, results in misleading confidence intervals. Researchers must carefully document and provide rationales for adaptations resulting from interim analysis. Failure to do so will indicate that results should be viewed with extreme caution. Finally, when all adaptations are considered, the overall results of the endpoint analyses may actually be invalid, providing inaccurate support for treatment effects. Consumers of research are urged strongly to consider these factors when interpreting and evaluating research using adaptive designs.

Statistical Techniques

❼ *The decision of which statistical test to employ is based on several factors—research question, study design, DV and IV considerations, and assumption violations—all of which are interconnected.* The next section describes the application and assumptions of the statistical tests most commonly used in the biomedical sciences applicable to designs with one measured DV. Within each section, a description of the statistical test is provided as well as an example with an associated results section as it will appear in the literature. Then the assumptions of each test are provided. It is incredibly important to take careful note of the assumptions for each statistical test, as these are vital in determining whether the correct statistical test was used when evaluating biomedical literature.

The discussion of statistical techniques begins with a brief introduction to degrees of freedom. Then, tests for nominal and categorical data are discussed, followed by statistical tests for evaluating group differences or relationships. Also, note a brief statistical decision tree has been provided at the end of this section to assist in determining the appropriate statistical test based on several factors including the distribution of the DV, repeated measurements, key assumption violations, covariates, and so on (see Table 8–2).

DEGREES OF FREEDOM

Degrees of freedom (df) are a vital component of all statistical tests, as most probability distributions, and, thus, statistical significance, are based on them. In all published research, degrees of freedom are provided for all statistical tests and are a useful indicator of adequate sample size in the presence of assumption violations. For example, reconsider the central limit theorem. The central limit theorem states that the distribution of sampling means is approximately normal with degrees of freedom for error greater than 20 (this will become apparent in the sections below), or with a sample greater than 30. Thus, the central limit theorem operates independently of the distribution of the actual raw data. Therefore, if an author presents the mean and standard deviation of a variable that is clearly skewed (but without outliers), and degrees of freedom for error of the statistical test is greater than 20, the results can typically be viewed as accurate.

The definition of degrees of freedom is obscure and beyond the scope of this chapter; however, a brief description is provided. Degrees of freedom equal the number values that are free to vary prior to the last value being fixed. For example, consider a group of three participants with a mean age of 50. Here, the mean is the fixed value. Because the mean is 50, any two of the participants can be of almost any age greater than zero (as long as the sum of their ages is not equal to or greater than 150 because age cannot take on a negative value). The third participant, however, must be the age that creates the mean of 50.

TABLE 8–2. DETERMINING THE APPROPRIATE STATISTICAL TEST

	DV Scale	Distributional Assumptions Met	Repeated Measures (#)	Number of IV(s) (scale)	Covariate(s)	Statistical Test
Differences from Population	Continuous	Yes	No	None	No	One sample z test
	Continuous	Yes	No	None	No	One sample t test
	Dichotomous		No	None	No	Binomial test
	Continuous		No	None	No	Kolmogorov-Smirnov test
Between-Group Differences	Continuous	Yes	No	One (Dichotomous)	No	Independent samples t test
	Ordinal or higher	No	No	One (Dichotomous)	No	Mann-Whitney test
	Ordinal or higher	No	No	One (Dichotomous)	No	Median test
	Continuous	Yes	No	One (Categorical)	No	One-way ANOVA
	Ordinal or higher	No	No	One (Categorical)	No	Kruskal-Wallis test
	Continuous	Yes	No	One (Categorical)	Yes	ANCOVA
	Continuous	Yes	No	>= Two (Categorical)	No	Factorial ANOVA
Within-Group Differences	Continuous	Yes	Yes (2)	None	No	Paired samples t test
	Ordinal or higher	No	Yes (2)	None	No	Signed-rank test
	Ordinal or higher	No	Yes (2)	None	No	Sign test
	Continuous	Yes	Yes (>= 2)	None	No	One-way RM ANOVA
	Ordinal or higher	No	Yes (>= 2)	None	No	Friedman test
	Continuous	Yes	Yes (>= 2)	One (Categorical)	No	Two-way mixed ANOVA
	Dichotomous		Yes (2)	None	No	McNemar test
	Dichotomous		Yes (> 2)	None	No	Cochran Q test

continued

TABLE 8–2. DETERMINING THE APPROPRIATE STATISTICAL TEST (*Continued*)

	DV Scale	Distributional Assumptions Met	Number of IV(s) (scale)	Covariate(s)	Statistical Test
One Sample	Categorical	Yes	None	No	Chi square test
Association	Categorical	No	None	No	Fisher's exact test
	Categorical		None	Yes	Mantel-Haenszel test
	Continuous	Yes	One (continuous)	No	Pearson's correlation
	Continuous	No	One (continuous)	No	Spearman's rank order correlation
Relationship or	Continuous	Yes	One (any)	No	Simple linear regression
Association	Continuous	Yes	Multiple (any)	Yes	Multiple linear regression
	Dichotomous		One (any)	No	Simple logistic regression
	Dichotomous		Multiple (any)	Yes	Multiple logistic regression
	Categorical		Multiple (any)	Yes	Multinomial logistic regression
Time-to-Event	Continuous		Multiple (any)	Yes	Cox regression
Reliability	Nominal	Yes	None	No	Kappa

400

Thus, if participant A is 40 and participant B is 45, participant C must be 65. If instead, participant A is 75 and participant B is 40, then participant C must be 35, because this value is determined specifically by the mean. In this case, there are two degrees of freedom.

Degrees of freedom become increasingly complex in accordance with the complexity of the statistical test. That is, degrees of freedom for bivariate tests are easier to conceptualize than multivariate tests. For the analyses described below, calculation of degrees of freedom is not explained, but it is important to note the distribution, probability, and statistical significance of all statistical tests are based primarily on their values. Further, in all published studies, degrees of freedom are subscripted next to the test statistic for all parametric tests (e.g., $F_{1,30}$ or t_{98}) and some nonparametric tests (e.g., χ^2_1).

TESTS FOR NOMINAL AND CATEGORICAL DATA

Nonparametric Tests

Pearson's chi square test

Pearson's chi square test (or simply the chi square test) is one of the most common statistical tests used in the biomedical sciences. It is used to assess for significant differences between two or more mutually exclusive groups for two variables measured on nominal, dichotomous, or categorical scales. Note that the data may also be ordinal, if the number of ranks is small; however, the test does not consider rank order. The chi square test assesses for differences between observed (i.e., actual) and expected frequencies (i.e., the frequencies that would be expected if there actually was no difference).

For example, consider a study to determine whether a significant difference in gender exists between three treatment groups. In most journal articles, a 2×3 (i.e., gender by treatment group) contingency table (similar to Table 8–1, but obviously larger) containing the observed frequency counts within each cell will typically be presented. Next, a chi square (χ^2) statistic will follow, with appropriate degrees of freedom, either in a footnote under the table or described in the narrative. If the probability of the difference is less than alpha—that is, if the actual frequencies are different from the expected frequencies—the test is considered statistically significant indicating a significant gender difference between the groups. The results of a statistically significant gender difference are presented as follows:

Statistically significant gender differences were indicated between the three treatment groups ($\chi^2_2 = 11.59$, $p < 0.05$).

When the chi square test is based on a contingency table larger than 2×2, the test is considered an omnibus test. That is, in the example above for the 2×3 table, the chi square test indicated that a statistically significant gender difference existed between treatment groups, but failed to indicate which treatment groups differed. In these situations, Bonferroni-corrected *post hoc* chi square tests (or Fisher's exact tests if expected frequencies are low) are used to determine where statistically significant differences occurred. A Bonferroni correction reduces the probability of committing a Type I error by maintaining the appropriate experiment-wise alpha (i.e., the overall alpha for all statistical tests; again, typically 0.05). The Bonferroni correction adjusts alpha by dividing it by the total number of *post hoc* tests.

For example, in the 2×3 chi square above, three 2×2 *post hoc* chi square test are required (i.e., gender compared between groups A and B; gender compared between groups A and C; gender compared between groups B and C). Thus, if alpha for the omnibus test is set at 0.05, then the Bonferroni-adjusted alpha becomes 0.017 (i.e., 0.05/3).

Following the Bonferroni-corrected *post hoc* tests, the additional information provided is added to the result described above:

Statistically significant gender differences were indicated across the three treatment groups ($\chi^2_2 = 11.59$, $p < 0.05$). Bonferroni-corrected post hoc *chi square tests indicated statistically significant gender differences between groups A and B ($\chi^2_1 = 6.54$, $p < 0.017$) and between groups B and C ($\chi^2_1 = 10.26$, $p < 0.017$), with group B including significantly more males compared to both groups A and C. Further, no statistically significant gender difference was indicated between groups A and C.*

The assumptions of the chi square test include:

1. Data for both variables being compared must be categorical.
   a. Note that continuous data can be categorized; however, information will be lost via categorization as discussed earlier.
2. The categories must be mutually exclusive.
   a. That is, each individual can fall into one, and only one, category.
3. The total sample size must be large.
   a. The expected frequencies in each cell must not be too small. For chi square tests with degrees of freedom greater than 1 (i.e., when the number of columns and/or rows are greater than 2), no more than 20% of the cells should have expected frequencies less than 5. Further, no cell should have an expected frequency less than 1.[31] This is a difficult assumption to verify, outside of calculating the expected frequencies by hand. However, if an article fails to indicate this assumption was tested, view results with caution.

Fisher's exact test

Fisher's exact test is ubiquitous in the biomedical literature. The test can only be applied to 2×2 contingency tables, however, and is most useful when the sample size is small (i.e., it is used when assumption 3 of the chi square test is violated). Conceptually, Fisher's exact test is identical to the chi square test, in that, the two variables being compared must be discrete and have mutually exclusive categories.

For example, consider a study assessing for differences in cardiac events in dialysis patients who initiated beta blocker therapy compared to patients who did not initiate therapy. Note, both variables are dichotomous (event versus no event; beta blocker versus no beta blocker). Fisher's exact test provides the exact probability of observing this particular set of frequencies within each cell of the contingency table. Results of a statistically significant Fisher's exact test are presented as follows (notice only a p value is provided):

The results of a Fisher's exact test indicated patients initiating beta blocker therapy had significantly fewer cardiac events compared to patients failing to initiate therapy ($p < 0.05$).

The assumptions of Fisher's exact test include:

1. Data for both variables being compared must be dichotomous.
   a. Note that continuous data can be dichotomized; however, information will be lost via categorization as discussed above.
2. The dichotomous categories must be mutually exclusive.
   a. That is, each individual can fall into one, and only one, category.

Mantel-Haenszel chi square test

The Mantel-Haenszel chi square test (or Cochran-Mantel-Haenszel test or Mantel-Haenszel test) measures the association of three discrete variables, which usually consists of two dichotomous IVs and one categorical confounding variable or covariate. The covariate is then used as a stratification variable.

For example, consider a study assessing the presence or absence of lung cancer in smokers and nonsmokers (the IVs) after stratifying for frequent exposure to secondhand smoke (the dichotomous covariate; exposure versus no exposure). A 2×2 contingency table is created at each level of secondhand smoke. That is, a contingency table for exposure and another for no exposure. This test produces a chi square statistic (χ^2_{MH}), with a statistically significant result indicating a significant difference in the presence of lung cancer for smokers and nonsmokers across the levels of the covariate (i.e., exposed versus unexposed). A statistically significant result is presented as follows:

The results of a Mantel-Haenszel chi square test indicated the proportion of nonsmokers developing lung cancer was significantly greater for those exposed to secondhand smoke ($\chi^2_{MH} = 29.67$, 1 df, $p < 0.05$).

The assumptions of the Mantel-Haenszel chi square test include:

1. Data of the IVs must be dichotomous.
   a. Note that continuous data can be dichotomized; however, information will be lost via categorization as discussed above.

2. The dichotomous categories must be mutually exclusive.

   a. That is, each individual can fall into one, and only one, category.

3. Data of the covariate must be categorical.

   a. Again, note that continuous data can be dichotomized; however, information will be lost via categorization as discussed above.

The kappa statistic

The kappa statistic (also known as Cohen's kappa or κ) is a measure of inter-rater reliability (i.e., agreement) for a categorical variable measured on a nominal scale. Kappa provides the proportion of agreement corrected for chance and ranges from 0 (i.e., no agreement) to 1 (i.e., perfect agreement). The larger the kappa value, the better. However, there is no agreement as to what is a good kappa value. The literature contains various benchmarks for kappa values, and the reader is referred to additional readings on the subject. Because this statistic corrects for chance agreement, it is more appropriate than simply calculating overall percent agreement.[32] In fact, percent agreement should rarely be used, and published results using percent agreement should be viewed with caution. Kappa can be applied to a variable with any number of categories, with the understanding that as the number of categories increases, overall agreement will probably decrease. That is, the more choices two raters have, the less likely they are to agree.

For example, consider 100 professional school applicants, who each interview with two faculty members. After the interview is complete, each faculty member rates the applicant as accept, deny, or waitlist. Kappa is then used to calculate the agreement between faculty members. Results using the kappa statistic are presented as follows:

Cohen's kappa was employed to measure the agreement between faculty members in determining whether applicants should be accepted, denied, or waitlisted. Results indicated good agreement between faculty members (κ = 0.75).

The assumptions of the kappa statistic include:

1. Each object (e.g., the applicant in the example above) is rated only one time.

2. The outcome variable is nominal with mutually exclusive categories.

   a. That is, each individual can fall into one, and only one, category.

3. There are two independent raters.

   a. That is, each rater provides one, and only one, response for each applicant.

TESTING FOR DIFFERENCES FROM THE POPULATION

Parametric Tests

One sample z test

The one sample z test is used to assess for a difference between the mean of the study sample and a known population mean. For example, consider data collected from a random sample of 1000 patients with borderline high cholesterol, for which their mean serum total cholesterol was 210.01 mg/dL. The researcher is interested in determining whether the total cholesterol of this sample is significantly higher than the mean total cholesterol within the general population. The 2007-2008 National Health and Nutrition Examination Survey (NHANES) has determined the mean serum total cholesterol level for individuals in the United States aged 6 years and older is 186.67 mg/dL with a standard deviation of 42.15.[33] A one sample z test provides a z-score indicating how many standard errors the sample mean is from the known population mean, and if this difference is large enough it is considered statistically significant. Results of a statistically significant one sample z test with no assumption violations are provided as follows:

Results of a one sample z test indicated a statistically significant difference in total cholesterol between the study sample and population ($z_{999} = 2.10$, $p < 0.05$), with the study sample having significantly higher total cholesterol compared to the population (210.01 mg/dL versus 186.67 mg/dL, respectively).

Assumptions of the one sample z test include:

1. The DV is measured on an interval or ratio scale.
2. The sampling distribution of means for the DV is normal.
   a. This can be assured by assessing the individual group sample distributions or by applying the central limit theorem.
3. The population mean and standard deviation are known.
4. The observations are independent.
   a. That is, each participant provides one, and only one, observation (i.e., data or response).

One sample t test

Only in rare cases is the population standard deviation known; thus, test statistics often must be based on sample data (i.e., standard deviation and sample size). The one sample t test is used in situations where only the population mean is known, or can at least be estimated by very large amounts of data. For example, consider a study to compare the mean total cholesterol of a random sample of 1000 adults aged 20 years or older with borderline high cholesterol (e.g., 231.26 mg/dL) to the mean total cholesterol of the general population. In 2006, the National Center for Health Statistics determined the mean serum total cholesterol for adults in the United States aged 20 years and older was 199 mg/dL.[34] Notice, no population standard deviation is available; thus, a one sample t test is required. Note that this test produces a t statistic, which can be considered similar to a z-score when samples are large. The result of a statistically significant one sample t test with no assumption violations is presented as follows:

Results of a one sample t test indicated a statistically significant difference in total cholesterol between the study sample and population ($t_{999} = 2.23$, $p < 0.05$), with the study sample *having significantly higher total cholesterol compared to individuals aged 20 or older in the general population (231.26 mg/dL versus 199.00 mg/dL, respectively)*

Assumptions of the one sample *t* test include:

1. The DV is measured on an interval or ratio scale.
2. The sampling distribution of means for the DV is normal.
   a. This can be assured by assessing the individual group sample distributions or by applying the central limit theorem.
3. The population mean is known.
4. The observations are independent.
   a. That is, each participant provides one, and only one, observation (i.e., data or response).

Nonparametric Tests

Binomial test

The binomial test is used when the DV is dichotomous (e.g., inpatient or outpatient, male or female) and all of the possible data (or outcomes) fall into one, and only one, of the two categories. The binomial test uses the binomial distribution to test the exact probability of whether the sample proportion differs from the proportion expected by chance (i.e., the expected population proportion). Further, the binomial test is often used in the literature when sample sizes are small and violate the assumptions of the chi square test; that is, low expected frequencies.[17]

For example, consider the binomial distribution example presented previously. Briefly, a fair coin (i.e., equal probability of flipping a head or tail) is flipped 10 times, and lands on heads 6 of the 10 flips. The expected population proportion is 0.50; that is, if the coin is fair, as the number of flips increases the coin should land on heads 50% of the time. Because the coin landed on heads 6 of the 10 flips, the statistical test is whether this proportion (i.e., 6/10 or 0.60) is statistically different from the expected proportion (i.e., 0.50). In this case, the binomial test indicates the difference between these proportions is nonsignificant and results are presented as follows:

Results of the binomial test indicated the probability of flipping 6 heads in 10 flips was not statistically different from the expected population proportion of 0.50 (p > 0.05).

The assumptions of the binomial test include:

1. Data for both variables being compared must be dichotomous.
   a. Note that continuous data can be dichotomized; however, information will be lost via categorization as discussed above.
2. The dichotomous categories must be mutually exclusive.
   a. That is, each individual can fall into one, and only one, category.
3. The population proportion is known.

4. The observations are independent.
    a. That is, each participant provides one, and only one, observation (i.e., data or response).

Kolmogorov-Smirnov one sample test

The Kolmogorov-Smirnov one sample test is a goodness-of-fit test used to determine the degree of agreement between the distribution of a researcher's sample data and a theoretical population distribution.[17] That is, it allows researchers to compare the distribution of their sample data against a common probability distribution (e.g., the normal distribution).

For example, consider a study where HbA1c data was collected for a random sample of 100 patients with diabetes. The researcher is interested in determining whether the distribution of HbA1c data was sampled from a population of patients with an underlying normal distribution. That is, the researcher is interested in whether the sample data is normally distributed.

A nonsignificant Kolmogorov-Smirnov test indicates the sample distribution and the hypothesized (or theoretical) normal distribution are not statistically different; that is, the distribution of sample data can be considered normally distributed. Results of the Kolmogorov-Smirnov test are presented as follows:

Results of the Kolmogorov-Smirnov test indicated HbA1c variable had a nonsignificant departure from normality ($p > 0.05$); thus, the data are considered to result from a normal distribution.

The assumptions of the Kolmogorov-Smirnov one sample test include:

1. The DV is measured on an interval or ratio scale.
2. The underlying population distribution is theorized or known.
    a. That is, the researcher must specify the correct probability distribution to test the sample data against. If the distribution is unknown, the test is inappropriate.
3. The observations are independent.
    a. That is, each participant provides one, and only one, observation (i.e., data or response).

TESTING FOR BETWEEN-GROUP DIFFERENCES

Parametric Tests

Independent samples t test

The independent samples t test (also referred to as Student's t test) is used to assess for a statistically significant difference between the means of the two mutually exclusive (i.e., independent) groups. For example, consider testing for a mean difference in a methacholine challenge, measured by a 20% decrease in forced expiratory volume in 1 second

(FEV1; PC20), in two groups of asthma patients receiving either rosiglitazone or placebo at the end of an 8-week study period. The independent sample t test provides the t statistic and probability of obtaining a difference of this size based on specific degrees of freedom. Results of a statistically significant independent samples t test with no assumption violations are presented as follows:

The results of an independent samples t *test indicated a statistically significant difference between groups* ($t_{31} = 9.654$, $p < 0.05$), *with asthma patients receiving rosiglitazone displaying significantly better lung function compared to placebo (mean PC20 = 10.7 mg/mL versus 3.8 mg/mL, respectively).*

The assumptions of the independent samples t test include:

1. The DV is measured on an interval or ratio scale.
2. The sampling distribution of means for the DV within each level of the IV (i.e., group) is normal.
   a. This can be assured by assessing the individual group sample distributions or by applying the central limit theorem.
3. The IV is dichotomous.
   a. Note that continuous data can be dichotomized; however, information will be lost via categorization as discussed above.
4. The IV categories are mutually exclusive.
   a. That is, each individual can fall into one, and only one, category.
4. Homogeneity of variance is assured.
   a. That is, the variance within each group is similar. A crude indicator of a violation of this assumption (i.e., heterogeneity) is the ratio of the largest variance to smallest variance being greater than 10:1.[12] For example, most studies do not provide the variance for each variable; however, the standard deviation is reported consistently. Remember, variance is simply the standard deviation squared. Now, consider two variables with standard deviations of 4 and 13. The homogeneity of variance assumption can be tested by squaring the standard deviations (i.e., 16 and 169, respectively) and finding their ratio (i.e., 169/16 = 10.56). In this case, the ratio is greater than 10:1; thus, the assumption is violated.
5. The observations are independent.
   a. That is, each participant provides one, and only one, observation (i.e., data or response).

One-way analysis of variance

A one-way analysis of variance (ANOVA) is an extension of the independent samples t test to situations where researchers want to assess for mean differences between three or more mutually exclusive groups. For example, consider the rosiglitazone example from above, but in addition to the placebo group, include two groups receiving different doses of rosiglitazone (e.g., 4 mg and 8 mg). The use of three independent samples t tests to test for mean differences between groups (i.e., 4 mg versus placebo, 8 mg versus placebo, 4 mg versus 8 mg) is inappropriate due to the increased probability of committing a Type I error. Instead, one-way ANOVA is used to partition the variance between and within groups to determine if a statistically significant group difference exists. The result of a statistically significant one-way ANOVA with no assumption violations is presented as follows:

Results of a one-way ANOVA indicated a statistically significant difference between groups ($F_{2,27} = 6.89$, $p < 0.05$).

ANOVA provides an omnibus F test; that is, an overall test assessing the statistical significance between the three (or more) group means. A statistically significant F test indicates a statistically significant difference between at least two group means. Thus, similar to the omnibus chi square test described above, a series of adjusted *post hoc* tests are conducted to determine where significant differences occurred. The *post hoc* tests can be viewed as a series of independent samples t tests with the alpha level adjusted (i.e., reduced) to control for Type I error. Thus, the significant one-way ANOVA in the example above required three adjusted *post hoc* tests (i.e., 4 mg versus placebo, 8 mg versus placebo, and 4 mg versus 8 mg). The most commonly used *post hoc* tests in the literature include the Tukey and Scheffé tests. It should be noted the Scheffé test is the most conservative *post hoc* test available (i.e., greatest adjustment); however, some authors indicate it may be too conservative (that is, may not find statistically significant differences) and support the use of Tukey tests, which is conservative to a lesser degree. In most cases, the two tests will indicate similar results and both are viewed as acceptable.

The results of a statistically significant one-way ANOVA including *post hoc* tests are presented as follows:

Results of a one-way ANOVA indicated a statistically significant difference between groups ($F_{2,27} = 6.89$, $p < 0.05$). Post hoc Tukey tests indicated statistically significant differences ($p < 0.05$) between placebo (3.8 mg/mL) and 4 mg dose of rosiglitazone (10.7 mg/mL) as well as between placebo and the 8 mg dose of rosiglitazone (12.2 mg/mL). No statistically significant differences were indicated between the 4 mg and 8 mg doses of rosiglitazone.

The assumptions for one-way ANOVA include:

1. The DV is measured on an interval or ratio scale.
2. The sampling distribution of means for the DV within each level of the IV is normal.
   a. This can be assured by assessing the individual group sample distributions or by applying the central limit theorem.

3. The levels of the IV are mutually exclusive.
   a. That is, each individual can fall into one, and only one, category.
4. Homogeneity of variance is assured.
   a. That is, the variance within each group is similar. A crude indicator of a violation of this assumption (i.e., heterogeneity) is the ratio of the largest variance to smallest variance being greater than 10:1. For example, most studies do not provide the variance for each variable; however, the standard deviation is reported consistently. Remember, variance is simply the standard deviation squared. Now, consider two variables with standard deviations of 4 and 13. The homogeneity of variance assumption can be tested by squaring the standard deviations (i.e., 16 and 169, respectively) and finding their ratio (i.e., $169/16 = 10.56$). In this case, the ratio is greater than 10:1; thus, the assumption is violated.
5. The observations are independent.
   a. That is, each participant provides one, and only one, observation (i.e., data or response).

Factorial between-groups ANOVA

A factorial between-groups ANOVA (or simply factorial ANOVA) is an extension of the one-way ANOVA to a study with more than one IV. For example, consider a study to evaluate differences in heart rate (measured by beats per minute, bpm) between gender following either a 25 mg dose of synephrine or placebo. In the literature, this may be described as a 2×2 factorial design indicating two IVs (i.e., gender and treatment) each with two levels (i.e., male versus female; synephrine versus placebo). This type of design produces two main effects (one for gender and one for treatment) and an interaction effect between gender and treatment; thus, three separate F tests are provided. Note that statistical significance is determined separately for main effects and interaction effect.

It is extremely important to note that if the interaction effect is statistically significant, the results of the main effects (i.e., effect of gender and the effect of treatment) cannot be interpreted directly, as the IVs are dependent on each other. This situation is similar to the order effects discussed above for a crossover study. From the example, a statistically significant interaction effect indicates treatment effects differ depending on the gender of the participant (i.e., synephrine had a different effect for males than it did for females). However, if the interaction effect is nonsignificant, main effects can be interpreted appropriately. When interpreting the main effect of an IV, the levels of the other IV are collapsed. That is, interpreting the main effect of gender is done irrespective of whether the participants received synephrine or placebo. Likewise, interpreting the main effect of treatment is done irrespective of the participant's gender.

Similar to one-way ANOVA, following a statistically significant main effect or interaction, *post hoc* tests may be required to identify where statistically significant differences occurred. There are a number of *post hoc* tests available depending on whether the inter-action or main effects are statistically significant, including the Tukey and Scheffé tests, realizing there are many more that are beyond the scope of this chapter.[35] Each *post hoc* test adjusts alpha differently (i.e., more or less conservatively) to reduce Type I error. *Post hoc* tests for factorial ANOVA used in the literature are often termed simple compari-sons, simple contrasts, simple main effects, or interaction contrasts. These tests are essentially formal names for a collection of adjusted Tukey tests or Bonferroni-corrected independent samples *t* tests.

In the biomedical sciences, the results of a nonsignificant interaction effect for a 2×2 factorial ANOVA with no assumption violations are presented as follows:

Results of a 2 (gender; male versus female) × 2 (treatment; synephrine versus placebo) factorial ANOVA indicated a nonsignificant interaction effect between gender and treat-ment ($p > 0.05$). However, the main effect for gender was statistically significant ($F_{1,26} = 21.36$, $p < 0.05$), with males having significantly higher heart rates than females (91.6 bpm versus 84.3 bpm, respectively). Further, the main effect of treatment was statistically signifi-cant ($F_{1,26} = 15.24$, $p < 0.05$), with synephrine resulting in a significantly higher heart rate compared to placebo (70.3 bpm versus 65.2 bpm, respectively).

The results of a 2×2 factorial ANOVA with a statistically significant interaction and no assumption violations are presented as follows:

Results of a 2 (gender; male versus female) × 2 (treatment; synephrine versus placebo) factorial ANOVA indicated a statistically significant interaction effect between gender and treatment ($F_{1,26} = 15.42$, $p < 0.05$). Simple main effects, using Bonferroni-corrected indepen-dent samples t tests, were assessed to identify at which treatment level gender differed. Results indicated synephrine increased heart rate significantly higher for males compared to females (90.5 bpm versus 82.4 bpm, respectively). No statistically significant gender difference in heart rate was indicated for the placebo group.

The assumptions of factorial between-groups ANOVA include:

1. The DV is measured on an interval or ratio scale.
2. The sampling distribution of means for the DV within each level of the IV is normal.
   a. This can be assured by assessing the individual group sample distribu-tions or by applying the central limit theorem.
3. The levels of the IVs are mutually exclusive.
   a. That is, each individual can fall into one, and only one, category.
4. Homogeneity of variance is assured.
   a. That is, the variance within each group is similar. A crude indicator of a violation of this assumption (i.e., heterogeneity) is the ratio of the largest variance to smallest variance being greater than 10:1. For example, most studies do not provide the variance for each variable; however, the standard

deviation is reported consistently. Remember, variance is simply the standard deviation squared. Now, consider two variables with standard deviations of 4 and 13. The homogeneity of variance assumption can be tested by squaring the standard deviations (i.e., 16 and 169, respectively) and finding their ratio (i.e., $169/16 = 10.56$). In this case, the ratio is greater than 10:1; thus, the assumption is violated.

5. The observations are independent.

   a. That is, each participant provides one, and only one, observation (i.e., data or response).

Analysis of covariance

Analysis of covariance (ANCOVA) in an extension of ANOVA (both one-way and factorial) where main effects and interactions are assessed after statistically adjusting for one (or more) confounding variables called covariates. That is, ANCOVA adjusts all group means to create the situation as if all participants scored identically on the covariate.[12] For example, consider a study comparing vitamin D to placebo (IV) and assessing their effects on systolic blood pressure (SBP) (DV). The researchers note, however, that previous research has shown SBP and BMI to be highly correlated.[36] Thus, the study will include BMI as a covariate assessing the effect of vitamin D on SBP over and above the effect of BMI on SBP. If the vitamin D group has greater BMI values compared to the placebo group, ANCOVA will adjust the SBP within both groups to account for this initial difference in BMI.

In ANCOVA, covariates are typically continuous, measured before the DV, and correlated with the DV. It should be noted that ANCOVA is closely related to linear regression (discussed in detail below, and, although not completely necessary, it may be useful to revisit this section after reading the section on linear regression). In ANCOVA, group means are statistically adjusted by the magnitude of the association (i.e., slope) between the DV and covariate.[39] That is, the greater the association, the more useful the covariate and the better the adjustment. Thus, the goal of the covariate(s) is to reduce error, thereby increasing the statistical power of the test. From the example, the group means (i.e., SBP for the vitamin D and placebo groups) are adjusted by the association between BMI and SBP, and because previous research has shown the association between systolic blood pressure and BMI to be considerable, the statistical power of this test will be increased.

When presenting the results of ANCOVA, researchers should provide adjusted means; that is, the mean of the DV at each level of the IV after adjusting for the covariate. Published research that does not present adjusted means should be viewed with caution. Further, the effect (or relationship) of the covariate must also be presented, which provides information regarding the effectiveness of the covariate in adjusting group means. Finally, it should be noted that ANCOVA is more suited for experimental design in which participants are randomized to groups, as opposed to nonexperimental designs without randomization. Remember, ANCOVA is used to adjust group means as if all participants had identical covariate values. However, in nonexperimental research, important covariates may have been missed and causality is difficult to infer—a characteristic intrinsic to all nonexperimental work. Thus, the limitations may be significant when applying ANCOVA to nonexperimental designs, and results must be viewed cautiously.[21]

In the biomedical sciences, the results of a statistically significant ANCOVA with no assumption violations are presented as follows:

Results of a one-way ANCOVA indicated a statistically significant group difference in SBP *after adjusting for BMI ($F_{1,17} = 7.98$, $p < 0.05$), with patients receiving vitamin D having significantly lower* SBP *compared to placebo (adjusted means = 118 mm Hg versus 141 mm Hg, respectively). The relationship between* SBP *and BMI was also statistically significant after adjusting for group ($F_{1,17} = 39.85$, $p < 0.05$) with a pooled within-group correlation of 0.61.*

The assumptions of ANCOVA include:

1. The DV is measured on an interval or ratio scale.
2. The sampling distribution of means for the DV and covariate(s) within each level of the IV is normal.
   a. This can be assured by assessing the individual group sample distributions or by applying the central limit theorem.
3. The levels of the IV are mutually exclusive.
   a. That is, each individual can fall into one, and only one, category.
4. Homogeneity of variance is assured.
   a. That is, the variance within each group is similar. A crude indicator of a violation of this assumption (i.e., heterogeneity) is the ratio of the largest variance to smallest variance being greater than 10:1. For example, most studies do not provide the variance for each variable; however, the standard deviation is reported consistently. Remember, variance is simply the standard deviation squared. Now, consider two variables with standard deviations of 4 and 13. The homogeneity of variance assumption can be tested by squaring the standard deviations (i.e., 16 and 169, respectively) and finding their ratio (i.e., 169/16 = 10.56). In this case, the ratio is greater than 10:1; thus, the assumption is violated.
5. Homogeneity of regression is assured.
   a. Briefly, this means the association (i.e., slope) between the DV and covariate are the same within each level of the IV. A violation of this assumption renders ANCOVA inappropriate. However, violation is difficult to detect, as most authors fail to provide the appropriate information in the narrative. Thus, when reading a journal article employing ANCOVA, if the

author fails to indicate whether this assumption was tested, results must be viewed with extreme caution.

6. The covariate(s) is measured reliably.
   a. For example, make sure the instrumentation used to measure the covariate is working properly or that the covariate does not vary over short periods of time.
7. The observations are independent.
   a. That is, each participant provides one, and only one, observation (i.e., data or response).

Nonparametric Tests

Mann-Whitney test

The Mann-Whitney test is the nonparametric alternative to the independent samples *t* test and is one of the most powerful nonparametric tests.[17] It is used when the distribution of a continuous DV is not normal or when the DV is measured on an ordinal scale. The Mann-Whitney test is based on ranked data. That is, instead of using the actual values of the DV, as an independent samples *t* test does, each participant's DV value is ranked with the highest value receiving the highest rank and the lowest value receiving the lowest rank. The ranks within each group are then summed, and the test assesses whether the difference in ranked sums between groups is statistically significant.

For example, consider a performance improvement study assessing gender differences in patient satisfaction of hospital stay following total hip replacement surgery. The measurement instrument uses a Likert-type scale with four possible responses anchored from strongly disagree to strongly agree. Note that neutral and not applicable responses were removed prior to analysis to maintain an ordinal scale of measurement. That is, the neutral response was removed because in most analyses, this response, which essentially indicates no opinion, is given a higher ranking than a response where the respondents provide an opinion (e.g., strongly disagree). Further, a large number of neutral responses indicates that the question was written poorly and failed to discriminate well. A statistically significant Mann-Whitney test indicates gender differences in patient satisfaction, with the group with the highest-ranked sums indicating higher DV scores. The results of the Mann-Whitney test are presented as follows:

The results of a Mann-Whitney test indicate a statistically significant gender difference in patient satisfaction following total hip replacement surgery ($z = 2.65$, $p < 0.05$), with males indicating higher satisfaction scores compared to females.

The assumptions of the Mann-Whitney test include:

1. The DV is measured on an ordinal, interval, or ratio scale.
2. The IV is dichotomous.

a. Note that continuous data can be categorized into a dichotomous variable; however, information will be lost as discussed above.
3. The levels of the IV are mutually exclusive.
a. That is, each individual can fall into one, and only one category.
4. The observations are independent.
a. That is, each participant provides one, and only one, observation (i.e., data or response).

Median test

The median test is used to assess whether two mutually exclusive groups have different medians. There is no parametric alternative to the median test; however, the non-parametric Mann-Whitney test can be used as an adequate alternative. The test calculates the medians within each group and then classifies the data within each group as either above or below the respective group median. Further, because the test is based on the median, it can be used appropriately for skewed data or data containing outliers.

For example, consider a study evaluating gender differences in childhood autism as measured by the Childhood Autism Spectrum Test (CAST).[37] The CAST measures difficulties and preferences in social and communication skills using the total score from a 37-item questionnaire, with lower scores indicating fewer symptoms. Because autism is a relatively rare disorder, the distribution of CAST scores is expected to have severe positive skewness. That is, most children will score low, while a few autistic children will have high scores. The median test was used to determine whether statistically significant gender differences existed in CAST scores.

The results of a statistically significant median test are presented as follows.

The results of the median test indicated gender differences in CAST scores ($p < 0.05$), with boys having a significantly higher median score compared to girls (median = 5 versus median = 4, respectively).

Assumptions of the median test include:

1. The DV is measured on an ordinal, interval, or ratio scale.
2. Samples sizes are sufficiently large.
a. If sample sizes are small, and when the expected frequency within a cell is less than 5, Fisher's exact test can be used. From the example, this means using a 2 (group; male versus female) × 2 (median; above versus below) contingency table.
3. The observations are independent.
a. That is, each participant provides one, and only one, observation (i.e., data or response).

Kruskal-Wallis one-way ANOVA by ranks

The Kruskal-Wallis one-way ANOVA by ranks (or simply, the Kruskal-Wallis test) is the nonparametric alternative to the one-way ANOVA. The test is an extension of the Mann-Whitney test to assess group differences between three or more mutually exclusive groups. The Kruskal-Wallis test is typically used when the distribution of a continuous DV is not normal or when the DV is measured on an ordinal scale. Further, the Kruskal-Wallis test is based on rank sums, where the DV scores are ranked from highest to lowest. Similar to the Mann-Whitney test, statistically significant group differences are evaluated based on these rank sums.

For example, consider a study evaluating regional differences in whether volunteer preceptors believe they have adequate time available to dedicate to their experiential pharmacy students.[38] In this study, the DV was measured on a 4-point Likert-type scale; thus, the Kruskal-Wallis test was used in lieu of one-way ANOVA. The results of the statistically significant Kruskal-Wallis test are presented as follows:

Results of the Kruskal-Wallis test indicated regional differences regarding whether volunteer preceptors believe they have adequate time to dedicate to experiential students (χ^2_6 = 33.07, p < 0.05).

Similar to a one-way ANOVA, the Kruskal-Wallis test is an omnibus test; that is, the test will determine whether an overall statistically significant difference exists between groups, but will not indicate where statistically significant differences occurred. Thus, Bonferroni-corrected *post hoc* tests are required. In this situation, the Mann-Whitney test is used to compare all two-group combinations (e.g., West versus Midwest, West versus South, West versus Northeast, and so on totaling six *post hoc* tests). Thus, the Bonferroni-corrected alpha used for the *post hoc* tests is (.05/6) 0.008. The results of the Kruskal-Wallis test including adjusted Mann-Whitney *post hoc* tests are presented as follows:

Results of the Kruskal-Wallis test indicated regional differences regarding whether volunteer preceptors believe they have adequate time to dedicate to experiential students (χ^2_6 = 33.07, p < 0.05). Bonferroni-adjusted post hoc Mann-Whitney tests indicated preceptors in the West disagreed more compared to preceptors located in the Midwest (p < 0.008) and agreed less with preceptors in the South (p < 0.008). No other statistically significant group differences were indicated.

The assumptions of the Kruskal-Wallis test include:

1. The DV is measured on an ordinal, interval, or ratio scale.
2. The IV is categorical.
   a. Note that continuous data can be categorized; however, information will be lost as discussed above.
3. The levels of the IV are mutually exclusive.
   a. That is, each individual can fall into one, and only one category.

4. Each group has approximately the same distribution.
    a. Although the Kruskal-Wallis test does not assume data are distributed normally, if the distribution for one level of the IV is skewed negatively and the other levels are skewed positively, the results produced by the test may be inaccurate.
5. The data do not include a large number of ties.
    a. Tied values are given average ranks. Typically, if less than 25% of the data are ties, the test is unaffected.[17]
6. The observations are independent.
    a. That is, each participant provides one, and only one, observation (i.e., data or response).

TESTING FOR WITHIN-GROUP DIFFERENCES

Parametric Tests

Paired samples t test

The paired samples t test (also known as the matched t test or nested t test) is used when one group of participants is measured on the DV twice, or two groups of participants are matched on specific characteristics. In both cases, the assumption of independence, or mutually exclusive groups, is violated. When one group of participants is measured twice, it is known as a repeated measures design. Repeatedly measuring participants is a valid method for reducing error and increasing statistical power, which requires fewer participants. This highlights why a crossover design often requires fewer participants than a parallel-groups design; that is, in a crossover design all participants serve as their own control by receiving all treatments.

When two groups of participants are matched on specific characteristics, it is called a matched design. For example, when studying the effects of a new statin medication on hyperlipidemia, researchers would identify a group of patients to receive the statin and then identify a matched control group by matching individuals based on age, race, gender, BMI, and years with diagnosis. Note that the matched control group does not receive any medication. Matching participants serves the same purpose as repeated measures (i.e., reduce error variance), but is often more difficult because as the number of matching criteria increases the probability of finding a suitable match decreases.

The simplest design requiring a paired samples t test is called a pretest-posttest design. For example, consider measuring the therapeutic knowledge of 20 fourth-year pharmacy (P4) students prior to clinical rotations (i.e., pretest) and following rotations (i.e., posttest) to assess for increases in therapeutic knowledge. Therapeutic knowledge was measured using a well discriminating 20-question test. The paired samples t test assesses for a statistically significant mean difference (i.e., change) in correct responses from pretest to posttest. Results of a statistically significant paired samples t test with no assumption violations are presented as follows:

The results of a paired samples t *test indicated a statistically significant difference in therapeutic knowledge between pretest and posttest scores ($t_{19} = 3.25$, $p < 0.05$). Therapeutic knowledge increased significantly following clinical rotations (mean = 10.4 correct responses at pretest to a mean of 16.5 at posttest).*

The assumptions of the paired samples t test include:

1. The DV is measured on an interval or ratio scale.
2. The two DV measurements are associated.
3. The sampling distribution of means for both DV measurements is normal.
   a. This can be assured by assessing the individual group sample distributions or by applying the central limit theorem.
4. Homogeneity of variance for both DV measurements is assured.
   a. That is, the variance within each group is similar. A crude indicator of a violation of this assumption (i.e., heterogeneity) is the ratio of the largest variance to smallest variance being greater than 10:1. For example, most studies do not provide the variance for each variable; however, the standard deviation is reported consistently. Remember, variance is simply the standard deviation squared. Now, consider two variables with standard deviations of 4 and 13. The homogeneity of variance assumption can be tested by squaring the standard deviations (i.e., 16 and 169, respectively) and finding their ratio (i.e., $169/16 = 10.56$). In this case, the ratio is greater than 10:1; thus, the assumption is violated.

One-way repeated measures ANOVA

A one-way repeated measures ANOVA (or simply repeated measures ANOVA) is an extension of the paired samples t test to situations where the DV is measured three or more times. Again, this can occur when the same participants are measured repeatedly or when three or more matched groups are measured once. A repeated measures ANOVA is used to indicate whether statistically significant differences exist between the repeated measurements.

For example, reconsider the pretest-posttest design described above for the paired samples t test. Briefly, a researcher is interested in testing whether therapeutic knowledge of 20 P4 students differs (i.e., changes) before and after clinical rotations. To be applicable to repeated measures ANOVA, students would be tested on a third occasion 6 months after posttest to assess knowledge retention. That is, the design measures therapeutic knowledge at pretest, posttest, and 6-month follow-up (i.e., three repeated measures). The repeated measures ANOVA is then used to test whether a statistically significance difference exists between any of the repeated measurements.

It should be noted that some researchers prefer to use repeated measures ANOVA over paired samples *t tests* when participants are only measured twice (e.g., pretest and posttest). This is an appropriate use of repeated measures ANOVA, and in this situation (i.e., only two repeated measures) the results would be identical to the paired samples *t* test. That is, repeated measures ANOVA can be used in any situation when a paired samples *t* test is appropriate. However, note that the test statistic from the repeated measures ANOVA will be an F value instead of a *t* value produced by the paired samples *t* test. This is a nonissue, as the F value in this situation is simply t^2.

In most cases, repeated measures ANOVA has more statistical power than a paired samples *t* test. This has been alluded to in the sections above discussing the analysis of clinical trials and paired samples *t* test. In general, increasing the number of repeated measures (i.e., three or more) further reduces error, which allows for more precise measurement and decreases the overall probability of committing a Type I error. With that said, increasing the number of repeated measurements has diminishing returns in statistical power. That is, for most studies, statistical power will increase drastically by adding a few additional repeated measures, but the magnitude of this increase weakens rapidly between four and six repeated measurements, with little to no increases in statistical power beyond seven repeated measurements.[39] Finally, if a study has more than 10 repeated measurements, the repeated measures ANOVA may be the incorrect analysis, as a time series analysis may be more appropriate. Thus, studies employing repeated measures ANOVA with more than seven repeated measurements should be viewed with caution.

In addition, a brief discussion of the key assumption to repeated measures ANOVA is useful as a basic understanding of this assumption will assist in determining whether the test statistics produced from the analysis are correct. This key assumption, known as sphericity, states that all repeated measurements must have a similar association (i.e., correlation) to one another. For example, consider a study with four repeated measurements. For the sphericity assumption to be satisfied, the association between the first and second measurements must be similar to the association between the first and third, first and fourth, second and third, and so on. However, this assumption is incredibly restrictive, as most measurements closer in time tend to have a stronger association than measurements further apart in time. That is, in most situations, the first and second measurements will have a stronger association than the first and fourth measurements. When reading a journal article, if the authors fail to provide information regarding the assurance or violation of the sphericity assumption, results and interpretations must be viewed with caution.

Briefly reconsider the example above where 20 fourth-year pharmacy students have therapeutic knowledge measured before clinical rotations (i.e., pretest), once immediately after rotations (i.e., posttest), and at a 6-month follow-up. That is, therapeutic knowledge is measured on three separate occasions. A statistically significant repeated measures ANOVA with no assumption violations will be presented as follows:

The results of a one-way repeated measures ANOVA indicated a statistically significant difference in therapeutic knowledge between pretest, posttest, and 6-month follow-up ($F_{2,38}$ = 9.87, p < 0.05).

It must be noted that with more than two repeated measurements the one-way repeated measures ANOVA is an omnibus test. That is, the F test will identify whether a statistically significant difference exists between repeated measures, but will not identify which repeated measurements differ. Thus, adjusted *post hoc* tests, known as pairwise comparisons, are required. Similar to other analysis requiring *post hoc* tests, there are numerous adjusted pairwise comparisons available, with the most common being the Bonferroni correction. Each type of pairwise comparison adjusts alpha differently, with some being more conservative. It may be simpler to think of these comparisons as a series of paired samples t tests with adjusted alpha values. That is, adjusted paired samples t tests comparing the first and second repeated measurements, the first and third, the second and third, and so on. The additional information required to present results of a statistically significant one-way repeated measures ANOVA with no assumption violations are presented as follows:

The results of a one-way repeated measures ANOVA indicated a statistically significant difference in therapeutic knowledge between pretest, posttest, and 6-month follow-up ($F_{2,38}$ = 9.87, p < 0.05). All pairwise comparisons were assessed using the Bonferroni correction to adjust alpha (i.e., p < 0.017 to indicate statistical significance). Results of the pairwise comparisons indicated a statistically significant increase in therapeutic knowledge from pretest to posttest (mean = 5.50 versus 15.90, respectively, p < 0.017). Further, no statistically significant difference was indicated from posttest to 6 month follow-up (mean = 15.90 versus 15.50, respectively) indicating therapeutic knowledge was retained 6 months following clinical rotations.

The assumptions of the one-way repeated measures ANOVA include:

1. The DV is measured on an interval or ratio scale.
2. All DV measurements are associated.
3. The sampling distribution of means for all DV measurements is normal.
   a. This can be assured by assessing the individual group sample distributions or by applying the central limit theorem.
4. Homogeneity of variance for all DV measurements is assured.
   a. That is, the variance within each group is similar. A crude indicator of a violation of this assumption (i.e., heterogeneity) is the ratio of the largest variance to smallest variance being greater than 10:1. For example, most studies do not provide the variance for each variable; however, the standard

deviation is reported consistently. Remember, variance is simply the standard deviation squared. Now, consider two variables with standard deviations of 4 and 13. The homogeneity of variance assumption can be tested by squaring the standard deviations (i.e., 16 and 169, respectively) and finding their ratio (i.e., 169/16 = 10.56). In this case, the ratio is greater than 10:1; thus, the assumption is violated.

5. Sphericity is assured for designs with three or more repeated measurements.
   a. This is a complex assumption discussed briefly above. In general, sphericity is violated when the associations between all repeated measurements are not similar.

Two-way mixed ANOVA

A two-way mixed ANOVA (also known as a factorial ANOVA with repeated measures, mixed between-within ANOVA, or split-plot ANOVA) is a combination of factorial ANOVA and repeated measures ANOVA. The mixed terminology highlights this combination, and indicates that the design considers two or more levels of the IV (i.e., mutually exclusive groups) when the DV is measured repeatedly. The simplest case is a 2×2 pretest-posttest design, using two mutually exclusive treatment groups measured on two separate occasions. The primary advantage of this analysis is that it allows researchers to assess the interaction effect (i.e., do the two groups respond differently across time) in addition to between-subjects main effect (similar to the one-way ANOVA; the overall effect irrespective of measurement) and within-subjects main effect (similar to the one-way repeated measures ANOVA; the overall effect irrespective of group).

For example, consider a study examining the effectiveness of a relatively new FDA-approved tricyclic antidepressant (TCA) compared to amitriptyline over a 12-week study period. The researcher hypothesizes that the new TCA is more effective than amitriptyline in reducing symptoms of clinical depression. Prior to initiating treatment, 20 patients with diagnosed clinical depression are measured on the Beck Depression Inventory II (BDI-II).[40] Following this pretest or baseline measurement, each patient is randomized to receive one of two treatment options (the new TCA or amitriptyline) with 10 patients in each group. Patients then initiate the prescribed medication therapy and, at the end of the 12-week study period, BDI-II scores are measured again (i.e., posttest). A two-way mixed ANOVA provides researchers with three separate F tests (i.e., interaction, between-groups main effect, and within-groups main effect), each evaluated with specific degrees of freedom. Within this example, the primary effect of interest is the interaction effect, evaluating whether BDI-II scores changed differently from pretest to posttest for the new TCA group compared to the amitriptyline group.

Similar to factorial ANOVA discussed above, only if the interaction effect is nonsignificant can the researcher evaluate the statistical significance of overall group mean difference (between-group main effect) and the overall change in BDI-II scores (within-group main effect). That is, a statistically significant interaction effect indicates that the change in BDI-II scores from pretest to posttest changed differently in the group receiving the new TCA group compared to the group receiving amitriptyline (reconsider Figure 8–11). Or, said another way, the reduction in symptoms from pretest to posttest was dependent on whether the patient received the new TCA or amitriptyline. In this example, the researcher's hypothesis would be supported by a statistically significant interaction effect; that is, the new TCA was more effective at reducing the symptoms associated with clinical depression compared to amitriptyline.

Although the example above was for a 2 (group: new TCA versus amitriptyline) × 2 (repeated measures: pretest versus posttest) design, a two-way mixed ANOVA can be used for a design with any number of IVs (or levels of the IVs) and repeated measures. This is often seen in the literature. For example, consider the pretest-posttest study evaluating the effectiveness of three treatment groups (e.g., new TCA, amitriptyline, and placebo) in reducing symptoms of clinical depression (i.e., a 3 × 2 design), or consider the same study evaluating gender differences within these three treatments (i.e., a 3 × 2 × 2 design). It must be noted that as the number and levels of the IVs increase (e.g., 3 or more treatment groups or adding another IV such as gender), so does the complexity of interpreting results. Thus, extreme care must be taken when interpreting results and implementing suggestions supported by these types of designs. Consultation with an individual well versed in research methodology and statistical analysis is advised prior to implementing findings into an evidence-based practice.

Because a two-way mixed ANOVA is an extension of factorial ANOVA and repeated measures ANOVA, *post hoc* tests or pairwise comparisons may be required for any IV with three or more levels. That is, when there are more than three levels of the between-groups IV (e.g., new TCA, amitriptyline, and placebo), the between-groups main effect is an omnibus test. A statistically significant between-groups main effect indicates that a statistically significant difference in BDI-II scores exists, but does not indicate which groups have a statistically significant difference. Further, with three or more repeated measures, a statistically significant within-groups main effect indicates a difference between repeated measures, but fails to indicate where the statistically significant difference occurred. The *post hoc* tests and pairwise comparisons for factorial between-groups ANOVA and repeated measures ANOVA, respectively, are also appropriate for a two-way mixed ANOVA.

The results of a 2 × 2 two-way mixed ANOVA with no assumption violations for a nonsignificant interaction effect, but with statistically significant main effects (both between- and within-groups) is presented as follows:

The results of a 2 (treatment group: new TCA versus amitriptyline) × 2 (measurements: pretest versus posttest) two-way mixed ANOVA failed to indicate a statistically significant *interaction ($F_{1,18}$ = 1.215, $p > 0.05$). However, both main effects were statistically significant. Overall, patients receiving the new TCA had lower BDI-II scores compared to patients receiving amitriptyline ($F_{1,18}$ = 27.97, $p < 0.05$; mean = 29.41 versus 47.50, respectively). Further, an overall decrease in depressive symptoms was indicated from pretest to posttest ($F_{1,18}$ = 24.74, $p < 0.05$; mean = 49.86 versus 35.72, respectively).*

With a statistically significant interaction effect, results of the two-way mixed ANOVA with no assumption violations are presented as follows:

The results of a 2 (treatment group: new TCA versus amitriptyline) × 2 (measurements: pretest versus posttest) two-way mixed ANOVA indicated a statistically significant interaction effect ($F_{1,18}$ = 10.37, $p < 0.05$). Simple main effects, using Bonferroni-corrected independent samples t tests, were assessed to identify statistically significant treatment differences at pretest and posttest individually. Results indicated no statistically significant difference between the new TCA and amitriptyline at pretest (mean = 48.53 versus 50.23, respectively). However, at posttest, a statistically significant difference was indicated, with the new TCA having significantly lower BDI-II scores compared to amitriptyline (mean = 24.63 versus 47.53, respectively).

The assumptions of a mixed between-within ANOVA include:

1. The DV is measured on an interval or ratio scale.
2. All DV measurements are associated.
3. The sampling distribution of means at each level of the IV(s), collapsed across the repeated DV measurements, is normal.
    a. This can be assured by assessing the individual group sample distributions or by applying the central limit theorem.
4. Homogeneity of variance for all DV measurements within each level of the IV(s) is assured.
    a. That is, the variance within each group is similar. A crude indicator of a violation of this assumption (i.e., heterogeneity) is the ratio of the largest variance to smallest variance being greater than 10:1. For example, most studies do not provide the variance for each variable; however, the standard deviation is reported consistently. Remember, variance is simply the standard deviation squared. Now, consider two variables with standard deviations of 4 and 13. The homogeneity of variance assumption can be tested by squaring the standard deviations (i.e., 16 and 169, respectively) and finding their ratio (i.e., 169/16 = 10.56). In this case, the ratio is greater than 10:1; thus, the assumption is violated.
5. Sphericity is assured for designs with three or more repeated measurements.
    a. This is a complex assumption discussed briefly above for one-way repeated measures ANOVA. In general, sphericity is violated when the associations between all repeated measurements are not similar.

Nonparametric Tests

Wilcoxon signed-rank test

The Wilcoxon signed-rank test (or simply signed-rank test) is the nonparametric alternative to a paired samples t test. The test is used typically when the distribution of the DV is not normal or when the DV is measured on an ordinal scale to assess for differences between two repeated measurements (or two matched groups). The signed-rank test is based on ranked difference scores (e.g., difference between pretest and posttest), with the highest difference score receiving the highest rank and the lowest difference score receiving the lowest rank.

For example, consider a one-time (i.e., one group) pretest-posttest study evaluating the secondary effect of weight loss (in pounds) while on exenatide therapy in a sample of 20 IDDM patients. Prior to initiating exenatide therapy, all patients are weighed (i.e., pretest). At the end of a 1-year study period, patients are weighed again (i.e., posttest). For this study, the DV (i.e., weight in pounds, which is a continuous variable and normally would be assessed using parametric testing) has severe negative skewness due to outliers; thus, the signed-rank test is used in lieu of paired samples t test to assess for a change in patient weight from pretest to posttest. The result of a statistically significant signed-rank test is presented as follows:

The results of the signed-rank tests indicated a statistically significant decrease in body weight from pretest to posttest ($z = 2.32$, $p < 0.05$).

The assumptions of the signed-rank test include:

1. The DV measured repeatedly on an ordinal, interval, or ratio scale.
2. The two DV measurements are associated.
3. The two samples (i.e., measurements) come from populations with the same median.
4. There should not be a large number difference scores equal to zero.
   a. That is, the number of participants having no change (i.e., difference score of zero) should be low.

Friedman two-way ANOVA by ranks

The Friedman two-way ANOVA by ranks test (or simply the Friedman test) is the nonparametric alternative to the one-way repeated measures ANOVA and is an extension of the signed-rank test to a situation with three or more repeated measurements. Similar to the other nonparametric tests, it is most often used when the distribution of the DV is not normal or the DV is measured on an ordinal scale. The Friedman test is based on ranked data, with higher scores receiving higher ranks, and is used to assess for statistically significant differences between repeated measurements.

For example, reconsider the exenatide example described above. Briefly, the example consisted of a one-time pretest-posttest study evaluating the secondary effect of weight loss (in pounds) while on exenatide therapy in a sample of 20 IDDM patients. To extend this design to the Friedman's test, consider a study where patients are weighed prior to initiating exenatide therapy (i.e., pretest), 6 months after initiation, and 1 year after initiation. Thus, each patient is weighed on three occasions (i.e., three repeated measurements). Because the distribution of weight has severe negative skewness due to outliers, the Friedman test is employed. The results of a statistically significant Friedman test are presented as follows:

The results of the Friedman test indicated statistically significant differences between the three repeated measurements ($\chi^2_2 = 15.21$, $p < 0.05$).

Similar to the one-way repeated measures ANOVA, the Friedman test is an omnibus test. That is, it assesses whether a statistically significant difference exists between the repeated measurements, but does not indicate which measurements differ. Thus, adjusted *post hoc* tests are required, which consist of Bonferroni-corrected signed-rank tests with alpha equal to (.05/3) 0.017. For the example above, three adjusted signed-rank tests are required to test for differences between measurements: pretest versus 6 months, pretest versus 1 year, and 6 months versus 1 year. The results of a statistically significant Friedman test including the additional *post hoc* tests are presented as follows:

The results of the Friedman test indicated statistically significant differences between the three repeated measurements ($\chi^2_2 = 15.21$, $p < 0.05$). Bonferroni-corrected signed-rank tests indicated a statistically significant decrease in body weight from pretest to 6 month follow-up ($z = 2.65$, $p < 0.017$), with no statistically significant difference between the 6 month and 1 year follow-up ($z = 0.51$, $p > 0.017$). Thus, results suggest weight loss occurred rapidly, within 6 months of initiating exenatide therapy, and was sustained through 1 year of therapy.

The assumptions of the Friedman test include:

1. The DV is measured repeatedly on an ordinal, interval, or ratio scale.
2. All DV measurements are associated.
3. The DV measurements come from populations with the same median.

The sign test

The sign test is another nonparametric alternative to the paired samples *t* test. Similar to the signed-rank test, the sign test is used typically when the distribution of the DV is not normal or when the DV is measured on an ordinal scale. The sign test is used to assess for differences between two repeated measurements (or two matched groups). It must be noted that the sign test can be used in any situation that is appropriate for the signed-rank test; however, the sign test is typically less powerful, as the signed-rank test uses more information from the data to calculate the test statistic. Nevertheless, the sign test is presented here because it is seen in the literature; however, in most situations, the signed-rank test should be used.

For example, consider a pretest-posttest study to evaluate change in BMI following a physical activity intervention in a sample of 20 third grade students. In this study, BMI was measured at the beginning of the school year (i.e., pretest) and again after school year was complete (i.e., posttest). The sign test assesses whether a statistically significant difference (i.e., change) between repeated measurements. The results of a statistically significant sign test are presented as follows (note, no test statistic is presented, only a p value):

The results of the sign test indicated a statistically significant decrease in BMI from pretest to posttest ($p < 0.05$).

The assumptions of the sign test include:

1. The DV is measured repeatedly on an ordinal, interval, or ratio scale.
2. The two DV measurements are associated.

The McNemar test of change

The McNemar test of change (or simply the McNemar test) is an extension of the chi square and Fisher's exact test when participants are measured on two separate occasions and assesses the statistical significance of observed changes between the two repeated measurements. The McNemar test is a bit limited, in that it is only applicable to a DV measured on a dichotomous scale; however, continuous variables can be artificially dichotomized, with the understanding that information will be lost (as discussed regarding discrete variables).[17,41]

In the biomedical sciences, the McNemar test is often used for pretest-posttest studies to assess change following an intervention or treatment. For example, consider a study to determine the effectiveness of a swine flu vaccination across two consecutive flu seasons. At the beginning of the first flu season, 20 participants are randomized to receive either vaccination or placebo (i.e., 10 in each group). At the end of the first flu season, participants are asked whether they were diagnosed with the swine flu or not (a dichotomous outcome). Then, at the beginning of the second flu season, participants who received the vaccination originally will receive placebo and those who received placebo originally will receive the vaccination. At the end of the second flu season, participants are asked again whether they were diagnosed with swine flu. The McNemar test is used in this study to statistically test whether the swine flu vaccination was effective, where participants diagnosed with swine flu while taking placebo should not have developed swine flu with the vaccination. That is, the participant's outcome changed depending on the treatment received.

A critically important caveat is that the McNemar test only considers participants who changed between the two repeated measurements, with participants who did not change removed from analysis. Thus, if a researcher believes that change will be rare, the McNemar test may be inappropriate because the statistical power of this test may be extremely reduced due to the sample size decrease from removing participants who did not change.

Based on the example above, the results of a statistically significant McNemar test are presented as follows (note only the p value is provided):

The results of a statistically significant McNemar test indicated a statistically significant change between treatment and placebo ($p < 0.05$), with the vaccination significantly reducing swine flu diagnoses compared to placebo.

The assumptions of the McNemar test include:

1. The DV is measured repeatedly on a dichotomous scale.
2. The two DV measurements are associated.

The Cochran's Q test

The Cochran's Q test (or simply Cochran's Q) is an extension of the McNemar test to situations where participants are measured repeatedly on three or more separate occasions.[17] Similar to the McNemar test, the DV must be measured repeatedly on a dichotomous scale.

In the biomedical literature, Cochran's Q is often used to assess stability of a treatment over time or to compare the effectiveness of several treatments. For example, consider a study evaluating the effectiveness of the combination treatment sildenafil and psychotherapy in reducing symptoms of erectile dysfunction (ED).[42] Eight patients with psychogenic ED attended weekly psychotherapy sessions and ingested 50 mg of sildenafil citrate orally as needed over a 6-month period. Symptoms of ED were assessed at baseline, 6-months (i.e., end of treatment), and at a 3-month posttreatment follow-up (i.e., month 9 of the study). For this study, Cochran's Q was used to evaluate a change in the stage of remission for patients dichotomized into ED and no ED. A statistically significant finding indicated change from baseline and the possibility of sustaining effects at posttreatment follow-up. That is, all patients were diagnosed with ED at baseline, thus a statistically significant change indicates patients indicated remission of ED symptoms.

In the literature, the results of the Cochran's Q test may be presented with a χ^2 statistic and a p value; however, in other studies, the results may only present a p value. Although failing to include the test statistic provides less information, it does not necessarily damage the integrity of results. The result of a statistically significant Cochran's Q for the example above is presented as follows:

The results of the Cochran's Q test indicated a statistically significant change in psychogenic ED symptoms from baseline ($p < 0.05$) suggesting a combination of psychotherapy and 50 mg sildenafil are effective in reducing ED symptoms.

Because Cochran's Q is used to assess change over three or more repeated measures, it is an omnibus test. That is, the test will determine whether a statistically significant change exists between the repeated measurements, but will not indicate where the change occurred. Thus, adjusted *post hoc* tests are required, which for the Cochran's Q test consist of Bonferroni-corrected McNemar tests comparing each repeated measurement. In this example, three McNemar tests are required (i.e., baseline versus 6-month, baseline versus posttreatment follow-up, and 6-month versus posttreatment follow-up) with alpha equal to $0.017(0.05/3)$. The results of a statistically significant Cochran's Q including results of adjusted *post hoc* McNemar tests are presented as follows:

The results of the Cochran's Q test indicated a statistically significant change in psychogenic ED symptoms from baseline ($p < 0.05$). Bonferroni-corrected McNemar tests indicated statistically significant changes from baseline at 6-month as well as at posttreatment follow-up (all $p < 0.017$). These results suggest the combination of psychotherapy and sildenafil are effective in reducing ED symptoms, and this effect may continue to reduce ED symptoms up to 3 months following treatment completion.

The assumptions of the Cochran's Q test include:

1. The DV measured repeatedly on a dichotomous scale.
2. All DV measurements are associated.

Case Study 8–2

Consider a randomized, two-arm, crossover comparison of antiplatelet effects following a 75 mg/day or 150 mg/day dose of clopidogrel in 50 healthy participants. At the initial visit, a baseline blood sample was drawn to assess percent inhibition of platelet aggregation. Participants were then randomized to receive either 75 mg/day or 150 mg/day of clopidogrel for 7 consecutive days. On the seventh day of clopidogrel dosing, participants had blood drawn to assess for platelet aggregation inhibition. A 2 week washout period followed this assessment. At the end of the washout period, a second baseline blood sample was drawn to assess platelet aggregation inhibition. Participants were then crossed over to the alternate dose of clopidogrel for 7 consecutive days. On the seventh day of the alternate clopidogrel dose, blood was drawn again to assess platelet aggregation inhibition.

1. What is the DV in this study? On what scale is the DV measured?
2. The authors used an independent samples *t* test to assess whether the washout period was effective. Is this appropriate? Why or why not?

3. The authors did not test to assess for differences following randomization. Was this appropriate? Why or why not?

4. The author tested for order effects using a two-way mixed ANOVA. Was this appropriate? Why or why not?

5. When testing for order effects, the interaction effect was statistically significant. What does this indicate? Can the study be analyzed as is?

6. No statistically significant order effects were indicated. For the final analysis the authors used a paired samples t test. Was this appropriate? Why or why not?

7. Consider the distribution of the DV to be normal. Further, no statistically significant group differences were identified following randomization. The authors used an ANCOVA to test for differences at the posttest measurement (i.e., platelet inhibition following the second dose of clopidogrel) after statistically controlling for the first baseline measurement. Did this analysis add value to results?

TESTING FOR RELATIONSHIPS OR ASSOCIATIONS

When exploring the association or relationship between two or more variables, two specific types of analyses are employed—correlation or regression. These analyses are applied to determine the magnitude and direction of an association or relationship. Correlation analysis indicates the co-relationship of two variables (i.e., how one variable changes in relationship to the other). It is critically important to note that correlation does not imply causation. For example, consider the positive association between serum creatinine and BUN. In most cases, as creatinine increases so does BUN, but increasing creatinine does not cause BUN to increase and vice versa. Instead, they both may be increasing due to renal failure (i.e., the cause).

Regression analysis is a type of correlational analysis used to predict the value of one variable from the value of another variable. In this type of analysis, researchers attempt to determine the amount of variance in the DV that is explained by the IV(s) or covariates. Note that regression analysis can also permit multiple IVs and/or covariates measured on any scale. This type of analysis is referred to as a multivariate or multivariable analysis. While the definition of an IV and covariate is not always concrete, it is easier to think of an IV as the primary variable of interest and a covariate as a variable correlated with the DV, but not of specific interest. For example, consider a multivariate analysis assessing the effect statin use (IV) had on all cause mortality due to heart failure (DV) during a 5-year study period after statistically controlling for age, gender, race, comorbid conditions, and concurrent medications (covariates; which may explain the reason a patient died, but are not of specific research interest). These types of analyses are discussed in detail below.

This section begins by discussing bivariate (i.e., the relationship between two variables) techniques followed by multivariate techniques (i.e., the relationship between more than two variables). The discussion in this section will progress in a similar fashion to the tests of group differences above; that is, parametric tests will be discussed first, followed by the nonparametric alternatives.

Parametric Tests

Pearson's product-moment correlation

Pearson's product-moment correlation (or simply Pearson's correlation or Pearson's r) is one of the most commonly used correlation measures. It measures the direction and strength of a linear relationship between two variables measured on a continuous scale. Pearson's r ranges from -1 and $+1$, with r of 0 indicating no relationship. That is, as the correlation approaches -1 or 1, the relationship becomes stronger. A positive correlation (e.g., 0.30 or 0.99) indicates that as the values of one variable increase so do the values of the other variable, while a negative correlation (e.g., -0.50 or -0.80) indicates that as the values of one variable increase, the values of the other variable decrease. Pearson's r tests whether the correlation of two variables is different from zero (i.e., no relationship); thus, a statistically significant r indicates the slope of the linear relationship is not horizontal.

For example, research has shown a moderate, but statistically significant, positive correlation ($r = 0.25$) between weight (kilogram) and platelet count in men aged 20 to 55.[43] Thus, in men, as weight increases, so does platelet count. However, the magnitude of this increase may vary from person to person, which is why this correlation is not 1. That is, for any individual man, a one-kilogram increase in body weight may indicate an increase in platelet count that is different from the platelet count increase for another man. It should be noted the value of r is dimensionless because it is based on standardized scores. That is, measuring weight in pounds or kilograms in the example above will not change the value of the correlation. Finally, it must be noted that r is substantially affected by outliers, so researchers must identify and remove them from analysis or transform the data to draw the outliers in toward the rest of the distribution (see the Data Transformations section earlier).

The relationship between two variables can be assessed visually by plotting the data on a scatterplot. In fact, this practice is highly recommended.[5] The magnitude (i.e., value) of the correlation is directly related to the strength of the linear relationship. Take a moment to consider Figures 8–13 and 8–14. In Figure 8–13, the value of Pearson's r is approximately 1. Notice the dots on the scatterplot lie almost along the best fit line and that the slope of this line is fairly steep (i.e., not horizontal). The positive correlation coefficient indicates that as the values of variable 1 increase so do the values of variable 2.

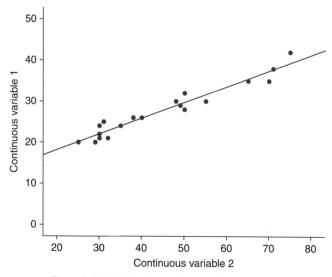

Figure 8–13. Scatterplot showing a positive correlation.

In Figure 8–14, Pearson's *r* is approximately 0. Here, notice the dots are scattered all over the plot with no real direction, and the best fit line (a straight line that passes as close as possible to the most points on a scatterplot and best represents the data on that scatterplot) is almost perfectly horizontal, which indicates no relationship between the two continuous variables.

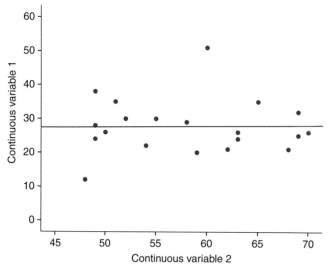

Figure 8–14. Scatterplot showing no correlation.

To highlight the substantial effect outliers have on Pearson's r, take a moment to draw an outlier on Figure 8–13, say, a value of 45 for variable 1 and a value of 25 for variable 2. What effect does this outlier have on the previously strong positive correlation? Which direction does this outlier pull the best fit line? The answers are that the outlier will essentially pull the line toward horizontal and the correlation will essentially approach 0.

Finally, the result of a statistically significant Pearson's product-moment correlation with no assumption violations for the example above is presented as follows:

The results of a Pearson's product-moment correlation indicates a statistically significant moderate relationship between body weight (in kilograms) and platelet count, (r_{81} = 0.252, p < 0.05) indicating body weight increased in concordance with platelet count.

Assumptions of the Pearson's product-moment correlation include:

1. Both variables are measured on an interval or ratio scale.
2. The sampling distribution of means for both variables is normal.
   a. This can be assured by assessing the individual group sample distributions or by applying the central limit theorem.
3. There are no outliers.
4. The relationship between the variables is linear.
5. Homoscedasticity is assured.
   a. The assumption states that the variability around the best fit line of the linear relationship is the same for all data. A violation of this assumption can be seen within the scatterplot. For example, consider a scatterplot where the lower values for a variable fall near the best fit line and higher values for this same variable fall far from the best fit line. In this situation, the variability around the line is not constant.
6. The observations are independent.
   a. That is, each participant provides one, and only one, observation (i.e., data or response) for each variable.

Simple linear regression

As stated above, the magnitude of the correlation is directly related to the strength of the linear relationship. The pattern of this linear relationship is typically identified by the regression line (i.e., another name for the best fit line in Figures 8–13 and 8–14). The regression line is a best fit line describing how a continuous response variable, also known as the DV, changes as the explanatory variable, also known as the IV, changes. Similar to Pearson's r, the statistical test in simple linear regression is whether the slope of the regression line is statistically different from zero (i.e., no slope or horizontal). Simple linear regression, however, takes Pearson's r one step further, where the regression line is used to predict values of the DV for a given value of the IV.[11] This is incredibly useful to evidence-based practitioners looking to implement findings into their practice. The algebraic linear regression equation (i.e., $\hat{y} = a + bx$) is based on the regression line's intercept with the y-axis (a) and slope (b), and is used to estimate (i.e., predict) values of the DV ($\hat{y}$) from a value of the IV (x). Note the intercept is interpreted as the predicted value of the DV when the value of the IV is zero, and the slope is interpreted as the overall change in the DV for a one-unit increase in the IV. Further, while not described in detail here, note that the value of the correlation between the DV and IV (i.e., Pearson's r) is incorporated into the equation for slope.

For example, consider the relationship between SBP (mm Hg) and height (cm) in 100 children aged 5 to 7 years.[44] The results of this study indicated a positive correlation between height and SBP ($r = 0.33$). In addition, simple linear regression analysis was used to determine the intercept of the regression line with the y-axis (46.28 mm Hg) and the slope (0.48) for SBP. That is, for a child with height of 0 cm, systolic blood pressure is 46.28 mm Hg (i.e., the intercept); while a one-cm increase in height increases SBP 0.48 mm Hg (i.e., the slope). It should be noted that a child with a height of 0 cm is impossible. This is a prime example of the awareness readers must have when interpreting the intercept. That is, unless it makes theoretical sense to have a meaningful zero point for the IV, the interpretation of the intercept is rarely useful. Thus, in situations, similar to above where a zero value is meaningless, the intercept simply serves as a starting point for prediction. For example, using the linear regression equation, by imputing the intercept and slope values provided, SBP can be predicted for a child 115 cm tall (i.e., predicted SBP = 46.28 + 0.48*115), which equals 101.48 mm Hg.

It is important to note that the predicted values of the DV are rarely identical to the actual observed values. That is, a child 115 cm tall in this sample may actually have a SBP of 105 mm Hg, but have a predicted value of 101.48 mm Hg. The difference between the actual and predicted scores is referred to as a residual value (or error), which for this participant is 3.52 mm Hg. Residual values are calculated for all participants included in the regression analysis, and one of the primary assumptions of linear regression is that the distribution of these residual values be normal. This assumption is a key indicator of the reliability of the results. Thus, if a study fails to describe the distribution of residuals, the study should be read and interpreted with extreme caution.

In addition, note that the interpretation of slope used in the above example is only appropriate for IVs measured on a continuous scale (e.g., height). If instead the IV is categorical, interpretation is slightly different. For example, consider replacing height in the example above with the dichotomous IV gender (i.e., male versus female). In this situation, the researcher must specify which level of gender will serve as the reference (or comparison) category. That is, specify which level of the IV the calculated slope represents. Therefore, if females are specified as the reference category, the slope for gender provides the overall difference in predicted SBP for males compared to females.

Interpretation follows this logic. For example, reconsider the example with females considered the reference category and the slope for gender calculated to be 0.48. This slope indicates that any predicted value of SBP will be 0.48 mm Hg higher for males compared to females. This is a confusing topic, but is a critically important detail to consider when interpreting a study. Every published study should indicate which group served as the reference category, and if the authors fail to provide a reference category, interpretation becomes impossible.

The primary test used in simple linear regression is an omnibus ANOVA (without going into detail, note that linear regression and ANOVA are mathematically equivalent). The omnibus ANOVA provides an F test indicating whether the IV explains a statistically significant amount of variance in the DV. That is, does the IV reliably predict the DV? Only if the ANOVA is statistically significant is the slope of the individual IV interpreted. Most research studies will provide the results of the ANOVA prior to presenting the slope of the IV. Further, the ANOVA results presented in simple linear regression will be presented identically to the one-way ANOVA examples discussed earlier. The statistical significance of the IV will most often be presented as the regression coefficient (i.e., slope) with associated p value. However, sometimes authors present an associated t value. If a t value is presented in the narrative portion of the study (i.e., results section), the slope should be presented in a table (often referred to as regression coefficient or B). If the slope is not presented in the narrative portion or in a table, complete interpretation of the regression analysis is impossible, and the study is essentially rendered useless.

Finally, the amount of variance in the DV explained by the IV must be considered. That is, how much of the reason a participant has a particular value on the DV is attributable to the IV value. As a side note, the word *explained* should not and does not imply causality, as causality in correlational studies is extremely difficult to determine. The amount of variance explained in simple linear regression is quantified by the coefficient of determination. This coefficient is calculated by squaring the Pearson's r between the IV and DV (i.e., r^2), and in the literature it will often be referred to simply as r^2, or identically as R^2. Note that how this value is referred to in a study is dependent on the researcher, but regardless of whether r^2 or R^2 is reported, their values will be identical and, thus, interpreted identically. The coefficient will often be presented as a proportion, ranging from 0 to 1, with higher values indicating more reliable prediction. From the example above, remember the correlation between a child's height and SBP was 0.33. Thus, approximately 0.11 (i.e., 0.33^2) of the child's measured SBP can be explained by the child's height. Said another way, approximately 11% of the reason a child has a particular SBP value is attributable to his or her height.

In the literature, the result of a statistically significant simple linear regression analysis with no assumption violations will be presented as follows:

The results of a simple linear regression analysis indicated a child's height significantly predicts SBP ($F_{1,98} = 12.03$, $p < 0.05$, $r^2 = 0.11$), with a 1 cm increase in height resulting in a 0.48 mm Hg increase in SBP.

The assumptions of simple linear regression include:

1. The DV is measured on an interval or ratio scale.
2. The sampling distribution of means for the DV is normal.
   a. This can be assured by assessing the individual group sample distributions or by applying the central limit theorem.
3. There are no outliers.
4. The relationship between the DV and IV is linear.
5. Homoscedasticity is assured.
   a. The assumption states that the variability around the regression line is the same for all data. A violation of this assumption can be seen within a scatterplot. For example, consider a scatterplot where the lower values for a variable fall near the regression line and higher values for this same variable fall far from the regression line. In this situation, the variability around the regression line is not constant.
6. Residuals are distributed normally.
   a. Remember, residuals are the difference between the actual and predicted values.
7. The observations are independent.
   a. That is, each participant provides one, and only one, observation (i.e., data or response) for each variable.

Multiple linear regression

Multiple (sometimes called multivariate or multivariable) linear regression is an extension of simple linear regression for designs with one continuous DV and multiple IVs or covariates. Remember, an IV is defined as an explanatory variable of specific research interest, while a covariate is a nuisance variable that is significantly associated with the DV but not of specific research interest. That is, covariates are typically included because they are related to the DV or because previous research has indicated they are important. In multiple linear regression, IVs can be any combination of continuous or discrete variables (e.g., height, gender, HbA1c). Further, this analysis is often a better option than simple linear regression because the inclusion of additional IVs often explains a higher percentage of variance in the DV. That is, higher R^2 values.

For example, previous research has shown a statistically significant negative Pearson's correlation ($r = -0.28$) between serum 25-hydroxyvitamin D (25OHD; ng/ml) and serum parathyroid hormone (PTH; pg/ml).[45] PTH is an important indicator of bone production.

Based on this correlation, the percentage of variance in serum PTH explained by serum 25OHD is 8% (i.e., -0.28^2). That is, 8% of the reason a participant has a predicted serum PTH value is due to their serum 25OHD level. In an effort to increase this percentage of variance explained, a new study is designed to determine the effect serum 25OHD (i.e., IV) has on serum PTH (i.e., DV) after statistically adjusting for covariates known to significantly affect PTH (i.e., age, BMI, total calcium intake, and serum creatinine). Thus, a multiple linear regression analysis will be used to determine whether there is an effect of serum 25OHD on serum PTH over and above the effect of the covariates. That is, multiple linear regression assesses the unique correlation between 25OHD and serum PTH after removing the effects already accounted for by age, BMI, total calcium intake, and serum creatinine.

The percentage of variance explained in multiple linear regression is always referred to as R^2 (as opposed to r^2 in simple linear regression), where the R indicates the multiple correlation. That is, R is the multivariate extension of Pearson's r and is defined as the combined correlation between all IVs and the DV. Similar to Pearson's r, R ranges from -1 to 1, with 0 indicating no relationship. Thus, as R approaches -1 or 1, the association between the IVs and DV becomes stronger. In addition, most studies will also present an adjusted R^2 value (i.e., adjusted R^2 or R^2_{adj}). Adjusted R^2 is interpreted exactly the same as R^2, but it is adjusted for the sample size of the study. When reading a study, comparing R^2 and adjusted R^2 is incredibly useful to interpretation, as large differences between the two indicate significant issues with the analysis (e.g., inadequate sample size), which essentially render the regression model useless (i.e., not generalizable to the population). Finally, it should be noted a multiple linear regression model will never explain 100% of the variance in the DV. However, do not disregard studies reporting low values of R^2. This is because the definition of what constitutes a large R^2 value varies by research arena. That is, lower R^2 values are expected when using human participants because measurement error is usually high (e.g., consider a study using participant self-reported daily calorie intake). Whereas, high R^2 values are expected for bench research studies because in a well-conducted study measurement error is typically not an issue (e.g., think biomedical research using analytic chemistry).

In general, the results of a multiple linear regression model are interpreted in an almost identical fashion to simple linear regression. As a result, please consider the section on simple linear regression carefully. Similar to simple linear regression, multiple regression produces a regression equation allowing for prediction of DV values based on the y-intercept and slope of the regression line for individual IVs and covariates. Briefly, the intercept is the predicted value of the DV when all values of the IVs and covariates are 0, while the slope quantifies the change in the predicted DV with a 1 unit increase in the IV or covariates. Again, the regression equation is incredibly useful to evidence-based practitioners looking to implement findings into their practice. For example, consider the multiple regression example above, where serum PTH was predicted from

25OHD and a set of covariates. Based on the regression equation from this study, the practitioner can provide the patient with empirical evidence regarding which variables (i.e., age, BMI, total calcium intake, serum creatinine, and serum 25OHD) to increase or decrease in an effort to optimize serum PTH levels and increase bone production.

The overall test of the multiple linear regression model is an omnibus ANOVA, which indicates at least one of the IVs or covariates are significantly predicting the DV. However, this omnibus test fails to indicate which specific variables (whether the IVs or covariates) are significantly predicting the DV. Thus, the statistical test for each IV or covariate is considered. Each of the statistical tests for the IVs and covariates can be considered similar to a *post hoc* test; however, unlike the other *post hoc* tests already discussed, alpha typically remains unadjusted. In most studies, the results of the individual IVs or covariates are presented as regression coefficients (i.e., slope) or t values. Note that regardless of which result an author presents, the p values will be identical. Interpretation of the slopes for the individual coefficients is also slightly different compared to simple linear regression; the interpretation of a particular IV or covariate is statistically adjusted for all other IVs and covariates in the regression model (similar to ANCOVA).

An example may help clarify this information. Consider a situation where the result of a statistically significant multiple linear regression analysis based on the example above indicates 25OHD has a statistically significant slope of -1.5 pg/ml. Because the analysis is multivariate, this slope must be interpreted considering all covariates included in the model. Thus, the slope of -1.5 pg/ml indicates that with age, BMI, total calcium intake, and serum creatinine held constant, a 1-ng/ml increase in 25OHD decreases serum PTH 1.5 pg/ml. Note that *held constant* indicates that the values of the covariates do not change with increases in 25OHD. Authors often forget to highlight this important fact when interpreting their results; thus, diligence is required when reading and basing clinical decisions on studies using multiple linear regression techniques.

Based on the example, the results of a statistically significant multiple linear regression analysis with no assumption violations are presented below. Notice the effects of statistically significant covariates (i.e., BMI and serum creatinine) are also described; however, authors will vary on which covariates (if any) they interpret.

The results of a multivariate linear regression analysis indicated age, BMI, total calcium intake, serum creatinine, and 25OHD significantly predicted serum PTH ($F_{5,472} = 21.82$, $p < 0.05$, adjusted $R^2 = 0.18$). After adjusting for covariates, 25OHD significantly predicted serum PTH (regression coefficient $= -1.5$, $p < 0.05$). That is, with all else held constant, a 1-ng/ml increase in serum 25OHD resulted in a 1.5 pg/ml decrease in serum PTH. Regarding the individual covariates, after adjustment, increases in BMI and serum creatinine (regression coefficients $= 0.75$ and 2.12, respectively, both $p < 0.05$) resulted in higher serum PTH levels. Finally, after adjustment, age and total calcium intake were not associated with serum PTH.

The assumptions of multiple linear regression include:

1. The DV is measured on an interval or ratio scale.
2. The sampling distribution of means for the DV is distributed normally.
   a. For multiple linear regression analysis, the distribution of the IVs and covariates are not considered too important; however, statistical power can be increased by using normally distributed IV(s).[4] Nevertheless, the assumption can be assured by assessing the individual group sample distributions or by applying the central limit theorem.
3. Absence of multicollinearity is assured.
   a. That is, no Pearson's r between any IVs and covariates should be greater than 0.90, as correlations this high indicate the variables are redundant. That is, high correlations indicate the variables may be measuring the same facet. Including redundant variables will significantly bias results. However, most published studies provide all correlations (i.e., Pearson's r) between the DV, IVs, and covariates; thus, a violation of this assumption is easy to identify.
4. There are no outliers.
5. The relationship between the DV and IVs and between the DV and covariates is linear.
6. Homoscedasticity is assured.
   a. The assumption states that the variability around the regression line is the same for all data. A violation of this assumption can be seen within a scatterplot. For example, consider a scatterplot where the lower values for a variable fall near the regression line and higher values for this same variable fall far from the regression line. In this situation, the variability around the regression line is not constant.
7. Residuals are distributed normally.
   a. Residuals are the difference between the actual and predicted values.
8. The observations are independent.
   a. That is, each participant provides one, and only one, observation (i.e., data or response) for each variable.

Nonparametric Tests

Spearman rank-order correlation coefficient

The Spearman rank-order correlation coefficient (r_s), also known as Spearman's rho (ρ), is the nonparametric alternative to Pearson's r. This correlation is used when the two variables being considered are not normally distributed, when the variables are measured on an ordinal scale, or when the relationship between the two variables is nonlinear.

Similar to the other nonparametric statistical tests discussed above, this correlation is based on rank-ordered data as opposed to the actual values. Because of this fact, Spearman's correlation can handle data containing outliers. That is, disconnected values are a nonissue because higher values simply receive higher ranks and lower values receive lower ranks. Finally, the values of r_s range from −1 to 1, with 0 indicating no association. Thus, as r_s approaches −1 or 1, the association between the two variables becomes stronger. A statistically significant r_s indicates that the association is significantly different from 0 (i.e., no association).

For example, consider a study assessing the association between triglyceride content and lag time in LDL oxidation in a sample of 18 renal transplant patients.[46] Spearman's rank-order correlation was used in this study because outliers were identified in the sample. Further, because the sample was small, removing outliers was not considered. The study found a statistically significant negative r_s of −0.502, suggesting that as triglyceride content increased, LDL oxidation decreased.

Based on the example above, the result of a statistically significant Spearman rank-order correlation coefficient is presented as follows:

The Spearman rank-order correlation analysis was employed in lieu of Pearson's correlation due to the presence of outliers and small sample size. Results indicated a statistically significant negative association between triglyceride content and lag time in LDL oxidation ($r_{s\ 16} = -0.502$, $p < 0.05$), which suggest increases in triglyceride content translates into decreases in LDL oxidation.

The assumptions of the Spearman rank-order correlation coefficient include:

1. The two variables are measured on an ordinal, interval, or ratio scale.
2. The relationship between the two rank-ordered variables is linear.
   a. Although the relationship between the two variables based on their actual values may be nonlinear, the relationship based on rank-ordered data must be linear. This assumption typically cannot be tested by what the authors provide in the narrative. Thus, when authors fail to indicate whether the assumption was tested, results should be viewed with caution.
3. The observations are independent.
   a. That is, each participant provides one, and only one, observation (i.e., data or response) for each variable.

Logistic regression

The interpretation of a logistic regression analysis is similar to linear regression; thus, a basic understanding of the interpretation of simple and multiple linear regression is extremely useful. Please consider reading these sections, as much of this material discussed here is simply an extension of the material described in detail previously.

Logistic regression is used when the DV is measured on a discrete scale and the relationship between the DV and IV is nonlinear. This analysis, especially with a dichotomous DV, is ubiquitous in the biomedical sciences. It is important to note that in any logistic regression analysis, the measurement scale of the DV is always considered unordered. That is, the categorized DV is always considered measured on a nominal scale. While the logistic regression analyses discussed here are only for a dichotomous DV, an extension of logistic regression is available for a DV with three or more categories. This analysis is termed multinomial logistic regression, with the definition of multinomial being multiple nominal categories. Interpretation of results from this analysis is similar to the analyses discussed in this section and interested readers are encouraged to consider obtaining the recommended readings referenced at the end of the chapter.

As an example of a design requiring a simple logistic regression analysis, consider a 5-year study designed to assess the effect that the duration of statin use (i.e., IV; measured as percentage of time on any statin during the study period) has on all-cause mortality (i.e., DV) in a sample of Veteran Administration (VA) patients previously suffering congestive heart failure. Note that the DV is dichotomous (i.e., dead or alive). Further, a simple logistic regression analysis can be extended to a multivariate analysis by including additional IVs and covariates in an effort to explain more of the reason why patients experienced the outcome of interest. For example, consider a multivariate extension to the study above where the effect that duration of statin use (i.e., IV) has on all-cause mortality (i.e., DV) is assessed after statistically controlling for age, race, gender, concurrent medications, and comorbid conditions (i.e., covariates).

For all logistic regression models, researchers must choose a reference category within the DV. This is a topic similar to the one discussed within the section on simple linear regression. When identified, the reference category is used as a comparison group for the primary outcome of interest. In most situations, the reference category is typically the category determined by the researcher to be of less specific interest. For example, consider all-cause mortality, a dichotomous DV (i.e., dead versus alive). Most studies are interested in the individuals who died; essentially the researcher wants to identify the primary reasons for death. Thus, because patients alive at the end of the study period are considered to be the reference category, all regression coefficients (i.e., slopes) are calculated for patients who died compared to patients who lived. Thus, the first step in properly interpreting the results of logistic regression analysis is to identify the primary outcome of interest and the reference category within the DV. It should be noted that most authors will not explicitly identify the primary outcome of interest or the reference category; however, this information can be obtained easily as all results and interpretations are typically written in relation to the primary outcome of interest.

Similar to linear regression, a logistic regression analysis provides a regression equation that can be used to predict the primary outcome of interest. Briefly, the regression equation contains a y-intercept and slope values for all IVs included in the analysis. This equation is interpreted slightly different from linear regression because the relationship between the DV and IV is nonlinear. However, the usefulness of the equation is the same. That is, the equation can be used to assist evidence-based practitioners in instructing patients regarding what changes need to be made to optimize (or prevent) a specific outcome.

The primary statistical test in logistic regression determines whether the logistic model including all IVs or covariates better predicts the probability of experiencing the outcome of interest compared to the model with no IVs or covariates (often referred to in the literature as the constant-only model). That is, a logistic regression analysis determines whether the IVs significantly predict the primary outcome of interest. Similar to linear regression, this overall test is an omnibus test, which in this case is a chi square test. If this omnibus chi square test is statistically significant, the statistical significance of each IV or covariate is assessed and interpreted. These tests of individual predictors can be thought of as *post hoc* tests, and typically no adjustment to alpha is considered. When interpreting the results for individual predictors, authors typically provide two values, the slope and odds ratio.

The slope is interpreted similar to linear regression; however, slopes in logistic regression indicate changes in the log-odds of experiencing the outcome of interest. That is, a one-unit increase in the IV indicates a change in the log-odds of experiencing the primary outcome. For example, reconsider the 5-year study assessing the effect duration of statin use (measured as percentage of time on any statin during the study period) has on all-cause mortality. Say, the slope for statin use is −0.25. With death considered the primary outcome of interest (i.e., alive is the reference category), this slope suggests that a 1% increase in statin use during the study period resulted in a 0.25-unit decrease in the log-odds of dying (a decrease because the slope was negative). Based on this interpretation, an important question is, what does a 0.25-unit decrease in log-odds mean? While the slope is integral in producing the regression equation, the interpretation in log-odds is fairly convoluted and beyond the scope of this chapter. Thankfully, logistic regression provides an alternative value that is easier to interpret—the odds ratio.

The odds ratio produced by a logistic regression analysis is calculated and interpreted similarly to the odds ratios discussed in the section on epidemiologic statistics above. Briefly, odds ratios can range from 0 to infinity, with 1 indicating no association. Therefore, an odds ratio above 1 indicates an increase in the odds of experiencing the primary outcome of interest, while an odds ratio below 1 indicates a decrease in the odds of experiencing the primary outcome of interest. For example, reconsider the example above with a slope of −0.25. The associated odds ratio for this slope is 0.78. Because the odds ratio is below 1, a 1% increase in statin use is associated with a 22% (i.e., 1 − 0.78) decrease in the odds of dying during the study period.

It is important to consider that authors vary the information they present in journal articles, as one article may only provide slopes, while another article may only provide odds ratios. This is not an issue because there is a direct relationship between slopes and odds ratios. That is, the slope is simply the natural log of the odds ratio (i.e., ln 0.78 = –0.25), whereas the odds ratio is simply the exponentiated slope (i.e., $e^{-0.25} = 0.78$). Thus, if an author only provides slopes, the odds ratio can be easily calculated to ease interpretation. Also, note that regardless of which value the authors present, the associated p value will be identical. That is, a statistically significant slope will have a statistically significant odds ratio, and vice versa.

Finally, similar to linear regression, the primary reason a researcher includes additional IVs and covariates in a multivariate logistic regression model is to increase the amount of variance explained in the primary outcome of interest. That is, multivariate logistic regression models aim to better identify the reason why participants experienced the outcome of interest. However, unlike R^2 in linear regression, there is no unanimously accepted measure for quantifying explained variance in logistic regression. Thus, when reading a journal article, several pseudo-R^2 values may be presented, with the most common including the Nagelkerke R^2 and the Cox and Snell R^2. These pseudo-R^2 values are used to approximate R^2 from linear regression and are interpreted in an identical fashion. For example, reconsider the 5-year study assessing the effect of statin use on all-cause mortality. Say the Nagelkerke R^2 value from the logistic regression analysis was 18%. This value indicates that 18% of the reason why patients died was due to their statin use. Again, it is important to note that these pseudo-R^2 values will never be near 100%; however, the definition of a large or small pseudo-R^2 value is determined by the specific research arena, as discussed in the section on multiple linear regression.

Based on the example described above, the result of a simple logistic regression analysis is presented as follows:

The results of a simple logistic regression analysis indicated a statistically significant association between duration of statin use and all-cause mortality. ($\chi^2_1 = 13.65$, $p < 0.05$, Nagelkerke $R^2 = 0.06$) where a 1% increase in duration of statin use resulted in a 22% decrease in the odds of dying during the study period.

An example of a multivariate logistic regression analysis, with the addition of age, race, gender, concurrent medications, and comorbid conditions as covariates is presented below. Notice in this example, the researcher is not interested in the individual effects of the covariates, as they are not interpreted.

The results of a multivariate logistic regression analysis indicated a statistically significant overall association between the variables as a set and all-cause mortality ($\chi^2_1 = 156.02$, $p < 0.05$, Nagelkerke $R^2 = 0.23$). After controlling for age, race, gender, concurrent medications, and comorbid conditions, duration of statin use significantly predicted all-cause *mortality (OR = 0.62, p < 0.05). Thus, holding all variables constant, a 1% increase in statin use resulted in a 38% decrease in all-cause mortality.*

The assumptions of logistic regression include:

1. The DV is discrete with mutually exclusive categories.
2. The sample size is large.
    a. A basic rule is to have at least 50 participants per variable included in the model. This is required so that the parameters (e.g., slopes, standard errors) are estimated accurately.[47] Thus, a model with 10 IVs and covariates requires at least 500 participants (i.e., 10*50 = 500).
3. Adequacy of expected frequencies is assured.
    a. This assumption applies only to categorical IVs and is the same assumption as the chi square test. That is, no more than 20% of cells can have expected frequencies less than 5. This is a difficult assumption to verify, outside of calculating the expected frequencies by hand. Thus, if an article fails to indicate this assumption was tested, view results with caution. However, most studies using logistic regression will have large sample sizes, and this assumption is rarely violated.
4. Linearity in the logit is assured.
    a. This is a convoluted assumption, and difficult to explain without getting into mathematical detail. However, the logit is defined as the nonlinear transformation of probability. This assumption is tested by determining whether the relationship between continuous IVs or covariates and the DV is linear. Briefly, the initial relationships between continuous variables and the DV are nonlinear because the DV is dichotomous; thus, a link function is used to make these relationships linear. There are numerous link functions available, and researchers often vary in which one they use. However, this is a key assumption, and a violation severely biases results. Thus, if authors do not mention that the assumption was assured in the methods or results sections, view results with caution.
5. Absence of multicollinearity assured.
    a. That is, no Pearson's *r* between any continuous IVs and covariates should be greater than 0.90, as correlations this high indicate the variables are redundant. That is, high correlations indicate the variables may be measuring the same facet. Including redundant variables will significantly bias results.
6. There are no outliers.
7. The observations are independent.
    a. That is, each participant provides one, and only one, observation (i.e., data or response) for each variable.

Survival analysis

Survival analysis (or failure analysis) consists of two of the most commonly used statistical techniques in the biomedical sciences—the Kaplan-Meier method and Cox regression. In general, survival analysis is concerned with time-to-event data; that is, the time to experience an outcome of interest. For example, consider a study designed to examine whether a new hormone therapy, in comparison to chemotherapy, prolongs remission in women previously diagnosed with breast cancer over a 20-week study period.

In survival analysis, participants who do not experience the outcome of interest (which for survival analysis is called the event) are considered to survive, while those who experience the event are considered to fail. Although this is fairly grim terminology, survival and failure do not necessarily imply living or dying. For example, in the example above, failure was defined as breast cancer recurrence, not death. In survival analysis, the outcome will typically be dichotomous (e.g., recurrence versus no recurrence), patients do not need to enter the study at the same time (i.e., enrollment can be continuous), and patients are followed until the study ends (known as end of follow-up).

Patients who do not experience the event by the end of follow-up, who are lost to follow-up, or who drop out of the study are termed censored. The key advantage survival analysis has over the analyses presented above (particularly logistic regression) is that it can handle censored data, which is essentially incomplete data. That is, censored data are considered incomplete because the researcher does not know when these participants experienced the event. Briefly, survival analysis can handle censored data because the DV is time, which is a continuous variable allowed to vary for each participant. Thus, as long as participants have a survival time indicated, they are included in analysis. The key point here is that survival time for censored participants is the time until they were censored (i.e., left the study for reasons other than suffering the event). Thus, all participants who entered the study are included in analysis regardless of whether they experienced the event or are censored because the analysis specifically considers their time in the study.

This section will cover two techniques for assessing time-to-event data—life tables and the Cox proportional hazards model (also known as Cox regression).

Life tables present time-to-event data in table format. That is, a life table tabulates the time that has elapsed until the event is experienced. Life tables are used to indicate the proportion of individuals surviving (i.e., not experiencing the event) based on fixed or varying time intervals. For example, reconsider the example examining the effectiveness of the new hormone therapy in preventing recurrence of breast cancer. A life table allows the researcher to tabulate the cumulative proportion of women who are surviving (i.e., no breast cancer recurrence) at any interval (e.g., 6-month, 1-year, or 3-year).

As stated above, life tables can be based on fixed or varying time intervals. Life tables based on fixed time intervals have a significant weakness, because they do not consider the exact time within the specified interval when the patient experienced the event (e.g., when breast cancer recurred). Thus, depending on the length of the time interval, a great amount of information is lost regarding the exact time the event was experienced. That is, the longer the time interval, the less precise a researcher can be regarding the exact moment the event occurred.

Alternatively, the Kaplan-Meier method is an extension of the life-table using varying time intervals. Using this method, the cumulative proportion surviving is recalculated every time an event occurs.[48] It is noted that the Kaplan-Meier method is the most widely used in the biomedical sciences.[49] For example, instead of assessing the total number of women who have a breast cancer recurrence at fixed intervals of 6 month, the Kaplan-Meier method recalculates the proportion of women surviving every time a woman in the study has a recurrence. In most studies, Kaplan-Meier data is presented as a graph of the cumulative survival over the study period known as a Kaplan-Meier curve. The Kaplan-Meier curve presents either a survival or hazard functions, where the survival function is the cumulative frequency of participants not experiencing the event, while the hazard function is the cumulative frequency of participants experiencing the event. A Kaplan-Meier curve is provided in the vast majority of published literature using survival analysis and will appear similar to the survival function presented in Figure 8–15. Note that the curve in Figure 8–15 only presents data for the sample of women initiating the new

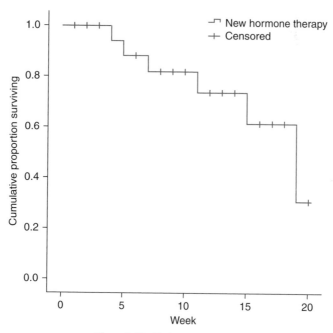

Figure 8–15. Kaplan-Meier curve.

hormone therapy and does not include data for women initiating chemotherapy. Notice the *y*-axis indicates the cumulative proportion of women surviving, while the *x*-axis indicates the total number of weeks of the study. The solid line presents the survival function. That is, the cumulative proportion of women not experiencing the event (i.e., surviving) at any specific time. The survival function indicates when a woman experienced the event when the function steps down. For example, by week 5, two women have experienced the event, indicated by the two steps in the survival function. Further, notice the vertical dashes throughout the survival function. These dashes indicate individual women who were censored. That is, women who dropped out of the study for reasons other than experiencing the event (e.g., side effects, moved out of the area). Few studies provide information regarding censored participants on the Kaplan-Meier curve because most survival analyses involve large samples. Thus, the dashes in Figure 8–15 are usually omitted from the curve; however, censored participants are always described within the narrative or in table format.

The Kaplan-Meier curve can also be presented for multiple groups. For example, consider the overall survival of women initiating the new hormone therapy compared to women initiating chemotherapy. Figure 8–16 presents a Kaplan-Meier curve where the survival functions for both treatment groups are presented simultaneously. Interpretation

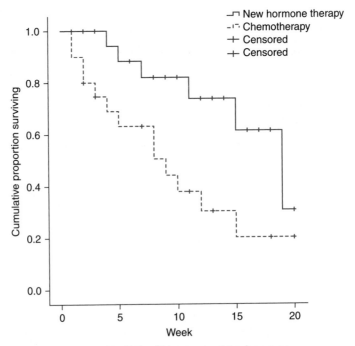

Figure 8–16. Kaplan-Meier curve—comparing groups.

of these survival functions is identical to the methods described above for Figure 8–15. However, with two or more treatment groups, a statistical test can be conducted to assess for a statistically significant group difference in survival rate. The most common test in the biomedical literature is the log-rank test (also known as the Mantel-Cox test).[4] A statistically significant log-rank test indicates there is a significant difference in survival rate between the groups. However, it is important to note that a Kaplan-Meier curve and associated log-rank test have no way of indicating why the breast cancer recurred beyond the possibility of the therapy being ineffective.

Based on the survival functions presented in Figure 8–16, the results of a statistically significant log-rank test are presented as follows:

The results of the log-rank test indicated a statistically significant difference in duration of breast cancer remission between the new hormone therapy and chemotherapy groups ($\chi^2_1 = 5.68$, $p < 0.05$), with women initiating the new hormone therapy experiencing significantly longer breast cancer remission.

It should be noted that when more than two treatment groups are being compared the log-rank test is an omnibus test. That is, with three or more groups, a statistically significant log-rank test will indicate that a statistically significant difference exists between groups, but will not indicate which groups differ specifically. Thus, Bonferroni-corrected *post hoc* log-rank tests are required to determine where a significant difference in survival occurred. For example, consider the addition of another treatment group to the breast cancer example, say, women who do not want to initiate any therapy. Three Bonferroni-corrected log-rank tests are required using an adjusted alpha of 0.017 (0.05/3). These adjusted *post hoc* tests determine whether statistically significant differences in survival rate occurred between hormone therapy versus chemotherapy, hormone therapy versus no therapy, and chemotherapy versus no therapy.

The results of statistically significant *post hoc* tests are presented as follows:

The results of the log-rank test indicated a statistically significant difference in breast cancer recurrence between the three treatment groups ($\chi^2_2 = 9.76$, $p < 0.05$). Bonferroni-corrected post hoc log-rank tests indicated women initiating the new hormone therapy experienced significantly longer breast cancer remission compared to women receiving chemotherapy or women choosing not to receive therapy (both $p < 0.017$). No statistically significant difference was indicated between women initiating chemotherapy and women receiving no therapy.

Although the Kaplan-Meier method is effective in assessing for overall differences in survival, the analysis is unable to identify the association between covariates and survival. That is, the Kaplan-Meier method cannot identify whether the IV significantly predicts survival. For many studies, this is a far more important consideration. Thus, a form of regression analysis is required. The Cox proportional hazards model (or simply Cox regression) is a semiparametric method (i.e., includes parametric and nonparametric components) used to predict the time (i.e., DV) to experience a discrete outcome (known as the event). Note that the event is usually a dichotomous variable (e.g., dead versus alive). In addition, all predictor variables in a Cox regression are termed covariates. That is, in the literature, authors will not identify a distinction between IVs and covariates. Finally, it should also be noted that most published studies progress from Kaplan-Meier curves and log-rank tests to Cox regression analysis. That is, the Kaplan-Meier curve will first present the survival functions for the covariate of interest as well as associated log-rank tests, and then authors will present the results of a Cox regression assessing for the relationship between covariates and the event of interest.

The interpretation of Cox regression can be considered a combination of linear and logistic regression; however, the primary difference is that in Cox regression, results are considered to be time dependent. That is, Cox regression is concerned with the time-dependent risk of experiencing the event (remember, the DV is time) instead of the overall occurrence of events as in logistic regression. Consider the example presented in the section on logistic regression for a study designed to assess the effect duration of statin use (i.e., IV; measured as percentage of time in any statin during the study period) has on all-cause mortality (i.e., dead versus alive) in a sample of VA patients previously suffering from congestive heart failure. If the researchers were interested in the effect that duration of statin use had on prolonging the time until death during the study period, a Cox regression is the analysis of choice. Again, the primary consideration in Cox regression is time-to-event, not the overall probability of the event.

Similar to the other forms of regression already discussed, Cox regression can be simple or multivariate. For example, in the example above a simple Cox regression analysis was required because only one covariate (i.e., statin use) was used to predict the risk of death. However, if the study was extended to statistically control for age, gender, race, comorbid conditions, and concurrent medications, a multivariate Cox regression is appropriate. That is, assess the effects that duration of statin use had on the risk of death over and above the effects of the other covariates.

Similar to logistic regression analysis, the researcher must choose the primary event of interest and the associated reference category. When identified, the reference category is used as a comparison group for the event of interest. In most situations, the reference category is typically the category determined by the researcher to be of less specific interest. For example, consider all-cause mortality, a dichotomous outcome variable (i.e., dead versus alive). Most studies are interested in the individuals who died. Thus, patients who lived are usually considered the reference category, and all regression coefficients (i.e., slopes) are calculated for patients who died compared to patients who lived. Therefore, the first step in properly interpreting the results of a Cox regression analysis is to identify the event and the reference category. If an author does not explicitly state the reference category, this information can be obtained easily, as all results and interpretations are typically written in relation to the primary event of interest.

It is critically important to note that in the literature authors will report using one of two different Cox regression analyses with or without time-varying covariates. The use of Cox regression with time-varying covariates is based on a violation of the primary assumption of Cox regression, termed the proportionality of hazards assumption. This assumption typically applies to all categorical covariates (e.g., new hormone therapy versus chemotherapy) and states that, although events can begin to occur at any time during the study period, when events do begin, the rate at which events occur between levels of a categorical covariate must remain constant over time. That is, when events begin to occur, the survival functions for the groups must be the same (i.e., roughly parallel).

For example, reconsider Figure 8–16. Here, the proportionality of hazards assumption is not violated. Notice women initiating the new hormone therapy did not begin experiencing breast cancer recurrence (i.e., the event) until week 4, as indicated by no steps in the curve until week 4, while women in the chemotherapy group began experiencing the recurrence at week 1, steps occurred immediately. However, when events began to occur, they occurred at approximately the same rate. That is, the slopes of the survival functions are roughly parallel. Thus, proportionality of hazards assumption is assured, and the treatment group covariate is assumed to have constant survival rates over time (i.e., the use of this covariate in a Cox regression without time-varying covariates is appropriate). By contrast, a violation of the proportionality assumption is provided in Figure 8–17. Notice that in this figure, events began occurring at roughly the same time (weeks 3 and 4) within both treatment groups. However, the survival functions are drastically different, and, in fact, intersect twice. That is, any time the survival functions intersect, the proportionality of hazards assumption can be viewed as violated, which indicates survival within each group varies across time. Thus, Cox regression analysis with time-varying covariates is required.

When reading a journal article, take careful notice of the Kaplan-Meier curves presented prior to the Cox regression analysis. Clear violation of this assumption is apparent whenever survival functions intersect. If a violation is observed, identify whether the appropriate Cox regression analysis was employed. That is, if a violation is indicated, Cox regression with time-varying covariates must be used. If Cox regression without time-varying covariates was used in the presence of a violation, results and interpretations are extremely misleading.

Similar to the other forms of regression discussed, Cox regression allows researchers to produce a regression equation useful in determining the overall risk score for a patient based on specific characteristics. The primary difference in Cox regression, however, is that there is no y-intercept (i.e., baseline hazard function). Thus, overall risk is calculated simply by using the slopes for the covariates. However, this regression equation remains useful for evidence-based practitioners when consulting their patients on the changes required to decrease their risk of experiencing a unfavorable event.

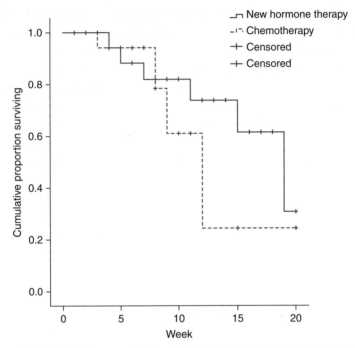

Figure 8–17. Kaplan-Meier curve showing violation of proportionality of hazards assumption.

Identical to logistic regression, the overall statistical test in Cox regression is whether the model including the covariates predicts the time elapsed prior to experiencing the event significantly better than the model with no covariates (again termed the constant-only model). That is, a Cox regression analysis determines whether the covariates significantly predict the time elapsed prior to experiencing the primary event of interest. Again, this overall test is an omnibus test, and similar to logistic regression, it is a chi square test. Only if this omnibus chi square test is statistically significant does the researcher evaluate the significance of each covariate. The tests of individual predictors can be considered *post hoc* tests, but typically without adjustment to alpha. When interpreting the results for individual predictors, authors typically provide two values, the slopes and/or hazard ratios.

In Cox regression, slopes are interpreted similar to linear regression. However, for this analysis, a 1-unit increase in a covariate results in an increase or decrease in the risk of experiencing the event. For example, say the slope for women initiating the new hormone therapy was –0.65. That is, women initiating chemotherapy served as the reference (or comparison) group. Thus, the slope represents a 0.65-unit decrease (i.e., because the slope is negative) in the risk of breast cancer recurrence for the new hormone therapy compared to chemotherapy. A 0.65-unit decrease is complicated to explain and beyond the scope of this chapter; thus, the presentation and interpretation of hazard ratios are a useful alternative.

The hazard ratio produced by a Cox regression analysis is calculated a similarly to the relative risk discussed in the section on epidemiologic st However, it is important to note that a hazard ratio is not identical to relative risk. Briefly, hazard ratios can range from 0 to infinity, with 1 indicating no association. Therefore, a hazard ratio above 1 indicates an increase in the risk of experiencing the event, while a hazard ratio below 1 indicates a decrease in the risk of experiencing the event. For example, reconsider the example above where the slope for the new hormone therapy was –0.65. The associated hazard ratio for this slope is 0.52. Because the hazard ratio is below 1, initiating the new hormone therapy resulted in a 48% (i.e., 1 – 0.52) decrease in the risk of breast cancer recurrence compared to chemotherapy.

It is important to consider that authors vary the information they present in journal articles, as one study may only provide slopes, while another study may only provide hazard ratios. This is not an issue because there is a direct relationship between slopes and hazard ratios. That is, the slope is simply the natural log of the hazard ratio (i.e., ln 0.52 = –0.65), whereas the hazard ratio is simply the exponentiated slope (i.e., $e^{-0.65}$ = 0.52). Thus, if an author only provides slopes, the hazard ratio can be easily calculated to ease interpretation. Also, note that regardless of which value the authors present, the associated p value will be identical. That is, a statistically significant slope will have a statistically significant hazard ratio, and vice versa.

Finally, no pseudo-R^2 exists for Cox regression. Although several have been suggested, they are not interpreted as the percentage of variance explained. That is, these values do not indicate how much of the overall reason why a participant experienced the event.[49] Thus, when reading a journal article, do not be discouraged by authors failing to provide this information.

Based on the breast cancer example, a statistically significant multivariate Cox regression analysis is presented below. Note that this will typically be presented in addition to the results of the Kaplan-Meier analysis.

No violation of the proportionality of hazards assumption was indicated (see Figure 8–16); thus, a Cox regression without time-dependent covariates was conducted to assess the effectiveness of a new hormone therapy compared to chemotherapy in preventing breast cancer recurrence after adjusting for age, concurrent medications, and comorbid conditions. Results indicated the covariates, as a set, significantly predicted time to breast cancer recurrence (χ^2_8 = 63.12, p < 0.05). Holding age, concurrent medications, and comorbid conditions constant, women initiating the new hormone therapy experienced a 48% decrease in the risk of breast cancer recurrence compared to women initiating chemotherapy.

The assumptions of Cox regression include:

1. Time is measured on an interval or ratio scale.
2. Sample size must be large.

    a. A basic rule is to have at least 50 participants per variable included in the model. This is required so that the parameters (e.g., slopes, standard errors) may be estimated accurately.[47] Thus, a model with 10 IVs and covariates requires at least 500 participants (i.e., 10*50 = 500).

3. Proportionality of hazards is assured.

    a. The survival functions for all categorical covariates must be similar.

4. No differences between withdrawn and remaining cases exist.

    a. Because Cox regression can handle censored (i.e., incomplete) data, those who are lost to follow-up must not differ from those whose outcome is known. That is, participants who dropped out of the study must not be different from those who completed it. For example, women who dropped out of the new hormone group because they were experiencing unbearable side effects that do not occur in the chemotherapy group.

5. Absence of multicollinearity is assured.

    a. That is, no Pearson's r between any continuous covariates should be greater than 0.90, as correlations this high indicate that the variables are redundant. High correlations indicate that the variables may be measuring the same facet. Including redundant variables will significantly bias results.

6. There are no outliers.

7. Observations are independent.

    a. That is, each participant provides one, and only one, observation (i.e., data or response) for each variable.

Case Study 8–3

Consider a health care resource utilization study to determine if the higher cost (in dollars) of nicardipine compared to other antihypertensive agents (e.g., labetalol, esmolol, fenoldopam) can be offset by the overall reduction in cost of the hospital stay for patients in the intensive care unit (ICU). The analysis statistically controlled for a number of confounding variables including age, gender, race, concomitant antihypertensive agents, inpatient complications, systolic and diastolic blood pressure, coronary artery disease, and diagnosis of a noncardiac event.

    Prior to analysis, the researchers identified severe positive skewness for hospital cost and moderate positive skewness for SBP. Further, moderate negative skewness was indicated for DBP. For the primary analysis, multiple linear regression analysis was conducted. Results indicated an omnibus F test of $F_{16, 286} = 14.22$, $p < 0.05$ with adjusted $R^2 = 0.146$. Further, the slope for the nicardipine group was -5.29, $p < 0.05$.

1. Is the multiple linear regression analysis appropriate to answer the research question? Why or why not?
2. Is a data transformation required for hospital cost? (Hint, see section on Data Transformations earlier.) If the hospital cost is not transformed, can the analysis be interpreted appropriately?
3. Is a data transformation required for systolic and diastolic blood pressure measures? If the variables are not transformed, can the analysis be interpreted appropriately?
4. Assume that the test statistics provided are correct. What does the omnibus F test indicate? Is the overall multiple regression model statistically significant?
5. Can the researcher interpret the slopes of the individual IV and covariates?
6. Assume the test statistics are correct. Interpret the adjusted R^2 value.
7. Assume that the test statistics are correct. With the group taking any other antihypertensive medication serving as the reference category, interpret the slope for the nicardipine group. Would you consider this statistically significant result clinically significant?

Conclusion

A thorough understanding of statistical methods is integral to effectively evaluating medical literature. Being cognizant of the effect study design has on results, interpretation, and generalization is incredibly important when implementing evidence-based practice. Statistical analyses are simply a piece of the puzzle when evaluating literature, since the design and research question determine the appropriate analyses. It must be noted that simply because a study is published this does not define it as a quality study. Further, all research has flaws, some trivial, others significant. A reader's task is to determine whether these flaws prevent the research from being credible.[50] Thus, when reviewing an empirical study, the following steps must be considered carefully:

1. Thoughtfully consider the study design (see Chapters 4 and 5). This includes, but is not limited to, the theory, specific research question(s), randomization, sample characteristics, data collection methods, variables, and outcomes. A poor design will lead to inaccurate or biased estimates, leading to an inferior study.
2. Evaluate the statistical test. Is it appropriate for the research question? Did the author test for assumption violations? If no assumption tests are stated, can

violations be determined from the descriptive statistics provided? Was the test interpreted properly? Were effect size (i.e., clinical significance) measures provided?

3. Evaluate the discussion section. Are the results interpreted within the context of the sample and population? Are generalizations accurate? What were the limitations? How does the study lend itself to future research?

Finally, this chapter is by no means exhaustive of all statistical tests, nor does it provide a complete overview of statistical tests. Interested readers are encouraged to consult any of the recommended readings below for a more thorough treatment of the topics discussed.

Self-Assessment Questions

1. You want to design a study to evaluate whether the effect on heart rate of a newly FDA-approved calcium channel blocker differs by an individual's race. You decide you want to assess two dosages of the medication in addition to placebo. What is the most appropriate method to achieve a representative and generalizable sample?
   a. Convenience sample
   b. Cluster sample
   c. Stratified random sample
   d. Multi-stage sample

2. What is the independent variable in the question above?
   a. The individual's race.
   b. Treatment group.
   c. Heart rate.
   d. There is no IV.

3. The definition of mutually exclusive groups is:
   a. The DV is not related to the IV.
   b. The data for a level of the IV is related to data in other levels of the IV.
   c. Participants and data in one level of the IV cannot be considered in another level of the IV.
   d. Participants are measured repeatedly on the same DV.

4. An example of a continuous variable is:
   a. Data measured on an interval level
   b. Years with diabetes diagnosis
   c. Age in months
   d. All of the above

5. The most appropriate measure(s) of central tendency for a positively skewed continuous variable is:
   a. The median
   b. The mean
   c. The mode
   d. The mean and median

6. The standard deviation is the appropriate measure of variability for a continuous variable when:
   a. It is appropriate in all situations with continuous variables.
   b. It is appropriate if the distribution is normally distributed.
   c. It is not appropriate for continuous variables.
   d. It is appropriate when a variable has been z-score standardized.

7. Z-score standardization normalizes a skewed distribution.
   a. True
   b. False

8. What is the difference between incidence and prevalence?
   a. Incidence quantifies the occurrence of an outcome with respect to time; prevalence quantifies the number of individuals who have already experienced the outcome.
   b. Prevalence quantifies the occurrence of an outcome with respect to time; incidence quantifies the number of individuals who have already experienced the outcome.
   c. Incidence is assessed with the binomial distribution; prevalence is assessed by the Poisson distribution.
   d. They are the same thing, they just use two words to confuse us.

9. The gold standard of research design is:
   a. A randomized control trial
   b. An experimental design with proper control of error variance
   c. An observational study
   d. Both a and b

10. The central limit theorem states:
    a. With degrees of freedom for error greater than 5, the distribution of sample means is normally distributed.
    b. The population distribution is always normal.
    c. With a sufficiently large sample (greater than 30) the distribution of sampling means is normally distributed as long as there are no outliers.
    d. The central limit theorem and law of large number is a lie.

11. Statistical significance at $p < 0.05$ indicates:
    a. The study will replicate 95% of the time.
    b. The probability of Type I error assuming the null hypothesis is true.
    c. The statistical test is significant, and reliably establishes the theory or hypothesis as true.
    d. The probability that the null hypothesis is true.

12. If the DV is measured on an ordinal scale, you will use which of the following to analyze the data:
    a. A nonparametric test
    b. A parametric test
    c. A parametric test if the ordinal scale contains enough rank-ordered values to be considered continuous
    d. Either a or c

13. How many *post hoc* tests are required following a statistically significant one-way ANOVA with 4 levels of the IV?
    a. 3
    b. 4
    c. 6
    d. 9

14. You are evaluating a study that used multivariate linear regression assessing the effect of age on prostate-specific antigen (PSA) doubling time (a continuous variable, measured in weeks) after controlling for race and comorbid conditions. The slope (i.e., regression coefficient) for age is 1.50. This slope indicates that
    a. The average PSA for all men in the sample is 1.50.
    b. Holding race and comorbid conditions constant, for every 1-unit increase in age, PSA doubling time increases 1.50 units.
    c. It does not matter, the analysis is inappropriate based on the scale of measurement for the DV.
    d. Age is a statistically significant predictor of PSA doubling time.

15. You are evaluating an observational study to assess the effect beta blocker therapy has on time to cardiac event in hemodialysis patients for a 5-year study period. The outcome variable is whether patients suffer a cardiac event, and the IV is whether they initiate beta blocker therapy or not. In addition, the analysis is statistically adjusted for several important covariates, which include age, gender, race, years with kidney failure, comorbid conditions, and concurrent medications. The authors conducted a multivariate logistic regression analysis. Was this the appropriate statistical test?

a. No. The authors should have conducted a multivariate Cox regression.

b. Yes. The multivariate logistic regression was correct.

c. No. The authors should have conducted a linear regression analysis.

d. No. Observational studies are never correlational in nature.

REFERENCES

1. United States Census Bureau [database on the Internet]. Census regions and divisions of the United States. [cited 2010 June 24] Available from: http://www.census.gov/geo/www/us_regdiv.pdf.

2. Stevens SS. On the theory of scales of measurement. Science. 1946;103(2684):677-80.

3. Hockenberry MJ, Wilson D. Wong's Essentials for Pediatric Nursing. 8th ed. St. Louis (MO): Mosby; 2009.

4. Tabachnick BG, Fidell LS. Using Multivariate Statistics. 5th ed. Boston (MA): Pearson Education Inc.; 2007.

5. Tukey JW. Exploratory Data Analysis. Reading (MA): Addison-Wesley; 1977.

6. McCaffery M, Beebe A. Pain: Clinical Manual for Nursing Practice. Baltimore (MD): V.V. Mosby Company; 1993.

7. DeCarlo LT. On the meaning and use of kurtosis. Psychol Methods. 1997;2(3):292-307.

8. Gordis L. Epidemiology. Philadelphia (PA): Saunders Elsevier; 2009.

9. Hennekens CH, Buring JE, Mayrent SL, editors. Epidemiology in Medicine. Philadelphia (PA): Lippincott, Williams, and Wilkins; 1987.

10. Friis RH. Epidemiology 101. Sudbury (MA): Jones and Bartlett Publishers; 2010.

11. Moore DS. The Basic Practice of Statistics. 2nd ed. New York (NY): W. H. Freeman and Company; 2000.

12. Tabachnick BG, Fidell LS. Experimental Design Using ANOVA. Belmont (CA): Duxbury Press; 2007.

13. Cohen J. Statistical Power Analysis for the Behavioral Sciences. 2nd ed. Hillsdale (NJ): Lawrence Erlbaum Associates Inc.; 1988.

14. Nickerson RS. Null hypothesis significance testing: A review of an old and continuing controversy. Psychol Methods. 2000;5(2):241-301.

15. Cumming G, Finch S. Inference by eye: confidence intervals and how to read pictures of data. Am Psychol. 2005;60(2):170-80.

16. Cumming G, Finch, S. A primer on the understanding, use, and calculation of confidence intervals that are based on central and noncentral distributions. Educ Psychol Meas. 2001;61(4):532-74.

17. Siegel S, Castellan NJ. Nonparametric Statistics for the Behavioral Sciences. 2nd ed. New York (NY): McGraw-Hill Inc.; 1988.

18. Sheskin DJ. Handbook of Parametric and Nonparametric Statistical Procedures. 3rd ed. Boca Raton (FL): CRC Press; 2000.

19. Feinstein AR. Epidemiologic analyses of causation: the unlearned scientific lessons of randomized trials. J Clin Epidemiol. 1989;42(6):481-89.

20. Ioannidis JP, Haidich AB, Pappa M, Pantazis N, Kokori SI, Tektonidou MG, et al. Comparison of evidence of treatment effects in randomized and nonrandomized studies. JAMA. 2001;286(7):821-30.

21. Campbell DT, Stanley JC. Experimental and Quasi-Experimental Designs for Research. Boston (MA): Houghton Mifflin Company; 1966.

22. United States National Institutes of Health [database on the Internet]. Understanding Clinical Trials. Available from: http://clinicaltrials.gov/ct2/info/understand#Q18. Accessed June 25, 2010.

23. Hopewell S, Dutton S, Yu L-M, Chan A-W, Altman DG. The quality of reports of randomized trials in 2000 and 2006: Comparative study of articles indexed in PubMed. BMJ. 2010;340(c723):1-8.

24. Everitt BS, Pickles A. Statistical Aspects of the Design and Analysis of Clinical Trials. 2nd ed. River Edge (NJ): Imperial College Press; 2004.

25. Chow S, Liu J. Design and Analysis of Clinical Trials: Concepts and Methodologies. 2nd ed. Hoboken (NJ): John Wiley & Sons; 2004.

26. International Conference on Harmonisation of Technical Requirements for Registration of Pharmaceuticals for Human Use (ICH) [database on the Internet]. Statistical Principles for Clinical Trials E9. [cited 2010 June 26]. Available from: http://www.ich.org/LOB/media/MEDIA485.pdf.

27. United States Department of Health and Human Services [database on the Internet]. Guidance for industry: Adaptive design clinical trials for drugs and biologics. [cited 2010 June 18]. Available from: http://www.fda.gov/downloads/Drugs/GuidanceComplianceRegulatoryInformation/Guidances/UCM201790.pdf.

28. Lachin JM. Statistical considerations in the intent-to-treat principle. Control Clin Trials. 2000;21(3):167-89.

29. Enders CK. A primer on the use of modern missing-data methods in psychosomatic medicine research. Psychosom Med. 2006;68(3):427-36.

30. Rubin DB. Inference and missing data. Biometrika. 1976;63(3):581-92.

31. Cochran WG. Some methods for strengthening the common χ^2 tests. Biometrics. 1954;10(4):417-51.

32. Cohen J. A coefficient of agreement for nominal scales. Educ Psychol Meas. 1960;20(1):37-46.

33. United States Centers for Disease Control and Prevention [database on the Internet]. National Health and Nutrition Examination Survey. [cited 2010 June 24]. Available from: http://www.cdc.gov/nchs/nhanes/nhanes2007-2008/lab07_08.htm.

34. Schober SE, Carroll MD, Lacher DA, Hirsch R. High serum total cholesterol—an indicator for monitoring cholesterol lowering efforts; U.S. adults, 2005–2006. NCHS data brief no. 2. Hyattsville (MD): National Center for Health Statistics; 2007.

35. Keppel G. Design and Analysis: A Researcher's Handbook. 3rd ed. Englewood Cliffs (NJ): Prentice Hall; 1991.

36. Hardy R, Kuh D, Langenberg C, Wadsworth ME. Birthweight, childhood social class, and change in adult blood pressure in the 1946 British birth cohort. Lancet. 2003;362(9391): 1178-83.

37. Williams JG, Allison C, Scott FJ, Bolton PF, Baron-Cohen S, Matthews FE, et al. The Childhood Autism Spectrum Test (CAST): Sex differences. J Autism Dev Disord. 2008;38:1731-9.

38. Skrabal MZ, Jones RM, Walters, RW, Nemire RE, Soltis DA, Kahaleh AA, et al. National volunteer preceptor survey of experiential student loads, quality of time issues, and compensation: differences in responses based on region, type of practice setting, and population density. J Pharm Prac. 2010;23(3):265-72.

39. Vickers AJ. How many repeated measures in repeated measure designs? Statistical issues for comparative trials. Br Med Res Methodology. 2003;3(22):1-9.

40. Beck AT, Steer RA, Brown GK. Manual for Beck Depression Inventory-II. San Antonio (TX): Psychological Corporation; 1996.

41. Jekel JF. Epidemiology, Biostatistics, and Preventative Medicine. 3rd ed. Philadelphia (PA): Asunders Elseiver; 2007.

42. Melnik T, Abdo CHN. Psychogenic erectile dysfunction: comparative study of three therapeutic approaches. J Sex Marital Ther. 2005;31(3);246-55.

43. Siebers RWL, Carter JM, Wakem PJ, Maling TJB. Interrelationship between platelet count, red cell count, white cell count and weight in men. Clin Lab Hematol. 1990;12(3);257-62.

44. Petrie A, Sabin C. Medical Statistics at a Glance. 2nd ed. Malden (MA): Blackwell Publishing Ltd.; 2005.

45. Need AG, Horowitz M, Morris HA, Nordin BEC. Vitamin D status: effects of parathyroid hormone and 1,25-dihydroxyvitamin D in post menopausal women. Am J Clin Nutr. 2000; 71(6):1577-81.

46. Sutherland WH, Walker RJ, Ball MJ, Stapley SA, Robertson MC. Oxidation of low density lipoproteins from patients with renal failure or renal transplants. Kidney Int. 1995;48(1):227-36.

47. Aldrich JH, Nelson FD. Linear Probability, Logit, and Probit models. Sage University Paper series on Quantitative Applications in the Social Sciences, series no. 07-045. Newbury Park (CA): Sage Publications, Inc.; 1984.

48. Kleinbaum DG, Klein M. Survival Analysis: A Self Learning Text. 2nd ed. New York (NY): Springer; 2005.

49. Allison PD. Survival Analysis using the SAS System: A Practical Guide. Cary (NC): SAS Institute Inc; 1995.

50. Simon SD. Is the randomized clinical trial the gold standard of research? J Androl. 2001;22(6):938-43.

SUGGESTED READINGS

The recommended readings below are for interested readers to gain further insight into some of the topics covered in this chapter. Note that most of the information provided in the Basic Concepts section can be obtained in any introductory statistics textbook, regardless of the specific field of study (e.g., medicine, psychology, business).

Epidemiological Statistics

1. Gordis L. Epidemiology. Philadelphia (PA): Saunders Elsevier; 2009.

Clinical Significance and Effect Size

1. Cohen J. Statistical Power Analysis for the Behavioral Sciences. 2nd ed. Hillsdale (NJ): Lawrence Erlbaum Associates Inc.; 1988.

Experimental and Nonexperimental Design

1. Campbell DT, Stanley JC. Experimental and Quasi-experimental Designs for Research. Boston (MA): Houghton Mifflin Co.; 1966.

Randomized Controlled Trials

1. Chow S, Liu J. Design and Analysis of Clinical Trials: Concepts and Methodologies. 2nd ed. Hoboken (NJ): John Wiley & Sons; 2004.

Nonparametric Statistical Tests

1. Siegel S, Castellan NJ. Nonparametric Statistics for the Behavioral Sciences. 2nd ed. New York (NY): McGraw-Hill, Inc; 1988.

ANOVA Designs

1. Keppel G. Design and Analysis: A Researcher's Handbook. 3rd ed. Englewood Cliffs (NJ): Prentice Hall; 1991.

Linear and Logistic Regression, Survival Analysis

1. Tabachnick BG, Fidell LS. Using Multivariate Statistics. 5th ed. Boston (MA): Pearson Education Inc.; 2007.
2. Stevens J. Applied Multivariate Statistics for the Social Sciences. 4th ed. Mahwah (NJ): Lawrence Erlbaum Associates, Inc.; 2002.
3. Cohen P, Cohen J, West SG, Aiken LS. Applied Multiple Regression/Correlation Analysis for the Behavioral Sciences. 3rd ed. Mahwah (NJ): Lawrence Erlbaum Associates Inc.; 2003.
4. Hosmer DW, Lemeshow S. Applied Logistic Regression. 2nd ed. New York (NY): John Wiley and Sons; 2000.
5. Kleinbaum DG, Klein M. Survival analysis: A Self-Learning Text. 2nd ed. New York (NY): Springer; 2005.

9

Chapter Nine

Professional Writing

Patrick M. Malone

Learning Objectives

● *After completing this chapter, the reader will be able to*

- State reasons both for and against writing professionally.
- Describe the various steps of professional writing.
- Identify the order for authors in a professional paper.
- Describe the importance of knowing the audience.
- Describe the various writing styles and their differences.
- Explain where to find a publication's requirements for submission.
- Describe what an article proposal consists of and why it is used.
- Explain the need to practice to develop good writing skills.
- List the components of both a research and review paper.
- Explain the general guidelines for writing.
- Describe the peer-review process.
- Explain the absolute importance of revision.
- Explain the steps in creating a newsletter or Web site.
- Describe how to prepare audiovisual materials for a poster or platform presentation and place those items on a Web site.
- Describe techniques for creating an abstract for an article.
- Describe how to correctly cite an article in a bibliography.

Key Concepts

① Essentially, anytime a professional takes pen, pencil, chalk, typewriter, word processor, or any other writing implement in hand to fulfill professional duties, it is considered professional writing.

② When writing, it is best to keep things as simple and direct as possible.

③ With the probable exception of policy and procedure documents, the two most important paragraphs in any document are the first and last.

④ If the information is taken from a particular source, even if it is reworded, the original author should be given credit via endnotes.

⑤ In many cases, revision of a document will be necessary.

⑥ Instead of concentrating on the technology, it is best to concentrate on the message.

⑦ Professional writing is a skill necessary for every pharmacist.

Introduction

A common thought when considering the topic of professional writing is "That doesn't apply to me, I'm not writing for a journal." But professional writing is certainly not limited to journal articles or books. It includes writing evaluations of medications for consideration on a hospital formulary, preparing written policies and procedures for the preparation of an intravenous admixture, reporting the results of the latest sale to the home office, preparing a written evaluation of a technician or clerk, writing in a chart, writing a term paper for a class, preparing slides or posters for presentation, and many other things. ① *Essentially any time a professional takes pen, pencil, chalk, typewriter, word processor, or any other writing implement in hand to fulfill professional duties, it is considered professional writing.* Although the format changes, the general principles remain the same. So whether the object is to write the ultimate book on the practice of pharmacy or to type a label, a pharmacist must know how to write professionally.

Although some may say the purpose of writing is to keep my job or to pass this course, there are, generally, four larger purposes for the existence of written material: that material serves to inform, instruct, persuade, or entertain. The first three items are those usually considered in professional writing, although including the fourth, whenever possible, will help convince people to read what has been written.

There are also some advantages to professional writing, besides those mentioned above. For example, writing is often good for promotion in many jobs. In academia, there is always the concept of publish or perish. Even pharmacy technicians are encouraged to write as a means of advancement.[1] Also, writing gives the authors the opportunity to share their knowledge or ideas,[2] obtain gratification or satisfaction,[3] and improve their knowledge. It may even lead to some fame or notoriety in a field.

Unfortunately, there are disadvantages to professional writing, too. The major problem is that any significant amount of writing often involves a lot of potentially frustrating work, because few people are natural writers. The author must practice to become proficient at writing, which will involve false starts, numerous drafts, roadblocks, and other problems.[4] If that is not enough, writing exposes a person to criticism and possible rejection. Although at one time authors were paid to publish articles, today it is not unheard of that authors may actually have to pay to have their article published.[5,6] At best, the direct financial rewards are likely to be few, unless a best-selling novel is produced. Indirectly, writing may lead to pay increases and promotions. However, because writing is a professional necessity, it can be made easier by following the correct procedures, which will be covered in this chapter.

Steps in Writing

As each of the steps in professional writing are covered in this section, the emphasis will be on writing items likely to be encountered in a practice setting, although additional steps that are necessary when writing for publication will be mentioned.

PREPARING TO WRITE

The first step in writing is to know the purpose—why something needs to be written in the first place. It is necessary at this time to have a good idea of the expected endpoint, which is important, no matter what is being done. For example, someone learning to plow a field with a tractor may be concentrating on the ground near the tractor and end up wandering all over the field, thinking he or she is going straight. However, by concentrating on going to a specific point on the far end of the field, rather than looking just in front of the tractor, the row will probably be plowed fairly straight. Throughout this whole process it is necessary to keep in mind that endpoint, to keep from wandering all over the place. If the item being written is for publication, rather than something required for work, it will also be necessary to pick the topic and, perhaps, submit an article proposal (Figure 9–1). Although the writing is considered to be more important than the idea, it is still important to have a good idea or important topic before starting.[7] It should also be pointed out that in the case of clinical trial results, it can be important to publish articles showing that something did not work, although in the past such topics have often been avoided.[8]

Although relatively few professionals write articles for journals or books, those who do need to follow an occasional step in addition to those outlined in the main text of this chapter. One difference is the potential need to write an article proposal to the publisher. This simply is a letter asking the publisher whether there would be any interest in possibly publishing something on a particular topic written by the person who is inquiring. As might be expected, this step is generally not necessary if writing a description of original research, but would be important when writing a review article or even a descriptive article. The letter should contain certain information, which will be described below, and be addressed to an appropriate editor. If at all possible, it is also a good idea to talk to an editor before submitting your proposal. For example, the proposal for the first edition of this book originated after a discussion with the editor at the Appleton & Lange booth in the ASHP Midyear Clinical Meeting Exhibitor's Area.

In the written proposal, the prospective author should first briefly explain the basic idea that is to be covered in the article or book, including a working title. Similarly, a description of the approach the author wishes to take in covering the subject should be described. Although this description should be kept brief, it must provide enough information for the publisher to determine whether the topic and approach are even appropriate for their journal, etc. In the case of a book, it is important to include a table of contents that is descriptive enough to be useful to reviewers who will be advising the publisher on the need for such a book. Related to that need, it is also necessary to describe why the proposed article or book will be important to the publisher's customers. This is the sales pitch. It is necessary to briefly show that there is nothing similar, or as good, currently available in the literature for the audience being addressed.

Although the above is the meat of the proposal, there are several other items that should be included. These include the time necessary to complete the article/book (be realistic), the approximate length of the work, and a statement of the authors' qualifications, including any previous publications. There are several good reasons for submitting a proposal. The first is simply to avoid work if the editor decides that there is no need for such a publication (although an author should not hesitate to send the proposal to another publisher, if it still seems that the topic is important). Second, and perhaps most important, it allows the editor(s) to make suggestions. By following those suggestions, an author is more likely to be successful in getting work published. Finally, if the idea is accepted, the acceptance letter will provide motivation.

Figure 9–1. Article proposal to publishers.

The topic should be of interest and/or importance to prospective readers. It can even cover an old topic, as long as the topic is covered in greater depth, in a new way, or is addressed to a different group.

It is also necessary to decide whether there needs to be a co-author. This may be easy to resolve, depending on who is working on the project. However, even if no one else has been involved, it may be a good idea to look for a co-author. An inexperienced writer would benefit from working with an experienced author, and working with someone will give a different perspective and, hopefully, lessen the work for each person. Finally, it is sometimes a necessity to include co-authors for political reasons (as in "Would you prefer to share the credit or work nights and holidays for the rest of your life?"). Although this last reason should not exist, it does. A variety of other problems with authorship credit are also seen.[9,10] The best that may be fought for under the circumstances may be that everyone must do part of the writing[11] and that authors be listed in the order of their contributions to the project. This does not always happen.[12,13] In some cases, pharmaceutical manufacturers may want ghost writers to write an article for the researchers, but even they agree that original authors must prepare the first draft of editorials or opinion pieces, although non–English speaking authors may be assisted by others after that.[14] The ghost writers should also be appropriately acknowledged.[8] Although arguments may be made,[15-21] there is no valid reason for people to be listed as an author in excess of their contribution to the writing and submission of the work for publication.[22-26] The only exception would be if the publisher has specific other rules. For example, some journals may want to list contributors with an explanation of what they contributed (e.g., writing, origination of study idea, data collection). Generally, all of the following must be met for an individual to be given credit as an author:[25]

- Conception and design of the study, or analysis and interpretation of the data in the study
- Writing or revising the article
- Final approval of the version that is published

Things that do not qualify a person to be listed as an author include:[24,25]

- Acquisition of funding
- General supervision of the research group

Individuals that do not meet the first qualifications should be listed in the acknowledgments section. Also, the primary author should be able to explain the order the authors are listed in, and journals may require one or more authors to be guarantors, who will be taking responsibility for the work as a whole.[26]

It should also be mentioned that there can be too many authors and acknowledgements.[27] Some scientific papers list many, many authors for a particular paper, and the number of authors has grown over the years.[28] It is obvious that 20 authors could not have written a 3-page paper. Some of this may be a result of job requirements that include publishing a certain number of articles, leading to demands by individuals to get their name listed on any article they can. Again, authors should contribute to the written work in some significant way, as defined above. In some cases it may be necessary to just name the group performing the research, with a few of the most responsible individuals specifically named, and to list others as acknowl-edgments, sometimes by group, institution, or type of contribution.[23,27,29] Others may be listed as clinical investigators, participating investigators, scientific advisors, data collectors, or other appropriate titles.[26]

Before the first word is written, it is necessary to know the audience, which involves knowing the type of person who will be reading the final document and where it will be published. Keep in mind that the word *published* was picked for a specific reason. Whether the final product appears in *New England Journal of Medicine,* the *IV Room Policy and Procedure Book,* or even the label on a prescription vial, it is published. It is necessary to aim the work at the audience. At a broad level, written work should not be submitted for possible publication in a journal that does not cover the topic; it is no more appropriate to submit an article on preparation of cardioplegic solutions to the *Journal of Urology* than it is to type a monthly fiscal report on prescription labels. So, be sure to review a journal and its Instructions for Authors before attempting to write an article for submission to that journal.[30]

More specifically, it is necessary to aim both the writing style and depth of informa-tion toward the audience. If something is written for physicians, it is not likely to be under-stood by lay people. Conversely, items written for lay people may not satisfy the needs of physicians. It is certainly appropriate to have a secondary audience in mind. For example, a report written for physicians may be of interest to pharmacists and nurses. However, make sure the secondary audience is not served at the expense of the primary audience.

In regard to writing style, there are three types normally used by pharmacists and other health care professionals: pure technical style, middle technical style, and popular technical style (Table 9–1).[31]

Pure technical style is used by business or technical professionals when they are writing for other professionals in the same or similar fields. For example, an article pub-lished in *American Journal of Health-Systems Pharmacy* would normally be written in this style. There are several characteristics of this style. First, the authors can use technical jargon, because they can expect the readers will understand it. Second, it is written in formal English. Third, it is written in the third person; words such as I, we, us, and you are eliminated. Finally, there is a general lack of slang or contractions. The great majority of writing done by pharmacists will be in this style, because it is usually other pharmacists who will be reading their work.

TABLE 9–1. TYPES OF TECHNICAL WRITING

Pure technical style—used by professionals addressing other professionals in the same field
Middle technical style—used by professionals addressing professionals in other fields
Popular technical style—used by professionals addressing lay people

Middle technical style is very closely related to pure technical style. This style is used by authors when they are writing for readers with a variety of technical backgrounds, with everyone having some unifying factor. For example, a report regarding a Pharmacy Department's quality assurance activities might be presented to the hospital's pharmacy and therapeutics committee. That committee is made up of physicians, nurses, hospital administrators, and other professionals. Although each has a background that makes their membership on the committee appropriate, not all of them would understand what a HEPA filter is, as would most hospital pharmacists. Therefore, it is necessary to better explain, or sometimes avoid, some technical areas. Otherwise, this writing style is very similar in most respects to pure technical style.

Finally, popular technical style is used in anything meant for the general public. Common language is used throughout. For example, a patient information sheet would need to be written in this style. A widely available example would be the articles on medical subjects that have appeared in *Reader's Digest* over the years. Information that is written in this style will use less complicated words and be less formal in its presentation.

It should be pointed out that usual technical writing differs greatly from what most people learn in high school English class or college composition courses. Although there is often a tendency to protest the formality of professional writing styles at first, the reality of the situation is that those styles must be followed for a piece of written material to be accepted.

The next step is to know the requirements of the publisher. Whether the work is for the department's policy and procedure manual or a journal, chances are that there is a format that needs to be followed. In the case of a journal, directions on the format to follow will be published at least once a year, usually in the first issue of the year. Also, specific guidelines are followed by a number of professional journals, both for general format and statistical reporting. Many journals have approved those guidelines and expect that all work submitted for publication will follow them. They are referred to as the "Uniform Requirements for Manuscripts Submitted to Biomedical Journals."[26] This standardization makes it easier on the prospective author; one style can be learned and followed, regardless of the journal. Other publications that can be helpful are *Scientific Style and Format: The CBE Manual for Authors, Editors, and Publishers* prepared by the Council of Biology Editors (CBE—now known as the Council of Science Editors, although the book uses the old name), *The American Medical Association Manual of Style, The MLA Style Manual*, and the *Publication Manual of the American Psychiatric Association*.

In the case of reports, policy and procedure manuals, and similar documents, it is best to see what has been done in the past. If this is the first time a particular item is being prepared, it is advisable to try to see what has been done in other places, and prepare something similar that meets the perceived needs. If writing something for work, do not be afraid to try to improve the format to make it more usable. However, be aware that it may be necessary to get any changes in format approved by the appropriate individual(s) or committee(s). Whenever possible, follow the Uniform Requirements[26] format used by the medical journals, because it is the standard for biomedical writing.

GENERAL RULES OF WRITING

Once the preparation is completed, it is time to start writing. Unfortunately, there is no easy way to learn how to write professionally; it just requires a lot of practice. However, a number of rules can be followed (Table 9–2). This section covers some of the general rules, with information on how to prepare specific items (e.g., introduction, body, conclusion, references, abstracts) being covered later. The first step is to organize the information before starting to write. At risk of sounding like a high school English teacher, it is still true that this step should include preparing an outline.[4] In the past, that was an onerous task that few performed. However, with modern word processing software, the outline actually becomes part of the finished product, so it does not amount to any significant extra work. Minimally the different sections should be listed to create some order to the layout of the work (remember, keep in mind the endpoint). Overall, the goal is to prepare a document that is clear, concise, complete, and correct. The two latter items depend, to a large part, on preparation. The former items, however, can be helped by following some simple rules.

The first two rules actually apply to the organization step. First, do sufficient research before getting started. Research in this regard, means obtaining whatever information— whether records, articles, performance evaluations, or anything else—necessary to

TABLE 9–2. CHECKLIST IN PREPARATION OF WRITTEN MATERIALS

Do research first
Put yourself in the reader's position
Use proper grammar and spelling
Make the document look professional
Keep things simple and direct
Keep the document short
Avoid abbreviations and acronyms
Avoid the first person (e.g., I, we, us)
Use active sentences
Avoid slash construction (e.g., he/she, him/her)
Avoid contractions
Cite other references wherever appropriate (and get permission to do so where appropriate)
Cover things in whatever order is easiest
Get everything down on paper before revising
Edit, Edit, Edit!

prepare the item. Although, it is likely that additional research will be necessary to fill in the fine points at some point in the process, most information should be gathered ahead of time. It is impossible to be organized if there is nothing collected, and a document that is not organized will generally not be worth much. The second rule is to put yourself in the reader's position. What does that reader want and how does he or she want it presented?

Although it should not need to be stated, it is very important to use proper spelling and grammar. This is easier than in the past, because word processing programs check both; however, it is still necessary to double check, because the computer is likely to overlook things. For example, a properly spelled, but incorrect, word will be missed (e.g., *two* instead of *to*, *trail* instead of *trial*, *ration* instead of *ratio*). Unfortunately for some writers, appearances count greatly. The writer may know more about a particular subject than anyone else, but if poor grammar and spelling permeate the document, it is unlikely that anyone will read or believe the information presented.[32] It will be dismissed as probably wrong, based on grammar and spelling alone. In a case where the finished product will be published in a language other than the writer's native language, the writer should have the work read and edited by someone for whom the language is the first language. It should also be mentioned that the writing should try to be entertaining. Although professional writing tends to be a bit dry, an attempt should be made to make it as enjoyable and easy to read as possible, although it is necessary to be cautious with humor and stay within limits of professionalism and good taste. It should also be unpretentious, direct, and accurate.[33]

Related to this, the document should look presentable. Some students are well known for turning in papers that are crumpled, creased, torn, dirty, or, at least prior to the common use of computers, practically dipped in correction fluid. That is not professional and must be avoided. Fortunately, that problem appears to been lessened with the use of word processors. The sad truth is that people will assume that if an author was sloppy with the appearance of the document, he or she was probably sloppy with the information. That may not be so, but that assumption will kill a good, but sloppy, document.

❷ *When writing it is best to keep things as simple and direct as possible.*[34-37] This has been referred to as the KISS (Keep It Simple, Stupid) principle. There is a temptation to use big words that sound impressive, but doing so is more likely to confuse than impress. Related to that, keep the paper as short as possible.[38] Also, consider whether tables, figures, or graphs would make the document simpler and easier to understand. This can be particularly useful with documents containing a great deal of data that may be organized through the use of tables.

When writing, avoid using abbreviations or acronyms. If it is necessary to do so, state the full form of the word or term the first time it is mentioned in the document, followed by the abbreviation in parenthesis (e.g., acquired immunodeficiency syndrome [AIDS]).

The only exceptions to this rule are units of measurement (e.g., mL, mg). Units of measurement should be expressed in the metric system. Clinical chemistry and hematologic measurements should be in terms of the International System of Units (SI). If a document is long, subheadings should be used. This can be part of the outline step, mentioned earlier.

- Several rules apply to the wording that is used in professional writing.[31] First, completely avoid writing in the first person, and avoid the second person wherever possible. It is not a bad idea, at least at first, to ask the word processor to find all occurrences of *I, we, us,* and *you.* If those words are found, try to rewrite the sentence to avoid them. Also, it is preferable to avoid using the passive voice throughout;[39] again, a grammar checker can help. Avoid both contractions and slash construction (i.e., *and/or, he/she* [use *he or she*], *this/that*). Finally, in this politically correct era, avoid sexism. That includes words like *he* or *she,* although it is not always appropriate or desirable to delete those terms. For example, using *he* in a case report of a patient with testicular cancer is quite appropriate. It is also inappropriate to use *their* instead of *his or her* to get around the problem.

- When writing, be sure to give credit where it is due. This just does not mean making sure the listed authors wrote part of the document. It includes endnoting all information obtained from one or a limited number of sources. If there is extensive quoting, permission to do so should be obtained by writing to the person or organization holding the copyright on the material. Endnoting was something everyone dreaded in the past. They waited until the end, because the articles should be cited in the order they appear in the document. By that time it was difficult to go back and do it. Now, however, this chore is much easier with word processors; it is possible to insert the citations as the document is prepared and let the software worry about making sure they are in the correct order.

- Related to the endnotes, everything that is stated should be supported by objective evidence. When writing a paper based on scientific literature, that evidence must be shown in the endnotes. To reemphasize, any unreferenced statement of fact is for all practical purposes worthless. However, it is necessary to make sure information is extracted from the original article and expressed properly. Some writers will improperly twist facts, whether inadvertently or not, to support their assertions.[40]

- Finally, work through the document in whatever order seems easiest.[4] In preparing a drug evaluation for a pharmacy and therapeutics committee, a stack of 50 articles might be used. At first, the stack may look like an impossible task, but after sorting the articles into groups that correspond to the sections, start with the shortest stack or the easiest information. By the time the document is finished, the writer may be surprised to find out that they were all fairly short, easy stacks.

- At first, a writer should simply try to make sure that all of the information is down on paper.[4] Once that occurs, go back and revise, and perhaps reorganize the document. Waiting a few days before revising the document can be very beneficial. After some time away from the project, errors practically jump off the page. It is also a good idea to have someone else who has not been involved with the writing read the document. Something that seems quite clear to the author may not actually be clear at all. Also, the author may be mentally inserting words or even sentences that were inadvertently omitted. Having someone edit the document can be humbling but helpful. Be sure to provide the product in a format that will make things easier for the person reviewing the document. A typed, double-spaced manuscript will make it easy to read and provide room for comments. Even better, send electronic versions of a document out for review directly from the word processor. The reviewer can put in comments or suggested wording changes electronically and then return the document. The writer can then go through the document making changes or simply accepting proposed changes with the click of a mouse. Often, the use of the electronic reviewing mechanism will be quicker, easier, and provide much clearer suggestions.

The three most important things in real estate may be location, location, location, but the three most important things in writing are edit, edit, edit. Also, remember editing includes paring out unnecessary words, sentences, and larger sections. It is not sufficient to settle for good enough—do your best. Look at it this way: the boss or editor is only going to do so much editing before giving up. The trick is to make sure that the document is well prepared and does not need that much editing.

SPECIFIC DOCUMENT SECTIONS

A typical document consists of three main parts—the introduction, body, and conclusion. In the case of a clinical study, it is recommended to follow the IMRAD structure, which divides a paper into Introduction, Methods, Results, and Discussion.[26] Other parts, such as references, tables, figures, and abstracts may also be necessary. These will be discussed in later sections and in the appendices of this chapter. It should also be noted that a number of the points in Chapters 5, 6, and 9 are applicable to writing of journal articles, as are the contents of the Web sites for the International Committee of Medical Journal Editors (http://www.icmje.org), Consolidated Standards of Reporting Trials (CONSORT) statement (contains checklist for contents of clinical trial) (http://www.consort-statement. org),[41-51] referred Reporting Items for Systemic Reviews and Meta-Analysis (PRISMA)[52,53] (http://www.prisma-statement.org), Conference on Guideline Standardization (COGS) standards (http://gem.med.yale.edu/cogs/), and the Good Publication Practice for Pharmaceutical Companies (http://www.gpp-guidelines.org), and should be considered along with this material. An example question layout is show in Appendix 9–1.

Introduction

❸ *With the probable exception of policy and procedure documents, the two most important paragraphs in any document are the first and last.* It is vital to start out strong, to encourage the reader to continue reading. Otherwise, the work will end up in that stack of articles all professionals have that they intend to read someday. That first paragraph should also inform readers of what they can expect in the rest of the document; it should be similar to a road map that shows what is to be accomplished in the document. The introduction should have a clear objective for the existence of the document. Many people neglect the need for a clear objective, which leaves the reader to flounder and wonder whether there really is a purpose to the document. In a research article, the introduction will also contain the hypothesis being investigated. In a policy and procedure document, it may simply be a description of what the remainder of the document will cover. The introduction should also contain background information about the topic that provides a good information base for the reader. The amount of background information has to be a balance—enough to show the reader that the writer has done an appropriate amount of research, but yet not so exhaustive as to bore or overwhelm the reader with unnecessary details.[54] Overall, the introduction should be short but contain properly referenced background material and show the reader where the document is headed.

The introduction should generally not be a conclusion; some people are so anxious to jump to the end that they put the conclusion first. Admittedly, the BLOT concept (bottom line on top) has its purpose in some documents (e.g., policy and procedures, formulary monographs), but that should be a conscious decision. If the introduction amounts to a conclusion, many people will read no further, making the remainder of the document a waste of time and paper.

Body

The body of the document contains all of the details. In a research article, the body may be divided into the methods, results, and, possibly, discussion sections, although the latter section may be incorporated into the conclusion. Details of what should be included are covered in Chapter 5. In other documents, the body will probably be divided into whatever sections are appropriate or logical. A number of rules can be followed in preparing the body of a document.

The first rule is that, while it is important to be concise, all necessary information must be presented. Again, keep an eye on the desired endpoint, and do not stray from the subject unless it is absolutely necessary. Including unnecessary information, even if it is interesting, will tend to confuse or obscure the important points. Also, be sure to provide a balanced coverage of the material and avoid unsupported bias.[8]

It is important to cover the information in a logical order, so that it flows easily from one point to another. A common mistake, when learning to write professionally, is to skip back and forth between subjects. For example, someone might insert a point about dosing in the middle of indications, when dosing is discussed at another point in the document.

Material that can identify patients should be left out of any work, unless it is absolutely necessary to include. If that is not possible, informed consent must be obtained,[26] and pertinent legal procedures must be followed (see Chapter 10). The authors should also disclose any approval of the study by institutional review boards and their following of other rules related to protection of study subjects (both human and animal).[26]

Writers should also put the information in their words. Perhaps out of lack of confidence, a number of professionals are tempted to simply quote other authors word for word. However, by presenting the information in their own words, writers demonstrate that they actually understand the topic. ❹ *Remember, though, that if the information is taken from a particular source, even if it is reworded, the original author should be given credit via endnotes.*

It is necessary to expand on the topic discussed in the previous paragraph, because there seems to be much confusion about it, and there are many cases where the rules against copyright infringement and plagiarism are broken. Plagiarism can be considered the copying of another's words or ideas, without properly giving credit. Copyright violations consist of copying another's work, even with appropriate quotations and citation, without permission. They are similar; however, it is possible to commit either plagiarism or copyright violations without committing the other. It appears that plagiarism is becoming more frequent and many people do not understand that it is wrong to copy work without proper attribution, even something from a source written by many anonymous people (e.g., Wikipedia).[55]

Sometimes those infractions are rather blatant, such as the cases documented in the newspapers about students downloading papers from the Internet and presenting them as their own or simply retyping a previously published article (an attempt to prevent this can be seen on the Internet at http://www.plagiarism.com, http://www.plagiarism.org, or http://www.turnitin.com).[56,57] Interestingly, although there might be suspicions that this is more prevalent with online classes, a study found that it was more likely to occur with traditional campus students.[58] Other times, the infringement is quite accidental. For example, it was once brought to the attention of the famous science fiction writer, Isaac Asimov, that a short story he wrote was similar to an article that had been published 10 years previously.[59] Dr. Asimov went back and found the article and read it, realizing as he did so that he had read it when it first came out and had forgotten about it. When he wrote his story 10 years later, he did not at all realize that portions of it could be considered plagiarism. Although he had no intention of infringing upon the other author's work, Dr. Asimov made sure that the story was never reprinted and even wrote an article discussing the problem. This shows how easy it is to inadvertently cross the line into copyright infringement or plagiarism, and there are many examples that would fall in between the extremes given above.[60] Therefore, it is necessary for the author to be on guard and to try to prevent the problem in the first place. A few general rules can act as a guide.

- When copying wording directly from another's work, it should be in quotations (or otherwise shown to be a quote), and a citation should appear to give credit to the original author(s). Also, if a significant amount of a work published in the last 100 years is quoted, it is probably necessary to get permission from the copyright holder, which may require paying a fee.[61] Exactly what is a significant amount is debatable; however, it would be best to err on the side of asking for permission if a quotation is more than a few sentences. Reproducing an entire chart, table, figure, and so on should normally require asking for permission. A letter to the copyright holder will solve problems; publishers often also have forms to request permission. Some special cases need to be mentioned. First, U.S. government documents are not copyrighted, so only quotation marks and citations are necessary. Second, if it is impossible to locate a copyright holder (e.g., the publisher went out of business without transferring copyrights), the writer should at least be able to document a thorough effort to obtain permission. Finally, there are special legal requirements for use of copyrighted materials in online education, covered in the Technology, Education and Copyright Harmonization (TEACH) Act. Further information on this can be found in Chapter 10.

- Extensive quotations should be avoided. After all, if writers cannot put something in their own words, do they truly understand the material? In any writing, there really is very little reason to provide quotations. Authors should try to put things in their own words whenever possible.

- Paraphrased information should have the original publication(s) cited, if it comes from one or a limited number of sources.

- Extensive paraphrasing, particularly without citations, may be considered plagiarism (i.e., copying the ideas of others).

- When citing an article, cite the one that the material comes from. If the material came from a review article, cite that article, not the original study that was not consulted. It is worth mentioning that in the case of unusual information, reading and citing the original study is preferable to just using a review article, because the review may be inaccurate.

- Be sure to follow publishers' rules or licenses, which may be stricter and may not allow any reproduction of material.

- Remember that it is necessary to always cite others work, even on slides.[62]

In preparing certain documents (written answers to questions, for example), there may be very little information available. Perhaps only one or two research articles will have been written on the topic. If so, it will often be desirable to summarize the articles in detail, including most of the information presented in an abstract (see

Appendix 9–2). In general, the information presented will summarize how many and what type of patients (i.e., inclusion and exclusion criteria), the drug or procedure being investigated, the results (e.g., efficacy, adverse effects), and the author's conclusions. It is also important to point out any noticeable flaws in the paper. An example would be:

> Smith and Jones performed a double-blind, randomized comparison of the effects of drug X and drug Y in patients with tsutsugamushi fever. Patients were required to be between 18 and 70 years old, and could not have any concurrent infection or disorder that would affect the immune response to the disease (e.g., neutropenia, AIDS). Twenty patients received 10 mg of drug X, three times a day for 15 days. Eighteen patients received 250 mg of drug Y, twice a day for 10 days. The two groups were comparable, except that the patients receiving drug X were an average of 5 years younger ($p < 0.05$). Drug X was shown to produce a cure, both in terms of symptoms and cultures in 85% of patients, whereas drug Y only produced a cure in 55.5% of patients. The difference was statistically significant ($p < 0.01$). No significant adverse effects were seen in either group. Although it appears that drug X was the better agent, it should be noted that drug Y was given in its minimally effective dose, and may have performed better in a somewhat higher or longer regimen.

A list of material to be covered in a review of an article similar to that above is found in Table 9–3.

TABLE 9–3. ITEMS TO INCLUDE IN WRITTEN REVIEW OF A JOURNAL ARTICLE

Items to Include	Examples
Main author of article and a reference number	Johnson et al.[2] Smith and associates[24]
Type of article	Clinical study, case report, case series, review, meeting abstract
Research design (if appropriate)	Blinding, randomization, experience report, descriptive report
Purpose of the report	
Description of group studied	Size of groups, age, sex, disease state(s), other pertinent demographic characteristics
Any important confounding factors	Smoking, age, general health
Description of treatment being studied	Drug, dose, administration route, dosing interval, treatment duration
What was measured as an indicator of effect	
Results	Efficacy, adverse effects
Author conclusions	
Strengths and weaknesses of the study	See Chapters 4 and 5

Conclusion

● A conclusion should be placed at the end of the body of the document, except for certain documents (e.g., policy and procedures). This conclusion should follow logically from the information presented and should serve to summarize that information. Remember, the conclusion should also correspond with the objective stated in the introduction.[63] It is also worth noting that in clinical consultations, a common mistake is to write the conclusion in a general manner, rather than addressing the specific patient in question, which is what the reader wants to hear about. The author must remember to address the specific patient's situation.

Many writers are tempted to avoid formulating a conclusion. Various reasons include not feeling qualified to make a conclusion for the reader, not wanting to restate what has already been stated, laziness, and so on. This is improper. The readers need something to bring their thoughts together at the end, and the author is in the perfect position to provide this closure. However, the author should also be careful to avoid extrapolating beyond the information available.

Other Items

If items are endnoted, the references should be found following the conclusion (see Appendix 9–3 for more information on how to prepare a bibliography). Use of bibliographic software, such as Reference Manager (ISI ResearchSoft, Carlsbad, CA, http://www.refman.com), ProCite (ISI ResearchSoft, Carlsbad, CA, http://www.procite.com), or EndNote (ISI ResearchSoft, Carlsbad, CA, http://www.endnote.com) can be helpful in this process.[14] Other items may also be necessary, depending on the document, such as tables, graphs, figures, and so forth. They will not be dealt with here, other than to say that those items should supplement or clarify (not distort or misrepresent), and not duplicate material in the text portion of a piece of written work. Also, it is worth mentioning that many computer programs make the preparation of professional quality graphs and figures easy and often allow embedding the artwork in the word processing document itself, when allowed by the circumstances.

SUBMISSION OF THE DOCUMENT

● Once the document is completed, proofread, and edited, it is ready to be submitted, whether to a boss or a journal. In the latter case, you will need to include a cover letter that serves as an introduction to the document. In the former case, it will be possible to be less formal. Also, it should be noted that when submitting an item to a journal it may be necessary to include transfer of copyright forms, conflict of interest disclosures (including financial)[11,64-66] or other items, which will be found in the directions for authors for that journal (usually found in the first issue of each year and on the publication's Web site). The conflict of interest may be reported by the publisher in the final publication, but that is variable.[67] In addition, be sure to precisely follow the journal's Instructions for Authors to improve chances for acceptance.[68] It is also worth a word of warning that articles should very rarely, if ever, be submitted to more than one journal at the same time (note: prior publication of an abstract does not mean that submission of a full article is duplication and publication in a second language is often considered acceptable).[8,11,69] If duplicate submission is felt to be appropriate and/or necessary, the rules outlined in the Uniform Requirements must be followed.[26] Also, the article should not be broken down into many small articles and submitted over time, unless submission as a whole would result in a publication that would be too long or complex.[70]

REVISION

⑤ *In many cases, revision of the document will be necessary.* This may be due to a difference in opinion or different perception of need. Although author should never change a document to say something they believe is wrong, minor revisions are often necessary to improve clarity or make the document more appropriate in some other manner. The comments given with the request for revision are likely to be helpful,[71] and they should be taken seriously. Even if it is felt that the person who read and commented on the paper is wrong, all concerns should be addressed. If a comment is truly wrong, it may still indicate that the work was not clear in a particular area and needs some other appropriate revision to clarify the material. Changes should be made, based on the comments and completed within the time limits necessary.

Sometimes, however, a document may be rejected entirely. This can be for any of the following reasons:[31]

- The document is not up to standards (too much work for the boss or editor to correct).
- The idea or research the document is based on is too weak.
- The idea is inappropriate for that forum of publication.
- A similar article has been recently prepared (and possibly published) by someone else in that forum.

In the case of the first item, major revisions would be necessary before resubmitting to the boss or a journal. The second reason may also prompt major revisions, or even cause an author to stop working on the document. An article submitted to a journal but rejected for the last two reasons is not necessarily bad. It may be possible to submit it to another journal after only minor changes.

GALLEY PROOFS

A term well known to authors who have published articles or books is galley (or page) proofs. This is a copy of the final article, as it is to appear when published. It is the responsibility of the author(s) to carefully check to make sure there have been no mistakes made in typesetting. Although it may seem like a lot of work, everything must be checked, including the references, which frequently contain errors.[72-77] This step is necessary to prevent problems later. Although documents ready for the copy machine at work are generally not referred to as galley proofs, it is still necessary to carefully check those items.

Referees

Although this term is more familiar to sports fans, referees (also referred to as reviewers) are used in writing. These are the individuals to whom journals send submitted articles for review and comment. This is also referred to as the peer-review process. On a local level, reviewers are the people that a writer may ask to look at a report before the boss gets it. Whatever arena, whether local or international, a person should also be willing to be a reviewer at that level. To be a reviewer for a journal, a person usually can simply write a letter stating interests, qualifications, and experience to the editor of the journal, and ask to be considered for the journal's reviewer list. If the person has adequate credentials, the journal will usually be happy to have that person as a reviewer.

Anyone who is a reviewer should be up front about such things as lack of expertise, conflict of interest,[66] or inability to complete a review within a reasonable time, and should be willing to step aside as a reviewer of a particular paper if those are problems.[78] Also, reviewers should treat anything submitted to them as a confidential document.

It should be pointed out that people who act as a reviewer for a paper should follow the procedures discussed in Chapters 4 and 5. Specific directions will also be received from the editor and may involve preparing comments for both the editor (to discuss matters, such as ethics, with the editor alone) and for the author (this latter document is also used by the editor). It may be required that the latter be signed or unsigned. Also, as with any quality assurance procedure, the reviewer should treat it as an opportunity to provide constructive, as opposed to destructive, criticism.[79] Finally, for those who are reviewers for journals, it is recommended to get new people involved in the process, such as residents or new practitioners, so that they can learn how to be a reviewer.[80]

It is beyond the scope of this chapter, but if further information is needed on being an editor of a biomedical journal, the reader should consult the Web site of the World Association of Medical Editors, http://www.wame.org.

Case Study 9–1

Your boss comes to you and lets you know that you are assigned to write a new policy and procedure for a product that is to be added to the formulary, but which requires specific safety precautions when administered to patients (e.g., premedication of the patient, availability of resuscitation equipment, unusual preparation for administration). This is to be available for approval at the next pharmacy and therapeutics committee meeting.

1. What are your first steps?
2. You have progressed to the point where you have the material gathered to prepare your policy and procedure. What should be done at this stage?
3. Once the document is written, what needs to be done next?

Specific Documents

NEWSLETTERS AND WEB SITES

Newsletters have been considered to be a part of any pharmacy practice, but have probably been encountered most frequently in hospitals as a method for communicating pharmacy and therapeutics committee actions and other drug-related topics to the medical, pharmacy, nursing, and other health care provider staffs. Newsletters have also been seen from community pharmacies[81,82] (addressed to patients and/or physicians), nursing homes, drug companies, pharmacy organizations, and government or regulatory bodies. Wherever newsletters are found, their reason for existence is likely to be one or more of the following reasons: to communicate information to a target group, advertisement, and/or compliance with legal/accreditation standards.

In many cases, newsletters are now replaced by a Web site. Such sites can serve the same purposes, but can also have some specific advantages and disadvantages. For example, Web sites require very little effort for distribution, because all they take is a computer on the Internet, which can actually be provided by an Internet service provider (ISP) for a few dollars a month. Also, the material can take a greater variety of forms, including audio and video. The Web site can actually be used to sell products, including prescriptions. Within institutions, the material can be kept available for health care providers to review for an indefinite time period, thereby preventing problems when somebody wants another copy of some old article or when the nurses are trying to make sure they have all of the publications for an accreditation visit. As for disadvantages, it must be noted that consulting a Web site does take more effort, because it does not just fall into people's hands when they open their mailboxes. Also, some people do not use the Internet and would, therefore, not be able to consult the site.

Whatever the reason for setting up a newsletter or Web site, the same set of steps generally apply to their preparation.[83-87] These steps will be covered individually in the remainder of this section.

Define the Audience

Who will be, or at least should be, reading the newsletter or accessing the Web site? It may be physicians, pharmacists, nurses, other health care professionals, the lay public, other groups, or some combination of these. The target group(s) will have an effect on decisions made in the other steps.

Define the Goals of the Newsletter

The goal can be any of the reasons mentioned previously, but generally includes informing and educating the reader, and also to report news (including changes in policies and procedures, laws, etc.). With Web sites, the goal can also be to directly sell products or gather information.

Identify Constraints

No matter what kind of newsletter or Web site is produced, there are always going to be constraints that will limit what it can contain and how good it will be. One of the first constraints is time. It seems as though every year people are busier and have less time to do things that they want or need to do. This includes preparing a newsletter or keeping up a Web site (must be done continuously), which can take a significant amount of time if it is done right. It will be necessary to have time to write, type, edit, typeset, and perform other functions in publishing the newsletter—and all of those things have to be done in time to get the finished result to the printer, so that it can be ready for distribution on time. With a Web site, it is necessary to write the material, figure out the layout or organization, and prepare it on the computer. It is generally best, when beginning publication of a newsletter, to have it come out at longer intervals. If the newsletter is well received and it is found that there is enough time and sufficient material, publication frequency can be increased. Overall, it is better to find it necessary to speed up publication frequency, rather than spread it out (people might get the idea the newsletter has ceased publication).

- Another constraint is the people that will be involved with publishing the newsletter or Web site, particularly the editor-in-chief and/or webmaster. This is a case where the phrase, "many hands make light work" may be applicable. If a group of dependable people are willing to work together to make sure the articles get written, the job may be easier. Generally, there are two extremely hard parts to publishing a newsletter or Web site, neither of which is the actual writing. One of them is coming up with topic ideas; the other is to make it look good. If others are at least willing to help here, it can be a great aid to the editor of the newsletter. If at all possible, people from all groups served by the newsletter should be asked for topics, if not entire articles. If a pharmacist is in charge of the newsletter or Web site, some other possible places for help include an institution's public relations department, if available, and clerical help (to do the typing, formatting, copying, distribution, etc.). Keep an eye on the time necessary for pharmacy staff to produce the newsletter or Web site, because this is likely to be the most costly item.

- The third constraint is financial. "There is no such thing as a free lunch." This also applies to newsletters and Web sites. There is always some cost involved. Although personnel costs are likely to be the largest expense, the computer equipment and printing or duplication charges (for newsletters) can be significant. If the printing is to be done by an outside agency it is best to check on such items as the effect of order size (number of copies) and type of paper (e.g., plain versus glossy, 8½ × 11 versus 11 × 17 versus A4, colors), stapling or binding on the cost. It is preferable to get bids from at least three printers. Another item to consider is method of delivery (e.g., personal versus first-class mail versus second-class mail). All of these items add up and, depending on the budget, it may be necessary to sell advertising space to cover the costs.

- Finally, it is necessary to look at what equipment is available. If at all possible, the use of a high-end word processing program or desktop publishing program with a laser or inkjet printer will allow production of a high-quality, professional newsletter quicker and at a lower cost. This equipment may be all that is necessary for a Web site, assuming that the computer has some type of Internet connection. Although a number of Web programs are now available for little cost, and are the preferable solution, many times it is possible to just use a word processor or Web browser to create and maintain the Web site.

Newsletter/Web site Design

For children of the 1960s, it was easy during and shortly after college to believe substance was more important than appearance. For older and (hopefully!) wiser (or at least more cynical) people, it now is noticeable that many people do not bother looking at the substance if the appearance is poor or unprofessional. Therefore, one of the most important things is to make the publication look appealing.[88,89] People tend to throw away newsletters that look sloppy or unprofessional, and do not bother with Web sites that are not exciting, easy to use, and neat. Even if the publication looks good, it may[90-92] or may not[93,94] have any impact on physicians; but without looking professional it is highly unlikely to even have a chance.

A few general rules can help to make a newsletter or Web site more appealing. These will be covered in the remainder of this section. However, for a more in-depth look at this subject, the reader is directed to references specializing in the subject.[95,96] A particularly detailed book is available on the Internet at http://www.usability.gov/guidelines/.

- One of the first rules is to keep the publication consistent. This means not only from month to month, but also from page to page. This does not mean that improvements cannot be made from time to time. Nor does it mean that each page has to look exactly like the previous one. Instead, it means that it should have its own style that is recognizable by the reader, and that the various pages must fit with one another. The easiest way to do this, with either a newsletter or Web site, is to create a template, style sheet, or theme (these terms overlap somewhat). Many pieces of software make this possible for either type of publication. A *template* is a file that contains material that appears the same from issue to issue—the term is often associated with a newsletter. Examples of this can be the newsletter's masthead (first page heading), the listing of editors, footers at the bottom of each page, number of columns, and so on. A *theme* should be similar to a template, but may be used more frequently when discussing a Web site. *Style sheets* are a definition of how specific paragraphs or other parts of the newsletter or Web sites will look (they would often be incorporated into the template or theme). For example, a style might be called "Heading 1," and by using this style for each article's title, the look remains the same from page to page, and issue to issue. This style can include such items as what the font looks like (e.g., typeface, font size, bold, italic, underlined, superscript, subscript, etc.), and what the paragraph looks like (e.g., left justified, right justified, centered, line spacing, space before or after, etc.), in addition to other items (e.g., whether the section is to be located in a particular part of the page, borders, etc.). A style manual should be established or at least a commercially available style manual, such as the *American Medical Association Manual of Style,* should be used. Whatever the editor(s) establish should be reasonably simple and elegant (i.e., do not get carried away—a couple of different fonts on a page are fine, but 10 fonts look terrible). In the case of Web sites, it might be useful to consult the publication *Elements of E-text Style,* which is available at http://www.cets.sfasu.edu/PastPort/Introduction/e-StyleSheet.htm.

- A second rule is to use appropriate software and equipment. A high-end word processor or desktop publishing program and a laser printer can be used to produce the master copy of the newsletter for reproduction.[97,98] This can allow a pharmacy to turn out a product that looks typeset at a fraction of the cost. As mentioned, there are a variety of low (or no) cost Web site software tools. Some are specific, whereas others are incorporated into word processors, Web browsers, or other software. Also, just using a text editor is possible, although that tends to be much more difficult.

●   A third rule is to make the newsletter or Web site look good. For example, use white space properly. Do not just crowd in as much material as possible on the page. The reader will have a hard time following if the text is too crowded, and may just give up. Layout is really a difficult problem, and requires at least a little artistic ability to do well. If lack of artistic ability is a problem, it is probably a good idea to look over other newsletters or Web sites from various sources to try to come up with ideas concerning what looks good. Minimally, most newsletters should at least be set up in two columns to allow easier reading. Other, more artistic, items to consider are asymmetrical layout (not having the two sides of each page look the same from a distance, perhaps using a narrow column for graphics or titles along one edge), different column widths, teasers (statements taken from the text that may pique the curiosity of the reader enough to read the article), surrounding boxes and columns with rules, and artwork/graphics.[99] The programs used to prepare either newsletters or Web sites can also have samples that can be used to prepare a professional-looking end product.

●   Next on the list for newsletters is to design a masthead. The masthead is essentially the part of the first page of the newsletter that gives the name of the publication, volume, issue, date, and so on. This may be at the top of the page or down one side of the first page. It is a good idea to consider having this done professionally, because it is a one-time expense and can be a major factor in the appearance of the newsletter. Sometimes it is good to have a multicolored masthead that is preprinted on blank stock paper. The newsletter text can then just be photocopied onto the paper and look much more professional. Material to be put into the masthead, or at least be included somewhere in the newsletter includes the newsletter name (be descriptive, but do not get cute—remember this is a professional newsletter), name and address of the pharmacy/organization, names of editor and editorial staff (give credit or blame where it is due), and frequency of publication. The name of the publication, along with some way of identifying the issue and page, should be placed on every page of the newsletter, so that the source of information can be identified if the page is photocopied or torn out.

●   Much of the material in a masthead should also be contained on the home page, if not every page, of a Web site. Again, getting professional design help, at least at first, may be of value. Also, following the guidelines of the Health on the Net Foundation Code of Conduct, http://www.hon.ch/HONcode/Conduct.html, in designing the web page is appropriate.

In general, software themes available will help create a professional-looking site, if professional help is not available. However, some specific items that need to be considered for a Web site include[100,101]:

- Provide information that is good, credible, timely, and original. Share everything possible.
- Custom tailor information to take into account user preferences.
- Break up tables for readability.
- Use graphics effectively, but sparingly (they may take too long to download, annoying the reader). Graphics should be no more than 20 kilobytes in size, if at all possible. In any case, they should be as small as possible.
- Related to the previous item, optimize the other aspects of the page to improve download times.
- Make the page easy to read—good contrast between the text and background, not too busy.
- Use self-generating content—make the site interactive.
- Web pages should be well organized—both the pages by themselves and how the pages are interconnected on the site.
- Consider selling things, if appropriate.
- Make sure everything works, from all likely browsers.

In designing the newsletter or Web site, effort should also be placed in deciding on a name. A local or institutional newsletter will often have a name related to the organization and the purpose of the newsletter. A Web site may be similarly named, but there is an opportunity to go farther. In this case, the Uniform Resource Locator (URL) should be considered. This is the address of the Web site on the intranet and/or the Internet. An institution may already have a registered URL, and the pharmacy web page may simply be under that name (e.g., http://www.yourorganizationname.org/pharmacy). However, independent community pharmacies can also register an unused name on the Internet and have that address (e.g., http://www.johnspharmacy.com).

It is necessary to make a very specific decision on how the newsletter is to be printed. While typesetting still produces the best-looking newsletter, it is quite easy to get a good-looking final product using a good photocopy machine. Also, even if the pharmacy produces the original copy on its computer, the file can be taken to a service bureau that can essentially produce a typeset copy. It is necessary to determine the paper to be used (do not use glossy paper if photocopying). Most newsletters are $8\frac{1}{2} \times 11$ in in size, but that does not mean the paper is that size. It is better to use 11×17 paper for multipage newsletters and just fold the sheets. That looks much better than simply stapling the corner. Also, it is possible to take a CD-ROM with the newsletter file on it to some professional printers for them to print good-looking final copies.

Newsletter/Web Page Content

Before getting into items that a newsletter or Web site should or can contain, it is necessary to discuss some general rules that deal with any article.[102]

First, it is a good idea to have a number of short articles, rather than one long article.[89,103] People will take a look at a short article and mentally decide they have the time to read it, whereas a long article may be dismissed immediately ("If I'm going to read something that long, it will be out of *New England Journal of Medicine!*") or put aside to read when I have time. (Does house dust actually come from publications on the bottom of that read-someday pile as they disintegrate from old age?) As a matter of fact, some recommend that newsletters should not exceed two pages (one sheet, front and back),[102] and one hospital cut their newsletter to one page (for P&T News) and replaced the remaining articles with a page to fit into a Drug Therapy Pocket Guide that consisted of useful tables (e.g., sodium content and neutralizing capacity of different antacids).[104] Related to the above, use catchy titles to draw the reader into reading the article right then.

Use proper writing techniques, as described earlier in this chapter. Be clear, concise, and complete—do not waste the reader's valuable time. Also, be unbiased—support the article with facts. Be positive—talk about 90% compliance, rather than 10% noncompliance.

Finally, be sure the newsletter or Web site is properly edited. Have multiple people read and edit the newsletter or Web pages before publication. Having more people read it makes it more likely that simple mistakes will be noticed and corrected. In particular, the editors should check for spelling, grammar, and readability. Also, it is a good idea to have people from each target group as editors, particularly physicians.[105]

The actual content of a newsletter or Web site is one of the two most difficult areas for the editor that were mentioned in the Identify Constraints section (the other being that the newsletter should look good). Coming up with new ideas on a regular basis can be rather difficult. A list of possible areas to cover are included in Table 9–4. If at all possible, material that was prepared for a different audience can be recycled for the newsletter or Web site readers. For example, material from the pharmacy and therapeutics committee meeting might be turned into a short review of a drug. Whenever possible, the material presented should be topics that are not available to the audience from another source, or material that is prepared in a format that will be of greater value to the readers than that same topic area as presented by other publications. Whatever the topics used, it is a good idea to survey readers on a regular basis to make sure their needs are being met.

Newsletter Distribution

All of the above work will be for nothing if the readers do not get the newsletter. A good distribution system must be developed. Sometimes it can be as simple as sticking the newsletters in individual mailboxes, setting out piles of newsletters, or using interorganizational mail systems. If it is necessary to use the post office, it would be a good idea to check on the possibility of second class or bulk mail, which can save money. Newer innovative

TABLE 9–4. NEWSLETTER OR WEB SITE TOPICS

Adherence
Adverse drug reactions
Calendar of events
Clinical pearls
Compliance
Effects of external events on jobs
Job-related information
New information sources
New legal or regulatory requirements
New services
News from other departments
Organization's stand on issues
Patient safety
Personnel policies
Pharmacoeconomics
Pharmacogenomics
Pharmacy and therapeutics committee actions and news (major area to be covered)
Productivity improvement
Professional announcements
Review of drugs/drug classes
Quality assurance

Data from references 83,84,89, and 102.

distribution methods are by electronic mail[106] or other computerized methods.[107] Community pharmacies may also distribute their newsletters by providing copies to physician waiting rooms or noncompeting businesses (e.g., banks, barber shops, beauty shops, daycare centers), or even including them with monthly statements.[82] Whatever method used, it is important to make sure the readers actually get the newsletter. Also, make sure they get the newsletters on a regular cycle, so that they know when to anticipate the arrival of the publication.

Case Study 9–2

Your boss comes and lets you know that you are in charge of a new Web site for your pharmacy/pharmacy department.

1. What are the first steps to do?

PRESENTATIONS

A pharmacist may have the opportunity to give a formal presentation at some point in a career. This could be simply where the pharmacist works or at a national meeting. Although it is well known that fear of public speaking is extremely common, a speaker who prepares should do well. The problem may simply be fear of the unknown. Having some simple directions may be of immense help. Overall, the main concern should be to know the topic. If someone knows enough to be asked to talk, chances are that person will know quite a bit about a topic, or will be able to learn enough about the topic. Alternately, the potential presenter may volunteer to give a presentation on an interesting topic or one in which the person has done a lot of work (e.g., a new method to practice or a new practice area). After that, most of the concern will deal with looking good. This includes a variety of items, many of which involve professional writing, and will be dealt with in the remainder of this section.

In cases where a person is asking to speak, a proposal will need to be submitted. This describes the proposed topic, which should be of interest to the target audience. The directions given by the organization preparing the meeting will need to be followed. Beyond that, the skills described earlier in this chapter or appendices will need to be used.

Next, it may be necessary to write an abstract that the organization providing the presentation forum will use to inform potential attendees about the presentation. Each organization may have a format to be followed in creating the abstract, which should be followed. As to what should appear in the abstract, the writer might use the information presented in Appendix 9–2. Admittedly, an abstract should usually be prepared after the presentation is done to best reflect what was said. However, abstracts may be requested more than 6 months before the presentation, so in this case it will serve more as a planning document. Actually, it is probably best to create a brief outline of the presentation (at least the topics to be covered) and then write the abstract.

Along with the abstract, it may be necessary to prepare learning objectives to describe what the attendee will be able to do as a result of participating in the program. The objectives should state these goals in objective, measurable terms. For example, an objective may state that the attendee can explain, list, or identify something. It will not say that the attendee knows, understands, or learns, because those are not measurable. The objectives should relate directly to the program and should be adequately broken down to cover the different areas of the presentation. Refer to the beginning of any of the chapters of this book for examples of objectives. Also, refer to *Bloom's Taxonomy of Educational Objectives and Appropriate Verbs* for more details.[108] Also, this information could be used for objectives written for other documents.[109]

Occasionally, the presenter may be requested to provide self-assessment questions. Often these will be multiple-choice or true/false, to simplify assessment. Those questions should be clearly stated and measure whether the attendee has met the objective. Efforts should be made to make the questions clear. Also, they should avoid the use of not or except, because these terms can lead to confusion. Writing good questions can be extremely difficult, so testing the questions out on others before the presentation may help improve the quality.

The speaker may also have to prepare a brief biography to be used in the introduction. This includes a few items about the speaker's background, such as title and current position. Also, some information that gives the audience an idea of why that speaker is qualified to make a presentation is useful.

Presentations can usually be broken down into platform or poster presentations. The former is a more formal, oral presentation that typically requires some sort of audiovisual component and is often presented in a room set up for an audience. The latter requires the presenter to place a summary of the material to be presented on a poster (or series of small posters) that will be displayed on a bulletin board-type display (usually provided by the organization) that will be 3 to 4 ft high and 6 to 8 ft wide. In that situation, the attendees can walk through a group of such presentations, stopping to look at any that appeal to them and ask the presenter questions.

Many of the rules described in the main part of this chapter relate to preparing the information to be presented, including slides, posters, and other audiovisual materials. However, a few other rules need to be mentioned.

- The presenter should learn the circumstances under which the presentation is to be given. That includes whether it is a platform or poster presentation.
- The presenter should learn what equipment is to be provided (e.g., computer projector, microphone, size of poster presentation).
- If the presenter needs other items, they should be made clear to the organization. For example, it is common for presenters to want to use computer slide projection equipment, which may present certain technical requirements for both the equipment and support people. Also, the presenter may need such things as power outlet strips, extension cords, wireless microphones (many good speakers prefer to move about on the stage or in the audience and are frustrated by a podium microphone that requires them to stand in one place behind a podium), Internet connection, connections from a computer to the room sound system, BlueTooth, USB connection, CD-ROM, videotape player, cables, audience response systems, and other items. The presenter's own needs and desires should be taken into account, in addition to those of the audience. It is necessary to be very specific, since the people organizing the meeting may not understand the requirements. For example, a speaker requesting an Internet connection may arrive to find a connection that is too slow or one that has

security restrictions preventing access to necessary Internet sites. Also, even the resolution of a computer projector or type of connector for a network may need to be specified.

- If the speaker is doing a poster presentation, it is necessary to remember to bring pushpins to mount the poster on the provided display board.
- The audience should be taken into account. One common complaint when speakers fly in for a presentation is that they may not know anything about local circumstances, including simple social skills that are expected (e.g., foreign countries). It is best if the speaker tries to find out more about the audience and the situation, adjusting the presentation to take those items into account.[110]
- If necessary, the setup of the room should be specified (e.g., theater-style, discussion tables, screen placement).

All of the above should be double-checked at the location of the presentation after arrival, but in plenty of time to correct any problems. Speakers may also want to take advantage of a Speaker Ready Room that many organizations offer to check out slides, and so on. As a side note, checking in with those arranging the presentation is necessary so that they will not be worried about your arrival and they will be able to clear up any last-minute items.

The speaker then needs to prepare the presentation, doing appropriate research and preparation, using skills described earlier in this chapter and in the following sections. The presentation should also be rehearsed adequately. The next steps will discuss preparation of audiovisual materials, which can help the audience understand and retain the material.[111,112]

Platform Presentations

When giving platform presentations it is usually necessary to prepare audiovisual materials and, possibly, handouts. This was once rather difficult and expensive. Often a graphic artist would be necessary to prepare good-looking slides. Presenters might have settled for slides prepared by a drug company or may have tried to type and photograph simple slides. In some cases, simple handwritten overhead projector transparencies would be used. However, the availability of presentation programs has made the preparation of professional-quality audiovisual materials a much easier task. There really is no good excuse any longer to have less than professional-looking slides because of these programs. Overhead slides should only be used to allow recording of items during a discussion; there is little, if any, reason to use them in a formal presentation.

Most office software suites (e.g., Microsoft Office, Google Docs) have very powerful tools to create slides and other materials. These also have professionally designed templates that provide good layouts for materials, including color and background choices. The programs may also guide the user to follow general rules, such as avoiding a busy slide that will be unreadable from the back of a large room.[113] Also, the programs can be used to do everything from creating simple slides to multimedia extravaganzas—the former being learned in a few minutes, with the more advanced features available for those who need or desire them. Be aware, however, that it is necessary to use only those features that truly add to the presentation and to avoid having fancy effects in slides just for the sake of the effects.[113] ⑥ *Instead of concentrating on the technology, it is best to concentrate on the message.*[114] That will also have the advantage of having fewer things that might go wrong in a presentation.

When starting to prepare audiovisuals, it is necessary to determine what type of equipment and situation will be available at the presentation. The most desirable type of audiovisual is the use of a computer with a projector and appropriate software to give the presentation. It is also possible to project slides from a personal digital assistant (PDA) or smartphone that is properly equipped,[115] although the presentation will likely be unable to use any advanced features, such as the embedding of multimedia items.[116] The use of computers equipped with presentation software poses various advantages, including lower cost for the presenter, the ability to make last-minute changes to slides before the presentation, the ability to include audio and video in the presentation slides, and the capability to embed Internet links into the presentation. When information or software is available on the network or the Internet, it can be demonstrated. Also, in cases where a discussion ensues, it is possible for the presenter to use a word processor, presentation program, or other software to record items on the screen for users to read during or after the session. It is even possible, using a Web creation program (e.g., Microsoft FrontPage) or specific presentation programs (e.g., Elluminate) to not only record the information on the screen during the presentation, but to also make it immediately available on the Internet at the end of the program. Some disadvantages include the cost of the equipment for the organizing group, the need for greater technical skills by both the presenter and organizing group, the potential for technological problems (e.g., a computer that refuses to boot, a corrupted data disk, an Internet connection that does not work), and it may be necessary for the presenter to bring a notebook computer with appropriate software and data. Fortunately, the technical support people for professional meetings are familiar with the equipment, and the equipment itself is often more dependable.

When preparing the slides themselves, the presenter will have to prepare an outline to guide what is to be presented and determine the information to be presented in each slide. Some general rules can be mentioned.

- Limit each slide to a particular topic. Sometimes this will be an overview, but specifics should be limited to a discrete topic. One or two minutes of presentation material per slide is appropriate. If it is necessary to refer back to a previous slide, just make a duplicate that is inserted at the appropriate location.

- Keep things simple. The program may be able to do many things (e.g., 20 fonts in 16 million colors), but they may not be desirable. Typically use one font (perhaps with bold or underline in a few specific places for emphasis) and limited graphics.
- Limit the amount of information presented on each slide.[113] A rule of thumb is no more than about five bulleted points per slide and no more than about five words per bulleted point. Any more than that quickly becomes confusing or unreadable. Generally, if someone in the back of the room has to squint or it takes more than 10 seconds to take in a slide, there is too much information on it.[117] It has been theorized that a portion of the blame for the loss of the space shuttle, *Columbia*, was due to the information necessary for NASA engineers being hidden in small print on an extremely busy slide.[118] While the consequences for most presentations are not nearly as large, it is still important that slides enhance the provision of the appropriate information, rather than obscure it.
- Consider using a theme in the program that will provide colors that go together well and contrast enough to be legible. Colors and color combinations have to be carefully considered, because they may have emotional overtones or, in cases of color-blind attendees, may not even be distinguishable.[119]
- Consider graphics. They can make the slide more pleasing to the eye, but they also need to be as simple as possible. If cartoons are included to entertain the audience, make sure they are related to the talk and, preferably, help to make a point. Also, pictures of landscapes or the presenter's institution may be desired by the presenter, but serve only to distract from the presentation and should be avoided. Also, remember that if copyrighted material is to be used, it is necessary to get permission to reproduce the material.
- Consider embedding sound or video in the presentation, if it adds to the presentation. That sounds difficult, but may be done with a few clicks of the mouse.
- Embed links to appropriate Web sites in the presentation.
- Save the presentation several ways. Even if it is on the computer hard drive, it may become corrupted or the computer can break. Perhaps also bring it on a USB drive, so that someone else's computer can be borrowed if necessary. It is often useful to consider burning the presentation to a recordable (or read/write) CD-ROM or DVD, which will not be sensitive to magnetic fields that might have affected the original disk. Also, in case the computer to be used in the presentation does not have presentation software, it might be necessary to use the feature in many presentation software packages that creates a run-time presentation that does not require the actual software. In some cases, putting the slides on a Web server in presentation format may work, although accessing the slides and Web pages over the Internet can be a risky proposition. Also, as mentioned previously, the presentation might be given using a PDA/smartphone device.

Other items to consider include the following:

- Make sure to carry the presentation materials personally and do not check them as luggage, since they may be lost. Also, be careful not to damage the materials being carried.
- Make the presentation interactive—ask the audience questions and take input. This is now a requirement of continuing education programs.
- In all but a very small room, be sure to use the microphone. Speakers may not want to be bothered or may feel it is a sign of weakness to use a microphone, but they need to remember that the microphone is there to help the audience, not the speaker, and should be used so that everyone in the back of the room can hear over the ventilation system, etc.
- Keep to the slides, if at all possible, but do not read the slides—use the slides as a jumping point to the oral presentation information and to organize your thoughts.[113]
- Do not read a prepared script. Actors and politicians can read such scripts and sound natural, but most speakers cannot. Instead use the slides (preferable) or a simple outline. The presentation program will allow easy preparation of handouts and speakers notes that can be used.
- Consider the delivery of the material, including pitch, power, pace, poise, and confidence.[120]
- Be prepared for technological disaster.[113] Even when using something as simple as a projector, the bulb can burn out. When using more equipment and more complex equipment, the potential for equipment failure rapidly increases. Whenever possible, have backup equipment, but also have a backup plan so that the presentation can proceed without any equipment

It may be desirable to prepare a handout for the audience, in which case, the presenter can consider the following styles:[121]

- *Outlines*—A reference document that gives the audience a guide to where the speaker is going in text form. This can often be prepared by importing the slide content from the presentation software to a word processor. Some presentation programs will also prepare the document itself.
- *Full-text handouts*—This is essentially a transcription of the speech. While helpful as a reference document, it is probably of more use to politicians when they wish to avoid being misquoted. This is seldom seen in pharmacy presentations, because the presenter will not be able to make last-minute changes, and the audience will likely read ahead and become bored. Interestingly, a comment heard when such documents are presented is that the speaker did not know the material, because all the person did was read the handout, even though the speaker was the one who wrote it!

- *Slide reproductions*—This is becoming more popular and easy; presentation pro-grams allow easy slide handout preparation. This does give the attendee all of the information, including graphics, but will likely require more paper.
- *Partial text handouts*—This can be something of a combination of the above, where only a portion of the talk is on the handouts.

In any of the above, it is good to consider the following:[121]

- Consider whether it is necessary to provide references or supplemental read-ings.
- Make sure the handout follows the order of the presentation. If it does not, the attendee may become confused and annoyed.
- Make it look good, using skills mentioned elsewhere in this chapter. By all means, allow plenty of room for the attendee to take notes.

The speaker may also use the handout as a set of speaker notes, but care should generally be taken to avoid just reading the handout to the audience, except in the case of full-text handouts, for the reasons previously mentioned.

The skills necessary to give the presentation itself are beyond the scope of this chapter, deals with the preparation and distribution of written material. New presenters may wish to read a book or pamphlet on how to give effective talks. Also, Toastmasters International (http://www.toastmasters.org) is a group that will help individuals develop their speaking skills. Many organizations have a chapter of this organization. These aids will provide guid-ance on such skills as what level of sophistication to use in speaking, how to stand (e.g., do not hide behind the podium, making eye contact), what language to use, how to use humor and other techniques to entertain the audience, how to address questions (including so-called sniper questions that tend to disrupt speakers due to level of difficulty and how they are thrown into the middle of the presentation),[122] how to avoid distractions by having every-one turn off phones and pagers,[123] and so forth. Also, some of the references used in prepa-ration of this chapter provide many additional suggestions.[111,121]

Case Study 9–3

You are preparing a platform presentation for the American Society of Health-System Pharmacists Midyear Clinical Meeting for the first time.

1. What are some things that should be considered in slide preparation?

Poster Presentations

Preparing a poster requires the presenter to first determine what is to be included. Typically, the information will be similar to that found in an abstract, but with an expansion of the various sections. There are likely to be tables, bulleted points, and figures. Overall, the information to be presented must be brief, so that it can be read within a couple of minutes by an individual passing by the display. Therefore, large amounts of text are undesirable. A poster presentation will not likely contain nearly as much information as a formal journal article, but will contain many of the same sections. It will serve as a place for discussion to begin between the presenter and interested individuals.

Preparing posters was at one time a very difficult prospect. This has changed with the availability of presentation and high-end word processing/publishing software on computers. It is now possible to upload materials to Web sites on the Internet and have a very professional, color poster arrive in the mail within a few days.

Some people prefer to use essentially the same presentation programs as would be used for slides. The individual slides, which may be longer than could possibly fit on a typical 2×2 slide, will then be printed on a color printer and mounted on poster board. An assortment of these slides will then be pinned to the board provided at the meeting. This is easy to do, but does require carrying and mounting many individual pieces. Also, it tends to limit the size of items on the presentation and may not lend itself to allowing the most professional-looking presentation. A final disadvantage is that any one-page handout will have to be prepared separately.

Another possibility is the preparation of a large, one-piece poster that is typically about 3×6 feet. Although the final poster must be printed by a graphics firm (e.g., printer, architectural drawing firm), the cost can be reasonable for a very good-looking poster. As mentioned previously, this may be done over the Internet. The initial preparatory work can also be done by such firms, but it is less expensive to do this yourself. The software necessary would be either desktop publishing software (e.g., Adobe PageMaker, Microsoft Publisher) or a high-end word processor (e.g., Microsoft Word). Essentially, what needs to be done is to lay out the page in these programs so that it is in landscape format (i.e., sideways from the normal typed page). The top of the page will have a centered title in large print, with the author names, institution, city, and so on, centered in a smaller font below the title. Often, it is desirable to place graphics to one or both sides of that information, such as the symbol for the authors' institution(s). Under that, the page may be divided up into three or so columns and the information laid out in a logical order, including tables and figures. It may be desirable, once finished, to print out the final copy. One can produce a copy that fits on typical $8\frac{1}{2} \times 11$ in paper that can be reproduced and distributed to interested individuals at the meeting. It may also be on larger paper (e.g., 11×17 in), if there is a suitable high-quality printer available.

Whatever method is used, the final product will need to be transported to the meeting (poster tubes are available for little or no cost from many graphics firms). It is preferable to carry such posters on airplanes, because they may be crushed in the baggage areas. The presenter should also remember to bring pushpins to mount the presentation at the meeting. The presenter should show up early enough for the presentation to have the material mounted to the bulletin board before meeting attendees are allowed in the area, and presenters will be expected to remain with the presentation to answer questions for the assigned time. Although many people may be the authors of a presentation, it is not uncommon that only one or two actually attend the meeting and give the presentation.

Web Posting

After a presentation, consider making the material available on the Internet. Some organizations are now making at least some presentation materials available that way. Of course, copyright restrictions may prevent individuals from posting the material, but technology makes it easy when it is allowable. Text documents, such as posters, are easily placed on a Web site. However, even full slide presentations can be placed on a Web site, using streaming audiovisual. A variety of software can be used to prepare such streaming presentations that can include slides and an audiovisual recording of the presenter. This can even be done concurrently with the presentation (live streaming), with a recording being made for later viewing. The equipment needs are relatively minor (i.e., modern computer, presentation software, microphone, inexpensive computer video capture device). For the actual Internet streaming, the appropriate streaming software, running on a file server, is necessary. For those who do not have the appropriate streaming software, just placing the slides themselves, as a downloadable file or in presentation format, can be an easy process using the original software used to prepare the slides. Even the simplest Web site can then be used to give access to the material.

Conclusion

➐ *Professional writing is a skill necessary for every pharmacist. It simply consists of following the accepted rules for writing that have been established by the profession to prepare a written item that is clear, concise, complete, correct, and in the appropriate format.*

Self-Assessment Questions

1. Which of the following items are considered to be a type of professional writing?
   a. An article published in *American Journal of Health-System Pharmacy*
   b. A budget report
   c. A label for a prescription vial
   d. A performance evaluation of a new pharmacy technician
   e. All of the above

2. Which of the following is considered to be adequate for credit as an author?
   a. Acquisition of funding for the study
   b. Conception and design of the study
   c. Provision of equipment used in the study
   d. Supervision of the research group
   e. All of the above

3. When writing a document that is intended for an audience of physicians, pharmacists, nurses, and other health care practitioners, which style of writing should be employed?
   a. Pure technical style
   b. Middle technical style
   c. Popular technical style

4. Which guideline tends to be used the most in writing for medical and pharmacy journals?
   a. *American Medical Association Manual of Style*
   b. *MLA Handbook for Writers of Research Papers*
   c. *Publication Manual of the American Psychiatric Association* (APA)
   d. *Scientific Style and Format: The CBE Manual for Authors, Editors, and Publishers*
   e. *Uniform Requirements for Manuscripts Submitted to Biomedical Journals*

5. It is necessary to only define unusual abbreviations in a document, since nearly every reader will understand common abbreviations, such as the use of AIDS for acquired immunodeficiency syndrome.
   a. True
   b. False

6. When writing a document, it is not necessary to provide a citation to a source like Wikipedia, since that only contains information that is considered to be common knowledge.
   a. True
   b. False

7. In most cases, when writing up an answer to a question for another health care practitioner, the first paragraph of the paper should contain the summary of the information contained in the body to make things simpler and faster to read.
   a. True
   b. False

8. Copyright violations and plagiarism are not the same. It is possible to commit one while avoiding the other.

a. True
b. False

9. Health on the Net Foundation provides what?
   a. A code of conduct for Web sites
   b. A web hosting site for medically related Web sites
   c. General drug information references
   d. b and c
   e. All of the above

10. Which of the following is an appropriate objective for a presentation? The attendee will:
    a. Explain the steps for preparation of the intravenous form of drug X.
    b. Know the steps for preparation of the intravenous form of drug X.
    c. Learn the steps for preparation of the intravenous form of drug X.
    d. Understand the steps for preparation of the intravenous form of drug X.
    e. None of the above are appropriate.

11. When preparing slides for presentations, it is best to provide as many details on each slide as possible, even if the font has to be smaller than normal.
    a. True
    b. False

12. You are going to provide a 1-hour CE presentation. How many slides should you likely be preparing?
    a. 10
    b. 50
    c. 100
    d. 150

13. Which of the following is true when giving a presentation?
    a. It is best to avoid the use of a microphone, if possible, since most people do not know how to use them for the best effect and they are just another technology that may fail. Most of the time speaker can just raise their voice so that everyone can hear.
    b. Microphones are placed in a room for the convenience of the audience, not the presenter. If there is a microphone present, the speaker should always use it.

14. Presentation handouts should:
    a. Follow the order of the presentation.
    b. Provide the full text of the speech.
    c. Supplement, but not replace the presentation.

    d. a and c.

    e. All of the above.

15. It is necessary to always send an article proposal to a publisher, prior to sending in an article.

    a. True

    b. False

REFERENCES

1. Thordsen DJ. Preparing an article for publication. J Pharm Technol. 1986; Nov/Dec:268-75.
2. Generali JA. Why publish? Hosp Pharm. 2008;43(11):868.
3. Moghadam RG. Scientific writing: a career for pharmacists. Am J Health-Syst Pharm. 2003 Sept 15;60:1899-1900.
4. Armbruster DL. Starting the writing process. J Pediatr Pharmacol Ther. 2003;8(3):210-1.
5. Fye WB. Medical authorship: traditions, trends, and tribulations. Ann Intern Med. 1990; 113:317-25.
6. Gannon F. Ethical profits from publishing. EMBO Rep. 2004;5(1):1.
7. Nahata MC. Publishing by pharmacists. DICP Ann Pharmacother. 1989;23:809-10.
8. Wager E, Field EA, Grossman L. Good publication practice for pharmaceutical companies. Curr Med Res Opin. 2003;19(3):149-54.
9. Wilcox LJ. Authorship. The coin of the realm, the source of complaints. JAMA. 1998; 280:216-7.
10. Hoen WP, Walvoort HC, Overbeke AJPM. What are the factors determining authorship and the order of the authors' names? A study among authors of the Nederlands. Tijdschrift voor Geneeskunde (Dutch Journal of Medicine). 1998;280:217-8.
11. Committee on Publication Ethics (COPE). Guidelines on good publication practice. Cope Report. 2002:48-52.
12. Shapiro DW, Wenger NS, Shapiro MF. The contributions of authors to multiauthored bio-medical research papers. JAMA. 1994;271:438-42.
13. Flanagin A, Carey LA, Fontanarosa PB, Phillips SG, Pace BP, Lundberg GD, et al. Prevalence of articles with honorary authors and ghost authors in peer-reviewed medical journals. JAMA. 1998;280:222-4.
14. Wager E. Raising the quality of publications: now we have GPP! Qual Assur J. 2003;7:166-70.
15. Peterson AM, Lowenthal W, Veatch RM. Authorship on a manuscript intended for publication. Am J Hosp Pharm. 1993;50:2082-5.
16. Carbone PP. On authorship and acknowledgments. NEJM. 1992;326;1084.
17. Hart RG. On authorship and acknowledgments. NEJM. 1992;326;1084.
18. Pinching AJ. On authorship and acknowledgments. NEJM. 1992;326;1084-5.
19. Canter D. On authorship and acknowledgments. NEJM. 1992;326;1085.
20. Rennie D, Yank V, Emanuel L. When authorship fails. A proposal to make contributors accountable. JAMA. 1997;278:579-85.

21. Fathalla MF, VanLook PFA. On authorship and acknowledgments. NEJM. 1992;326;1085.
22. The International Committee of Medical Journal Editors. Statement from the International Committee of Medical Journal Editors. JAMA. 1991;265:2697-8.
23. Hasegawa GR. Spurious authorship. Am J Hosp Pharm. 1993;50:2063.
24. Rennie D, Flanagin A. Authorship! Authorship! Guests, ghosts, grafters, and the two-sided coin. JAMA. 1994;271:469-71.
25. International Committee of Medical Journal Editors. Uniform requirements for manuscripts submitted to biomedical journals. Med Educ. 1999;33:66-78.
26. International Committee of Medical Journal Editors. Uniform requirements for manuscripts submitted to biomedical journals: writing and editing for biomedical publication [Internet]. Philadelphia (PA): International Committee of Medical Journal Editors. 2009 Nov. [cited 2010 Nov 16]. Available from: http://www.icmje.org/index.html/.
27. Kassirer JP, Angell M. On authorship and acknowledgments.NEJM. 1991;325:1510-2.
28. Drenth JPH. Multiple authorship. The contribution of senior authors. JAMA. 1998;280: 219-21.
29. Kassirer JP, Angell M. On authorship and acknowledgments. NEJM. 1992;326;1085.
30. Foote MA. How to write a better manuscript. Drug Inf J. 2009;43:111-4.
31. McConnell CR. From idea to print: writing and publishing a journal article. Health Care Supervisor. 1984;2:78-94.
32. Burnakis TG. Advice on submitting papers. Am J Hosp Pharm. 1993;50:2523.
33. Higa GM. Scientific publications and scientific style. W V Med J. 1995;91:198-9.
34. Crichton M. Medical obfuscation: structure and function. NEJM. 1975;293:1257-9.
35. Jones DEH. Last word. Omni. 1980;2(12):130.
36. Hamilton CW. How to write effective business letters: scribing information for pharmacists. Hosp Pharm. 1993;28:1095-100.
37. Albert T. The fear of writing—it's not as hard as pharmacists seem to think. Pharmaceut J. 2003 Jan 11;270:55-6.
38. Baker SJ. Getting published. Aust J Hosp Pharm. 1994;24(5):410-5.
39. Hamilton CW. How to write and publish scientific papers: scribing information for pharmacists. Am J Hosp Pharm. 1992;49:2477-84.
40. Ingelfinger FJ. Seduction by citation. NEJM. 1976;295:1075-6.
41. Moher D, Schulz KF, Altman D. The CONSORT statement: revised recommendations for improving the quality of reports of parallel-group randomized trials. JAMA. 2001;285: 1987-91.
42. Moher D, Hopewell S, Schulz KF, Montori V, Gøtzsche PC, Devereaux PJ, et al. CONSORT 2010 explanation and elaboration: updated guidelines for reporting parallel group randomized trials. BMJ. 2010;340:c869doi: 10.1136/bmj.c869.
43. Campbell MK, Elbourne DR, Altman DG for the CONSORT Group. CONSORT statement: extension to cluster randomized trials. BMJ. 2004;328:702-8.
44. Piaggio G, Elbourne DR, Altman DG, Pocock SJ, Evans SJW for the CONSORT Group. Reporting of noninferiority and equivalence randomized trials. An extension of the CONSORT Statement. JAMA. 2006;295:1152-60.

45. Gagnier JJ, Boon H, Rochon P, Moher D, Barnes J, Bombardier C for the CONSORT Group. Reporting randomized, controlled trials of herbal interventions: an elaborated CONSORT Statement. Ann Intern Med. 2006;144:364-7.

46. Boutron I, Moher D, Altman DG, Schulz KF, Ravaud P for the CONSORT Group. Methods and processes of the CONSORT Group: example of an extension for trials assessing non-pharmacologic treatments. Ann Intern Med. 2008;148:W-60-W-66.

47. Ioannidis JPA, Evans SJW, Gøtzsche PC, O'Neill RT, Altman DG, Schulz K, et al. Better reporting of harms in randomized trials: an extension of the CONSORT Statement. Ann Intern Med. 2004;141:781-8.

48. Hopewell S, Clarke M, Moher D, Wager E, Middleton P, Altman DG, et al. CONSORT for reporting randomized controlled trials and conference abstracts: explanation and elaboration. PLoS Med. 2008;5(1): e20. Doi:10.1371/journal.pmed.0050020.

49. von Elm E, Altman DG, Egger M, Pocock SJ, Gøtzsche PC, Vandenbroucke JP for the STROBE Initiative. The Strengthening the Reporting of Observational Studies in Epidemiology (STROBE) Statement: guidelines for reporting observational studies. Ann Intern Med. 2007;147:573-7.

50. Vandenbroucke JP, von Elm E, Altman DG, Gøtzsche PC, Mulrow CD, Pocock SJ, et al. Strengthening the Reporting of Observational Studies in Epidemiology (STROBE): explanation and elaboration. Ann Intern Med. 2007;147:W-163-W-194.

51. Zwarenstein M, Treweek S, Gagnier JJ, Altman DG, Tunis S, Haynes B, et al. Improving the reporting of pragmatic trials: an extension of the CONSORT Statement. BMJ. 2008;227:a2390 doi: 10.1136/bmj.a2390.

52. Moher D, Cook DJ, Eastwood S, Olkin I, Rennie D, Stroup DF. Improving the quality of reports of meta-analyses of randomised controlled trials: the QUOROM statement. Lancet. 1999;354:1896-900.

53. Moher D, Liberati A, Tetzlaff J, Altman DG. The PRISMA Group (2009) preferred reporting items for systematic reviews and meta-analyses. The PRISMA Statement. PLoS Med. 2009;6(7):e1000097. Doi:10.1371/journal.pmed.1000097.

54. Talley CR. Perspective in journal publishing. Am J Hosp Pharm. 1993;50:451.

55. Gabriel T. Plagiarism lines blur for students in digital age. New York Times. 2010 Aug 1 [cited 2010 Aug 2]:[4 p.]. Available from: http://www.nytimes.com/2010/08/02/education/02cheat.html?_r=1&scp=1&sq=plagiarism%20lines%20blur&st=cse /.

56. Mapes D. Net's plagiarism "cops" are on patrol. MSNBC [Internet]. 2009 Sept 10 [cited 2009 Sept 11]: [3 p.]. Available from: http://www.msnbc.msn.com/id/32657885/ns/technology_and_science-tech_and_gadgets/ .

57. Ware J. Cheat wave. Yahoo! Internet Life. 1999;5(5):102-3.

58. Stuber-McEwen D, Wiseley P, Hoggatt S. Point, click, and cheat: frequency and type of academic dishonesty in the virtual classroom. Online J Dist Learning Admin. 2009 Fall [cited 2009 Sept 17];XII(III):[10 p.]. Available from: http://www.westga.edu/~distance/ojdla/fall123/stuber123.html/.

59. Asimov I. Gold. The final science fiction collection. New York (NY): HarperPrism; 1995.

60. Willful infringement. [cited 2004 Aug 9]. Available from: http://www.willfulinfringement.com/.

61. Ardito SC, Eiblum P, Daulong R. Conflicted copy rights. Online. 1999 May/June:23(3):91-5.

62. Crawford M. Are you committing plagiarism? Top five overlooked citations to add to your course materials [Internet]. Message to: Patrick M. Malone. 2010 Sept 29. [4 p.].

63. Gousse G. Advice on submitting papers: I. Am J Hosp Pharm. 1993;50:2523.

64. World Association of Medical Editors. WAME policy statements [Internet]. Chicago: World Association of Medical Editors; 2004 April 7 [cited 2004 Apr 14]. Available from: http://www.wame.org/wamestmt.htm/.

65. International Committee of Medical Journal Editors. Conflict of interest. Am J Hosp Pharm. 1993;50:2398.

66. Davidoff F, DeAngelis CD, Drazen JM, Hoey J, Højgaard L, Horton R, et al. Sponsorship, authorship, and accountability. Lancet. 2001 Sept 15;358:854-6.

67. Krimsky S, Rothenberg LS. Financial interest and its disclosure in scientific publications. JAMA. 1998;280:225-6.

68. Laniado M. How to present research data consistently in a scientific paper. Eur Radiol. 1996;6:S16-S18.

69. DeAngelis CD. Duplicate publication, multiple problems. JAMA. 2004;292:1745-6.

70. Stead WW. The responsibilities of authorship. J Am Med Inform Assoc. 1997;4:394-5.

71. Garfunkel JM, Lawson EE, Hamrick HJ, Ulshen MH. JAMA. 1990;263:1376-8.

72. Evans JT, Nadjari HI, Burchell SA. Quotation and reference accuracy in surgical journals. JAMA. 1990;263:1353-4.

73. Roland CG. Thoughts about medical writing. XXXVII. Verify your references. Anesth Analg. 1976;55:717-18.

74. Biebuyck JF. Concerning the ethics and accuracy of scientific citations. J Anesthesiol. 1992;77:1-2.

75. McLellan MF, Case LD, Barnett MC. Trust, but verify. The accuracy of references in four anesthesia journals. Anesthesiology. 1992;77:185-8.

76. de Lacy G, Record C, Wade J. How accurate are quotations and references in medical journals. BMJ. 1985;291:884-6.

77. Doms CA. A survey of reference accuracy in five national dental journals. J Dent Res. 1989;68:442-4.

78. Hasegawa GR. How to review a manuscript intended for publication. Am J Hosp Pharm. 1994;51:839-40.

79. Hoppe S, Chandler MJJ. Constructive versus destructive criticism. Am J Health-Syst Pharm. 1995;52:103.

80. Baker DE. Peer review: personal continuous quality improvement. Hosp Pharm. 2004;39:8.

81. Seltzer SM. Desktop publishing in a drug store? Am Druggist. 1987;196:64, 66.

82. Srnka QM, Scoggin JA. 10 ways to distribute newsletters to build sales volume. Pharm Times. 1984;50;71-2, 74.

83. Making the media. The pharmacy newsletter. Hosp Pharm Connection. 1986;2(3):11-12.

84. Kaldy J. Effectively creating a pharmacy newsletter. Consult Pharm. 1992;7(6):697-8, 700.

85. Goldwater SH, Haydon-Greatting S. How to publish a pharmacy newsletter. Am J Hosp Pharm. 1991;48:2121, 2125.

86. Almquist AF, Wolfgang AP, Perri M. Pharmacy newsletters—the journalistic approach. Hosp Pharm. 1988;23:974-5.

87. Schultz WL, Dendiak ST. Pharmacy newsletters: a needed service. Hosp Pharm. 1975;10(4):146-7.

88. Plumridge RJ, Berbatis CG. Drug bulletins: effectiveness in modifying prescribing and methods of improving impact. DICP Ann Pharmacother. 1989;23:330-4.

89. Appearance and content attract newsletter audience. Drug Utilization Review. 1988; 4(4):45-8.

90. Lyon RA, Norvell MJ. Effect of a P&T Committee newsletter on anti-infective prescribing habits. Hosp Formul. 1985;20:742-4.

91. Fendler KJ, Gumbhir AK, Sall K. The impact of drug bulletins on physician prescribing habits in a health maintenance organization. Drug Intell Clin Pharm. 1984;18:627-31.

92. May JR, Andrusko KT, DiPiro JT. Impact and cost justification of a surgery drug newsletter. Am J Hosp Pharm. 1984;41:1837-9.

93. Ross MB, Volger BW, Bradley JK. Use of "dispense-as-written" on prescriptions for targeted drugs: influence of a newsletter. Am J Hosp Pharm. 1990;47:2519-20.

94. Denig P, Haaijer-Ruskamp FM, Zijsling DH. Impact of a drug bulletin on the knowledge, perception of drug utility, and prescribing behavior of physicians. DICP Ann Pharmacother. 1990;24:87-93.

95. Parker RC. Looking good in print. 4th ed. Scotsdale (AZ): The Coriolis Group, LLC; 1998.

96. Baird RN, McDonald D, Pittman RK, Turnbull AT. The graphics of communication. Methods, media and technology. 6th ed. New York (NY): Hartcourt Brace Jovanovich College Publishers; 1993.

97. Don't let cost prohibit publication of pharmacy-related newsletter. Drug Utilization Review. 1988;4(4):48-9.

98. Utt JK, Lewis KT. Using desktop publishing to enhance pharmacy publications. Am J Hosp Pharm. 1988;45:1863-4.

99. Pfeiffer KS. Award-winning newsletter design. Windows Mag. 1994;5(8):208-18.

100. What makes a great web site? [cited 1999 May 13]:[1 screen]. Available from: URL: http://www.webreference.com/greatsite.html/.

101. Tweney D. Don't be a slow poke: keep your site up to speed or lose visitors. InfoWorld. 1999;22;21(12):64.

102. Tullio CJ. Selecting material for your newsletter. Hosp Pharm Times. 1992;Oct:12HPT-16HPT.

103. Journalism pro offers editing tips for effective pharmacy newsletters. Drug Utilization Review. 1988;4(4):49-50.

104. Mitchell JF, Cook RL. Pharmacy newsletters: time for a new approach. Hosp Formul. 1985;20:360-5.

105. Ritchie DJ, Manchester RF, Rich MW, Rockwell MM, Stein PM. Acceptance of a pharmacy-based, physician-edited hospital Pharmacy and Therapeutics Committee newsletter. Ann Pharmacother. 1992;26:886-9.

106. Craghead RM. Electronic mail pharmacy newsletters. Hosp Pharm. 1989;24:490.

107. Mok MP, Castile JA, Kowaloff HB, Janousek JR. Drugman—a computerized supplement to a hospital's drug information newsletter. Am J Hosp Pharm. 1985;42:1565-7.

108. Bloom BS, editor. Taxonomy of Educational Objectives, Handbook 1: Cognitive Domain. New York: David McKay; 1956.

109. Medina MS. Using the three e's (emphasis, expectations, and evaluation) to structure writing objectives for pharmacy practice experiences. Am J Health-Syst Pharm. 2010 Apr 1;67:516-21.

110. Speaking abroad. How to prepare when you're presenting over there. Presentations. 1999;13(6):A1-A15.

111. Spinler SA. How to prepare and deliver pharmacy presentations. Am J Hosp Pharm. 1991;48:1730-8.

112. Simons T. Multimedia or bust? Presentations. 2000;14(2):40-50.

113. Buchholz S, Ullman J. 12 commandments for PowerPoint. Teaching Prof. 2004;18(6):4.

114. Zielinski D. Technostressed? Don't let your gadgets and gizmos get you down. Presentations. 2004 Feb: 28-35.

115. Malone PM. Slides, files and keeping up. Adv Pharm. 2004;2(2):175-80.

116. Goldstein M. PDA presenting has come a long way, but still has drawbacks. Presentations. 2003 Nov:22.

117. Endicott J. For the prepared presenter, fonts of inspiration abound. Presentations. 1999;13(4):22-3.

118. Bullet points may be dangerous, but don't blame PowerPoint. Presentations. 2003 Nov:6.

119. The psychology of presentation visuals. Presentations. 1998;12(5):45-51.

120. DeCoske MA, White SJ. Public speaking revisited: delivery, structure and style. Am J Health-Syst Pharm. 2010 Aug 1;67:1225-7.

121. Engle JP, Firman SC. Perfecting pharmacist presentation skills. Am Pharm. 1994; NS34(7):60-4.

122. Simons T. For podium emergencies. Presentations. 2003 Nov:24-29.

123. Hill J. The attention deficit. Presentations. 2003 Oct:27-32.

Chapter Ten

Legal Aspects of Drug
Information Practice

Martha M. Rumore

Learning Objectives

● *After completing this chapter, the reader will be able to*

- Describe the legal issues related to the provision of drug information (DI).
- Determine the applicability of various legal theories that impose liability on pharmacists providing DI.
- Describe how pharmacists can help protect themselves from malpractice claims resulting from the provision of DI.
- Explain the Doctrine of Drug Overpromotion as it pertains to the 1997 Food and Drug Administration (FDA) Modernization Act (FDAMA).
- Identify the liability concerns inherent with off-label drug use and informed consent.
- Describe U.S. copyright law as it pertains to the provision of Drug Information.
- Identify copyright, liability, and privacy issues arising from the Internet.
- Formulate a plan to deal with the major provisions of the Health Insurance Portability and Accountability Act (HIPAA) of 1996.
- Explain the legal issues involved with industry support for pharmaceutical educational activities.

Key Concepts*

① Currently, most litigation concerning pharmacists involves negligence.

② There are a number of ways in which tort liability can attach to the provision of DI: incomplete information, inappropriate quality information, outdated information, and inappropriate analysis or dissemination of information.

③ There are at least three key areas of labeling and advertising liability: the learned intermediary rule, which is a defense to failure-to-warn actions; the doctrine of overpromotion, under which adequate warning is alleged to have been diluted by communications failing to adequately convey the full impact of the warning; and promotion of off-label use or non-FDA-approved indications.

④ DI is currently being obtained from a number of Wikis, blogs, and search engines, and there is possibility of DI liability for information obtained from the Internet and electronic journals.

⑤ Pharmacists providing DI must have a working knowledge of copyright law both to avoid liability and to protect their own literary works.

⑥ The HIPAA Privacy Rule is not intended to disrupt or discourage adverse event reporting or DI in any way.

⑦ The FDA, the American Council for Continuing Medical Education (ACCME), and the Pharmaceutical Research and Manufacturers of America (PhRMA) have established educational policies, guidelines, or guidances that allow communication between industry and the Continuing Medical Education (CME) providers.

Introduction

There are myriad legal issues confronting the various facets of DI. These legal issues cross over a number of traditional legal specialties, including computer law, advertising law, privacy law, intellectual property law, telecommunications law, and tort law. This chapter provides an overview and discussion of the key legal issues involving intellectual property rights, torts, privacy, and advertising and promotion that may arise in the provision of DI.

Decades after the genesis of drug information services, the legal duties of pharmacists providing DI are still evolving. Today, most pharmacy curriculums and PGY-1

---

*An understanding of the legal aspects of DI can help practitioners in day-to-day practice, as well as provide some possible ways to protect oneself in the legal system. This chapter is intended to examine legal issues and should not be considered legal advice.

residencies include DI, realizing that whether a student specializes in DI or not, it is an integral part of pharmacist-supervised patient care. Pharmacists can and will be held liable for their conduct relating to DI. This chapter begins with an examination of the expanded liability of the DI specialist, which is defined as those pharmacists who either work in DI centers or who spend the majority of their working day providing DI (e.g., Clinical Managers, Drug Information Specialists, PGY-1 and PGY-2 residents). The liability inherent in the provisions of DI to patients as an integral component of pharmacist-supervised patient care is then examined, and recommendations for prevention and mitigation of liability are provided for the non-DI specialist. The chapter then explores copyright, privacy, unique legal issues pertaining to the Internet, direct-to-consumer advertising, off-label use, as well as industry support for educational activities.

Tort Law

DI is a specialized discipline of pharmacy practice. Specialists are held to the highest degree of care by the law. Because of the DI pharmacist's greater expertise in the area of DI, it is likely that the courts would expand their legal and professional liability beyond that of other pharmacists. The liability of the DI specialist versus generalist differs for a number of reasons, the most obvious of which are the nature of the information provided and the recipients of the information. The DI specialist is most often providing DI to other health professionals and often has the title "Drug Information Specialist or Manager."[1]

Functions such as online searching; monitoring or recommending drug therapy; preparing Drug Alerts and Pharmacy Bulletins; participating in pharmacy and therapeutics (P&T) committees; conducting medication use evaluation (MUE); writing and revising medication policies; training pharmacy students, staff pharmacists, and residents; and identifying adverse drug events entail legal obligations of proper performance.

Minimal practice standards for specialists have been put forth to delineate functions and activities that may be considered essential to the provision of DI services and the expected competencies of DI specialists. Position papers and standards of the American Society of Health-System Pharmacists (ASHP) and The Joint Commission, as well as DI curriculum standards, and literature regarding appropriate management of DI requests DI remove any doubt about the level of expertise needed for DI specialists and standards for DI centers.[2-4] Minimal standards of performance and a consistent level of competence must be assured by pharmacists promoting or offering this service regardless of the practice site. Although there are no standards to accredit DI centers, professional standards of performance may be used by courts as an objective measuring tool for the standard of care.

In the latter part of the nineteenth century the locality rule or community rule was followed. This doctrine stated that local defendant practitioners would have their standard of performance evaluated in light of the performance of other peers in the same or similar communities.[5] This is no longer the case, and a DI center in a rural area will be held to the same standard as one in New York City. Creation of standards of practice and the disappearance of the "locality rule" make it easier for plaintiffs to prevail.

In addition to the DI specialist, the pharmacy profession is assuming an increased legal responsibility to provide DI in the daily practice of pharmacist-supervised patient care. The physician has been considered the learned intermediary, responsible for communicating the manufacturer's warnings to the patient. However, "failure to counsel or warn" cases are showing a trend in pharmacist liability.[6] Although most cases still maintain the pharmacist has no duty to warn, a minority of cases in various jurisdictions demonstrate the pharmacist's duty to warn of foreseeable complications of drug therapy is becoming a recognized part of the expanded legal responsibility of pharmacists. Courts have been more willing to apply a duty to warn where the pharmacist voluntarily assumes the duty, or has special knowledge about a patient, or the prescription is dangerous as written.[7]

Where the patient is at higher risk than the general population, the courts have uniformly found liability. There are many such cases against physicians for failure to disclose material risks of medical procedures or treatments to their patients.[8-10] Today pharmacists providing DI, be they generalists or DI specialists, are more likely to be held to the same standards as physicians when determining standard of care.

❶ *Currently, most litigation concerning pharmacists involves negligence.* Traditionally, physicians remain responsible for their patients and must exert "due care"; that is, a physician who knows or should have known that the information provided was improper may be held liable for negligence. Therefore, it is safe to assume that a legal cause of action pertaining to the provision of DI will be founded on the theory of negligence as the direct or proximate cause of personal injury or death. Malpractice liability based on negligence refers to failure to exercise the degree of care that a prudent (reasonable) person would exercise under the same circumstances. Elements of negligence include the four Ds: (1) duty breached, (2) damages, (3) direct causation, and (4) defenses absent. To establish a negligent failure, actual conduct must be compared to what is considered standard professional conduct. Typically, this is accomplished by introducing evidence of the relevant professional standards or testimony from expert witnesses, such as pharmacy school faculty or other DI practitioners. Once the duty of care is established, the plaintiff would need a preponderance of evidence to prove that (1) the information provided was materially deficient, (2) the deficient information was a proximate cause of injury suffered (or at least a substantial contributing factor), (3) the recipient reasonably relied on the information provided, (4) the information deficiency was due to failure to exercise reasonable care, and (5) the pharmacist knew or should have known that the safety or health of another may have depended on the accuracy of the information provided.

Expanding on the first element of negligence, duty breached, it is important to be aware of the fact that the duty must be a legal duty, not a moral or ethical duty. Although there are many ethical dilemmas pertaining to the provision of DI by pharmacists and they can sometimes give rise to a cause of action, an ethical breach is not necessarily a legal breach. Similarly, conduct that is considered unprofessional in the broad sense (e.g., rudeness) is distinct from legal duty. An example of an ethical breach that could result in liability for the pharmacist would be a breach of patient confidentiality, if that disclosure caused damages (e.g., loss of employment or the misuse of information gained in the course of employment).

In a study of DI requests, calls from consumers raised more ethical issues than calls from health professionals.[11] For example, should a pharmacist respond to a drug identification request for someone else's medication? Is the situation different if the medication is a drug of abuse and the inquiry is from a parent, relative, teacher, or police officer? Current law provides little guidance for disclosure of DI for questionable purposes, and pharmacists must exercise independent professional judgment and assume legal responsibility for that judgment when exercised.

It is necessary to expand on the fourth element of negligence, which is reasonable care. Reasonable care is that which would be considered acceptable and responsible. Suppose a patient develops a reaction that is believed to be caused by a drug, and the pharmacist is consulted to find any case reports of this drug causing the reaction. If the case is available online, but not in print, and the pharmacist had access to online databases, but did not consult them, was the pharmacist required to do so? Did the pharmacist exert reasonable care? What if the pharmacist searched MEDLINE, but not EMBASE databases, or vice versa, and thereby failed to retrieve the case? Should the pharmacist have searched both? There are no clear answers here. Who can say what a reasonable search might have been on a given day? However, using outdated references or old editions of textbooks would more likely constitute an inadequate search. In a German case, a court held a patent information service to be responsible for not having used updated materials.[12]

Case Study 10–1

The following case study and questions are provided for the reader to consider the information presented in this section.

The anticoagulation clinical pharmacist receives an order for enoxaparin in a patient who is receiving warfarin. The patient's current INR is 5.2. The anticoagulation pharmacist is a board-certified specialist. The pharmacist dispenses the enoxaparin and the patient is harmed.

- What factors favor finding the pharmacist liable for negligence?
- Is the prescription dangerous as written?
- Is the specialist more liable than the generalist?
- Who may be liable in this situation—the pharmacist, the physician, the clinic?

In a highly publicized case involving a clinical trial being conducted at Johns Hopkins University, a researcher conducted an incomplete search for lung damage from hexamethonium on PubMed, which was searchable only back to 1966, and an open Web search.[13] Although articles published in the 1950s and other sources such as TOXLINE and POISINDEX warned of such dangers, the researcher had not consulted these references, resulting in a patient's death.

Recent cases against pharmacists have held that pharmacists who gain information about the unique susceptibility of a patient are liable for failure to warn of the risks. In *Dooley v. Everett,* the court held the pharmacist liable for failing to warn a patient on theophylline of the interaction with erythromycin that produced seizures and consequent brain damage.[14] Similarly, in *Hand v. Krakowski,* the pharmacist failed to alert either the patient or physician of the drug interaction between the patient's psychotropic drug and alcohol.[15] The fact that the medication profile indicated that the patient was an alcoholic created a foreseeable risk of injury and, therefore, a duty to warn on the part of the pharmacist.

Case Study 10–2

The health-system pharmacist receives a prescription order for metformin 500 mg twice daily for a 55-year-old male patient who has severe renal impairment. The pharmacist dispenses the drug without checking the patient's renal function in the computer. The policy for metformin in the pharmacy department's manual on medication use requires the pharmacist to check and document the patient's creatinine clearance prior to dispensing metformin.

- If the patient is harmed, did the pharmacist fall below the standard of care? Could the pharmacist be judged negligent?

In *Baker v. Arbor Drugs, Inc.,* the court ruled that by advertising its drug interaction software, the defendant pharmacy voluntarily assumed a duty to use its computer technology with due care. The pharmacy technician had overridden the drug interaction between tranylcypromine sulfate (Parnate) and clemastine fumarate/phenylpropanolamine hydrochloride (Tavist-D) that the system detected from the patient's medication profile. The patient committed suicide after suffering a stroke from the combination.[16] In a very recent case, the pharmacist chose to override the computer alert regarding an interaction between tramadol and methadone, resulting in the patient's death. A $6 million verdict was returned against the pharmacy for failure to warn.[17]

❷ *There are a number of ways in which tort liability can attach to the provision of DI: incomplete information, inappropriate quality information, outdated information, inappropriate analysis or dissemination of information.*

INCOMPLETE INFORMATION

Is the pharmacist liable when the DI provided is incomplete? Should the pharmacist provide all the medication information, via a DI sheet or patient package insert (PPI)? There have been several cases against pharmacists for failure to dispense mandatory PPIs for certain drugs that later caused harm. In *Parkas v. Saary,* the court addressed the issue of whether the pharmacist's failure to dispense the Food and Drug (FDA)-mandated PPI for progesterone was the proximate cause of the congenital eye defect that occurred.[18] Because congenital defects, but not eye deformities, were specified in the PPI, failure to provide the PPI could not be proven to be the proximate cause. Therefore, judgment was in favor of the pharmacy. In *Frye v. Medicare-Glaser Corporation,* the pharmacist counseled the patient regarding drowsiness with Fiorinal, but failed to provide a warning not to consume alcohol. The patient died presumably as a result of combining the drug with beer. Here, the DI provided was incomplete. The trial court did not find the pharmacist had a duty to warn in this instance.[19] Although this case was decided before Omnibus Budget Reconciliation Act of 1990 (i.e., OBRA '90), with its mandatory patient counseling provisions in effect, its outcome would not seem to have changed as a result.

In a number of cases where the plaintiffs asserted that the pharmacist breached a duty to warn as required under OBRA '90, the courts have held that OBRA does not create an independent or private cause of action.[20-22]

Other cases are finding pharmacists have a responsibility for patient counseling and drug therapy monitoring.[23] In *Sanderson v. Eckerd Corporation,* the pharmacist was liable for "voluntary undertaking" to act in the absence of a duty, where the pharmacy's computer was inappropriately used by the pharmacist in detection of an adverse reaction and the pharmacist failed to warn the patient of the potential for an adverse reaction.[24] In *Horner v. Spalitto,* the court imposed a duty on a pharmacist to alert the prescriber when the dose prescribed is outside the therapeutic range.[25] In *Happel v. Wal-Mart Stores,* the pharmacy's computer system was overridden, and the pharmacist failed to warn a patient allergic to aspirin and ibuprofen of the potential for cross-allergenicity with ketorolac.[26] The court found the pharmacist has a duty to warn when a contraindicated drug is prescribed. In *Morgan v. Wal-Mart Stores*, where the plaintiffs alleged that the pharmacist's failure to properly warn of the known dangers of desipramine was the proximate cause of the patient's death, the court held that pharmacists have a duty beyond accurately filling a prescription "based on known contraindications, which would alert a reasonably prudent pharmacist to a potential problem."[27] However, the court did not find for the plaintiff, opining that pharmacists do not have knowledge that desipramine may cause hypereosinophilic syndrome.

Clearly, these cases demonstrate an expansion of pharmacist's duties from the non-discretionary standard of technical accuracy to a discretionary standard that requires pharmacists to perform professional functions; that is, from a technical model to a pharmacist-supervised patient care model. Knowledge of, or access to, DI is becoming an important factor that courts consider in determination of the pharmacist's duty to warn.

In a case of first impression, a court decided whether a hospital pharmacist contacting a physician regarding the dosage of colchicine had a duty of care to the physician to provide complete DI.[28] While the pharmacist advised what a correct oral dosage would consist of, he did not advise of the correct dose in a renally impaired patient. The plaintiff alleged that the hospital pharmacy's voluntary undertaking to provide DI, and the pharmacist's voluntary intervening between the patient and physician, created a duty on the part of the pharmacist "to the physician." This is different from other duty-to-warn cases where plaintiff alleges the pharmacist has a duty to warn "to the patient." In the present case, the plaintiff alleged the hospital's pharmacy voluntarily undertook to be a DI resource and that the hospital pharmacist voluntarily intervened between the patient and physician, thereby creating a duty on the part of the pharmacist to the physician. The court, however, rejected the argument that a "voluntary undertaking of a duty to a physician" was created based on a pharmacist's interaction with the patient's physician. The court further held that the learned intermediary doctrine forecloses any duty of care on the part of the pharmacist to the patient, based on the pharmacist's statements to the physician. Significantly, the court commented that even if such a duty were placed on the pharmacist, the duty was not breached inasmuch as the pharmacist correctly followed the hospital's intervention policy.

While pharmacists are in a position to provide DI, providing the patient with all information may have a detrimental effect. In fact, it is the FDA's position that the information contained in professional labeling can be safely used only under the supervision of the licensed prescriber. It has, therefore, been the practice not to provide the patient with the professional labeling unless the patient specifically requests it. With regard to the duty to disclose to the patient low percentage risks, the court rulings have been inconsistent. One court has allowed strict liability against a pharmacy. In *Heredia v. Johnson,* the pharmacist dispensed an otic solution without warning of the risk of tympanic membrane rupture and the need to discontinue the drug if certain symptoms appeared. The plaintiff claimed that because of the lack of warning he suffered from severe and permanent injury including brain damage.[29] However, in *Marchione v. State,* a prison inmate alleged lack of informed consent based on the failure of the prison doctor to inform him about the side effects of prazosin (Minipress), which caused permanent impotence. The physician argued that his duty was only to warn of severe or frequent side effects. The *Marchione* court concluded that the physician need not disclose a laundry list of 31 remote drug side effects. The side effect had a reported incidence of only two or three cases out of several million prescriptions and was, therefore, rare. The plaintiff also did not have any unique risk factors that would increase the likelihood of the reaction occurring.[30] The courts seem to look at risk factors unique to the patient in deciding whether the health professional is required to indicate the likelihood of occurrence of the risks.

Brushwood and Simonsmeier[31] delineate two responsibilities with regard to patient counseling: risk assessment and risk management. Risk assessment is judgmental and occurs before prescribing when a decision is made to accept or forgo drug therapy. Although this has traditionally been the responsibility of the physician, the current scope of pharmacy practice is expanding, as many states permit independent, dependent, and collaborative prescribing.[32] Each level of prescriptive authority is characterized by a specific level of liability. For example, independent prescribers are professionally accountable for their own prescribing decisions. Dependent prescribing, which involves the delegation of authority from an independent prescriber, as is typical of therapeutic interchange and drug therapy management protocols in health care facilities, involves a shared accountability. Similarly, in collaborative prescribing, where there is a collaborative practice agreement that allows pharmacists to initiate and/or modify patients' medication regimens pursuant to an approved protocol, both the physician and pharmacists share accountability.[33] In addition, employers remain vicariously liable for the actions and decisions of their staff.

Risk management occurs after prescribing, is nonjudgmental, and assists the patient in proper drug use to maximize benefits and minimize potential problems.[34,35] Drug risk management, but not drug risk assessment information, should be provided to patients. The drug management information provided to patients should be accurate and in a form that the patient understands.

Hall and Honey[36] divided the risks associated with a particular drug into two groups, inherent or noninherent. Inherent risks are unavoidable, unique to the drug, and are usually identified in the package insert (PI), but do not include probable or common side effects. However well a drug is researched, manufactured, and prescribed, it still may have the ability to produce certain side effects. Examples of inherent drug risks are stroke from oral contraceptives or teeth discoloration from tetracyclines. Noninherent risks are created by the particular drug in combination with some extrinsic factor about which the pharmacist should reasonably know, and include maximum safe dosages, interactions, patient characteristics influencing pharmacokinetics, and probable or common side effects. Examples of noninherent risks would be nephrotoxicity from aminoglycosides in patients with renal impairment. The responsibility of the pharmacist to provide DI about noninherent risks is expanding.

What liability does the pharmacist incur for information outside of the PI? Physicians may prescribe drugs as they see fit, without adhering to the specific therapeutic indications or dosing guidelines within the labeling. The FDA regulates the manufacture and promotion of drugs, not the practice of medicine. However, it has been held that a physician's deviation from the PI was *prima facie* (i.e., not requiring further support to establish validity, on its face value) evidence of negligence if the patient's injury resulted from the failure to adhere to the recommendations.[37] However, the states appear to be split on whether recommendations in a PI are *prima facie* evidence of the standard of care. It would be prudent for the pharmacist to consult the PI when responding to an inquiry and include such information in the response, especially if the response is contrary to what is contained in the PI.

A disciplinary action by a state pharmacy board highlights the importance of checking the PI or literature concerning the proposed use of a product. In *In re Michael A. Gabert,* a pharmacist received a prescription for 5% silver nitrate for bladder instillation. The pharmacist contacted a DI center and was told there was no literature supporting the proposed use of the product. The pharmacist then asked the physician what support he had for such use and the physician referred to a published Mayo Clinic Newsletter. The pharmacist did not ask to see a copy of the letter, or have a copy of it for the pharmacy records. Significant patient harm resulted when the solution was instilled into the patient's bladder. The Mayo Clinic Newsletter pertained to silver argyrol, not silver nitrate.[38]

INAPPROPRIATE QUALITY INFORMATION

It has long been recognized by law that false information provided to another could result in harm to the recipient if the recipient acted relying on the false information. Although negligent misrepresentation has not been applied to DI, there is no guarantee that it will not be in the future.[39] The relevant law is the *Restatement (Second) of Torts, §311, Negligent Misrepresentation Involving Risk of Physical Harm*, which states:

> One who negligently gives false information to another is subject to liability for physical harm caused by action taken by the other in reasonable reliance upon such information.... Such negligence may consist of failure to exercise reasonable care in ascertaining accuracy of the information, or in the manner in which it is communicated.[40]

Thus, the DI itself may be faulty for one or more reasons: it may be dated; it may simply be wrong; it may be incomplete and, therefore, misleading; or none may have been provided because of an incomplete search or incompetent searcher. Information negligence may occur because of: (1) parameter negligence (failure to consult the correct source) or (2) omission negligence (consulting the correct source, but failure to locate the correct answer[s]). A study evaluated the accuracy of a drug identification response by 56 DI centers. Approximately 30% correctly identified the investigational drug product; 67% could not make the identification; most importantly, 3.6% (two DI centers) made an incorrect identification. The study found inconsistencies in responses of DI centers.[41] Another study evaluated the quality of DI responses provided by 116 DI centers to multiple queries. The correct response rates varied from 5% for a question pertaining to erythromycin for diabetic gastroparesis to 90% for a drug interaction question pertaining to didanosine-dapsone. For each of three patient-specific questions, the percentages of centers eliciting vital patient data were 5%, 27%, and 86%. The findings suggest that many DI centers continue to fail to elicit patient-specific information necessary for informed responses and focus instead on procedural and technical matters.[42] As an illustration, recently, despite the peer-review process all too familiar to authors, the structure of bilirubin was found to be incorrect in an article as well as the three leading biochemistry textbooks in the United States.[43]

Inappropriate quality information may be the result of ghostwriting or publication marketing. Ghostwriting is when a pharmaceutical company develops the concept for an article to counteract criticism of a drug or embellish its benefits, hires a professional writing company to draft the article, retains a health professional to sign off as the author, and finds a publisher to unwittingly publish the work. In a recent product liability case, the court ordered the pharmaceutical company to disclose its documents pertaining to its ghostwriting practices.[44] In some instances, posters and meeting abstracts may actually be generated by the pharmaceutical industry or are incomplete and lacking in peer review. For example, the reader has no way of knowing whether the abstract results are reflective of the entire study population or merely a small subset.

Can pharmacists providing DI be held responsible for retrieving information that is itself inaccurate? What responsibility does the information producer incur for errors in information sources? An unskilled searcher or one with insufficient searching knowledge may not find correct or complete information, which can lead to the wrong answer. The fault can lie anywhere in the information dissemination chain; publication, collection, storage, retrieval, dissemination, or utilization. Errors are often encountered in DI databases.[45] Although very few cases have been brought before courts concerning the liability of print or online information sources, there is some case law to guide. The issue concerns strict liability.

Strict liability applies where a defective product proximately causes physical harm. Where the service rendered is deemed to be a professional service, the courts exhibit a reluctance to impose strict liability. With exceptions, persons physically injured because of their reliance on defective and unreasonably dangerous information have only negligence as a cause of action, and only against the author, not the publisher;[46] only if the publisher is negligent or offers intentionally misleading information could it be held liable. This was tested in *Jones v. J.B. Lippincott Co.,* where a nursing student was injured after consulting and relying on a nursing textbook that recommended hydrogen peroxide enemas for the treatment of constipation. The courts rejected the plaintiff's claim that strict liability should be applied to the publisher.[47] Similarly, in a German case, a misprint in a medical textbook resulted in the injection of 25% rather than 2.5% sodium chloride solution, injuring a patient. Again, the court rejected strict liability for the publisher on the basis that any medically educated person should have noticed the misprint.[48] In *Roman v. City of New York,* the plaintiff sued for an alleged misstatement in a booklet distributed by a Planned Parenthood organization that resulted in a "wrongful conception." The court found that "a publisher cannot assume liability for all misstatements, said or unsaid, to a potentially unlimited public for a potentially unlimited period."[49] In *Winter v. G.R Putnam's Sons,* two persons required liver transplants after collecting and eating poisonous wild mushrooms. They had relied on an *Encyclopedia of Wild Mushrooms* in choosing to eat the mushrooms that caused this severe harm.[50] The court refused to hold the publisher liable and found that a publisher has no duty to investigate the accuracy of the information it publishes.

In *Delmuth Development Corp. v. Merck & Co.,* the plaintiff claimed lost sales because of the publication of erroneous information in the *Merck Index.* The court considered the duty of a publisher to a reader to publish accurate information in a compendium.[51] The court noted a publisher's right to publish without fear of liability is guaranteed by the First Amendment and societal interest. It further held that even if it had a duty to publish with care, the plaintiff could not claim it suffered damages because of reliance on this information.

What liability is incurred by an author or publisher for publication of product comparisons? Recently, a pharmacy journal publisher and article author were sued for defamation by a device manufacturer where the publication compared and opined on the performance of devices for compounding sterile products.[52] The court granted the defendants' motion to dismiss stating lack of actual malice (a necessary element of defamation). In this ruling, the court protected the First Amendment rights of scientists to report product comparisons and the rights of publishers regarding the peer-review process and publication of such comparisons.[53]

In *Libertelli v. Hoffman La Roche, Inc. & Medical Economics Co.,* the plaintiff became addicted to diazepam (Valium) and sued the publisher of the *Physician's Desk Reference* (PDR).[54] The claim was based on the absence of warnings in the PDR regarding the addictive nature of the drug. The court dismissed the case against the publisher. Under a long line of cases, a publisher is not liable for matters of public interest if it has no knowledge of its falsity. Although some effort should be made to verify search results, the pharmacist cannot be held responsible for knowing and verifying the contents of all sources, whether in print or online. However, checking a second reference to verify information is prudent.

Strict liability would appear applicable to software that is licensed without significant modification as a standard packaged system, as has been found with defective medical computer programs.[55] Pharmacists providing DI should be aware of computer-related lawsuits that have arisen involving defects (or bugs) in software that caused erroneous results. These cases result in greater damage awards based on consequential (i.e., special as opposed to actual) damages suffered. An example of consequential damages would be damage to a firm's reputation. Perhaps the most widely cited software-related accidents involve malfunctioning computerized radiation machines where overdosages have caused patient deaths.[56] Radiation overdosages from faulty software continue to occur today; grim reminders of the problems faced by reliance on software.[57] In one particularly relevant case, the court held that the National Weather Service was liable for the deaths of four fishermen off Cape Cod, Massachusetts. The Weather Service had forecasted calm weather because of faulty software. Although the verdict was overturned on technical grounds, the U.S. District Court let stand the precedent holding an entity liable for information it provides.[58]

In another case, Jeppesen, an information provider, was held liable for an airplane crash caused by faulty data from the Federal Aviation Administration on flight patterns. A pilot used one of the faulty charts and crashed into a mountain, killing the crew and destroying the plane. The company paid $12 million in damages.[59] The court held the information provider strictly liable because the charts were considered a "product." In *Jeppesen,* the mass production and mass marketing of the charts rendered them a product. Similarly, in *Greenmoss Builders v. Dun & Bradstreet,* the issue involved the erroneous listing of Greenmoss Builders as a company in bankruptcy in Dun & Bradstreet Business Information Report database. A jury awarded $350,000, including $300,000 in punitive damages. The case was appealed all the way to the Supreme Court, where Dun & Bradstreet lost the case.[60]

In *Daniel v. Dow Jones & Co., Inc.,* where a subscriber brought action against a provider of a computerized database alleging that he relied on a false news report in making investments, the court found that the subscriber did not have a "special relationship" with the database provider necessary to impose liability for negligent misstatements. First Amendment guarantees of freedom of the press also protected the provider from liability.[61]

As mentioned previously, D.I. provided may be inaccurate because it is dated, incomplete, or wrong. For example, inappropriate quality information may occur because references are updated differently. Even electronic references are updated differently—some monthly, others weekly. Most DI services require documentation of an answer in at least two different sources. The "double check" procedure is common practice when preparing chemotherapy and avoiding drug administration errors. In many of the cases described above, liability could have been prevented by checking the information in more than one reference or source. Thus, checking a DI response in several references is the standard of practice.

INAPPROPRIATE ANALYSIS/DISSEMINATION OF INFORMATION

Is liability for providing DI a rhetorical supposition or a real possibility? The responsibility of pharmacists providing DI goes beyond that of mere information intermediary, the person in between the information producer and the user. Published studies for DI centers have reported that 41% to 83% of requested information is patient-specific or judgmental in nature.[62] In addition to liability for the negligent information retrieval and dissemination, the pharmacist's role involves information interpretation, evaluation, and giving advice. This role falls into a consultative model and differs greatly from that of librarians. Librarians are not equipped to give advice. The pharmacist's role as evaluator and interpreter of the information creates a duty sufficient to sustain liability.

The paucity of case law in the area does not negate liability. The issue deserves consideration because of the potential for harm caused by the DI provided by the pharmacist. There have only been two cases involving poison information centers, one of which also was a DI center. In *Reben v. Ely,* the plaintiffs filed suit against the DI center for injuries sustained by inadvertent administration of cocaine solution instead of acetaminophen to a 10-year-old patient. The local pharmacy had colored the 10% cocaine solution red and labeled it "red solution" to thwart abuse. When the nurse realized the mistake, she contacted the Arizona Poison and DI Center. The DI pharmacist described the symptomatology of cocaine overdose, but did not go far enough in recommending that the patient seek emergency care. The patient developed seizures and cardiopulmonary arrest with brain damage that will require lifetime nursing care. At the trial, the expert witness testified that the DI center operated below the standard of care. The issue was not erroneous information, but whether the center went far enough in its responsibility in handling the call. The plaintiff was awarded $6.5 million; the DI center was held liable for $3.6 million.[63]

In another case, a lawsuit named a poison information center that was called for assistance when a student died after swallowing a toxic substance during a laboratory experiment. The poison center was named in the $2.5 million suit because it refused to release proof of its claim that the person who called had given the wrong name for the solution that the student drank.[64]

From a liability standpoint, there are disadvantages to the formal combination of poison control and DI centers. For example, poison inquiries usually require immediate answers in critical situations without written documentation and sometimes without supporting references.[65,66] The outcomes of poisonings (e.g., overdoses and suicide attempts) are more likely to result in patient morbidity and mortality and require medical backup for acute treatment decisions. Some states (e.g., Arkansas, Oregon, Washington, Arizona, New Jersey) have statutory provisions for joint poison control and DI centers. In several of these states, such as Arkansas, immunity from personal liability in judgment (in contrast to carelessness or inadvertence) would not be actionable as malpractice unless a lack of due care can be shown. However, not all DI centers are protected from liability. Additionally, there have been other lawsuits involving poison control centers but these have mostly involved medical toxicologists serving as poison control center consultants, not DI pharmacists.[67]

Defenses to Negligence and Malpractice Protection

Even if the plaintiff can establish all the necessary elements of negligence, legal defenses can avoid or reduce liability. Some defenses might include a statute of limitations, comparative or contributory negligence, informed consent, or governmental immunity. It is important to keep in mind that there may be differences in both types of defenses to negligence and insurance coverage for individuals and employers. Further information on defenses will be described in the following sections.

DEFENSES FOR INDIVIDUALS

Assumption of the risk via informed consent and comparative or contributory negligence are defenses to negligence for individuals. Under informed consent, the defendant could assert that the patient knowingly assumed the risk for a new or experimental therapy or regimen. However, the risks the patient assumes does not include negligence on the part of the physician or pharmacist. There is no assumption of the risk for negligent behavior.

Comparative negligence is the allocation of responsibility for damages incurred between the plaintiff and defendant, based on the relative negligence of the two. Concurrent negligence is the wrongful acts or omissions of two or more persons acting independently, but causing the same injury. Under comparative or concurrent negligence, the pharmacist may also be held liable, either alone or together with the information requestor (e.g., physician and nurse), for inaccurate information or information that does not ensure maximal protection for the patient.

In the landmark case *Harbeson v. Parke Davis,* a federal court ruled that the doctrine of informed consent required a physician to furnish a patient contemplating pregnancy with information concerning the teratogenicity of the phenytoin she was taking. The physician had a duty to provide information reasonably available in the medical literature, but failed to do so. Even though the physician was not aware of the potential effects of phenytoin, studies were reported in the medical literature.[68] This case represents the only case in which a lack of a literature search resulted in liability.

Cases of vicarious liability are not new to medical malpractice. Vicarious liability is the attribution of liability upon one person for the actions of another. Through the doctrine of vicarious liability, a pharmacist could become associated with professional liability actions as part of a case against a hospital or physician. Physicians have been found negligent for the negligence of nurses, therapists, and others working under their supervision. Significantly, no cases were found where physicians were found negligent from the negligence of pharmacists working under them. If physicians request DI, they would also be held liable if a patient suffers because the search was deficient or the information incorrect. For example, in the *Harbeson* case, if the physician had requested the pharmacist to search for information about the teratogenicity of phenytoin and no references were found because of a faulty search, the pharmacist would share in the negligence together with the physician. The institution would probably also be named as a party in such legal action.

Delegation of authority does not mean abdication of responsibility. Under vicarious liability, a pharmacist who has not been personally negligent could be held responsible for the negligence of others. Supervision and adequate training of subordinates (e.g., interns, pharmacy technicians, other employees) are essential. Incompetence and substandard training of these individuals can lead to liability. An example might include a breach of confidentiality (e.g., revealing someone has a loathsome disease) by one of these employees.

From a legal standpoint, does charging a fee increase liability for the DI provider? Fee-based providers would appear to be at greater malpractice risk, especially if the relationship is a contractual one. If any of the contractual expectations are not met, the client has a contractual cause of action against the DI center. The courts will look to the terms of the agreement and the reasonable expectations of the parties. However, where bodily injury results, tort law may impose liability even where the defective information is given gratuitously and the DI provider derives no benefit from giving it.

Does providing DI services to consumers increase liability exposure? Many DI centers provide services to consumers; some via a hotline or health information lines, some via the Internet. Several studies have reported that more ethical questions to DI centers arise from consumers than from any other group.[69-71] Such ethical questions may involve drug abuse and toxicologic effects, the safety of drugs in pregnancy or nursing, experimental therapy, or the appropriateness of prescribing decisions. A decision to comment on a physician's therapeutic recommendations, even if factually correct and in the patient's best interest, may result in a legal liability. The answers to this and other questions that the pharmacist providing DI encounters are not found in the legal precedent.

DEFENSES FOR EMPLOYERS

Is the provider the hospital or university where the DI center is located, or the pharmacist providing the DI? The vast majority of DI centers are located in hospitals and universities. In addition, many pharmaceutical companies have DI departments staffed by pharmacists who handle inquiries on the company's products. There also exist independent information brokers who have liability under contract law, as well as tort law. The employer-employee relationship is a significant factor under either common law *respondeat superior* doctrine or, alternatively, a theory of negligent hire or supervision. *Respondeat superior* refers to the proposition that the employer is responsible for the negligent acts of its agents or employees. The injured party may also sue the employer for its negligence in hiring or supervising the employee. Under a negligent hire theory, it must be shown that the employee was unfit for the position and that a reasonable, pre-employment interview or postemployment supervision would have discovered this fact.[72]

Although the person who provides the information is liable for the harm caused by it, the employer may also be held liable in the absence of sovereign or charitable immunity. For pharmacists providing DI employed by the government (e.g., Veteran's Administration [VA] or Public Health Service [PHS]), there are statutes providing governmental immunity, also called sovereign immunity, from civil liability. Such immunity, however, will not protect an intentionally or grossly negligent person.

Even if the lawsuit is nonmeritorious, DI centers affiliated with hospitals or universities provide another deep pocket for contribution to the settlement. With exceptions, suing the pharmacist alone would fail to provide a windfall settlement for plaintiffs. The board of directors/trustees of the hospital or university or director of the DI center or pharmacy department where the DI center is located would be jointly liable. Joint and several liability refers to the sharing of liabilities among a group of people collectively and also individually. If the defendants are jointly and severally liable, it means that the injured party may sue some or all of the defendants together, or each one separately, and may collect equal amounts or unequal amounts from each. In states where joint and several liability applies, the pharmacist provides additional assurance that there will be sufficient assets to recover. The DI provider will be held responsible for the standard of care in the response to DI inquiries and may be found negligent.

PROTECTING AGAINST MALPRACTICE

Methods to protect against lawsuits include contracts covering financial arrangements, adequate documentation, disclaimers, and insurance.[73] For example, a disclaimer can be placed on results of online searches stating that the data being provided are from a source believed to be reliable and factually correct.[74] The best way to avoid omission negligence is to learn from experience, anticipate mistakes that may appear in databases, and keep abreast of changes in DI sources. Even if the delivery of false information is the result of inaccurate information itself, the pharmacist would likely be named as a defendant if the database producer were sued.

Adequate documentation may spell the difference between refuting or not refuting an unfounded claim of malpractice. Such documentation includes responses to inquiries, as well as a record of steps taken in a search. Designing and following procedures to document the research process can help avoid negligence. In *Fidelity Leasing Corp. v. Dun & Bradstreet, Inc.,* the court looked at the operation procedures and adherence to them in the particular instance to determine liability for providing false information.[74]

The key to provision of quality DI in an information service is the availability of current, objective information. Procedures should be in place to ensure that data is continually reviewed and updated. Quality assurance (QA) standards for the timeliness, thoroughness, and accuracy of information could also insulate against liability. QA programs, although they exist, are inconsistent among DI centers.

Problem areas common to DI centers regardless of practice site include files not updated and incomplete documentation of responses to requests. With regard to inquiries about adverse reactions, details of the adverse event should be taken and reported to the FDA reporting program. Cases may be clinically urgent, and the physician or nurse may have a patient waiting. Response via e-mail, even with alerts attached, is not prudent in such situations as there is no guarantee that callers are at their desk to receive such e-mails. All statements made should be traceable to the literature. Additionally, information should be confirmed with other references to ensure consistency between various resources. DI centers should address at least some of the items in Table 10–1.

Insistence on a good educational background for entry-level positions, followed by the continuing education of DI professionals, certification in online training courses, and good interpersonal communication skills, may also protect against malpractice. Several studies have shown that physicians who were sued frequently had poor interpersonal skills; that is, patients did not like them.[75] It is also important to keep abreast of changes in sources of DI via regular advanced training, conferences, and reading. All courses in DI should teach situations in ethical conflict that will assist in the decision making and value judgments encountered in the provision of DI.

Under the tort law doctrine of *respondeat superior*, both the pharmacist providing DI and the employer are jointly and severally liable for the damages. This enables the plaintiff to have access to the pharmacist's personal assets where the employer's assets are not sufficient to cover an adverse judgment. Professional liability insurance provides protection to cover exactly this kind of liability. Consideration should be given to obtaining professional indemnity insurance for the DI pharmacist.

Most policies now provide coverage on either an occurrence or claims-made basis. Occurrence means any incident that occurs during the policy period, no matter when the

TABLE 10–1. QUALITY ASSURANCE AS A LIABILITY-REDUCING FACTOR

Identify scope of activities and personnel requirements.

Develop and follow policies and procedures or formal call triaging protocols.

Keep standard operating procedure manual available for consultation.

Avoid violations of statutes and regulations.

Unapproved uses or doses should be well documented, and if a use or dose differs from the labeling, the requestor must be so notified.

Do not recommend a use or dose of a drug based solely on foreign literature or animal studies or questionable resources or references that are not peer-reviewed.

Never extrapolate pediatric or geriatric dosages from usual adult dosages.

Maintain knowledge of the current literature, new drug applications and supplemental approvals, labeling changes, and new warnings.

Do not present inadequate data or ignore contrary data.

Avoid overly enthusiastic or exaggerated efficacy and safety claims.

Do not attempt to diagnose or treat acute poisoning—direct such inquiries to a poison control center or an emergency room.

Know the circumstances of the case and appropriate background information (e.g., knowledge of causality assessment scales [e.g., Naranjo], laboratory findings, concurrent drugs that are necessary for adverse drug reaction inquiries).

Exert special care for drug identification questions in view of the growth of counterfeit drugs.

Responses of new employees, students, residents should be checked—document, document, document. Maintain reasonable response time; if necessary, prioritize requests.

Obtain peer concurrence or outside professional consultation, if necessary.

Develop a QA mechanism to ensure that service is maintained at a high level of quality (e.g., periodic audits or surveys).

Maintain up-to-date files and reference texts (e.g., paper files should be randomly checked to be sure they contain articles at least as recent as 2 years old).

For Internet-specific data, check currency, authorship, publisher, length of time site has existed, site reviews, links to and from other sites, biases/objectiveness, intended audience, quality of the writing, references provided, who maintains the site. (See Chapter 3 for further information regarding evaluating Internet Web sites.)

claim is filed, within the applicable statute of limitations. Claims-made policies cover only claims that are filed while the policy is active. To cover claims that are filed after a claims-made policy is terminated, the DI pharmacist can purchase tail coverage from the insurer. It is important to be aware of the limitations and exclusions in these policies. Many do not require the carrier to obtain the consent of the insured before settling a claim. In these policies, the right to protect one's reputation may conflict with the economic interest of the insurer to dispose of the claim as inexpensively as possible. Therefore, it is imperative that individuals obtain insurance coverage policies separate from those of their employers. Most common exclusions are coverage for dishonest, fraudulent, criminal, or malicious acts; property damage; and personal injury coverage. In these cases, the pharmacist faces such liability alone, and in certain situations can be ruined financially.

Finally, limiting language in subscriber contracts (i.e., exculpatory clauses) may serve to restrict monetary awards in certain circumstances. Such clauses could be included in either contracts for subscribers or signed on acceptance of responses to inquiries. A provision could be included that specifically disclaims any responsibility to a third party who might rely on the information. Written information, such as a bulletin, should carry a disclaimer specifying that the information provided is issued on the understanding that it is the best available from the resources available to the service at a particular time.

An attorney could draft a standard agreement providing that the application of the research by the recipient would not be subject to any implied warranty of fitness for that purpose. However, certain jurisdictions have held that contracts that purport to exculpate a party from negligence will be subjected to strict judicial scrutiny. Courts in certain jurisdictions have declared contracts that attempt to exempt a party's willful or grossly negligent conduct to be void. Further, no exculpatory clause will protect a pharmacist who is grossly or intentionally negligent.

Labeling and Advertising

The FDA defines labeling as written or oral information used to supplement or explain a product, regardless of whether the information accompanies the product. As such, even literature, textbooks, reprints of articles, and scientific seminars may constitute labeling. Labeling requires full disclosure. Advertisements, on the other hand, require a fair balance, meaning there must be a discussion of both benefits and risks, so as not to be misleading, and substantial evidence from clinical trials must be included for comparative claims.[76]

❸ *There are at least three key areas of labeling and advertising liability: the learned intermediary rule, which is a defense to failure to warn actions; the doctrine of overpromotion, under which adequate warning is alleged to have been diluted by communications failing to adequately convey the full impact of the warning; and promotion of off-label use or non-FDA-approved indications.*

DIRECT-TO-CONSUMER (DTC) DRUG INFORMATION AND EROSION OF THE LEARNED INTERMEDIARY RULE

In 1997, the FDA relaxed the standards for DTC television advertising.[77] DTC advertising involves magazine, television, Web-based, cell phone, and text advertisements, suggesting the use of various prescription drugs for medical conditions the viewer might experience and also suggesting viewers ask their physician if the medication would be appropriate for them.

Today, prescription drug advertising is a multibillion dollar industry. Prescription drug advertising is governed by the Food, Drug, and Cosmetic Act (FDCA) and 21 U.S.C. §331, which prohibits the misbranding of a prescription drug.[78] The primary regulation aimed at pharmaceutical product advertising is found at 21 C.F.R. § 202.1, which pertains to all "advertisements in published journals, magazines, other periodicals, newspapers, and other advertisements broadcast through media such as radio, television, and telephone communication systems." These implementing regulations specify that prescription drug advertisements cannot omit material facts and must present a fair balance between effectiveness and risk information. Further, for print advertisements, the regulations specify that every risk addressed in the product's approved labeling must also be disclosed in the advertisements. The regulations further require that the advertisement contain a summary of "all necessary information related to side effects and contraindications" or provide convenient access to the product's FDA-approved labeling and the risk information it contains. DTC advertising of off-label uses of prescription drugs is prohibited.[79]

There is evidence that DTC advertising is becoming more aggressive.[80] The FDA has cited unsubstantiated safety claims and minimization of risk, including "Web sites that omit or bury important safety information," as areas of particular concern.[81] In some cases, the advertising does not focus on a product but rather on patient education. One company has developed a campaign to bring mental health educational forums to college campuses featuring free screenings for depression. In another case, a 24-hour television network directed to a captive audience (i.e., hospitalized patients) was launched. As federal regulations require patient education, this programming may be used by hospitals for patient education. Other manufacturers offer monetary rewards or gifts (e.g., free exercise video) to patients who visit their physician regarding the product or offer a rebate or sweepstakes opportunity if the patient completes a questionnaire. Manufacturers are also sending out video press releases about drugs that are often aired as news stories. Many advertisements provide an 800 number to encourage consumers to seek additional information about the products; others offer free videotapes, brochures, and information packets discussing the product.[82] There also exist DI search tools for use directly by consumers, such as PDR.net, http://www.pdr.net.[83]

Another popular DTC vehicle is Blog posts. For example, YouTube videos about products from patients are being posted on pharmaceutical company Web sites without review. Often these patient testimonials go well beyond what a company is permitted to advertise about the product. In general, patient testimonials minimize product risks and adverse events and are unbalanced. However, the FDA has yet to establish formal regulations or guidance on such activity, even where the pharmaceutical company is hosting the Blog.[84]

The advent of DTC advertising bypasses the advice of the physician. In 1999, the first lawsuit was brought against a pharmaceutical company in connection with DTC advertising. Other DTC cases have followed where attorneys for plaintiffs have made some footholds in convincing courts to abandon the learned intermediary doctrine, greatly impacting pharmaceutical product liability law.[85]

In *Perez v. Wyeth Laboratories Inc.*,[86] the New Jersey Supreme Court created an exception to the learned intermediary doctrine on the ground that foundational tenets of the doctrine are no longer applicable in the context of DTC advertising. The court wrote, "...we believe that when mass marketing of prescription drugs seeks to influence a patient's choice of a drug, a pharmaceutical manufacturer that makes direct claims to consumers for the efficacy of its product should not be unqualifiedly relieved of a duty to provide proper warnings of the dangers or the side effects of the product." *Perez* involved Norplant, an implantable contraceptive which provided contraception for up to 5 years, but was removable. The plaintiffs alleged personal injury and failure to warn of the contraceptive's side effects, including removal complications, which resulted in pain, and scarring. The plaintiffs asserted that based on the mass advertising campaign directly to women that the pharmaceutical manufacturer had a duty to warn patients directly. According to the majority in *Perez,* the learned intermediary doctrine has four theoretical premises: (1) a reluctance to undermine the doctor-patient relationship, (2) an absence for the need for the patient's informed consent, (3) the inability of drug manufacturers to communicate with patients, and (4) the complexity of the subject matter. The court asserted that each of these bases, except the fourth, is obviated in DTC advertising of prescription drugs. According to *Perez*, when direct advertising influences a patient to request a particular drug, and the physician does not adequately consult with the patient, "neither the physician nor the manufacturer should be entirely relieved of their respective duties to warn."[87]

It is important for pharmacists providing DI to be aware of the emerging legal issues relating to DTC advertising, such as erosion of the learned intermediary doctrine and the shifting of liability to pharmaceutical manufacturers.[88] Additionally, the erosion of the learned intermediary rule, as demonstrated in *Perez*, and the shifting of liability away from physicians has broad implications for pharmacists. Increasingly, the courts are holding that the pharmacist has a duty to warn patients and intervene on their behalf. In 1991, Pharmacists Mutual reported no claims involving drug utilization review. In 1999, drug review claims accounted for 9% of all pharmacist liability claims. A 2002 study by the same firm found that drug review claims were continuing in a straight-line increase.[89] In 2008, drug review claims at 9.6% represented the largest category of intellectual errors (as opposed to mechanical or dispensing errors).[90]

Multiple constitutionality issues have been raised regarding any government interference with DTC advertising of prescription drugs. In *Thompson v. Western States Medical Center*, the U.S. Supreme Court upheld the rights of pharmacists to advertise compounded prescription drugs.[91] In doing so, the Court held that the Food and Drug Administration Modernization Act (FDAMA) prohibition of the promotion or advertisement of compounded drugs by pharmacists violated the First Amendment and that proposed restrictions would limit the First Amendment rights of pharmaceutical manufacturers as well as the implied constitutional right of patients to receive the information.

In any event, pharmacists must remain vigilant to ensure that DTC advertising does not promote false expectations. Clearly, DTC advertising achieves its goals of encouraging consumerism, whereby patients go to seek prescription information from health professionals. DTC advertisements increasingly lead patients to seek information that will confirm or refute the manufacturer's claims that differentiate a product from its competitors. When confronted with the influences of such advertising, pharmacists are on the front lines educating patients regarding these products, including the cost effectiveness of prescription drug options. Pharmacists have a responsibility to provide objective information, to educate the patient, and to serve as a DI resource.[92]

DOCTRINE OF DRUG OVERPROMOTION

The doctrine of overpromotion is based on liability where an adequate warning is alleged to have been diluted by communications that do not adequately convey the full impact of the warning and are so overpromoting of a drug that members of the medical profession prescribe it when it was not warranted. In other instances, overpromotion involves promoting a drug to a group for an off-label use. Recent examples include promoting an opioid indicated for cancer pain to non-oncologists; promoting a birth control pill to treat premenstrual syndrome and/or acne; promoting an antipsychotic approved for bipolar disorder and schizophrenia for anxiety, obsessive compulsive disorder, dementia, and autism.

On August 9, 2003, Prescription Access Litigation Project filed the first class action lawsuit against a pharmaceutical company in connection with DTC ads. The class action was brought for allegedly deceptive advertising and overpricing of Claritin.[93] Plaintiffs alleged that the company's DTC advertisements overstated the limited efficacy of its product and that the company deliberately left out any unfavorable information about the drug's efficacy.

In yet other cases, the overpromotion failed to warn of the potential for serious side effects. While product liability laws vary by jurisdiction, counts of fraud/intentional misrepresentation, negligent misrepresentation, and breach of warranty are often found in the lawsuit pleadings. Another DTC lawsuit involves Paxil, one of the top-selling drugs in the world.[94] Plaintiffs allege the drug causes withdrawal symptoms, such as severe nausea and psychological problems, and that the company failed to tell plaintiffs, their physicians, or the public of this adverse effect.[94] If the adverse reaction is not listed in the labeling, the health care prescriber (e.g., the physician) is exonerated, leaving the pharmaceutical company liable. Recent cases have involved tendon rupture from fluoroquinolone antibiotics, amputation from inadvertent promethazine intravenous extravasation,[95] and neuropathy and polyneuropathy from 3-hydroxy-3-methylglutaryl-coenzyme A (HMG-CoA) reductase inhibitors.[96]

As evidenced by these DTC cases, there is no doubt that there has been a narrowing of the learned intermediary doctrine in pharmaceutical liability litigation and the use of the doctrine in failure-to-warn claims.

OFF-LABEL USE AND INFORMED CONSENT

Off-label use involves use for indications not specifically approved by the FDA. It is an accepted principle that once FDA approves a drug for marketing, a physician's discretionary use of that product is not restricted to the uses indicated on FDA-regulated labeling. This is particularly important in the areas of oncology and acquired immunodeficiency syndrome (AIDS), where a significant portion of drug use is off label. While patients and medical innovation, in general, benefit from having doctors informed about off-label uses, off-label use information from manufacturers has been restricted. In fact, manufacturer promotion of off-label use constitutes misbranding under the Food, Drug, and Cosmetic Act (FDCA).[97]

Under the 1997 FDAMA, specifically Section 401, the FDA attempted to strengthen regulation of information pertaining to off-label uses.[98] One requirement under FDAMA was FDA review of material to be disseminated to ensure that it does not pose a significant risk to public health and is not false and misleading.[99] However, the authority of the FDA under the FDAMA to regulate the promotion of off-label uses was successfully challenged and Section 401 ceased to be effective on September 30, 2006.[100] In favoring the commercial free speech doctrine, the court ruled that the FDA had to permit drug company–sponsored advertisements for off-label use, as long as they were directed at physicians and not consumers.[101] In 2009, FDA released a guideline allowing for distribution of reprints about off-label uses from peer-reviewed publications.[102] Major provisions of that Guideline which refer to what is considered "Good Reprint Practices" are found in Table 10–2. FDA agrees that off-label uses by unbiased researchers in bona fide published literature should be discussed.

Moreover, medical science liaisons are permitted to provide off-label information in response to unsolicited medical inquiries. The types of nonpromotional information that can be provided include general education, report of a clinical trial, follow-up to a question originally posed to a sales representative, and advice for formularies. Problematic are responses to inquiries that are not really unsolicited or formulary advice that borders on preapproval promotion (known as new product "seeding").[103] Additionally, pharmaceutical companies may freely distribute to health professionals copies of articles from peer-reviewed professional journals or reference textbooks containing discussions of off-label product usage. However, sales representatives are not permitted to use this information to promote the company's products.

Researchers continually conduct studies to determine new uses for already marketed drugs and effective combinations of drugs for new indications with the results being

| TABLE 10–2. **MAJOR PROVISIONS OF FDA GUIDANCE FOR INDUSTRY—GOOD REPRINT PRACTICES FOR THE DISTRIBUTION OF MEDICAL JOURNAL ARTICLES AND MEDICAL OR SCIENTIFIC REFERENCE PUBLICATIONS ON UNAPPROVED NEW USES OF APPROVED DRUGS**

- Articles should:
  - Be published by an organization with an editorial board.
  - Be peer-reviewed.
  - Be an unabridged reprint, copy of an article, or reference publication.
  - Be accompanied by the approved labeling and, when such information exists, a comprehensive bibliography of well-controlled clinical studies.
  - Be disseminated with a representative publication which reaches contrary or different conclusions.
- Articles should not:
  - Be a special supplement or funded by a manufacturer of the product that is the subject of the article.
  - Be primarily distributed by a manufacturer, but should be generally available via other distribution channels.
  - Be written, edited, excerpted, or published specifically at the request of a manufacturer or edited or influenced by someone having a significant financial relationship with the manufacturer.
  - Be false or misleading or discuss a clinical trial that FDA has indicated is not adequate and well-controlled.
  - Post a significant risk to public health, if relied upon.
  - Be marked, highlighted, summarized or characterized by the manufacturer.
- Not consistent with Good Reprint Practices are:
  - Letters to the editor.
  - Abstracts of a publication.
  - Reports of phase I trials in healthy subjects.
  - Reference publications with little or no substantive discussion of relevant investigation or data.
- Articles should be distributed separately from information that is promotional.
  - They may not be distributed in exhibit halls or during promotional speakers' programs.
- Articles should be accompanied by a prominently displayed and affixed statement disclosing:
  - That the uses are off-label.
  - The manufacturer's interest in the subject drug of the article.
  - Any person known to the manufacturer that has funded the study.
  - All significant risks or safety concerns known to the manufacturer.
  - Any author who has received financial compensation from the manufacturer and the nature and amount of same.

published in the literature. Additionally, with up to 40% of all prescriptions being for off-label use, off-label use comprises a large component of providing DI.[104] These queries are often from physicians seeking evidence to support a particular off-label use. Problems arise when the off-label use is not really off-label, but rather, crosses the line and is experimental (in which case an investigational new drug application[IND] and/or institutional review board [IRB] approval for study is required).[104]

Unfortunately, once an off-label use becomes rampant, the market drives it, and there remains little incentive for the pharmaceutical company to provide more data or conduct further research regarding that off-label use. This disincentive arises not only because of the expense involved in conducting clinical trials but also because trial results could actually have an adverse effect on sales by showing lack of efficacy or safety. For example, it was a study of rofecoxib (Vioxx) for an off-label use that first uncovered the cardiovascular risks that eventually led to market withdrawal.[105]

- Medicare Part B is required to cover off-label uses of drugs in cancer treatment when the use is supported by a citation in at least one of the following references: the *AHFS Drug Information (AHFS-DI)*, *The National Comprehensive Cancer Network's NCCN Drugs and Biologics Compendium*, *Thompson MICROMEDEX DRUGDEX*, or *Clinical Pharmacology* and two or more peer-reviewed articles published in respected medical journals.[106] When providing drug information, it should be realized that not all compendia include revision dates for the monographs. Moreover, a recent study revealed that update policies were not followed, certain off-label indications were excluded without rationale, and for common off-label cancer treatments, old literature and scanty and inconsistent evidence was found in the compendia.[107] Under the Medicare Improvements for Patients and Providers Act of 2008 (MIPPA), the criteria for medically-accepted off-label cancer

- uses are now the same for both Medicare Part B and Part D.[108] For non-cancer Part D drugs, the off-label coverage criteria remain unchanged, that is, limited to indications listed in DRUGDEX and AHFS-DI. Peer review literature still may not be used to support off-label use for non-cancer drugs.

- Following these guidelines for DI queries pertaining to an off-label use would appear to be a prudent practice. Similarly, in providing responses to DI requests pertaining to off-label uses (including usages of off-label dosages), it is prudent to provide complete information, so that a decision may be made whether the information is enough to warrant a particular off-label use. For example, letters to the editor or abstracts would not be complete information. When there is another drug on the market with an approved-label use for the same indication that the off-label product is being considered, the response to the DI request should mention that labeled alternative.[109] Moreover, it is also important to be cognizant of the implications of disseminating off-label information could have in the

- context of patient safety and liability. Responding to consumer requests for information about off-label uses is not advised, simply because, unlike health professionals, most often they are not in a position to evaluate the literature and extrapolate to a particular situation.

Off-label use of pharmaceuticals has resulted in liability. Recently, for example, physicians have been the target of lawsuits involving coadministration of insulin with rosiglitazone (Avantia) before the combination was approved by FDA, and included in the labeling.

While there is no question that patients should be advised if a proposed treatment is truly investigational or experimental, off-label use is not necessarily experimental or investigational, and informed consent is not necessary whenever an off-label use is proposed.[110] Federal-informed consent regulations governing investigational drugs do not apply to off-label use.[111] State-informed consent laws vary but usually require discussion of the nature, risks, benefits, and alternative modes of treatment. For example, the New York statute states:

> Lack of informed consent means the failure to the person providing the professional treatment or diagnosis to disclose to the patient such alternatives thereto and the reasonably foreseeable risks and benefits involved as a reasonable medical...practitioner under similar circumstances would have disclosed, in a manner permitting the patient to make a knowledgeable evaluation.[112]

Actions for informed consent are, therefore, limited to the nondisclosure of medical information. However, failure to disclose FDA status does not raise a material issue of fact as to informed consent.

Liability Concerns for Web 2.0 Information

❹ *DI is currently being obtained from a number of Wikis, blogs, and search engines and there is possibility of DI liability for information obtained from the Internet and electronic journals.* Google Scholar, Wikipedia, Rx Wiki, PubDrug, and Web citations in general are increasingly being accessed for handling DI queries. Recently, these sources have appeared as references in publications.[113] More than 25% of the Internet's content involves health care and medical information.[114] The surfer can now expect to find full prescribing information for most heavily marketed drugs. The situation is complicated by links to investigational products or investigational uses and vice versa. The question is whether this is promotion of off-label uses.[115]

Liability concerns arise in the area of whether a manufacturer's Web site content is considered labeling or advertising. It appears to be necessary to distinguish between Internet promotion directed to health professionals and consumers. DTC advertising on the Internet is considered labeling, rather than advertising and, as such, FDA has principal authority to regulate it.[116]

On February 2004, the FDA issued new industry guidelines, entitled *Help-Seeking and Other Disease Awareness Communications by or on Behalf of Drug and Device Firms* and *Brief Summary: Disclosing Risk Information in Consumer-Directed Print Advertisements*. While these guidelines are intended to improve the brief summaries of side effects that must be included in DTC advertising, they do not address Internet ads. The FDA has not issued guidelines on DTC advertising via the Internet. In fact, the FDA has stopped work on a planned guidance on Internet drug promotional activities because the Internet is changing so rapidly. FDA now believes existing regulations can be followed.[79] For example, a drug's black box warning should be configured "prominently" on the Internet. A person should not have to click multiple times to get this important information. Additionally, there are liability risks inherent in DTC advertising via the Internet, mainly because the risks are ill-defined by sparse FDA guidance and judicial precedence commingled with jurisdictional and extraterritoriality issues.

QUALITY OF INFORMATION

Not all Web sites are reputable and currently there is no way to discriminate which sites providing DI are authoritative and which are not. Problems have arisen such as hyperlink obsolescence, defunct Web sites, broken links, altered content, and an inability to determine currency.[113] Moreover, it is common for Web sites to change or move. Entries in Wikipedia, an encyclopedia project, recently ranked as one of the top 10 sites visited, can be the subject of erroneous entries, fraud, conflict of interest, or even criminal mischief.[117] For example, pharmaceutical companies may edit or delete their product information as the site is user edited. Thus, sites such as Wikipedia are not authoritative and can only be supplementary to, rather than the sole source of, drug information.[118] Google Scholar includes both published and nonpublished (hence not peer-reviewed) information and, unlike PubMed, it may not contain the latest literature. However, as the number of Internet-only journals not indexed in PubMed increases there will be increased reliance on Google Scholar as an easy-to-use source for locating primary literature. In fact, in a recent comparison with PubMed, no significant differences were found regarding the number of primary literature articles. PubMed did retrieve more specific articles.[119]

What about DI liability for information obtained from the Internet and electronic journals? Is there a possibility of pharmacist liability occurring via cyberspace? As mentioned above, the Internet contains a growing hodgepodge of sources with little organization and uneven credibility. In fact, material on the Internet may contain innocent mistakes and/or deliberate fraud, as well as outdated material. Several situations may result in search results that are not comprehensive. Examples include faulty search strategies and failing to search for historical information. Many databases including PubMed do not contain material prior to the 1940s. Searchers may not even be aware that pre-Internet or old non-electronic material exists. Old Medline articles from 1949 through 1965 may not be updated with MESH terms and may not contain searchable abstracts.[120] For e-books (e.g., online textbooks) with their own built-in search engine (e.g. Merck Manual), there is a possibility of patient harm occurring where the computer malfunctions.

● Currently, there are no laws pertaining to, and no means for, ensuring the accuracy of information posed on the Internet. It is possible for information on the Internet to be false, misleading, corrupted by an outside source, or otherwise harmful to the reader to apply it to their specific situation. There is a potential for misinformation to be disseminated, while the reader unknowingly assumes the information to be accurate and true via the Internet and related technologies.

The Health Summit Working Group, which consists of professional societies including ASHP, and the Health on the Net Foundation (HON) are currently working to improve
● the quality of DI on the Internet. The Health Summit Working Group is developing an interactive tool to use in evaluating quality of DI on the World Wide Web available at http://www.ahrq.gov/data/infoqual.htm. HON has developed a code for quality and reliability, which, if displayed, increases the likelihood that the information is reliable. The *Journal of Medical Internet Research* requires authors to archive their Web references at http://www.webcitation.org before including them in manuscripts. Also, the application of the National Information Infrastructure to consumer health information is one of the priorities of the federal government. Examples of Web site QA criteria are included in Table 10–1 and are found in Chapter 3.

Another venue where the quality of drug information may be suspect is e-mail communication. Both the American Medical Association and the American Medical Informatics Association have issued guidelines for physicians using e-mail to communicate
● with patients.[121] These guidelines, available at https://www.amia.org/mbrcenter/wg/ kim/docs/email_guidelines.html and http://www.ama-assn.org/ama/pub/about-ama/ our-people/member-groups-sections/young-physicians-section/advocacy-resources/ guidelines-physician-patient-electronic-communications.shtml, encourage physicians to be cautious when using e-mail because of the possibility of liability due to misunderstanding and privacy concerns.[122] Perhaps in the near future, health insurers will cover calls made to online pharmacists providing DI, much the same way as Medicare now covers teleconferencing.

The Internet is at the forefront of future practice, where pharmacists will consult with each other, thereby learning from one another and benefiting their DI clients and patients.[123] Web 2.0 is the term commonly associated since 2004 with Web applications that facilitate interactive information sharing, such as wikis, blogs, hosted-services, and networking sites. Specific examples include the University Health System Consortium
● and Google Scholar. In the fast-paced practice of DI, Web 2.0 information may provide a quick starting point for an answer to a query. However, other non-Web-based references should also be consulted. DI professionals should never rely solely on a Google Scholar retrieved search to respond to a DI query. Additionally, when using Web citations, it is recommended to include the date accessed to provide readers with some indication of how current the information is (refer to Appendix 9–3).

TELEMEDICINE AND CYBERMEDICINE

Legal issues are emerging from e-health technologies, such as telemedicine and cyber-medicine programs. Telemedicine is defined as the use of telecommunications and inter-active video technology to provide health care services to patients who are at a distance. Cybermedicine is a broader concept that includes the marketing, relationship creation, advice, prescribing, and selling pharmaceuticals and devices in cyberspace. Therefore, *telepharmacy* is a subset of *telemedicine*, and the terms are used interchangeably here. As telemedicine and cybermedicine expand, questions regarding liability for pharmacists providing DI on the Internet will need to be addressed. For example, health professionals, such as pharmacists, are licensed by states. Which state law applies when the pharmacist is located in New York, the patient is in Florida, and the Web site is maintained by a com-pany in California? Who is liable for technical problems that make it impossible for the information to be received in a timely manner or for breaches of confidentiality caused by those who would invade private files? Already some sites offer fee-based live physician offices and nurse triage services (e.g. OptumHealth Care Services) for self-diagnosis and health screening. Additionally, some DI centers provide information over the Internet.

Although the courts have yet to test liability for medical malpractice involving the practice of pharmacy or medicine on the Internet, such a case is bound to surface soon. The most important determination of whether there is such malpractice is whether or not a health care provider-patient relationship has been created by the consultation in the absence of physical contact. Hard copy printouts of Internet discussions would be discov-erable before trial and could be uncovered in the defendant's computer files by a plaintiff's attorney. It is likely that where a physician consults with a pharmacist for DI via telemedi-cine, the pharmacist will not be deemed to have established a pharmacist-patient relation-ship. Telephone consultations between physicians are most analogous and have not been held to create a physician-patient relationship.[124] Similarly, as previously mentioned, no pharmacist-physician relationship has been found based on a provision of DI to the physi-cian.[28] This is largely because of the public policy interest of promoting consultations, professional association, and education, as well as the assumed limited information con-veyed to the consulting physician. However, in view of advancing technology where the patient's entire medical history and test results are available on the computer, this situa-tion may change, especially where a consultation fee is involved. Also, where a pharmacist posts a Web site and is paid to provide drug information, the courts will surely find such cybermedical consultation to create a pharmacist-patient relationship.

Although there have been several lawsuits for false information on online bulletin boards (e.g., USENET News, CompuServe), the basis of these lawsuits has been defama-tion, not malpractice.[125,126] The offering of general medical advice and judgments online (e.g., chat rooms) does not appear to be creating a formal physician-patient relationship.

Nor does it appear that the giving of generic advice will generate liability for either the provider or the publisher. If, however, the information is fraudulent or quackery, then courts do have authority under both state and federal computer statutes to stop the activity. Similarly, Internet (or telephone) medical call centers, or triage services used by some health care plans can expect to be held liable when misdiagnosis occurs. On the other hand, liability is lessened where Internet discussions resemble an academic conference between health care providers, rather than a formal consultancy. Similarly, the issuance of a disclaimer in writing with the original subscription and with each message written may help insulate from any liability.

Some Web sites now carry disclaimers to protect the authors from liability. The limitation of the remedies available should be displayed prominently. A cap equal to the price of the service sold may be included. The following is an example: "Please read this agreement entirely and carefully before assessing this Web site. By accessing the site, you agree to be bound by the terms and conditions below. If you do not wish to be bound by these terms and conditions, you may not access or use this site. Our maximum liability to you under all circumstances will be equal to the purchase price you paid for any goods, services, or information." This statement is then followed by disclaimers pertaining to accuracy, currency, copyright, no medical advise, no warranties, a disclaimer of endorsement, disclaimer regarding liability for third-party content, and a general disclaimer of liability including negligence with a statement that the user assumes all responsibility and risk for use.[127] It may also be desirable to include a provision that any dispute will be brought in the city of the site owner's principal place of business.

FRAUD AND ABUSE

Another consideration pertains to fraud and abuse laws, such as the antikickback laws.[128] The antikickback statute prohibits physicians participating in the Medicaid and Medicare programs from submitting any false remuneration, "including any kickback, bribe, or rebate" to induce referrals of patients.[129] Certain aspects of e-health promotional and marketing tools, such as per click payment arrangements, are particularly susceptible to violation of the antikickback statute. The violation occurs because the health care provider is receiving remuneration based on the referral rate provided by the fee charged per click. Likewise, promotional banners on a health care organization or pharmacist's Web site that link to a pharmacy or other type of patient care items are most likely in violation because the referring provider is receiving a benefit (i.e., per click arrangements involve the payment of a fee based on the clicking on a particular link on a Web site) in exchange for referrals.[130] Similarly, the provision of free e-mail services, online publications, computer equipment, or other types of computer ventures are in violation of the antikickback statute when these companies sell items or services reimbursable under Medicaid or Medicare programs.

Another area of uncertainty pertains to the handling of links between Web pages. A link is any component of a Web page that connects to another Web page. The issue of whether pharmaceutical manufacturers will be liable for material posted on sites they have not sponsored, but have merely linked to their own, is yet to be decided in the courts.

At least according to cases over the past few years, mere hyperlinking does not constitute copyright or trademark infringement.[131] Copyright law does not require that permission be obtained for linking, but if there is copyrighted graphic material, you will be reproducing and displaying copyrighted material you do not own. You need the copyright owner's permission to use the graphic image, unless your use is fair use (fair use is discussed further under the section for copyright law). Where the information being linked to is violating the copyright law, it is also possible that a Web site owner who links to a site containing infringing material may be liable for contributory copyright infringement. Contributory copyright infringement is established when a defendant, with knowledge of another's infringing activity, causes or materially contributes to the infringing conduct.

Moreover, whether deep linking (i.e., bypassing the homepage and linking to an internal page of the linked site) is copyright infringement is currently unclear.[132] However, if a Web page specifically states, "ask permission before linking," it is possible that linking to the site without the owner's permission may be trespass or breach of contract where there are terms of use that were agreed to.[133]

Additionally, certain businesses, who do not want their valuable content associated with or connected to certain sites, have brought legal action under theories of trademark, defamation, disparagement, unfair competition, false advertising, invasion of privacy, and other laws. In *Playboy Enterprises, Inc. v. Universal Tel-A-Talk, Inc.*, an X-rated Web site linked to the Playboy Web site.[134] Playboy sued and proved that users of the site may be confused as to whether Playboy sponsored or endorsed the adult site. Playboy also proved that its trademark bunny logo would be blurred or tarnished by the association with the adult site. Also, in *Coca-Cola Co v. Purdy*, the court entered judgment for several well-known trademark owners on their infringement claims where an antiabortionist used a host of domain names incorporating their famous marks.[135] The antiabortionist linked the domain names (e.g., *mycoca-cola.com*) with a Web site associated with *abortionismurder.com*. According to the decision, the "quick and effortless nature of 'surfing' the Internet makes it unlikely that consumers can avoid confusion through the exercise of due care."[136]

The practice of using framing to incorporate third-party content into a Web site is also an area of unsettled law. The framing site can surround the framed pages with its own advertising, logos, or promotions. Framing may trigger a dispute under copyright and trademark law theories because a framed site arguably alters the appearance of the content and creates the impression that its owner endorses or voluntarily chooses to associate with the framer.[137] However, liability for framing has not been fully or clearly resolved by the courts.[138]

Advances in technology may render this dilemma moot. Technology now exists to keep undesired links or frames off a Web site. In any event, it is advisable not to link to or frame another Web site without the express permission of that site. However, if a Web site owner is concerned about liability for links or frames, a prominently placed disclaimer may be added. Additionally, if you want to obtain permission before linking to your site, post a request permission notice and require users to agree to the terms by clicking "I agree" on your homepage.

The Internet raises a variety of legal issues, most of which are unresolved but evolving. Future goals should be for pharmaceutical manufacturers to promote their products to consumers more responsibly, for the FDA to regulate DTC advertising more effectively, and for the medical and pharmacy communities to educate the public about prescription drugs more constructively.

Intellectual Property Rights

COPYRIGHT

The current copyright law is codified at 17 U.S.C.A. § 101 *et seq*. A copyright is a property right in an original work of authorship that is fixed in tangible form.[139] It is a statutory requirement that literary, dramatic, and musical works, for example, must have been recorded or produced in some physical object (or fixed) before copyright can subsist. A copyright holder in a work is granted certain exclusive rights to control use of the work created. A work of authorship must be original in order to qualify for copyright protection. This requirement has two facets. First, the author must have engaged in some intellectual endeavor of his own, and not just have copied from a preexisting source. Second, the work must exhibit a minimal amount of creativity. Copyright protection covers both published and unpublished works. Also, the fact that the previously published work is out of print does not affect its copyright. Works of authorship under copyright and items not entitled to copyright are found in Table 10–3.

❺ *Pharmacists providing DI must have a working knowledge of copyright law both to avoid liability and to protect their own literary works.* Under the 1976 Copyright Act, an author is protected as soon as a work is recorded in some concrete way. The process of registering for a copyright involves depositing material with the Copyright Office to be reviewed by an examiner, followed by publication with a copyright notice, usually the symbol ©. Under the Copyright Term Extension Act (CTEA) of 1998, such work is protected until 70 years after the death of the author or for 95 years for corporate copyright holders.

TABLE 10–3. COPYRIGHT PROTECTION

Works of authorship entitled to copyright protection include the following:
Literary works
Musical works, including any accompanying words
Dramatic works, including any accompanying music
Pantomimes and choreographic works
Pictorial, graphic, and sculptural works
Motion pictures and other audiovisual works
Sound recordings
Architectural works
The following are not entitled to copyright protection:
Ideas, concepts, principles, or discovery
Procedures, processes, systems, methods of operation
Mere compilations of facts

In effect, the CTEA retroactively extended copyright terms by twenty years.[140] The constitutionality of CTFA has been challenged and upheld by the Supreme Court. The author or copyright owner has the exclusive right to make copies of the work, control derivative works or adaptations, and sue for damages and injunctive relief (an injunction is a judicial remedy issued in order to prohibit a party from doing or continuing to do a certain activity) against infringers. Public domain works may be copied and distributed without copyright permission. Works of the U.S. government (e.g., General Accounting Office [GAO] reports, Congressional Record, FDA releases) are considered part of the public domain.

Ownership of copyright usually rests with the author at the time the work is created. The exception is a work made for hire (i.e. "a work prepared by an employee within the scope of the employment relationship, or is a work specially ordered or commissioned for use as a contribution to a collective work, as part of a motion picture or other audiovisual work, as a translation, as a supplementary work, as a compilation, as an instructional text, as a test, as an answer material for a test, or as an atlas, if the parties expressly agree in a written instrument signed by them that the work shall be a work made for hire").[141] Another exception is the first-sale doctrine, which in effect, permits intralibrary loan of materials. Under the first-sale doctrine, a person who legitimately owns a copy of a work is one who purchased the work or otherwise acquired ownership of the work with the permission of the copyright owner, and has full authority to "sell or otherwise dispose of the possession of that copy."[142]

Since the Berne Convention in 1989, the copyright formalities of registration and notice have lost almost all their legal significance. Registration, although not mandatory, affords the copyright claimant certain advantages. For example, it prevents an infringer from pleading innocent infringement. Similarly, the only substantive legal effect of copyright registration is that attorney fees and statutory damages are only recoverable for postregistration infringements. That is, U.S. authors must register before bringing suit. But for works prior to 1989 and the Berne Convention, copyright can be lost if notice was omitted and that omission was not cured within 5 years of publication by registration and affixation of notice to the remaining copies.

Under the fair use provision of the 1976 Copyright Act, if a use is fair, permission of the copyright owner need not be received, nor royalties paid. Fair use is determined by a four-pronged test: (1) nature and character of use, (2) nature of the work, (3) the proportional amount copied, and, most importantly, (4) the effect on the market for the copied work.[143]

The first factor in the fair use analysis is the nature and character of the use. Uses for research, teaching, scholarship, and news reporting are more likely to be considered fair than strictly commercial uses. In addition, there is a narrow special exemption for educators. The mere fact that the use is educational and not for profit does not insulate the use from a finding of infringement.

The second factor in the fair use analysis is the nature of the work. This factor centers on whether a copyrighted work is creative or informational, and whether it is published or unpublished. The scope of fair use is greater when the copyrighted work is informational, because it is generally recognized that there is a greater need to disseminate factual material than works of fiction or fantasy.[144] An unpublished work is given greater copyright protection than a published work and is, therefore, less likely to be subjected to a valid assertion of fair use.[145] In *Harper & Row Publishers, Inc. v. Nation Enterprises, Nation* obtained an unauthorized manuscript of former President Ford's memoirs before they were published in a book form under a contract with Harper & Row. The fact that President Ford's memoirs had not yet been published by the time *Nation* published them was a deciding factor.[146] That is, in looking at the nature of the work, an unpublished work seems to be entitled to greater protection than a published work.

The third factor is the amount copied. There does not appear to be a minimal amount or threshold quantity (e.g., five sentences) standard where fair use will be presumed. Although the statute itself does not set the maximum standards for educational fair use, Classroom Guidelines have been agreed upon by educational, author, and publisher organizations.[147] Multiple copies for classroom use, but not to exceed in any event more than one copy per pupil in a course, are permissible, provided each copy bears a copyright notice and meets the test of (1) brevity, (2) spontaneity, and (3) cumulative effect. For example, to meet the test of brevity the Classroom Guidelines prohibit multiple copying of complete articles longer than 2500 words. They prohibit copying excerpts longer than 1000 words or 10% of the work, whichever is shorter. For motion media, up to 10% or 3 minutes, whichever is shorter. For motion media, up to 10% or 3 minutes, whichever is less, in the aggregate of a copyrighted motion media work may be reproduced or otherwise incorporated as part of an educational multimedia project. To meet the test of spontaneity, the copying must be at the instance and inspiration of the individual teacher, where the teacher's decision to use the work in class does not allow for a timely reply to request for permission. To meet the cumulative effect requirement, the copying must be for only one course in the school, and except for current news periodicals, newspapers, and current news sections of periodicals, only one article or two excerpts therefrom may be copied from the same author, or three excerpts from the same collective work or periodical volume. Additionally, the copying must be for only one class term; and no more than nine instances of such multiple copying for one course during one class term. In other words, the copied material may only be used for one semester and permission for longer use must be obtained. Further, students may not be charged for the copy beyond the actual cost of photocopying.

Case Study 10–3

You are publishing a guide regarding "do not crush" drugs for which you will receive compensation. You are merely listing all drugs which should not be crushed. However, the material for this publication is derived from a number of published references, all of which are copyright protected. You adopt an entire table from one of the articles without permission. You also take several direct sentences without providing any source reference. One of the references you are using is out of print.

- Which of these acts would constitute a violation of the copyright law? What steps should have been taken to avoid copyright violation?

In *Association of American Publishers v. New York University* the issue was the production and distribution of custom-made anthologies sold to students. Although the classroom guidelines allow students to make single copies for personal use, the court found infringement when anthologies were sold for profit.[148] The action was settled with the adoption of certain procedures by New York University.

The fourth factor in a fair use analysis is the impact the infringing work will have on the market or potential market of the copyrighted work. The Supreme Court has decided that all four factors of the fair use test should be given equal weight.[149] Under the Copyright Act of 1976, these four fair use factors provide a broad and flexible defense against copyright infringement.

Fair use is an equitable defense to copyright infringement, determined by the courts on a case-by-case basis. Unfortunately, in court decisions on educational photocopying to date, the ruling in almost every case has been against fair use. Copying by nonprofit medical libraries has been held to be a fair use where the photocopying of medical journals by federal nonprofit institutions was made solely for the purpose of medical research. In *Williams & Wilkins Co. v. United States*, the library was copying a single copy for each request, and the court found that "medical science would be seriously hurt if such library photocopying were stopped."[150] In *Williams & Wilkins*, the copying of medical journals was by two governmental libraries: the National Institutes of Health and the National Medical library, a repository of much of the world's medical literature.[151] The public benefits of fair use apparently held considerably more weight than any commercial considerations presented before the courts. However, where the photocopying of medical journals by scientists occurred in a large for-profit company, the court decided the making of unauthorized copies of copyrighted articles published in scientific journals for use by research scientists was not fair use. The court determined that the publishers had created through the Copyright Clearance Center, Inc., a viable market for institutional users to obtain licenses to allow photocopying of individual articles. However, in *Princeton University Press v. Michigan Document Services, Inc.,* the court held that a copy shop selling coursepacks, which are compilations of various copyrighted and uncopyrighted materials such as journal articles, sample test questions, course notes, and book excerpts, infringed the copyrights of several publishers.[152] In deciding this was not a fair use, the court noted that the copying was substantial and commercial. Similarly, in *Basic Books v. Kinko's Graphic Corp.,* the court held that a copy shop's reproduction and sale of coursepacks to students was not a fair use of the copyrighted material.[153]

Course management systems and digital coursepacks that post copyrighted articles, book excerpts, and research data are used today by 90% of U.S. colleges and universities. Simply because the material is online does not mean it is free from copyright protection. Unless fair use or some other exemption applies, permission is required before posting.[154] When fair use does not apply, the institution must obtain permission from the rights-holder, who may charge a fee for such permission based on the amount of content and the number of people, usually students, who will view the content. Additionally, reporting of the same material for use in a subsequent semester requires a new permission. Moreover, it violates the intent and spirit of copyright law to use course management systems as a substitute for the purchase of books, subscriptions, or other materials when substantial portions of the material are required for educational purposes. When scanning in paper materials (such as textbooks) to create electronic copies, be sure you are using legally obtained copies of the work, either purchased or owned by the institution. All posted materials in a course management system should contain both the copyright notice from, and complete citation to, the original material, as well as a caution against further electronic distribution.[154] Instant permission may be obtained at http://www.copyright.com though the Copyright Clearance Center for use in course management systems, coursepacks, e-reserves, classroom handouts, and other formats.

The court has also ruled that there is only a limited copyright protection available to a compilation of works written by another author. In *Silverstein v. Penguin Putnam*, the plaintiff had compiled a collection of 122 unpublished Dorothy Parker poems.[155] He presented the compilation to Penguin, which rejected it and subsequently inserted the poems into a new edition of Parker's work published by Penguin. The court held that Silverstein would not be entitled to injunctive relief as he did not hold the copyrights on the poems, as his efforts to gather the poems were not protectable in copyright. Additionally, the court looked at Silverstein's arrangement of the poems and found that Penguin did not copy his arrangement.

Recently, in *Warner Bros. Ent'mt, Inc. v. RDR Books*, a lexicon of terms from the *Harry Potter* series of books, initially posted on a free Internet Web site and then scheduled for publication, was held as copyright infringement.[156] The legal issues involved were whether there is a distinction in the law between digital and printed copyright and what is a third party's right to create a new reference book designed to help others better understand the original work, that is, a study guide. The court held the print version of the lexicon was not a derivative work, especially in view of the number of places where copying was deemed excessive. However, the court explicitly stated that authors do not have the right to stop the publication of reference guides and companion works.

Copyright infringement requires a showing of copying, which can be proven circumstantially by demonstrating that the defendant had access to the copyrighted work and that the defendant's work is substantially similar to that work. Copyright infringement for purposes of commercial advantage or private financial gain is punishable under 18 U.S.C. §2319. Although the Act allows for damages of as much as $100,000 per infringement, innocent infringers (e.g., educators and universities) may be entitled to a remission of statutory damages. They are only liable for actual damages, such as profits earned by the infringer or profits denied to the copyright holder. This provision lowers the incentive for the publishing industry to sue. Recently, publishers have resorted to unsavory tactics in their attempts to control educational copying, such as the sending of letters threatening to sue copy shops for infringement unless they agree to pay royalties.

Newsletter copying is strictly prohibited, and violators risk not only the statutory damages ($100,000) but can also be subject to criminal penalties. These newsletters require a fee to be paid to the Copyright Clearance Center even for internal or personal copying and offer rewards to those who report violations. Washington Business Information, Inc. has won major payments in infringement actions against pharmaceutical manufacturers for photocopying its *Food & Drug Letter*.

Section 201(c) of the Copyright Act has produced electronic copyright issues for freelance articles and photography in electronic databases. Specifically, a series of cases involves whether or not permission is required from authors to place their articles on commercial databases or in the electronic public domain (e.g. MEDLINE). In *New York Times v. Tasini*, the U.S. Supreme Court ruled that publishers cannot republish printed works on CD-ROMs and in electronic databases without obtaining permission from authors.[157] *Tasini* should not have much impact on new work as most publisher agreements now address electronic publication rights. Problematic, however, are older works published without a written agreement. The publishers argued unsuccessfully that the use of the articles in a database was no different from issuing a microfilm or microfiche copy of a newspaper. However, permissibility of electronic republication of an entire issue of a newspaper, magazine, newsletter without further payment to authors remains unresolved.[158] Rather than attempt to contact freelancers and offer compensation for articles, some database producers have already begun to purge their databases of freelance contributions.

Photocopies fall within the territory of the Copyright Act. When sending copies of original articles, a statement to the effect that the copies are only for personal or private use must be made. The most effective way for any DI facility to protect itself against copy infringement lawsuits is to copy the page with the copyright notice and stamp the first page of the copies with a statement that the enclosed document is protected by copyright, thus putting the burden of responsibility on the recipient of the one copy. Such a notice might state, *"This material is subject to the United States Copyright Law (17 U.S. Code): unauthorized copying may be prohibited by law."*

The Computer Software Act of 1980 amended the Copyright Act to extend protection to computer software. However, copyright laws do not provide sufficient protection for information transmitted over the Internet and other information networks. Although copyright protection applies when copyrighted material is converted into a digital form, the havoc that cyberspace can wreak on copyright owner's rights cannot be overestimated. A debate is currently raging over whether existing copyright law can successfully adapt to the Internet.

Google recently settled two class action lawsuits regarding application of copyright protection to the indexing of scanned documents.[159] The lawsuits involve the Google Library Project where in 2004, the company announced it has entered into agreement with several libraries to digitalize books and other documents from those libraries' collections. The books and documents were also to be indexed for search purposes. Thus, the legal question arises of whether indexing for search purposes is fair use. Google was sued by publishers and authors when attempting to create an unprecedented extensive digitalized library of books. The authors and publishers claimed the scanning and indexing was not fair use but commercial in nature.[160] Since the case was settled and not decided by

TABLE 10–4. MAJOR PROVISIONS OF THE TEACH ACT

- Expanded range of allowed works. (e.g., nondramatic literary works; nondramatic musical works; audiovisual works).
- Expanded receiving locations. Educational institutions may now reach students through distance education at any location.
- Storage of transmitted content. Allows retention of the content and student access for a brief period of time especially with regard to digital transmission systems.
- Allows for digitalizing of analog works but only if the work is not already available in digital form.
- Educational institutions must now institute policies regarding copyright, although the details of content of those policies are not provided.
- Transmission of content must be made solely to students officially enrolled in a course for which the transmission is made. Technological restrictions on access are required.

a court, the question of the legal fair defense of unauthorized copying of the works remains unresolved.

On October 3, 2002, Congress enacted the Technology, Education, and Copyright Harmonization (TEACH) Act, fully revising §110(2) of the U.S. Copyright Act governing the lawful uses of existing copyright materials in distance education. The TEACH Act defines the conditions and circumstances on which educators may clip pieces of text, images, sound, and other works and include them in distance education. Table 10–4 outlines the key provisions of the TEACH Act. If a particular use does not fit these conditions, one may still consider whether the use is a fair use.[161]

Access to works on the Internet does not automatically mean that these can be reproduced and reused without permission or royalty payment, and, furthermore, some copyrighted works may have been posted on the Internet without authorization of the copyright holder. With the ease of electronic retrieval of material, copyright holders are likely to uncover those who are violating their copyright. Publishers who did not previously press for royalty payments of small segments of works can now trace the borrowing of snippets of text and create systems of payment and collection. Research downloading, with deletion of material after use, appears to be a fair use of the material. However, downloading to create a personal database and avoid payment of connect fees and higher user fees is illegal unless covered under special agreements between the database owner and subscriber. Further, although the Berne Convention is the principal copyright treaty, there is no such thing as an International copyright. The treaty obligates signatory countries to extend the protection of their copyright law to foreigners whose works are infringed within their borders.[162]

Current copyright law denies protection to compilations of facts unless such facts are arranged or organized with some minimal element of originality. Even then, it is the creative aspect of such arrangements or organization that may be protected and not the underlying facts themselves. Legislation has been repeatedly introduced, advocated primarily by large database companies, aimed at codifying into law a new unique form of intellectual property protection for databases. The situation is different in Europe where the European Union (EU) 1996 Database Directive grants copyright protection for the selection and arrangement of information in a European database, and calls downloading and hyperlinking unfair extraction of information.

Related to copyright infringement is plagiarism and fictitious reporting. Plagiarism is a legal offense or crime. The owner of a copyright (e.g., author) could sue the plagiarist in federal court for violation of the copyright. Fictitious reporting may simply constitute poor journalism, or it may rise to the level of fraud or libel. Plagiarism involves not citing material while fictitious reporting involves citing things that do not exist.

The definition of *plagiarism* is subjective and vague. History, facts, and ideas are not copyrighted, although they may be plagiarized. The addition of original material by the plagiarist in no way excuses the act of plagiarism. In fact, trivial changes in copies of text in an attempt to avoid copyright infringement are specifically prohibited by the copyright law. Additionally, there is no fixed number or percentage of words that can be used without exposure to charges of plagiarism.[163] Verbatim quotes are permitted, provided they fall within the fair use protection. Software and Web-based technologies (e.g., Turnitin) now exist that can scan millions of documents almost instantly to compare what has been written before to what is being written today. Further information on plagiarism is contained in Chapter 9.

Privacy

HEALTH INSURANCE PORTABILITY AND ACCOUNTABILITY ACT OF 1996

6 *It is important to keep in mind that the HIPAA Privacy Rule is not intended to disrupt or discourage adverse event reporting or DI in any way.*

Information security concerns are at the forefront of legal issues involved in electronic communications, specifically, questions of authenticity of medical or pharmacy records and confidentiality or privacy of the contents of medical and personal information of patients. Today an individual's health information is often used for payment, QA, research, peer-review, accreditation, and a multitude of other purposes. In realizing that this creates significant privacy and security concerns, Congress enacted the Health Insurance Portability Act of 1996 (HIPAA).[164] HIPAA's security standards are intended to protect the security of the environment in which health care information is maintained and transmitted. For pharmacies, the security standards are applicable only to electronic protected health information, not paper, facsimile, nor telephone transmissions. HIPAA's privacy standards govern the use and disclosure of protected health information. Many aspects of HIPAA fall outside the scope of this chapter. In any event, reasonable steps should always be taken to ensure that fax transmissions are sent to and received by the intended recipient. Examples of such steps include confirming with the intended recipient that the receiving fax machine is located in a secure area or the intended recipient is waiting by the fax machine; pre-programming and testing fax numbers for frequent recipients of DI faxes to avoid errors associated with misdialing; double-checking the recipient's fax number prior to transmission; using a fax cover sheet with statement of procedures to follow in case of an erroneous transmission and advising the erroneous recipient to notify the sender immediately and arrange for return or destruction of the fax; promptly checking all fax confirmation sheets to determine that faxed material was received at the intended fax number.

Individually identifiable health information is information, including demographic data, that relates to the individual's past, present, or future physical or mental health or condition; the provision of health care to the individual, or the past, present, or future payment for the provision of health care to the individual; and that identifies the individual or for which there is a reasonable basis to believe it can be used to identify the individual.[165] Individually identifiable health information includes many common identifiers such as name, address, birth date, and Social Security number.

However, there are no restrictions on the use or disclosure of de-identified health information.[166] De-identified health information neither identifies nor provides a reasonable basis to identify an individual. There are two methods for de-identifying protected health information: the statistical method and the safe-harbor method via removal of certain identifiers.[167] De-identified data sets, which separate individuals' identities from their protected health information, are becoming increasingly available through the Centers for Medicare and Medicaid Services and the National Institutes of Health.[168] These data are proving useful for outcomes and medical error research not associated with the original data collection protocol.

Under HIPAA, a covered entity may engage in research activities in four ways: (1) by using or disclosing only de-identified information, (2) by obtaining an authorization from the individual to use and disclose the information for research purposes, (3) by obtaining a waiver of an authorization from an IRB, or (4) by representing that the use or disclosure is solely of the protected health information of a deceased individual. Clinical investigators are most likely to choose option 3.[169]

HIPAA specifically permits covered entities such as pharmacists, physicians, or hospitals to report adverse events and other information related to the quality, effectiveness, and safety of FDA-regulated products to both the manufacturers and directly to FDA. Under this exception, a pharmacist need not obtain an authorization from a patient before notifying a pharmaceutical company and FDA that the patient had an adverse reaction to a drug manufactured by the drug company.[170]

In responding to DI questions it is of utmost importance to obtain specific patient identification information including, but not limited to, patient name, age, height, weight, or medical record number. Nothing in HIPPA would diminish or affect that responsibility. In the DI arena, HIPPA allows disclosure of patient information for treatment, payment, and health care operations. Examples of health care operations include quality management, QA, outcomes evaluation, development of clinical guidelines, peer-review, and credentialing. While not specifically mentioned, DI would appear to fall under both treatment and health care operations. In most instances, HIPPA should not affect DI requests from health care providers as patient identity is usually not required or is provided via medical record number only. However, when patient identifying information is communicated, protection of information within the DI center (or pharmacy) is an important HIPPA requirement. Policies and procedures governing use and disclosure of confidential information should be in place. These policies should include guidance on training and strategies for mitigating risks during all stages of the DI request processing (receipt, triage, and response). For example, procedures should be in place to verify the identity of the requestor of information. Patient information security safeguards should be in place, for example, requiring personal identifiers to be removed as soon as feasible, physical controls, software controls, and formal oversight.[171]

Case Study 10–4

A drug information question involves a patient who has a socially stigmatic disease. In responding to the question, the pharmacist needs to share the patient's personally identifiable health information with the laboratory and pharmacokinetic services. However, in sharing this information the pharmacist discusses it as well as the diagnosis in an area where it was easily overheard by others not entitled to know. Additionally, the patient's personal information is faxed by the pharmacist to a fax machine in an unsecured area where many people had access to the fax machine.

- Does HIPPA prohibit any of the pharmacist's actions?
- What safeguards should be taken when discussing the patient and the patient's information?
- What reasonable steps are necessary to ensure that fax transmissions are sent and received by the intended recipient?

There are several other situations in pharmacy practice where HIPAA compliance issues may be triggered. For example, in clinical case reports, whether for publication or teaching purposes, the patient should only be referred to by initials, age, or sex (e.g., RM, a 35-year-old female). HIPAA permits a pharmacist to counsel individuals other than the patient (e.g. a friend, family member, or neighbor picking up the patient's prescription) even though some of the patient's protected health information may be revealed in such a situation. However, the regulation is clear that such disclosures must be limited and should only be made when the provider believes it is in the patient's best interest. For example, there can be no doubt that disclosing that the medication picked up is for treatment of HIV infection would not be necessary. Under HIPAA, personal representatives, defined as individuals legally authorized, under state or other applicable law, to make health care decisions on behalf of a patient, are to be treated in the same way as a patient. However, in some cases the personal representatives' authority is limited to a specific matter, such as treatment for a life-threatening illness. In these cases, the personal representative may only access protected health information directly related to that illness. Additionally, many states have enacted laws that protect persons with illnesses that are seen as particularly stigmatizing, such as HIV, mental illness, and drug addiction. The Public Health Service Act and implementing regulations govern the confidentiality of substance abuse records maintained by federally assisted drug and alcohol abuse programs.[172]

Similarly, parents are considered the personal representative of a minor child and can access the minor's health records. Exceptions exist when the minor consents to health care and consent of the parent is not required under state or other law, or when the minor obtains health care at the direction of a court, or when the minor is emancipated. Other exceptions exist if a provider believes that patients or minors are subject to abuse, neglect, or domestic violence by their personal representative.[173]

HIPAA also requires that pharmacies make a good faith effort to obtain patients' acknowledgement that they have received a copy of the Notice of Privacy Practices. The Notice describes how the pharmacy uses and discloses protected health information to carry out treatment, payment, or health care operations and to protect the patient's rights. The Notice is to be distributed to patients on or before the first treatment encounter. Where the prescription is being picked up by someone other than the patient, the pharmacy must attempt to deliver the notice to the patient. Examples of a good faith effort include providing the notice in the prescription bag or mailing the notice to the patient together with some type of return receipt means. However, the pharmacy is not in violation if the return receipt is not returned. The pharmacy needs it only to document its efforts. [174]

Under HIPPA, pharmacists will be held accountable for handling confidential information properly. Civil and criminal penalties for violating patient confidentiality exist.

COMMUNICATION PRIVACY

The Telephone Consumer Protection Act sets rules prohibiting unsolicited commercial faxes. A Federal Communication Commission (FCC) regulation implementing the Act requires businesses and nonprofit groups to get signed written permission from clients or members before faxing unsolicited materials containing advertisements.

Privacy is also an issue on the Internet (e.g., e-health sites) where the dominant privacy issue arises from the growing practice of data collection. Some Web sites are interactive; that is, they may require the patient to complete a survey or will send visitors a prescription refill reminder. These sites then link to privacy policies that address any concerns prospective patients may have about filling out an online survey. Disclosure of an online privacy policy together with an opt out feature can provide assurances about the protection of consumer privacy and personal information. The policy should also address passive disclosure of information, for instance, from cookies (a feature that allows Web servers to recognize a specific user or computer to access the Web site) or Web server logs. Unfortunately, e-health sites were not included under HIPPA. Some of these e-health Internet sites violate their own privacy policies and transfer patient-identifiable information to third parties.[175]

E-mail use in health care has developed without encryption, and HIPPA does not directly address e-mail in any of its standards. However, because e-mail may involve protected health information in electronic form, both HIPPA's privacy and security rules apply. The security of unencrypted e-mail is low. Passwords, firewalls, and other conventional network security should exist to secure electronic DI communications.[176]

A number of broad consumer privacy bills have been introduced in Congress aimed at consumer surveys, mandated opt-in consents, and other privacy enhancing technological features.[177] Many of these bills implicate DTC advertising such as interactive Web sites, which inherently have invasion of privacy liability issues.

There has also been litigation in this area. In *re Pharmatrak Inc. v. Privacy Litigation* the plaintiffs alleged that numerous pharmaceutical companies secretly intercepted and accessed their personal information through the use of computer cookies and other devices,[178] in violation of state and federal laws such as the Electronic Communications Privacy Act.[179]

Industry Support for Educational Activities

Many pharmacists attend conferences, sometimes funded by pharmaceutical companies to further their professional education. Dialogue between health professionals and the pharmaceutical industry is an opportunity to pass along scientific and educational information, and product risks and benefits. Such dialogue encourages and supports medical research, while providing the health professional with an opportunity to address questions, discuss issues, and offer expertise.

GUIDELINES AND GUIDANCE

❼ *The FDA, the American Council for Continuing Medical Education (ACCME), and the Phamaceutical Research and Manufacturers of America (PhRMA)*[180] *have established educational policies, guidelines, or guidances that allow communication between industry and the Continuing Medical Education (CME) providers with the proviso that the final decisions and control rest with the accredited provider.* Recently, the Office of Inspector General (OIG) issued a Guidance that prohibits the pharmaceutical industry from direct communication with CME providers and calls for an intermediary organization to develop CME programs.[181] The following factors are provided in the OIG Guidance: Does the arrangement skew clinical decision-making? Is the information complete, accurate, and non-misleading? Does the arrangement have the potential to be a disguised discount or result in inappropriate over- or underutilization? Does the arrangement raise patient safety, quality, or care concerns? Importantly, for pharmacists providing DI as industry clinical education consultants or medical liaisons, the Accreditation Council for Pharmacy Education (ACPE) no longer accredits pharmaceutical and biomedical manufacturers.[182] However, not all states actually require all of a pharmacist's continuing education activities to be accredited by the ACPE.[183]

The PhRMA Code, which became effective in July 2002, and updated in January 2009, is the most specific and stringent and deals with various interactions between industry and health care professionals, such as informational presentations, professional meetings, consultant activities, scholarships and educational funds, and educational and practice-related items.[184] Scholarships for pharmacists, students, and residents to attend selected educational conferences may be provided. Salient features of the latest PhRMA Code are found in Table 10–5 and at http://www.phrma.org/sites/default/files/108/phrma_marketing_code_2008.pdf

The FDA Guidance seeks to draw a distinction between educational activities that the FDA considers nonpromotional and those it considers promotional. The distinction is important, especially with regard to off-label uses, which can be an important component of educational activities. FDA's Factors to Determine Independence of the Educational Activity are found in Table 10–6.[185]

Some health care institutions have established their own best practices approach to developing ethical guidelines for pharmaceutical industry support. The practice involves a process similar to weighing the risks and benefits of a particular medication

TABLE 10–5. PHRMA CODE ON INTERACTIONS WITH HEALTH CARE PROFESSIONALS

- Gifts
  - Generally prohibited.
  - Exceptions: $100 or less that benefits patients or educates health care professionals; e.g., medical textbooks or anatomical models permitted, but not stethoscope which are primarily used for treating patients—fine distinction.
  - Pens, pads, etc. no longer permitted.
  - Product samples allowed.
- Meals
  - Modest meals accompanying informational presentations.
  - Can only be offered occasionally.
  - Can only be directly provided in office or at hospital (no restaurants or resorts).
- Entertainment
  - Prohibited.
  - May sponsor meals or reception at conferences.
- Spouses
  - Never appropriate for lodging, travel, meals, entertainment.
- Consultants
  - Must be *bona fide* via written contract, appropriate venue, selection criteria related to purpose of service, must exclude spouses.
  - Special disclosure requirements for health care professionals that set up formularies or develop clinical practice guidelines (disclosure requirements extend 2 years beyond the terms of any speaker or consultant arrangements).
  - Legitimate need identified in advance of entering into agreement required.
  - Number of consultants cannot be greater than number reasonably needed to achieve purpose.
- Financial sponsorship of educational conferences
  - Support should be provided to CPE sponsor, not individual pharmacist.
  - Sponsor should control selection of content, faculty, educational materials, venue.
  - Faculty, but not attendees or spouses, may be paid/reimbursed for time, travel, and lodging.
  - Exception: companies may pay for travel/lodging for students to attend educational conferences; educational institution must select individual students.
- Informational presentations
  - Should be modest by local standards.
  - Should occur in a venue and manner conducive to informational communication.
  - Should provide scientific or educational value.
  - Can comment to CE providers topics of interest manufacturer would sponsor.

or therapeutic intervention, whereby each proposal for support can be viewed as having potential value, which may or may not outweigh any potential drawbacks inherent in the involvement of funding from a for-profit company. Often a committee assesses proposals based on the apparent balance between these factors and a set of guidelines developed by the institution.[186]

In general, most policies and procedures prohibit acceptance of commercial support of educational activities if such acceptance would appear to (1) create an atmosphere limiting academic freedom and the free exchange of ideas and information, (2) introduce bias or otherwise threaten objectivity, (3) create a conflict of interest, or (4) be in conflict with the mission and profit status of the health care organization.[187]

TABLE 10–6. FACTORS USED BY FDA TO DETERMINE INDEPENDENCE

- Control of content and selection of faculty: Is there scripting or other actions designed to influence the content by the supporting company?
- Disclosures: Do they include company funding the program, relationship between provider(s) and presenters to the supporting company, off-label discussion?
- The focus of the program: Does the title accurately represent the presentation; is there fair-balanced educational discussion?
- Relationship between provider and supporting company: Is there a legal, business, or other relationship between the parties?
- Provider involved in sales or marketing: Are provider employees also doing marketing or promotional programs?
- Provider's demonstrated failure to meet standards: Does the provider have a history of biased programs?
- Multiple presentations: Do they serve public health interests?
- Audience selection: Is the audience generated by sales or marketing departments to influence marketing goals?
- Opportunities for discussion: Is there an opportunity for meaningful discussion?
- Dissemination: Is the supporting company distributing additional information after the activity, unless requested by participant and then through an independent provider?
- Ancillary promotional activities: Are promotional activities taking place in the educational meeting room?
- Complaints: Are provider(s), faculty, or others complaining about the supporting company?

RELATIONSHIP TO THE ANTIKICKBACK STATUTE

Particular arrangements between pharmacists and the pharmaceutical industry pose potential risks under the antikickback statute. The antikickback statute makes it a criminal offense to knowingly and willfully offer, pay, solicit, or receive any remuneration (in cash or in kind) to induce (or in exchange for) the purchasing, ordering, or recommending of any good or service reimbursable by any federal health care program.[188] Funding that is conditioned, in whole or in part, on the purchase of product implicates the statute, even if the educational or research purpose is legitimate. Several cases hold that intent is improper if one purpose, not the sole or even primary purpose, is to induce the purchase or recommendation of a company's goods or services.[189,190] When a grant is provided to a customer or potential customer, it may violate the antikickback statute if one purpose is to induce the customer to buy the company's product. Educational grants, for example, were at the heart of the $161 million Caremark settlement,[191] and research grants were at the heart of the $450,000 Hoffman La-Roche settlement.[192] Furthermore, to the extent that the manufacturer has any influence over the substance of an educational program or the presenter, there is a risk that the educational program may be used for inappropriate marketing purposes.

In the area of DI, specific practices that may be problematic under the antikickback statute include gifts, use of pharmacist customers as consultants or members of speaker's bureaus, and questionable research grants. Problems under the antikickback statute could arise where the DI pharmacist participates in any of these activities and also advises on formulary choices or is a member of a formulary committee or subcommittee or is involved with purchasing decisions. If you recommend a product or service and you stand to make financial gain from it, and that service is paid for in part or in whole by the federal government, you may be violating the antikickback statute. Similarly, no gifts should be accepted if there are strings attached.

Educational activities or speakers can be funded by the pharmaceutical industry, whereas promotional marketing activities that purport to be of an educational purpose but serve no direct patient benefit are prohibited. Hiring DI pharmacists under the guise of a consultant or advisor, or focus group participant or advisory board member, or even as a speaker at a meeting, could be considered payments for referrals. Similarly, compensating DI pharmacists as consultants, when all they do is attend conferences primarily in a passive capacity, is suspect. Other suspect activities include compensation for speaking, researching, listening to marketing pitches, or providing preceptor, shadowing, or ghost-writing services. However, where the pharmacist is compensated for actual, reasonable, and necessary services, the activities may be considered legitimate.

The antikickback statute prohibits involvement with research contracts that come through a pharmaceutical company's marketing department, research not reviewed by the manufacturer's scientific or medical department, research that is unnecessarily duplicative or not needed for any purpose other than the generation of business, and postmarketing research used as a pretense for product promotion.[193] Manufacturers should use Chinese walls (i.e., ethical barriers prohibiting exchange of confidential information between different departments of an organization) for marketing and grant-funding activities to demonstrate that grants are bona fide and not improperly influenced by marketing considerations. The antikickback statute requires that grants be given in exchange for fair market value research consideration. This is often difficult to accomplish, since the precise costs and schedules of research activities are not knowable in advance and sometimes not conducive to being reduced to written agreements.

Conclusion

By now the reader has undoubtedly discovered that the liability aspects of DI include more than just negligence. Liability for off-label uses, consumer advertising, copyright infringement, liability issues unique to the Internet, privacy concerns, and industry support for educational activities are all connected to DI practice. The DI practitioner must at least have a working awareness of these areas. DI services provide a foundation for the provision of pharmacist-supervised patient care. To date, pharmacists providing DI have only speculated about and not actually faced malpractice lawsuits. Hopefully, this chapter has shed some light on how courts would react to malpractice suits against pharmacists for negligent provision of DI. However, legal precedents cannot be relied upon to predict the future. There is no way to predict how a court will rule in a particular case. What can be done to avoid malpractice and other causes of action? First, be good at what you do. Second, have good relations with requestors and make sure they are aware of alterations or modifications in information systems and sources. Third, make no outrageous claims about the accuracy and thoroughness of the information provided. Finally, carry your own malpractice insurance policy.

The future of DI pharmacists clearly lies in their ability to provide consultative DI services. While in the past, most of the reported appellate decisions against pharmacists have involved routine dispensing errors, not mistakes in DI or other expanded practice areas, in the future this situation may change. Pharmacists should not be preoccupied with the risk of incurring liability, but they should take the necessary steps to limit exposure and develop an appreciation of modern legal philosophy. Definitive guidelines need not emerge only through court decisions. It remains most important that DI be recognized as a liability-reducing factor for the institution and personnel who provide health care to patients.

REFERENCES

1. Brand KA, Kraus ML. Drug information specialists. Am J Health-Syst Pharm. 2006;63:712-4.
2. American Society of Health-System Pharmacists. ASHP supplemental standard and learning objectives for residency training in drug information practice. Practice standards of ASHP. 1995-1996. Bethesda (MD): American Society of Health-System Pharmacists; 1995.
3. Southwick AF. The law of hospital and health care administration. 2nd ed. Ann Arbor, MI: Health Administration Press; 1988.
4. Nathan JP, Gim S. Responding to drug information requests. Am J Health-Syst Pharm. 2009;66:706, 710-11.
5. Dobbs DB, Hayden PT. Torts and compensation. 3rd ed. St. Paul (MN): West Publishing Co.; 1997. p. 336.
6. Baker K. OBRA '90 mandate and its impact on pharmacist's standard of care. Drake Law R. 1996;44:503, 508.
7. Burns K, Spies A. A pharmacist's duty to warn: trying to make sense of all the legal inconsistencies. Rx Ipsa Loquitur. 2008;35:1-2.
8. Rosenberg v. Equitable Life Insurance Society of the United States, 595 N.E.2d 840 (N.Y. 1992).
9. Keller v. Manhattan Eye, Ear & Throat Hospital, 563 N.Y.S.2d 88, 89 (2nd Dept. 1990).
10. Kashkin v. Mt. Sinai Medical Center, 538 N.Y.S.2d 686 (Sup. Ct. 1989).

11. Kelly WN, Krause EC, Krowinski WJ, Small TR, Drane JF. National survey of ethical issues presented to drug information centers. Am J Hosp Pharm. 1990;47:2245-50.

12. Doppelparker Case, OLG Karllsrule GRUR 1979 P267.

13. Perkins E. Johns Hopkins' tragedy: Could librarians have prevented a death? [cited 2010 Jan 17]. Available from: http://www.newsbreaks.infotoday.com//nbreader.asp?ArticleID=17534.htm.

14. 805 S.W.2d, 380 (Tenn. Ct. App. 1991).

15. 453 N.Y.S.2d 121 (1987).

16. 544 N.W.2d 727, 731 (Mich. Ct. App. 1991).

17. Fink JL. Overriding a computer alert leads to liability. Pharmacy Times. 2009:84.

18. 191 A.D.2d 178, 594 N.Y.S.2d 195 (1993).

19. 579 N.E.2d 1255 (Ill. App. 1991) *rev'd* by 605 N.E.2d 557 (Ill. 1992).

20. Moore v. Memorial Hospital & Winn Dixie, 825 So.2d 658 (Miss. 2002).

21. Deed v. Walgreens, 2004 WL 2943271 (Conn. Super. Ct.).

22. K-Mart v. Chamblin, 612 S.E.2d 25 (Ga. Ct. App. 2005).

23. Brushwood DB, Belgado BS. Judicial policy and expanded duties for pharmacists. Am J Health-Syst Pharm. 2002;59:455-7.

24. 780 So.2d 930 (Fla. App. 2001).

25. 1 S.W.3d 519 (Mo. App. 1999).

26. 737 N.E.2d 650 (Ill. App. 2000).

27. 30 S.W.3d 455 (Tex. App. 2000).

28. Larrimore v. Springhill Mem. Hosp. LEXIS 38:008 WL 54 2000 (Ala. 2008). CV-02-3205, 1051748.

29. 827 F. Supp. 1522 (D. Nev. 1993).

30. 598 N.Y.S.2d 592 (App. Div. 1993).

31. Brushwood DB, Simonsmeier LM. Drug information for patients. J Leg Med. 1986;7:279.

32. Howe A. Are independent prescribing rights for pharmacists set to increase in 2004? Prescr Pract. 2004;1 (2 Suppl 1):5-6.

33. Canadian Society of Hospital Pharmacists [homepage on the Internet]. Information paper on pharmacist prescribing within a health care facility. Canada; 2001 Aug [cited 2005 Mar 2]: [about 17 p.]. Available from: http://ww.cshp.ca/.

34. Abood RR. Pharmacy practice and the law. 6th ed. New York: Aspen Pub.; 2011. p. 388.

35. Berry M. The Canadian pharmacist's duty to counsel. Pharm Law Annual. 1992;19-75.

36. Hall M, Honey W. The evolving legal responsibility of the pharmacist. J Pharm Market Manage. 1994;8:27-41.

37. Brushwood DB. The pharmacist's drug information responsibility after McKee v. American Home Products. *Food Drug L J.* 1993;48:377-410.

38. In re Michael A. Gabert, No. 92 PHM 21 (Wis. Pharmacy Examining Bd., Dec. 14, 1993).

39. Rees W, Rohde NF, Bolan R. Legal issues for an integrated information center. J Am Soc Info Sci. 1991;42:132-6.

40. Restatement (second) of torts, Section 311, 1982.

41. Beaird S, Coley R, Blunt JR. Assessing the accuracy of drug information responses from drug information centers. Ann Pharmacother. 1994;28:707-11.

42. Calis KA, Anderson DW, Auth DA, Mays DA, Turcasso NM, Meyer CC, et al. Quality of pharmacotherapy consultations provided by drug information centers in the United States. Pharmacother. 2000;20:830-6.

43. McDonagh, AF, Lightner, DA. Attention to stereochemistry. Chem & Engin News. Feb. 3, 2003;2.

44. In re Prempro Products, 03-CV-015070-WRW, U.S. Dist Ct., E.D. Ark., July 17, 2009.

45. Clauson KA. Pharmacists: Are your drug information databases accurate? U.S. Pharmacist. Sept. 2008;54-63.

46. Gray JA. Strict liability for the dissemination of dangerous information? Law Lib J. 1990;82:497-517.

47. 694 F. Supp. 1216 (D. Md. 1988).

48. Bundesqe Richtsaf. *Neue juristische Wochenschrift* (1970), 1973.

49. 110 Misc.2d 799, 442 N.Y.S.2d 945 (N.Y. Sup. 1981).

50. 938 F.2d 1033 (9th Cir. 1991).

51. 432 F. Supp. 990 (E.D.N.Y. 1977).

52. Containment Technologies v. ASHP, 2009 U.S. Dist. LEXIS 25421 (March 26, 2009), 2009 U.S. Dist. LEXIS 76270 (August 26, 2009).

53. Talley CR. Affirming science and peer-review publishing. Am J Health-Syst Pharm. 2009;66:896.

54. Prod. Liab. Rep (CCH), Section 8968 (S.D.N.Y.Feb. 20, 1981).

55. Brannigan & Dayhoff. Liability for personal injuries caused by defective medical computer programs. Am J L & Med. 1981;122:132-3.

56. Joyce EJ. Software bugs: a matter of life and liability. Datamation. 1987; May 15: 88-92.

57. Gage D, McCormick J. Case 108...we did nothing wrong. Panama's Cancer Institute. Baseline. 2004;28:32-47.

58. Cuzamanes PT. Automation of medical records: the electronic superhighway and its ramifications for health care providers. J Pharm & Law. 1997;6:19.

59. Brocklesby v. Jeppesen, 767 F.2d 1288 (9th Cir. 1985), *cert. denied*, 474 U.S. 1101 (1986).

60. 472 U.S. 749 (1985).

61. 137 Misc.2d 94, 520 N.Y.S.2d 334 (N.Y. Civ. Ct. 1987).

62. Amerson AB. Drug information centers: an overview. *Drug Info J.* 1986;20:173-8.

63. 705 P.2d 1360 (Ariz. Ct. App. 1985).

64. Rumore MM, Rosenberg JM, Costa JG. The pharmacist and the law: legal aspects of providing drug information. Wellcome Trends in Hosp Pharm (Dec). 1989;6-8.

65. Gough AR, Healey KM, Rupp SR. Poison control centers, from aspirin to PCBs and the scarlet runner beam: a study of legal anomaly and social necessity. Santa Clara L R. 1983;23:791-809.

66. Brushwood DB, Simonsmeier LM. Drug information for patients...duties of the manufacturer, pharmacist, physician, and hospital. J Leg Med. 1986;7:279-341.

67. Curtis JA, Greenberg MI. Legal liability of medical toxicologists serving as poison control center consultants: a review of relevant legal statutes and survey of the experience of medical toxicologists. J Med Toxicol. 2009;5(3):144-8.
68. 656 P.2d 483 (Wash. 1983).
69. Sigell LT, Bonofiglio JF, Siegel EG, McCray EA, Tsipis GB. The role of drug information centers with consumers. Drug Info J. 1987;21:201-8.
70. Arnold RM, Nissen JC, Campbell NA. Ethical issues in a drug information center. Drug Intell Clin Pharm. 1987;21:1008-11.
71. Okasas RM. Hospital drug information centers: a new role in patient counseling. Pharma-Guide to Hospital Med .1988;2:1-4.
72. Gray JA. The health sciences librarian's exposure to malpractice liability because of negligent provision of information. Bull Med Libr Assoc. 1989;77:33-7.
73. Mintz AP. Information practice and malpractice. Libr J. 1985:38-43.
74. Fidelity Leasing Corp. v. Dun & Bradstreet, Inc., 494 F. Supp. 786 (E.D. Pa. 1980).
75. Baker KR. Do people sue people who counsel? Drug Topics. Dec 3, 2007, p. 4.
76. Food & Drug Administration [homepage on the Internet]. Center for Drug Evaluation and Research, Office of Medical Policy, Division of Drug Marketing, Advertising and Communications, Comparative Advertising, Fair Balance, and the Patient-Consumer; c2003 [cited 2005 Mar 2]. Available from: http://www.fda.gov.
77. Food & Drug Administration. Guidance for industry: consumer-directed broadcast advertisements, August 8, 1997.
78. 21 U.S.C. § 352(n).
79. 21 C.F.R. § 202.1(e).
80. Wilkes MS, Bell RA, Kravitz RL. Direct-to-consumer prescription drug advertising: trends, impact, and implications. Health Aff. 2000;19:110-28.
81. Anon. FDA officials describe agency actions on problematic drug promotion activity. BNA Pharm Law & Indus Rep. 2003 Sept 19;1(3):1006.
82. Schwartz TM. Consumer-directed prescription drug advertising and the learned intermediary rule. Food Drug L J. 1991;46:829-37.
83. Available at http://gettingwell.com/drug_info/index.html.
84. Anon. FDLI Panel cautions firms on new media use. FDC Reports. The Pink Sheet. Sept. 15, 2008, p. 24.
85. Lyles A. Direct marketing of pharmaceuticals to consumers. Ann Rev Public Health. 2002;23:73-91.
86. 161 N.J. 1, 734 A.2d 1245 (N.J. 1999).
87. Ferrelli JJ. Perez creates exceptions to learned intermediary doctrine, N.J.L.J. (1999).
88. Heather JL. Liability for direct-to-consumer advertising and drug information on the internet: while the learned intermediary doctrine still lives, drug manufacturers can take some precautionary measures if it is ruled inapplicable. Defense Counsel J. 2001.
89. Gebhart F. Here comes the judge. Drug Topics. 2005 Jan 24;26-32.
90. Pharmacist's Mutual Web Page. [cited 2010 Jan 17]. Available from: http://www.phmic.com/phmc/services/RM/profliab/claimsstudy/Pages/DrugReviewClaims.com.

91. 122 S..Ct. 1497 (2002).

92. Rumore MM. Direct-to-consumer advertising of prescription drugs: emerging legal and regulatory issues. Hosp Pharm. 2004;39:1058-68.

93. Prescription Access Litigation Project. Claritin lawsuit [home page on the Internet] [cited 2005 Mar 2]. Available from: http://www.prescriptionaccesslitigation.org/Claritin.htm.

94. Anderson v. SmithKline Beecham Corp., W.D. Wash. No. CV 03-2886-L, September 22, 2003.

95. Wyeth v. Levine 129 S. Ct. 1187, 1200 (2009).

96. Patsy BM, Furburg CD, Ray WA, Weiss NS. Potential for conflict of interest in the evaluation of suspected adverse drug reactions: cerivastin and risk for rhabdomyolysis. JAMA. 2004;292:2585-90.

97. FDC Act § 312.7.

98. 21 U.S.C. §§ 360.999, 403 (1998).

99. 21 C.F.R. § 99.101(a)(3)-(4).

100. Ward SM. WLF and the two-click rule: The First Amendment inequity of the Food and Drug Administration's regulation of off-label drug use information on the Internet. Food Drug L J. 2001;56:41-56.

101. Kennedy D. The old file-drawer problem. Science. 2004;305:451.

102. Good reprint practices for the distribution of medical journal articles and medical-scientific reference publications on unapproved new uses of approved drugs and approved or cleared medical devices. Dept. HHS, Food and Drug Administration, Office of the Commissioner, Jan. 2009.

103. The Medical Science Liaison: Examining the role. CME Briefing, July-Sept 2002, pp. 3, 5.

104. American Academy of Pediatrics. Policy Statement 2002;110-1, 2002: July 181-3.

105. Fugh-Berman A, Melnick D. Off-label promotion, on-target sales. PLoS Med. 2008;5(10). Available from: www.Medscape.com. Accessed January 16, 2010.

106. Understanding the approval process for new cancer treatments. Bethesda (MD): National Cancer Institute [homepage on the Internet]; c.2004 [cited 2004 Mar 3]. Available from: http://www.nci.gov/clinicaltrials/learning/approval-process-for-cancer-drugs/page 5.

107. Abernethy A, Raman G, Balk EM, Hammond JM, et al. Systematic review: reliability of compendia methods for off-label oncology indications. Ann Intern Med. 2009;150: 336-43.

108. P.L. No. 110-275. Medicare Improvements for Patients and Providers Act of 2008. July 15, 2008.

109. Vivian JC. Off-label use of prescription drugs. US Pharm. 2003;28:508.

110. Beck JM, Azari ED. FDA, off-label use, and informed consent: debunking myths and misconceptions. Food Drug L J. 1998;53:71-103.

111. 21 C.F.R. pt. 50.

112. N.Y. Pub. Health L. § 2805-d(1) (McKinney 1993).

113. Edmunds MW, Scudder L. Using web citations in professional writing. J Prof Nursing. 2008;24:347-351.

114. Wood JM, Dorfman HL. Dot.com medicine...Labeling in an Internet age. Food Drug L J. 2001;56:143-178.

115. Moberg MA, Wood JW, Dorfman HI. Surfing the Net in shallow waters: product liability concerns and advertising on the Internet. Food Drug L J. 1998;53:213-24.

116. 21 U.S.C. §§ 351-354 (1994).

117. Deugan L, Powe N, Blakey B, Makary M. Wiki-Surgery? Internal validity of Wikipedia as a medical and surgical reference. J Am Coll Surg. 2007;205(Suppl):576-7.

118. Clauson KA, Poten HH, Boulos MK, Dzeno Wagis JH. Scope, completeness, and accuracy of drug information in Wikipedia. Ann Pharmacother. 2008;42:1814-21.

119. Freeman MK, Lauderdale SA, Kendrach MG, Woolley TW. Google Scholar versus PUBMED in locating primary literature to answer drug-related questions. Ann Pharmacother. 2009;43:478-84.

120. Adams SR. Information quality-liability and corrections. Online. Sept/Oct. 2003, p. 16-22.

121. Kane B. Guidelines for the clinical use of electronic mail with patients. White paper. JAMA. 1998;5:104-11.

122. Gulick PG. E-health and the future of medicine: the economic, legal, regulatory, cultural, and organizational obstacles. Alb L J Sci & Tech. 2002;12:351-60.

123. Engstrom P. Can you afford not to travel the Internet? Med Econ. 1996;73:173-80.

124. Lopez, et al. v. Aziz, 852 S.W.2d 303, 304 (Tex. App. 1993).

125. Cubby v. Compuserve, 776 F. Supp. 135,140 (1990).

126. Stratton Oakmont Inc. and Daniel Porush v. Prodigy Services Co. & Others (NY Sup. Ct. 1995).

127. Medivision. [cited 2010 Jan 18]. Available from: http://www.medivision.ch/rechtliche_infos-en.asp.

128. Kalb PE, Bass IS. Government investigations in the pharmaceutical industry: off-label promotion, fraud and abuse, and false claims. Food Drug L J. 1998;53:63-70.

129. 42 U.S.C. § 1320a-7b(b)(1) (1994).

130. Huntington S. Emerging professional liability exposures for physicians on the Web. Presentation to the American Bar Association Health Law Section. 2001 June 8.

131. Warnecke M. Tested IP litigation storm of '04: fair use principles prove their pluck. Patent, Trademark, Copyright J. 2005;69:369.

132. Ticketmaster Corp. v. Tickets.Com, Inc., 2003 U.S. Dist. LEXIS 6483 (C.D. Cal. 2003).

133. eBay, Inc. v. Biddder's Edge, Inc., 100 F. Supp. 2d 1058 (N.D. Cal. 2000).

134. 1998 U.S. Dist. LEXIS 17282 (E.D. Pa. 1998).

135. D Minn., No. 02-1782 ADM/JGL, 2005 Jan 28.

136. Warnecke M. Effortless nature of Web surfing makes it unlikely consumers can avoid confusion. Patent, Trademark Copyright J. 2005;69:363-4.

137. Millstein JS, Neuberger JD, Weingart JP. Doing business on the Internet. Law Journal Press; 2004, §3.02[17][a][iii].

138. Futuredontics, Inc. v. Applied Anagramics, Inc., 1998 U.S. App. LEXIS 17012 (9th Cir. 1998).

139. 17 U.S.C. § 102.

140. Eldred v. Ashcroft, 239 F. 3d 373 (D.C. Cir. 2001).

141. 17 U.S.C. § 106.

142. 17 U.S.C. § 109(a).

143. 35 U.S.C. § 107.

144. College Entrance Examination Boar v. Pataki, 889 F. Supp. 554, 568 (N.D.N.Y. 1995).

145. Epstein E, Zulieve AJ. The Fair Use doctrine: commercial misappropriation and market diversion. Isaacson Raymond [homepage on the Internet] [cited 2005 Feb 8]. Available from: http://www.isaacsonraymond.com/fair_use_doctrine.html.

146. 471 U.S. 539 (1985).

147. Guidelines for Classroom Copying in Not-for-Profit Educational Institutions. H.R. Rep. No. 1476, 94th Cong., 1st Sess. § 68-70 (1976).

148. Latman A, Gorman R, Ginsberg JC. Copyright for the nineties. 3rd ed. Charlottesville (VA): Michie;1989. p. 655-6.

149. Campbell v. Acuff-Rose Music, 510 U.S. 569, 578 (1994).

150. 420 U.S. 376 (1975).

151. Perlman R. Williams & Wilkins Co. v. United States; photocopying, copyright, and the judicial process, 1975 Sup. Ct. Rev. 1976;355.

152. 74 F. 3d 1512 (6th Cir. 1996).

153. 758 F. Supp. 1552 (SDNY 1991).

154. Copyright Clearance Center. Using Course Management Systems. Guidelines and Best Practices for Copyright Compliance. Available from: www.copyright.com. Accessed January 18, 2010.

155. 2004 WL 1008314 (2d Cir., May 7, 2004).

156. No. 07 Civ. 09667 (S.D.N.Y. Sept. 8, 2008).

157. Available from: http://laws.findlaw.com/us/000/00-201.html .

158. Greenberg v. National Geographic, 201 U.S. App. LEXIS 4270 (11th Cir. 2001).

159. Google Book Search Copyright Class Action Settlement. Available from: www.googlebook-settlement.com.

160. Persky AS. Paper or plastic? Google's plan to digitalize materials pits book lovers v. book innovators. Wash Lawyer. June 2009:35-40.

161. American Libraries Association [homepage on the Internet]; c 2004 [cited 2005 Feb 10]. Crews KD. New Copyright law for distance education: The meaning and importance of the TEACH Act. Am Libr Assoc. Available from: http://www.copyright.iupui.edu/teach_summary.htm.

162. Smedinghoff TJ (ed). Online law. New York: Addison Wesley Press; 1996:139.

163. Pack R. Honest writers. Washington Lawyer. Sept 2004:21-6.

164. Health Insurance Portability and Accountability Act of 1996, Pub. L. No. 104-191, 110 Stat. 1936 (1996) (codified as amended in scattered sections of 18, 26, 29 and 42 U.S.C.A.); 42 U.S.C.A. § 1320d to 42 U.S.C.A. § 1320d-8.

165. 45 C.F.R. § 160.103.

166. 45 C.F.R. §§ 164.502(d)(2), 164.514(a) and (b).

167. Daniels JG. Health care privacy and HIPAA. In: Cronin KP, Weikers RN, editors. Data security and privacy law. West Group; 2002.

168. Clause SL, Triller DM, Bornhorst CP, et al. Conforming to HIPAA regulations and compilation of research data. Am J Health-Syst Pharm. 2004;61:1025-31.

169. 45 C.F.R. § 164.512(i)(1)(i).

170. 45 C.F.R. § 164.512(b)(1)(iii).

171. Car J, Sheikh A. Email consultation in health care: 2. Acceptability and safe application. *BMJ*. 2004;329:439-42.

172. 42 U.S.C.A. § 290dd-2.

173. Bishop S. Interactions with individuals other than the patient, Part 2: Caregivers, personnel representatives, and minors. Pharm Today. 2003 July [cited 2010 Jan 18]. Available from: http://www.pharmacist,com/articles/h_hi_ 0013.cfm.

174. Bishop S. Interactions with individuals other than the patient, Part 1: Notice of privacy practices and medication counseling. Pharm Today. 2003 July. Available from: http://www. pharmacist.com/articles/h_hi_0012.cfm [cited 2010 Jan 17].

175. E-health privacy policies. Oakland (CA): California health care foundation; 2000.

176. Baker DB. Provider-patient e-mail: with benefits come risks. J Am Health Info Mgmt Assoc. 2003;74:22-9.

177. ANA Compendium of Legislative Activities, p. 9.

178. D. Mass, No. 00-11672-JLT, Nov. 6, 2003.

179. 18 U.S.C. § 2510 *et seq.*

180. Pharmaceutical Research and Manufacturers of America Code on Interactions with Healthcare Professionals. July 2002, Updated Jan 2009.

181. Health and Human Services, OIG Compliance Program for Pharmaceutical Industry, April 2003.

182. Accreditation Council for Pharmacy Education [home page on the Internet]. Accreditation Standards and Criteria; c2005 Jan [cited 2010 Jan 17]. Available from: http://www.acpeaccredit.org/ceproviders/standards.asp.

183. 2008 National Association of Boards of Pharmacy (NABP) Survey of Pharmacy Law. Mount Prospect (IL); NABP; 2008.

184. Cutting the strings on gifts and other questionable marketing practices: PhRMA takes a stand. CME Briefing. July-Sept. 2002, p. 1-6.

185. FDA Guidance for Industry-Supported Scientific and Educational Activities, 1997.

186. Steiner JL, Norko M, Devine S, Grottole E, Vinoski J, Griffith EE. Best practices: developing ethical guidelines for pharmaceutical company support in an academic health center. Psychiatr Serv. 2003;54:1079-89.

187. Rosner F. Pharmaceutical industry support for continuing medical education programs: a review of current ethical guidelines. Mt. Sinai J Med. 1995;62:427-30.

188. 42 U.S.C. § 1320a-7b(b).

189. U.S. v. Greber, 760 F.2d 68 (3d Cir. 1985).

190. U.S. v. LaHue, 261 F.3d 993 (10th Cir. 2001).

191. *In re* Caremark Int'l, Inc. Derivative Litig., 698 A. 2d 959 (1996).

192. Drug firm settles kickback charges. Palm Beach Post, Sept. 6, 1994.

193. Astrue MJ, Szabo DS. Pharmaceutical marketing and the anti-kickback statutes. Food Drug Cosmet Med Device Law Dig. 1993;10(2):57-60.

11

Chapter Eleven

Ethical Aspects of Drug Information Practice

Linda K. Ohri

Learning Objectives

● *After completing this chapter, the reader will be able to*

- Explain characteristics that differentiate an ethical deliberation from other types of decision making.
- Interpret and make use of ethics rules, principles, and theories to analyze identified ethical dilemmas.
- Identify and analyze examples of ethical dilemmas that may arise for health professionals when providing drug information, in various practice settings and for various types of clients and circumstances.
- Identify "micro," "meso," and "macro" levels of ethical decision making that may occur during the provision of drug information
- Use the described process of ethical analysis in order to propose and justify a specific decision or course of action in an ethical dilemma case.
- Describe structures that can prepare, guide, and support clinicians faced with ethical dilemmas during the course of providing drug information.

Key Concepts

❶ Ethical deliberations may be differentiated by three characteristics: they are ultimate (fundamental), the issue is universal, and the welfare of all affected parties is considered.

❷ Ethical judgments may occur at micro, meso, or macro levels of health care decision making.

❸ Professional ethics is different from the law.

❹ A primary focus will be on the health professional's identification, interpretation, specification, and balancing of pertinent ethical rules and principles.

❺ The application of a proposed process of ethical analysis when identifying, analyzing, and resolving ethical dilemmas that may arise during health professionals' provision of drug information.

❻ The first process step requires the identification and evaluation of pertinent background information to insure that the facts of the specific case are understood.

❼ Application of ethical theory can be used to rank or balance pertinent rules and principles in order to carry out ethical decision making.

❽ Health care professionals need training, resources, and support to prepare them to effectively address ethical dilemmas they confront.

What Is Ethics and What Is Not

The Ethics Course Content Committee of the American Association of Colleges of Pharmacy (AACP) described ethics as "the philosophical inquiry of the moral dimensions of human conduct."[1] They mentioned that Aristotle taught ethics as "an eminently practical discipline [dealing] with concrete judgments in situations in which action must be taken despite uncertainty."[1] These authors indicated that the term ethical is often used synonymously with the term moral to describe an action or decision as "good" or "right." They further stated that ethics is not the study of moral development, and it is not the law.

Veatch stated that "an ethical, or moral, issue involves judgments between right and wrong human conduct or praiseworthy and blameworthy human character."[2] This author indicated that an **❶** *ethical deliberation may be differentiated from other endeavors by three characteristics: (1) it is ultimate or fundamental, there is no higher standard against which to measure the rightness of the decision or action; (2) the issue is universal, the parties involved in the dilemma do not consider it simply a difference of opinion or taste—each party believes there is a right or wrong answer—even if they disagree about what the answer is; and (3) the deliberation takes into account the welfare of all involved or affected by the judgment at hand.*

Those engaged in the practice of pharmacy and other health professions typically rely on an intuitive sense of these characteristics. They have the feeling that the situation being confronted is a big deal, and somehow anticipate that they should address not only personal preference in the matter at hand.

Over the past two decades an evolving literature has described ethical issues within a framework of three levels of decision making in health care:[3-15]

❷ 1. *A traditionally recognized micro level of health care–related decision making involves decisions made at the individual professional–patient level of health care;*

2. *A less commonly discussed meso level of decision making (with some literature using the term organizational for similar purposes) is variably described as occurring at the institutional/organizational level or at community/regional levels; and*

3. *Macro-level decision making often sets policy for the health system, as a standard established for an entire profession, or through government as law/regulation for the society as a whole.*

Health care providers may be involved in ethical decision making at each of these levels related to the provision of or access to drug information. Primarily micro-level ethical decision-making scenarios will be presented in this chapter. However, certain scenarios involving meso- and macro-level ethical decision making will also be addressed. For example, a physician, nurse, and pharmacist may all be participating on a pharmacy and therapeutics committee that is developing an organizational policy regarding the use of pharmaceutical samples within hospital clinics. The policy also addresses the use of in-house professionals versus industry detailers to provide information about new drug products. Each of these professionals may have competing priorities and concerns that add ethical dimensions to their decision making on this proposed policy.[11] This constitutes a meso level of ethical decision making for these professionals. A clinician participating on a national task force charged with developing policy related to medication therapy management services (with inherent drug information access) as part of a health care reform model will have macro-level ethical decisions to make relative to balancing patient needs, professional identity, and societal economic constraints.[10]

❸ *Professional ethics is different from the law.* Law might be defined as rules of conduct imposed by society on its members. By contrast, professional ethics has been defined as "rules of conduct or standards by which a particular group in society regulates its actions and sets standards for its members."[16] Both constitute macro-level policy making, across society or across an entire profession. Law involves written rules set by the whole society (or its representatives) that address responsibilities of that society's members. Professional ethics focuses on explicit or implicit rules and standards set by a professional subgroup of society, and addresses the responsibilities of only those who are members of that subgroup. Certain ethical standards of a given profession may be institutionalized as law by society as a whole. However, professional ethical standards (e.g., do no harm or preserve life) are often impossible to fully regulate by law. Meeting an ethical standard also goes beyond legal requirements; indeed, our ethical beliefs may on occasion command our civil disobedience. On the other hand, as will be discussed further below, law represents one aspect of the culture within which ethical decisions are made. In considering the cultural perspectives of a given dilemma, relevant legal requirements must be identified and considered when one seeks to make an ethical decision.

Ethical Dilemmas When Providing Drug Information

This chapter will present case scenarios representing ethical dilemmas. These scenarios may be utilized to demonstrate a specific method for analyzing ethical dilemmas confronted by the pharmacist or other health professionals providing drug information. The discussion will address ethical dilemmas encountered by generalist and specialist patient care providers providing drug information, as well as provide examples drawn from the experiences of drug information specialists. All pharmacists and many other health professionals provide drug information and must address the ethical dilemmas that arise in the course of providing this service. Many of these scenarios represent examples of micro-level ethical dilemmas that primarily involve an interaction between a drug information provider and the direct recipient of the information. Other scenarios where health professionals may be providing or determining access to drug information occur at meso (organizational) or macro (societal) levels of ethical decision making. Although perhaps less immediately obvious than an ethical dilemma to the individual involved, these may constitute dilemmas that have even farther-reaching impacts for both individual professionals and impacted groups. These larger-arena dilemmas may often seem beyond the scope of individual decision making, but indeed ultimately are primarily addressed through the contributed actions/decisions of individuals, typically as they interact in some group process. Of course, it should also be recognized that all ethical dilemmas, by definition, have some implications beyond the welfare of the most immediate individuals involved. The list of example dilemmas provided in Table 11–1 includes scenarios from each of these levels. These dilemmas might arise in a wide variety of settings and circumstances where health care is practiced or health care policy is set. Please identify the level of ethical decision making that each example seems to represent, and consider what ethical issues might exist for each scenario.

TABLE 11–1. EXAMPLE ETHICAL DILEMMAS

- The hospital practitioner is asked to provide information that might be used to speed the ending of a terminal patient's life.
- The community pharmacist or physician is requested by a patient to critique another health care provider's drug therapy recommendations.
- The emergency room nurse is asked to tell the patient's significant other that the administered medication is for other than the sexually transmitted disease being treated.
- The drug information specialist is confronted by a physician or an administrator pressuring for a certain formulary recommendation that is possibly more cost containment than evidence based.
- A home health care practitioner is asked to positively present questionably substantiated information on the efficacy of a given therapy in order to support insurance reimbursement for a truly needy patient.
- A practitioner working in industry is asked to prepare two versions of a consumer product education and promotion piece: One meets U.S. regulatory requirements to describe key safety issues; the other version, for use in a country without such legal requirements, omits all safety information.
- A health professional practicing in any patient care setting experiences another episode (in a repetitious pattern) where his or her patients would benefit from additional drug information, but finds workload demands to be an impossible barrier to providing more than the minimum, legally required information.
- A health professional is enrolled by her professional organization to testify against a proposed health reform policy that mandates her profession to provide verbal drug information whenever dispensing a prescription refill, but does not set any requirements for third-party payer reimbursement of this service.

In the fifth edition of their foundational text, *Principles of Biomedical Ethics*,[17] Beauchamp and Childress address the following aspects of the moral life: principles and rules; rights, character, and virtues; and moral emotions. The responsibilities (based on principles and rules) and rights of the health care provider and other involved parties will be addressed briefly in this chapter as considerations that must be dealt with in the course of responding to a specific dilemma. While acknowledging their importance, this chapter will not address the roles of character, moral virtue, or emotions in ethical decision making by health professionals. One might say that they constitute the provider's inherent moral perspective that will direct and support his or her decision making. The interested reader is referred to the text referenced previously for a fascinating discussion of these factors;[17] this discussion is continued in the 2008 edition of the same text for those wishing to review updated coverage of this material.[18] The remainder of this chapter is intended to prepare and assist the pharmacist and other health professionals providing drug information to analyze and address dilemmas, such as those listed previously. ❹ *The primary focus here will be on the health professional's identification, interpretation, specification, and balancing of pertinent ethical rules and principles* as the health professional seeks to justify what he or she considers to be the right decision or the best course of action.

Basics of Ethics Analysis

This section briefly presents relevant terminology and definitions used in the field of ethics, as well as an overview of a specific process of analysis that may be used in assessing ethical dilemmas. In the section following this one, specific case scenario demonstrations of this process for analysis will be presented.

DEFINITIONS USED IN THE FIELD OF ETHICS

Beauchamp and Childress[19] defined ethics as "a generic term for several ways of examining the moral life." These authors described a process of deliberation and justification that is necessary when confronting a moral dilemma. They stated, "When we deliberate . . . we are considering which judgment is morally justified . . . ." They indicated that "particular judgments are justified by moral rules, which in turn are justified by principles, which ultimately are defended by an ethical theory." These authors presented a hierarchical diagram that depicts this approach to analysis (Figure 11–1). A later article by Beauchamp further addresses the need to consider these principles and rules within the specific context of the case at hand, in order to fully realize their action-guiding potential.[20]

The authors referred to these hierarchical levels of analysis (particularly rules and principles) as action-guides, which are utilized to justify a particular judgment. They describe a rule of ethics as specific to context and relatively restricted in scope; for instance, the moral rule about confidentiality that specifically addresses a patient's right to consent prior to the release of privileged information.[19] Principles are more broad and fundamental in scope; for example, the principle of respect for autonomy, which is the patient's right to decide on personal issues. They describe ethical theories as "integrated bodies of principles and rules . . . that may include mediating rules that govern cases of conflicts." The prominent rules and principles guiding ethical decision making by health care professionals can generally be placed within one of two broad ethical theories: consequentialist theory or deontological (derived from the Greek word *deon*, meaning duty)

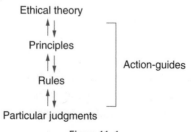

Figure 11–1

theory.[19] Multiple versions exist of each of these broad categories. Consequentialist theories describe actions or decisions as morally right or wrong based on their consequences, rather than on any intrinsic features they may have. The two cardinal principles of consequentialist theory are beneficence (do that which promotes a good outcome) and nonmaleficence (do that which minimizes bad outcomes). Consequentialist theories focus on this one feature of an act—its consequences. For example, an informed-consent ethical rule can be of value within consequentialist theory because consent generally results in improved compliance and outcome—good consequences. However, if informed consent were likely to result in a bad outcome, it would not be justifiable within consequentialist theory. A mediating rule utilized by many advocates of consequentialist theory is to hold nonmaleficence as more important, or more foundational, than beneficence.

Duty-driven (deontological) theories look more to intrinsic qualities of an act or decision to assert its moral rightness or wrongness. Deontological theory considers other inherent features of an act, besides consequences, as also relevant and often of greater importance. For example, in various forms of deontological theory, the act is considered inherently wrong if it is dishonest or breaks confidentiality, or if it does not respect individual autonomy. Conflicts between different rules are mediated by appealing to more foundational, underlying principles such as adherence to justice or to respect for persons.

Conscious recognition of the pertinent action-guides and understanding mediating rules that operate within the health professional's preferred ethical theory or theories can help providers honestly and equitably analyze the ethical dilemma, and better comply with the required characteristics of ethical deliberation (see the beginning of this chapter).

OVERVIEW OF A SUGGESTED PROCESS OF ANALYSIS TO BE USED WHEN AN ETHICAL DILEMMA ARISES

• In the article, "Hospital Pharmacy: What Is Ethical?," Veatch[2] indicated that often we reach a particular ethical decision without a great deal of conscious deliberation, through our moral intuition, and without subsequent challenge from any external party. However, on occasion, when pondering a certain ethical judgment, we are called on (internally or externally) to analyze and justify the basis for our conviction. He suggested that when this occurs, it is first important to understand the facts of the specific case. He then described progression through three additional process stages of reflection (on ethical rules, principles, and theories) by which we may identify, analyze, and present reasons for our judgment. In the same report, the author also emphasized the importance in one's reflection of taking into account the points of view of all parties. As stated earlier in this chapter, this is one of the key characteristics distinguishing an ethical deliberation. A survey of the text

Cross-Cultural Perspectives in Medical Ethics (2nd ed)[21] demonstrates that there are many commonalities but also important differences across the ethical perspectives of different cultures. These cultural perspectives must be considered if all parties' points of view are to be taken into account.

This section addresses ❺ *the application of a proposed process of ethical analysis when identifying, analyzing, and resolving ethical dilemmas that may arise during health professionals' provision of drug information.* These steps of analysis are derived from the writings of Veatch, Beauchamp, and Childress, as well as other authors.[2,19,21-23] The process may be summarized as follows:

I. Identification of relevant background information.
   A. Factual details of the issue at hand.
   B. Consideration of who is affected by the ethical issue.
   C. Learn and respectfully address the cultural perspectives (including applicable legal requirements) for those affected by the dilemma.
II. Identification and justification of the relevant moral rules and principles (action-guides) pertinent to the case.
III. Deliberation, through the use of moral intuition and application of ethical theory, on how to rank/balance the rules and principles pertinent to the case in order to resolve the ethical dilemma.

Step I. Identification of Relevant Background Information

❻ *The first process step requires the identification and evaluation of pertinent background information to insure that the facts of the specific case are understood.* This first step deserves careful consideration and research. Once the facts of a case are known, the moral concerns may be resolved. This step is divided into three parts: (A) data gathering, (B) consideration of the welfare of all affected parties, and (C) respect for the cultural perspectives of these parties.

Health professionals already use data gathering when they apply a systematic approach to answering any drug information question (see Chapter 2). When addressing a potential ethical dilemma, the providers must learn about the factual details of the issue, who is directly involved, and whether there is conflict in factual understanding among the parties involved in the issue. For example, does the parent who calls to ask about the medication recently prescribed for her teenager already know that the teenager is taking a birth control pill prescribed by a gynecologist (rather than a dermatologist for acne) and simply wants to know the name of the product?

If the matter seems still to involve an ethical dimension once data gathering clarifies the facts, the next step is to consider the rights and responsibilities of all affected parties. As previously mentioned, this has been described as an essential component of

• any ethical deliberation.[2] The health care provider, direct client (patient), other indirect but individual clients (e.g., any existing or unborn children, or spouse), other health professionals (e.g., the patient's physician), other societal groups (e.g., other patients who might be harmed by an incompetent practitioner), and any higher power recognized by the health professional have rights and/or responsibilities that should be considered.

• Finally, during first consideration of any potential ethical issue, the provider should take into account the cultures of the affected parties.[22] In his reviews of the foundations of modern medical ethics theories, Veatch[21,23] described how the unique perspectives of Western, Chinese, Hindu, Jewish, Catholic, Protestant, and other cultural groups have affected the formulation of their dominant medical ethics traditions. Other cultural classifications might include socioeconomic status, political affiliation, age category, and racial or ethnic group. A report by Najjar et al.[24] demonstrates some important similarities (e.g., requests to assess physicians' recommendations) and differences (e.g., requests to serve as a primary health care provider) in the types of ethical dilemmas that are identified by drug information specialists functioning within the cultural environment of Saudi Arabia, compared to those reported at U.S. centers.

In a very interesting case study, Carrese et al.[25] discussed the ethical obligations of medical professionals in caring for those of a different ethnic culture. In this case, a young Laotian mother had utilized a traditional Mien folk cure to treat her infant. The treatment involved placing several small burns on the child's abdomen to treat "gusia mun toe," an apparently transient, but very distressing, colic-like ailment. The cure resulted in several small scars, but no other obvious ill effects. The mother indicated that the cure worked. The physician recognized the value in supporting the positive impacts of the woman's attachment to her cultural support group. However, the physician was confronted with the dilemma of how to respond to this mother's revelation of a culturally promoted treatment measure that was not scientifically supported and could be danger-

• ous. Sometimes, culturally based actions may conflict with the professional's goal to avoid harm and promote benefit. However, failing to consider a cultural perspective may also have harmful effects. An extended discussion of how differing cultural perspectives affect ethical decision making is beyond the scope of this chapter. However, the health professional should strive to be aware of and respect the cultural perspectives of the affected parties when contemplating an ethical dilemma. The interested reader is encouraged to refer to the resources cited here and previously for further discussion of cultural factors in ethical analysis.[21,23]

• One final issue should be addressed relative to cultural considerations. The legal requirements of the society within which an ethical dilemma occurs are part of the culture and must be identified. A specific ethical decision will not always exactly conform to the existing legal requirements of society. The ultimate nature of ethical deliberations may result in decisions that are more demanding than the legal requirements and, unfortunately, may even occasionally involve perceived or true conflict with specific legal requirements. This may involve, for instance, a decision not to divulge confidential communications between a professional and client, which may or may not be acceptable within the law. In another case, the health professional may decide not to provide information related to abortion or capital punishment, even though these activities are acceptable within the law. Obviously, legal requirements cannot be ignored or dismissed lightly when making a specific ethical decision.

Step II: Use of Rules and Principles (Action-Guides) to Assist in the Analysis of an Ethical Dilemma

If the dilemma persists, once the available background information has been identified and considered, the process of full ethical deliberation should proceed. Veatch suggests that the involved party/parties can proceed as far as necessary through successive stages of general moral reflection, assessing at the level of moral rules and then at the level of ethical principles, within their accepted ethical theory.[2] These might be described as the action-guides referred to by Beauchamp and Childress.[19] This second process step of analysis will look at moral rules that may apply to the specific case and more general pertinent ethical principles. Definitions are provided at the end of this section for a number of ethical rules and principles that are considered particularly relevant to decision making by pharmacists and others providing drug information.

It should be noted that specific action-guides may be considered a rule within one ethical theory and a principle within another. For example, veracity (truth telling) as mentioned previously, may be considered by some ethicists to be a specific moral rule and by others to be a general principle, depending on which ethical theory is followed. For the practitioner immediately involved in analyzing a specific ethical dilemma, defining the relevant action-guides as rules or principles is important only to the extent that this helps in assessing which are more fundamental to the issue at hand. Therefore, in this chapter, both rules and principles will be included within the same process step of ethical analysis.

Examples of moral rules within biomedical ethics include a confidentiality rule dictating that patient-entrusted information should not be disclosed or an informed-consent rule that addresses the individual's right to information before agreeing to a specific medical procedure. Unfortunately, there is no definitive list universally defining all moral rules, and sometimes multiple pertinent rules can be in conflict. Furthermore, there are acceptable exceptions to most moral rules. For instance, disregarding the informed-consent rule might be justifiable in an acute situation to protect the life of the client; suffering may be necessary in order to achieve cure of serious disease; and many consider killing justified under certain circumstances. Therefore, there may not be a specific rule that resolves a particular ethical dilemma.

When such a circumstance arises, the practitioner may begin a more general level of analysis by looking at the ethical principles that apply to the case. Sometimes, the involved parties can reach an acceptable resolution to an ethical dilemma once they recognize the more broad relevant ethical principles. In a given dilemma, the professional may decide that the primary principle is to respect the autonomy of the client, which requires providing complete information that enables the client to make an informed decision. In another dilemma, if *do no harm* is considered the most fundamental ethical principle, decisions or acts that deny this principle would be considered unethical. It becomes immediately obvious, however, that relevant ethical principles such as these may also come into conflict. This problem can be demonstrated by the following example: The professional may believe that full disclosure will result in nonadherence by the patient, with significant risk of resultant harm. The practitioner therefore confronts two conflicting principles: respecting client autonomy versus the duty to do no harm.

Step III: Ethical Theory as a Means to Clarify or Resolve Ethical Dilemmas

This third step of ethical analysis reveals how relevant moral rules and principles interact within the preferred ethical theory to address the given dilemma. When confronted with conflicting ethical rules or principles, the practitioner may simply resolve the dilemma through his or her moral intuition of the right thing to do, even if unconsciously this reflects the individual's at least temporary affiliation to some theory of what constitutes good versus bad or right versus wrong. ❼ *Sometimes, the professional will find it necessary and valuable to more consciously deliberate on how various ethical theories suggest that the relevant rules and principles should be prioritized or balanced.* According to Veatch,[2] this process step can lead to more rational and honest decision making or action taking. He suggests that these ultimate deliberations at the level of ethical theory will be affected by our most basic religious and/or philosophical commitments. It is important that the practitioner recognizes and acknowledges the impact on decision making of his or her own personal ethical perspective. Those dilemmas that cannot be fully resolved can at least be viewed with greater clarity.

Veatch[23] states that "the components of a complete theory will answer such questions as what rules apply to specific ethical cases, what ethical principles stand behind the rules, how seriously the rules should be taken, and what constitutes the fundamental meaning and justification of the ethical principles." In this reference and another text, the author reviews the foundations of consequentialist, deontological, and other ethics theories particularly relevant to health professionals, including the Hippocratic tradition; Judeo-Christian and other religious-based traditions; the philosophies of the modern secular West; and medical ethics theories outside the Anglo-American West, including Socialist, Islamic, Hindu, African, Chinese, and Japanese traditions.[21,23] Frequently, versions of the broad consequentialist and deontological theories are expressed in various ways across these traditions. Particular note should be given to the core of the various Hippocratic Oaths, because this has been the central ethical tradition of Western medicine: "Those who have stood in that [Hippocratic] tradition are committed to producing good for their patient and to protecting that patient from harm."[23] In Hippocratic tradition, there is also a special emphasis placed on the responsibility of the medical professional to the specific patient versus obligations to other less directly affected parties or to society in general. A contract theory of medical ethics has also been proposed, which describes an implicit (unwritten) contract between professionals and patients.[23] This modern theory is of special relevance to the pharmacist providing drug information as a service within an implicit pharmaceutical care contract.[23,26] First of all, this theory represents a shift in thinking for those pharmacists who might have considered their primary obligation to be to the prescriber rather than to the patient. Furthermore, this contract between patient and professional suggests an obligation for more substantive communication with patients and a higher level of care-giving than some pharmacists have previously felt obligated to offer. The reader is referred to foundational writings by Veatch, as well as those of Beauchamp and Childress, for a more in-depth discussion of various medical ethics theories.[18,19,21,23]

AN ANNOTATED LISTING OF RULES AND PRINCIPLES (ACTION-GUIDES) APPLIED IN MEDICAL ETHICS INQUIRY

The following rules and principles of ethical conduct will be described and subsequently used in the analysis of case scenarios provided in the next section. Their description will necessarily be brief. The reader is referred to other sources to read more about these rules and principles.[19,23]

1. *Nonmaleficence*—A basic principle of consequentialist theory; encompasses the duty to do no harm. This tenet has a long history as part of the Hippocratic tradition, where it has often been described in terms of the health care provider's duty to the individual patient. The principle is also cited as justification for actions benefiting all. Sometimes, application of the principle requires addressing conflicts between the needs of one and all.[18]

2. *Beneficence*—Another basic principle of consequentialist theory that expresses the duty to promote good. Again, conflict can arise between what constitutes good for one individual versus the larger societal group. Good or bad consequences are also of importance within deontological theories, but are evaluated along with other principles that may be considered of equal or greater importance.[18]

3. *Respecting the patient-professional relationship*—A moral rule, often referring to respect for the physician–patient relationship, but also applicable to other

professional–patient relationships, as well. This rule has been mentioned in published reports of ethical dilemmas arising during the provision of drug information.[24,27-29] As expressed in Hippocratic traditions, this rule indicates that the physician's primary duty is to the patient and tends to give the physician, rather than the patient, control in the relationship. This rule is particularly noted in duty-driven (deontological) ethical theories that consider the professional's duty to the patient, but also supports consequentialist theory to the extent that good outcomes are enhanced.

4. *Respect for autonomy*—A principle described particularly within deontological theory. This principle is founded on a belief in the right of the individual to self-rule. It speaks to the individual's right to decide on issues that primarily affect self.

5. *Consent*—A moral rule related to the principle of autonomy, which states that the client has a right to be informed and to freely choose a course of action, for example, informed consent to receive a therapy or procedure.

6. *Confidentiality*—A moral rule, also related to the principle of autonomy, which specifically addresses the individual client's right to give or refuse consent relative to the release of privileged information.

7. *Privacy*—Another rule within the principle of autonomy, more generally relating to the right of the individual to control his or her own affairs without interference from or knowledge of outside parties. This rule has been addressed in deliberations on the rights of individuals with AIDS versus those of their potential contacts.

8. *Respect for persons*—A principle expressing duty to the welfare of the individual, particularly described within religion-based deontological theories. This principle may also be expressed within dignity-of-life or sanctity-of-human-life principles. It has common elements with the respect-for-autonomy principle, but addresses more directly a belief in the inherent value of human life, independent of characteristics or abilities of the specific human being.

9. *Veracity*—This term addresses the obligation to truth telling or honesty. Veracity is considered an ethical principle within deontological theory. However, it is considered a useful rule within consequentialist theory, to the extent that it promotes good.

10. *Fidelity*—Another principle of moral duty in deontological theory that addresses the responsibility to be trustworthy and keep promises. This principle also relates to a duty of reciprocity—consideration of the other's point of view. Descriptions of pharmaceutical care have spoken of the need to develop an ethical covenant between pharmacist and client.[26] This covenant details the characteristics of a relationship requiring fidelity and reciprocity, in which

each party takes on certain responsibilities and gives up certain rights in order to achieve specific good outcomes (consequentialist theory). Success of this contract depends in good measure on consideration by each party of the other's point of view.

11. *Justice*—This concept has been presented within various principles that relate to fairness and tendering what is due, resource allocation, and providing that to which the individual is entitled. A number of justice theories have also been developed to connect and justify these various principles.[18,19] Moral decision making at the meso and macro levels will frequently cite justice as a main justification for particular decisions. A more thorough discussion on justice-related principles and theories is beyond the scope of this chapter. However, recent texts that address this topic can provide much assistance to those health professionals preparing for roles at these levels of ethical decision making, or to those who teach these professionals.[18,30,31]

These are certainly not the only relevant rules or principles, nor are they necessarily universally accepted definitions. However, these action-guides seem particularly pertinent to medical ethics inquiry. Furthermore, several of these rules and principles have been specifically discussed in published reports that describe ethical dilemmas encountered by drug information specialists.[27,28] Such dilemmas have also been described in situations where pharmacists are providing drug information directly to patients, either from a formal drug information center or during the process of providing patient care.

Demonstration of the Process for Analyzing Ethical Dilemmas

The following example demonstrates an ethical dilemma that might arise for a pharmacist providing drug information to consumers in the course of dispensing prescriptions. This case will be utilized to demonstrate the aforementioned process of analysis for the pharmacist encountering an ethical dilemma occurring at the micro level of health care.

DEMONSTRATION OF CASE ANALYSIS

Case Study 11–1

Mrs. Green, a new patient at the medical center, calls the drug information (DI) center (which the medical center advertises as a resource for both patients and professionals) and asks Dr. John Smith, the information specialist, a question. She is concerned about whether she should take the metronidazole just prescribed for her by Dr. Raymond Mack, her family practitioner (who practices at the center where the DI center is located).

■ ANALYSIS

Step 1: Identification of relevant background information

A. Factual details of the issue at hand. The drug information practitioner learns the following information through discussion with the patient:

1. Mrs. Green is approximately 8 weeks pregnant; she wonders if this medication is safe for the baby.
2. She says she is being treated for a recently acquired vaginal infection.
3. She states that this is the first vaginal infection that she has had in several years.
4. She mentions that she has only recently begun seeing Dr. Mack as her family just moved into town about 3 months ago.
5. Mrs. Green indicates that Dr. Mack knows she is pregnant: He is managing her pregnancy.
6. She states that she asked him about the drug's safety, but he rather impatiently brushed off her questions by asking, "Don't you trust me?"
7. The provider may decide that it is necessary to consult professional resources to evaluate whether the therapy appears to be appropriate. The provider should not hesitate to ask the patient for some reasonable time period in which to investigate the pertinent information before providing an answer.
8. The provider will need to consider whether any identified risks are likely to be known to the physician.
9. The provider may decide that further facts must be obtained through direct discussion with the prescriber.

B. Identification of who is affected by the ethical issue. As the drug information provider reflects on this patient's inquiry, it is helpful to consider who might be impacted by his response:

1. Himself, relative to his own desire to do "right"; any relationship between him and his patient, any relationship between him and the physician.
2. The woman, relative to the consequences of any harm to her infant or of inadequate treatment of the infection, and relative to her future relationships with both the physician and the drug information provider.
3. The woman's infant, relative to the consequences of any harmful or beneficial effects of the drug, or of inadequate treatment of the woman's infection.
4. The physician, relative to the consequences of prescribing a potentially inappropriate therapy during the woman's pregnancy, and relative to the effects of any drug information provided on the patient-physician relationship.

5. The woman's family, significant others, and society in general relative to the impacts of either delivery or abortion of a child with harm from the therapy, or from inadequate treatment of the woman's infection.

C. Consideration for the cultural perspectives of those affected by the dilemma. The DI professional will consciously or unconsciously act within his own cultural and religious framework, and his understanding of his legal obligations. Awareness of his own perspective, as well as consideration of the cultural perspectives of others who may be affected, is important if he is to pursue a truly ethical course of action. To repeat Veatch's words differentiating ethical deliberations, "The deliberation takes into account the welfare of all involved or affected."[1] Each involved party's welfare is affected by his or her cultural perspective. Cultural, religious, and legal perspectives that the pharmacist must be aware of in this case might include

1. Perspectives regarding parental responsibility to the unborn infant versus self

2. Perspectives and legal requirements relative to both the DI provider's and the physician's obligations to the patient and to her infant

3. Perspectives about the role and authority of the physician and of the DI provider

D. Consideration of the level of decision making involved in responding to any ethical dilemma recognized by the DI practitioners.

Within the context of this DI professional's job description, or the charge of the particular case, it should be fairly obvious whether micro-, meso-, or macro-level decision-making activities are involved. However, a clinician may be involved in micro-level decision-making activities related to individual patients, but also have obligations to the pharmacy and therapeutics committee within the health organization (meso level), or perhaps even beyond as a policy committee member for his or her national professional organization (macro level). By definition, all ethical dilemmas tend to have implications beyond the context of just two individuals (note from the first page of this chapter that ethical deliberation takes into account the welfare of all involved or affected by the judgment at hand), but meso- and macro-level decision making will always affect various population groups, as well as the individuals within those groups.

Step 2: Identification and justification of the relevant moral rules and principles (action-guides) pertinent to the case at hand

If the background facts of Mrs. Green's inquiry do not dismiss the DI provider's ethical concerns, Dr. Smith will find it helpful to consider the various rules and principles discussed previously in order to clarify the dimensions of his concern. It is most useful to first identify all potentially pertinent action-guides and seek an understanding of how fundamentally each applies to the situation.

Ethical action-guides that seem pertinent to this inquiry include the following:

1. *Informed consent*—A moral rule supporting Mrs. Green's right to be informed and freely choose whether to take the metronidazole in relation to other available options.

2. *Respect for the patient-professional relationship*—This rule addresses Dr. Smith's obligation to support the professional relationship between Mrs. Green and Dr. Mack. It also requires Dr. Smith to respect his own professional relationship with the patient. Increasingly, professionals within all health care professional groups are interpreting this ethical rule to define their obligation to the patient as primary. Such an interpretation represents a departure for many health care providers from a historical orientation of their primary obligation being to the physician.

3. *Veracity*—Addresses Dr. Smith's responsibility to tell the truth to Mrs. Green. This may be considered a basic principle of obligation within deontological theory, or a useful rule within consequentialist theory (to the extent that it promotes good).

4. *Nonmaleficence*—A basic principle of consequentialist theory that would base a decision to divulge information on minimizing the potential for harm.

5. *Beneficence*—This consequentialist principle would base the decision regarding what information to divulge on the potential to promote good. Beneficence and nonmaleficence can be considered together in judging the ethical response to Dr. Smith's dilemma. Dr. Smith must consider the potential benefits of the prescribed therapy for Mrs. Green and address the potential harm resulting from exposure of her infant to the metronidazole. Consideration of other available alternatives for therapy is also pertinent. Frequently such consideration takes place, at least initially, in the face of inadequate and conflicting information. Dr. Smith will also need to decide what constitutes harm and good for Mrs. Green versus all others who may be affected.

6. *Fidelity/reciprocity*—A principle of obligation to an ethical covenant between Dr. Smith and Mrs. Green (within deontological theory), which may suggest a requirement for full disclosure of information. However, to the extent that this covenant asks that each party take on certain responsibilities and give up certain rights in order to achieve specific good outcomes, full disclosure of potentially harmful information may not be required. For instance, if Dr. Smith were concerned that Mrs. Green may decide to forgo any treatment, this could have strong potential for negative consequences for both Mrs. Green and her infant.

7. *Justice*—This principle is considered of intrinsic value within certain deontological theories and addresses Mrs. Green's (and other affected parties') right to be given

what is due—entitlement to information may be considered justice in this case. Certainly, Dr. Smith's time and expertise might be legitimately considered due to his patient.

8. *Autonomy*—This principle is directly applicable to Dr. Smith's dilemma, as was the related rule of informed consent, based on a belief in Mrs. Green's right to decide on issues that primarily affect her. The principle of autonomy has support within both deontological (as an intrinsic good) and consequentialist (if it is likely to promote good consequences) theories. However, competing interests (e.g., Mrs. Green's and her child's) and the individual's capability to be truly autonomous (e.g., the infant in this case) are factors that often complicate the application of this principle in medical ethics.

The reader may believe that other ethical rules or principles are pertinent to this case. If so, these should also be considered as the analysis proceeds.

Step 3: How should these rules and principles be ranked or balanced against each other in order to resolve the ethical dilemma?

This step may sometimes be accomplished rather easily through the use of moral intuition. At other times, careful consideration of ethical theory can suggest which are the more fundamental action-guides to be applied. In some cases, it may be necessary to balance similarly weighted principles against each other, identifying when the weight of one versus another might be considered greater.

The rules and principles that Dr. Smith considers pertinent to his dilemma over how to respond to Mrs. Green's inquiry could be ranked as shown in Figure 11–2.

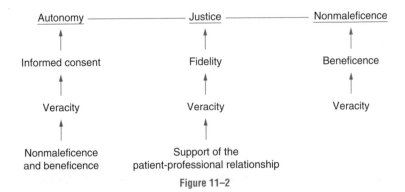

Figure 11–2

SUMMARY

In the case of Dr. Smith and Mrs. Green, autonomy, justice, and nonmaleficence could be considered the primary principles that must be balanced against each other. Autonomy and justice are both valued principles within various deontological theories. Nonmaleficence and beneficence are the cornerstone principles of consequentialist theory. The principle of justice also seems to be inherent in the contract theory of medical ethics described by Veatch.[2] The other relevant rules and principles described previously support these primary principles and inform how they apply to specific ethical dilemmas. The Code of Ethics for Pharmacists (see Appendix 11–1) approved in 1994 provides further support for these fundamental principles and clearly indicates that Dr. Smith's primary obligation is to Mrs. Green rather than to Dr. Mack.[16,17] It may be surmised that all of the fundamental principles seem to support honestly discussing the benefits and risks of the therapy with the patient. However, if there were no good alternative therapies for Mrs. Green's infection, and Dr. Smith was concerned that probable noncompliance constituted a greater risk to her and/or her baby, the decision would become more difficult. Once Dr. Smith has considered the facts of the case, who will be affected by his action, the cultural perspectives and legal requirements for the affected parties, and the relevant action-guides, he should have more clarity on what constitutes the ethical action. Finally, Dr. Smith's personal beliefs and values relative to these principles of patient autonomy, promotion of justice, and the importance of potential consequences will all affect his ultimate ethical decision. It must be emphasized that he will make some response, even if only by avoiding the patient's question.

It is not likely that all will agree on the provided ranking or balancing of the pertinent rules and principles in this case, nor will there be universal agreement about what constitutes the right resolution to the ethical dilemma presented. It is necessary to remember that an ethical issue has been defined as one where most agree that there is a right answer, but cannot always agree on what that answer is.

The reader is encouraged to apply this process of analysis to two additional case scenarios, found in Case Studies 11–2 and 11–3 of this chapter. Imagine a set of circumstances that might provide the background context behind each case and carry out your ethical analysis in light of this context. Perhaps you might then vary some important aspect of the background context to determine whether this affects your analysis of the ethical dimensions of the case. As you consider each case, also assess at what level of health care (micro, meso, or macro) does the ethical decision making seem to apply?

Resources for Use by Professionals Seeking to Learn More About Medical Ethics

8 *Health care professionals need training, resources, and support to prepare them to effectively address ethical dilemmas they confront.* The first goal in learning more about medical ethics should be to learn to recognize opportunities for ethical deliberation when they confront us. Situations will arise where ethical judgments will be made that have moral consequences—with or without the conscious understanding of the parties involved. It is just as important for professionals to be prepared to deal with these situations as it is for them to learn how to address efficacy and safety concerns relative to drug therapies. This section of the chapter offers a survey of medical ethics resources that can assist practitioners who personally desire to learn how to better recognize ethical situations and how to respond to them, or who will be teaching others in formal settings or informally in the workplace.

Formal coursework, in-services, or continuing education opportunities can teach skills that will aid professionals in handling ethical dilemmas related to work responsibilities that involve the provision of drug information. Thornton et al.[22] discussed what should be taught in basic ethics education that takes place within and outside the academic environment. Their review of important elements to be included in ethics education is worthwhile reading for anyone who may desire to participate in these teaching activities. They also refer the reader to other useful resources on the topic. In Davis's manual on patient-practitioner interactions, the author presents an easy-to-understand description of the stages of moral development, comparing two commonly identified models proposed by Piaget and Kohlberg.[32] This information is valuable to assist in gaining insight into one's personal moral development, as well as that of others. This workbook, published by a physical therapist for the purpose of assisting in the professional socialization process, also offers a description of moral values associated with development as a professional. The author goes on to present a framework for resolving ethical dilemmas that has similar elements to those presented in this chapter; she also provides exercises that could be readily adapted for use in various health care professionals' education or in-services. Haddad et al.[1] provided a comprehensive guideline on pharmacy ethics course content; this is also valuable reading for those wishing to address ethics topics in continuing education of the pharmacist or other practitioners. This guideline describes examples of educational methods including case presentation and debate; scenario building, with identification and discussion of potential ethical issues; and role-playing activities. The authors indicate that such educational methods should involve group participation to conduct the analysis of sample cases for the ethical issue being discussed. Writing techniques, such as a 5-minute-write exercise prior to discussion, can serve to focus the participant's ideas and facilitate the resultant discussion.[33] The guideline also provides an extensive bibliography of resource materials. Two other texts, one edited by Haddad[34] and the updated second edition of *Case Studies in Pharmacy Ethics* by Veatch and Haddad,[35] provide further discussion of teaching methods and many case examples of ethical dilemmas confronted by pharmacists. Pirl[16] described the use of role-playing assignments for pharmacy students. This article also listed case scenarios that could be used in continuing education programs for practitioners who are exploring ways to resolve ethical dilemmas arising in their practice. Smith et al.[36] wrote a book on pharmacy ethics that also provides background discussion and case examples that relate to many target areas of pharmacy practice. This resource can be very useful for the pharmacy practitioner who wishes to address ethical issues in a particular area of practice. Such activities should always respect the privacy of individual practitioners and patients who have been involved in any specific case with ethical dimensions.

Information technology is an integral part of the provision of drug information by pharmacists or other practitioners. Sometimes technology is utilized as a tool to access literature and other information sources utilized by the professional responding to an inquiry. In other cases, the professional may utilize the Internet to offer drug information to various target audiences, both professional and the lay public. Anderson and Goodman authored a text, *Ethics and Information Technology: A Case-Based Approach to a Health Care System in Transition.*[37] This text addresses many ethical issues of pertinence to health care professionals, related both to Web-based services and drug information. Case studies on topics such as provision or use of inaccurate information, conflicts of interest, issues of confidentiality and data sharing, and ethical standards that have been set for health Web sites are presented.

Poirier and Laux[38] discussed the redesign of a drug information resources course to meet the needs of nontraditional PharmD students; this report describes the addition of a course section where ethical issues associated with drug information questions received at the author's practice site were utilized to demonstrate how to deal with such situations. The authors utilized self-study, computer-assisted instruction, and recitations to teach the course. Published descriptions of ethical dilemmas arising during the provision of drug information may be utilized to build case discussions; these scenarios are helpful for educators of both traditional and nontraditional students, as well as for in-services aimed at practicing pharmacists and other health care practitioners.[24,27-29]

Structures That Support Ethical Decision Making

Berger describes the need for an ethical covenant between the pharmacist and the patient who is being provided pharmaceutical care.[26] This term suggests an implicit contract between client and health care provider that broadly describes the relationship involved whenever a pharmacist provides drug information. Within this contract, the service recipient has a right to receive competently provided information as well as respectful treatment. He or she also has the obligation to provide background information needed by the pharmacist. Likewise, the provider pharmacist has the right to adequate background information (and respectful treatment as well), and the obligation to give competent, trustworthy, and caring service. Recognition of this implicit contract can occasionally suggest corrective action to resolve or avoid perceived ethical dilemmas. Such recognition is especially helpful when there has been a failure to adequately communicate, or there has been a lack of mutual respect in the interaction. Pharmacists also have a revised Code of Ethics for Pharmacists available to them since 1994, which may serve as a general guide to those obligations implicit to the patient-pharmacist relationship.[39,40] The text of this Code is provided in Appendix 11–1.

It is also important to establish organizational structures that guide and support the practitioner providing drug information (in any setting) when he or she is faced with an ethical dilemma. Some formal structures, such as ethics committees[41,42] and other policy-setting bodies, are generally available in larger hospitals. Formal attention to education and anticipatory planning activities on how to address ethical conflict situations is also needed within smaller institutions, the chain pharmacy setting, or in smaller organizations such as the independent community pharmacy. A report on a survey of medicine information pharmacists, conducted in the United Kingdom, assessed perceptions of possible ethical scenarios involving lay callers and asked about respondents' training to address such situations.[43] The authors described considerable variation in how specific scenarios were addressed, and a minority of the respondents had received training in this area. It is also imperative that pharmacists and other practitioners participate in policy setting that may affect how they are expected to practice. Both the organization and the individual practitioner have an obligation to plan in advance how they will handle situations where ethical conflict might arise, particularly relative to compliance with any policy affecting the employee's patient care obligations. A February 2004 Associated Press news story demonstrates this message very clearly (and was one source for an example case analysis presented in this chapter for the third edition of this text).[44] The story describes an incident where a pharmacist on duty at a branch of the Eckerd pharmacy chain declined to fill a prescription written for an emergency contraception product for a rape victim. (Apparently all three pharmacists on duty refused to fill the prescription or to refer the patient to someone who would fill the prescription.) One pharmacist was fired for the action by Eckerd. His stated reason for declining the prescription was that he believed the product could cause an abortion if fertilization had already occurred, expressing his unwillingness to participate in such action. A spokesman for the Eckerd chain indicated that their employment manual was clear that their pharmacists could not decline to fill a prescription for moral or religious reasons. The pharmacist claimed that he was not aware of the policy until he was fired; his attorney protested that such a policy violated part of the Civil Rights Act. The attorney said that this Act "prohibits private companies from forcing employees to do something that violates their religious beliefs." Yet, another article, "Promising, Professional Obligations, and the Refusal to Provide Service," by Alexander maintained that the professional "may not override the obligations derived from a prior act of promising to abide by the values, norms, and procedures that define their professional roles as instantiated within a specific practice," suggesting that the professional should leave the organization if he or she cannot conform to the expectations of his or her role within that practice.[45]

In practice, pharmacists and other practitioners may have to deal with a specific ethical dilemma very rapidly and alone in order to decide or act in a timely manner. Policies and procedures to inform and support the clinician in overall client interactions, and in ethical analysis and decision making, can better prepare the practitioner to address the real-life dilemmas he or she will encounter. The emergency contraception case makes it clear that practitioners must also be involved early (whatever their side in the issue) to make their voices heard during initial policy development (a meso-level activity within the organization, or perhaps a macro-level one if contributing to policy development for the whole profession or in law). They must also keep themselves informed about existing organizational policies in order to protect themselves and their patients. In the opinion of this author, after-the-fact controversy over unfamiliar policies does not serve the needs of practitioners, patients, or organizations.

Organizations can assist professionals by sponsoring the creation of explicit policies addressing certain issues that have demonstrated a history of ethical controversy. For example, a written policy might state that clinicians may refer questions (perhaps at a minimum back to the prescriber), where provision of an answer would violate their personal ethics. This could at least partially resolve a potential dilemma for the practitioner who has been asked to provide information that involves ethical conflict. A policy that states that practitioners are not required to answer questions from a client who refuses to provide required background information could guide response in the dilemma of dealing with an unidentified client who wants to know how long amphetamine can be detected in the urine. Another policy might address adequate staffing requirements to ensure that the community pharmacist has adequate time to perform counseling services. Of course, the legal and ethical rights of clients have to be recognized during the development of such policies. This author believes that, as professionals, pharmacists should demand the right to a major role in organizational policy development that affects their practice, preferably with input from client/patient representatives. To be useful, organizational policies must be developed with attention to avoiding what constitutes infringement on the domain of personal ethics (such as a personal prohibition against euthanasia).

Finally, institutions engaged in the professional education of health care practitioners must provide foundational education in the area of ethics, and organizations employing these practitioners should continue this education through the use of various continuing education programs that foster increasing skills in the application of ethical principles to practical decision making.[46]

Summary

Many health care practitioners will be called on to provide drug information. On occasion they will encounter ethical dilemmas regarding what information, if any, should be provided. It is important that the professional approach such moments prepared to (often quickly) identify the pertinent facts, analyze relevant points of the situation, and rank or balance the pertinent ethical rules and principles that are involved. The individual professional must recognize his or her rights and responsibilities relative to the client, to other involved individuals and populations, to society as a whole, and to any higher power to whom the practitioner feels accountable. Organizations can assist employee clinicians by formal identification and orientation on certain implicit and explicit policies. Furthermore, opportunities for the deliberate study and rehearsal of important analytic steps are important to help practitioners be prepared to address ethical dilemmas that arise when providing drug information.

Case Study 11–2

A nurse (a member of the hospital's pain management team) on one of the medical-surgical units of your hospital calls a drug information pharmacist with a question. She has a patient who she believes is being undertreated for pain. He is a young man who was admitted from the emergency room (ER) the previous evening after a motorcycle accident. He is a frequent patient in the ER, known to have a drug problem, with use of a variety of street products. She does not believe that he is in withdrawal, but does think he is getting inadequate pain medications for severe bruises, scrapes, and a broken leg. However, the admitting physician (coincidentally, the rather testy chair of the pharmacy and therapeutics committee) is quite adamant that he will not enable the patient's drug habit, and maintains that perhaps living with some pain will encourage the patient to mend his ways. The nurse asks the pharmacist to intervene with the physician to convince him that additional pain therapy is indicated, medically and ethically, for this patient.

■ ANALYSIS

1. Assess whether this drug information request constitutes a potential ethical dilemma, based on the three characteristics that differentiate such a situation.
2. What background information might you want to obtain to clarify this information request? (Imagine a background with details that might establish this as an ethical dilemma for you.)

3. If you can imagine this scenario to constitute an ethical dilemma for the pharmacist, identify whether you consider it a situation requiring decision making at a micro, meso, or macro level.
4. If, as a practitioner, this question constitutes an ethical dilemma, consider what moral rules and principles are likely to apply to this issue.
5. Assuming that some of these relevant action-guides conflict with others, describe further deliberations by which the clinician might prioritize or balance these conflicts in order to reach a decision on how to respond to the information request.
6. What organizational strategies might best prepare this pharmacist to most effectively respond to ethical dilemmas such as this one?

   Refer to the article, "Ethical Dilemmas: Controversies in Pain Management," by Janet Brown to read the analysis of a similar case.[47]

Case Study 11–3

Dr. Rich, who develops drug information materials for a managed care organization, is asked to review and is strongly encouraged to recommend a policy to routinely deny coverage for an expensive drug therapy (infliximab) for an unlabeled indication to treat celiac sprue.

■ ANALYSIS

1. Assess whether this drug information request constitutes a potential ethical dilemma, based on the three characteristics that differentiate such a situation.
2. What background information might you want to obtain to clarify this information request? (Imagine a background context with details that might establish this as an ethical dilemma for you.)
3. If you can envision this scenario to constitute an ethical dilemma for this health care professional, identify whether you consider it a situation requiring decision making at a micro, meso, or macro level.
4. If, as a practitioner, this question constitutes an ethical dilemma, consider what moral rules and principles are likely to apply to this issue.

5. Assuming that some of these relevant action-guides conflict with others, describe further deliberations by which the clinician might prioritize or balance these conflicts in order to reach a decision on how to respond to the information request.

6. What organizational strategies might best prepare this pharmacist to most effectively respond to ethical dilemmas such as this one?

Self-Assessment Questions

1. Three characteristics that differentiate an ethical deliberation from other decision-making endeavors include all *but* which of the following?
   a. The issue is universal, with any parties involved agreeing that there is a right or wrong answer.
   b. The issue has been addressed in law, with penalties identified for failure to comply with the legal directive.
   c. The welfare of all parties affected by the judgment at hand is taken into account.
   d. The issue is fundamental, with no higher standard against which to measure the rightness of the decision.

2. A nurse at the poison control center receives a call from someone indicating that a friend fed him several brownies earlier that evening that contained marijuana. The caller asks if this could be dangerous, but states that he is feeling all right. He then notes that he has an appointment the next day for a drug test related to a new job, and asks for the name of a chemical that he understands will interfere with tests for marijuana in the blood or urine. The nurse is nearly convinced that this is a legitimate call, but feels ethical qualms about how to deal with the information request. What level of ethical decision making would this constitute?
   a. Micro level
   b. Meso level
   c. Macro level
   d. None of the above

3. While picking up a prescription, a patient requests detailed information about the medication, which she must begin immediately. Twelve other clients are waiting for service, and there are only 30 minutes remaining until closing (a time strictly enforced by the nationwide corporate administration). If this constitutes

an ethical dilemma for the practitioner, what level of ethical decision making does it require?
a. Micro level
b. Meso level
c. Macro level
d. None of the above

4. A physician on the local hospital's pharmacy and therapeutics committee is asked to sign on to a proposed policy that will prohibit patients from bringing homeopathic remedies in for administration during their hospitalization. The physician is not a proponent of many such remedies, but does believe that some are beneficial, and has ethical concerns about dictating such a policy to patients being admitted to the institution. What level of decision making would this ethical dilemma require?
a. Micro level
b. Meso level
c. Macro level
d. None of the above

5. A practitioner is asked by administration to present an in-service for department colleagues on a recently approved drug product that may have applicability for use in the department's target population. The clinician is expected to present a set of materials provided by the administrator. What would be a first step in determining whether this is an ethical dilemma for the presenter?
a. Considering who might be affected by the dilemma
b. Considering the cultural perspectives of those attending the presentation
c. Determining what ethical rules seem to be at play in this situation
d. Seeking the factual details relative to the content provided by the administrator

6. Which of the following statements are *true* when describing ethics?
a. Philosophical inquiry on the moral dimensions of human conduct.
b. The terms ethical and moral have substantially different meaning.
c. Ethics involves the study of moral development.
d. Ethics involves concrete judgments on the legal aspects of situations.

7. Ethical issues might arise around which of the following kinds of issues in relationship to the provision of drug information?
a. Decisions by the health professional on whether to provide drug information.
b. Decisions on policies related to access to drug information.
c. Both answers in a and b may involve ethical issues.
d. Neither answer in a nor in b is likely to involve ethical issues.

8. Identification of relevant background information when analyzing an ethical dilemma includes all of the following statements *except*:
   a. A determination of the applicable moral rules in the case
   b. Determining the factual details of the issue at hand
   c. Consideration of who is affected by the ethical issue
   d. Identifying the cultural perspectives of the dilemma

9. The purposes for identifying relevant background in analyzing a potential ethical dilemma include all of the following *except*:
   a. Knowledge of available background information sometimes alleviates any moral concerns about the issue.
   b. Background information typically clarifies what parties might be affected by decisions made or actions taken.
   c. Background information often leads to the resolution of a recognized ethical dilemma without further analysis.
   d. Background information normally facilitates the drug information provider in addressing the dilemma in a culturally sensitive manner.

10. A hospital hotline nurse is contacted by a patient inquiring about a medication his physician has recently prescribed for him called Obecalp (placebo spelled backwards). Which of the following moral rules will likely be of concern if the nurse has any ethical qualms about this situation?
    a. Beneficence
    b. Veracity
    c. Consent
    d. Respect for autonomy

11. A primary care physician is told by the mother of his 5-year-old patient that she regularly gives the child ground rhino horn in order to help him grow to be a strong man. What background information should this practitioner consider while addressing any ethical concerns he may have about this situation?
    a. The source of the product
    b. Any cultural reasons for the mother's use of this product
    c. The dose and frequency of administration
    d. All of the above

12. In considering the case identified in question 11, what ethical principle do you think the physician should most consider when considering the ethical implications of the situation?
    a. Privacy
    b. Consent

c. Veracity

d. Respect for persons

13. A physician in the endocrinology department of the hospital asks the pharmacist clinician in the department to assist with the development of a report for presentation to the pharmacy and therapeutics committee that supports the use of growth hormone in children to treat short stature. It is generally known that there is a shortage of this expensive agent at the current time. If concern over resource allocation is the major ethical concern for this practitioner, which action-guide (rule or principle) is likely to be prioritized?

a. Beneficence

b. Respecting the patient-professional relationship

c. Justice

d. Veracity

14. Educational methods intended to prepare professionals to effectively and efficiently address ethical dilemmas that might confront them in their work should include:

a. Opportunity for group activity including case analysis and debate

b. Role-playing activities to critique the handling of cases that staff have confronted

c. Both of the activities listed above

d. Neither of the activities listed above

15. Preparation of health care professionals to address ethical dilemmas that may occur during the course of their providing drug information should generally include:

a. Clear communication of the company's policy that the customer is always right

b. Involvement of the professionals in developing policies under which they will be practicing

c. Both of the actions above

d. Neither of the actions above

REFERENCES

1. Haddad AM, Kaatz B, McCart G, McCarthy RL, Pink LA, Richardson J. Report of the ethics course content committee: curricular guidelines for pharmacy education. Am J Pharm Educ. 1993;57(Winter Suppl):34S-43S.

2. Veatch RM. Hospital pharmacy: what is ethical? (Primer). Am J Hosp Pharm. 1989;46:109-15.

3. Wilson R, Rowan MS, Henderson J. Core and comprehensive health care services: 1. Introduction to the Canadian Medical Association's decision-making framework. Can Med Assoc. 1995;152(7):1063-6.

4. Smith L, Morrissy J. Ethical dilemmas for general practitioners under the UK new contract. J Med Ethics. 1994;20:175-80.

5. Dierchx de Casterle B, Meulenbergs T, van de Vijver L, Tanghe A, Castmans C. Ethics meetings in support of good nursing care: some practice-based thoughts. Nurs Ethics. 2002;9(6):612-22.

6. Kirby J, Simpson C. An innovative, inclusive process for meso-level health policy development. HEC Forum. 2007;19(2):161-76.

7. Martin D, Singer P. A strategy to improve priority setting in health care institutions. Health Care Anal. 2003;11(1):59-68.

8. Pentz RD. Expanding into organizational ethics: the experience of one clinical ethics committee. HEC Forum. 1998;10(2):213-21.

9. Goold SD. Trust and the ethics of health care institutions. Hastings Cent Rep. 2001;6:26-33.

10. Nunes R. Evidence-based medicine: a new tool for resource allocation? Med, Health Care Phil. 2003;6:297-301.

11. Coyle SL, for the Ethics and Human Rights Committee, American College of Physicians— American Society of Internal Medicine. Physician-industry relations. Part 1: Individual physicians. Ann Intern Med. 2002;136:396-402.

12. Kenny N, Joffres C. An ethical analysis of international health priority-setting. Health Care Anal. 2007;16:145-60.

13. Ruger JP. Ethics in american health 1: Ethical approaches to health policy. Am J Pub Health. 2008;98(10):1751-6.

14. Ruger JP. Ethics in american health 2: An ethical framework for health system reform. Am J Pub Health. 2008;98(10):1756-63.

15. Khushf G. The case for managed care: reappraising medical and socio-political ideals. J Med Phil. 1999;24(5):415-33.

16. Pirl MA. An ethics laboratory as an educational tool in a pharmacy law and ethics course. J Pharm Teach. 1990;1(3):51-68.

17. Beauchamp TLC, Childress JF. Principles of Biomedical Ethics. 5th ed. New York, (NY): Oxford University Press; 2001.

18. Beauchamp TLC, Childress JF. Principles of Biomedical Ethics. 6th ed. New York, (NY): Oxford University Press; 2008.

19. Beauchamp TLC, Childress JF. Principles of Biomedical Ethics. 4th ed. New York, (NY): Oxford University Press; 1994.

20. Beauchamp TL. Principles or rules? In: Kopelman L, editor. Building Bioethics. Great Britain: Kluwer Academic Publishers; 1999:15-24.

21. Veatch RM. Cross-Cultural Perspectives in Medical Ethics. 2nd ed. Sudbury (MA): Jones and Bartlett Publishers; 2000.

22. Thornton BC, Callahan D, Nelson JL. Bioethics education: expanding the circle of participants. Hastings Cent Rep. 1993;23(1):25-29.

23. Veatch RM. A Theory of Medical Ethics. New York, (NY): Basic Books Publishers; 1981.

24. Najjar TA, Al-Arifi MN, Gubara OA, Dana MH. Ethical requests received by drug and poison information center in Saudi Arabia. J Soc Adm Pharm. 2000;17(4):234-7.

25. Carrese J, Brown K, Jameton A. Culture, healing, and professional obligations. Hastings Cent Rep. 1993;15:7.

26. Berger BA. Building an effective therapeutic alliance: competence, trustworthiness, and caring. Am J Hosp Pharm. 1993;50:2399-403.

27. Arnold RM, Nissen JC, Campbell NA. Ethical issues in a drug information center. Drug Intell Clin Pharm. 1987;21:1008-11.

28. Kelly WN, Krause EC, Krowsinski WJ, Small TR, Drane JF. National survey of ethical issues presented to drug information centers. Am J Hosp Pharm. 1990;47:2245-50.

29. Schools RM, Brushwood DB. The pharmacist's role in patient care. Hastings Cent Rep. 1991;12:7.

30. Powers M, Faden R. Social Justice. The Moral Foundations of Public Health and Health Policy. New York, (NY): Oxford University Press; 2006.

31. Bayer R, Gostin LO, Jennings B, Steinbock B, editors. Public Health Ethics. Theory, Policy and Practice. New York, (NY): Oxford University Press; 2007.

32. Davis CM. Patient–Practitioner Interaction: An Experiential Manual for Developing the Art of Health Care. Thorofare (NJ): Slack; 1989.

33. Coach R. 5-minutes to monitor progress. Teaching Prof. 1991;5(9):1-2.

34. Haddad AM, editor. Teaching and Learning Strategies in Pharmacy Ethics. 2nd ed. Binghamton (NY): Pharmaceutical Products Press; 1997.

35. Veatch RM, Haddad AM. Case Studies in Pharmacy Ethics. 2nd ed. New York, (NY): Oxford University Press; 2008.

36. Smith M, Strauss S, Baldwin HJ, Alberts KT. Pharmacy Ethics. New York, (NY): Pharmaceutical Products Press; 1991.

37. Anderson JG, Goodman KW. Ethics and Information Technology: A Case-Based Approach to a Health Care System in Transition. New York, (NY): Springer-Verlag; 2002.

38. Poirier TL, Laux R. Redesign of a drug information resources course: responding to the needs of nontraditional PharmD students. Am J Pharm Educ. 1997;61:306-9.

39. Vottero LD. Code of ethics for pharmacists. Am J Health-Syst Pharm. 1995;52:2096-131.

40. American Pharmacists Association. Code of ethics for pharmacists. [Internet]. Washington: American Pharmacists Association. [cited 2010 March 26]. Available from: http://www.pharmacist.com/AM/Template.cfm?Section=Search1&template=/CM/HTMLDisplay.cfm&ContentID=2903.

41. Mappes TA, Zembaty JS, editors. Biomedical Ethics. 3rd ed. New York, (NY): McGraw-Hill; 1991.

42. Mappes TA, Degrazia D, editors. Biomedical Ethics. 5th ed. Boston, (MA): McGraw-Hill; 2001.

43. Wills S, Brown D, Astubry S. A survey of ethical issues surrounding supply of information to members of the public by hospital pharmacy medicines information centres. Pharm World Sci. 2002;24(2):55-60.

44. Austin L. Emergency contraception denial raises moral, legal issues. Associated Press State and Local Wire. 2004 Feb 21.

45. Alexander JK. Promising, professional obligations, and the refusal to provide service. HEC Forum. 2005;17(3):178-95.

46. Gettman DA, Benson B, Nguyen V, Luu SN. Use of motivational techniques by drug information center personnel to respond to calls involving perceived ethical dilemmas [Abstract]. ASHP Midyear Clinical Meeting; 2000: PCM-4.

47. Brown J. Ethical dilemmas: controversies in pain management. Adv Nurse Pract. B1997:69-72.

SUGGESTED READINGS

Beauchamp TLC, Childress JF. Principles of Biomedical Ethics. 6th ed. New York, (NY): Oxford University Press; 2008.

Kelly WN, Krause EC, Krowsinski WJ, Small TR, Drane JF. National survey of ethical issues presented to drug information centers. Am J Hosp Pharm. 1990;47:2245–50.

Veatch RM, Haddad A. Case Studies in Pharmacy Ethics. 2nd ed. New York, (NY): Oxford University Press; 2008.

Wills S, Brown D, Astbury S. A survey of ethical issues surrounding supply of information to members of the public by hospital pharmacy medicines information centres. Pharmacy World and Science (Netherlands). 2002;24(Feb):55-60.

Chapter Twelve

Pharmacy and Therapeutics Committee

Patrick M. Malone • Nancy L. Fagan
• Mark A. Malesker • Paul J. Nelson

Learning Objectives

After completing this chapter, the reader will be able to

- Describe the pharmacy and therapeutics (P&T) committee.
- Describe the attributes and structure of a P&T committee likely to promote its ability to function successfully.
- Define the functions of the P&T committee.
- Describe where and how the P&T committee fits into the organizational structure of a health care institution or other groups.
- Describe how the pharmacy department participates in P&T committee activities.
- Describe and explain the concepts of drug formularies and drug formulary systems, and how pharmacy participates in their establishment and maintenance.
- Describe how P&T committee activities contribute to the quality improvement of medication use.
- Describe how to develop policies and procedures for the process of medication use.

Key Concepts

❶ A pharmacy and therapeutics (P&T) committee oversees all aspects of drug therapy within an institution.

❷ Although it is not uncommon for pharmacists to downplay or misunderstand the importance of P&T committee support in comparison to other clinical activities, such support is vital for pharmacy to impact patient care.

❸ A P&T committee may find it necessary to create ad hoc committees to address various issues, depending on their complexity and size.

❹ Typically, P&T committee functions include determining what drugs are available, who can prescribe specific drugs, policies and procedures regarding drug use (including pharmacy policies and procedures, standard order sets, and clinical guidelines), quality assurance activities (e.g., drug utilization review/drug usage evaluation/medication usage evaluation), adverse drug reactions/medication errors, dealing with product shortages, and education in drug use.

❺ A variety of topics regarding the quality of medication use are normally part of the activities of a P&T committee.

Introduction

When considering how a pharmacist can have an impact on a patient's drug therapy, it is common to consider the individual practitioner dealing with a specific patient or, perhaps, a small group of patients. Certainly the clinician can have a deep impact this way, but it does have the disadvantage of dealing with a very limited number of patients. In order for pharmacists to efficiently impact a great number of patients, a different approach is necessary. Fortunately, one approach pharmacists can take is to participate in the activities of a **❶** *P&T committee or its equivalent, which generally oversees all aspects of drug therapy in an institution.* Physicians and pharmacists have collaborated to implement cost-effective prescribing practices and assess clinical outcomes through educational initiatives, administrative programs to restrict ordering practices, the use of formularies and prescribing guidelines, and financial incentives.[1] There are data to show that P&T committee actions are useful.[2,3]

Before proceeding, it must be stated that although this chapter deals with the P&T committee, which is usually the group responsible for overseeing all aspects of drug therapy in an institution, there is sometimes a similar body referred to as the formulary committee. This latter group deals strictly with determining which drugs are carried within an institution or organization, whereas the P&T committee has numerous other tasks, covering all aspects of drug therapy (e.g., adverse drug reaction [ADR]/medication error monitoring, quality assurance, policy and procedure approval), although the exact group of functions may vary from place to place.[4] Some institutions use a formulary committee, because other bodies may perform the additional P&T committee tasks described later in this chapter. Also, some health care groups may use both committees, with one body addressing the issues for the group as a whole, while the other is located separately at various institutions to address issues specific to that location (e.g., only one institution in the group has an oncology unit; therefore, the committee for that individual institution will consider specific antineoplastic agents that are not of much use for the rest of the group). In this chapter, anything discussed regarding which drugs are available within an institution or group applies to both bodies, whereas all other items are for the P&T committee only.

It should be noted that although P&T committees have normally been associated with institutional pharmacy, other organizations have increasingly used P&T-type committees in an attempt to improve drug therapy while lowering costs. Some places where such committees are seen include managed care organizations (MCOs),[5] insurance companies, pharmacy benefit management (PBM) companies, unions, employers,[6] state Medicaid boards, state departments of public institutions,[7] Medicare,[8] long-term care facilities,[9] ambulatory clinics,[10] and even community pharmacies.[11] Much of this chapter will use examples from institutional pharmacy and managed care, simply because much of the published literature deals with those areas of practice and it is the most likely setting in which a pharmacist will be directly involved in P&T committee activities. However, the concepts covered are applicable to any P&T-type committee and comply with the recommendations of the American Medical Association (AMA),[12,13] the American Society of Health-System Pharmacists (ASHP),[14] The Joint Commission (formerly the Joint Commission for the Accreditation of Health Care Organizations) (TJC),[15] and the Academy of Managed Care Pharmacy (AMCP).[16]

❶ *The role of the P&T committee has been continuously expanded over the years and now encompasses a great number of functions and activities that cover all aspects of overseeing drug therapy.* As some of these are of sufficient size and importance, they are covered separately in other chapters (e.g., drug monographs and quality assurance). In addition, there are a number of areas (e.g., investigational drugs) in which P&T committees play a secondary role, and these too are covered in other chapters. This chapter serves to provide a base to tie together discussions of all of these areas and a number of smaller functions or activities that will be covered as a portion of this chapter. The information is appropriate both for those just learning about the concepts and also for those individuals who are involved with P&T committee activities.

Organizational Background

The concept of a P&T committee represents a unique niche within the structure of the hospital. The current role of a hospital in Western countries[17] began about 200 years ago, at a time when very few efficacious medications were available, although drug formularies had been developed during the Revolutionary War to list the drugs available.[18] It has also been noted that a drug formulary was developed for all municipal hospitals in New York City at Bellevue Hospital in 1868.[19] The original hospital was a place to receive basic health care when a person had no extended family to provide the basic needs of good health. After infection control became a recognized concept, and anesthesia for surgery evolved around 1900, the value of the modern hospital progressively became a recognized need for all segments of society. The origins for standards of how a hospital functioned subsequently developed during the first half of the twentieth century. This began with the early efforts of the American College of Surgeons in the United States to develop the first accreditation standards for hospitals. Later, the Joint Commission on Accreditation of Hospitals (JCAH), now known as TJC, evolved to centralize the basic requirements for the functional character of a U.S. hospital. The concept of the P&T committee originated and evolved to help hospitals meet various standards regarding drug therapy. The first P&T committee was formed at Bellevue Hospital in New York City in the mid-1930s.[18,20] Although it dealt with true compounding formulas, it was originally founded to ensure the quality and efficacy of those products, which is still a portion of the functions of P&T committees.

In keeping with the social origins of the hospital, the legally sanctioned or licensed privilege of being a professional health care provider evolved.[17] Both the physician and pharmacist were considered unique for the needs of society. Minimum standards evolved, including the accreditation of their training as a basis for being licensed. Originally, physicians and pharmacists functioned primarily as independent professionals. The nature of a physician's independence was legally defined to further support their obligations to a patient. Many states in the United States legally prohibited a physician from being employed by a corporation. Eventually, these laws were all repealed, but they had the effect of creating the basis for a medical staff as being a separate legal entity within a hospital. The medical staff reflected the legally evolving traditions of a physician, and indirectly the pharmacist, as being independent professionals committed only to the care of a patient without unnecessary outside influences. This evolution has had a major impact on the organizational structure of hospitals.

A typical hospital organization is shown in Figure 12–1. The board of directors divides the functions of its organization into two entities. First, the administration of the hospital operates as a typical business with a chief executive officer, chief operating officer, and so

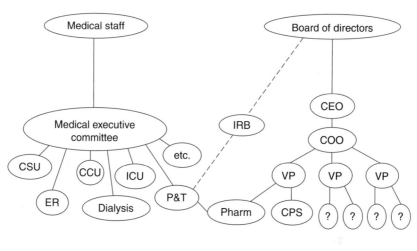

CCU   Coronary Care Unit Committee

CEO   Chief Executive Officer

COO   Chief Operating Officer

CPS   Central Processing & Supply

CSU   Cardiac Surgery Unit Committee

ER   Emergency Room Committee

ICU   Intensive Care Unit Committee

IRB   Institutional Review Board

Pharm   Pharmacy Department

P&T   Pharmacy & Therapeutics Committee

VP   Vice President

?   Other Hospital Departments

Figure 12–1. Hospital organization.

forth. Second, the board of directors authorizes that a medical staff be formed that reports separately to the board of directors. Although the medical staff as a whole is ultimately in charge of all clinical aspects of care in the hospital, in most institutions this is unworkable without an administrative structure of some kind. Therefore, the medical staff may elect officers and either elect or appoint somebody to oversee all aspects of patient care. In this example, the term medical executive committee is used for that body, although the name and exact function may vary. The medical staff functions to certify the credentials of its members, establish their scope of practice where appropriate, monitor the quality of health care provided by its members, and maintain the means to collaborate with the administration of the hospital.

In modern medicine, there are so many clinical areas to consider that it is unrealistic for one committee to adequately oversee all aspects of patient care, except in very small institutions. For this reason, various subcommittees of the medical executive committee are usually necessary, as can be seen in Figure 12–1. As a means to coordinate the needs of the medical staff and the operation of the hospital pharmacy, the modern P&T committee developed. From the traditions established by TJC and ASHP, the P&T committee developed as a function of the medical staff's responsibilities. This committee or related committees may have other names, such as the drug and therapeutics committee in Australia,[21] but the functions are the same. Although the P&T committee has been referred to in TJC accreditation standards in the past, it is no longer specifically required and may be replaced by some other committee or body,[15,22,23] although the P&T committee concept is supported by many national and professional organizations.[24] Given the continuing growth in the number, complexity, and expense of medications, both the importance and number of functions of the P&T committee have continued to increase. Policy and procedures to set up a P&T committee are described in Appendix 12–1, but the following will serve as a general description of P&T committees and their actions.

In some cases, the P&T committee may be part of a corporation of hospitals and medical centers, rather than just being for a specific institution. Although the philosophy of operating one P&T committee within this corporate structure seems reasonable, this is not often accomplished without problems, and decentralization of these efforts may be better.[25] Different patient populations, medication needs, cross-hospital physician participation, meeting time, length and location of meetings, and differing clinical cultures within a specific institution are examples of barriers that may be present. The P&T model may need to be revised to work with these challenges.[26-31]

Although it is easy to assume from its name that the P&T committee is organizationally a part of the pharmacy department, such is not the case, as was mentioned previously. Instead, it is usually a medical staff entity and, perhaps, only one or two pharmacists may actually be members of the committee (possibly *ex officio* members without voting privileges). Commonly, the pharmacy director or clinical coordinator, serving as the committee's secretary (e.g., taking minutes, collating, and arranging the agenda), may be the sole official pharmacy representative. Other pharmacists may also attend to act as consultants to the committee, often having great impact on the committee's decisions, even if they cannot officially vote. Fortunately, in larger hospitals, it appears that more pharmacists are now becoming members of the P&T committee.[32]

Typically, the voting members of an institutional P&T committee are limited to members of the medical staff. Membership is mostly physicians (preferably a wide variety of physicians from different areas of practice), but usually includes at least one pharmacist and often members from other areas of the hospital (e.g., nursing, administration, quality assurance, medical records, laboratory, and risk management).[33] A pharmacoeconomist also can be extremely helpful. There have also been recommendations to include other individuals, such as a medical ethicist or community pharmacist.[34] It may be best to try to keep down the number of physician members to encourage a smaller group to participate more fully, while taking care of addressing the wide variety of issues by calling in physicians to consult with the committee on an as-needed basis.[35] In some cases, the pharmacy department is asked to recommend physicians for the committee. If possible, the pharmacy department should suggest physicians who are noted for their commitment to rational drug therapy.[36] As an example, the U.S. Department of Defense has procedures for the appointment of members, including nonphysician members, of the P&T committee that are available on the Internet.[37] Also, efforts should be made to ensure that the physician chosen to be chairman of the committee is an advocate of the pharmacy department. It is possible for the medical executive committee of the medical staff to pass a resolution to approve a policy broadening the voting members of the P&T committee (e.g., director of pharmacy or hospital vice president) or delegating the functions of the P&T committee to the hospital. In this latter arrangement, the medical staff would reserve the right to terminate the policy if the P&T committee fails to support the needs of the medical staff. If the P&T committee is a hospital committee, rather than a medical staff committee, a pharmacist or nurse might more easily obtain voting privileges, given appropriate physician quorum requirements in the authorizing policy.

The P&T committee of MCOs and government bodies often have similar membership to that in institutional committees; however, there may need to be a requirement for at least some of the members to be independent practitioners and retail pharmacists (i.e., having no financial ties to the organization or group that sponsors the P&T committee).[33,38,39] In accordance with the 2003 Medication Modernization Act, the use of formularies is an essential component to the PBM.[33]

Once the general organizational setting of the P&T committee has been determined, the operating policy of the P&T committee requires careful attention to two key issues. The first key issue is obvious—to whom does the P&T committee report and to what degree can the decisions of the P&T committee be overturned by another segment of the organization? It is important to point out that the P&T committee may act only as an advisory body to the medical executive committee. Decisions of the P&T committee may not be considered final (and therefore not be implemented) until they are reviewed and approved by the medical executive committee. In this situation, a report is forwarded from the P&T committee after each meeting to the medical executive committee. In addition, an annual report of the P&T committee may be prepared for both internal review and review by the medical executive committee. This annual report is time-consuming to prepare, but is a very important means of tracking P&T activities and action over time.

The second issue is that the P&T committee will likely be successful based on the leadership qualities of its members and the chairperson. The role of the chairperson includes developing the respect and involvement of all members.

PHARMACY BENEFIT MANAGEMENT (PBM) P&T COMMITTEE ORIGIN

The origin of the PBM organizations dates back to the late 1960s. Their primary focus was on claims administration for insurance companies. Later, it became a challenge for the insurance companies to efficiently manage the increase in drug coverage in the private sector when the prescription volume was high and the cost per claim was low.[40] The plastic drug benefit card began in the 1970s and changed the way many prescriptions were bought and paid for by the insurance company and employee. From then on, any employee with an ID card, using a pharmacy network, only had a small copayment.[40] In addition, administrative costs for the third-party payer (whether it is the insurance company, health plan, or employer) were reduced, with the PBM creating pharmacy networks and mail service benefits. Pharmacy networks are a group of pharmacies that are under contract with the insurance company, health plan, and/or their contracted PBM partner to promote prescription services at a negotiated discounted fee.[41] Mail service is a program offered by the PBM, whereby pharmaceutical agents, both prescription and nonprescription, are offered through the mail.[41]

The introduction of real-time electronic claims processing came in the late 1980s. Not only was there two-way communication between the pharmacy and the PBM for claims processing, but also for clinical information. In the 1990s, the PBMs moved toward a greater emphasis on patient health by offering a variety of new services in addition to the claims processing. Since 2000, there has been an emphasis on consumer behavior modification, enhanced patient interventions, physician connectivity, clinical consulting, disease management, and retrospective drug utilization review (DUR; see Chapter 14 for further information) to name a few.[40]

One of the key functions of a PBM is to design, implement, and administer outpatient drug benefit programs for employers, MCOs, and other third-party payers. PBMs manage prescription drug benefits separate from other health care services (i.e., physician and hospital services).[41] Determining which medications are most cost-effective, without compromising patient care, is one of the key elements for controlling the cost of a prescription drug benefit.[6,42] PBMs accomplish this by developing drug formularies.[6] Formularies define what medications are covered (i.e., paid for) and provide the main component of the pharmacy benefit. Specific PBM drug payment and management activities occur within this formulary structure, such as therapeutic interchange and disease management programs. Eighty to one hundred percent of most PBM-covered patients receive some type of formulary management service.[6,41] The use of drug formularies is in flux due to the advantages and disadvantages identified over the last decade or so; however, they are likely to be continued for at least the foreseeable future, particularly due to the Medicare drug formulary requirements.[43]

The development and maintenance of drug formularies for third-party payers is an ongoing process. The formulary must be continuously updated to keep pace with new drugs, therapies, prices, recent clinical research, changes in medical practice, evidence based-treatment guidelines, and updated Food and Drug Administration (FDA) information.[44] PBMs use a panel of experts called the P&T committee to develop and manage their drug formularies. Many times individuals with special clinical expertise are consulted when considering medications within a specific therapeutic class.[44] Meetings are usually held on a quarterly basis, and not only are drug formulary recommendations made, but this group also provides input into other clinical areas, such as the development of disease management programs.[6,40,41,43,44]

Many PBMs establish their own P&T committee to evaluate the efficacy, safety, uniqueness, cost of therapeutic equivalent drugs, and other appropriate criteria. In addition, PBMs work with the health plan, employer, or insurance company P&T committee to develop drug formularies using the same evaluation process. In either case, if the P&T committee determines that one drug provides a clear medical benefit over the other therapeutically equivalent drugs in that same therapeutic category, the drug is usually added to the formulary.[6] However, if there are drugs in the same therapeutic category that have very similar efficacy and safety profiles and no unique properties that would make it a better drug, then the net cost becomes a deciding factor as to which drug should be added to the formulary.[6] There has been some discussion as to whether drug costs are weighted too heavily, while drug efficacy and other clinical information is weighted too lightly when it comes to drug formulary decisions.[40,41] The committee leadership needs to recognize the potential for conflicts of interest between efficacy and the economic interests of the PBM and to establish means of resolving conflicts that arise.

Me-too drugs are drugs that are structurally very similar to an already known drug that has only minor differences. For example, many drugs come in two versions: an L isomer (left) and an R isomer (right). An example of a me-too drug is esomeprazole (Nexium), the L-isomer of omeprazole (Prilosec, the R- and L-isomers). Both drugs are used to treat gastroesophageal reflux disease (GERD). When a comparative analysis was conducted looking at drugs approved for marketing between January 2007 and July 2008, those that had a different chemical entity and a separate mechanism of action accounted for 69%; however, they offered no clinical improvement over those already on the market. Forty-four percent offered some type of new convenience, but only 13% offered greater efficacy.[45]

In the case of a health plan, employer, or insurance company's own P&T committee, the drug formulary recommendations made by the PBM P&T committee are presented and reviewed by the organization's P&T committee. The PBM recommendations regarding drug formulary recommendations can be either accepted or denied by the organization's P&T committee and the organization's own decision made regarding formulary inclusion.

PHARMACY SUPPORT OF THE P&T COMMITTEE

❷ *Although it is not uncommon for pharmacists to downplay or misunderstand the importance of P&T committee support in comparison to other clinical activities, such support is vital for pharmacy to impact patient care.* P&T committee support and participation can have far-reaching effects on the overall quality of drug therapy in an institution and must be given a great deal of attention. Although such attention is time-consuming,[46] it can be of value to the pharmacy because this is an opportunity to present recommendations to a decision-making body, and P&T committees often accept pharmacy recommendations;[47,48] therefore, pharmacy departments can have a great and far-reaching impact on drug therapy through this mechanism.

Some pharmacists who participate in P&T committee activities feel they are serving their function by just providing information requested by physicians and considering drugs for formulary approval only following physician requests. This can rapidly deteriorate into crisis management, where the pharmacy department reacts to problems, fighting each fire as it occurs. It is much better for a pharmacy to be proactive,[49,50] seeking to address issues (e.g., changes in drugs carried on the formulary, new policies and procedures, quality assurance activities, and so forth) before they become problems. TJC accreditation requirements include annual evaluation of all drugs and/or drug classes.[15] Through prospective actions with the P&T committee it is possible for the pharmacy to get physician support for their clinical activities.

In the specific instance of P&T committee support, one or more pharmacists must be identified to conduct the necessary planning. This may consist of a pharmacy-based steering committee and might include administrators, purchasing agents, or clinicians, and, particularly, drug information specialists. These people must develop and regularly evaluate data sources to anticipate physicians' needs[51] (see Table 12–1). For example, it is necessary to find out what drugs have recently been FDA approved in order to identify drugs for possible formulary inclusion. FDA approval often occurs about 3 months before commercial availability and is published on the FDA Web site (http://www.accessdata.fda.gov/scripts/cder/drugsatfda/index.cfm). Therefore, there is time for the drug to be considered for formulary addition before the first orders arrive from the nursing units, which necessitates a review of some sort under TJC standards.[15] In a case where it is not possible to consider a drug before it is commercially available, it has been suggested by some that drugs rated P (priority) by the FDA be made available to physicians until the drug can be fully considered (the FDA classification codes are found in Table 12–2 and Table 12–3, with the priority versus standard explanation found in Table 12–3).[52] This latter procedure may be effective, but considering the drug before commercial availability is preferable, because if the ultimate P&T committee decision is to leave the drug off the drug formulary, there may be difficulties in getting physicians to stop use of the product. It is also a good idea to track older drugs. For example, the use of nonformulary drugs

TABLE 12–1. AREAS WHERE PHARMACISTS SHOULD BE SUPPORTING A PHARMACY AND THERAPEUTICS COMMITTEE

- Planning future agendas (including medications, policies and procedures, quality assurance, and other subjects to be addressed)
- Gathering data to create drug monographs and other necessary documents
- Evaluating medications for formulary adoption or deletion
- Preparing and conducting quality assurance programs (including drug usage evaluation and monitoring of adverse effects and medication errors)
- Preparing policies and procedures
- Communicating information from the P&T committee to other areas of the institution
- Creating hardcopy and electronic versions of the formulary

may be tracked within the hospital (please note: a nonformulary drug may be a product that has not been approved for use within an institution, but it may also be a drug that has been approved for use, but has been prescribed in a particular situation for a use other than what was approved by the P&T committee when it was added to the drug formulary).[53-55] If patterns of increased use are noted, it is best to identify a reason for that use. If the use is inappropriate, the physician(s) should be contacted and given information

TABLE 12–2. FDA CLASSIFICATION BY CHEMICAL TYPE*

Type	Definition
1	New molecular entity not marketed in the United States
2	New salt, ester, or other noncovalent derivative of another drug marketed in the United States
3	New formulation or dosage form of an active ingredient marketed in the United States
4	New combination of drugs already marketed in the United States
5	New manufacturer of a drug product already marketed by another company in the United States
6	New indication for a product already marketed in the United States
7	Drug that is already legally marketed without an approved NDA
	• First application since 1962 for a drug marketed prior to 1938.
	• First application for Drug Efficacy Study Implementation (DESI)-related products that were first marketed between 1938 and 1962 without an NDA.
	• First application for DESI-related products first marketed after 1962 without an NDA. In this case, the indications may be the same or different from the legally marketed product.
8	Over-the-counter switch

*Drugs@FDA Frequently Asked Questions [Internet]. Washington, DC: Food and Drug Administration, [updated 2010 Jun 25; cited 2010 Oct 19]. Available from: http://www.fda.gov/Drugs/InformationOnDrugs/ucm075234.htm#chemtype_reviewclass.

TABLE 12–3. FDA CLASSIFICATIONS BY THERAPEUTIC POTENTIAL

Type	Definition
P	Priority handling by FDA—before 1992 this was two categories: A—Major therapeutic gain B—Moderate therapeutic gain
S	Standard handling by FDA—before 1992 this was referred to as Class C, which indicated that the product offered only a minor or no therapeutic gain
O	Orphan drug

*Drugs@FDA Frequently Asked Questions [Internet]. Washington, DC: Food and Drug Administration, [updated 2010 Jun 25; cited 2010 Oct 19]. Available from: http://www.fda.gov/Drugs/InformationOnDrugs/ucm075234.htm#chemtype_reviewclass.

about alternative formulary agents. In some cases, new information may be available showing a new advantage or use for an old agent, which can lead to its reconsideration for formulary adoption. Related to this is the necessity to regularly consider the material being promoted by the drug company representatives. It is worth mentioning that some hospitals will restrict drug representative access to the institution or restrict the drugs that may be promoted by those representatives to only items approved for use in the hospital in order to prevent this problem. There may also be new indications or other information that will increase demand for nonformulary items. If there are sufficient changes noted in the use(s) of a particular class of drugs, it is useful to review the class as a whole to decide which drug(s) are to be retained on the formulary. TJC now requires annual review of all medications,[10-15] which is useful because there may be new information not otherwise noted that necessitates changes in formulary items in a particular class, both additions and deletions. However, the situations noted previously may necessitate moving up the review. Other items, such as trends in reported ADRs in the institution or published data for new products with little information in the literature on first approval, may also be useful in determining products for P&T committee consideration or reconsideration.[56] Although there must be a mechanism by which physicians can request that drugs be added to the formulary, all of the methods mentioned and others can help the pharmacy anticipate physician needs, allowing time for information gathering, evaluation of products, and P&T committee consideration before the need becomes too urgent to permit proper consideration.

To guide the clinician in considering the logic of requesting the addition of items to the drug formulary, a specific request form may be useful. Items that a physician may be required to fill out or attach to the form are listed in Table 12–4.[57] An example form can be found in Appendix 12–2.

The P&T committee should be kept advised by the above-mentioned pharmacy-based steering committee of future plans, so that it can be aware that a rational planning process is governing its agenda. Also, it is a good idea for one or more representative(s) of this steering committee to meet with the pharmacy director, chairman of the P&T

TABLE 12–4. ITEMS THAT MAY BE ON A REQUEST FOR FORMULARY CONSIDERATION FORM

- Date and time of request
- Name of product (e.g., generic, trade, chemical)
- Source of product (e.g., manufacturer, distributor)
- Specific information about drug product (e.g., class of drug, mechanism, adverse effects, clinical studies)
- Anticipated use of drug (e.g., what type of patient, how often)
- Comparable drugs already on the formulary
- Why the product is needed
- What drugs could be removed from the formulary
- What restrictions, policies, cautions, etc., are necessary
- How the drug fits into any clinical guidelines
- Action requested (e.g., addition, deletion, restriction)

committee, and a representative of the hospital administration on a regular basis to assist with planning and ensure that their concerns are addressed. This meeting could be held shortly before the P&T committee actually meets to present preliminary formulary evaluations, drug usage evaluation (DUE) material, and policy and procedure documents for an initial review, allowing modifications addressing physician and administration concerns to be made before formal committee review and action. During this meeting, plans for future months can be made or adjusted as the circumstances dictate. Other appropriate physicians or groups should also be consulted in order to ensure that their concerns are addressed. For example, if changes to the cephalosporins carried on the drug formulary or their permitted uses (e.g., restrictions to particular uses or prescribing groups) are considered, the infectious disease specialists should be contacted to provide input. (Note: This does not mean that recommendations are changed to account for physician preferences, but that their options and concerns are specifically addressed in the evaluation.)

Regarding quality assurance activities, the pharmacy department should obtain data to guide the selection of upcoming quality assurance programs. This will be covered in greater detail in Chapter 14.

The pharmacy should also investigate what medications may need specific policies and procedures developed to guide their use and monitoring. This may be done when the drug is first being evaluated for formulary addition or later if problems (e.g., increased ADR reports, medication errors, and overuse) are noted. For example, concerns about a new thrombolytic agent leading to increased morbidity and mortality through improper use might prompt the P&T committee to approve specific protocols for the use of the agent. Policy and procedure documents are covered later in this chapter and also in Chapter 18.

Finally, it is extremely important for the P&T committee to make sure that physicians are informed about the actions taken. Often the pharmacy is heavily involved in providing this information to physicians. Although a great deal of effort is placed on communication within the committee itself, it is also necessary to keep the entire medical staff informed. This may be accomplished through medical department meeting presentations, newsletters and Web sites (refer to Chapter 9), or other mechanisms.

AD HOC COMMITTEES

❸ *A P&T committee may find it necessary to create ad hoc committees to address various issues, depending on their complexity and size.* Some of the common committees are discussed in the following. Institutions may or may not use these committees (sometimes referred to as subcommittees) and their exact use varies from place to place, depending on their needs or desires.[4]

Adverse Reactions

A comprehensive ADR monitoring and reporting program is an essential component of the P&T committee (see Chapter 15 for further information about ADRs and how they are handled). A subcommittee may be helpful to review the entire ADR data for trends and any necessary actions that need to be taken. The P&T committee will usually report the ADR data on a monthly or quarterly basis. Following approval of this report, the P&T committee is responsible for the dissemination of information to the medical staff and other health professionals in the institution. This includes recommending processes to cut the rate of preventable ADRs. This subcommittee may be combined with the medication errors subcommittee.[15,58]

Anticoagulation

The anticoagulation subcommittee is responsible for policies and procedures to maintain compliance with TJC Goal 3E, now called the TJC National Patient Safety Goal 03.05.01.[15] This goal is to reduce the likelihood of patient harm associated with anticoagulation therapy. The subcommittee can also participate in improvement processes to maintain standards with quality organizations such as the National Quality Forum (NQF) and the Surgical Care Improvement Project (SCIP). Standard orders and policies to follow evidence-based guidelines of the American College of Chest Physicians (ACCP) are also developed by this subcommittee. Pharmacists have an important role on this committee. Most hospitals have pharmacists dedicated to anticoagulation monitoring and education.

Antimicrobials/Infectious Disease

Antibiotics can represent the largest category of formulary medications.[59] Frequent category review and revision is necessary and complex.[60] Cunha has defined five factors to consider when reviewing antimicrobial agents for formulary inclusion: microbiologic activity,[61] pharmacokinetics and pharmacodynamics profiles,[62] resistance patterns,[63,64] adverse effects,[65] and cost to the institution.[66] The P&T committee or a subcommittee of the P&T may be responsible for developing appropriate antibiotic selection and use in both inpatient and outpatient settings.[67,68] Some institutions may rely on input from the infection control committee regarding antibiotic formulary management and appropriate utilization. Multidisciplinary antibiotic use committees have limited inappropriate prescribing of antimicrobials and increased the medical staff's knowledge on appropriate antibiotic use.[66,69,70]

The main purpose of the antimicrobial/infectious disease subcommittee is to promote antimicrobial stewardship to ensure cost-effective therapy and improve patient outcomes. Antimicrobial stewardship promotes and optimizes antimicrobial therapy consistent with the hospital's/health system's antibiograms. Guideline development and education is provided to the medical staff as well as to other health care professionals. The subcommittee is also involved in the enforcement of formulary agent use, substitution policies, and restrictions for antibiotics. In addition, review and feedback on prescribing patterns is provided to the medical staff regarding antibiotic therapy.[71-73]

Medication Safety

A medication safety committee (sometimes called safety committee or medication misadventure subcommittee) should be multidisciplinary in nature. This subcommittee will review medication misadventures and medication errors that occur within the institution or health care system. They may also review adverse drug reactions (instead of an adverse reaction committee), drug-drug interactions, drug dispensing processes, medication errors (see Chapter 16 for more information), look-alike/sound-alike medications, and communication errors. A report will commonly be presented to the P&T committee on a quarterly or semiannual basis. Following approval of this report, the P&T committee is responsible for the dissemination of information to the medical staff and other health professionals in the institution. This includes recommending processes to cut the rate of preventable medication safety issues. In some places, a medication error reduction plan (MERP) is prepared to identify process improvements that have been made and those that are planned. When evaluating drug cost strategies, patient safety should always be a priority.[74] The 2010 Joint Commission Accreditation Process Guide for Hospitals addresses the potential for adverse drug events.[15] Also, as will be explained in the next chapter, patient safety will be evaluated whenever a product is considered for formulary addition.

Medical Devices

The P&T committee or a subcommittee may be responsible for the approval of some medical devices within an institution. This subcommittee is often multidisciplinary and is given the opportunity to review medical devices before purchases are made or contracts are signed. The committee is also responsible for reviewing the safety information associated with these devices because adverse medical device events are an important patient safety issue. The committee may also review devices that contain medications, such as topical hemostats that contain thrombin.

Nutrition

As nutrition of the hospitalized patient evolved and became more complex, the role of pharmacists on a nutrition support team became more justified. Their role started out improving the ordering process for parenteral nutrition and communicating these changes to the pharmacy staff for proper preparation. Today, pharmacists on the nutritional team assist in the clinical management of parenteral nutrition patients, parenteral nutrition research, and continual involvement with improving the safety of parenteral nutrition use.[75] TJC, in their National Patient Safety Goals (NPSG), addresses the safe use of parenteral nutrition feeding solutions.[76] One of the responsibilities of the P&T committee is to oversee and approve the components of the parenteral nutrition solutions.

Quality Assurance of Medication Use

A subcommittee of the P&T committee may be placed in charge of planning and overseeing the plan for quality assurance regarding drug therapy. Details about this activity are found in Chapter 14. This committee may develop criteria for a drug use evaluation, collect the data, interpret the data, and recommend acting when necessary regarding the appropriate use of medication.

Many times departments or service lines (e.g., oncology, cardiology, psychiatry/mental health, radiology, anesthesiology, women's health) are asked for input regarding the formulary management within their specialty area of practice.

P&T COMMITTEE MEETING

Before beginning the description of a typical P&T committee meeting, it is important to note that a smoothly functioning P&T committee has certain needs. The committee will need the support of its parent organization. A room for the meetings should be carefully selected (see Appendix 12–3). The agenda for the meeting should be prepared in advance by the committee's secretary and sent to the members. Most often, as mentioned previously, an informal meeting of the supporting pharmacists and others is required between P&T committee meetings to plan the activities necessary to support the agenda. The chair of the committee may also attend such planning meetings to ensure that issues are addressed before the meeting. Formulary reviews represent a special concern when sending out an agenda, because they may trigger the outside influences of dedicated pharmaceutical marketing efforts if companies learn from committee members that their products or their competitors' products are being evaluated. Efforts must be made to make sure the committee is not distracted by outside influences, such as the pharmaceutical industry and advertisements. This consideration should be reflected in the selection of members, and it might be necessary to avoid sending out some materials ahead of time, to lessen the chance of them being obtained by pharmaceutical company representatives. Also, if it is possible to prevent pharmaceutical representatives from knowing the membership of the committee, many of these problems may be avoided. If materials are sent out, it may be found that sending minutes from the previous P&T committee meeting is not always appropriate, because it may be difficult to adequately describe the full basis of a decision in a set of minutes. As a result, the minutes might be open to inappropriate projection regarding the basis for the P&T committee decision process. Some institutions simply make the minutes a pure recording of the decisions, eliminating any information about the discussion, to avoid this problem. A sample set of minutes is provided in Appendix 12–4. Along with sending an agenda to members, a reminder phone call, fax, and/or e-mail may be useful to facilitate attendance. Each P&T committee meeting will require extensive preparation by the pharmacists involved in its affairs. Specifically, management of the formulary requires extensive background research and the preparation of written reports for any addition or deletion. Similarly, quality-related functions require time-consuming review of patient records. Finally, the P&T committee functions will be peripherally related to other affairs of the parent organization, e.g., the standard order set preparation by other segments of a hospital. This requires special attention in order to prevent the use of nonformulary products. These items will be discussed in greater detail in the next section. Finally, the chairperson should be skilled at guiding an efficient meeting (see Appendix 12–5). In respect of the time commitment for members, meetings should always start and end at the scheduled times.

P&T Committee Functions

❹ *Typically, P&T committee functions include determining what drugs are available, who can prescribe specific drugs, policies and procedures regarding drug use (including pharmacy policies and procedures, standard order sets, and clinical guidelines—see Chapter 7 for the latter), quality assurance activities (e.g., DUR/DUE/medication usage evaluation—see Chapter 14), ADRs/medication errors (see Chapters 15 and 16), dealing with product shortages, and education in drug use.*[15,77,78] Many of those functions are quality-assurance-type activities, because they are designed to improve the quality of drug therapy. Because the functions may improve drug therapy quality, they may actually provide some legal protection for an institution, as long as the reason for decisions is not strictly based on financial considerations.[79] P&T committee functions can also include investigational drug studies; however, that is often delegated to the institutional review board (IRB) that oversees all investigational activities in the hospital (see Chapter 17). In addition, some P&T committee functions may be delegated to subcommittees (e.g., quality assurance, antibiotic, and medication errors subcommittees);[80] however, this can be cumbersome and is often avoided, except in larger institutions. P&T committees should recognize principles of epidemiology and pharmacoeconomics in the decision making whenever possible.[81-83] A standardized safety assessment tool has been developed to evaluate potential formulary agents.[84]

According to the TJC, the medical staff, pharmacy, nursing, administration, and others are to cooperate with each other in carrying out the previously mentioned functions.[15] Although the medical staff normally takes overseeing drug therapy very seriously and expects to approve all activities of the P&T committee, it is common for the pharmacy department to do much of the preparation work for the committee. Although it is tempting to say that the reason pharmacies are charged with all of the work is that they are the drug experts, which is often true, the more realistic reason is probably that pharmacists are paid to do this as part of their salary, whereas physicians often do not obtain any direct monetary compensation for this committee's preparatory work, although such compensation may be considered by an institution to encourage more physician participation.

Case Study 12–1

You are the clinical pharmacist assigned to be the Secretary of the Pharmacy and Therapeutics (P&T) Committee. You are asked to develop an agenda for each monthly meeting, prepare each agenda topic, present each agenda item in a presentation, take notes, and provide follow-up to the meeting.

1. What steps do you need to take to prepare an agenda?
2. What steps are needed to prepare a medication monograph, including the summary page?
3. What methods are used to disseminate the information once approved by the committee?

FORMULARY MANAGEMENT

Drug Formulary

Wherever a drug formulary system is in place, there is usually a drug formulary published as a hardcopy book and/or in electronic format (e.g., Web site or intranet). In its simplest form, the drug formulary contains a list of drugs that are available under that formulary system, which reflects the clinical judgment of the medical staff.[85,86] This list will be arranged alphabetically and/or by therapeutic class (American Hospital Formulary Service [AHFS] classification, usually), and usually contains information on the dosage forms, strengths, names (e.g., generic, trade, and chemical), and ingredients of combination products. Many drug formulary publications contain a great deal more material related to the drugs, including a summary of indications, side effects, dosing, use restrictions, and other clinical information.[87] Formularies may also be referred to as preferred medication lists or preferred drug lists.[18]

A related term, the formulary system, can be thought of as a method for developing the list, and sometimes even as a philosophy.[88] In theory, a well-designed drug formulary can guide clinicians to prescribe the safest and most effective agents for treating a particular medical problem, at the most reasonable cost.[89-94] Some people argue that the formulary system itself does not work because it is not properly implemented and recommend replacing it with counter-detailing by pharmacists or computers at the time a prescription order is written.[95] However, whether or not that is true has yet to be determined. The most well-known article indicating that formularies may ultimately result in higher patient costs was written by Horn and associates.[96] Although this may be one of the best articles on the topic and the author has defended criticism of the article,[97] there are nevertheless various deficiencies in the study that make it uncertain whether it was truly the drug formulary or other factors that led to increased costs.[98-101] Horn and associates[102] also published a similar study conducted in the ambulatory environment, which appears to have similar results and deficiencies. In the case of national drug formularies, there has been a positive[103] effect on prescribing habits shown in Canada. Further research is needed before a definite conclusion may be reached on the effectiveness of formulary management.[104] For now, a well-constructed formulary is still believed to improve patient care while decreasing costs.

The goal of the formulary system is to provide a decision-making process leading to the selection of medications necessary for the treatment of any disease states likely to be seen in that institution.[90] In some cases, decisions for formulary addition can be made for entire groups of institutions, for example, the U.S. Veteran's Administration has combined the formularies of all of its component parts.[105] These formulary medications should be the most efficacious and cost-effective agents with the fewest side effects or drug interactions.[15] Other factors should also be taken into consideration, such as the variety of dosage forms available for the medication, estimated use, convenience, dosing schedule, compliance, abuse potential, physician demand, ease of preparation, storage requirements, and risks.[106] Economic factors should not be the sole basis for this evidence-based process.[90] Typically, only two or perhaps three drugs from any drug class are added to the formulary. Some people would argue that only one agent is necessary from any class; however, some individuals will not respond and/or tolerate certain agents, so at least one secondary agent is usually desirable. Therapeutic redundancy must be minimized, however, by excluding superfluous or inferior preparations. This should improve the quality of prescribing and also lead to improved cost-effectiveness, both by eliminating less cost-effective agents that do not improve patient care and by assisting patients to become well faster. To analyze potentially conflicting literature and strength of recommendation, a grading system has been developed for the review of potential formulary additions.[107]

Whether an institution has a very strict formulary with a minimum number of items or a less-restricted formulary that excludes items that are significantly inferior is sometimes a matter of philosophy. The former will cut down the pharmacy department's inventory and often save money through the avoidance of highly priced products, but may only be practical in closed health maintenance organizations (HMOs) where the same formulary is used in both the inpatient and ambulatory environments. In cases where physicians are free to prescribe whatever products they prefer in the ambulatory environment, they have been shown to have difficulty in remembering what products are contained in the formularies of third-party payers.[108] Therefore, the increased time necessary for pharmacists to contact physicians for order changes may lead to the disruption of patient care. As a result, a less-restricted formulary may be more practical. As an example, a patient is admitted to the hospital on a nonformulary medication. While there would be other satisfactory medications in the same therapeutic category on the formulary, it may be best to simply allow the use of the nonformulary product, rather than adding another complicating factor to the patient's hospital treatment by attempting to change therapy. Pharmacist and physician time would also be saved.

Even in cases where an institution has a strict and enforced drug formulary, it should be noted that there are occasions when it is necessary to prescribe a drug that is not on the drug formulary. This might be due to a patient with a rare illness, a patient who does not respond or has intolerable side effects to the formulary drugs, a patient stabilized on a nonformulary medication where it would be difficult or dangerous to change, a conflict between the institutional formulary and the patient's insurance company formulary,[109] or some other valid reason. A mechanism must be in place to promptly obtain the particular drug when it is shown to be necessary (the National Committee for Quality Assurance [NCQA] requires such a mechanism for HMOs,[110] as does TJC for other hospitals,[15] but it must try to prevent physicians ordering nonformulary drugs "because I said so!"). Some institutions require specific request forms to be filled out (see example in Appendix 12–2), sometimes with a cosignature from the physician's department head, or at least require a consultation between a pharmacist and the physician before the drug is obtained. Also, patients may be charged more for the nonformulary medications. In some HMOs and insurance company plans, the physicians or pharmacies may be financially penalized for the use or overuse of nonformulary medications.[111] Whatever mechanism is used, it is important to make it easy to obtain necessary nonformulary medications, but difficult to obtain unnecessary medications; otherwise, the benefits of the formulary system may be negated.[54] Also, it is necessary to track which nonformulary drugs are being used regularly and why that is happening, because it may be worthwhile to add some of those agents to the drug formulary.[112]

Some physicians feel that a drug formulary serves only to keep costs down, at the expense of good patient care.[113] These physicians must be reassured that there is evidence to support that a good formulary does keep expenses down[114] without negatively affecting care,[115] although in some cases the costs are merely transferred to other hospital expenses.[116,117] One study demonstrated that a well-controlled formulary or therapeutic substitution (substituting a different medication that is effective for the disease being treated for the one ordered by the physician) results in 10.7% lower drug costs per patient day, and both a well-controlled formulary and therapeutic substitution together could result in 13.4% lower drug costs per day.[118] Some physicians do not like formularies because they consider them to be a limitation to their authority.[113] It is necessary to keep in mind that when physicians become a part of a medical staff or sign up to participate in some managed care group they are given privileges, not rights. The privileges generally do include limitations on what medications they can prescribe, and when and how they can prescribe them. If a drug formulary system is run well there is little reason to feel that there are inadequate drugs available; however, it does take some effort for the physician to learn to use the drugs available rather than the drugs he or she normally prescribes. An effort must be made to help physicians in this regard and to reassure them that every effort is being made to ensure that the best drugs are available for the patients. Additionally, all changes to the drug formulary must be quickly and effectively communicated to the physicians to avoid confusion. A lack of such communication can negate some of the benefits of the formulary and lead to poor physician/pharmacist relations.[116] Also, it is important for physicians to be aware that it is the medical staff that makes these decisions, in order to avoid pharmacy being perceived as the policeman who is waiting to jump on the unsuspecting physician.[119] Increasingly, physicians will enter prescription orders into the computer, which can quickly inform the physician of formulary drug choices and guide therapeutic decisions. Currently, however, pharmacists often have to tactfully contact the physician about nonformulary drugs in order to make a formulary system work.

Similarly, pharmacies filling prescriptions for an HMO must be kept informed of the formulary status of drugs. One suggestion is to have a help desk to answer pharmacist questions and to provide information.[120]

Oftentimes, the drug formularies will have a number of other sections that may include information about the P&T committee and pharmacy department, policy and procedure information (e.g., how to obtain nonformulary drugs, how to request that a drug be placed on the formulary), laboratory test information, dietary supplement charts, pharmacokinetics information, approved abbreviations, sodium content, nomograms, dosage equivalency charts, apothecary/metric equivalents, drug-food interactions, skin test directions, cost data, antimicrobial therapy charts, and any other brief clinical information tables felt to be necessary. Use of linking in Web sites can make such information much more readily available and usable, because users can navigate back and forth between these tables and the drug list. MCOs may need to include the procedure they use to limit choice of drugs by physicians, pharmacists, and patients.[16,121]

In institutional pharmacies, a hardcopy book was normally published once a year. Often it was published in a pocket-sized format that could be carried in lab coats by physicians, pharmacists, and nurses. There may also have been a larger loose-leaf binder published that could be updated regularly throughout the year. Such a book is no longer justified.[122] It is now common for this reference to be available electronically. The electronic form can be made more widely available and can be kept continually up-to-date by making changes, as necessary, at one central location. Also, the electronic formulary coupled with physician order entry may lead to the most efficient and effective way to encourage or enforce the use of formulary items,[123-125] although there is some evidence that electronic messages may be ignored by physicians.[126] Also, other information can be included to improve drug therapy. For example, this may include a requirement for a consultation by a specialist or pharmacokinetic monitoring. For outpatient drug formulary books this may include quantity level limits and requirements for prior authorizations.

The publication of a hardcopy drug formulary can be a very time-consuming process. If at all possible it is best if the pharmacy can download the information about drug products carried in the institution from their computer system or a separate database management program to a word processing or other suitable program.[127] This list can then be manipulated to a more readable and understandable format without a big problem in transcription errors, and the other clinical information can easily be placed into the document (particularly if it is just being updated from a previous year). Almost any high-end word processing program or desktop publishing program can be used to do this, producing a printer-ready copy that can be more inexpensively reproduced, in both time and dollars, than a typeset copy. Later, using colored paper and an edge index can make use of the final product easier. Even with the availability of computer technology, the production of a drug formulary is a very time-intensive effort, requiring a few weeks to several months of work. Fortunately, technical and clerical personnel can do much of the work. One or more pharmacists, however, should carefully proof all material to ensure it is correct. Often, this task will be divided up so that somebody involved with purchasing will check the drug list, an administrator will review the policies and procedures, and a clinician will update the clinical information. Even if an electronic drug formulary is produced, rather than the hardcopy, this checking of the material is necessary on a regular basis.

Pharmacies can also use commercial vendors who will take their drug lists and prepare a professional-looking formulary (hardcopy and/or electronic). These commercial formularies can also include condensed monograph information (e.g., indications, dosing, side effects, and so forth), which can be of value to the prescriber.

Preferably, the pharmacy can use the information on its computer system to create a formulary that is constantly up-to-date. The information can be accessed as part of the prescription order software and/or it may be interfaced with Web software.[128] The latter makes it possible to embed other information easily, but may take further work by the pharmacist. In any case, this information should be available to the physician and other health care professionals wherever necessary—even by wireless connection. As a side note, many institutions do not want information about their formularies readily available to individuals not directly associated with the institution (e.g., pharmaceutical manufacturers), but this should not be a problem using Virtual Private Network (VPN) software and firewalls to secure the data—allowing access to only qualified individuals. Increasingly, it should be expected that physicians will access this information using iPads or Google Android devices.

PBMs, in conjunction with an organization, may publish a patient pocket formulary in addition to the formulary published for physicians and provided online for pharmacies. These patient pocket formularies may contain the top therapeutic categories and other information as well. Within these categories are the key drugs in that specific therapeutic class as well as the designated preferred products and the associated patient cost index. Patients are encouraged to take these pocket formularies on their physician visits as a means of ensuring formulary compliance when discussing therapeutic options. Physicians may also have the capability of prescribing online, whereby the physician enters the prescription in an electronic device and instant messaging occurs, alerting the physician to potential drug interactions or formulary status of the prescription, allowing the physician to change the prescription immediately, and eliminating the need for a pharmacist to call.[41,129]

In addition to pocket formularies, one method whereby the pharmacist educates the physician about formulary drugs is academic detailing. Through mailings, phone conversations, and personal visits the pharmacist discusses with the physician his or her prescribing patterns and, using evidence-based medical literature, supports the rational for preferred formulary product selection and clinically appropriate, cost-effective prescribing without compromising quality.[41]

Evaluating Drugs for Formulary Inclusion

The establishment and maintenance of a drug formulary requires that drugs or drug classes be objectively assessed based on scientific information (e.g., efficacy, adverse effects, cost, contribution to some critical treatment pathway,[130] ease of preparation/use, and other appropriate items), not anecdotal physician experience.[88,131] Medication selection and procurement were specifically added to the TJC accreditation process under medication management in the 2009 standards.[132] There is an emphasis in the literature that P&T committee activities should be a result of evidence-based decisions.[90,133] Regarding the formulary process, 2010 TJC standard MM.02.01.01 calls for written criteria for the addition or deletion of medications.[15] Any health care practitioner who is involved with ordering, dispensing, administering, and monitoring medications needs to be involved with the development of the criteria.[15,132] A process must also be in place to monitor patient responses to a new medication. All formulary medications are to be reviewed at least annually based on safety and efficacy information. This means that in addition to new formulary additions, all categories of the AHFS therapeutic classification should be reviewed at least yearly.

According to the 2010 TJC, the criteria used for approving the addition of a drug to a formulary need to minimally include the following:[15]

- Indications for use
- Effectiveness
- Risks (e.g., adverse effects, drug interactions, and potential for medication errors)[134]
- Cost

A procedure for preparing the written evaluation of drug products is found in the next chapter; however, this section will go further into how the P&T committee should use that information and other items to do the actual evaluation.

When a P&T committee considers a drug for formulary adoption, it is quite common for the discussion to include statements such as, "In my clinical experience . . .," which leads the discussion into rather subjective areas. It must be kept in mind that physicians are most likely to request drugs if they have met with the pharmaceutical company representative or received money from the drug company (e.g., speaking fees and travel funds to a meeting).[126,135] Valid formulary decisions should be based on objective evidence, particularly clinical studies,[136] rather than a few cases of clinical experience by a physician attending a meeting.[90] Efforts must be made to guide discussions to scientific information when it wanders into vague subjective areas.[89] In some cases, this is rather difficult because many new drugs have limited published information when they are first commercially available. The information that is available is generally placebo-controlled studies that are funded by the manufacturer. In situations such as this, the decision on formulary addition may need to be postponed until adequate information is available. It may be recommended that consideration of any new product be delayed until it has been on the market at least 1 year, unless it is a treatment that is significantly different from those already available.[137] In at least one case, it has been bluntly stated that a P&T committee should show leadership by restricting the availability of a drug product if there is no convincing evidence that the product offers meaningful benefits over other available products.[138] Sometimes the decision cannot wait, as is the case with many managed care companies, which need to review a drug before a patient picks up the drug from the pharmacy so that appropriate coverage determination can be made, or in hospitals in response to the new TJC accreditation standards.[15,132]

Then the P&T committee's decision-making process needs to be structured in a manner that is very objective and data driven, and takes into account the lack of data.[90] In these cases, a committee may make a decision and then place the product on a 6-month follow-up for an additional review, after which time additional prescribing and patient use data or clinical trial data may be available.

Although there is a temptation to think that anything new is better, which is an attitude that is certainly pushed by drug company representatives with new products to sell, it cannot be assumed and must be proven. In some cases, experts have determined that the new products pose no significant advantages to the patients to justify the costs.[139-141] The rate at which the new chemical entities are approved by the FDA has been declining from that of the past,[142] although there was a slight increase in 2003.[143] The FDA approved 24 new or first-of-a-kind drugs in 2008.[144] Often, manufacturers are trying to get products approved and on the market that may be in a different strength or dosage form, a single isomer of a product, a new indication for a product, or even an extended-release version of a product (sometimes several different extended-release versions).[145] All of the products potentially need to be given consideration by a P&T committee. However, with a lack of published trials and, in many cases, objective and reliable data, the P&T committee faces the challenge of creating a sound drug formulary that represents the needs of an organization or patient population in an objective manner that encompasses current clinical practice, established guidelines of patient care, and a thorough risk-benefit analysis of the drug product.[24] Some places have even tried computerized methods to make more objective decisions;[146,147] however, there does not seem to be any data demonstrating the superiority of such a method. Similarly, there are processes called System of Objectified Judgment Analysis (SOJA), which uses a computer program to score different aspects of drugs in the same class to determine the best product,[148,149] and multi-attribute utility technology.[150] A Web-based tool for designing pediatric vaccine formularies has been developed (http://www.vaccineselection.com).[151]

The 2010 Joint Commission Accreditation Process Guide for Hospitals also addresses the elements of performance for selecting and procuring medications.[15] Elements of this performance that provide additional information to that already covered are the following:

1. Members of the medical staff, licensed independent practitioners, pharmacists, and staff involved in the ordering, dispensing, administering, and/or monitoring of the effects of medications develop written criteria for determining which medications are available for dispensing or administering to patients.

2. Before using a new medication, the hospital establishes processes to monitor patient response (see MM.07.01.01, EP 2).

Conflict of Interest

Also, it is necessary to determine whether people involved in the discussion and decision about a drug's formulary status have some conflict of interest (i.e., would receive some direct or indirect compensation from having a drug available, e.g., stock in a company, honoraria for speaking, consulting fees, and gifts or grants from a company)[78,137,152-154] and avoid that biasing factor. Nationally, this is considered to be a significant problem.[155] The P&T committee has the responsibility to identify and address conflict-of-interest issues in the decision-making process.[90] Perhaps a conflict-of-interest policy, requiring regular disclosure of any possible conflicts, needs to be established.[24,156,157] An example form to gather information about conflicts of interest is provided in Appendix 12–6. In certain cases, regular voting P&T committee members may have to abstain from the vote if they disclose a possible conflict of interest, or the committee may vote to determine whether the conflict is considered to be significant enough to prevent voting by the individual in question. There is concern at a federal, state, and institutional level regarding potential conflict of interest. In 2009, some drug manufacturers made public their financial relationship with healthcare providers.[158] There is also concern that the PBMs P&T committees may be financially influenced by drug manufacturers.[159] Unlike the traditional health insurers, the U.S. Department of Defense solicits input from various providers and beneficiaries. In addition, they provide beneficiaries and their representatives an opportunity to comment on the committee recommendations prior to final approval. However, this has not deterred their placement on the tier 3, which is where they will provide the lowest reimbursement for the product.[160]

Other Aspects of Formulary Evaluation

Several other areas need to be considered, which will be explained in the following.

Patent expiration is a common question that should be considered for all products or drug classes undergoing formulary review, because the introduction of generic products after that date may lead to decreasing prices. Patent expiration information can be found at http://www.fda.gov/cder/ob/default.htm.

The TJC Medication Management Standards for 2010 are focused on medication safety. The definition of a medication goes beyond prescription products and the FDA classification as drugs. Also considered medications in the 2010 standards are herbal/alternative therapies, vitamins, nutraceuticals, nonprescription products, vaccines, diagnostic and contrast agents, radioactive agents, respiratory treatments, parenteral nutrition, blood derivatives, intravenous (IV) solutions, anesthetic gases, sample medications, and anything else deemed by the FDA to be a drug.[132,161] The pharmacist is required to review the appropriateness of all medication orders before a medication is dispensed.[15,132,161,162]

Although it is now necessary to evaluate herbal or other alternative medicine products,[163-165] some institutions may instead handle them as nonformulary requests or investigational drugs.[166] Although alternative and herbal medications seem somewhat unusual to the P&T committee, they can still be treated much the same way as any drug product, perhaps with additional evaluation of the purity and composition of the products (see Dietary Supplement Medical Literature section of Chapter 5 for additional details regarding how to evaluate for these products).[167] Some pharmacies also have other policies and procedures,[168] perhaps some that are highly restrictive,[169] including requiring pharmacists to verify labeled product ingredients.[170]

The possibility of a new drug product leading to medication errors should also be considered in the evaluation of products. Such things as difficulty in dosing or administration, black box warnings, look-alike and sound-alike names, the need for extra monitoring, unusual storage requirements, and other issues may be considered.[171]

In addition to considering the cost of drug products in the institution, it is necessary to consider the cost to the patient, once he or she returns home. If a product is so expensive that an uninsured or underinsured patient cannot afford it in the ambulatory environment, it may not be good to place the patient on that drug in the hospital. However, in some cases pharmaceutical companies may offer assistance to this type of patient.

Open Versus Closed Formularies

When setting up a drug formulary there are several things to consider. First is whether there will be an open or closed formulary.[172] The open (or voluntary) formulary essentially means any drug on the market is available, and some would argue that the term open formulary is really an oxymoron.[89] One exception to this definition is that the NCQA states that an open formulary for an MCO can be a list of recommended drugs, as long as there are no requirements concerning its use.[173] A closed (or restricted) formulary means that only a limited number of agents are available.[85] This is certainly preferable, because such agents should be chosen by objective evidence in the scientific literature that supports the superiority of the agents over other similar drugs, and because closed formularies can result in cost savings.[174] Closed formularies are becoming much more common in HMOs.[175,176] In some instances of closed formularies, patients may have access to these nonformulary or nonpreferred drug products by paying a substantially higher copayment, by paying the difference between the formulary and nonformulary products in addition to the copayment, or by paying for the nonformulary drug in its entirety unless there is a prior authorization to allow this drug.[40]

Issues may arise with a closed or restricted formulary in that it may be too restrictive for those patients who cannot afford the drug, even though the drug is still available in a closed formulary. A growing health policy concern is the ability to successfully appeal for coverage of a nonformulary product. Newer breakthrough medications and biotechnology products are making their way onto the market. Although clinically valuable, they are very expensive. In addition, PBMs have managed or preferred formularies. In a managed or preferred formulary, interventions may be used to encourage physicians to use the preferred products. Some of these interventions for physicians include academic detailing, prior authorizations, and coverage rules. For pharmacies this may mean a higher dispensing fee for formulary compliance. For the patient this may mean higher copayments if the formulary or preferred product is not used.

Unlike hospitals, PBMs along with their clients (i.e., health plans) place their formulary and nonformulary medications into tiers with an associated copayment with each tier. This tier copayment structure came about in response to the rising cost of prescription drugs. The first tier is generally reserved for generic drug products. This tier usually has the lowest copayment (e.g., $10). The second tier is usually reserved for those name-brand drugs that are formulary. This tier has a higher copayment (e.g., $15) than the first tier due to the added cost of the brand-name drug. The third tier is reserved for those drug products that are nonformulary brand names. This copayment is significantly higher than the other two tiers (e.g., $30). However, some third-tier copayments may be calculated as a proportion of the drug cost, even as much as one-third as a form of coinsurance, or require paying for the drug in its entirety. The reason for the copayment structure is to encourage the patient to use the most clinically appropriate, cost-effective drug without compromising quality care.[40]

The closed formulary can also be broken down into what is referred to as positive or negative formularies. This is the method by which the formulary is developed. A positive formulary effectively starts with a blank sheet of paper and specifically adds agents. While this is probably the best method to limit the number of drugs available, it is often not very popular when first implementing the formulary because every agent must be considered. That means the physicians must make specific decisions even on whether they should add such things as acetaminophen and amoxicillin to the formulary. Therefore, in hospitals just establishing a formulary, it is often more popular and easier to use a negative formulary system. This essentially starts with the current hospital drug stock, with each drug class being evaluated to eliminate agents that are not necessary.[177] The first steps in this process may be as simple as eliminating multiple salts/esters of the same drug. Then classes of drugs with multiple similar products could be addressed (e.g., analgesics, antacids, laxatives, vitamins, and topical steroids). Although in some ways this process is easier, it is also likely to result in a much bigger formulary, because the decision will be made as to what drugs are definitely not needed, rather than which drugs the institution definitely needs. However, the specific institution's situation will need to be assessed before deciding on the method of determining the formulary items. Overall, the goal is to provide the optimal agents. It is easy to end up with too many duplicative agents; however, having a greater number of agents to choose from can lead to better patient care in some areas.[178,179]

Therapeutic Interchange

The AMA[12,172] defines therapeutic interchange as "authorized exchange of therapeutic alternatives in accordance with previously established and approved written guidelines or protocols within a formulary system." An example would be the use of cefazolin in specific doses whenever any other first-generation injectable cephalosporin is ordered. Therapeutic interchange is used in nearly 90% of U.S. hospitals[180] for reasons that include cost savings,[181,182] improved patient outcomes, decreased adverse effects, decreased inventory, fewer medication errors,[183] or other benefits. Therapeutic interchange has been shown to decrease costs without adversely affecting patient outcomes.[50,184] There is even reason to believe that when therapeutic interchange is properly performed, and not entirely based on financial considerations, it may produce lower legal liability for an institution,[79] although there are no published legal cases regarding therapeutic interchange to demonstrate either increased or decreased legal liability.[185] The concept of therapeutic interchange through collaborative interactions with interdisciplinary teams to develop protocols and comprehensive therapeutic assessments has been described. Several medication classes may be the target of therapeutic interchange and an aggressive intravenous-to-oral conversion may be part of this process.[186] The most common classes of drugs for therapeutic interchange are, in order, H_2 antagonists, proton pump inhibitors, antacids, quinolones, potassium supplements, cephalosporins, and hydroxymethylglutaryl-coenzyme A reductase inhibitors.[187] Some drug classes, such as low-molecular-weight heparins, that at first glance may appear to be possible places for therapeutic interchange to take place, may be found to be unacceptable after a closer inspection.[187]

Therapeutic interchange is considered acceptable to the AMA, unlike therapeutic substitution, which it defines as the "act of dispensing a therapeutic alternative for the drug product prescribed without prior authorization of the prescriber" (note: prior authorization may be a blanket authorization, not a specific authorization for each case).[188,189] Therapeutic interchange has also been found to be acceptable by other organizations, including the American College of Clinical Pharmacy (ACCP), American College of Physicians (ACP) (they require immediate prior consent by the physician),[190] ASHP, American Pharmacists Association (APhA), American Association of Colleges of Pharmacy (AACP), AMCP,[191] and the American Society of Consultant Pharmacists (ASCP).[192,193] The ACCP spells out the concept of therapeutic interchange in great detail and suggests that it not only be conducted under the auspices of a P&T-type committee, but also that it specifically include DUE, a set method for informing the physicians and other staff that interchange is taking place (should be well planned and thorough[194]), and a mechanism under which the therapeutic interchange policies may be overridden in specific cases. Evaluations for therapeutic interchange should also consider medical, legal, and financial evaluations.[187] Other practical aspects, such as communication forms, policies and procedures, medical staff bylaw changes, and other items, may need to be addressed by the institution.[195]

Electronic means to provide authorization for interchange may be seen more in the future.[196] Outside of an institution (e.g., ambulatory environment), therapeutic interchange may not be as easy to implement due to practical procedure methods and because patients are not as closely monitored; however, it may still be possible.[197,198] In the ambulatory situation, the AMA states that therapeutic interchange recommendations must be approved by the majority of physicians affected and must otherwise follow similar standards to that described for inpatient settings.[172]

The consideration of certain therapeutic agents for interchange may result in strong differences of opinion among medical staff members regarding their appropriate use. The process for evaluating any product, especially those for which physicians have deeply held opinions, should be followed, along with efforts being made by committee members to actively approach appropriate influential individuals before a crisis occurs. Through anticipatory, structured negotiation, it is more likely that rational and balanced decisions will be made. Also, it is necessary to take into consideration whether a short-term interchange of products, while the patient is in a hospital, may cause confusion or other difficulties when the patient returns to the outpatient environment and may be restarted on the original agent.[199] Working with the physicians to resolve this issue is a necessity for the long-term care of patients.

Generic substitution is also considered by the P&T committee in some cases, but many pharmacies consider generic substitution to be one of their responsibilities and do not take such decisions to the P&T committee for approval. The one exception may be drugs with narrow therapeutic indexes (e.g., anticonvulsants), where a P&T committee may determine that a list of products where generic substitution is not allowed,[200] although the FDA insists that such precautions are unnecessary.[201] In relation to generic substitution, it must be mentioned that pharmacies must determine quality suppliers. The ASHP has guidelines for this function.[202] Also, states may have a variety of laws governing generic substitution. They may also publish so-called positive and negative formularies, which differ in definition from those terms used elsewhere in this chapter in that they are lists of drugs that may or may not be substituted for one another, respectively.[185]

In some instances, physicians may prefer that no generic substitution or therapeutic substitution occur on a written order or prescription by indicating "Dispense as Written" on that document. This can occur in the inpatient setting as well as the outpatient setting. Depending on the state, dispense as written is synonymous with the following: no substitution, do not substitute, medically necessary, brand necessary/medically necessary, no drug product selection, brand medically necessary, substitution prohibited without permission of physician or patient, or no substitution/brand necessary.

In most states, the law provides that pharmacists can use a generic version of any medication on a prescription or medication order if the physician has not precluded that action by indicating dispense as written. In the outpatient setting, in general, if patients want a generic medication, they should be sure that their pharmacist knows of their desire.

In some benefit plans, if the physician requests a brand-name medication when a generic equivalent is available, the patient member may be responsible to pay the difference in cost in addition to the generic copayment. In some instances, members may not be required to pay this cost difference, if their physician documents that the brand-name medication is necessary.

Nonformulary Usage

Many institutions track the drug-use patterns of prescribers, as mentioned previously in describing the tracking of nonformulary drug products.[203] Annually, a listing of nonformulary products and expenses should be made available to the P&T committee. It is helpful if the pharmacy director can report the total cost of nonformulary items as a percent of the total budget, particularly because the cost can exceed the cost of carrying the nonformulary product on the formulary.[204] Also, as part of this, it is good to check on whether nonformulary drug usage has led to medication errors, because there was at least one report that such nonformulary use resulted in a 28% error rate.[203] Ideally, a report of the number involved and costs of nonformulary orders will be made available to each prescriber. This process is helpful in improving the appropriate use of medications and has also been linked to the prescriber credentialing process.[205] The process can also be used to reevaluate whether nonformulary items should be made available on the drug formulary.

Unlabeled Uses

While some third-party payers may attempt to limit the use of drugs to only FDA-approved indications, this may unnecessarily restrict the use of products for indications that may have significant literature support. This should not be supported.[206] However, as will be discussed in more detail in Chapter 13, it is sometimes necessary for institutions to specifically restrict drugs to specific uses when they may be used inappropriately. Although at first glance this seems to be the same, in reality such restrictions may be totally unrelated to approved labeling. In this situation, it may be found that products are permitted to be used for unlabeled indications where there is adequate literature support and, conversely, may not be permitted to be used, at least without special approval within the institution, for FDA indications when there may be more appropriate drugs available.

New Product Introductions

When new drug products are added to the formulary, it is best to prepare physicians, nurses, and others.[126] To begin with, it is necessary to inform affected individuals that the drug will be available as of a specific date. That could be immediately or at some time in the near future. There are various reasons for a delay. For example, a drug may have been approved by both the FDA and the P&T committee, but the company may not have made it commercially available yet because they have not yet produced a sufficient supply or they are not yet ready to start their marketing efforts. In some cases, it is necessary for specific equipment to be obtained and installed. Such was the case a number of years ago when Fluosol-DA was made available for a limited period of time. This parenteral product required a very specialized preparation method involving a warm-water bath and percolating a mixture of gases through an IV bag under sterile conditions. Few, if any, pharmacies had the necessary equipment at the time of introduction, and it would have taken some time to get the equipment, set it up, and train pharmacists and technicians in its use, requiring a delay in making the product available in an institution. Most commonly, the reason for the delay is likely to be the time it takes to inform all individuals likely to be involved in the prescribing, preparing, and administering of the drug that the drug will be available and to educate them in the proper use, including applicable policies and procedures. These education efforts may be provided through newsletters, Web sites, portals, e-mail, memos, educational programs, RSS (Really Simple Syndication) aggregators (programs that pull together information from a variety of sources, such as news resources, an example being Google Reader), or other methods. The method chosen should generally be a standard method used within the institution and should be appropriate for the specific medication product introduction. In cases where a product is particularly complicated, dangerous, or prone to misuse, several methods of instruction, perhaps along with prescribing restrictions, should probably be employed. Further information about newsletters and Web sites is found in Chapter 9.

Case Study 12–2

You are the only pharmacist assigned to work the evening shift in the main pharmacy doing electronic order entry. The physician writes an order for desloratadine. From the order you cannot tell if the desloratadine is a patient home medication or a new order. The clinical pharmacist on that particular floor has gone home for the day. The hospital where you practice has a closed formulary. Your formulary agent is loratadine. Your hospital has a policy and procedure for nonformulary drug orders as well as a therapeutic interchange program that includes this class of drugs. You call the physician and explain to him that loratadine is the formulary agent. He states that desloratadine is what he prefers for this patient.

1. In order for desloratadine to be dispensed, what form does the physician have to fill out?
2. Upon receiving the nonformulary request, you notice that the reason for the desloratadine order is efficacy. Is this consistent with what you know about the products?

3. You call the physician and explain what you found and the approved therapeutic interchange. You inform the physician that per the nonformulary medication policy it may take 24 hours to obtain the nonformulary medication. The physician approves the interchange this time, but wants a formal review of the drug at P&T. How would you document the therapeutic interchange?
4. Knowing that the physician wants a formal review of desloratadine, how do you proceed with the request in the pharmacy records or medical records?

POLICIES AND PROCEDURES

Occasionally, policies and procedures must be developed to support the rational use of medications. Although the pharmacy department may decide that it needs to have its own policies and procedures for internal functions, that is not the focus of this discussion.[207] Instead, policies and procedures for the use of medications in an institution, clinic, and so forth will be discussed, because that is often provided through a P&T committee.

TJC has specifically stated that it expects policies and procedures for the following types of orders:[161]

- As needed (prn) medications
- Standard order sets
- Automatic stop
- Titrating
- Taper
- Range
- Compounded or admixed drugs
- Medication-related devices
- Investigational medications
- Herbal/natural products
- Discharge medications
- Anticoagulation dosing[53]

Some examples of policies and procedures can be found on the Internet at http://www.hosp.uky.edu/pharmacy/departpolicy/departmentalpolicies.html.

To begin this discussion, the definitions for policies and procedures should be considered.[208] A policy is a broad, general statement that describes the goals and purposes of the document. The procedures are specific actions to be taken. In some ways, policies and procedures may resemble a cookbook-type approach, in that a set of steps to be accomplished is described in order. Taken together, these policies and procedures may be a logical, step-by-step explanation of why and where a product may be used, how to use it, and who is to follow the policy (i.e., there may be different portions of the document addressed to pharmacists, technicians, nurses, and prescribers),[209] along with a brief introductory statement describing why the process is necessary.

Before developing a specific policy and procedure, the first step should be deciding whether it is necessary at all. In other words, is there a good reason for the existence of that particular policy and procedure, and is it likely to be used? This can be looked at as a risk-benefit decision. For example, is there sufficient risk that a particular medication will be used incorrectly (e.g., prepared wrong, administered wrong, and used for an inappropriate indication) to make it worthwhile to develop a policy and procedure? Generally, the answer will be no, but in a certain number of cases, policies and procedures may be necessary. Examples of where a policy and procedure may be necessary include thrombolytic agents (where the drug can cause serious or fatal effects if used improperly), antibiotics (where it is found that expensive, broad-spectrum antibiotics are being used where amoxicillin should suffice), injectable drugs (where specific individuals who will administer the medication and the process will be defined),[210] and even for drugs where reimbursement may be a problem.

Once a decision is reached to develop the policy and procedure, a logical and orderly course should be followed. It is undesirable to wait until after problems occur before deciding that policies and procedures are necessary. This process should follow the drug formulary process, where a mechanism is set up to help determine that a policy and procedure is necessary. In many cases, a policy and procedure for the use of drugs likely to be misused may be developed in conjunction with its consideration for addition to the drug formulary.

As in any process, it is first necessary to decide who will be coordinating the effort and the likely endpoint. That person, or designee, will then need to investigate various sources for background material necessary to develop the policy and procedure. This might include doing a literature search, talking to experts in the field, talking to other institutions that have already developed policies on the same topic, reviewing published professional (e.g., http://www.ashp.org/Import/PRACTICEANDPOLICY/PolicyPositions GuidelinesBestPractices.aspx) or clinical guidelines (e.g., http://www.guideline.gov), and checking the institution's requirements for developing policies and procedures. If the policy and procedure is for a hospital group, other institutions in the group must also be involved. In particular, it is necessary for the person developing the policy and procedure to have good communications with those who will be affected. After all, if the final product is looked at as being more trouble than it is worth, it is not likely to be followed. Where the policy and procedure fits in relation to other institutional policies and procedures will also have to be evaluated. Finally, a document should be written, reviewed, and revised, using many of the skills outlined in Chapter 9.

As part of the process of preparing the policy, it is important to be clear as to when it is applicable and where there may be exceptions. For example, institutions have policies for the automatic stop of specific medications (e.g., stopping an antibiotic after seven days). Only applying that policy in cases where it will be likely to improve drug therapy needs to be carefully considered. There also needs to be a mechanism to make sure that such an automatic stop, which may be programmed into the computer system, may not cause harm to particular patients[211] (e.g., patients with osteomyelitis receiving antibiotics for an extended period of time).

Once the policy and procedure is finished, it will need to be approved by the same mechanism that drug formulary changes go through (i.e., P&T committee, medical executive committee, and so forth). The approval and/or effective date for the policy and procedure should be recorded on the document itself to ensure that it is not confused with earlier or later documents. A plan for implementing the policy and procedure will need to be developed. Forms may need to be prepared and distributed. Copies of the policy and procedure will have to be distributed to those affected (preferably on the computer network), and educational programs will need to be planned and given. At that point, the policy and procedure can be implemented, perhaps in conjunction with the first appearance of a particular agent on the drug formulary. That is not the end of the process, however. At some point, the policy and procedure should be evaluated to determine if it is being properly followed and having the desired effect as a part of a quality assurance plan. A method to enforce compliance with the policies and procedures is required and it is necessary for legal reasons to demonstrate that this enforcement method is used.[209] Also, the policy and procedure will need to be reviewed, revised (if necessary), and reapproved on a regular basis (probably once a year). As part of that process, the actual need for the policy and procedure should be reconsidered. The policy and procedure should be eliminated if no longer needed. One way to determine whether the policy and procedures are consulted is if they are on a Web server, where the number of times the specific page is opened is recorded. Superseded copies (i.e., previous versions) of the policies and procedures should be kept on file for background and for legal purposes.

It is also necessary to have policies and procedures for the operation of the P&T committee itself (see Appendix 12–1 for policies and procedures for setting up a P&T committee). Some examples of other policies and procedures that may need to be developed include how new drugs are requested for addition to the formulary, how nonformulary drugs can be used, what procedure is used to evaluate new drugs,[132] the composition of the committee, and other committee functions (e.g., conflict of interest). These are discussed elsewhere in the chapter and will not be dealt with further. For more information on writing policies and procedures, please refer to Chapter 18.

Clinical Guidelines

P&T committees may be involved with the development, alteration (to fit local circumstances), and/or approval of evidence-based clinical guidelines. The reader is directed to Chapter 7 to obtain further information.

Standard Order Set Development

Many prescribers, both in their offices and in institutions (e.g., hospital and nursing home), make use of something called standard orders. This usually consists of some sort of form, preprinted hardcopy, or electronic checklist that lists various orders that are often written for specific patients under certain circumstances. This can include medications, laboratory tests, x-rays, other diagnostic tests, diet restrictions, preoperative preparation, restrictions, and many other things. For example, there may be a specific set of orders for all patients a prescriber admits to the hospital in general or for a specific diagnosis, or a set of orders for a patient who is scheduled to undergo a specific procedure, such as an operation. Standard order sets are commonly used for some medications, such as total parenteral nutrition solutions and oncology agents, where the order can be complex and confusing, perhaps resulting in potential medication errors. The prescribers using the standard order sets can simply indicate which of the items they wish their patients to receive and provide various necessary details, such as dose or duration. The use of standard order sets can be a very good practice, because they act like checklists used by pilots or astronauts—saving time and ensuring that important items are not inadvertently missed or misused. This can be particularly important in the use of drugs that can be dangerous or ineffective if not properly used, such as chemotherapeutic regimens in oncology patients. However, the disadvantage is that the standard order sets do take time to establish and maintain, and may not keep up with actual practice standards, therefore contributing to the perpetuation of outmoded or inappropriate practices. Although many P&T committees do not address standard order sets directly, leaving them to the individuals or groups that use them, it is something that still needs to be considered for several reasons.

First, P&T committees are responsible for overseeing all things related to medication use in an institution. Second, the standard order sets may contain medications that might be removed from the formulary for various reasons. This requires the P&T committee to make a special effort to communicate with those individuals or groups with standard order sets that contain drugs that may be eliminated from the formulary. This communication should begin prior to recommendation for removal of a product from the formulary, in order to find out the reason for the use of the product and the acceptability of available substitutes. By maintaining copies of standard order sets, the pharmacy department can help facilitate this process. Also, once it has been decided that a particular product on standard order sets is to be removed from the formulary, that decision must be quickly communicated to the affected individuals and groups, with enough time allocated before the removal becoming effective for the standard order sets to be updated and the new ones to be put into use. This process may be delayed by the frequency of meetings of the groups affected, the time it takes to have new standard order set sheets either printed or put on the computer system, and the necessity to adequately train personnel in the use of the replacement products. In all likelihood, it may take several months after a decision by the P&T committee before the changes can be put into effect. Finally, P&T committees may find that products on standard order sets may be used in ways that are not supported by the medical literature and/or hospital policy, which means that they need to make sure the prescribers or groups that use those orders make necessary changes.

Optimally, individuals or groups using standard orders should be required to review and reapprove their use on a regular basis (probably at least once a year). It may also be necessary to have standard order sets go through an institutional standard order sets committee. In any case, the TJC requires a specific policy and procedure for how institutions handle standard order sets.[132] Any changes should be reported to both the affected groups (e.g., nursing units, pharmacy, and information technology) and to the P&T committee in cases where the standard order sets include drugs. All printed sets of the standard order sets must include their revision date, to make sure that that old copies are not inadvertently used. Old copies of the orders must be maintained for medicolegal purposes, with the length of time for keeping such records to be determined by the institution's legal counsel.

Credentialing and Privileges

Health care institutions are required by various groups to verify that physicians and other health care professionals have the credentials to practice.[212] This can include degrees, licenses, training, and experience. Based on the credentials, professionals may be given privileges to practice within that institution and perform certain activities.[213] Note that the term is privilege, not right. For example, although all physicians may have the same license, only those trained in surgery may be allowed to do more than very minor surgical procedures (e.g., suturing lacerations and removing minor skin growths). There may be even more-specific rules, such as those preventing a chest surgeon from performing neurosurgery. These privileges can also extend to drugs. For example, it may be decided within the P&T committee that only oncologists have privileges to prescribe most antineoplastic agents. This type of policy and procedure is the basis for some restrictions that may be placed when a drug is considered for formulary addition. In addition to restrictions placed within an institution, restrictions may be enforced from outside the institution. For example, the use of dofetilide (Tikosyn) requires the credentialing of both the prescriber and hospital by the company (see http://www.tikosyn.com/ for details).

It also must be mentioned that policies and procedures may be in place within an institution to require pharmacists to perform certain operations, whether that is the preparation of particular agents or performing specific clinical functions (e.g., pharmacokinetics and warfarin dosing).[212] Institutions may have a method by which pharmacists are credentialed to perform such services.

Quality Improvement Within the P&T Committee—Internal Audit

❺ *A variety of topics regarding the quality of medication use are normally part of the activities of a P&T committee.* Many of these activities are covered in Chapter 14; however, the items described in the following sections may be considered to be specific to the P&T committee.

MEDICATION QUALITY ASSURANCE

In addition to determining which medications are available and providing direction in their use, it is required that the quality of use is regularly measured in whatever areas are felt to be necessary, including medication use evaluation (MUE), drug use evaluation (DUE), and other similar activities. The P&T committee will likely be involved in this, although coordination of such efforts, including preparing an annual plan of quality assurance activities, may occur through other groups, such as a quality assurance committee. Pharmacists may develop the initial plan, but multidisciplinary feedback is essential before the focused areas of evaluation are finalized. Ideally, all practice areas of the medical staff are given an opportunity to provide input into these focused evaluations. The project list should be continually reviewed and allow for special urgent projects when necessary. If a project is not completed during the year, it may be reconsidered for the next year. DUE criteria should be selected that can be used for continuous improvements that meet TJC accreditation requirements. DUE activities may be used to identify ADRs, contain cost, and expand clinical pharmacy activities.[214] Even if the P&T committee does not direct quality assurance efforts, it must be kept informed of the information gathered and the medication-related quality improvement efforts that are being instituted. This way the P&T committee can be supportive of such efforts directly (e.g., making changes to the drug formulary or policies and procedures to improve medication use) or less directly (e.g., providing statements supporting such activities). Quality assurance is a large topic and further information is available in Chapter 14.

ADVERSE DRUG REACTIONS

The P&T committee has a responsibility to review adverse reaction data in an institution to identify trends. One tool it can employ is to monitor the use of medications, sometimes referred to as tracer drugs, to treat the symptoms and side effects of other medications,[215] for example, the monitoring of epinephrine, flumazenil, phytonadione, or protamine to try to detect allergic responses, benzodiazepine overdoses, warfarin overdoses, or heparin overdoses, respectively. The topic of ADRs is covered further in the Chapter 15.

MEDICATION ERROR INCIDENTS

Data collected regarding medication errors may be reported to the P&T committee and, probably for investigational drugs, to the IRB. A systematic method to collect data about medication errors must be set up within an institution, perhaps using internal incident report forms employed by the institution to track all unusual occurrences regarding patients. All incidents are reviewed by severity (none, minimal, moderate, major, death) and by process (prescribing, transcription, dispensing, administration, other). A multidisciplinary review of all incidents should take place and trends in the specific quality indicators should be shared with the entire professional staff. High-alert medications (e.g., narcotics, patient-controlled analgesia, insulin, anticoagulants, electrolytes, neuromuscular blockers, thrombolytics, and chemotherapy) should be benchmarked and followed to identify trends to improve the medication management system and ultimately enhance patient safety.

Another monitoring consideration is related to errors with medical devices and may also be monitored by these committees. A study completed in a 520-bed tertiary teaching institution demonstrated that more intensive surveillance methods yielded higher rates of medical device problems as compared to voluntary reporting.[216]

The topic of medication errors is covered in more detail in Chapter 16.

ILLEGIBLE HANDWRITING, TRANSCRIPTION, AND ABBREVIATIONS

It is important to work with the medical staff and all other health professionals regarding illegible handwriting and transcription errors. Typically, a task force assigned by the P&T

committee is given the charge of evaluating and trending illegible handwriting, followed by developing process improvement measures. A report can be made to the P&T on an ongoing or quarterly basis. An education process must be in place for those individuals who consistently demonstrate poor handwriting. Hands-on reminders have been helpful or, in some extreme cases, handwriting school is recommended. In addition, institutions have adapted the TJC unapproved abbreviation list.[15] Unacceptable abbreviations may have an intended meaning but often are potentially misinterpreted and can lead to serious complications. In many institutions, the nurse or pharmacist must clarify the order with the prescriber when an unapproved abbreviation is written. In some cases, the only effective prevention of this problem has been when the medical staff has determined through the P&T committee that orders containing unapproved abbreviations are invalid and must be rewritten by the physician.[217] The addition to the formulary of look-alike, sound-alike medications is discouraged.[218-221] Increasingly, institutions are implementing computerized physician order entry (CPOE), which eliminates the problem of illegible handwriting and decimal point errors, thus reducing medication errors,[222] although implementation costs are considerable and some institutions may currently feel that it is not yet worth the effort and expense.[223]

TIMELINESS

The time for medication orders to be filled and sent to the floor may be tracked by the P&T committee. One area of importance is the response time sequence for a stat (immediate) order. The time should be evaluated from the time the order was written, to when the order was filled, to when the patient receives the medication. There are many obstacles in the order process and getting the medication to the patient. Each institution should have a standard expectation of the turnaround time for stat orders and a policy that will ensure that the medication is dispensed and administered promptly. Benchmarking should be done to make sure the policy is followed.

Although not quite as imperative, the timeliness of ordinary order fulfillment must also be evaluated for appropriateness.

COUNTERFEIT DRUG PRODUCTS

Counterfeit drugs can be considered to be those that do not contain the ingredients claimed on the labeling, perhaps having no active ingredients, incorrect dose, or even other drugs.[224] Counterfeit drugs appear to be an increasing problem, although the actual incidence is unknown.[225] The ASHP announced in February 2004 that it would partner with the FDA in a program to keep pharmacists informed about the entrance of counterfeit drug products into the nation's drug supply. The ASHP planned to provide rapid alerts to hospital pharmacy departments about counterfeit drug incidents.[226] Also, there are methods being developed or implemented that will help to ensure the pedigree of products, particularly those imported from foreign countries, to help avoid counterfeit products. This may include the use of radio frequency identification (RFID) tags to help track products.[227]

The FDA Web site may be consulted at http://www.fda.gov/Safety/MedWatch/SafetyInformation/SafetyAlertsforHumanMedicalProducts/default.htm for an updated list of counterfeit products. Because of the potential problems associated with counterfeit drug products, the P&T committee must be kept informed of any situations that affect the institution, as should the medical staff as a whole.[225] This topic also may be handled with medication errors, because it leads to such errors.

SAFETY ALERT

A variety of other safety-related items are also important to P&T committees, including recalls, black box warnings, risk evaluation and mitigation strategies (REMS), and product shortages, which will be covered in the following subsections. The items covered in this section can also be considered related to ADRs and medication errors, because some portions fit under those categories.

Recalls

The 2010 Joint Commission Accreditation Process Guide for Hospitals requires that a policy and procedure be in place, and be implemented when necessary, to retrieve recalled or discontinued medications. This policy must involve notification of prescribers and patients.[161] The pharmacy department constantly reviews medication products recalled by the manufacturer or the FDA due to a safety issue.[228] This information is provided to the pharmacy by the wholesaler and the manufacturer. If a product lot number involved in the recall is found in the pharmacy inventory, that product should be removed from the inventory immediately and recalled from other areas of the institution that may stock it.[132] In the outpatient environment, a recall from consumers may be necessary. A report of medications that have been pulled from the pharmacy inventory should be made available to the P&T committee and the committee may need to decide whether or not to identify patients who may have been affected by the safety issue. Further actions would be based on these findings. The P&T committee chair should be contacted when a patient has significant consequences in relation to a product recall. When a product recall requires the removal of a product for treating a disease with limited alternative treatments from the pharmacy inventory, therapeutic alternatives must be made known to the prescribers.[10]

The safety of medications is under constant evaluation, and the safety of new agents cannot be known until the product has been on the market for a period of time.[229]

Some newly reported serious adverse effects result in black box warnings being inserted in the product labeling or REMS, due to requirements of the FDA, which may necessitate action up to the withdrawal of the medication from the market, as was recently done with propoxyphene.[230] The reason for the name black box is that the warning is set off from the rest of the information in the package insert by a thick black box that is drawn around it. It is the responsibility of the P&T committee to review safety data for every medication on the formulary. Many P&T committees have a standing agenda item to review all new black box warnings or newly released FDA safety alerts for medications. The P&T committee needs to review the safety data and make any formulary, policy and procedure, and/or other changes as required. The black box safety data of formulary products need to be disseminated to the medical staff, including any special restrictions or actions taken on a specific product. The 2010 TJC Standard MM.02.01.01 addresses the hospital's role in selecting and procuring medications and their annual review for safety and efficacy.[161]

PRODUCT SHORTAGES

Product shortages should be continuously monitored by the pharmacy department in an organized fashion; this is a TJC requirement.[78,132,228] Information on this can be found at http://www.fda.gov/Drugs/DrugSafety/DrugShortages/default.htm. It is possible to get a free e-mail of these shortages from that site. There is a trend of more frequent medication shortages in recent years.[231] In some cases, the evaluation of information may show that acceptable alternative products or treatments may be interchanged for products affected by a shortage. The appropriate health care professionals (e.g., physicians, drug information service, pharmacy director, and buyer) need to be immediately notified of product shortages that may have an effect on therapeutic outcomes, along with plans or recommendations on how to address the situation.[232] In some instances, the chief of the medical staff and even the ethics committee may need to be consulted when policies need to be put into place to ration drug supplies. The shortage of intravenous immunoglobulin (IVIG) in the 1990s necessitated a complete medical staff and pharmacy department agreement for appropriate patient selection for treatment.[233] This shortage required product rationing with the available supply. Unfortunately, no therapeutic alternatives were available for the IVIG shortage. Methods of alerting medical staff of shortages include personal communication, the use of posters or message boards in key areas of the hospital (e.g., medical staff lounge, dictation area, parking garage, and high traffic areas), e-mail, computer notification during physician order entry, and the use of newsletters or faxes. A guideline is available from the ASHP to aid in determining how to handle various types of shortages.[228]

In today's health care environment, it is essential to keep medication shortages as a standard agenda item for each P&T meeting. Products with limited availability and products that are not available need to be evaluated constantly. Formulary alternatives for these product shortages then need to be communicated to the medical staff.

Case Study 12–3

You are the pharmacist medication buyer for the health system. Your wholesaler has notified you that there is a product shortage of intravenous furosemide and there is no timeframe when it will be available. You check the Food and Drug Administration (FDA) Web site as well as the American Society of Health-System Pharmacists (ASHP) Web site for further information. Information is available for estimated resupply dates, implications for patient care, safety and alternative agents, and management of this shortage. You are asked to develop a plan to manage this shortage.

1. What health care personnel should be notified of this shortage?
2. What methods should be used to alert the medical staff?
3. What information should you provide regarding this drug shortage?
4. What steps are needed to develop a plan to manage this shortage and ensure that patient care is not compromised?

Communication Within an Organization

INVESTIGATIONAL REVIEW BOARD ACTIONS

While P&T committees are generally responsible for overseeing all aspects of medication use in a hospital, they often turn the major responsibility for overseeing investigational drug use over to an IRB. The IRB should provide a regular overview of its actions to the P&T committee for review, but oftentimes this is all that is done. Further information about IRBs can be found in Chapter 17.

COST, BUDGET, AND FORECASTING

How does the P&T committee actively balance its quality-promoting activities as well as the economic requirements of its parent organization? For an individual hospital, this is probably an easier task as long as the economic pressures on the hospital's margin are manageable. As previously mentioned, a closed formulary can result in lowered costs within an institution.[174] However, the P&T committee decisions will be more difficult for the PBM function of a health insurance company or HMO. In the latter situation, the pressures of cost containment, the contents of an insurance plan's Certificate of Benefits, and the applicable payer regulations represent formidable obstacles for building broad support for the decisions of a PBM's P&T committee. In comparison to institutional formularies, PBMs have instituted tier-based formularies that encourage the use of more cost-effective agents to control prescription costs and improve therapy.[234,235] In spite of the economic influences on the P&T committee functions of a PBM, there is no end to opportunities for quality improvement by a PBM because there is no other organization that has the ability to access outpatient medication use to the same extent. Regardless of the organizational setting, the requirements for quality as a basis for decisions should be the chief focus of a P&T committee. Obviously, this is a potentially moving target because of the need to achieve a balance between the ethical standards involved in health care. The vested interests of the parent organization; the patient's needs and expectations; the professional activities of physicians, pharmacists, and nurses; the pharmaceutical companies; and the requirements of society may be very difficult to reconcile.

National drug expenditure projection data and the factors likely to influence drug costs for a particular year can be reviewed by the P&T committee on a yearly basis. Also, it is necessary to keep hospital administrators informed of drug costs.[236] An understanding of current trends is essential for formulary management.[142,237,238]

LIAISON WITH OTHER ELEMENTS OF THE ORGANIZATION

Within any organization, it is often found that the root of problems is communications or, perhaps more often, lack thereof. Unfortunately, the solution is not simply an increase in communication efforts in general. Instead, the need is for increasing appropriate communication, along with decreasing inappropriate communication. Some specific things have to be kept in mind.

First, make sure that everyone involved in any way in drug therapy receives some communication about medication-related matters.[154] Often, this may simply be a list of new drugs available being given to practitioners, along with any policies and procedures. Newsletters and educational presentations may also be valuable, depending on the circumstances.

Second, make sure the amount of material is not overwhelming, otherwise it will be ignored. A news program on television a number of years ago described a situation that the military found regarding its pilots in Vietnam. They had a tape from the cockpit of an aircraft that had been shot down. Those listening to the tape could clearly hear the warning alarm letting the pilot know that a radar missile was locked on his aircraft and posing an imminent danger; however, it was also clear that the pilot did not even realize that warning was happening because of everything else going on. He mentally tuned out the warning and was shot down as a result. It became clear to those training pilots that it was necessary to limit the amount of information to whatever is most important, so that those items were noticed. This is also important in communicating P&T committee materials.

In addition, it is important to keep certain materials confidential for various reasons. In the case of quality assurance materials, keeping materials suitably confidential may protect that data from legal discovery in court (see Chapter 10 and consult attorneys for specifics). Also, some P&T committees keep the agenda and handouts confidential by not sending them to committee members in advance and by collecting the materials at the end of the meeting in order to destroy them. By doing so, they can often avoid pressure put on the committee by pharmaceutical company representatives, who may be trying to have their products included on the formulary while having their competitors' products excluded. The disadvantage, of course, is that committee members are not able to prepare for a meeting in advance. In relationship to this, it is often a good idea to make sure the pharmaceutical company representatives do not know the members of the committee and who is preparing the evaluation of a particular product, because that can lead to the evaluator being pressured to sway his or her opinion about a particular product.

Finally, an annual report of the P&T committee may be prepared for both internal review and review by the medical executive committee. This annual report is time-consuming to prepare but is a very important means of tracking P&T activities and actions over time.

Overall, it is necessary for the chairman and secretary of the P&T committee to work in cooperation with other appropriate individuals and groups to make sure that essential information is provided wherever needed, while minimizing the amount of extraneous material.

Conclusion

The pharmacy department can have a major impact on the quality of drug therapy in an institution through participation in P&T committee functions and activities described in this chapter, many of which are related to the management of information or are commonly performed by drug information practitioners. Although there are many appropriate ways that may be used in addition to those outlined in this chapter, those described can be successfully used to improve drug therapy.

Acknowledgment

Donald R. Fagan, PharmD, and Debra L. Lee, PharmD, from Creighton University Medical Center are acknowledged for their assistance in preparing this chapter.

Study Questions

1. What is the P&T committee, what are its functions, and how does the committee relate to a pharmacy department?
2. How should a pharmacy/pharmacist be involved in supporting a P&T committee?
3. Define drug formulary and formulary system. How do those items relate to one another?
4. Define open versus closed formularies, including the specific types of closed formularies.
5. How does a P&T committee improve the quality of medication use in a hospital?
6. a. Define policy. b. Define procedure.
7. What are the steps in preparing a policy and procedure?
8. Name and briefly explain four policies and procedures that may be implemented by a P&T committee.
9. How does an institutional P&T committee differ from one in a PBM?
10. With whom must a P&T committee communicate? What should they communicate and how should they communicate?
11. What is considered a conflict of interest?

Self-Assessment Questions

1. A pharmacy and therapeutics (P&T) committee can be defined as:
   a. A committee that oversees all aspects of medication therapy in an institution
   b. A committee that oversees all procedures of the institution
   c. A committee that oversees only the medications that are carried in a hospital
   d. A committee that oversees only the quality of medication utilization

2. The P&T committee may act only as:
   a. An advisory body to the medical executive committee
   b. An advisory body to the administration
   c. An advisory body to the board of trustees
   d. An advisory body to the pharmacy

3. The functions of a P&T committee include:
   a. Determining what medications are available
   b. Quality assurance activities
   c. Policies and procedures regarding drug use
   d. All the above

4. Pharmacy/pharmacists support the P&T committee by:
   a. Having the P&T committee be part of the pharmacy department
   b. Serving as chairperson
   c. Involvement in the rational planning process for each meeting agenda
   d. Only addressing medications to be carried on the formulary

5. A drug formulary and a formulary system relate to each other in that:
   a. A drug formulary is a list of available medications under the formulary system, which is the method for developing the drug list that reflects the clinical judgment of the medical staff.
   b. A drug formulary comes before a formulary system.
   c. The formulary system provides for a drug formulary that serves only to keep costs down at the expense of patient care.
   d. Where there is a drug formulary system in place there is never a drug formulary published.

6. A closed formulary differs from an open formulary in that:
   a. A closed formulary includes all medications on the market.
   b. Closed formularies may not result in cost savings.
   c. Only certain medication classes are available in a closed formulary.
   d. It is restrictive.

7. Which of the following does not describe the benefits of a therapeutic interchange:
   a. Decreased cost
   b. Improved patient outcomes
   c. Decreased inventory
   d. Increased medication errors

8. The P&T committee improves the quality of medications used in the hospital by:
   a. Objectively assessing medications based upon the scientific evidence
   b. By anecdotal physician experience
   c. By manufacturer-sponsored information
   d. Occasional review of formulary medications

9. A policy differs from a procedure in that a policy:
   a. Is a broad, general statement that describes the goals and purpose of a document
   b. Provides specific action to be taken
   c. Is usually developed after a problem occurs
   d. Is not required by The Joint Commission

10. Taken together, policies and procedures may be a logical, step-by-step explanation of why and where a product may be used, how to use it, and who is to follow the policy.
    a. True
    b. False

11. Policies and procedures that may be implemented by the P&T committee include:
    a. As needed (prn) medications
    b. Hold medications
    c. Resume medications
    d. All of the above

12. A conflict of interest is considered when people involved in the drug decision process:
    a. Receive direct or indirect compensation from having the drug available
    b. Have stock in the company
    c. Receive honoraria for speaking, consulting fees, and gifts or grants from the company
    d. All the above

13. A pharmacy benefit management (PBM) P&T committee differs from an institutional P&T by the following:
    a. Members consist of physicians, pharmacists, and nurses.
    b. It works with health plans, insurers, and employers to develop drug formularies.
    c. It meets on a monthly basis.

14. Pharmacy networks are a group of pharmacies that are under contract with insurance companies, health plans, and/or contracted PBM parties to promote pharmacy services at negotiated discount fees.
    a. True
    b. False

15. PBMs place their formulary and nonformulary medications into tiers with an associated copayment with each tier.
    a. True
    b. False

REFERENCES

1. Shulkin DJ. Enhancing the role of physicians in the cost-effective use of pharmaceuticals. Hosp Formul. 1994;29:262-73.

2. Nair KV, Ascione FJ. Evaluation of P&T committee performance: an exploratory study. Hosp Formul. 2001;3:136-46.

3. Zellmer WA. Dr. Avorn's wake-up call to pharmacy. Am J Health-Syst Pharm. 2004;61:2010.

4. Nair KV, Coombs JH, Ascione FJ. Assessing the structure, activities, and functioning of P&T committees: a multisite case study. P&T. 2000;25(10):516-28.

5. Redman RL, Mays DA. Data analysis. Drug information services in the managed care setting. Drug Benefit Trends. 1997;9:28-40.

6. Sroka CJ. CRS Report for Congress: Pharmacy Benefit Managers. Washington, DC: Library of Congress; 2000 Nov 29.

7. Gourley DR, Halbert MR, Hartmann KM, Malone PM. Development and implementation of a P&T committee for state institutions. Hosp Formul. 1981;16(2):143-4, 149-51, 154-5.

8. McCutcheon T. Medicare Prescription Drug Benefit Model Guidelines. Washington, DC: United States Pharmacopeial Convention; 2004.

9. Stefanacci RG. The expanding role of P&T committees in long-term care. P&T. 2003;28:720-3.

10. Feldman L. Pharmacists' role in the pharmacy and therapeutics committee. Pharm Times. February 2004:26.

11. Jenkins A. Formulary development by community pharmacists. Pharmaceutical J. 1996;256:861-3.

12. AMA Board of Trustees. Drug Formularies and Therapeutic Interchange. Recommendations adopted at the American Medical Association (AMA) House of Delegates Interim Meeting 1993. Chicago (IL): American Medical Association; 1993.

13. H-125.991 Drug Formularies and Therapeutic Interchange. Chicago (IL): American Medical Association; 2000 [cited 2004 Mar 9]. [2 p.]. Available from: http://www.ama-assn.org/apps/pf_new/pf_online?f_n=browse&doc=policyfiles/HnE/H-125.991.HTM.

14. Formulary Management (Medication-Use Policy Development). Bethesda (MD): American Society of Health-System Pharmacists; 2004 [cited 2004 Mar 9]. 1 p. Available from: http://www.ashp.org/bestpractices/formulary.cfm?cfid=497523&CFToken=39106216.

15. CAMH Comprehensive Accreditation Manual for Hospitals: The Official Handbook. Oakbrook Terrace (IL): The Joint Commission; 2010.

16. Format for Formulary Submissions. Version 3.0. Alexandria (VA): Academy of Managed Care Pharmacy; 2009.

17. Raffel MW, Barsukiewicz CK. The US Health System: Origins and Functions. Albany (NY): Delmar; 2002.

18. Balu S, O'Connor P, Vogenberg FR. Contemporary issues affecting P&T committees. Part 1: The evolution. P&T. 2004;29:709-11.

19. Worthen DB. The amazing Charles Rice and Bellevue Hospital. Pharm Pract News. 2010;37(06): [2 p.]. Available from: http://pharmacypracticenews.com/index.asp?section_id=402&show=dept&issue_id=643&article_id=15339.

20. Millano C. Bellevue Hospital: the birthplace of formulary medicine? Pharm Pract News. 2004;31:14.

21. Plumridge RJ, Stoelwinder JU, Rucker TD. Drug and therapeutics committees: the relationships among structure, function, and effectiveness. Hosp Pharm. 1993;28:492-3, 496-8, 508.

22. Doherty EC. The JCAHO agenda for change: what changes in pharmacy and P&T activities do you need to prepare for in 1994. Hosp Formul. 1994;29:54-68.

23. The Joint Commission on Accreditation of Healthcare Organizations. 1995 Comprehensive Accreditation Manual for Hospitals. Oakbrook Terrace (IL): Joint Commission on Accreditation of Healthcare Organizations; 1994.

24. Academy of Managed Care Pharmacy. Principles of a sound drug formulary system. 2000 [cited 2004 Mar 18]. Available from: http://www.amcp.org/data/nav_content/drugformulary%2Epdf.

25. Eavy GR, Swinkey NJ, Rehan A. Decentralizing the P&T committee: rationale and successes. Formulary. 2000;35:752-69.

26. Mubarak-Shaban H, Billups SJ. The pharmacy and therapeutics committee within a hospital corporation: challenges and solution. P&T. 1998;23(6):309-10, 332.

27. Herbert WJ, Mahaney LM. Consolidating P&T committees in an integrated health care system. Formulary. 1996;31:497-504.

28. Cano SB. Formularies in integrated health systems: Fallon health care system. Am J Health-Syst Pharm. 1996;53:270-3.

29. Rizos AL, Levy E, Furnier J, Crowley K. Formularies in integrated health systems: Sharp HealthCare. Am J Health-Syst Pharm. 1996;53:274-8.

30. Barkley GL, Krol G, Anandan JV, Isopi M. An integrated health care system's attempt to create a unified formulary. Formulary. 1997;32:60-74.

31. Jarry PD, Fish L. Insights on outpatient formulary management in a vertically integrated health care system. Formulary. 1997;32:500-14.

32. Mannebach MA, Ascione FJ, Gaither CA, Bagozzi RP, Cohen IA, Ryan ML. Activities, functions, and structure of pharmacy and therapeutics committees in large teaching hospitals. Am J Health-Syst Pharm. 1999;56:622-8.

33. Balu S, O'Connor P, Vogenberg FR. Contemporary issues affecting P&T committees. Part 2: Beyond managed care. P&T. 2004;29:780-3.

34. Solow BK. P&T committees today: ensuring they bring value to your organization. Am J Pharm Benefits. 2009;1(4):189-90.

35. Teagarden JR. How many members should be on a P&T committee. P&T Society. Fall 2003.

36. Miller WA. Making the pharmacy and therapeutics committee more effective. Curr Concepts Hosp Pharm Manage. Summer 1986:10-15.

37. Christopherson GA. Policy for implementation of the DoD pharmacy and therapeutics committee [Internet]. Washington, DC: 1998 Mar 23 [cited 2004 Jan 23]. [4 p.]. Available from: http://www.tricare.osd.mil/policy/fy98/dptc9825.html.

38. Barlas S. Role of P&T committees in Medicare: how much authority, accountability? P&T. 2004;29:678.

39. Cross M. Increased pressures change P&T Committee makeup. Managed Care. 2001;10(12):18-30.

40. The ABCs of PBMs. A discussion featuring Peter D. Fox, Ph.D; Terry S. Latanich; Chris O'Flinn, J.D. LLM; and Phonzie Brown. Washington, DC: The George Washington University. National Health Policy Forum. Issue Brief No. 749; 1999 Oct 27.

41. Lipton HL, Kreling DH, Collins T, Hertz KC. Pharmacy benefit management companies: dimensions of performance. Annu Rev Public Health. 1999;20:361-401.

42. Cross M. Do P&T committees have enough power? Managed Care. 2007;16(4):28-30.

43. Teagarden JR. Perspectives on prescription drug benefit formularies. Hosp Pharm. 2004;39:1102-25.

44. PricewaterhouseCoopers. The Value of Pharmacy Benefit Management and the National Cost Impact of Proposed PBM Legislation. Washington: Pharmaceutical Care Management Association; 2004 July.

45. Carroll J. Plans look askance at me-too medications. Managed Care. 2008;17(1):37-42.

46. Butler CD, Manchester R. The P&T committee: descriptive survey of activities and time requirements. Hosp Formul. 1986;21:89-98.

47. Chi J. When R.Ph.s talk P&T committees listen. Hosp Pharm Rep. 1994;8(5):1, 7-8.

48. Gannon K. More power to you. Pharmacists flex their muscles and exert greater influence on P&T committees. Hosp Pharm Rep. 1998;12(2):18-20.

49. Chase P, Bell J, Smith P, Fallik A. Redesign of the P&T committee around continuous quality improvement principles. P&T. 1995;20(10):25-26, 29-30, 32, 34, 37-8, 40.

50. Croft CL, Crane VS. Redesign of P&T committee functions and processes: a model. Formulary. 1998;33:1105-22.

51. Crane VS, Gonzalez ER, Hull BL. How to develop a proactive formulary system. Hosp Formul. 1994;29:700-10.

52. Poirier TI, Vorbach M, Bache T. Linking a policy on nonformulary drugs to the FDA's therapeutic-potential classification system. Am J Hosp Pharm. 1994;51:2277-8.

53. Rich DS. Pharmacies' noncompliance with 2009 Joint Commission hospital accreditation requirements. Am J Health-Syst Pharm. 2009;66:e27-e30.

54. Green JA, Chawla AK, Fong PA. Evaluating a restrictive formulary system by assessing nonformulary-drug requests. Am J Hosp Pharm. 1985;42:1537-41.

55. Hailemeskel B, Kelvas M. Nonformulary drug requests as a guide in formulary system management. Am J Health-Syst Pharm. 1999;56:818, 820.

56. Cohen MR. Adding drugs to the formulary: your work is never done. Hosp Pharm. 1999;34(7):828.

57. Shea BF, Churchill WW, Powell SH, Cooley TW, Maguire JH. P&T committee overview: Brigham and Women's Hospital. Pharm Pract Manag Q. 1998;17(4):76-83.

58. McCain J. P&T Committees in position to reduce medication errors. Managed Care. 2004;13(6):39-42.

59. Cunha BA. Principles of antibiotic formulary selection for P&T committees. P&T. 2003;28(6):396.

60. Empey KM, Rapp RP, Evans ME. The effect of an antimicrobial formulary change on hospital resistance patterns. Pharmacotherapy. 2002;22(1):81-7.

61. Cunha BA. Principles of antibiotic formulary selection for P&T committees. Part 1: Antimicrobial activity. P&T. 2003;28(6):397-9.

62. Cunha BA. Principles of antibiotic formulary selection for P&T committees. Part 2: Pharmacokinetics and pharmacodynamics. P&T. 2003;28(7):468-70.

63. Cunha BA. Principles of antibiotic formulary selection for P&T committees. Part 3: Antibiotic resistance. P&T. 2003;28(8):524-7.

64. Polk RE. Antimicrobial formularies: can they minimize antimicrobial resistance? Am J Health-Syst Pharm. 2003;60(Suppl 1):S16-S19.

65. Cunha BA. Principles of antibiotic formulary selection for P&T committees. Part 4: Antimicrobial side effects. P&T. 2003;28(9):594-6.

66. Cunha BA. Principles of antibiotic formulary selection for P&T committees. Part 5: The cost of antimicrobial therapy. P&T. 2003;28:662-5.

67. Motz JC. Influence of the P&T committee on antibiotic selection in a staff model HMO. P&T. 1998;23(8):411-8.

68. DiLiegro N, Groves AJ, Caspi A. Cost savings from an antimicrobial-monitoring program. P&T. 1998;23(8):419-24.

69. Carlson JA. Antimicrobial formulary management: meeting the challenge in a health maintenance organization. Pharmacotherapy. 1991;11(1 pt 2):32S-35S.

70. Quintiliani R, Quercia RA. How to create a therapeutics committee that is scientifically and economically sound. Formulary. 2003;38:594-602.

71. Owen RC, Shorr AF, Deschambeault AL. Antimicrobial stewardship: shepherding precious resources. Am J Health-Syst Pharm. 2009;66(Suppl 4):S15-S22.

72. Lesprit P, Brun-Buisson C. Hospital antibiotic stewardship. Curr Opin Infect Dis. 2008;21:344-9.

73. Drew RH. Antimicrobial stewardship programs: how to start and steer a successful program. J Manag Care Pharm. 2009;15(2)(Suppl):S18-S23.

74. Culley CM, Carroll BA, Skledar SJ. Formulary decisions for pre-1938 medications. Am Health-Syst Pharm. 2008;65(15):1368-83.

75. Mirtallo JM. Advancement of nutrition support clinical pharmacy. Ann Pharmacotherapy. 2007;41:869-72.

76. The Joint Commission. 2010 provision of care, treatment and services. The Joint Commission Web. [cited 2010 Oct 21]. Available from: http://site.www.jointcommission.org.

77. ASHP statement on the pharmacy and therapeutics committee. Am J Hosp Pharm. 1992;49:2008-9.

78. Ventola CL. An interview series with members of the ASHP Expert Panel on Formulary Management. Part 1: Linda S. Tyler, Pharm.D. P&T. 2009;34(11):623-31.

79. Brushwood DB. Legal issues surrounding therapeutic interchange in institutional settings: an update. Formulary. 2001;36:796-804.

80. Mutnick AH, Ross MB. Formulary management at a tertiary care teaching hospital. Pharm Pract Manag Q. 1997;17(1):63-87.

81. Dore DD, Larrat EP, Vogenberg FR. Principles of epidemiology for clinical and formulary management professionals. P&T. 2006;31(4):218-26.

82. Suh D, Okpara I, Agnese WB, Toscani M. Application of pharmacoeconomics to formulary decision making in managed care organizations. Am J Managed Care. 2002;8(2):161-9.

83. Odedina FT, Sullivan J, Nash R, Clemmons CD. Use of pharmacoeconomic data in making hospital formulary decisions. Am J Health-Syst Pharm. 2002;59:1441-4.

84. Pick AM, Massoomi F, Neff WJ, Danekas PL, Stoysich AM. A safety assessment tool for formulary candidates. Am J Health-Syst Pharm. 2006;63:1269-72.

85. Barr B. Open and closed. Pharmaceutical Representative [Internet] 2007 May 1 [cited 2008 Jul 14]: [4 p.]. Available from: http://license.icopyright.net/user/viewFreeUse.act?fuid=MTI2ODQyMg%3D%3D.

86. ASHP statement on the formulary system. Am J Hosp Pharm. 1983;35:326-8.

87. ASHP technical assistance bulletin on drug formularies. Am J Hosp Pharm. 1991;48:791-3.

88. ASHP guidelines on formulary system management. Am J Hosp Pharm. 1992;49:648-52.

89. Rucker TD, Schiff G. Drug formularies: myths-in-formation. Med Care. 1990;28:928-42.

90. Tyler LS, Cole SW, May JR, Millares M, Valentino MA, Vermeulen LC Jr, Wilson AL. ASHP guidelines on the pharmacy and therapeutics committee and the formulary system. Am J Health-Syst Pharm. 2008;65:1272-83.

91. Grissinger M. The truth about hospital formularies Part I. P&T. 2008;33(8):441.

92. Lehmann DF, Guharoy R, Page N, Hirschman K, Ploutz-Snyder R, Medicis J. Formulary management as a tool to improve medication use and gain physician support. Am J Health-Syst Pharm. 2007;64:464-6.

93. ASHP statement on the pharmacy and therapeutics committee and the formulary system. Am J Health-Syst Pharm. 2008;65:2384-6.

94. Rubino M, Hofman JM, Koseserer LJ, Swendryznski RG. ASHP guidelines on medication cost management strategies for hospitals and health systems. Am J Health-Syst Pharm. 2008;65:1368-84.

95. Chi J. Hospital consultant foresees dim future for drug formularies. Drug Topics. 1999 April 19:67.

96. Horn SD, Sharkey PD, Tracy DM, Horn C, James B, Goodwin F. Intended and unintended consequences of HMO cost-containment strategies: results from the managed care outcomes project. Am J Manag Care. 1996;2:253-64.

97. Horn SD. Unintended consequences of drug formularies. Am J Health-Syst Pharm. 1996;53:2204-6.

98. Goldberg RB. Managing the pharmacy benefit: the formulary system. J Manag Care Pharm. 1997;3(5):565-73.

99. Formulary effectiveness: many questions, but few clear answers. Consult Pharm. 1996;11(7):635.

100. Curtiss FR. Drug formularies provide a path to best care. Am J Health-Syst Pharm. 1996;53:2201-3.

101. Formularies and generics drive up health resource use, study suggests. Am J Health-Syst Pharm. 1996;53:971-5.

102. Horn SD, Sharkey PD, Phillips-Harris C. Formulary limitations and the elderly: results from the managed care outcomes project. Am J Manag Care. 1998;4:1105-13.

103. Marra F, Patrick DM, White R, Ng H, Bowie WR, Hutchinson JM. Effect of formulary policy decisions on antimicrobial drug utilization in British Columbia. J Antimicrob Chemother. 2005;55:95-101.

104. Hepler CD. Where is the evidence for formulary effectiveness. Am J Health-Syst Pharm. 1997;54:95.

105. VHA Formulary Management Process. Washington, DC: Department of Veterans Affairs; 2009.

106. Kelly WN, Rucker TD. Considerations in deciding which drugs should be in a formulary. J Pharm Pract. 1994;7(2):51-7.

107. Corman SL, Skledar SJ, Culley CM. Evaluation of conflicting literature and application to formulary decisions. Am J Health-Syst Pharm. 2007;64:182-5.

108. Shih Y-C T, Sleath BL. Health care provider knowledge of drug formulary status in ambulatory care settings. Am J Health-Syst Pharm. 2004;61:2657-63.

109. Muirhead G. When formularies collide. Hospitals vs. health plans. Hosp Pharm Rep. 1994;8(10):1, 8.

110. 1999 accreditation standards address public concerns, says NCQA. Am J Health-Syst Pharm. 1998;55:2221, 2225.

111. Bruzek RJ, Dullinger D. Drug formulary: the cornerstone of a managed pharmacy program. J Pharm Pract. 1992;5(2):75-81.

112. North GLT. Handling nonformulary requests for returning or transfer patients. Am J Hosp Pharm. 1994;51:2360, 2364.

113. Davis FA. Formularies: a dangerous concept for patients. Priv Pract. 1991 Sept:11-17.

114. Palmer MA, Hartman SK, Gervais S. Introducing a formulary system in long-term care facilities: initial experience. Consult Pharm. 1994;9:307-14.

115. Shulkin DJ. Enhancing the role of physicians in the cost-effective use of pharmaceuticals. Hosp Formul. 1994;29:262-73.

116. Pearce MJ, Begg EJ. A review of limited lists and formularies. Are they cost-effective? Pharmacoeconomics. 1992;1:191-202.

117. Sloan FA, Gordon GS, Cocks DL. Hospital drug formularies and use of hospital services. Med Care. 1993;31:851-67.

118. Hazlet TK, Hu T-W. Association between formulary strategies and hospital drug expenditures. Am J Hosp Pharm. 1992;49:2207-10.

119. Pickette S, Hanish L. Dealing with demands for nonformulary drugs. Am J Hosp Pharm. 1992;49:2920, 2923.

120. Corliss DA. Computer-assisted help desk for handling drug benefits. Am J Health-Syst Pharm. 1997;54:1941-42, 1945.

121. NCQA draft accreditation standards for 2000 address formularies. Am J Health-Syst Pharm. 1998;55:1266-7.

122. Le AG, Generali JA. From printed formularies to online formularies. Hosp Pharm. 2004;38:1003.

123. Navarro RP. Electronic formulary control. Med Interface. 1997;10(8):74-6.

124. Drug czars, electronic formulary systems increase formulary compliance. Formulary. 1997;32:171-2.

125. Ukens C. Hospital finds computer carrot can save drug dollars. Hosp Pharm Rep. 1994;8(6):20.

126. Computerized drug cost information fails to sway physician prescribing. Am J Health-Syst Pharm. 1999;56:1183-4.

127. Sateren LA, Sudds TW, Tyler LS. Computer-based system for maintaining and printing a hospital formulary. Am J Hosp Pharm. 1987;44:1367-70.

128. Sears EL. Development and maintenance of an online formulary for a large health system. Am J Health-Syst Pharm. 2008;65:510, 2.

129. E-prescribing applications help physicians with Vioxx recall. Pharm Pract News. 2004;31(11):67.

130. McCaffrey S, Nightingale CH. How to develop critical paths and prepare for other formulary management changes. Hosp Formul. 1994;29:628-35.

131. Current formulary decision-making strategies and new factors influencing the process. Formulary. 1995;30:462-70.

132. Rich DS. New JCAHO medication management standards for 2004. Am J Health-Syst Pharm. 2004;61:1349-58.

133. Neumann PJ. Evidence-based and value-based formulary guidelines. Health Aff. 2004;23(1):124-34.

134. Murri NA, Somani S. Implementation of safety-focused pharmacy and therapeutics monographs: a new University Health System Consortium template designed to minimize medication misadventures. Hosp Pharm. 2004;39:654-60.

135. Chren M-M, Landefeld CS. Physicians' behavior and their interactions with drug companies. JAMA. 1994;271:684-9.

136. Haslé-Pham E, Arnould B, Späth H-M, Follet A, Duru G, Marquis P. Role of clinical, patient-reported outcome and medico-economic studies in the public hospital drug formulary decision-making process: results of a European survey. Health Policy. 2005;71:205-12.

137. Ventola CL. An interview series with members of the ASHP Expert Panel on Formulary Management. Part 3: Sabrina W. Cole, Pharm.D. P&T. 2010;35(1):24-8.

138. Shrank WH. Change we can believe in: requiring better evidence for formulary coverage. Am J Pharm Benefits. Fall 2009:134-6.

139. Asmus MJ, Hendeles L. Levalbuterol nebulizer solution: is it worth five times the cost of albuterol? Pharmacotherapy. 2000;20:123-9.

140. Desloratadine (Clarinex). Med Lett. 2002;44(W1126B):27-9.

141. Escitalopram (Lexapro) for depression. Med Lett. 2002;44(W1140A):83-4.

142. Hoffman JM, Shah ND, Vermeulen LC, Hunkler RJ, Hontz KM. Projecting future drug expenditures—2004. Am J Health-Syst Pharm. 2004;61:145-58.

143. FDA sees rebound in approval of innovative drugs in 2003 [Internet]. New York (NY): Science Daily; 2004 Jan 19 [cited 2004 Apr 22]: [4 p.]. Available from: http://www.sciencedaily.com/releases/2004/01/040116074839.htm.

144. FDA new drug approvals up in 2008. Itasca (IL): Putnam Media. C2004. [cited 2009 Feb 22]. 1 p. Available from: http://pharmamanufacturing.com/industrynews/2009/018.html.

145. Most medications approved in the 1990s not new, but modified versions of older drugs, report states [Internet]. Menlo Park (CA): kaisernetwork.org; 2002 May 29 [cited 2004 Apr 22]. Available from: http://www.kaisernetwork.org/daily_reports/print_report. cfm?DR_ID-11414&dr_cat=3.

146. Senthilkumaran K, Shatz SM, Kalies RF. Computer-based support system for formulary decisions. Am J Hosp Pharm. 1987;44:1362-6.

147. Computer tool lets P&T members assess Tx classes with their own weightings, product ratings. Formulary. 2000;35:603.

148. Janknegt R, Steenhoek A. The system of objectified judgement analysis (SOJA). A tool in rational drug selection for formulary inclusion. Drugs. 1997;53(4):550-62.

149. Janknegt R, van den Broek PJ, Kulberg BJ, Stobberingh E. Glycopeptides: drug selection by means of the SOJA method. Eur Hosp Pharm. 1997;3(4):127-35.

150. Zachry WM III, Skrepnek GH. Applying multiattribute utility technology to the formulary evaluation process. Formulary. 2002;37:199-206.

151. Jacobson SH. A web-based tool for designing vaccine formularies for childhood immunization in the United States. J Am Med Informatics Assoc. 2008;15(5):611-9.

152. Berghelli JA. Conflict of interest policy approved. P&T. 1995;20:497.

153. Alpert JS. Doctors and the drug industry: how can we handle potential conflicts of interest? Am J Med. 2005;118:88-100.

154. Ventola CL. An interview series with members of the ASHP Expert Panel on Formulary Management. Part 2: J. Russell May, Pharm.D. P&T. 2009;34(12):671-7.

155. Campbell EG. Doctors and drug companies—scrutinizing influential relationships. N Engl J Med. 2007;357(18):1796-7.

156. Palmer MA. Developing a conflict-of-interest policy for the pharmacy and therapeutics committee. Am J Hosp Pharm. 1987;44:2012-4.

157. Fredrick DS, Maddock JR, Graman PS. Hashing out a policy on conflicts of interest for a P&T committee. Am J Health-Syst Pharm. 1995;52:2791-2.

158. Campbell EG. A national survey of physician-industry relationships. N Engl J Med. 2007;356:1742-50.

159. Barlas S. Inspector General cautions PBMs on formulary decision making. P&T. 2003;28(6):367.

160. Trice S, Devine J, Mistry H, Moore E, Linton, A. Formulary management in the Department of Defense. J Manag Care Pharm. 2009;15(2):133-46.

161. 2010 Accreditation Process Guide for Hospitals. Chicago (IL): The Joint Commission; 2010.

162. JCAHO unveils medication-management standards. Am J Health-Syst Pharm. 2003;60:1400-1.

163. Cardinale V. Alternative medicine: the law, the marketplace, the formulary. Hosp Pharm Rep. 1999;13(7):15.

164. Is alternative medicine poised for hospital formularies. Drug Util Rev. 1999;15(5):65-8.

165. Brubaker ML. Setting up the herbal formulary system for an alternative medicine clinic. Am J Health-Syst Pharm. 1998;55:435-6.

166. Beal FC. Herbals and homeopathic remedies as formulary items. Am J Health-Syst Pharm. 1998;55:1266-7.

167. Johnson ST, Wordell CJ. Homeopathic and herbal medicine: considerations for formulary evaluation. Formulary. 1997;32:1166-73.

168. Malesker MA, Meyer RT, Kuhlenengel LJ, Galt MA, Nelson PJ. Development of an alternative medication use policy [abstract]. ASHP Midyear Clinical Meeting. 1998;33(Dec):P-406R.

169. Walker PC. Evolution of a policy disallowing the use of alternative therapies in a health system. Am J Health-Syst Pharm. 2000;57:1984-90.

170. Ansani NT, Ciliberto NC, Freedy T. Hospital policies regarding herbal medicines. Am J Health-Syst Pharm. 2003;60:367-70.

171. Pick AM, Massoomi F, Neff WJ, Danekas PI, Stoysich AM. A safety assessment tool for formulary candidates. Am J Health-Syst Pharm. 2006;63:1269-72.

172. H-125.911 Drug Formularies and Therapeutic Interchange [Internet]. Chicago (IL): American Medical Association [cited 2004 Apr 23]. Available from: http://www.ama-assn.org/apps/pf_new/pf_online?f_n=browse&doc=policyfiles/HnE/H-125.991.HTM.

173. NCQA draft accreditation standards for 2000 address formularies. Am J Health-Syst Pharm. 1999;56:846.

174. Chiefari DM. Effect of a closed formulary on average prescription cost in a community health center. Drug Benefit Trends. 2001;13:44-5, 52.

175. Survey reveals continued HMO shift toward closed and partially closed formularies. Formulary. 1997;32:781-2.

176. Survey finds HMOs, PBMs still moving to restricted formularies, quickly advancing in informatics. Formulary. 1998;33:622, 625.

177. Abramowitz PW. Controlling financial variables—changing prescribing patterns. Am J Hosp Pharm. 1984;41:503-15.

178. Open formularies improve oncology outcomes in capitated care system. Formulary. 1996;31:878, 881.

179. TennCare formulary restrictions hurt patient care, survey says. Formulary. 1996;31(6):443.

180. Schachtner JM, Guharoy R, Medicis JJ, Newman N, Speizer R. Prevalence and cost savings of therapeutic interchange among U.S. hospitals. Am J Health-Syst Pharm. 2002;59:529-33.

181. Bowman GK, Moleski R, Mangi RJ. Measuring the impact of a formulary decision: conversion to one quinolone agent. Formulary. 1996;31:906-14.

182. Chase SL, Peterson AM, Wordell CJ. Therapeutic-interchange program for oral histamine H2-receptor antagonists. Am J Health-Syst Pharm. 1998;55:1382-6.

183. Stoysich A, Massoomi F. Automatic interchange of the ACE inhibitors: decision-making process and initial results. Formulary. 2002;37:41-4.

184. Frighetto L, Nickoloff D, Jewesson P. Antibiotic therapeutic interchange program: six years of experience. Hosp Formul. 1995;30:92-105.

185. Vivian JC. Legal aspects of therapeutic interchange. 2004 Aug 15 [cited 2004 Oct 22]; [6 screens]. Available from: http://www.uspharmacist.com/index.asp?show=article&page=8_1129.htm.

186. Janifer AN, Chatelain F, Goldwater SH, Mikovich G. Reengineering hospital pharmacy through therapeutic equivalency interchange while maintaining clinical outcomes. P&T. 1998;23(2):78-82, 85-8, 90-2.

187. Merli GJ, Vanscoy GJ, Rihn TL, Groce JB III, McCormick W. Applying scientific criteria to therapeutic interchange: a balanced analysis of low-molecular-weight heparins. J Thromb Thrombolysis. 2001;11(3):247-59.

188. Reich P. Therapeutic drug interchange. Med Interface. 1996;9(5):14.

189. H-125.995 Therapeutic and Pharmaceutical Alternatives by Pharmacists [Internet]. Chicago (IL): American Medical Association [cited 2004 Apr 23]. Available from: http://www.ama-assn.org/apps/pf_new/pf_online?f_n=browse&doc=policyfiles/HnE/H-125.995. HTM.

190. American College of Physicians. Therapeutic substitution and formulary systems. Ann Intern Med. 1990;113:160-3.

191. AMCP position statement on therapeutic interchange. 1997 Sept 13 [cited 2000 Feb 4]: [1 screen]. Available from: http://www.amcp.org/public/legislative/position/therapeutic.html.

192. American College of Clinical Pharmacy. Guidelines for therapeutic interchange. Pharmacotherapy. 1993;13(2):252-6.

193. Massoomi F. Formulary management: antibiotics and therapeutic interchange. Pharm Pract Manag Q. 1996;16(3):11-8.

194. Heiner CR. Communicating about therapeutic interchange. Am J Health-Syst Pharm. 1996;53:2568-70.

195. Rosen A, Kay BG, Halecky D. Implementing a therapeutic interchange program in an institutional setting. P&T. 1995;20:711-7.

196. Kielty M. Improving the prior-authorization process to the satisfaction of customers. Am J Health-Syst Pharm. 1999;56:1499-501.

197. Carroll NV. Formularies and therapeutic interchange: the health care setting makes a difference. Am J Health-Syst Pharm. 1999;56:467-72.

198. Nelson KM. Improving ambulatory care through therapeutic interchange. Am J Health-Syst Pharm. 1999;56:1307.

199. D'Amore M, Masters P, Maroun C. Impact of an automatic therapeutic interchange program on discharge medication selection. Hosp Pharm. 2003;38:942-6.

200. Banahan BF III, Bonnarens JK, Bentley JP. Generic substitution of NTI drugs: issues for formulary committee consideration. Formulary. 1998;33:1082-96.

201. FDA comments on activities in states concerning narrow-therapeutic-index drugs. Am J Health-Syst Pharm. 1998;55:686-7.

202. ASHP guidelines for selecting pharmaceutical manufacturers and suppliers. Am J Hosp Pharm. 1991;48:523-4.

203. Pummer TL, Shalaby KM, Erush SC. Ordering off the menu: assessing compliance with a nonformulary medication policy. Ann Pharmacother. 2009;43(July/Aug):1251-7.

204. Sweet BV, Stevenson JG. Pharmacy costs associated with nonformulary drug requests. Am J Health-Syst Pharm. 2001;58:1746-52.

205. Tse CST, Roecker W, Benitez M, Musabji M. How to tie a drug therapy improvement program to physician credentialing. Hosp Formul. 1994;29:646-56.

206. ASHP statement on the use of medications for unlabeled uses. Am J Hosp Pharm. 1992;49:2006-8.

207. Steinberg SK. The development of a hospital pharmacy policy and procedure manual. Can J Hosp Pharm. 1980;33(6):194-5, 211.

208. Ginnow WK, King CM Jr. Revision and reorganization of a hospital pharmacy and procedure manual. Am J Hosp Pharm. 1978;35:698-704.

209. Van Dusen V, Pray WS. Issues in implementation and enforcement of hospital pharmacy policies and procedures. Hosp Pharm. 2001;36(4):398-403.

210. Piecoro JJ Jr. Development of an institutional IV drug delivery policy. Am J Hosp Pharm. 1987;44:2557-9.

211. Grissinger M. Eliminating problem-prone, automatic stop-order policies. P&T. 2004;29:344.

212. Galt KA. Credentialing and privileging for pharmacists. Am J Health-Syst Pharm. 2004;61:661-70.

213. Galt KA. Privileging, quality improvement and accountability. Am J Health-Syst Pharm. 2004;61:659.

214. Sass CM. Drug usage evaluation. J Pharm Pract. 1994;7(2):74-8.

215. Orsini MJ, Funk Orsini PA, Thorn DB, Gallina JN. An ADR surveillance program: increasing quality, number of incidence reports. Formulary. 1995;30:454-61.

216. Samore MH, Evans RS, Lassen A, Gould P, Lloyd J, Gardner RM, et al. Surveillance of medical device-related hazards and adverse events in hospitalized patients. JAMA. 2004;291:325-34.

217. Traynor K. Enforcement outdoes education at eliminating unsafe abbreviations. Am J Health-Syst Pharm. 2004;61:1314, 1317, 1322.

218. Baker De. Sound-alike and look-alike drug errors. Hosp Pharm. 2002;37:225.

219. Vaida AJ, Peterson J. Common sound-alike, look-alike products. Pharm Times. 2002;68:22-3.

220. Starr CH. When drug names spell trouble. Drug Topics. 2000;144:49-50, 53-4, 57-8.

221. Cohen M. Medication error update. Consult Pharm. 1997;12:1328-9.

222. Soulliard D, Hong M, Saubermann L. Development of a pharmacy-managed medication dictionary in a newly implemented computerized prescriber order-entry system. Am J Health-Syst Pharm. 2004;61:617-22.

223. First Consulting Group. Computerized physician order entry: costs, benefits and challenges. A case study approach. Long Beach (CA): First Consulting Group; 2003.

224. FDA's Counterfeit Drug Task Force Interim Report. Washington, DC: U.S. Department of Health and Human Services, 2003 Oct [cited 2004 Mar 8]. Available fom: http://www.fda.gov/oc/initiatives/counterfeit/report/interim_report.html.

225. Generali JA. Counterfeit drugs: a growing concern. Hosp Pharm. 2003;38:724.

226. Young D. FDA Urges Adoption of Anticounterfeit Technologies by 2007 [Internet]. Bethesda (MD): American Society of Health-System Pharmacists, 2004 Feb 19 [cited 2004 Mar 8]. Available fom: http://www.ashp.org/news/ShowArticle.cfm?cfid=497458&CFToken=73579785&id=4194.

227. Redwanski J, Seamon MJ. Impact of counterfeit drugs on the formulary decision-making process. Formulary. 2004;39:577-9, 583.

228. ASHP guidelines on managing drug product shortages. Am J Health-Syst Pharm. 2001;58:1445-50.

229. Lasser KE, Allen PD, Woolhandler SJ, Himmelstein DU, Wolfe SM, Bor DH. Timing of new black box warnings and withdrawals for prescription medications. JAMA. 2002;287:2215-20.

230. Gandey A. Propoxyphene withdrawn from US market. Medscape [Internet]. 2010 Nov 19 [cited 2010 Nov 19]: [2 p.]. Available from: http://www.medscape.com/viewarticle/732887_print.

231. Fox ER, Tyler LS. Managing drug shortages: seven years' experience at one health system. Am J Health-Syst Pharm. 2003;60:245-53.

232. Leady MA, Adams AL, Stumpf JL, Sweet BV. Drug shortages: an approach to managing the latest crisis. Hosp Pharm. 2003;38:748-52.

233. Schrand LM, Troester TS, Ballas ZK, Mutnick AH, Ross MB. Preparing for drug shortages: one teaching hospital's approach to the IVIG shortage. Formulary. 2001;36:52-9.

234. Huskamp HA, Deverka PA, Epstein AM, Epstein RS, McGuigan KA, Frank RG. The effect of incentive-based formularies on prescription-drug utilization and spending. N Engl J Med. 2003;349:2224-32.

235. Thomas CP. Incentive-based formularies. N Engl J Med. 2003;349:2186-8.

236. Crane VS, Hull BL, Hatwig CA, Teresi M, Croft CL. Presenting drug cost information to a board of directors: a case example. Formulary. 2001;36:857-64.

237. Shah ND, Vermeulen LC, Santell JP, Hunkler RJ, Hontz K. Projecting future drug expenditures—2002. Am J Health-Syst Pharm. 2002;59:131-42.

238. Shah ND, Hoffman JM, Vermeulen LC, Hunkler RJ, Hontz K. Projecting future drug expenditures—2003. Am J Health-Syst Pharm. 2003;60:137-49.After completing this chapter, the reader will be able to

Chapter Thirteen

Drug Evaluation Monographs

Patrick M. Malone • Nancy L. Fagan • Mark A. Malesker
• Paul J. Nelson • Linda K. Ohri

Learning Objectives

● *After completing this chapter, the reader will be able to*

- Describe and perform an evaluation of a drug product for a drug formulary.
- List the sections included in a drug evaluation monograph.
- Describe the overall highlights included in a monograph summary.
- Describe the recommendations and restrictions that are made in a monograph.
- Describe the purpose and format of a drug class review.

Key Concepts

1. The establishment and maintenance of a drug formulary requires that drugs or drug classes be objectively assessed based on scientific information (e.g., efficacy, safety, uniqueness, cost, and other appropriate items), not anecdotal prescriber experience.

2. The drug evaluation monograph provides a structured method to review the major features of a drug product.

3. A definite recommendation must be made based on need, therapeutics, side effects, cost, and other items specific to the particular agent (e.g., dosage forms, convenience, dosage interval, inclusion on the formulary of third-party payers, hospital antibiotic resistance patterns, and potential for causing medication errors), usually in that order.

④ The recommendation must be supported by objective evidence.

⑤ The most logical decision to benefit the patient and the institution should be recommended to the pharmacy and therapeutics (P&T) committee.

⑥ While some think that cost is emphasized too much in formulary decisions, it is still an extremely important item.

⑦ Preparation of a drug evaluation monograph requires a great amount of time and effort, using many of the skills discussed throughout this text to obtain, evaluate, collate, and provide information. However, the value of having all of the issues evaluated and discussed can be invaluable in providing quality care.

Introduction

① *The establishment and maintenance of a drug formulary requires that drugs or drug classes be objectively assessed based on scientific information (e.g., efficacy, safety, uniqueness, cost, and other appropriate items), not anecdotal prescriber experience.* The way to decide which drug is best for formulary addition is to rationally evaluate all aspects of the drug in relation to similar agents. In particular, it is necessary to consider need, effectiveness, risk, and cost (overall, including monitoring costs, discounts, rebates, and so forth)—often in that order. Some other issues that are evaluated include dosage forms, packaging, requirements of accrediting or quality assurance bodies, prescriber preferences, regulatory issues, patient/nursing convenience, advertising, and consumer expectations.[1] It is expected that in the future there will be more emphasis on evaluating clinical outcomes from high-quality trials, continuous quality assurance information, comparative efficacies, pharmacogenomics, and quality of life (QOL).[2] Even such a factor as the public image of the institution may have an impact on the decision to add a drug to the formulary. An in-depth drug evaluation monograph can be prepared to assist in this process as described in the following.

② *The drug evaluation monograph provides a structured method to review the major features of a drug product.* Once a monograph is prepared, it can easily be used as a structured template or overview of a drug product. That allows for easy comparison or contrast to other products that may be used for the same indication or that are in the same product class. Commercially prepared monographs can also be obtained from several sources that can be used as is or with modifications to suit the needs of the institution. If this latter method is used, be aware that the quality of the commercial monographs may vary, even from the same publisher, and they may need extensive updating. Often, writing a new drug evaluation monograph may be easier than improving a commercial monograph.

When a pharmacy and therapeutics (P&T) committee desires to review an entire class of drugs, the drug category review is often another method used. Drug class reviews are often more lengthy than a single-product drug evaluation monograph; however, they can also use a similar structure and format. Hospitals, health systems, and managed care organizations review an entire class of drugs on a scheduled basis, which must be at least annually, according to accreditation standards.[3] This allows an organization the opportunity to reevaluate the formulary status of products in light of new publications or trials or new products that have entered the market, or oftentimes reevaluate a drug class for possible deletion of particular products from the class. Samples of drug class reviews prepared by the Veterans Administration are available on the Internet at http://www.pbm. va.gov/DrugMonograph.aspx.

Whether the monograph is commercial or prepared by a member from within the organization, the material should reflect the local conditions or current prescribing practices and may be sent to P&T committee members at a reasonable time before the meeting in order to allow full consideration of the information. In order to prevent drug company representatives or others from obtaining the material, however, some institutions only distribute this material for review during the meeting and then require the materials to be returned at the end of the meeting. Some institutions even number each monograph with a unique numbering system to assist in tracking the return of P&T committee documents.

Although there are recommendations concerning monograph contents,[1,4] information that may be valuable and specific to an institution, and necessary for an objective review of the product, is commonly missing.[5] An outline of a sample monograph is found in Appendix 13–1. Each of the sections of this monograph will be discussed in the following. An example of some of the information found in the various parts of a monograph is shown in Appendix 13–2. This sample monograph meets or exceeds the recommendations of the American Society of Health-System Pharmacists (ASHP),[4] and should serve as a good example for most circumstances. Guidelines published by the Academy of Managed Care Pharmacy (AMCP)[1,6] and The Joint Commission (TJC)[3] are also noted and discussed for situational applicability. The AMCP format is actually the standard recommended by an organization for manufacturers to submit data to managed care organizations. It is designed to restrict the marketing impact of the company in providing information and, although it has applicability as to how an institution may evaluate a drug, it also has restrictions as to the amount of information that it can cover in some areas, which may make it undesirable in some cases. However, it may be very worthwhile for institutions or other organizations to request this information from the drug company, preferably well in advance of the time it is needed. Please note, in some cases this request may require signing a nondisclosure agreement, because it may contain proprietary information.[1]

Overall, the precise monograph should be tailored to the institution, organization, patient population, clinic, and so forth. Several sections not recommended by ASHP have been added to increase the utility of the monograph for other sites of practice, including ambulatory clinics, pediatric institutions, long-term care facilities, managed care or pharmacy benefit managers, or even Medicare or Medicaid formularies. Also, in some cases, the information has been divided into multiple sections or subsections to increase clarity. This format can also be used to evaluate whole classes of drugs. In most cases, a specific drug is compared to others in the same class. The only difference in a class review is that one drug is not receiving the greatest attention; all drugs are being compared with equal attention. Comparative charts and tables are often more prevalent in drug class reviews, as they can serve as a concise method to provide an overview of comparative features for the products in a particular drug class.

Specific formats, differing somewhat from the one presented here, may be required by organizations or governments. For example, Australia (http://www.tga.gov.au/industry/pm-argpm.htm),[7] Ontario, Canada (http://www.health.gov.on.ca/english/providers/pub/drugs/dsguide/dsguide_mn.html),[8] and the United Kingdom (http://www.nice.org.uk/aboutnice/howwework/devnicetech/technologyappraisalprocessguides/technology_appraisal_process_guides.jsp)[9] have very specific published guidelines that need to be followed for a drug product to be considered for their formularies. Where appropriate, features of these formats have been incorporated into the description presented in this chapter. Although the format described in this chapter does provide much of the information in those government standards, with the exception of details about product manufacturing and specific pricing for the particular country, the order and amount of information is often different and the reader is referred to those standards for details.

Before discussing details about monograph preparation, it should be emphasized that the drug monograph is a powerful tool for the pharmacy to guide the rational development of a drug formulary. Although the pharmacy department or an individual pharmacist may have few, if any, votes in the ultimate adoption of a formulary agent, the monograph guides the evaluation process and is likely to be a major factor in the final decision. Although monograph preparation can be very time-consuming, it is extremely important and should be given proper attention. The structured evaluation process of a drug monograph, in many cases, is the only time a full, fair, and balanced review of a drug may be presented to a practitioner. Pharmacists have a unique role in the preparation of a monograph in that they view the drug product from a whole and macroeconomic view—all aspects of the drug product are objectively reviewed in a monograph, whereas, oftentimes when prescribers are presented information about a new drug product, they may be basing their use or nonuse of the product on a single study, package insert data, pharmaceutical representative information, or some other microeconomic view of a drug product that may or may not represent the full utility of the drug product.[10,11]

In addition to United States Food and Drug Administration (FDA)-regulated drug products, pharmacists need to be aware of complementary/alternative medicine use, along with the responsibilities and implications that it has for pharmacy services. These products can only be marketed as dietary substances, since the FDA does not regulate herbal products, so manufacturers and distributors cannot make specific health claims. Although there may be minimal scientific evidence regarding the efficacy and safety of these products, pharmacists must provide information relating to all therapeutic agents patients are receiving, when preparing a drug monograph for the P&T committee, much the same as for any FDA-approved product. This can also follow the format described in this chapter.[12]

The following sections describe the parts of the drug monograph, as shown in the appendices. Please note that skills in information retrieval, drug literature evaluation, professional writing, and areas covered in various other chapters must be employed when preparing a drug evaluation monograph.

SUMMARY PAGE

The first page of the monograph is essentially a summary of the most important information concerning the drug and includes a specific recommendation of the action to be taken on the product. Some P&T committees only review this first sheet; however, the remainder of the document should be prepared in order to completely evaluate a drug product and to provide a record of all that was taken into consideration. The summary and recommendation could be placed at the end of the monograph, but it is probably best to keep it on the front to make it easier to refer to during the meeting.

The format of the summary page usually begins with general institutional information. Following the name header, specific introductory information about the product is included. The generic name, trade name, and manufacturer are self-explanatory, but the classification may require some explanation. This is meant to give the readers a very quick way of classifying the agent in their head. It includes the prescription/controlled substance status, American Hospital Formulary Service (AHFS) classification, and FDA classification. It may also contain other classification schemes used by particular organizations, such as the Veteran's Administration. Managed care organizations may use more detailed drug product identification schemes, such as those established by First Data-Bank (http://www.firstdatabank.com).

The AHFS classification can be found in the *AHFS Drug Information* reference book, published by the ASHP. This classification can help the reader determine where this new agent falls in therapy. Most of the time new drugs will be evaluated for possible formulary addition before they are actually placed in that book, so it will be necessary to consult the therapeutic classification table in the front of the *AHFS Drug Information* reference book or online at http://www.ahfsdruginformation.com/class/index.aspx to decide where the product fits. The classification of similar products listed in *AHFS Drug Information* can also be checked before deciding where to categorize the new product.

The FDA classification is given to nonbiologic products during the review process and is finalized when the new drug application (NDA) is approved. This classification gives some idea of the importance of the product. The classification consists of Chemical Type classification (Table 13–1) and Therapeutic Rating classification (Table 13–2). An FDA classification of 1P (or 1A prior to 1992) would indicate a drug that was given a priority review status by the FDA. This means that the product offered a therapeutic advance over existing products in the market, may be for a new disease state, or may represent a new drug class. The FDA generally reviews these products in an expedited manner, often not requiring as many clinical trials or a lower number of patients enrolled in the trials before the drug is approved to be on the market. In contrast, a classification of 3S (or 3C prior to 1992) is probably a me-too product, meaning that it is an additional product in a class of medications that is already on the market and is similar in many ways to the other products already marketed. These products are generally reviewed by the FDA in a standard review manner and do not receive an expedited review process. Knowing and understanding the FDA classification status of a product can assist a reviewer in preparing the drug evaluation monograph in several ways. First, if the reviewer knows that the product

TABLE 13–1. FDA CLASSIFICATION BY CHEMICAL TYPE*

Type	Definition
1	New molecular entity not marketed in the United States
2	New salt, ester, or other noncovalent derivative of another drug marketed in the United States
3	New formulation or dosage form of a active ingredient marketed in the United States
4	New combination of drugs already marketed in the United States
5	New manufacturer of a drug product already marketed by another company in the United States
6	New indication for a product already marketed in the United States
7	Drug that is already legally marketed without an approved NDA • First application since 1962 for a drug marketed prior to 1938 • First application for Drug Efficacy Study Implementation (DESI)-related products that were first marketed between 1938 and 1962 without an NDA • First application for DESI-related products first marketed after 1962 without NDAs. In this case, the indications may be the same or different from the legally marketed product.
8	Over-the-counter switch

*Drugs@FDA frequently asked questions [Internet]. Washington, DC: Food and Drug Administration, [updated 2010 Jun 25; cited 2010 Oct 19]. Available from: http://www.fda.gov/Drugs/InformationOnDrugs/ucm075234.htm#chemtype_reviewclass.

TABLE 13–2. FDA CLASSIFICATIONS BY THERAPEUTIC POTENTIALᵃ

Type	Definition
P	Priority handling by FDA—before 1992 this was two categories: A – Major therapeutic gain B – Moderate therapeutic gain
S	Standard handling by FDA—before 1992 this was referred to as class C, which indicated that the product offered only a minor or no therapeutic gain
O	Orphan drug

ᵃDrugs@FDA Frequently Asked Questions [Internet]. Washington, DC: Food and Drug Administration, [updated 2010 Jun 25; cited 2010 Oct 19]. Available from: http://www.fda.gov/Drugs/InformationOnDrugs/ucm075234.htm#chemtype_reviewclass.

he or she is reviewing has an FDA classification status of 1P, the reviewer will often have to compare the product to a drug outside of the class of the product being reviewed. For example, if a new class of antibiotics were developed called ketolides, the reviewer will not have any other drugs in the class to compare the product to, and therefore he or she may need to search for studies or review articles of products that fall in other classes of antibiotics, such as the macrolides. Oftentimes in cases in which cancer chemotherapy medications are approved for a treatment that was previously treated by nondrug therapy, a surgical procedure or radiation therapy may be the best comparator for the product. In the case of products that are given an FDA classification status of 3S, the reviewer generally will be able to prepare a head-to-head comparison of the product to another product that is in the same drug class. For example, if the FDA were to approve a new hydroxymethylglutaryl-CoA (HMG-CoA) reductase inhibitor, the reviewer would normally want to compare the product to other HMG-CoA reductase inhibitors. Usually, when 3S or standard review products enter the market, if there are already a number of similar products available in the market, the manufacturer will conduct trials with the product compared to others in the same class. This product is generally then referred to as the comparator or gold standard product. The reviewer will want to discuss the comparator product and any other similar agents in the class. This can assist the decision makers in the P&T committee in reviewing the new product if they are already familiar with other products in the class.

Additional product introductory information may include the product's patent exclusivity date and/or the product's patent expiration date. This information can generally be located on the FDA's Web site at http://www.accessdata.fda.gov/scripts/cder/drugsatfda/index.cfm. A particular institution may request additional or specific information that may be relevant to include in the introductory information. It is also common to provide a list of similar agents.

The summary itself is a brief overview of the important aspects of the drug product. If there are similar products or different drugs used for the same indication, it is important to state how the drug being reviewed compares to those products. If a comparison between the agent in question and some other treatment is possible, that comparison must make up the bulk of the section, just as the comparison must be a prominent feature in every other section of the document. The summary will include information on the efficacy, safety (e.g., adverse effects and drug interactions[13]), uniqueness, cost, and other factors, such as the likelihood that patients would be more compliant with one agent or another[14,15] or how the therapy fits into published clinical guidelines. Information should be limited in this section to those items where a drug has a definite advantage/disadvantage or, if products are similar, where there would be concern about the possibility of a clinically significant difference. Items that are not clinically significant and not likely to be of concern should be left out of the summary to avoid distractions. In cases where the new drug under evaluation is indicated for a disease that has normally received nondrug treatment (e.g., surgery, radiation, and physical therapy), the drug should be compared to that standard treatment. It is worth pointing out that the summary should be just that—a summary of the material presented in the body of the document. Similar to the conclusion of a journal article, this is not the place to put new material or, for that matter, to provide citations; both of those items belong in the body.

❸ *Finally, a definite recommendation must be made based on need, therapeutics (including outcome data and the use of evidence-based clinical guidelines), side effects, cost (full pharmacoeconomic analysis, if possible), and other items specific to the particular agent (e.g., dosage forms, convenience, dosage interval, inclusion on the formulary of third-party payers, hospital antibiotic resistance patterns, and potential for causing medication errors[16]), usually in that order.*[17,18] In hospitals, a new accreditation requirement makes it necessary to list the indications for use of the drug the P&T committee is approving; this must be a specific list, although it is okay to give a blanket authorization to FDA-approved indications in general.[19] (Please note: the requirement that drugs be approved for specific indications is likely to be practical only in hospitals where there is computerized order entry and the physician has to state the indication). When making a formulary recommendation as it pertains to third-party payers, consideration should also be given to the placement of the formulary agent into a multi-tiered copayment system where the copayment varies according to the cost of the drug and/or formulary status. The member is required to pay these varying amounts of copayment out of pocket at the time the prescription is filled. In general if the drug is a generic, the placement is at the first tier, which has the lowest copayment. If the drug is a brand-name drug preferred by the health plan, it is usually placed in the second tier with a higher copayment. All other brand-name, nonpreferred drugs are usually placed in the third tier with the highest copayment. Drugs in the third tier, the nonpreferred agents, usually have therapeutic alternatives in either the first or second tier. Members are encouraged to talk to their prescribers about switching to the more cost-effective, therapeutic alternative drugs in the lower tiers.[20,21] Tier designation or formulary status may change, based on the discretion of the health plan and/or pharmacy benefits management (PBM), in the absence of significant new clinical evidence.[22] QOL information and patient preferences should be considered, if possible. Recommendations for third-party payers may also include a step therapy approach, quantity limits on the prescription, prior authorization, and coverage rule criteria in order for the drug to be covered. Third-party payers may require some drugs to have a prior authorization before being dispensed. Prior authorization is usually required for those drugs that are high cost and/or are likely to be used inappropriately. Examples include appetite suppressants and growth hormones. Prior authorization requires that the member must meet predetermined guidelines before the drug can be covered by the third-party payer. As an example, the member may be required to try an established, less expensive drug therapy first. If this drug therapy proves to be ineffective or the patient is unable to tolerate the therapy, then the third-party payer may cover a newer, more expensive therapeutically equivalent drug.[23]

Recommendations should be specific to the circumstances in the institution, hospital system, third-party payer plan, and/or other organization in which it is being considered. In some cases, an institution may have a subformulary that is available for only a specific group of patients (e.g., Medicaid).[24] Recommendations to conduct drug use evaluation on the drug (see Chapter 14), clinical guidelines to be followed (see Chapter 7), how physicians are to be educated about the new drug, and other items may also be necessary. Education may range from a simple newsletter or Web page to a specific educational program and certification required before a physician can prescribe a drug product.[25]

Some people strongly object to the presence of specific recommendations being placed in the document. This may be because they do not feel it is appropriate for them to make these decisions; however, this should not be a concern if adequate research was done in preparing the evaluation. Sometimes, people have a philosophy that an unbiased decision should be reached only through a group consensus after discussing the matter in the P&T committee meeting; however, that too should not be a concern. For one thing, the person preparing the document, who also obtains input from other appropriate individuals, is in the best situation to advance a logical recommendation. Second, without a recommendation, the discussion does not have a foundation to begin with—allowing the discussion to wander aimlessly to some conclusion that may not make optimal sense. Third, the lack of a specific recommendation allows emotion and conjecture to overcome evidence and science. The provision of a specific recommendation is one of the best opportunities for pharmacists to have a deep and wide-ranging impact on patient care, and should not be neglected.

❹ *The recommendation must be supported by objective evidence (presented in the summary).* Subjective factors that are likely to be significant from the point of view of all involved parties (i.e., physicians, pharmacists, nurses, and patients) should also be considered. Decision analysis can be used to show the best drug at the least cost (effectively, this is pharmacoeconomic analysis—see Chapter 6 for details).[26-29] Other factors may also be considered and given weight to indicate importance (e.g., multiattribute utility theory[30]). These methods may be commonly seen in managed care.[31] They look at the possible decisions and their likely outcome, allowing a decision to be made that is likely to lead to the most desirable outcome. Meta-analysis may also find a place in the decision-making process[32]; however, it seems unlikely that most individuals evaluating products for formulary addition would have the skill or time to use that method. Tentative recommendations should be discussed with appropriate physicians and any clinical pharmacists specializing in that area of therapy before the recommendation is finalized. For example, if a cardiac medication is being evaluated, one or more cardiologists should be consulted to identify their concerns and desires. That does not mean the recommendation should necessarily be changed to what a prescriber wants. If the objective evidence supports the original recommendation, that is the one that should be made; however, it is necessary to demonstrate that the prescribers' concerns were addressed.

Overall, the items most likely to be added to the formulary include those that are unique, that serve the specific population, that are most cost-effective, and, unfortunately, those with the biggest marketing drive by the marketer. Multiple ingredient products or products that are the extended-release or other variations on the patent of a product are least likely to be added in the institutional setting.[33]

The recommendation should be whatever logical conclusion is supported by the objective evidence and the needs of the health care system, including health care staff needs, distribution concerns, drug administration, and drug availability. Whenever possible, at least in the case of recommendations prepared for an institutional pharmacy, it is best to follow the ASHP guidelines for recommendations, which would place the drug in one or a combination of the following groups[4]:

- Added for uncontrolled use by the entire medical staff.
- Added for monitored use—No restrictions placed on use, but the drug will be monitored via a quality assurance study (e.g., drug usage evaluation and medication usage evaluation) to determine appropriateness of use. This is a tie-in to the institution's quality assurance/drug usage evaluation process.[34] Please note: This category does not mean that the patient is monitored, because that is necessary for every drug. It means that the quality and appropriateness of how the drug is used is monitored.
- Added with restrictions—The drug is added to the drug formulary, but there are restrictions on who may prescribe it and/or how it may be used (e.g., specific indications, certain physicians or physician groups, and certain policies to be followed).
- Conditional—Available for use by the entire medical staff for a finite period of time.
- Not added/deleted from formulary.

Note, there may be different recommendations presented for specific strengths, forms, sizes, and so forth of a drug being reviewed; however, being that specific sometimes does not result in any real benefit and may only make things more complicated to manage, with little improvement in drug therapy or decrease in costs.[35] Also, remember that, in any of the above, there is now a requirement to provide a specific list of approved indications for which the drug may be used.[3]

Most drugs should be added for uncontrolled use or, at the other extreme, not be added, simply because the three other categories cause greater work for the pharmacy or other departments. As a side point, if a recommendation to not add the drug to the formulary is approved, it is often good to require a time period before the drug can be considered again (typically 6 months) to prevent heavy political action pushing through approval of a less-than-desirable drug, just because the P&T committee gets tired of having it requested every month. Monitored use is occasionally needed if there is concern that a drug might be used in some inappropriate manner or has a great risk for adverse events. A limited drug usage evaluation would be conducted until it is evident that the drug is being appropriately used or not causing adverse events. One example where monitored use might be considered is an expensive biotechnology product that only has one normal dose, but multiple investigational doses, where it could be inappropriately prescribed without an investigational protocol. Also, a very toxic product might be monitored to see if the prescriber appropriately addresses adverse effects. As electronic drug usage evaluation becomes standard, monitoring may be used to a greater extent, but is seldom justified in systems requiring the pharmacist to manually collect data. Conditional addition to the formulary is a recommendation of last resort, simply because it is much easier to keep a drug off the formulary rather than try to delete an inappropriate drug that is being used by a prescriber. This type of approval might be used when it is very difficult to clearly determine whether an agent will benefit the institution, if available data are limited at the time of the P&T meeting. If conditional approval is given, it is absolutely necessary to specify when the P&T committee will reconsider whether the drug should be retained on the formulary.

The added-with-restrictions choice deserves more explanation. Occasionally, there are drugs that should be added to a drug formulary, but are dangerous,[36] or prone to misuse or overuse. This could include agents such as antineoplastics, thrombolytics, and third- or fourth-generation cephalosporins.[37] In such cases, it may be desirable to limit the use of the drugs in some manner.[38] For example, the antineoplastics might be limited to prescriptions from oncologists or a defined group that might include a few physicians who are not oncologists (e.g., rheumatologists using methotrexate). Specific antibiotics might be limited to either infectious disease physicians or to specific, culture-proven diagnoses (this could be done in conjunction with the new TJC requirement to approve drugs for specific indications[3]). Often antibiotics may be restricted to a specific length of therapy, after which a new order must be written or the original order will automatically be discontinued. Other restrictions could include specific floors/areas of the institution or that the physician must receive counter-detailing by the pharmacist before the drug is dispensed.[39] Relatively new methods of restriction involve formularies for managed care organizations, where there may be a cap or limitation on the price, quantity, or on how many times a patient may receive a drug (e.g., one-time use for nicotine patches to quit smoking), or how much a patient may receive at one time (e.g., 3-month supply); a medication may be subject to prior authorization or precertification before the drug can be made available to a patient; there may be step therapy or medications that have to be tried and fail before a specific agent may be available for coverage for a patient; or whether the practitioners (e.g., prescribers and pharmacists) may receive financial or other incentives to cut back on the use of specific products.[40] Whenever possible, these types of restrictions should be based on objective data, such as the FDA recommended maximum dose limitations or prescribing contraindication that can be obtained from drug usage evaluation.

Some prescribers will object to restrictions, but remember that the prescribers are given privileges to prescribe specific drugs and not rights to do anything, which allows the use of restrictions. Usually, this is not much of a problem because good prescribers realize that there is a reason for the restrictions. The real problem, however, is the desire to use this category much too often in an attempt to ensure the proper use of all drugs. Although restrictions can be effective in changing the usage of specific formulary agents,[41] every time a restricted drug is prescribed, more time and effort by the pharmacy, managed care organization, and perhaps the prescriber is required to ensure compliance with restrictions. At the very least, a policy and procedure, and probably appropriate forms or computer restriction methods, will need to be developed or adapted and be presented as part of the drug recommendation to the P&T committee. A cost-benefit analysis may also need to be conducted to ensure that the restriction is valid, meaning that it really does assist in curbing inappropriate prescribing or use of an agent. A drug use evaluation may also be performed to assess the usefulness of the restriction. If the results of the drug usage evaluation suggest an acceptable level of appropriate use, the P&T committee may need to reconsider the restriction placed on the product, or the restriction could be costing the institution more to administer and monitor than it is saving or avoiding. Therefore, unless the computer system can eliminate much of the effort, great restraint needs to be used when deciding to recommend that a drug be added to the drug formulary with restrictions. Oftentimes, adding with monitoring may be a viable alternative. A twist to the restrictions or monitoring types of approval is the use of critical or clinical pathways.[42,43] In this case, a drug may be approved for use in a particular manner for the treatment of a particular disease. These critical pathways may be established for several target populations or target diseases, where additional guidance of patient treatments can result in significant improvement in patient care and/or significant decreases in costs. Because a great deal of time is necessary to develop and manage these critical pathways, they will most likely only be seen in a few areas of any institution at any given time. The recommendation should state if the drug is to be used as part of some clinical guidelines or disease state management (DSM) program.[44] The reader is referred to Chapter 7 for further information. In managed care organizations, critical pathways may be incorporated into the use parameters of a drug through prior authorization or precertification criteria. These are specific criteria that must be met, based on clinical guidelines, current medical practices, and product prescribing information, before a product is deemed medically necessary for use.

- Although the decision to add or delete a drug from the formulary is seldom black or white, a general guideline may be helpful. If the drug is less expensive or the same price as others, and is more efficacious or safer—add it to the formulary. If the drug is more expensive without added benefit, such as increased safety or effectiveness—do not add it to the formulary (or delete it from the formulary if it is already on it). The problem comes when the drug is more expensive and also has more benefits. In that case, the careful analysis of the literature and weighing of the institution's needs must be carried out. This is the gray area that has no right answer, but the most appropriate decision must be found. This latter decision may also involve conditional or monitored use.

- Whenever a recommendation is made to add a new agent, consideration should be given to the possibility of removing agents that will no longer be necessary or, in the case of a PBM , moving the agent to a different classification for reimbursement. This whole process can be used as a way of removing extraneous agents on the formulary; however, removal of agents can be difficult if the products are frequently prescribed. (Note: It is often worthwhile to annually review a list of products that have seen little or no use in the previous year in an attempt to remove these products from the formulary.) Whether removing agents individually or through a review of an entire therapeutic class, adequate information needs to be presented to the P&T committee to show that the product is no longer necessary. The reasons for removal may include superior agent(s) on the formulary, safety, low or no use, and high cost.[45] A timetable for deleting these agents from the formulary must then be developed and the physicians must be informed when the agent will no longer be available. The TJC, in their medication management standards, stated that as a requirement for accreditation, health care organizations should review medications that are available for dispensing or administration on at least an annual basis for safety and efficacy information.[3] Many managed care organizations, health systems, and individual hospitals accomplish this via the use of the drug class review on a scheduled basis. The drug classes may be placed on a schedule for review in which all classes are reviewed over the course of the year. No matter what system an institution chooses to use to delete or review agents, the use should be monitored and follow-up is necessary to

- ensure that the formulary deletions proceed smoothly.[46] Communication of these deletions can generally appear in newsletters/e-mails/Web sites/intranet or, if one is aware of

- a particular physician who is the only one utilizing a product, personal contact may be best to communicate the change as well as to provide information to the prescriber of alternative products.

- Finally, therapeutic interchange must be considered.[47,48] If this concept is acceptable to the institution, and legal in the state, it may be appropriate that the new drug be used to substitute for a less desirable agent, or vice versa. In that case, a separate policy and procedure for handling that interchange needs to be prepared and considered at the same time. Please refer to Chapter 12 for further information on this subject. Also, there may be other policies and procedures or clinical guidelines that may need approval as part of the recommendation, including the requirement for the availability and use of concomitant drug therapy (e.g., perhaps a requirement that antiemetic therapy needs to be given prophylactically prior to the administration of a new cancer chemotherapy agent).

- All of the material on recommendations presented here may be confusing. However, to state it simply, **❺** *the most logical decision to benefit the patient and the institution should be recommended to the P&T committee.*

BODY OF THE MONOGRAPH

Many parts of the body of the monograph are self-explanatory from their names and will not be discussed in detail. Some specific points, however, do need to be made about the body. First, the body may not always be reviewed by the P&T committee and, even if presented, it may be covered only briefly. The body needs to be written as a means to compile the information for reference and further information. Importantly, it serves as a way of bringing all of the information together in a logical order for preparation of the summary. Some P&T committees will want to review the data presented in the body of the monograph, but all need to know that the clinical data were reviewed adequately. Other times, an abbreviated monograph may be presented to the P&T committee and the full monograph is presented to the chairman.

- Second, efforts must be made to ensure that the drug in question has been adequately compared to other therapies (whether drug, surgical, radiation, or something else). The person preparing a monograph must go through each section and ask, "Have comparisons been made between this drug and the appropriate alternative therapy?" If not, there should either be a good reason for the lack of comparison or some explanation must be put in the section. Sometimes, there will be no published comparison with other drugs or therapies. For example, when anistreplase was first marketed there were only comparisons to streptokinase available, but physicians wanted to know how the drug compared to alteplase. In that case, information comparing both drugs to streptokinase was used to discern how the drugs would compare to each other. Scientifically, this leaves much to be desired, but sometimes there is no choice in the matter. Other indirect methods of comparison may also be necessary. If at all possible, studies directly comparing the drug being evaluated to the standard of therapy should be used. Also, if there are outcome studies data, that can be very important to put in the evaluation, including such hard-to-quantify items as QOL.[49]

Third, every item should be addressed, even if only to state that information was not available or that it is not applicable (absorption of intravenous [IV] drugs, for example). This follows the rule that "if it was not written down, it was not done," or in this case was not reviewed.

Finally, the source of the information should be mentioned—any important statement of fact must be referenced, or must be suspected of being inaccurate. The package insert (now often available from http://www.accessdata.fda.gov/scripts/cder/drugsatfda/index.cfm for newly approved products) will serve as a basis for some of the information, particularly to define what is the FDA-approved information, but other references must be used to fill in the gaps and to back up that information. Other information can be obtained from the manufacturer, as stated in the Format for Formulary Submissions, Version 3.0, by the AMCP[1] (an example letter requesting such information is available as a part of that document), but the person preparing the monograph should also personally do an adequate literature search.

The Pharmacologic Data section is often one of the shortest. A simple one-paragraph explanation of the proposed mechanism of action and how it differs from the comparator agent(s) usually will suffice for the drug in question. More may be needed if the agent is being compared to a drug with an entirely different mechanism of action (e.g., comparing a new angiotensin-converting enzyme [ACE] inhibitor to a calcium channel blocking agent). If the agent under consideration is an antibiotic, the spectrum of activity should be discussed, which will be much longer.

The Therapeutic Indications section normally requires the most work. This section may be broken into three main subsections. The first is a brief coverage of what indications the drug has been used to treat. It is necessary to clearly indicate which uses are FDA approved, non-FDA approved but reasonably supported and likely to be seen, and those that are early in investigation. Non-FDA-approved indications or possible uses may be difficult to find for new drugs; however, a literature search may be conducted to determine if any abstracts or case reports have been published for uses that were not approved by the FDA. It is important to note these non-FDA-approved uses as they may be helpful in determining possible restrictions to place on the drug in the Recommendations section of the monograph, and it will certainly be necessary to consider which, if any, of those uses will be approved for orders in an institutional pharmacy or health system. A current example is dabigatran (Pradaxa), which is approved as an anticoagulant to manage atrial fibrillation, but because it is a new alternative to warfarin, many prescribers may want to use it for investigational uses in patients in which warfarin is indicated but not tolerated.

Doses may be different in those indications. Also, this is vital when evaluating medications in a pediatric institution or various other subpopulations. Often, non-FDA-approved uses, if found to have therapeutic benefit, will be studied further and manufacturers will submit a request to the FDA to add indications for their product. So, their consideration is important when considering possible future use of the product. They can have an impact on the use of an agent for an institution. If, at the time the reviewer is researching the product, no off-label uses are noted, it is appropriate to note that fact in the evaluation.[50]

The second subsection will explain how the product and any comparison products fit into any published clinical guidelines. This should include methods for treatment of the condition, both pharmacologic and nonpharmacologic treatment approaches. An excellent source of these guidelines is the National Guidelines Clearinghouse (http://www.guideline.gov/). The reader may also consult Chapter 7 for further information. The use of clinical guidelines is important for a P&T committee's consideration. The inclusion of clinical guidelines allows the reader to see the product's anticipated place in therapy. If the product will be a new first-line agent, an agent should often be available for second- or third-line therapy after other agents have failed. The product's place in therapy for a particular disease or indication can play an important role in budgetary decisions when determining the usage potential of a particular product. A pharmacy department may want to increase its budget in anticipation of a new drug that will see a lot of usage for a particular condition. For example, if a new vaccine was developed to help reduce or prevent Alzheimer disease, a nursing home or long-term care pharmacy provider may want to increase its medication budget to allow for a larger supply of the product to be on hand. However, if a product is for an indication that occurs in less than 1% of a specific gender of a particular ethnic group, the recommendation for the product may be to not add it to the formulary.

The third subsection will be abstracts of clinical studies supporting the various uses (see Chapter 9 for further information on how to prepare an abstract of a study). In the rare case where a product only has one use, data from several studies on that use should be reviewed in the monograph. If there are multiple uses, at least one well-conducted study for each FDA-approved or likely-to-be-seen indication is usually reviewed; more can be added, but may be redundant and provide no added benefit. If there are several similar studies, one may be covered in depth with a statement at the end of the paragraph that the use is supported by other studies, providing citations. If one well-conducted study for a use cannot be found, several less-desirable studies may be needed to provide sufficient information. Whenever possible, clinical comparison studies should be used. When reviewing newly approved drugs, it is not unusual to find that no comparison studies have been published. In that case, a simple efficacy study should be used. In some cases, it may be necessary to use a meta-analysis, simply because the disease state is rare and a typical clinical study cannot be performed. In cases where no human trials are available, unless there are extenuating circumstances, the drug should generally not be added to a drug formulary until sufficient published information is available. An example of extenuating circumstances would be when a new drug is available for a previously untreatable illness. In that case, the philosophy of "anything is better than nothing" may apply.

The information should be presented in a manner that is similar to the description of abstracts given in the appendices to Chapter 9, making sure all information is covered. When reviewing the clinical study, the person writing the drug evaluation monograph should point out strengths and weaknesses of the studies, along with applicability of the information to the patients that are covered by the drug formulary. This evaluation may be vital in arriving at the final recommendation. In some cases, the quality, quantity, and consistency of the literature are formally graded and given a score, in a way similar to the described evaluation of articles in Chapter 7 on evidence-based clinical guidelines, which is then used in the final evaluation of the product.[51]

A new item to consider in this section is pharmacogenomics. Pharmacogenomics has been defined as the individualization of drug therapy based on individuals' genetic information.[52,53] Numerous articles have been cited showing the benefits of pharmacogenomics in potentially reducing adverse drug reactions.[54-56] If the genetic makeup of patients is a factor in how the medication is to be used,[57] such clinical study information should be presented in this section. In addition, where appropriate, pharmacogenomic information should be presented in other appropriate sections, such as Pharmacokinetics, Adverse Effects, Summary, and so forth. It has been postulated that by the year 2020 pharmacogenomics may become a standard of practice for many disease states and drugs. The FDA's Web site contains a table that includes 22 genes and 71 affected drug products.[58] The National Institutes of Health (NIH) and the FDA have announced a joint venture regarding the scientific and regulatory structure needed to support advancements in personalized medicine. Pharmacogenomic information can be placed in the therapeutic information section wherever it best fits. Quite often, if any information is available, it will be under all three subsections.

In cases of pediatric drug use, studies may focus on adult literature and the data for pediatric literature may be available in abstracts or poster presentations only. The situation may be the same in other areas where there may not be a great deal of information on the use of the product under review. For these cases, a summary of evidence table, such as the one in Table 13–3, may be beneficial to include in the product review, which should cover material whether it is positive or negative. This provides a concise overview of all the available literature, as well as a rating system for the weight of evidence that is available for a particular indication in the pediatric population. It also contains a comparative summary, in a tabular formation, of the literature and evidence available in the adult population. In cases in which published clinical trials are not available, the summary of evidence table serves to provide the P&T committee with an overview of the data available (see example in Table 13–4).

TABLE 13–3. SUMMARY OF EVIDENCE TABLE

Summary of Evidence [Place drug name here]		
Literature Type	Comments	Weight of Evidence*
Pediatric Evidence		
Efficacy		

Controlled trials
  Published reports
  Abstract		

Uncontrolled trials
  Published reports
  Abstract		

Experience reports
  Published reports
  Abstracts
  Local specialist experience		

Safety		
Published		
Abstract		
Local specialists' experience		
PK/Dosing		
Published		
Abstract		
Adult Evidence		
Efficacy		
Evaluative reviews		
Controlled trials		
Other		
Summary comments:		

Ra, randomized; DB, double-blind; PC, placebo controlled; F/U, follow-up studies.
*Levels of evidence: good, fair, poor, none.

Other information may also be covered in the Therapeutics section, including quality-of-life studies.

The Bioavailability/Pharmacokinetics section is similar to what would be found in most publications, but the information may be difficult to find for some new drugs. In some cases, a new dosage form may be considered in a drug evaluation. For example, when a drug is released in IV form, its use may be entirely different from the oral form, so the P&T committee might separately consider it. A change in route, however, does not necessarily mean that elimination is significantly different in the same patient population. Therefore, oral data may be more useful than no information. Whenever possible, a table comparing the drug in question to other products may be helpful.

TABLE 13–4. EXAMPLE SUMMARY OF EVIDENCE TABLE

Summary of Evidence Zonisamide (Zonegran)		
Literature Type	Comments	Weight of Evidence*
Pediatric Evidence		
Efficacy		
Controlled trials		
Published reports	2 trials; total n = 333 subjects; generalized and partial; intellectual disability and/or refractory	Good documentation of efficacy
Abstract		
Uncontrolled trials		
Published reports	1 review/study and 2 study reports on use for infantile spasms; total n = ~109	Good documentation for efficacy; poor for safety
Abstract	(Much of the pediatric literature is from Japan, with limited availability in the English language)14 prospective, open-label Japanese trials involving 1237 subjects were reviewed in an *Epilepsia* abstract. Direct study review available for some trials.	Poor documentation Response ($\downarrow$ by > 50%): Generalized 47%, 152/325 Partial: 63%, 578/912
Experience reports		
Published reports	2 reports; total n = 4 infants with infantile spasms	Good documentation for these cases
Abstracts	8 abstracts; total n = 135; most were pediatric	Poor documentation of varied experience from multiple independent groups
Local specialists' experience	Not indicated (NI)	
Safety		
Published	10 case/case series reports published, with extensive description of adverse events	Good documentation of ADR experience reports
Abstract	2 U.S. summaries of Japanese safety experience; First: 4 data sources, n = 2574; second: 14 studies, n = 1237. Likely overlap between 2 reports	Poor documentation; rather extensive experience
Local specialists' experience	NI	
PK/Dosing		
Published	2 reports; total n = 194; children and adults	Good documentation; limited data
Abstract	~6 reports; children and/or adults; drug interaction re: effects on PKs	Poor documentation of limited data

continued

TABLE 13–4. EXAMPLE SUMMARY OF EVIDENCE TABLE (*Continued*)

	Summary of Evidence Zonisamide (Zonegran)	
Literature Type	**Comments**	**Weight of Evidence***
Evaluative reviews	Cochrane Review of adjunctive use for refractory partial epilepsy in 3 Ra studies; total n = 499; 12-wk duration An assessment of Japanese experience was compared against clinical guidelines for AED use (established by the International League Against Epilepsy); n = 1008 (ped n = 403)	Reviewer conclusions: Effective as adjunctive treatment for refractory partial seizures. Authors concluded that zonisamide was effective against both partial and refractory generalized seizures.
Controlled trials	Deferred review; FDA approved for adjunctive therapy of partial seizures in adults	Good documentation, based on FDA approval
Other		
Summary Comments:	Extensive, independent pediatric reports of efficacy in a variety of seizure types, both published and abstracts; demonstrated benefit in refractory seizure types, including infantile spasms; substantial published experience literature on a variety of adverse events, generally documenting reversibility with dosage adjustment or discontinuation. Limitations in evaluation: multiple publications representing the same subjects.	

Ra, randomized; DB, double-blind; PC, placebo controlled; F/U, follow-up studies.
*Levels of evidence: good, fair, poor, none.

The Dosage Form section is a good place to point out the limitations in dosage forms available for some drugs. For example, perhaps the drug in question is available only as an oral solid, but the agent it is compared to is available in oral solid, oral liquid, and injectable forms, which could be an advantage to the second agent. This section can also be used to discuss unusual preparation directions or pointing out which product would be easier, quicker, and less expensive to prepare. Additionally, this section should state if the product has any limitations on access (i.e., the product is only available from a registry or available to select facilities), distribution, supply limitations, or possible anticipated shortages.[59] This section can also cover the handling of medications that have a high risk for serious injury if misused. In addition, the Dosage Form section should also address special provisions for the procurement, storage, ordering, dispensing, and monitoring of these high-risk agents. Medication error problems in this area are related to professional practice procedures describing product labeling and packaging, nomenclature, compounding and dispensing, education, administration, monitoring, and use. Specific recommendations are available regarding antineoplastic agents that address health care professionals, organizations, and patients.[60]

A problem often develops in presenting the information in the Known Adverse Effects/Toxicities section. Quite simply, some drugs have so many adverse effects listed that pages could be written. What should be done is to concentrate on the serious and/or common adverse effects for both the specific drug and the drug class. Whenever possible, incidence and severity should be included. An incidence comparison table listing the agent under consideration and other similar agents may be an efficient and informative method to show the material. If there are many rare, minor adverse effects, a statement to that effect can be listed at the end of the discussion. Conversely, other agents may have very little information available on adverse effects, simply because they are too new. In that case, it may be necessary to discuss adverse effects common to that class of agent, making it clear that they have not yet been seen with the new drug, but are possible. The new agent should be compared to other agents used for the same indication to determine whether there are any advantages. Keep in mind that these tables can be somewhat deceiving because older agents may have 20 years of side-effect reports, whereas a number of adverse effects of the new agent may not yet be discovered.

Also, TJC now requires patient safety information to be addressed in all monographs, including sentinel event advisories.[3] It has been recommended that a list of possible safety problems be compiled. This may include concerns in such areas as ordering, transcribing, order entry, storage, order verification, compounding, dispensing, administration, and monitoring.[61] It may be good in this section to consider Risk Evaluation and Mitigation Strategies (REMS) information from the FDA in this section.[62] Some drugs may be added to the formulary simply because of improved patient safety, even though that comes at an increased cost. Besides the package labeling, other sources of this information can be found at

- Institute for Safe Medication Practices: http://www.ismp.org
- MedWatch: http://www.fda.gov/medwatch
- FDA Patient Safety News: http://www.accessdata.fda.gov/scripts/cdrh/cfdocs/psn
- United States Pharmacopeia Patient Safety Program: http://www.usp.org/products/patientSafety.html

Once the list of possible safety concerns has been compiled, even a simple tally of the number of items can be helpful, but it also may be that specific items may cause an overriding concern. In response, P&T committees are implementing safety-focused drug monographs, which include information regarding medication errors.[63] In response to the public's concern about drug safety, the FDA has created a special advisory board to advise them.[64]

The Patient Monitoring Guidelines and Patient Information sections listed are items not suggested by ASHP. These sections were originally added for use in the ambulatory environment, although they can be quite informative in any practice area. The Patient Information section complies with the Omnibus Budget Reconciliation Act (OBRA) 1990 standards for prospective drug utilization review (DUR).

The final section to be discussed is the cost comparison, where the product being reviewed is compared in price to other similar products. Typically, three or four medications (possibly including both trade name and generic products) are compared, although sometimes it is necessary to compare a dozen or more products or dosage forms. Preferably, a pharmacoeconomic analysis should be prepared[65] (see Chapter 6), because the seemingly more expensive agent may turn out to be less expensive, overall, as it decreases the length of hospitalization, degree of monitoring, or number of adverse events that would otherwise occur.[66] Such an analysis is considered to be important by the majority of institutions[67] and managed care organizations.[68] It may, however, take a considerable amount of time to prepare, and sometimes attendees will challenge the assumptions made in preparing the analysis.[69] Sometimes it may even be necessary to provide a spreadsheet, which may be used during the meeting using a computer projector, to show what effect changes in assumptions may have on the economic analysis. In the case of reports prepared in the method of the AMCP guidelines, the information in this section may provide detailed abstracts of pharmacoeconomic studies, in a manner similar to that seen for clinical studies in the Therapeutics section.[1]

Often, a full pharmacoeconomic review is not practical because of lack of time or expertise, although most large hospitals do report doing a formal economic analysis of some kind for each drug reviewed for possible formulary addition.[70] With particularly expensive products, a comprehensive pharmacoeconomic analysis becomes much more necessary.[71,72] Even when a full pharmacoeconomic analysis is not practical, any pertinent information that could be used in a full analysis should be included. After all, it sometimes can be determined that the most expensive (per dose) drug product may actually be much cheaper in the long run because of increased or faster efficacy, decreased incidence of adverse effects, or lower monitoring costs.

In some cases, a simple price comparison can be prepared using just the cost of the drugs and the frequency of administration. Such a price comparison must consider that the patient may be getting medications both within an institution and after returning home, because institutional pharmacies may get considerable discounts. Therefore, both the institution's cost for the medication and the average wholesale price (AWP) price should be considered. Some medications are extremely inexpensive to the institution, making it tempting to include those agents on the formulary instead of similar therapeutic agents; however, if the AWP price is quite high, the patient may not be able to afford the product in the community, which could quickly lead to readmission to the hospital when the patient's disease is no longer being treated. In those cases, it may not be a good product to carry on the formulary. Also, the differences in package sizes and frequency of administration must be considered. In most cases, products can be compared on the cost of a typical day's therapy at a relatively normal dose; however, in some cases, a different approach may be necessary. For example, an antineoplastic agent may need to be compared with other agents based on a per-cycle or per-cost of therapeutic regimen basis. Another example that resulted in unusual cost comparisons in the past was Norplant (an implantable contraceptive agent that was effective for 5 years). The cost of both the drug and the implantation procedure needed to be compared to a 5-year supply of other contraceptive agents. In cases like this, over a period of years, it may be necessary to include calculations of inflation or other factors likely to change over the time period.[73] Other costs should also be considered when possible, such as drug preparation costs, administration costs, laboratory tests, monitoring requirements, and changes of length of stay/therapy—after all, it is not a savings overall if costs are simply shifted from the pharmacy (i.e., drug price) to the laboratory (i.e., monitoring costs).[74] In the future, theranostics (also known as pharmacodiagnostics—which is defined as the analysis of a patient's genome in order to personalize medical treatment using pharmacogenomics) will be a substantial cost that needs to be included in the analysis.[75] Some pharmacies even include such items as the cost to order and hold the drug, and the cost of preparing the evaluation of the drug for the P&T committee.[76] Also, it is becoming more common to take into account some items that are more difficult to assess, such as the probability and cost of therapeutic failure in comparison to other similar agents, impact of specific drug therapy on other health care costs (a drug may be cheaper, but require an increase in the cost of other nondrug therapy for the patient), and the cost of adverse drug effects.[77] Because these items may depend on the characteristics of the patients (e.g., age, socioeconomic status, and education level), the figures used are necessarily going to be uncertain. In some cases, however, they will be very important in the final formulary decisions; a drug that at first glance seems more expensive may be found to actually cost the institution less in the end.[66] Also, it is necessary to consider nondrug therapy (e.g., surgery, radiation therapy, and physical therapy) in the comparison, when they are legitimate alternatives to drug therapy. Overall, the goal is to ensure that the comparison makes sense and takes into consideration all of the relevant economic factors. ❻ *While some think that cost is emphasized too much in formulary decisions, it is still an extremely important item.* Some drugs cost thousands of dollars per dose, and that can quickly deplete a pharmacy department's budget and significantly affect the economic status of an institution.

Conclusion

❼ *Preparation of a drug evaluation monograph requires a great amount of time and effort, using many of the skills discussed throughout this text to obtain, evaluate, collate, and provide information. However, the value of having all of the issues evaluated and discussed can be invaluable in providing quality care.*

Case Study 13–1

You are a recent graduate who just completed a PGY1 residency. You have accepted a position at a local hospital medical center as a clinical pharmacist. One of your first assignments is to prepare and present a medication monograph on a new oral direct thrombin inhibitor that was just approved by the FDA. You will have 10 minutes to present at the next Pharmacy and Therapeutics Committee meeting that will be held next week. The only piece of information that you are given is the nonformulary request to add this drug to formulary. All medications are reviewed for the outpatient pharmacy as well.

1. Having reviewed the nonformulary request, what are the steps to add this drug to formulary?
2. What are the essential elements of a medication monograph?
3. What sources of information do you need to develop a complete, evidence-based medication monograph?

Case Study 13–2

Following the development of the drug evaluation monograph, you are then asked to prepare a concise, high-level summary page of this medication monograph.

1. What are the elements of a high-level summary page?
2. You are planning to use this monograph for the inpatient as well as the outpatient pharmacies. What information should be included as it relates to the outpatient dispensing of this medication?
3. What are the different types of formulary status recommendations and how do they differ?

Acknowledgment

Donald R. Fagan, PharmD, and Debra L. Lee, PharmD, from Creighton University Medical Center are acknowledged for their assistance in preparing this chapter.

Self-Assessment Questions

1. Medications or medication classes considered for a medication formulary should be objectively assessed based on:
   a. Scientific information
   b. Anecdotal prescriber experience
   c. Manufacturer information
   d. All of the above

2. Pharmacists have a unique role in the preparation of a medication monograph in that:
   a. Medications are viewed from a whole and macroeconomic view.
   b. Medications are viewed based on the package insert data.
   c. Medications are viewed based on pharmaceutical representative information.
   d. Medications are viewed from a microeconomic view.

3. Manufacturers of alternative/complementary medicines cannot make specific health claims because these products are considered:
   a. Medications
   b. Dietary supplements
   c. Orphan medications

4. The summary page of a medication monograph:
   a. Provides a summary of the most important information concerning the medication
   b. Completely evaluates a medication product
   c. Provides a record of all that was taken into consideration
   d. Includes items that are not clinically significant

5. Included on the summary page is a definite recommendation primarily based upon:
   a. Objective outcome data and the use of evidence-based clinical guidelines
   b. Cost
   c. Anecdotal prescriber experience
   d. Other items specific to the particular agent

6. Medications can be removed from formulary due to:
   a. Safety
   b. Cost
   c. No use
   d. All of the above

7. The body of the monograph does which of the following?
   a. Brings all the information together in a logical order
   b. Adequately compares the medication to other therapies
   c. Only addresses certain items
   d. Includes the source of the information
   e. a and b

8. Patient safety information is not considered essential by The Joint Commission and is not a required part of the monograph.
   a. True
   b. False

9. Hospitals and health systems review an entire class of medications on a scheduled basis, which must be at least annually according to The Joint Commission.
   a. True
   b. False

10. A medication monograph provides a tool for the pharmacy to:
    a. Guide the rational development of a medication formulary.
    b. Provide a full, fair, and balanced review of a medication.
    c. View medications from a whole and macroeconomic view.
    d. All the above.

11. Pharmacogenomics is the study of:
    a. Medication indication and off-label use
    b. Medication cost
    c. Medication tier placement
    d. Individualized drug therapy based on an individual's genetic makeup

12. Pharmacoeconomics is primarily the study of:
    a. Medication cost
    b. Medication indications
    c. Medication adherence
    d. All of the above

13. The therapeutic indications section in the body of the monograph primarily contains:

   a. Indications for use for both FDA and non-FDA-approved products as well as those in early investigation

   b. Product and comparison products

   c. Abstracts of clinical studies supporting the various uses

   d. Pharmacogenomic information

14. When making formulary recommendations as it pertains to third-party payers, consideration should be given to the placement of the formulary agent into a multi-tiered copayment system where the copayment varies according to the cost of the drug and/or formulary status.

   a. True

   b. False

15. Future medication monographs may be expected to include clinical outcomes, continuous quality assurance information, pharmacogenomics, and QOL issues.

   a. True

   b. False

REFERENCES

1. Format for formulary submissions, version 3.0. Alexandria (VA): Academy of Managed Care Pharmacy; 2009.

2. Wade WE, Spruill WJ, Taylor AT, Longe RL, Hawkins DW. The expanding role of pharmacy and therapeutics committees. The 1990s and beyond. PharmacoEconomics. 1996; 10(2):123-8.

3. CAMH Comprehensive Accreditation Manual for Hospitals: The Official Handbook. Oakbrook Terrace (IL): The Joint Commission; 2010.

4. ASHP technical assistance bulletin on the evaluation of drugs for formularies. Am J Hosp Pharm. 1991;48:791-3.

5. Majercik PL, May JR, Longe RL, Johnson MH. Evaluation of pharmacy and therapeutics committee drug evaluation reports. Am J Hosp Pharm. 1985;42:1073-6.

6. Academy of Managed Care Pharmacy. Therapeutic interchange. 2003 Feb. [cited 2010 Nov 5]: [2 p.]. Available from: http://www.amcp.org/amcp.ark?p=AA46FF1F.

7. Australian Regulatory Guidelines for Prescription Medicines. Woden, Australia: Australian Government, Department of Health and Ageing, Therapeutic Goods Administration; 2004.

8. Ontario Guidelines for Drug Submission and Evaluation. Toronto: Ministry of Health and Long-Term Care; 2000.

9. Technology appraisal process guides [Internet]. London: National Institute for Clinical Excellence; 2010. [cited 2010 Nov 5]. Available from: http://www.nice.org.uk/aboutnice/howwework/devnicetech/technologyappraisalprocessguides/technology_appraisal_process_guides.jsp.

10. Groves KE, Fanagan PS, MacKinnon NJ. Why physicians start or stop prescribing a drug: literature review and formulary implications. Formulary. 2002;37(4):186-8, 190-4.

11. Strite S, Stuart ME, Urban S. Process steps and suggestions for creating drug monographs and drug class reviews in an evidence-based formulary system. Formulary. 2008;43: 135-6, 139-40, 142, 144-5.

12. Cohen KR, Cerone P, Ruggiero R. Complementary/alternative medicine use: responsibilities and implications for pharmacy services. P&T. 2002;27(9):440-6.

13. Chan L-N. Consider potential for drug interactions during formulary review. Am J Health-Syst Pharm. 2000;57:391.

14. Feldman JA, DeTullio PL. Medication noncompliance: an issue to consider in the drug selection process. Hosp Formul. 1994;29:204-11.

15. Sesin GP. Therapeutic decision-making: a model for formulary evaluation. Drug Intell Clin Pharm. 1986;20:581-3.

16. Cohen MR. Adding drugs to the formulary: your work is never done. Hosp Pharm. 1999;34:828.

17. Hedblom EC. Pharmacoeconomic and outcomes data in the managed care formulary decision-making process. P&T. 1995;20:462-4, 468, 471-3.

18. Klink B. Formulary influences. Drug Top. 1998;142(20):72.

19. Rich DS. Pharmacies' noncompliance with 2009 Joint Commission hospital accreditation requirements. Am J Health-Syst Pharm. 2009;66:e27-30.

20. Abourjaily P, Kross J, Gouveia WA. Initiatives to control drug costs associated with an independent physician association. Am J Health-Syst Pharm. 2003;60:269-72.

21. Gleason PP, Gunderson BW, Gericke KR. Are incentive-based formularies inversely associated with drug utilization in managed care? Ann Pharmacother. 2005;39:339-45.

22. Reissman D. Issues in drug benefit management. Drug Benefit Trends. 2004;Dec:598-9.

23. Sroka CJ. CRS Report for Congress: Pharmacy Benefit Managers. Washington, DC: Library of Congress; 2000.

24. Tyler LS, Cole SW, May JR, Millares M, Valentino MA, Vermeulen LC Jr, et al. ASHP guidelines on the pharmacy and therapeutics committee and the formulary system. Am J Health-Syst Pharm. 2008;65:1272-83.

25. Dedrick S, Kessler JM. Formulary evaluation teams: Duke University Medical Center's approach to P&T committee reorganization. Formulary. 1999;34:47-51.

26. Kresel JJ, Hutchings HC, MacKay DN, Weinstein MC, Read JL, Taylor-Halvorsen K, et al. Application of decision analysis to drug selection for formulary addition. Hosp Formul. 1987;22:658-76.

27. Szymusiak-Mutnick B, Mutnick AH. Application of decision analysis in antibiotic formulary choices. J Pharm Technol. 1994;10:23-6.

28. Basskin L. How to use decision analysis to solve pharmacoeconomic problems. Formulary. 1997;32:619-28.

29. Kessler JM. Decision analysis in the formulary process. Am J Health-Syst Pharm. 1997;54 (Suppl 1):S5-S8.

30. Schumacher GE. Multiattribute evaluation in formulary decision-making as applied to calcium-channel blockers. Am J Hosp Pharm. 1991;48:301-8.

31. Barner JC, Thomas J III. Tools, information sources, and methods used in deciding on drug availability in HMOs. Am J Health-Syst Pharm. 1998;55:50-6.

32. Gibaldi M. Meta-analysis. A review of its place in therapeutic decision-making. Drugs. 1993;46:805-18.

33. Gannon K. Uniqueness of a drug key to formulary inclusion. Hosp Pharm Rep. 1996;10:27.

34. Chase P, Bell J, Smith P, Fallik A. Redesign of the P&T committee around continuous quality improvement principles. P&T. 1995;20(1):25-6, 29-30, 32, 34, 37-8, 40.

35. Ain KB, Pucino F, Csako G, Wesley RA, Drass JA, Clark C. Effects of restricting levothyroxine dosage strength availability. Pharmacotherapy. 1996;16(6):1103-10.

36. Limit potential dangers by restricting problem drugs on formulary. Drug Util Rev. 1997;13(4):49-51.

37. Anassi EO, Ericsson C, Lal L, McCants E, Stewart K, Moseley C. Using a pharmaceutical restriction program to control antibiotic use. Formulary. 1995;30:711-4.

38. Berndt EM. Drug expenditures. A medical center's experience with antibiotic cost-saving measures. Drug Benefit Trends. 1997;9:32-6.

39. McCloskey WW, Johnson PN, Jeffrey LP. Cephalosporin-use restrictions in teaching hospitals. Am J Hosp Pharm. 1984;41:2359-62.

40. Goldberg RB. Managing the pharmacy benefit: the formulary system. J Manag Care Pharm. 1997;3(5):565-73.

41. Hayman JN, Sbravati EC. Controlling cephalosporin and aminoglycoside costs through pharmacy and therapeutics committee restrictions. Am J Hosp Pharm. 1985;42:1343-7.

42. McCaffrey S, Nightingale CH. The evolving health care marketplace. How to develop critical paths and prepare for other formulary management changes. Hosp Formul. 1994;29:628-35.

43. Dana WJ, McWhinney B. Managing high cost and biotech drugs: two institutions' perspectives. Hosp Formul. 1994;29:638-45.

44. Armstrong EP. Disease state management and its influence on health systems today. Drug Benefit Trends. 1996;8:18-20, 25, 29.

45. Kelly WN, Rucker TD. Considerations in deciding which drugs should be in a formulary. J Pharm Pract. 1994;VII(2):51-7.

46. Lemay AP, Salzer LB, Visconti JA, Latiolais CJ. Strategies for deleting popular drugs from a hospital formulary. Am J Hosp Pharm. 1981;38:506-10.

47. Boesch D. Formularies and therapeutic substitution: gaining ground in long-term care. Consult Pharm. 1994;9:284-97.

48. Therapeutic Interchange [Internet]. Alexandria (VA): Academy of Managed Care Pharmacy; 2003 Feb [cited 2010 Nov 5]: [2 p.]. Available from: http://www.amcp.org/amcp.ark?p=AA46FF1F.

49. Lewis BE, Fish L. Drug approvals. Formulary decisions in managed care: the role of quality of life. Drug Benefit Trends. 1997;9:41-7.

50. ASHP statement on the use of medications for unlabeled uses. Am J Hosp Pharm. 1992;49:2006-8.

51. Corman SL, Skledar SJ, Culley CM. Evaluation of conflicting literature and application to formulary decisions. Am J Health-Syst Pharm. 2007 Jan 15;64:182-5.

52. Feero WG, Guttmacher AE, Collins FS. Genomic medicine—an updated primer. N Engl J Med. 2010;362:2001-11.

53. Hamburg MA, Collins FS. The path to personalized medicine. N Engl J Med. 2010;363:1092.

54. Philips KA, Veensta DL, Oren E, Lee JK, Sadee W. Potential role of pharmacogenomics in reducing adverse drug reactions: a systemic review. JAMA. 2001;286:2270-9.

55. Meyer UA. Pharmacogenetics and adverse drug reactions. Lancet. 2000;356(9242):1667-71.

56. Empey PE. Genetic predisposition to adverse drug reaction in the intensive care unit. Crit Care Med. 2010;38(6):S106-S116.

57. Morrow TJ. Implications of pharmacogenomics in the current and future treatment of asthma. J Managed Care Pharm. 2007;13(6):497-505.

58. U.S. Food and Drug Administration. Table of valid genomic biomarkers in the context of approved drug labels. August 18, 2009 [cited 2010 Aug 4]. Available from: http://www.fda.gov/Drugs/ScienceResearch/ResearchAreas/Pharmacogenetics/ucm083378.htm.

59. Leady MA, Adams AL, Stumpf JL, Sweet BV. Drug shortages: an approach to managing the latest crisis. Hosp Pharm. 2003;38:748-52.

60. ASHP guidelines on preventing medication errors with antineoplastic agents. Am J Health-Syst Pharm. 2002;59:1648-68.

61. Pick AM, Massoomi F, Neff WJ, Danekas PI, Stoysich AM. A safety assessment tool for formulary candidates. Am J Health-Syst Pharm. 2006;63:1269-72.

62. Milenkovich N. Ready or not, here come the REMS. Drug Top. 2009 Oct:65.

63. Murri NA, Somani S, University HealthSystem Consortium Pharmacy Council Medication Management/Quality Improvement Committee. Implementation of safety-focused pharmacy and therapeutics monographs: a new University HealthSystem Consortium template designed to minimize medication misadventures. Hosp Pharm. 2004;39(7):653-60.

64. Harris G. FDA to create advisory board on drug safety. New York Times. February 16, 2005 [cited 2005 Feb 16]: [about 3 p.]. Available from: http://query.nytimes.com/gst/abstract.html? res=F40916FF385E0C758DDDAB0894DD404482&incamp=archive:search.

65. Sanchez LA. Pharmacoeconomics and formulary decision-making. PharmacoEconomics. 1996;9(Suppl 1):16-25.

66. Heiligenstein JH. Reformulating our formularies to reflect real-world outcomes. Drug Benefit Trends. 1996;8:35, 42.

67. Odedina FI, Sullivan J, Nash R, Clemmons CD. Use of pharmacoeconomic data in making hospital formulary decisions. Am J Health-Syst Pharm. 2002;59:1441-4.

68. Suh D-C, Okpara JRN, Agnese WB, Toscani M. Application of pharmacoeconomics to formulary decision making in managed care organizations. Am J Manage Care. 2002;8(2):161-9.

69. McCain J. System helps P&T committees get pharmacoeconomic data they need. Managed Care [Internet]. April 2001 [cited 2007 Jul 17]: [14 p.]. Available from: http://www.managed-caremag.com/archives/0104/0104.amcp.html.

70. Mannebach MA, Ascione FJ, Gaither CA, Bagozzi RP, Cohen IA, Ryan ML. Activities, functions, and structure of pharmacy and therapeutics committees in large teaching hospitals. Am J Health-Syst Pharm. 1999;56:622-8.

71. Shepard MD, Salzman RD. The formulary decision-making process in a health maintenance organisation setting. PharmacoEconomics. 1994;5:29-38.

72. Johnson JA, Bootman JL. Pharmacoeconomic analysis in formulary decisions: an international perspective. Am J Hosp Pharm. 1994;51:2593-8.

73. Basskin L. Discounting in pharmacoeconomic analyses: when and how to do it. Formulary. 1996;31:1217-27.

74. Macklin R. Understanding formularies. Drug Store News Pharmacist. 1995;5:82-8.

75. Vogenberg FR, Barash CI, Pursel M. Personalized medicine. Part 1: Evolution and development into theranostics. P&T. 2010 Oct;35(1):560-2,565-7.

76. Myers CE, Pierpaoli P, Smith MA. Measurement of formulary inclusion costs. Hosp Formul. 1981;16:951-3, 957-8, 967-8, 970-1, 975-6.

77. Crane VS, Gonzalez ER, Hull BL. How to develop a proactive formulary system. Hosp Formul. 1994;29:700-10.

Chapter Fourteen

Quality Improvement and the Medication Use Process

Mark A. Ninno • Sharon Davis Ninno

Learning Objectives

After completing this chapter, the reader will be able to

- Explain the evolution of quality management in industry and health care.
- Describe the processes used to assess and improve quality.
- Define the role of the pharmacist in modern health care quality improvement initiatives.
- Explain the role of The Joint Commission in health care quality.
- Describe the basic principles behind continuous quality improvement, total quality management, and Six Sigma quality.
- Describe the role of medication use evaluation as a component of an organization's quality improvement program.
- Outline the general process of medication use evaluation.
- Describe the role of pharmacists and other health professionals in the medication use evaluation process.
- Discuss quality improvement techniques applied in drug information practice.

Key Concepts

1 Increasing competition in the health care marketplace, decreasing dollars with which to treat patients, and greater access to the availability of medical information through media outlets and the Internet have served to increase the public's awareness about the need to be more actively involved in the management of their health. As a result, there is an increasing demand for quality health care services at more affordable costs.

2 In more recent years, focus has shifted away from quality assurance and quality control to embrace a different discipline in the search for quality—total quality management (TQM). TQM takes a more investigative approach to identifying barriers to quality in the processes of providing goods or services.

3 Six Sigma is a data-driven, statistical process designed to eliminate defects and improve quality to a level of near perfection (99.99966% defect-free or six sigma).

4 Problems associated with quality in health care fall into one of three categories: overuse, underuse, and misuse. Overuse occurs when a service is provided but is not needed, and thus the risk of harm from that service outweighs the potential benefit. Underuse results when a needed service is unavailable or not provided. Misuse occurs when the correct service is provided so poorly that the full benefit is not seen.

5 The application of quality management techniques in health care is not very different than in other industries. Strong leadership, an open mind, willingness to put past differences or processes behind, and most importantly, a willingness to improve the existing system are required to ensure that quality goals are met.

6 Medication use evaluation (MUE) is often part of an organization's overall performance improvement program that uses definitions of safe and effective use of medications to assess components of the medication use process.

7 MUEs must reflect the scope of care provided by the organization and focus on high-volume, high-risk, or problem-prone medication-related processes.

8 Criteria used to conduct MUEs should be based on current standards of practice and supported by current literature. A multidisciplinary team should develop the criteria, and participation should be determined by the nature of the process under evaluation.

9 When the data collected as part of the MUE indicate that actual care provided to patients does not meet the standard of performance outlined within the criteria, intervention is necessary to improve performance.

Quality Improvement

"What is quality health care?" Answering this question has likely consumed more health care resources and public policy debate in the last two decades than any other health care–related topic. Health care providers, insurance payers, politicians, regulatory agencies, lawyers, and patients have all weighed in on what quality means to them. Despite the increased dialogue, policy, and regulation designed to improve the quality of the American health care system, few can agree on exactly how quality health care should be identified and measured. Much of the confusion relates to the fact that Americans have never really had to assess and quantify the quality of the health care they received. For many years, it was accepted that the quality of the American health care system was second to none, largely resulting from the relative ease of access to health care compared to other industrialized nations; the high regard for medical professionals, their training, and the institutions that trained them; and the significant advances in medical technologies and research generated in the United States each year. As a result, the consumer public was rather passive in their belief that the standard of health care in the United States was exceptionally high.[1,2] However, an undercurrent of question and doubt began to challenge these perceptions as access to health care became increasingly limited, if not entirely eliminated, for certain portions of the U.S. population, and an increasing number of reports of severe failures in the health care system began to surface. The quality of our health care system came into question as Americans observed, with growing alarm, nightly news reports of severe medication and medical errors resulting in disastrous consequences; recalls and black box warnings for approved medications they thought were safe; and the growing number of legal actions between patients, health care providers, hospitals, manufacturers, and others.

The release of the first Institute of Medicine report in 1999, *To Err Is Human*, altered many perceptions about not only the quality but the safety of the U.S. health care system.[3] (See Chapter 16 for more information on medication safety.) In fact, it was recognized that, similar to other high-risk industries, safety is the first and most basic marker of quality in the health care industry. Many Americans were shocked and dismayed that the health care industry they had trusted for so long had done so little over the years to define, monitor, and improve performance on even the most fundamental of quality markers—patient safety. The result of these revelations was an increasing array of regulatory and legal standards designed to push the health care industry to meet the quality standards it was not able, or willing, to do on its own. As such, the measurement of quality has shifted from a data-poor environment two decades ago, when few health care institutions monitored quality, to a data-rich environment, where quality indicators for a local hospital or physician can be accessed via a home computer. Despite this new-found wealth of quality data, health care consumers are still struggling to define quality, as the standard of care still varies significantly from state to state, institution to institution, practitioner to practitioner, and even patient to patient. ❶ *Increasing competition in the health care marketplace, decreasing dollars with which to treat patients, and greater access to the availability of medical information through media outlets and the Internet have served to increase the public's awareness about the need to be more actively involved in the management of their health. As a result, there is an increasing demand for quality health care services at more affordable costs.*[4] This demand is coming from all sectors of the community including health care providers, institutions, third-party payers, the government, and, most importantly, the consumer. More and more consumers are seeking information to compare health care providers and payers, and are shopping for health care services. Similarly, employers are seeking the best health care coverage for their employees while trying to reduce the costs associated with expanding medical technology. Balanced against all of these factors is an effort to ensure that all individuals, regardless of payer status, receive the same level, quality, and access to health care.

For the profession of pharmacy, the focus on quality of health care comes as both a great opportunity and a challenge. While in the past the assessment of quality was the domain of only a few pharmacy practitioners, today it has become an integral part of every pharmacy practice setting.[5] The use of quality management techniques in assessing therapy and influencing outcomes blends well with pharmacy's initiative to shed its traditional role in medication dispensing and become more involved in the provision of patient-focused care; however, determining "what is quality?" and "how is it measured?" has provided many hurdles in achieving this goal. Complicating matters are the numerous national, state, local, and private organizations, and regulatory bodies that each defines quality in their own terms. As a result, a survey that asks the question, "What is quality health care?" may be greeted with as many different responses as responders.

DEFINING QUALITY

The term quality has meant different things to different groups for as long as the term has been around. Compounding the confusion in defining quality has been the multitude of terms used to express the process of assessing quality in providing goods or services. Terms such as quality control, quality assurance, quality improvement, continuous quality improvement (CQI), total quality management (TQM), Six Sigma, and performance improvement have all been used, sometimes interchangeably, to define the process of determining and improving quality. In its most basic definition, quality is a degree or grade of excellence and can be applied to goods, services, processes, or even people.[6] Measures of quality can be applied to any service or good, but is most often associated with a physical product such as an automobile, computer, appliances, or other consumer products. Often, the association of quality is made with the service of a product and not the product itself (e.g., people may not be as aware of the quality in the construction of a dishwasher as they are the dishwasher repair service). More often, quality is associated with intangible items, such as friendliness or timeliness (e.g., people may not be as aware of the quality of the construction of the dishwasher or the repair service as they are of the friendliness of the person performing the repair).

Quality measures have been used for years in the industrial sector. Some quality assurance programs can be traced to J.C. Penney Company, Inc. as far back as 1913.[7] Walter Shewart is often viewed as the founding father of the American quality improvement initiative. Shewart and others at Bell Laboratories during World War II used quality improvement techniques in its zero-defect program.[8,9] Shewart, a statistician, recognized that quality could be best improved by preventing the defects that can be expected with any process. In order to prevent defects, one had to first identify them through a continuous analysis of data produced by the process. By continually reviewing these data, variations and defects can be anticipated and prevented, thus improving quality.[1,9] Shewart developed the simple model of Plan-Do-Check-Act (PDCA)—a model frequently employed in quality management today. This view of quality control as a statistical process is at the heart of modern quality management initiatives. The first real use of quality assurance techniques in large-scale industry can be traced back to the Japanese in the 1950s.[8,9] In an effort to rebuild their economy after World War II, the Japanese began to compete in markets traditionally dominated by the United States and Western Europe, such as automobile and electronics manufacturing. The Japanese had a limited infrastructure and few resources with which to begin manufacturing goods. Gaining insight from early quality pioneers, such as Deming and Juran, the Japanese employed quality improvement techniques to manufacturing. The Japanese recognized that to be competitive they needed to prevent defects because they did not have the resources to correct them after they had occurred, as was the practice in American manufacturing.[9] Early Japanese automobiles had a notorious reputation for being inferior in design and construction, and were held with little regard in the marketplace. Utilizing quality management techniques outlined by Shewart and others, the Japanese soon began to revolutionize the automotive industry with higher quality cars at competitive prices, much to the chagrin of many U.S. automobile manufacturers. The application of similar quality techniques ultimately led to Japanese dominance in other industrial fields.[8]

Having access to quality management techniques has not always proven to be the key to successful quality improvement. Many U.S. industries started to adopt quality assurance techniques when faced with stiff competition from abroad.[2,8] Unfortunately, many of these quality programs focused on measures of productivity and financial profitability without much regard to the final product or customer satisfaction. In this environment, individuals involved in the production of a good or service focused on identifying and changing the work habits of problematic departments or workers in an effort to improve quality. This practice is known as quality assurance or quality control and differs in practice from quality improvement. In most situations, quality assurance is retroactive, seeking to identify problems and those responsible for allowing problems to occur.[1,10] Additionally, quality assurance tends to focus only on the quality of a particular component within the process, but not the entire process. For example, individuals building the engine of a car may focus only on production of the engine, but not be empowered or feel responsibility for other aspects of the production of the vehicle. As a result, production falls into a silo without regard for the quality of the overall product. Silo production or processes occur when individuals within the process focus only on their specific role or function without a larger understanding or regard for the total product, process, and result. An example would be the pharmacist who focuses only on the preparation of an intravenous (IV) product, but does not take the steps needed to properly label the medication so that the nurse will understand how to administer the drug. Although the product was prepared correctly, the likelihood of a successful outcome is reduced because the pharmacist is not considering others involved in the medication use process. This failure to have ownership for the entire process leads to an environment of blame and conflict, which ultimately impacts the overall quality of the end product. Moreover, conflict within the production process most often results in one silo taking the role as authoritarian. In production industries, this authoritarian role usually falls to management or supervisor personnel. An authoritarian culture often fosters conflict between the different production and management silos and leads to the attitude that "it isn't my problem" or "that's not my responsibility." This is contrary to contemporary quality improvement techniques that stress that each member of the team has a stake in all aspects of production and the resulting quality of the final product. Additionally, an authoritarian culture often places one individual or group in a position of being able to override the concerns or decisions of the larger team. This aspect of quality management has often been problematic in health care as areas of expertise (e.g., physician, nurse, pharmacist, administrator) create natural barriers or silos that result in each individual focusing only on their part of the process as opposed to the process in total. For example, a surgeon may be viewed as the authority in the operating room. As such, the surgeon may override or dismiss concerns raised by nurses or other technicians in the operating room because they feel they have the final say on all decisions. Additionally, the surgeon's authoritarian behavior may create an environment in which others feel intimidated not to identify safety concerns or stop the surgery process in order to ensure patient safety. As a consequence, many quality assurance programs are retrospective and have an accusatory and punitive aspect for those individuals or departments that do not meet the established expectation of quality.[1] This shortsighted view of quality has led to the demise, or near demise, of many facets of the American industrial sector and represents a significant barrier to improving quality and safety in health care.

❷ *In more recent years, focus has been shifted away from quality assurance and quality control to embrace a different discipline in the search for quality—total quality management (TQM). TQM takes a more investigative approach to identifying barriers to quality in the processes of providing goods or services.*[1,9,10] TQM works under the basic principle that individuals are committed to quality; however, the processes under which they operate may not be conducive for allowing them to achieve that level of quality. In TQM, all participants are involved in the search for more efficient and cost-effective ways to improve the quality of services, products, and processes. TQM is a statistical, data-driven process that strives to improve quality by limiting variation in the processes involved in providing a good or service.[1] This contrasts with quality assurance, in which the assessment of quality and the plan to improve quality are managed by a limited few and focus on standards that may or may not be driven by data. A table comparing and contrasting the differences in approach and methodology between TQM and quality assurance is provided in Appendix 14–1.

Continuous quality improvement (CQI) is the term given to the methodologies used in the process of TQM. By using a systematic approach to identify internal and external factors that influence processes and functions, CQI seeks to remove the subjectivity from the assessment of quality and provide an ongoing mechanism for improving quality. CQI uses tools such as brainstorming, Pareto charts, scatter diagrams, cause-and-effect diagrams (also known as fishbone diagrams), run charts, control charts, and other statistical and investigational tools to provide insight into the barriers that are decreasing quality (or those processes that are improving quality) and to what extent those barriers exist.[10] Examples of these tools are provided in Appendix 14–2.

The shift in the global workplace from quality assurance to TQM has revolutionized many industries. Many companies now embrace these practices very zealously and have incorporated these techniques in their daily routine. While this change has come more quickly to some industries, health care is just now beginning to embrace these philosophies. Accrediting organizations such as The Joint Commission, the National Committee for Quality Assurance (NCQA), and the Center for Medicare/Medicaid Services (CMS) have been instrumental in bringing these philosophies to the forefront of contemporary health care. Despite this, many obstacles remain in place as health care seeks to improve quality. In the following sections of this chapter, changes and barriers to quality in health care as well as the expectations of quality set forth by some of the national health care accrediting bodies are reviewed. TQM, as it pertains to the medication use process, and steps to implement a medication quality program are outlined.

Beyond Total Quality Management: Six Sigma Quality

Over the past decade, a new approach to quality, based on the principles of TQM, has emerged and been embraced by many manufacturing and service industries. This principle is called Six Sigma quality and incorporates many of the tools used in TQM. Six Sigma quality derives its name from the statistical term sigma—a measure of deviation from a desired value. ❸ *Six Sigma is a data-driven, statistical process designed to eliminate defects and improve quality to a level of near perfection (99.99966% defect-free or six sigma)*. Originally developed by the Motorola Corporation, Six Sigma was created to describe a process that nearly eliminates defects in the all products being manufactured. A one-sigma process (one deviation from the mean) is a process in which only 31% of the products are defect-free. To perform the process at six-sigma (six deviations from the mean) would be to create a process in which 99.99966% of the products manufactured are defect-free. To better understand Six Sigma, it is of value to review an example familiar to most pharmacists: filling an automated medication-dispensing machine.[11]

For any given process, there exist opportunities for quality or defects in that process. In this example, each time the automated dispensing unit is filled, it can either be filled correctly or incorrectly. Thus, there is a chance for a defect with each opportunity. If the pharmacy fills the automated dispensing units 1 million times and does so at a level of accuracy of 99% (i.e., percent yield), then it can be expected that there will be 8800 defects per million opportunities (DPMO). That is to say, in 1 million attempts to fill the dispensing unit, the unit will be filled incorrectly 8800 times. A pharmacy functioning at this level would be achieving approximately four-sigma quality for the process of filling automated dispensing machines. What if the same pharmacy desired to achieve six-sigma quality in the same process? In order to accomplish this goal, the pharmacy would need to produce only 3.4 defects (incorrect fills) per 1 million opportunities (99.99966% defect-free yield). A pharmacy that performs this function at a three-sigma level (93.32% defect-free yield) can expect 66,800 defects per million opportunities. As demonstrated by this example, performing a process at 90% to 99% yield will still leave the potential for a significant number of defects. Most pharmacy managers would be pleased with 99% accuracy in any process; however, in the case of filling an automated dispensing machine, being 99% accurate will produce 8800 defects, each potentially leading to a dangerous medication misadventure. Beyond determining the percent yield and DPMO for a process, the Six Sigma discipline also utilizes a variety of tools and strategies to improve quality. Many of these strategies are similar to those employed in TQM and are based on the PDCA model. Six Sigma employs the strategies of DMAIC (define, measure, analyze, improve, control) and DMADV (define, measure, analyze, design, verify) to improve or incorporate quality into a given process or function.[11] The former (DMAIC) is used when improving an existing process that is performing below a desired standard; the latter process is employed when developing a new process. In the DMAIC strategy, a problem is *defined* and then the current process is *measured* to collect relevant data and risks. These data are then *analyzed* to determine cause-and-effect relationships. The process is then *improved* using any variety of process-improvement action steps, and finally the process is *controlled* (i.e., monitored to detect future problems before they occur). The DMADV strategy is similar but applies to a newly developed process. In this strategy, the first step is to *define* the goals of performance expectation (e.g. customer expectation) and then *measure* those characteristics of the product or process that are key to quality (referred to as critical to quality or CTQs). The next step is to *analyze* design plans to create high-performing processes and to develop alternative designs in case initial designs are not successful. The *design* details are then created including simulation to verify the performance of the process, and finally, the design is *verified* through the use of pilot evaluation. In health care, these methodologies could be applied to an existing process (e.g., medication fill of automated dispensing cabinets to reduce the error associated with placing a medication in the wrong drawer) or for new processes (e.g., implementing bedside barcode scanning of medications and patient identifiers to reduce the likelihood of administering a medication to the incorrect patient). The approach taken to facilitate these processes is very similar. A working group of all parties involved in the process (e.g., multidisciplinary group of pharmacists, nurses, and physicians) meet to define the process (e.g., how are automated dispensing units filled? by whom? when?) and measure the number of opportunities for that process (e.g., how many times is the automated dispensing unit filled? how many times is it filled incorrectly?). The data from the measurement process is analyzed (e.g., what is the current percent yield of accuracy and DPMO?) and steps to improve the process (e.g., reduce pharmacy technician workload or provide double-check methods) are identified and implemented. Lastly, control monitoring is used to verify that the process improvement has produced the desired result (e.g., determine if the changes improved accuracy). Many of the tools used in TQM and outlined in Appendix 14–2 (e.g., Pareto charts, flow charts, fishbone diagrams) are employed by the working group to better define the process, the nature and cause of the defects, and the most successful methods for improving performance. Although Six Sigma quality practices are being employed in an increasing number of industries, its application in the health care industry is relatively new and not well established. For Six Sigma techniques to be fully effective in the health care industry, industry leaders will need to develop the resources and personnel specifically trained in the techniques of Six Sigma quality.

QUALITY IN HEALTH CARE

In the industrial setting, assuring quality has often focused on materials, people, and processes to achieve a common goal of a quality product.[9] The measure of quality is usually associated with the final product and is often very tangible (e.g., car has no defects, it functions, and it has a low repair record). Health care is not different in that quality also focuses on materials, people, and processes; however, the end product or service is often much more difficult to quantify than a physical product.[12] Differences in diseases, treatments, facilities, and health providers all impact the level of quality. More importantly, differences in patients, their expectations, and their response to a given therapy significantly influence the perception of quality. Unlike the industrial sector, health care is also hampered by the complexity of its health systems and payer structure. While an automobile manufacturer may recognize the need to improve quality and can call upon all of its employees to contribute to obtain the desired goal, health care has many autonomous practitioners seeking to meet the clinical, quality, and financial expectations of numerous institutions, governmental agencies, third-party payers, and patients.

❹ *Problems associated with quality in health care fall into one of three categories: overuse, underuse, and misuse.*[13] *Overuse occurs when a service is provided but not needed, and thus the risk of harm from that service outweighs the potential benefit. Underuse results when a needed service is unavailable or not provided. Misuse occurs when the correct service is provided so poorly that the full benefit is not seen.* In the past, health care addressed these problems through quality assurance techniques. Traditionally, a committee or group would identify a standard that was thought to reflect quality (e.g., infection rate after surgery, cart fill errors, readmission rates) and would establish an acceptable threshold for performance of that standard. A review of the performance of a particular group or individual would be compared against the standard and some corrective action taken if variations existed. Often, such programs produced a very limited effect on quality and were perceived as punitive or judgmental. In an effort to avoid the drawbacks of quality assurance techniques, including the retrospective and punitive nature of quality assurance, many health care practices are employing the principles of TQM such as FOCUS (Find, Organize, Clarify, Understand, Select)-PDCA and Six Sigma methodology. However, utilizing these techniques is difficult work and is still facing many barriers in the health care setting.

Many health care practitioners take an isolated view of their role in providing care and do not consider how their actions and processes affect others involved in the care of the patient. For example, the pharmacy may only focus on decreasing the number of missing doses by getting the right drug into the right medication drawer, whereas it may be more appropriate to assist nursing in improving the documentation on the medication administration record to achieve the same goal. Additionally, a physician may view the delay of medication delivery as a quality issue among pharmacy and nursing, and not address the role that his or her illegible handwriting contributes to the process. This compartmentalized (or departmentalized) view is a barrier to quality in many health care systems and has unfortunately become entrenched in many practices.[10] The classic disagreement between pharmacy and nursing over missing doses is an excellent example of a system breakdown. Although it is easier to blame nursing for misplacing the dose or to lay blame on pharmacy for not sending the dose, it is more effective to apply the principles of TQM and systematically identify those process problems that contribute to poor quality (e.g., missing dose). The role of pharmacists in the TQM process is varied and determined by their role within the department and the institution. Most importantly, pharmacists must be willing to work within multidisciplinary groups and serve as leaders in identifying barriers to quality within pharmacy processes as well as in other processes that impact patient care.

QUALITY AND TEAMWORK

The process of quality improvement must include all practitioners involved in the aspect of care under assessment.[9,14] Within health care organizations, quality improvement functions are often coordinated through the pharmacy and therapeutics (P&T) committee or other similar multidisciplinary groups. The approach to quality improvement varies among organizations and is often specific to the opportunities for improvement identified. The section of this chapter discussing medication use evaluation outlines an example of how quality improvement activities can be conducted. Regardless of the process involved, there are some aspects of multidisciplinary group dynamics that are important to consider.

Working within multidisciplinary groups can pose significant challenges. Busy schedules, politics, and poor communication and planning can contribute to dysfunction. Often, physicians or other health practitioners are left out of quality improvement initiatives for a variety of reasons. Perceptions of aloofness or disinterest, fear of reprisal or admission of guilt, or previous conflicts may result in the exclusion of individuals or groups that are essential to the quality improvement process. Likewise, it is important when interfacing with a group charged with resolving quality issues that one goes about the process with an open mind. Understand where your current practices may provide a barrier to others and how you can change those practices without creating barriers for yourself. All groups or individuals involved in the process should be included as early as possible, preferably from the beginning.[15] One of the single greatest barriers to effective quality improvement is the addition of a new group or individuals once work has begun. This not only delays the process, but is likely to leave that group feeling slighted and its members are less likely to be cooperative.

Leadership is one of the most important aspects of a successful quality management initiative.[15] Most people can recall a committee that has seemingly met forever, always covering the same ground and seldom reaching closure on any issues. Strong leadership is essential to help keep working groups focused on the task at hand. It is important to establish which systems are contributing to the majority of problems and address only those that will have the biggest impact. It is of little benefit to expend a great deal of time and resources on a process that contributes little to the problem. Establishing clear goals, a timeline for completing tasks, and routine follow-up on progress will facilitate involvement and assist in bringing closure and documenting results. Although strong leadership is needed to facilitate any large working group such as a committee or quality improvement team, the leadership of that group should not override the group's ideas or present an accusatory or punitive image.[1,9,13,15] It is important that all involved with the quality initiative feel free to speak their minds and contribute to the process. The approach to developing and implementing a successful quality management program is varied and complex; however, some time-tested approaches such as FOCUS-PDCA, SMART (Statement, Measurement, Analysis, Remedy, Test) Problem-Solving Process, and the Ten-step method can be employed. Appendix 14-3 defines and outlines the key components of these quality management tools.

● ❺ *The application of quality management techniques in health care is not very different than in other industries. Strong leadership, an open mind, willingness to put past differences or processes behind, and most importantly, a willingness to improve the existing system are required to ensure that quality goals are met.* Often, it is most beneficial to examine programs or processes that work well and determine what makes them successful. Flow charts are useful in describing a process and can illustrate how a system is designed to work well. An example of a flow chart appears in Appendix 14-2. Applying these successes to processes that need improvement (e.g., problematic or high-risk processes) will often result in additional successes while making the most efficient use of time and resources. Determining the expectation of quality can often be the largest challenge facing a quality improvement initiative. For this reason, many national organizations and accrediting bodies have set out to establish benchmarks for quality in health care. This will be discussed in the next section of this chapter.

QUALITY AND THE JOINT COMMISSION

While this section will briefly address the role of The Joint Commission in establishing and accrediting health system quality, a detailed review of The Joint Commission's specific standards, methodology, and expectations for compliance are beyond the scope of this reference. As such, the reader is advised to consult the appropriate Joint Commission Accreditation Manual, Web site (http://www.jointcommission.org), and other published references for detailed information regarding The Joint Commission accreditation process.

Undoubtedly, the single most influential group directing quality improvement in the health system setting is The Joint Commission. Established in 1951 as the Joint Commission on the Accreditation of Hospitals, The Joint Commission has been a leader in assessing and promoting quality in the health care setting.[16] The Joint Commission currently oversees the accreditation of more than 5000 hospitals and 15,000 health care organizations including laboratories, home-care organizations, long-term care organizations, behavioral health organizations, and integrated health systems.[16] Accreditation by The Joint

Commission is an important component in maintaining eligibility for reimbursement from Medicare and Medicaid, and often serves as a means for comparison to similar health systems. The importance of accreditation to many health systems is so great that a significant number of resources are committed on an ongoing basis to meet their standards.

Prior to the early 1990s, The Joint Commission's standards on quality were divided into departmental areas, outlining the roles of those departments and the quality measures that should be expected from activities governed by those departments.[16] This departmental approach to quality focused more on function than outcome and did not meet the needs of modern health systems that were looking to improve quality and contain costs. As a result, The Joint Commission initiated its *Agenda for Change* in 1986, shifting the focus of quality away from departments and departmental roles to a more process-oriented quality assessment and performance structure.[17] For example, standards for pharmacy or specific mention of P&T committees, drug use evaluation, or formulary management were not included in the revised standards.[16] This initiative was designed to remove the responsibility of a particular activity away from a particular group or department, and increase the responsibility and ownership of all practitioners within the system for all aspects of patient care. The *Agenda for Change* reflected a significant philosophical transition from quality assurance to TQM and CQI.

In 1999, The Joint Commission continued the evolution of its accreditation services toward continuous quality improvement by reexamining the entire accreditation process. This reevaluation culminated with the launch of *Shared Visions—New Pathways* in January 2004. Shared Visions represented a radical restructuring of the Joint Commission accreditation process involving all components including application, standards, survey methodology, scoring, and follow-up. The goal of the restructuring was to move the accreditation process from a score-driven survey that is conducted once every 3 years to a continuous, systematic, quality-focused process with on-site surveys conducted at any time and without notice. As such, many of the standards used in previous accreditation manuals still exist; however, they have been reorganized and more clearly defined. Additionally, many of the old methodologies for the survey process and scoring were abandoned and new methodologies and requirements implemented. The goal of these changes was to improve the consistency, objectivity, and quality of the accreditation process and improve the quality of health care.

The Joint Commission continues to refine and remodel the accreditation process. In recent years, The Joint Commission has introduced the National Patient Safety Goals (NPSGs) as standard measures of quality performance for health care organizations. The NPSGs support performance measures in core clinical processes such as patient identification, communication among caregivers, health care–related infections, and patient falls. Significant to pharmacists are the NPSGs related to the safe administration of medications and medication reconciliation. The specific goals for these medication-related processes are by now very well known to most health-system pharmacists. Examples of NPSGs that have been incorporated into daily health-system practice include the identification of medications with look-alike/sound-alike names and action steps to reduce errors associated with incorrectly administering these medications; measures to reduce patient falls from medication and nonmedication-related causes; and improving the safety of anticoagulation therapy with agents such as warfarin and heparin through the use of standardized protocols and improved patient monitoring. Although an in-depth analysis of the NPSGs and recommendations for performance compliance is beyond the scope of this chapter, it is important to recognize the quality intent of these accreditation requirements. All of the NPSGs represent basic performance measures of patient safety such as reducing the likelihood of a patient fall or reducing errors by ensuring proper patient identification prior to procedures or drug therapy. In reality, the fact that such basic concepts of patient safety have to be assessed and evaluated at all provides some indication of the poor quality performance that many health care organizations have been able to achieve without external regulatory requirements. Moreover, the NPSGs represent processes for which collaboration among health care team members, administrators, and patients is essential in order to achieve ideal performance. To this end, The Joint Commission is addressing the most fundamental of health care quality indicators—patient safety.

The Future of Quality in Health Care

As the United States once again endeavors to overhaul national health care systems and infrastructure, there will be an increased emphasis on standards and measures to ensure the quality, safety, and cost-effectiveness of the care provided. This emphasis all but guarantees that regulatory agencies, such as The Joint Commission and others, will be active components of the national health care environment for years to come. Quality in health care will continue to be defined not only by consumer perception and service expectation, but also by agencies and organizations with a vested interest in improving the U.S. health care system. CMS, which mandates many patient safety and quality measures for the purposes of Medicare and Medicaid reimbursement, will be a significant driving force for health care quality in the future as it strives to reduce health care costs by improving the quality of care and decreasing the morbidity and mortality from medication errors. Organizations such as the Leapfrog Group (http://www.leapfroggroup.org/), a coalition of large companies with a significant number of insured employees (e.g., GE, Boeing, IBM, FedEx, and Toyota), will use its influence as a large purchaser of health care to promote advances in health care quality and improved transparency to the public, thereby increasing the public's ability to review, rate, and choose health care providers and systems based on the quality and safety of the care they provide. Increased competition resulting from this transparency will drive all health systems to focus on quality.

However, in order for the health care industry to truly make gains in the provision of high-quality health care services, there must be an industrywide effort to evaluate current practices and establish performance thresholds independent of outside regulatory agencies, accreditation bodies, or financial performance incentives (or disincentives). As with any industry, waiting until governmental or other bodies regulate change carries with it the possibility that the determination of quality may be influenced or completely determined by non–health professionals. Ultimately, those closest to the system, including physicians, nurses, and pharmacists, must create standards of performance for patient safety, therapeutic outcomes, and access to health care. Health care clinicians and administrators must be willing to create benchmarks that define quality, hold themselves and their organizations accountable to the standards, and share vital information with other institutions that can improve the overall quality of health care in the United States. Health care team members, including physicians, pharmacists, nurses, and patients, must be prepared to break down long-standing stereotypes, roles, and habits to better understand the risk points in our current health system infrastructure, and have the courage and vision to set performance benchmarks at a level that ensures that access to quality health care is available to all. Although patients are not always considered part of the health care team, their involvement and understanding of treatment options, outcomes, and risks is essential to providing dialogue that leads to informed decision making and facilitates successful outcomes through improved compliance, lifestyle changes, and an improved understanding of the scope of benefits and risks of modern pharmacotherapy. As with other industries that have made the quality transition, the most important step is recognizing key stakeholders in the process and reaching out to them in a collaborative fashion to formulate sound policy, performance expectations, and sufficient financial incentives to foster meaningful change in practice. In practical terms, this means that providers and consumers of health care, those with the greatest expertise and stake in the health care system, need to be the ones who redefine how the health care system performs with the goal of improving access, safety, and outcomes as their primary focus.

Pharmacists can, and should, play an instrumental role in the transition of the health care industry from a reactive quality culture that acts only in response to errors or regulatory requirements, to a proactive culture for patient safety and quality care that identifies, implements, and monitors best practices and risk reduction strategies. The pharmacists' unique knowledge of pharmacology, pharmacokinetics, and medication distribution systems are critical to improving the quality of health care and managing the costs associated with medication therapy. The pharmacist plays a vital role in many aspects of the medication use process. Beyond the traditional role of ensuring the proper preparation and distribution of medications, pharmacists play an active role as the medication auditor, ensuring that the therapy is appropriate for the patient's clinical condition, tailored to the patient's specific needs and requirements, and will not unnecessarily increase the risk of patient harm from adverse events, interactions, or safety problems related to the administration of the medication. Additionally, organizations that support the initial and ongoing training of pharmacists, including professional societies and colleges of pharmacy, will need to prepare current and future pharmacists with a strong understanding of the principles of quality management including TQM, CQI, and Six Sigma. Equipped with a working understanding of these principles and their traditional pharmacotherapy knowledge, pharmacists will be able to significantly shape health care policy in the United States and improve the quality and safety of our health care delivery system.

Drug Regimen Review and Drug Use Review

The next section of this chapter shifts from a broad discussion of quality to a review of a specific process called medication use evaluation (MUE). Examples of quality improvement activities occurring as part of the MUE process will be discussed. Although MUE is generally conducted in organized health systems, two other processes with similar names (drug regimen review and drug use review) focus on therapy provided within nursing facilities and for outpatients. Drug regimen review (DRR) is a requirement of the Health Care Financing Administration (HCFA) mandating pharmacist review of drug regimens for patients in nursing facilities. The intent of the regulation requiring DRR was to ensure that the drug therapy provided for each resident is reviewed monthly and that pharmacists are making appropriate recommendations to health care professionals to improve drug therapy. This requirement was implemented in 1974 through Medicare (Title XVIII) and Medicaid (Title XIX) regulations and was expanded in 1987 to include intermediate-care nursing facilities.[18,19]

The Medicare Catastrophic Coverage Act of 1988 required an assessment of medication prescribing in outpatient settings. Assessment included indication for use and evidence that prescribers were providing some degree of oversight of ongoing therapy. Most assessments were quantitative (e.g., involved counting the number of cases) and were weak assessments of prescribing. It was rescinded in early 1990. The Medicaid Anti-Discriminatory Drug Price and Patient Benefit Restoration Act (Pryor II), enacted in 1990, includes similar requirements. This bill mandates prospective and retrospective assessment of medication prescribing and utilization, and requires that each state establish educational outreach programs for outpatient pharmacy services. The intent of this provision is to ensure that prescription drugs are "appropriate, medically necessary, and not likely to result in adverse medical results." This legislation requires that drug utilization review (DUR) programs be designed to educate physicians and pharmacists in identifying and reducing the frequency and patterns of fraud, abuse, gross overuse, or inappropriate or medically unnecessary care and mandates patient counseling. Claims data are used as the primary source of information. Much of the data remain quantitative in nature, and the focus of interventions is usually on identified outliers whose use exceeds the norm or differs from what would be expected based on their practice. Although the Act did not specify the mechanism for education of health care professionals, the intent was that an assessment of prescribing patterns and patient medication compliance be used to reduce unnecessary or inappropriate medication use. Over time, the term DUR had also been adopted to describe an early version of what was referred to as drug use evaluation, and that has now evolved into a broader process referred to as MUE. These latter processes are largely employed in acute care settings and, unlike DUR, compare actual medication use to evidence-based standards adopted by the specific organization. These processes are further compared and contrasted within the following section. Long-term care facilities meeting the drug regimen review (DRR) requirements of the Department of Health and Human Services are exempt from the provision requiring DUR.[18-22]

MEDICATION USE EVALUATION

Medication use evaluation (MUE) is often included in the overall performance improvement programs within organizations to provide in-depth assessment of the medication use process. MUE programs should, over time, examine all aspects of medication use and require the direct involvement of pharmacists.[23,24] ⑥ *MUE is often part of an organization's overall performance improvement program that uses definitions of safe and effective use of medications to assess components of the medication use process.* These definitions are usually described as criteria and are endorsed by the organization within which they are to be applied. Criteria summarize an organization's definition of appropriate or acceptable use of the medication. The manner in which medications are actually used, administered, and monitored within the organization is compared to the criteria to determine if actual practice matches the best (or at least acceptable) practice as stated with the criteria. For example, based on evidence that slowing the infusion rate of an intravenous medication reduces the risk of serious adverse events, the criteria may state that the medication should be infused over at least 60 minutes. However, when actual practice is accessed as part of a MUE, results indicate that the medication is infused over 30 minutes or less in 50% of cases and adverse effects were noted in most of these cases. These results indicate that best practice is not occurring.

Case Study 14–1

In the situation described previously in which the antibiotic was administered more rapidly than recommended, what factors could be contributing to this problem?

Endorsement of criteria is usually provided by a multidisciplinary group that includes medical staff (e.g., the P&T committee). The goal of MUE is to provide all patients with the most rational, safe, and effective drug therapy through the assessment and improvement of specific medication use processes. MUE may focus on a specific medication (e.g., alteplase), a class of medications (e.g., thrombolytics), medications used in the management of a specific disease state or clinical setting (e.g., thrombolytics in acute myocardial infarction), medications related to a clinical event (e.g., drug therapy within the first 24 hours for patients admitted with acute myocardial infarction including aspirin, beta blockers, and thrombolytics), a specific component of the medication use process (e.g., time from admission to administration of thrombolytic), or can be based on specific outcomes (e.g., vessel patency following thrombolytic administration). MUE is not designed to address if-then questions (such as if one dose is used instead of another, will outcomes be effected?), but simply determines if the actual use of a medication is consistent with the standards established within the criteria. Although MUE is no longer explicitly addressed within the Joint Commission Standards, it remains an important component of broader requirements related to performance improvement within organizations. In order to be effective, challenges such as a lack of resources or authority, politics, difficulty in identifying issues (e.g., high-use, high-risk, or problematic medications or processes) or in acting upon data to improve performance, and cumbersome or ineffective reporting structure or processes must be addressed. For example, unless the organization has a functional process to use the information generated by MUE to improve patient care, outcomes are unlikely to improve. If a minority of prescribers or any single group (e.g., nursing, clinical laboratory, pharmacy, or respiratory therapy) can unilaterally disagree with the recommendations from a MUE and successfully block efforts to implement process improvement initiatives, efforts will fail. In order for MUE to effectively improve patient care, the organization must have a commitment to improving medication use and a committee structure that facilitates multidisciplinary collaboration and cooperation.

THE MEDICATION USE PROCESS

In 1989, a multidisciplinary task force was organized by The Joint Commission to describe the medication use process as a component of its effort to develop tools to assess medication use. The medication use process is the outline of the steps involved in providing medications to patients (e.g., prescribing, dispensing) and what happens after the medication is administered (e.g., monitoring). The original definition of the medication use process included prescribing, dispensing, administration, monitoring, and systems and management control (see Table 14–1 for the full definition). This description serves as the basis for contemporary MUE.[25,26] Currently, systems and management control is often not included within the description of the medication use process as it applies to virtually all

TABLE 14–1. DESCRIPTION OF THE MEDICATION USE PROCESS

Prescribing	Assessing the need for selecting the correct drug
	Individualizing the therapeutic regimen
	Designing the desired therapeutic response
Dispensing	Reviewing the order for correct dose and indication for use
	Processing the order
	Compounding/preparing the drug
	Dispensing the drug in a timely manner
Administering	Administering the right medication to the right patient
	Administering the medication when indicated
	Informing the patient about the medication
	Including the patient in administration
Monitoring	Monitoring and documenting the patient's response
	Identifying and reporting adverse drug reactions
	Reevaluating the drug selection, drug regimen, frequency, and duration
Systems/ Management Control	Collaborating and communicating among caregivers
	Reviewing and managing the patient's complete therapeutic drug regimen

aspects of patient care. Medication acquisition, storage, distribution, and disposal may also be assessed if pertinent.

It is important to note that this description outlines a process that is more multidisciplinary than the categories might imply. For example, although the prescribing category may imply a physician function, pharmacists are often involved as they assist in drug selection and individualization of the therapeutic regimen.

MEDICATION USE EVALUATION AND THE JOINT COMMISSION

The terminology used to describe MUE has changed over time and can be confusing. MUE, DUE (drug use evaluation), DUR, and AUR (antibiotic use review) are often used interchangeably, but are different in their approach and application. This section will attempt to provide some background as to how these terms developed and changed over time. Table 14–2 summarizes several key events in the development of MUE as it relates to The Joint Commission and governmental activities in the United States.[18,19,27,28]

Table 14–3 compares several of the acronyms applied to the evaluation of medications. As summarized within the table, the process has evolved from a retrospective evaluation of prescribing to a thorough assessment of how a medication is used within patient care provided throughout an organization. Early efforts to evaluate antibiotic use focused on how often a specific physician's patients received high doses of the antibiotic and how many patients experienced adverse effects. Contemporary evaluations looking at the same medication would examine how the computer prompts the prescriber to ensure that doses are appropriate and what action the prescriber is required to take to override these alerts; how the pharmacist reviews the order and the parameters used to determine when

TABLE 14–2. SUMMARY TIMELINE: THE EVOLUTION OF MEDICATION USE EVALUATION

1969	Task Force on Prescription Drugs (Department of Health, Education, and Welfare [DHEW]) Report calls for the development of programs to monitor drug use
1974	Health Care Financing Administration (HCFA) regulation mandates pharmacists' monthly review of medication for all residents of skilled nursing facilities; this was later (1987) expanded to include residents of intermediate-care nursing facilities
1978	Antibiotic utilization review standards included in Accreditation Manual for Hospitals
1980	Quality assurance standard included in Accreditation Manual for Hospitals
1986	Drug usage evaluation standard included in Accreditation Manual for Hospitals Agenda for Change initiated
1987	Omnibus Budget Reconciliation Act (OBRA): Required states to develop retrospective and prospective DUR programs
1994	Medication use evaluation standard included in Accreditation Manual for Hospitals
1996	Indicator Monitoring System (IMS) initiated
1997	Medication use evaluation standard included in PI.3.2.2 and TX.3.9 in the Joint Commission Accreditation Manual for Hospitals
2004	Specific reference to medication use evaluation removed from standards; considered a component of overall performance improvement; specific evaluation requirements added for high-alert medications, etc.

TABLE 14–3. ACRONYMS ASSOCIATED WITH THE EVALUATION OF MEDICATION USE

Term	Origin	Description
Drug use review (DUR)	1969 Task Force on Prescription Drugs	Retrospective evaluation to monitor medication use patterns. Usually quantitative and limited to trending.
	1990 Medicaid Anti-Discriminatory Drug Price and Patient Benefit Restoration Act (*Pryor II*)	Usually retrospective evaluation based on claims data. Results used to direct education and to reduce fraud, abuse, overuse, and inappropriate or unnecessary care.
Antibiotic use review (AUR)	1978 JCAHO Standards	Retrospective evaluation of antibiotic use. Usually quantitative and limited to identifying patterns of use.
Drug use evaluation (DUE)	1986 JCAHO Standards	Expansion of AUR to all drugs. Concurrent evaluation of prescribing and outcome only. Multidisciplinary involvement.
Medication use evaluation (MUE)	1992 JCAHO Standards	Expansion of DUE to include all medications and all aspects of medication use including prescribing, dispensing, administering, monitoring, and outcome.

to contact the prescriber to recommend alternative doses; how the prescriber responds to pharmacist recommendations; and how doses are adjusted based on laboratory results (e.g., drug levels, culture and sensitivity results). The focus has expanded from simply identifying issues to seeking systematic resolution to the issues identified and assessing the impact of these efforts to ensure that the use of the medication has improved. An early MUE may have identified a dosing issue and the action taken was to distribute a memo or newsletter on the topic. A contemporary MUE could identify the same dosing issue and a similar educational effort could be undertaken. In addition to education, a more direct action, such as implementation of dosing limits in the computer system, would also be undertaken to better ensure improved dosing. Also, a reassessment to ensure that dosing had actually improved as a result of these efforts would be required.

One of the first calls for a process to evaluate the use of medications appeared in the final reports of the Task Force on Prescription Drugs (U.S. Department of Health, Education, and Welfare).[27] This 1969 report called for the development of programs to monitor medication use. A retrospective evaluation process referred to as DUR was suggested.

The Joint Commission on Accreditation of Hospitals (JCAH), as The Joint Commission was known at the time, required AUR beginning in 1978. This assessment was largely retrospective, quantitative, and evaluated trends in antibiotic use. Retrospective review took place after the care had been provided and was often conducted by reviewing the documentation in the patient's medical record. The Joint Commission Standards evolved to include other medications in the mid-1980s. The number and specific type of evaluation was not specified, and patterns of drug use (versus a qualitative evaluation of individual cases) were often the focus. The term drug use review (DUR) was also used during this time period to describe the retrospective review of other drugs and should not be confused with the current use of DUR as discussed in the drug regimen review and drug use review section of this chapter. The requirement was expanded to include all drug therapy and the terminology was changed to DUE in 1986. The 1986 standards implied that concurrent evaluation of drug use was required. Concurrent evaluation occurs during the course of therapy and allows the use of information sources other than the medication record, such as interviewing caregivers and the patient. The responsibility for this function was shared by the medical, pharmacy, nursing, and other staff (as appropriate) and was assigned to the medical staff as a P&T committee activity. The activity was to be ongoing, planned, systematic, and criteria based using current knowledge and experience. Topic selection could not be based solely on hot topics from a recent professional meeting or the availability of prepared criteria from an outside source. Topic selection was to be based on the challenges seen within the organization. Over time, evaluations were to reflect the entire scope of care provided by the organization rather than focus on the same topics or same patient populations. Data from these activities were used in the process of medical staff reappointment and recredentialing within the organization.[28,29] The reappointment and recredentialing process is used to ensure that physicians (or other care providers) continue to meet the qualifications to practice in the organization and that the care they provide results in acceptable patient outcomes. If a prescriber's use of a medication has been identified as potentially problematic during a MUE and the prescriber has been counseled to modify his or her use of the medication and has refused to do so, the medical staff may elect to limit or suspend the prescriber's ability to practice within the organization.

An initiative called the *Agenda for Change* was adopted by The Joint Commission in 1986.[17,30] It was intended to improve standards by focusing on key functions of quality of care, to monitor the performance of health care organizations using indicators, to improve the relevance and quality of the survey process, and to enhance the accuracy and value of The Joint Commission accreditation. Indicators are quantitative measures of an aspect of patient care and are used to screen for potential problems (indicators are discussed in detail later in the chapter). The revised process was to focus on actual performance versus the capability to perform well. An organization could no longer hide behind having well-designed processes or policies and procedures on paper; The Joint Commission surveyors would now be looking at how processes were actually carried out. Within this initiative, The Joint Commission endorsed the concept of CQI and included CQI within its standards beginning in 1994. As part of this process, the Accreditation Manual for Hospitals (AMH) was significantly modified and much of the definition of expectations related to organization performance was deleted. Multidisciplinary involvement in the evaluation of medication use was emphasized. Eventually, the standards were moved from the Medical Staff Chapter of the AMH to the Care of Patients and Performance Improvement Chapters. In 1992, the terminology was also changed from drug use evaluation to medication use evaluation to reflect that all medications and all medication-related functions are included in the standard. This change also broadened the scope to reflect The Joint Commission's expanded reach into nonacute care settings (such as clinics and IV infusion centers) and clarified that the process did not focus on illicit drug use. This terminology is also consistent with the medication use process (described in Table 14–1) as defined by The Joint Commission as part of its *Agenda for Change*. Previously, the evaluation of medication use typically focused on only the prescribing and outcome components of the process. With this change, dispensing and administration were specifically included. MUE standards first appeared in the 1992 AMH and were required of all institutions beginning in 1994.

Current standards focus on performance improvement, but no longer require that a specific approach be used. The organization is allowed to select, based on its characteristics and structure, a performance-improvement approach (e.g., Six Sigma, FOCUS-PDCA, SMART) that best meets its needs and that of its patients. Appendix 14–3 briefly describes these approaches. Standards state that MUE should be a systematic, multidisciplinary process focusing on continual improvement in the medication use process and patient outcomes. The use of data for reappointment/recredentialing is still required, but the emphasis is on continuous performance improvement.

Priorities should be established based on

- Effect on performance and improved patient outcomes
- Selected high-volume, high-risk, or problem-prone processes
- Resources and organizational priorities

Evaluation of the use of high-cost medications is often a priority within organizations hoping to optimize the use of available financial resources. However, in the past, many organizations based their topic selection solely on cost-saving initiatives rather than on improving the quality of medication use. As a result, this category, when stated as a sole rationale for topic selection, is no longer considered to be consistent with the goals of MUE. Currently, high-cost medications continue to be a focus of evaluation, but organizations are careful to justify the evaluation based on other criteria, such as the use of the medication being problem-prone or its importance in determining patient outcome.

The pharmacist plays a key role within the multidisciplinary MUE process. Although not always involved in specific initiatives, all pharmacists should actively identify opportunities for improvement in processes.[4,31] Although many pharmacists within the organization will have some role in the MUE process, those responsible for the coordination and implementation of MUE initiatives are often those with drug information or performance improvement responsibilities, as well as those with specialized knowledge or experience in the component of medication use under assessment. The American Society of Health-System Pharmacists (ASHP, http://www.ashp.org) has developed guidelines for pharmacists' participation in MUE.[24] These guidelines can serve as a resource to those developing or revising a MUE program or for practitioners new to the process.

The MUE Process

Figure 14–1 outlines the process of medication use evaluation. This figure is an adaptation of the Ten-step process described by The Joint Commission in 1989.[32,33] The next section follows the major steps of the process and provides examples of what occurs within each step.

Responsibility for the medication use evaluation function

The Ten-step process begins with the organization defining which group or groups will participate in and be responsible for the evaluation of medication use. These groups oversee the process, since it has to be assumed that everyone will provide effort toward actually performing or implementing quality assurance activities. Although The Joint Commission standards no longer assign the responsibility for MUE to the P&T committee, nor do they require a P&T committee at all, the function is well suited to this group as

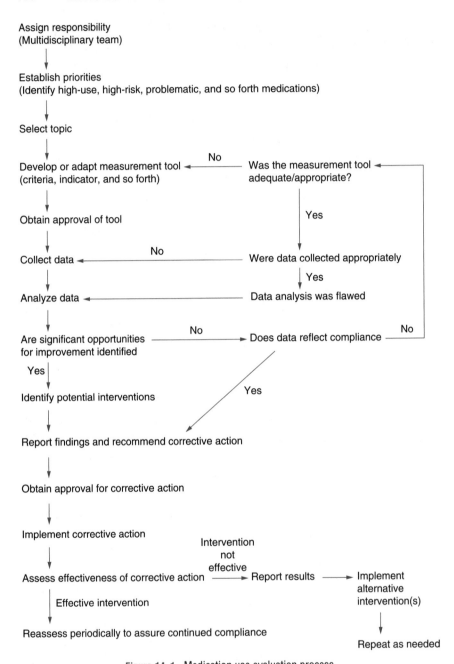

Figure 14–1. Medication use evaluation process.

well as to a Performance/Quality Improvement committee. Performance improvement committees are usually multidisciplinary but may lack medical staff participation. Their focus may be quite broad and may include oversight for a wide variety of performance-improvement functions throughout the organization. Some organizations have formed a MUE subcommittee to the P&T group, while others have distributed the responsibility for MUE along patient population or product lines. Subcommittees are generally assigned a specific set of responsibilities or information and report to the larger committee. They serve as a platform to work through the details of an issue or process and generate recommendations to parent committee. A patient safety committee may also play a role in the identification of topics, evaluation of findings, and implementation of corrective actions. The entire committee may participate in evaluations, or working groups, consisting of committee members, may be established; nonmembers may be appointed to address specific issues. The size, scope, and makeup of the health care organization and its approach to performance improvement should determine the approach to be used. The participants in the group charged with overseeing MUE must have a clear understanding that the purpose is to improve the quality of the medication use process and that each member is expected to actively participate.[15] Newly formed groups may benefit from an overview of the organization's overall approach to quality improvement and how MUE contributes to overall goals.

Topic Selection

❼ *Topic selection should be based on the mission and scope of care of the organization and should focus on high-volume, high-risk, or problem-prone medication-related processes. Topics may also focus on institutional priorities (e.g., initiation of new clinical programs or services).* Several sources of information are commonly used to identify these agents and issues. They include medication error reports, adverse drug reactions (ADRs), advances in patient care modalities that involve changes in optimal pharmacotherapy, disease- or diagnosis-based length of stay or cost outliers within an organization, purchasing reports indicating a significant increase in the use of an agent (without a related shift in patient population), medications that are a key component of a process or procedure (e.g., thrombolytics, glycoprotein 2b/3a receptor inhibitors), and so forth. It is essential that the topics selected reflect the overall scope of medication use throughout the organization, including inpatients, outpatients, emergency care, and short-stay settings.

The inclusion of specific requirements within The Joint Commission's Medication Management Standards and National Patient Safety Goals related to the identification and monitoring of medications described as high risk or high alert within the organization provides another mechanism to target specific medications for additional assessment. High-risk or high-alert medications are those that are most likely to result in adverse outcomes if used inappropriately or if errors are made.

Ideally, the group charged with MUE should develop an annual plan that will establish goals for new topics to be assessed and provide for follow-up on previous evaluations. Priorities should be reevaluated and the scope and breadth of recent evaluations should be assessed relative to the scope of care provided within the organization. For example, if recent MUE efforts focused primarily on issues related to antibiotic use, the plan for the upcoming year should deemphasize the assessment of this class in favor of a more balanced topic selection. The planning process can identify follow-up assessments (used to assess and document that previous efforts were successful in improving performance) that remain to be performed. The failure to perform and document these follow-up evaluations is problematic in many organizations, but they are a key component of the quality improvement process. The development of an annual plan also allows an opportunity to discontinue activities that are no longer useful, such as an ongoing assessment that has demonstrated sustained improvement and can now be replaced by periodic rechecks to ensure continued compliance.

Criteria, standards, and indicators

Criteria are statements of the activity to be measured, and standards define the performance expectations. For example, criteria for the management of patients with pneumonia might state that "the first dose of antibiotic must be administered within two hours." The standard for this criteria statement would be set at 100% if there were no acceptable exceptions to this timeframe. ❽ *Criteria should be based on current best or at least accepted practice or available organization-based clinical care plans, appropriate for the target patient population(s), and be supported by current literature. Ideally, a multidisciplinary group develops the criteria. The membership of this group (e.g., prescribers, nurses, pharmacists, respiratory therapists, social workers, clinical laboratory and information systems personnel, discharge planners) should be determined by the nature of the process under evaluation.* A flow diagram (see Appendix 14–2) outlining the process is often useful. Based on this diagram, additional disciplines should be invited to participate in the evaluation process as appropriate. Respiratory therapists, discharge coordinators, and social workers are a few of the disciplines not routinely represented as core members of medication-related committees. Inclusion of all involved disciplines initially will also facilitate the implementation of corrective actions, if deficiencies are identified. However, criteria are most often developed by one or two of the involved disciplines and are subsequently approved by a multidisciplinary group with representation from all applicable practice groups (e.g., prescribers, pharmacists, nurses). Explicit (objective) criteria are preferred in that they are clear-cut, based on specific measurable parameters, and are better suited for automation. Implicit (subjective) criteria require that a judgment be made and require appropriate clinical expertise to be effective. They are often too subjective to be consistently evaluated (i.e., different people would interpret them differently). Table 14–4

TABLE 14–4. EXAMPLES OF IMPLICIT AND EXPLICIT CRITERIA STATEMENTS

Implicit Criteria Statements	Explicit Criteria Statements
Blood work ordered	Pretreatment WBC with differential ordered and completed within 48 hours prior to the initiation of therapy
Renal function assessed routinely	Serum creatinine evaluated every 3 days during therapy
Neutropenic patients	Patients with WBC <1000/mm^3

compares implicit and explicit criteria statements. Appendix 14–4 provides an example of criteria. It is imperative that the appropriate oversight group approves the criteria prior to initiation of data collection.

_____ Case Study 14–2

The antibiotic that was being infused too rapidly is used to prevent surgical infections and for infections caused by gram-positive organisms. There is some evidence of other issues with the use of this antibiotic and a MUE is planned. The preoperative dose is given in the surgical area and the postoperative doses and treatment doses are given throughout the hospital and in home-care patients. Who would you invite to participate in an evaluation of the use of this antibiotic?

Criteria should be phrased in yes/no or true/false (along with _not applicable_ as appropriate) formats and should avoid interpretation on the part of data collectors. They should assess important aspects in the use of the medication or therapy under evaluation and focus on aspects most closely related to outcomes of the care provided. Definition of outcome should also be established within the criteria based on the scope of care provided by the organization. For example, in a truly acute care setting, the outcome assessment of antibiotic management of pneumonia may be limited to a decrease in clinical signs and symptoms indicating a response to therapy and the ability to be discharged on an oral antibiotic(s). However, in an integrated system that includes both acute and ambulatory or long-term care, the evaluation could continue through the entire treatment course and outcome could be assessed based on cure or control of the disease state at the conclusion of therapy.

As the criteria are finalized, it is helpful to consider how opportunities for improvement identified via a criteria statement could be addressed. For example, could the computer system be used as a tool to improve prescribing, would double-checks by a nurse and a pharmacist help to prevent errors, or could the dispensing process be modified to improve delivery time? If the corrective action would involve the participation of a group not represented in the development process, it may be wise to add them to the team at this point.

Validity should be assessed as part of the development process. Validity assessments consider how effective the criteria will be in providing the information necessary to obtain an actual comparison of what is happening to the expectations outlined in the criteria. Table 14–5 outlines several questions to test the validity of criteria or indicators.[34,35] A short pilot of data collection with an analysis of resulting information is often a good way to test the validity of criteria and its utility in assessing medication use.

Although general guidelines related to criteria are available, most texts providing example criteria are no longer published.[36-40] Many group purchasing organizations and other networks have systems to facilitate the sharing of MUE materials (e.g., criteria, data collection forms) and methods of comparing results with those from similar organizations. The advantages to using predeveloped criteria include prior expert review and assessment,

TABLE 14–5. TESTS OF THE VALIDITY OF CRITERIA OR INDICATORS

Face validity	Are they important to patient outcome?
	Do they assess a problematic area?
	Do they have some utility in improving patient care?
	Do they reflect systemwide performance?
	Are they appropriate, based on current practice standards and literature?
External validity	Have they been thoroughly reviewed by practitioners with expertise in the use of the medication?
	Are they applicable within the organization?
	Has the review process clarified and improved the criteria/indicators without weakening their intent?
Feasibility of data Collection and retrieval	Are they clear and not subject to interpretation?
	Are data available?
	How many cases will need to be evaluated in order to provide adequate data?
	How difficult or complex will the data collection process be?
	What benefits will be gained versus the effort associated with data collection?
	Will data collection methods be consistent?

and time savings. However, criteria developed outside the organization must be adapted to the practice setting and patient population as appropriate, and must be approved by the designated multidisciplinary group prior to data collection. For example, criteria intended for use in a general adult population may not be appropriate for geriatric patients without modification. Also, predeveloped criteria may include uses of a medication not applicable to certain settings or aspects of use that are not a priority for assessment within the organization. For example, criteria for the use of midazolam that address its use for conscious sedation in a setting where conscious sedation is not performed can be streamlined by eliminating criteria related to conscious sedation. Criteria related to the use of antibiotics to treat infection, when the concerns prompting the evaluation relate solely to perioperative use, should be streamlined to focus solely on perioperative use. Criteria may also be derived from guidelines for use developed or adopted within the organization. For example, the P&T committee may agree to add a medication to the formulary for specific indications and require that the use of the agent and patient outcomes be concurrently evaluated based on these guidelines. In this situation, the criteria for use of the medication would reflect the indications approved by the committee and the MUE would assess the desired outcomes as defined by the committee. Data collection would begin as the medication is first used with results reported to the P&T committee at specific intervals (e.g., quarterly) or after a defined period of time (e.g., for the first 6 months).

Case Study 14–3

Within your organization, warfarin is responsible for more adverse events than any other medication. The P&T committee wants to do a MUE to identify opportunities to reduce the number and severity of adverse effects associated with warfarin. How would you identify existing guidelines or standards for warfarin use to assist in drafting criteria for this MUE?

Performance indicators can also be used to evaluate medication use. An indicator is a quantitative measure of an aspect of patient care that is used as a screening tool to detect potential problems in quality.[37,41] For example, the number of doses of flumazenil administered to reverse the effects of benzodiazepines administered in a procedure area could serve as an indicator of the appropriateness of benzodiazepine dosing in the procedure area. If the number of flumazenil doses administered increased, it could reflect a new problem involving excessive benzodiazepine dosing, or it could reflect a push to move cases through the area more quickly by actively reversing the medication effects after the procedure. The indicator only serves as a trigger to prompt closer examination. (Table 14–6 provides additional examples of indicator.) Although the criteria used in MUE are focused and assess specific important components of medication use, indicators measure symptoms of a medication use system that could indicate that something is not working well, but there is no assurance that there really is a problem when an indicator is not met.

Indicators are not direct measures of quality and are not used in MUEs. They can serve as a tool to identify potentially problematic aspects of care, but require more focused assessment (such as a MUE) to identify the cause. Indicators can be used to monitor rate-based events (e.g., how often something does or does not occur, such as preoperative antibiotic administration within 2 hours of the first surgical incision) or sentinel events (events that occur rarely but are significant in impact, such as an adverse drug event that results in the patient's death). Indicators can assess structure, process, or outcome. Structure refers to the resources, tools, and other established attributes of the setting in which care is provided. Process refers to the activities that take place in giving and receiving care. Outcome denotes the effects of care on the health status of the patient or population. Indicators can be used as a mechanism to monitor the overall medication use system, either to screen for potential problems (e.g., to assess if a more comprehensive evaluation such as a MUE is needed) or to provide an ongoing monitor to ensure that performance improvement is sustained following the completion of an evaluation or intervention.[24] For example, the first indicator listed in Table 14–6 involves the estimation of creatinine clearance in patients older than 65 years of age. If an estimation of a patient's renal function is performed (e.g., if a creatinine clearance is calculated or measured) and is available to caregivers, they can use it to adjust therapy accordingly. The availability of an estimated creatinine clearance in the medical record of patients over the age of 65 suggests that the organization is systematically taking steps to adjust drug therapy in this population based

TABLE 14–6. EXAMPLES OF INDICATOR

Patients >65 years old in whom creatinine clearance (CrCl) has been estimated
Patients undergoing surgery who receive prophylactic antibiotics >X minutes before the first incision
Frequency of pharmacy stock outages
Frequency of discrepancies in automatic dispensing units
Patients with a diagnosis of acute myocardial infarction who are prescribed daily aspirin therapy at discharge
Patients with a diagnosis of congestive heart failure receiving an angiotensin-converting enzyme inhibitor
Patients discharged on >X number of prescription medications

on organ function. Of course, it cannot be certain that the information is used appropriately or even if it is used at all, but as an indicator, it does provide a useful screen related to patient-specific dosage adjustments. The lack of information related to renal function in elderly patients may indicate that the organization is not routinely making these assessments as part of its medication use system. In the past, some organizations assigned the responsibility to the clinical laboratory and posted estimated creatinine clearance values with laboratory data. Others assigned the responsibility to pharmacy either with automation of calculations and dose screening within the pharmacy dispensing system or requiring that pharmacists document creatinine clearance calculations in the medical record. Most organizations now automate creatinine clearance calculations (or an alternative estimate of renal function) within their clinical information system. The more contemporary challenge is to assess if this information is actively applied in patient care. For example, are medications appropriately selected in patients with reduced renal function? An updated indicator might be the number of patients who are prescribed a medication that is contraindicated (per organizational definition) based on diminished renal function and the availability of treatment alternatives (e.g., metformin or enoxaparin in severe renal dysfunction).

Within the MUE process, standards are used to define optimal performance and are usually set at 0% (should never happen) or 100% (should always happen). Thresholds are similar to standards, but they specify that an acceptable level of compliance or performance is usually set higher than 0% or lower than 100% based on acceptable variation, standards of practice, or benchmarks.[42] Thresholds are sometimes used instead of standards to allow limited noncompliance with the criteria when the clinical impact of noncompliance is felt to be of low risk. They should not be used to avoid intervention. Thresholds are useful when the group overseeing the MUE process is most interested in addressing performance that is clearly unacceptable, while allowing some variation from best practice.

Control limits can be used when measurements continue over an extended period of time (e.g., weeks or months). Unlike standards and thresholds, they are usually not applied in the initial MUE but can be used to follow a process over time. For example, a MUE was conducted and action taken to improve the use of the medication. Control limits could be used to monitor the ongoing use of the medication to ensure that the improvement was sustained over time. Control limits define the limits of allowable or expected variation in performance (often two to three times the standard deviation from the mean initially) and may be used to assess the results of ongoing monitoring. As long as performance remains between the upper and lower control limits, action is not necessary to address the variations that occur over time. However, performance above or below the control limits is referred to as special variation and prompts assessment as to what factor(s) resulted in the special variation and should result in actions being taken to

● address the impact of these factors over time. For example, within an organization training medical residents, the number of pharmacists' interventions as documented on a control chart might spike upward around July 1st, corresponding to the start date for the new residents. Although the organization may have limited opportunity to stagger starting dates, specific aspects of its orientation process could be enhanced to improve initial performance. As actions are taken to address factors resulting in special variations and the overall variability is reduced, control limits should narrow.[37] An example of a control chart with limits appears in Appendix 14–2.

● ❾ *Performance, as demonstrated by data collected in the performance improvement process, not meeting the defined standard or threshold, or falling outside the control limits (for ongoing or follow-up assessments) indicates that intervention to improve performance is necessary.* In some cases, performance outside the defined parameters may, upon review, be acceptable to the oversight group. This usually results from expectations being set too high (e.g., that the rate of adverse effects with any agent will be 0%) or when the criteria fail to include the appropriate exceptions. When this occurs, the multidisciplinary oversight group must agree that the level of performance is acceptable and that intervention is not necessary. These decisions must be clearly documented in meeting minutes or summaries of results. If this is not done, regulatory bodies may infer that the organization chose to ignore the findings of the evaluation, thus failing to meet the quality improvement requirements.

Data collection

● Prior to the initiation of data collection, the multidisciplinary oversight group must approve the topic selection, criteria, patient selection process, sample size, sampling method (e.g., all consecutive patients, intermittent sampling, random sampling), evaluation time frame, data collection method, and standards of performance.[24] It may be appropriate to distribute the approved criteria as an educational tool prior to data collection. Although this may address some performance issues prior to data collection and result in less dramatic results, it may support the ultimate goal of improving care and do so in a more expedient manner. In this situation, if there is a need to document the overall impact of a MUE effort, collection of baseline performance data, even as criteria are being final-

● ized and approved, can provide a more accurate representation of before and after. If at any point problems are identified in the criteria or indicators, or with any component of the evaluation, the issue should be brought back to the oversight group and modifications made as appropriate. Bringing necessary modifications back to the oversight group ensures that the MUE is conducted based on its guidance and approval and helps to ensure its support of the results and recommendations resulting from the MUE. This step is not unusual but can often be avoided through careful preparation and review of criteria early in the MUE process.

The timing of data collection can be influenced by seasonal variations in the types of care provided (e.g., increased frequency of pneumonia in the winter months), systems issues (e.g., construction, implementation of new computer systems, initiation of new services), and personnel issues (e.g., the influx of new health professional graduates and medical house staff that occurs during the summer months, staff absences during vacation or flu seasons). Therefore, the time frame for data collection, both in duration and time of year, should be considered in the planning process. For example, an assessment of care provided to patients with pneumonia is usually best performed during the winter months when this diagnosis is more frequent, while an assessment of the management of near-drowning may be more appropriate during the summer months. The longer the data collection period, the more likely various fluctuations in quality of care will be identified.

Retrospective data collection was used primarily in the era of AUR and DUR. This method involved reviewing the patient's medical record after discharge. It allowed data collection to be scheduled when convenient or when staff was available, but was totally dependent on documentation in the medical record. If an opportunity for improvement was identified, there was no opportunity to improve that particular patient's care; it would only help future patients.

Concurrent data collection occurs while the patient is still actively receiving the medication, but after the first dose is dispensed or administered. Data sources other than the medical record are available (e.g., staff or patient interviews) and there is an opportunity to improve patient care while the patient is receiving it. Based on complete information, results may be more complete as well as more accurate.[43] However, the need for data collection is constant and must occur within a specific time frame, which is not always convenient. This often results in an increased number of personnel being involved in the data collection process and increased inconsistency.

Prospective evaluation occurs before the patient receives the first dose of medication and is initiated whenever an order for the medication is generated. Simple prospective evaluations can be at least partially automated and are likely to become more common. An example of this is a clinical information system that generates a warning to the pharmacist or prescriber if the dose of a drug is outside the normal limits based on a patient's organ function. Clinical judgment must also be applied in many of these settings.

In systems with computerized prescriber order entry, the system itself can drive prescribing to comply with guidelines and standards by limiting prescribing options or directing users to specific therapy. In some cases, the system can report instances where prescribers attempt to prescribe a medication outside established limits. These limits are usually developed by the P&T committee, optimally as the agent is being considered for addition to the formulary, and fall into three general categories: diagnosis, prescriber, and medication specific. Diagnosis-based limits may define the allowable indications for use or may drive the use of an agent under a specific protocol approved by the committee.

Prescriber limits may restrict the use of an agent to a specific subset of prescribers (e.g., infectious disease or critical care specialists). Medication-specific limits can designate approved dosage regimens (e.g., disallow IV push promethazine), frequency of administration (e.g., once-daily dosing of ceftriaxone), and duration of therapy (e.g., no more than 10 doses or days of therapy).

Prospective evaluations that are not automated are the most cumbersome to implement because the evaluation must occur promptly every time an order is initiated to avoid therapy delays. This requires personnel to be available to collect data and report results at all times and force immediate interaction between practitioners. This approach offers the greatest opportunity for intervention and education, but also increases the risk for potentially negative interactions with prescribers and other health professionals, and can result in therapy delays. Furthermore, it is essential that the interventions made as part of the prospective evaluation are documented in order to evaluate workload, effectiveness of the interventions, and that outcomes are assessed in some manner.

Limiting the number of data collectors or automating data collection is valuable in maintaining consistency. When multiple data collectors are involved, it becomes even more important to have clear, explicit criteria that are not subject to interpretation.

The selection of patients or cases for inclusion in the evaluation should be determined and approved by the oversight group prior to data collection. It is essential that the selection be unbiased, consistent, and representative of the care provided. Sample size should be based on the size of the patient population. It has been suggested that for frequently occurring events a sample of at least 5% of cases be used, and for events occurring less frequently that a minimum of 30 cases be assessed.[44]

The term *target drug program* is often used to refer to programs that evaluate the use of a medication or group of medications on an ongoing basis. Within these programs, interventions are usually made at the time of discovery based on established criteria or guidelines. For example, it may be determined that one target drug program is set up to check whether patients being discharged from the intensive care unit have their medications switched from IV to oral, whenever possible. In that case, if the person checking on compliance with what has been done notes that a patient is still receiving IV medications, that person would contact the prescriber to try to get the medications changed to the oral route. It is important that these interventions are documented by practitioners and are periodically assessed by the multidisciplinary oversight group in order to determine the continued need for and appropriateness of the program.

Confidentiality is a key component of all quality improvement initiatives, including MUE.[15] It is important that the entire MUE program is identified as a performance-improvement activity. This helps to ensure that the information collected as part the program is legally protected and/or not discoverable. Although regulations vary from state to state (check with attorneys in your area), in most situations access by attorneys or courts to data generated from a performance-improvement initiative is restricted in legal cases. Within the program, individual patients and practitioners should usually be identified in some manner other than their actual name in order to ensure anonymous review, although it is necessary that identification data be available in cases where additional actions necessitate its use (e.g., checking charts for details, implementing corrective actions that involve discussing actions with practitioners who do something outside of the criteria). Many institutions use medical record numbers and codes assigned to individual prescribers within reports. It is also important not to inadvertently identify a practitioner. For example, if the results of an evaluation are reported by practitioner specialty (e.g., pediatrics, pediatric infectious disease) and there are only one or two practitioners in certain subspecialties, the practitioner has essentially been identified for the small subspecialty area.

Ultimately, practitioner-specific reports should be generated in most cases, as The Joint Commission requires that information related to medication use be considered in the reappointment/recredentialing of medical staff. Following peer review, the practitioner name may be revealed only to those responsible for the reappointment/recredentialing functions. Medical department chairpersons usually carry out this function. An example of a practitioner-specific report appears in Appendix 14–5.

Data analysis

The multidisciplinary oversight group should conduct the analysis of results. Reports should compare actual performance with expectations defined by the standards (or thresholds or control limits) established and approved prior to data collection. Performance not meeting standards (or threshold or control limits) may be considered opportunities for improvement. Alternatively, the oversight group may determine that the standards were too rigorous, that unforeseen exceptions were encountered, and/or that actual performance falls within current acceptable standards of practice. Specific corrective actions should be recommended for all identified opportunities for improvement (e.g., for all criteria statements for which the standard of performance was not met) whenever possible. The need for and nature of follow-up should also be assessed based on the frequency, prevalence, and/or severity of the issue. For example, if an evaluation of the management of pneumonia identified no issues with drug selection, but did identify an unacceptable delay in time to first dose of antibiotic (e.g., greater than 2 hours after admission), the follow-up evaluation could focus on the time to first dose and not assess antibiotic selection. Furthermore, if this issue was identified in patients admitted to a particular unit, then the follow-up could focus on assessing and documenting improvement in only that unit.

Often, a multidisciplinary group does not perform the actual data analysis. In this situation, the findings and actions must be reviewed and approved by the appropriate multidisciplinary group prior to the initiation of any corrective action or distribution of the results.

Computer software programs (e.g., relational databases and spreadsheets) can be very helpful in collecting data, managing data, and reporting results.[24,45-47] Handheld devices, bar code technology, proprietary software products, and computer systems used within the organization's clinical departments can be employed as tools to assist in patient identification, data collection and analysis, and documentation.[48]

The report to the oversight group should contain the rationale for the topic selection, team members involved in the evaluation, a description of the patient population evaluated, any selection criteria used, a copy of the criteria/indicators, discussion of the results, identification of likely causes for performance improvement opportunities identified, and recommendations for corrective action and follow-up evaluation. An example is provided in Appendix 14–6. In most settings, delineation of results on a practitioner-specific basis is not appropriate at this level. The exception would be if the practice of only a small subset of practitioners consistently fell outside the criteria. In this situation, some sort of code (e.g., Physician A or Physician 28) should be used instead of physicians' actual names.

Interventions and corrective actions

The key to quality improvement is improving the process and, ultimately, the results, not blaming an individual or group of individuals. Steps to improve performance or avoid similar outcomes in the future fall into three categories: educational interventions, restrictive interventions, and process changes. Educational interventions are most appropriate when knowledge deficits contribute to performance outside the criteria. They are most effective when they are directed personally, take place soon after the problem occurs, the educator is a peer or superior of the person being educated, and when the education is supported in the literature or by practice standards.[49] One-on-one or group discussion of results, letters, newsletters, computerized order-entry educational screens, protocols, or guidelines, and presentation via quality improvement channels are examples of educational approaches.[50,51] Generally, educational interventions incorporated into ongoing processes (e.g., education screens in computer order-entry systems) are more effective while one-time efforts (e.g., newsletters) may not have a sustained effect. In many situations, educational interventions are the most palatable.[52]

Restrictive approaches may involve special ordering procedures, compliance with guidelines for use, consultation with a specialty service, or formulary restrictions. The impact of restrictive interventions often reverses when the restrictions are removed.[53] Restrictive interventions are perhaps most effective when used to establish appropriate practice patterns when an agent is first made available for use within the organization.

Process changes incorporate the correction into routine practice. This approach may involve changes in policy or procedures, implementation of new services, acquisition of new equipment, changes in staffing, or generation of regular notifications, and so forth when practice does not appear to meet standards. As clinical information and physician order-entry systems become more sophisticated, process changes can be built directly into the prescribing, dispensing, and administering processes.

Disciplinary actions against individuals are not commonly employed as an intervention; however, when individuals refuse to modify their behavior, discipline may eventually be required. Discipline may include placing limits on an individual's activities and responsibilities or termination of employment. When possible, punitive actions should be avoided, because they can result in loss of acceptance of quality improvement efforts and fear of retribution.

Communication of MUE-related information is important and must be done carefully. Communication of the purpose of the evaluation and the significance of its outcomes should be reported to all groups involved in or impacted by the process. If a process is changed based on MUE results, the reason for the change should be explained. If, as a result of a MUE, prescribers will be required to change the way they prescribe a medication or nurses will no longer be able to access a medication as they had in the past, the reason for the change should be communicated along with the announcement of the change. Confidentiality of patient information (e.g., names and other identifiers) must be maintained. The identity of practitioners (physicians, pharmacists, nurses) must be revealed only in information provided for use by managers or designated peer-practitioners for assessment of personal performance.

Follow-up

Follow-up evaluation should occur within a reasonable time frame after completion of the initial evaluation and completion of the corrective action. Follow-up is designed to assess the effectiveness of the intervention. The same criteria, standards, and sample should be used for the follow-up assessment as in the initial evaluation. Exceptions to this rule should be made if there was a problem with the initial criteria, standards, and sample; the standard of practice changes in the interim; or there is an opportunity to focus on a subset of the original data elements or patient population. For example, if issues were only found in the administration component of the use of a medication (and not in the prescribing, dispensing, or monitoring components) or only in a specific age group, follow-up evaluation could focus on these issues or populations rather than repeating the broader assessment performed initially.

MUE has been criticized as being heavy handed and non-patient focused, and for not addressing the issue of accountability for provision of care based on a unique body of knowledge.[4] If the approach termed MUE is utilized in its true spirit, many of these challenges are addressed. MUE is a truly multidisciplinary, process-oriented approach to evaluate the quality of medication use. The process goes beyond numbers and percentages to identify opportunities for improvement and, more importantly, to improve the quality of care.

Quality in Drug Information

Quality standards for drug information practice have not been established to date, and quality assessment techniques used in drug information practice vary greatly among practice sites.[54-57] Several studies have found inconsistencies in the quality of drug information practice and have called for increased emphasis on quality and the development of practice standards.[58-60] Most drug information services conduct some form of quality assessment based on the scope of service provided by that center and preestablished levels of acceptable performance. Quality assessment is usually conducted on the responses provided to drug information requests, medical literature search and evaluation processes, availability, accuracy and timeliness of drug information resources, and the quality of materials produced by the drug information center staff (e.g., monographs, newsletters, continuing education programs). Although some quality assessment processes are conducted concurrently, most assessments are done retrospectively, often by randomly sampling drug information requests, monographs, and so forth. Furthermore, assessments may be performed via peer review or may be performed by the director of the service. Currently, no standards have been developed for this process.

Assessment of the quality of responses to drug information inquiries may include components such as timeliness, completeness, and appropriateness of response, and the method of communication of the response. Additionally, aspects such as documentation of search terms, references utilized, and the availability of appropriate background or patient-specific information may also be assessed. This assessment may be carried out internally based on standards of practice at the site. This usually offers the advantage of peer review by practitioners skilled in these functions. Another method is to poll those using the service about the quality of service and response received. This approach is hampered because consumers of the response are rarely able to assess the quality or appropriateness of the search strategy utilized to formulate the response they received in lieu of performing the search themselves or being present while the search is performed. An example assessment tool appears in Appendix 14–7. Questions that are often asked in the process of assessing drug information responses include

- Is the response correct and appropriate to the situation presented?
- Is the response provided promptly?
- Does the response completely address the question posed?
- Is the response communicated appropriately?
- Are search terms and references appropriately documented?
- Is the response clear, concise, and appropriate for the clinical situation?
- If follow-up was appropriate, was it provided?

The search process itself can be assessed by evaluation of the appropriate depth and breadth of resources used, the timeliness of the resources accessed, and the search strategy. This process can also assess documentation issues, the application of literature evaluation skills to the information, and resources used by the practitioner completing the search.

Drug information practitioners are often responsible for assessing and recommending drug information resources available within the organization. These resources may include printed references such as handbooks, textbooks, or educational materials, or electronic resources such as large search engines or Internet Web sites. This process should assess whether the appropriate information resources are available based on the scope of care provided and expertise of the practitioners, and whether the resources contain accurate and timely information that can be applied in clinical situations. Available primary, secondary, and tertiary resources should be evaluated based on established standards. The explosion of medical information on the Internet has created new challenges in evaluating drug and medical information resources. Because there are currently no regulations on the content of Internet sites, caution must be used when utilizing these resources to support clinical decision making. With the number of Web sites expanding faster than most practitioners can assess their content and editorial policies (if any), it has become increasingly difficult for drug information practitioners to stay abreast of those sites that offer legitimate and validated information compared to those offering only conjecture and opinion. Information obtained from other sources including manufacturers' drug information services should also be assessed. See Chapter 3 for further information on assessing information.

A final component of quality relates to material produced by the drug information service. This includes newsletters, drug monographs, and guidelines developed by the service. Most measure quality related to the accuracy, timeliness, and clinical applicability of such documents. Unfortunately, more time is often spent assessing the quality of grammar and writing style than devoted to clinical content and interpretation. Once again, Chapters 4 and 5 provide further information on assessing the quality of the material itself.

Conclusion

The focus on quality in health care has increased significantly in the past decade and has become a major initiative among governmental agencies and accreditation organizations. Within organizations, the emphasis has shifted from departmental efforts to multidisciplinary efforts related to key processes reflecting the move to continuous quality improvement. Within this context, the role of the pharmacist in quality improvement functions related to the medication use process has expanded. A practical working knowledge of total quality management principles is essential for pharmacists to contribute to and lead initiatives to improve patient care.

Self-Assessment Questions

1. The founding father of quality improvement is:
   a. J.C. Penney
   b. The Joint Commission
   c. Walter Shewart
   d. W. Edward Deming

2. The PDCA model of quality improvement stands for:
   a. Prepare, Develop, Calculate, Assess
   b. Produce, Design, Cost-Control, Act
   c. Plan, Develop, Check, Assess
   d. Plan, Do, Check, Act
   e. None of the above

3. Quality assurance or quality control is a proactive technique that is focused on the entire process.
   a. True
   b. False

4. Total quality management (TQM) can best be described as:
   a. Statistical
   b. Data driven
   c. People focused
   d. Improves quality by limiting variation
   e. a, b, and c
   f. a, b, and d

5. Examples of tools used in continuous quality improvement include:
   a. Brainstorming
   b. Pareto charts
   c. Scatter diagrams
   d. Control charts
   e. All of the above

6. In the Six Sigma quality method, defects are eliminated to improve quality to near perfection or:
   a. 90% defect-free
   b. 95% defect-free
   c. 99.837% defect-free
   d. 99.99966% defect-free
   e. 100% defect-free

7. Problems associated with quality in health care can fall into three main categories best described as:
   a. Overuse, underuse, and misuse
   b. Overuse, underuse, and lack of availability
   c. Overuse, practitioner error, and misuse
   d. Lack of availability, practitioner error, and high costs

8. The Joint Commission is a governmental agency charged with the legal enforcement of U.S. laws governing quality in health care.
   a. True
   b. False

9. Medication use evaluation (MUE) is primarily used to:
   a. Assess the quality of medication use within the organization based on established criteria.
   b. Compare the outcomes of different therapeutic alternatives.
   c. Compare the quality of care provided by two different physician teams.
   d. All of the above.

10. MUE topics are selected based on all of the following *except*:
    a. The potential to improve patient outcomes.
    b. The process to be assessed is known to be problem prone.
    c. The potential to directly impact the cost to the organization.
    d. The process to be assessed is known to be high risk.

11. You have been asked to conduct a MUE focused on the use of an inhaled medication used to treat asthma. Who should you ask to participate in planning and conducting the evaluation?
    a. Medical staff who are frequent prescribers
    b. Nursing personnel
    c. Respiratory therapists
    d. Emergency department staff
    e. All of the above

12. Identify the criteria statement(s) that could be problematic during data collection and analysis of results. "The antibiotic is":
    a. Initiated in a timely manner.
    b. Selected based on standards of practice.
    c. Changed from intravenous to oral on day 3.
    d. All of the above statements could be problematic.

13. All of the following are true *except*:
    a. Retrospective data collection offers no opportunity to improve care in the cases evaluated.
    b. During concurrent data collection, the medical record is the only source of information.
    c. Prospective evaluation takes place before the patient receives the first dose of the medication under evaluation.
    d. Prospective evaluation offers the greatest opportunity for intervention and education.

14. Which of the following is *true* regarding MUE interventions?
    a. Educational interventions work best when they take place long after the event.
    b. The impact of restrictive interventions does not reverse when the restriction is removed.
    c. Educational interventions are most effective when they are based on sound clinical evidence.
    d. None of the above.

15. The benefits of the oversight group developing an annual MUE plan include:
    a. There is the opportunity to redirect efforts based on changes in the scope of care.
    b. The group can ensure that a broad-spectrum antibiotic is evaluated at least twice a year.
    c. They can avoid completing follow-up evaluations resulting from prior MUEs.
    d. They can avoid performing evaluations that, over time, assess the breadth of care within the organization.

REFERENCES

1. Goldstone J. The role of quality assurance versus continuous quality improvement. J Vasc Surg. 1998;28(2):378-80.
2. Decker MD. The application of continuous quality improvement to healthcare. Infect Control Hosp Epidemiol. 1992;13(4):226-9.

3. Institute of Medicine. To Err Is Human: Building a Safer Health System. Washington, DC: National Academy Press; 2000.

4. Enright SM, Flagstad MS. Quality and outcome: pharmacy's professional imperative. Am J Hosp Pharm. 1991;48:1908-11.

5. Zellmer WA. Symposium: opportunity for pharmacy leadership in integrated health care systems. Am J Health-Syst Pharm. 1996;53(4):3S-4S.

6. Costello RB, editor. The American Heritage College Dictionary. Boston (MA): Houghton Mifflin Company; 1997.

7. Jablonski JR. Implementing TQM. Competing in the Nineties Through Total Quality Management. 2nd ed. Albuquerque (NM): Technical Management Consortium, Inc.; 1992.

8. Decker MD. Continuous quality improvement. Infect Control Hosp Epidemiol. 1992;13(2):165-9.

9. Chambers DW. TQM: the essential concepts. J Am Coll Dent. 1998;65(2):6-13.

10. Dorodny VS. Quality and caring: a fad or a religion? Hosp Pharm. 1997;32(3):316, 320, 325-6.

11. iSixSigma.com [home page on the Internet]. Bainbridge Island (WA): iSixSigma LCC; c2000-03 [cited 2010 June 10]. Avalable from: http://www.isixsigma.com/.

12. Relman AS. Assessment and accountability. The third revolution in medical care. N Engl J Med. 1988;319(18):1220-2.

13. Chassin MR. Quality improvement nearing the 21st century: prospects and perils. Am J Med Qual. 1996;11(1):4S-7S.

14. Cohen MR. Cooperative approaches to medication error management. Top Hosp Pharm Manag. 1991;11(1):53-65.

15. Tremblay J. Creating an appropriate climate for drug use review. Am J Hosp Pharm. 1981;38(2):212-5.

16. O'Malley C. Quality measurement for health systems: accreditation and report cards. Am J Health-Syst Pharm. 1997;54:1528-35.

17. Ente BH. The Joint Commission's agenda for change. Curr Concept Hosp Pharm Manag. 1989 (Summer):7-14.

18. Omnibus Budget Reconciliation Act of 1987. Section 843.60, Level A requirement; Pharmacy services. 54 FR1989:5359-69.

19. Omnibus Budget Reconciliation Act of 1990. Section 1903(I)10(B)(g) Drug Use Review and (A) Prospective Drug Review.

20. Navarro RP. DUR applications in managed care. Med Interface. 1995;8(3):67-8.

21. Briesacher D, DuChane J. Drug utilization review in the managed care environment. Med Interface. 1995;8(3):72-8.

22. Feinberg JL. Meeting the mandate for quality assurance through drug-use evaluation. Consult Pharm. 1991;6:611-20.

23. Stolar MH. Drug use review: operational definitions. Am J Hosp Pharm. 1978;35:76-8.

24. ASHP guidelines on medication-use evaluation. American Society of Health System Pharmacists. Am J Health-Syst Pharm. 1996;53(16):1953-5.

25. Nadzam DM. Development of medication-use indicators by the Joint Commission on Accreditation of Healthcare Organizations. Am J Hosp Pharm. 1991;48:1925-30.

26. Cousins DD. Medication Use: A Systems Approach to Reducing Errors. Chicago (IL): Joint Commission on Accreditation of Healthcare Organizations; 1998.

27. DHEW Task Force on Prescription Drugs: Final Report. Washington, DC: U.S. Department of Health, Education, and Welfare; 1969.

28. Gutshall EL, Davidson HE, Ninno SD, editors. Medication Usage Evaluation: Primer. 3rd ed. Norfolk (VA): Insight Therapeutics, LLC; 1999.

29. Todd MW, Keith TD, Foster MT. Development and implementation of a comprehensive, criteria-based drug-use review program. Am J Hosp Pharm. 1987;44:529-35.

30. New accreditation process model for 1994 and beyond. Am J Hosp Pharm. 1993;50:1111-2, 1121.

31. Flagstad MS, Williams RB. Assuming responsibility for improving quality. Am J Hosp Pharm. 1991;48:1898.

32. The Joint Commission on Accreditation of Hospitals. 1990 AMH. Accreditation Manual for Hospitals. Chicago (IL): Joint Commission on Accreditation of Hospitals; 1989.

33. Covington TR, Alexander VL. Drug Use Evaluation: The Fundamentals. Indianapolis (IN): Eli Lilly & Co.; 1991.

34. Schaff RL, Schumock GT, Nadzam DM. Development of The Joint Commission's indicators for monitoring the medication use system. Hosp Pharm. 1991;26:326-9, 350.

35. Bernstein SJ, Hilborne LH. Clinical indicators: the road to quality care? Jt Comm J Qual Improv. 1993:19(11):501-9.

36. Clark TR, Gruber J, Sey M. Revisiting drug regimen review, part III: a systematic approach. Consult Pharm. 2003;18:656-66.

37. Angaran DM. Selecting, developing, and evaluating indicators. Am J Hosp Pharm. 1991;48:1931-7.

38. Knapp DA. Development of criteria for drug utilization review. Clin Pharmacol Ther. 1991;50(Part 2):600-3.

39. Model drug use review criteria. Year one of HCFA project, model for developing strategies for outpatient drug use review. Center on Drugs and Public Policy, University of Maryland at Baltimore, Baltimore (MD). February 1991.

40. Screening criteria for outpatient drug use review. Final report of HCFA project, model for developing methodological strategies for outpatient drug use review. Center on Drugs and Public Policy, University of Maryland at Baltimore, Baltimore, MD. December 1992.

41. Melby MJ. A mid-sized hospital's experience in indicator data collection. Am J Hosp Pharm. 1991;48:1937-40.

42. Threshold vs. standards. QRC Advisor. 1988;5(2):5.

43. Makela EH, Davis SK, Piveral K, Miller WA, Pleasants RA, Gadsden RH Sr, et al. Effect of data collection method on results of serum digoxin concentration audit. Am J Hosp Pharm. 1988;45:126-30.

44. What is an adequate sample? QRC Advisor. 1985 (Aug);1:4-5.

45. Grasela TH, Walawander CA, Kennedy, Jolson HM. Capability of hospital computer systems in performing drug-use evaluations and adverse event monitoring. Am J Hosp Pharm. 1993;50:1889-95.

46. Zarowitz BJ, Petitta A, Mlynarek M, Touchette M, Peters M, Long P, et al. Bar-code technology applied to drug-use evaluation. Am J Hosp Pharm. 1993;50:935-9.

47. Burnakis TG. Facilitating drug-use evaluation with spreadsheet software. Am J Hosp Pharm. 1989;46:84-8.

48. Libby D, Grove C, Adams M. Collaborative use of informatics among hospitals to benchmark medication use processes. Jt Comm J Qual Improv. 1997;23:626-52.

49. Soumerai SB, McLaughlin TJ, Avorn J. Improving drug prescribing in primary care: a critical analysis of the experimental literature. Milbank Quarterly. 1989;67:268-317.

50. Avorn J, Soumeri SB, Taylor W. Reduction of incorrect antibiotic prescribing through a structured educational order form. Arch Intern Med. 1991;151:1825-32.

51. Kowalsky SF, Echols RM, Peck F. Preprinted order sheet to enhance antibiotic prescribing and surveillance. Am J Hosp Pharm. 1982;39:1528-9.

52. Pierson JF, Alexander MR, Kirking DM, Solomon DK. Physician's attitudes toward drug-use evaluation interventions. Am J Hosp Pharm. 1990;47:388-90.

53. Himmelberg CJ, Pleasants RA, Weber DJ, Kessler JM, Samsa GP, Spivey JM, et al. Use of antimicrobial drugs in adults before and after removal of a restriction policy. Am J Hosp Pharm. 1991;48:1220-7.

54. Restino MS, Knodel LC. Drug information quality assurance program used to appraise students' performance. Am J Hosp Pharm. 1992;49(6):1425-9.

55. Wheeler-Usher DH, Hermann FF, Wanke LA. Problems encountered in using written criteria to assess drug information responses. Am J Hosp Pharm. 1990;47(4):795-7.

56. Moody ML. Revising a drug information center quality assurance program to conform to Joint Commission standards. Am J Hosp Pharm. 1990;47(4):792-4.

57. Smith CH, Sylvia LM. External quality assurance committee for drug information services. Am J Hosp Pharm. 1990;47(4):787-91.

58. Halbert MR, Kelly WN, Miller DE. Drug information centers: lack of generic equivalence. Drug Intell Clin Pharm. 1977;11:728-35.

59. Beaird SL, Coley RM, Blunt JR. Assessing the accuracy of drug information responses from drug information centers. Ann Pharmacother. 1994;28(6):707-11.

60. Calis KA, Anderson DW, Auth DA, Mays, DA, Turcasso NM, Meyer CC, et al. Quality of pharmacotherapy consultations provided by drug information centers in the United States. Pharmacotherapy. 2002;20:830-6.

Chapter Fifteen

Medication Misadventures I: Adverse Drug Reactions

Philip J. Gregory • Zara Risoldi Cochrane

Learning Objectives

After completing this chapter, the reader will be able to

- Define adverse drug reactions.
- Explain methods for determining the probability and causality of an adverse drug reaction.
- Classify adverse drug reactions based on type and severity.
- Describe examples of adverse drug reaction monitoring systems that have been implemented successfully.
- Explain the use of technology in adverse drug reaction monitoring and reporting.
- Use The Joint Commission and the American Society of Health-System Pharmacists guidelines to implement an adverse drug reaction reporting program.

Key Concepts

1. An adverse drug reaction is any unexpected, unintended, undesired, or excessive response to a medicine.
2. One of the first steps in establishing an ADR program is to define what the institution or facility categorizes as ADRs.
3. Several algorithms have been published that try to incorporate information about an ADR into a more objective form.

④ ADR surveillance serves primarily to provide early signals about possible problems.

⑤ Communication is a critical component throughout the adverse drug reaction monitoring process.

⑥ Technology plays an important role in monitoring, identifying, and minimizing adverse drug reactions.

Introduction to Adverse Drug Reactions

The terminology surrounding adverse drug reactions (ADRs) is often confusing. All adverse drug events (ADEs), ADRs, and medication errors fall under the umbrella of medication misadventures. Medication misadventure is a very broad term, referring to any iatrogenic hazard or incident associated with medications. An *ADE* is the next broadest term and refers to any injury caused by a medicine. An ADE includes all ADRs, such as allergic or idiosyncratic reactions, as well as medication errors that result in harm to a patient.[1-5] ADRs and medication errors are the most specific terms.

① *ADRs refer to any unexpected, unintended, undesired, or excessive response to a medicine.* A medication error is any preventable event that has the potential to lead to inappropriate medication use or patient harm.[1] Figure 15–1 shows one way of graphically classifying these terms. Many of these concepts will be explored in greater depth elsewhere in this text. This chapter focuses only on ADRs, highlighting pertinent definitions, classifications, reporting systems, and methods to minimize such events.

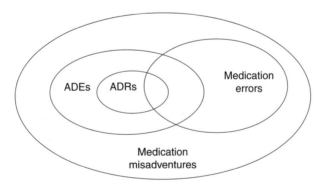

Figure 15–1. Relationship among medication misadventures, adverse drug events, medication errors, and adverse drug reactions. (*Adapted with permission from Bates DW, et al. Relationship between medication and errors and adverse drug events. J Gen Intern Med. 1995;April:10(4):199-205.*)

All medications, including the inactive ingredients of a product, are capable of producing adverse effects.[6] Adverse drug reactions account for about 5% to 15% of all hospital admissions, cause patients to lose confidence in their health care providers, and lead to a significant increase in morbidity and mortality.[7-11] This makes ADRs the fourth to sixth leading cause of death in the United States, just after heart disease.[9]

ADRs have economic consequences as well. These reactions result in an annual cost of $5 to $7 billion to the U.S. health care system. Each hospital in the United States spends up to $5.6 million annually as a result of adverse drug events. After experiencing an ADR, patients spend an average of 8 to 12 days longer in the hospital, increasing the cost of their hospitalization by $16,000 to $24,000.[11]

The incidence of ADRs for hospitalized patients has been reported to be as high as 28%. Of course, ADRs do not affect hospitalized patients alone. Approximately 20% of the ambulatory population receiving medications suffers from ADRs.[10] These outpatient events do not always result in hospitalization, but certainly affect morbidity and patient quality of life. Health care professionals agree that these estimates are somewhat conservative because many ADRs go undetected, unreported, and untreated.[10] One review concluded that only 2% to 4% of all ADRs, and fewer than 10% of serious ADRs, are ever reported.[11] One reason for these low percentages is that patients and health care professionals are not always adequately informed about medications and their potential for adverse events. Many countries, including the United States, have developed systems to encourage the reporting of ADRs. In addition, The Joint Commission, an accrediting body, requires hospitals to have a mechanism in place to monitor ADRs. Many hospitals have developed extensive programs that provide a foundation for the monitoring of adverse reactions, including a warning system to prevent further problems. The sharing of information about ADRs between health care practitioners and groups is vital to the success of these programs. In addition, the networking of ADR information can help in providing a useful database for the recognition or prevention of future ADRs.

Several agencies and professional organizations across the country contribute efforts to minimize the occurrence and impact of ADRs. Some of the key organizations include the Food and Drug Administration (FDA), The Joint Commission, the World Health Organization (WHO), and the American Society of Health-System Pharmacists (ASHP). See Table 15-1.

TABLE 15–1. ORGANIZATIONS INVOLVED IN PREVENTING ADVERSE DRUG EVENTS

Food and Drug Administration (FDA)	http://www.fda.gov
Joint Commission on Accreditation of Healthcare Organizations (JCAHO)	http://www.jcaho.org
World Health Organization (WHO)	http://www.who.int
Institute for Safe Medication Practices (ISMP)	http://www.ismp.org
The United States Pharmacopoeia (USP)	http://www.usp.org
American Society of Health-System Pharmacists (ASHP)	http://www.ashp.org

Despite the numerous organizations involved, efforts to minimize ADRs depend heavily on individual health care practitioners, including pharmacists, physicians, and nurses, to take measures to minimize ADRs and report events. Practitioners need to understand the potential for adverse drug reactions and be prepared to recognize and prevent such occurrences and minimize adverse outcomes.

Pharmacists play a pivotal role in the medication use process. Multiple studies have highlighted the tremendous impact individual pharmacists can have on minimizing ADRs.[12,13] In one study published in the *Journal of the American Medical Association*, pharmacists began participating in patient rounds in an intensive care unit. By implementing this measure, the hospital significantly reduced the incidence of ADRs and saved an estimated $270,000 per year.[12]

DEFINITIONS

❷ *One of the first steps in establishing an ADR program is to define what the institution or facility categorizes as ADRs.* There are many definitions for ADRs that have been described in the literature. Institutions, as well as clinicians, have used different definitions depending on their practice needs.

The WHO defines an ADR as "any noxious or unintended response to a drug that occurs at doses usually used for prophylaxis, diagnosis, or therapy of disease or for the modification of physiological function."[14]

The FDA definition of an ADR is any adverse event associated with the use of a drug in humans, whether or not considered drug related, including the following: adverse event occurring in the course of the use of a drug product in professional practice; an adverse event occurring from drug overdose, whether accidental or intentional; an adverse event occurring from drug abuse; an adverse event occurring from drug withdrawal; and any significant failure of expected pharmacologic action.[13] This definition is fairly broad and includes overdose situations as well as areas involving abuse.

The FDA goes on to define an unexpected drug reaction, which is what they would like to have reported, as one that is not listed in the current labeling for the drug as having been reported or associated with the use of the drug. This includes an ADR that may be symptomatically or pathophysiologically related to an ADR listed in the labeling, but may differ from the labeled ADR because of greater severity or specificity (e.g., abnormal liver function versus hepatic necrosis). An ADR may also be due to a drug interaction, defined as a pharmacologic response that cannot be explained by the action of a single drug, but is due to two or more drugs acting simultaneously.[13]

The use of unexpected in the language does limit the number of ADRs that the FDA would like health care professionals to report. This definition focuses on reporting the unusual, uncommon, or newly identified ADRs. Although the common or usual ADRs are relevant and important, they do not provide the FDA with additional information.

Edwards and Aronson propose another definition of ADRs: "An appreciably harmful or unpleasant reaction, resulting from an intervention related to the use of a medicinal product, which predicts hazard from future administration and warrants prevention or specific treatment, or alteration of the dosage regimen, or withdrawal of the product."[15]

Karch and Lasagna,[16] two prominent researchers in the area of ADRs, define a drug, an adverse event, and a patient drug exposure as

> Drug: a chemical substance or product available for an intended diagnostic, prophylactic or therapeutic purpose.
>
> Adverse Drug Reaction: any response to a drug which is noxious and unintended and which occurs at doses used in man for prophylaxis, diagnosis or therapy, excluding therapeutic failures. (As stated by the WHO, this definition excludes intentional and accidental poisoning as well as drug abuse situations.)
>
> Patient–Drug Exposure: a single patient receiving at least one dose of a given drug.

Many hospital programs use this definition because it excludes accidental poisonings as well as problems with drugs of abuse.

CAUSALITY AND PROBABILITY OF ADVERSE DRUG REACTIONS

One of the difficulties in defining an ADR is determining causality. Cause and effect is difficult to prove, in general, and ADRs are no exception. Many publications have dealt with this problem by developing definitions, algorithms, and questionnaires that try to determine the probability of a reaction. There are over 30 different published methods for assessing adverse drug reaction causality. They fall into three broad categories:[17]

1. Expert judgment/global introspection: This method involves the individual assessment of the event using previous knowledge and experience without using any form of standardized tool.
2. Algorithm: This method uses specific questions to assign a weighted score that helps determine the probability of causality in a given event.
3. Probabilistic: This method uses Bayesian approaches and epidemiological data to calculate and estimate the probability of causality.

To date, none of these attempts have been able to prove actual causality. These tools, however, are used to determine the probability that a particular drug caused an adverse event and are described in the following.

These algorithms and definitions use several key concepts.[15,18] Dechallenge and rechallenge are often discussed. Dechallenge occurs when the drug is discontinued and the patient is then monitored to determine whether the ADR abates or decreases in intensity. Rechallenge occurs when the drug is discontinued and, after the ADR abates, the drug is readministered in an attempt to elicit the response again. Dechallenge and rechallenge are effective means for establishing a strong case that the drug was responsible for the ADR. Unfortunately in clinical practice, a rechallenge may not be practical and may actually cause further harm to the patient. Patients who suffer a serious ADR may not be thrilled about experiencing the reaction again in the name of science. A rechallenge may not always be practical, but a dechallenge is often essential.

Another important factor to consider is the temporal relationship between the drug and the event. Does the time frame for the development of the ADR make sense? If there is literature on the ADR, does it describe a temporal relationship between the drug and the event? Medical literature and package inserts can be helpful in noting if a drug has been known to cause a certain type of reaction in a certain time frame in the past. Unfortunately, for rare or new ADRs the literature is not likely to be helpful, but this does not discount the fact that a reaction may have occurred.

Naranjo and associates[18] developed the following definitions to assist in determining the probability of an ADR:

> Definite ADR is a reaction that (1) follows a reasonable temporal sequence from administration of the drug, or in which the drug level has been established in body fluids or tissue; (2) follows a known response pattern to the suspected drug; (3) is confirmed by dechallenge; and (4) could not be reasonably explained by the known characteristics of the patient's clinical state.
>
> Conditional ADR is a reaction that (1) follows a reasonable temporal sequence from administration of the drug; (2) does not follow a known response pattern to the suspected drug; and (3) could not be reasonably explained by the known characteristics of the patient's clinical state.
>
> Doubtful ADR is any reaction that does not meet the criteria above.

❸ *Several algorithms have been published that try to incorporate information about an ADR into a more scientific form.* These algorithms determine the likelihood that the drug was responsible for the reaction and establish a rational and scientific approach to what previously required strictly clinical judgment. All of the algorithms are time-consuming and the results can vary according to the interpretation of multiple observers. In 1979, Kramer and coworkers[19] published a questionnaire composed of 56 yes or no questions (Appendix 15–1). This questionnaire includes sections about the patient's previous experience with the drug or related drugs, alternative etiologies, timing of events, drug concentrations, dechallenge, and rechallenge. Responses to each question are given a weighted value and these values are totaled. The total value then belongs to one of four categories: unlikely, possible, probable, or definite. One of the problems with this method is that clinicians can disagree on the weighted values because the user must make subjective judgments for some of the questions. Hutchinson and colleagues[20] evaluated the reproducibility and validity of the Kramer questionnaire. The authors concluded that although the questionnaire was cumbersome to use, the method described by Kramer was superior to clinical judgment alone. Another problem inherent with this questionnaire is that an unexpected ADR may not score well because of lack of literature or previous experience with the ADR. If the reaction is not universally accepted or is not in the most recent edition of the *Physicians' Desk Reference*, the reaction would score a zero in this section. Overall, however, the questionnaire provides professionals with the opportunity to use a standardized tool.

Naranjo and colleagues developed an alternative algorithm (Appendix 15–2). This algorithm has 10 questions. The questions involve the following areas: the temporal relationship, the pattern of response, dechallenge or administration of an antagonist, rechallenge, alternative causes, placebo response, drug level in the body fluids or tissue, dose-response relationship, previous patient experience with the drug, and confirmation by any other objective evidence. The answer to each question is assigned a score. The score is then totaled and placed into a category from definite to doubtful. The Naranjo algorithm also places emphasis on rechallenge and dechallenge, which may pose some problems in evaluating ADRs using this method. In the initial published report of this algorithm, Naranjo and colleagues tested the reproducibility and validity of the algorithm. Like the study by Kramer and associates, this algorithm was found to be a valid means of assessing ADRs. Today, this is one of the most commonly used methods to assess adverse drug reaction causality.

In 1982, Jones[21] published an algorithm that allows health care practitioners to answer a series of yes or no questions to determine if a true ADR occurred (Appendix 15–3). This type of format is similar to other published algorithms. The Jones algorithm is shorter and quicker to complete compared to Kramer's questionnaire.

All of the algorithms possess a certain degree of observer variability. However, all can be used to help determine whether an adverse event was precipitated by a certain drug or drug-drug combination. Michel and Knodel[22] compared the three algorithms by Kramer, Jones, and Naranjo. The study found that the Naranjo algorithm was simpler and less time-consuming, and compared favorably to the 56 questions asked by Kramer. The study found a higher correlation between the Naranjo algorithm and the Kramer questionnaire. Although there was agreement between the Naranjo and Jones algorithms, the correlation was not as high as that seen between the Naranjo and Kramer algorithms. The authors stated that more data were needed to support the use of the algorithm developed by Jones.

A Bayesian approach to assessing adverse reactions has also been developed by Lane.[23] Using the Bayesian approach, relevant information is collected and a quantitative measure of the odds that a particular drug caused a particular event is calculated. The Bayesian approach has the potential to be an outstanding tool for predicting populations that may be at higher risk for ADRs. The method needs further study, including determining whether the approach is applicable to the hospital environment.

In addition to these general methods for assessing adverse drug reaction causality, there are also methods for assessing specific types of adverse drug reactions. For example, different methods also exist for assessing drug-related liver toxicity.

Despite the abundance of tools available to help assess causality of adverse drug reactions, none of these methods have become the preferred or universally accepted method of assessment.

Case Study 15–1

A patient approaches you in the pharmacy. She explains that she recently began taking a dietary supplement called *ZygoControl Weight Loss*. She tells you that she began taking the product 6 weeks ago. Each time she took the product she says she felt like her heart was racing, she felt lightheaded, and her mouth felt dry. These symptoms last about 3 hours and then go away. She asks you if you think the product is causing these side effects. You research the product and find out that it contains high doses of caffeine and a stimulant called synephrine that is similar to ephedrine.

1. In this case, was there a dechallenge? If so, what happened when dechallenged?
2. Was there a rechallenge? Is so, what happened?
3. Was there a temporal relationship between taking this product and the reaction experienced?
4. Based on what you know about this product, is the reaction consistent with known pharmacology?
5. Do you think that this product *caused* this reaction?

CLASSIFICATION

Definitions and algorithms have also been used to classify the probability and severity of ADRs. Classification systems such as those developed by Naranjo, Kramer, and Jones have used the definite, probable, possible, and unlikely categories to establish the probability of ADRs. Other classification systems ranked the severity of ADRs from minor to severe.

One such classification system was developed by Karch and Lasagna, and classifies the severity of ADRs into minor, moderate, severe, and lethal as defined in the following.[15]

- *Minor:* no antidote, therapy, or prolongation of hospitalization required
- *Moderate:* requires a change in drug therapy, specific treatment, or an increase in hospitalization by at least one day

- *Severe:* potentially life threatening, causing permanent damage or requiring intensive medical care
- *Lethal:* directly or indirectly contributes to the death of the patient

The FDA classifies an ADR as serious when it results in death, is life threatening, causes or prolongs hospitalization, causes a significant persistent disability, results in a congenital anomaly, or requires intervention to prevent permanent damage.[24]

When developing an ADR monitoring program, these various systems can be used to determine probability (cause and effect) and severity of ADRs and help describe and quantify data.

MECHANISM OF ADVERSE DRUG REACTIONS

Karch and Lasagna also described various mechanisms for adverse drug reactions.[15] These mechanisms are related to the pharmacologic or pharmacodynamic aspects of drugs and can be used to classify the type of reaction that occurs.

- *Idiosyncrasy:* an uncharacteristic response of a patient to a drug, usually not occurring on administration
- *Hypersensitivity:* a reaction, not explained by the pharmacologic effects of the drug, caused by altered reactivity of the patient and generally considered to be an allergic manifestation
- *Intolerance:* a characteristic pharmacologic effect of a drug produced by an unusually small dose, so that the usual dose tends to induce a massive overaction
- *Drug interaction:* an unusual pharmacologic response that could not be explained by the action of a single drug, but was caused by two or more drugs
- *Pharmacologic:* a known, inherent pharmacologic effect of a drug, directly related to dose

When implementing an ADR program, these classifications can help health care practitioners to organize and present data. Potential causative drugs involved in ADRs can be listed, allowing trends to be followed over time. These trends can be used to change prescribing habits or alert the institution to potential problems. In addition, the data may also suggest the severity of reactions that are occurring and which medications cause the most severe reactions.

REPORTING

Well-designed programs that monitor ADRs, as well as network information to the medical community, are essential. ❹ *Gerald A. Faich, MD, MPH, Former Director, Office of Epidemiology and Biostatistics, Center for Drugs and Biologics, for the FDA, stated that*

"ADR surveillance serves primarily to provide early signals about possible problems." He further states: "Neither industry nor the FDA should consider its scientific job complete when a new drug is approved."[25] Faich explains the importance of postmarketing surveillance and the need to continually monitor drugs and report any adverse consequences. Postmarketing ADR reporting has been responsible for changes in prescribing as well as withdrawal of various drugs from the market.

FDA Reporting

Due to the limited size of studies required for the approval of a new drug entity, the FDA relies on postmarketing information to establish a better understanding of adverse events. Historically, some drugs have been approved by the FDA only to later be withdrawn from the market due to postmarketing adverse events. Pharmaceutical companies are required by the FDA to submit quarterly reports of all ADRs for the first 3 years that a drug is on the market as part of the postmarketing surveillance system.

The FDA was required to have a Spontaneous Reporting System (SRS) with the passage of the Kefauver-Harris Amendment of 1962 (due to limited numbers of study subjects, rare adverse effects could otherwise be missed). This program allows for an inexpensive monitoring system of ADRs for all drugs marketed in the United States.[26] All health care professionals and consumers can use this program to report ADRs.

The problem in the past has been the lack of voluntary reporting by the medical community. In a study of community-based physicians, only 57% were aware of the voluntary system of reporting.[27] In the past, the FDA utilized Form 1639 to allow anyone to report an adverse event through the SRS. However, in June 1993, the FDA switched to a new program called MedWatch: The FDA Medical Products Reporting Program. With this new program, the FDA receives reports via mailings, phone calls, faxes, and the Internet. Between June 1993 and September 30, 1993, the FDA received 1717 voluntary reports from pharmacists, physicians, nurses, risk managers, dentists, and other health and non-health professionals. Pharmacists provided 53% of the reports. Of the 1717 reports, 65% were ADEs and 3% were ADRs to biologics. To report a problem to the FDA, consumers and health care professionals can call 1-800-FDA-1088, fax a report to 1-800-FDA-0178, or enter a report via the Internet at http://www.fda.gov/medwatch. In addition, the Med-Watch Form, also known as FDA Form 3500, can be completed and mailed to the FDA (Appendix 15–4).[28] A unit of the FDA called the Central Triage Unit receives voluntary reports. This unit screens the reports and forwards them to the appropriate FDA program within 24 hours of receiving the report. In addition, they mail a letter to the sender acknowledging the report's receipt. The report becomes part of a database used by the agency to identify signals or warnings that would require further study or regulatory action. Like the previous FDA program, MedWatch is still interested in serious adverse events, which they describe as death, life-threatening events, hospitalization, disability, congenital anomaly, or requiring intervention to prevent permanent impairment or damage. The MedWatch program asks people to report an event even if they are not certain that the product was the cause.[29]

The MedWatch program does not overcome the lack of reporting due to a voluntary system. It is important to note that pharmaceutical manufacturers are required to report all adverse events to the FDA, whereas individual health care practitioners only do so voluntarily. Various explanations can account for the failure of practitioners to participate in the FDA program. Hoffman[29] best describes the lack of ADR reporting by physicians as follows:

1. Failure to detect the reaction due to a low level of suspicion
2. Fear of potential legal implications
3. Lack of training about drug therapy
4. Uncertainty about whether the drug causes the reaction
5. Lack of clear responsibility for reporting
6. Paperwork and time involved
7. No financial incentive to report
8. Unaware of reporting procedure or little understanding of it
9. Lack of readily available reporting forms
10. Desire to publish the report
11. Fear that a useful drug will be removed from the market or given a bad name
12. Complacency and lethargy
13. Guilty feelings because of patient harm
14. Reaction not worth reporting

Other explanations for the lack of reporting are that medical record personnel, whose job might be to categorize and report data, are not familiar with ADRs and/or their method of documentation. Therefore, the pharmacist can provide a valuable service by participating in the MedWatch program.

The FDA has recognized that voluntary postmarketing evaluations of drug safety data are not sufficient to identify serious adverse drug reactions. Recent drug-related adverse events related to drugs such as rofecoxib (Vioxx) and rosiglitazone (Avandia) are two prime examples of the insufficiency of the voluntary reporting system. The FDA, working with private companies as well as academic researchers, has developed new methodologies to get early detection signals about safety issues with medications. The FDA has developed additional pharmacovigilance methods as well as improving the spontaneous reporting system in order to apply these latest techniques. The FDA is using data mining approaches for more rapid identification of potential problems. Data mining is a statistical process that attempts to find a drug-associated event that appears more often in the databases than would normally be expected to occur in the general population. When a higher-than-expected event occurs, this is referred to as a signal detection. Again, statistics are used to identify these signals using both Bayesian and non-Bayesian methods. When an association is flagged in the system, the FDA then requires a clinical review involving experts to decide if any further action is needed for those events.[30]

With these new techniques, some hospitals have investigated pharmacovigilance methods for evaluating the safety profile of drugs at their institutions. The New York Presbyterian Hospital implemented a pharmacovigilance system that involved the electronic health record and used natural language computer processing with various statistical techniques that were used to establish associations between drugs and adverse events as well as cutoff thresholds. In the hospital's feasibility study, seven drug classes were evaluated for novel adverse events. The researchers believed that the use of a comprehensive unstructured data-monitoring program of electronic health records was a feasible option for computerized pharmacovigilance at a local health-system level. This study demonstrates that even local data mining and signal detection provide a mechanism for ADR reporting.[31]

The traditional randomized controlled clinical trial (RCT) is usually focused on efficacy implications of a therapy and not usually powered for relevant safety information. With this in mind, it is easy to see why adverse events may go undetected in these trials. It has been estimated that any adverse event that occurs in fewer than 1 in 10,000 people will not be detected with most RCTs. Therefore, some experts have recommended the use of what is known as a large, simple trial (LST) to increase sample sizes and to monitor larger numbers of participants. LSTs have less stringent eligibility criteria, and typically subjects are studied for shorter periods of time. LST designs still use randomization techniques and continue to have important safety monitoring thresholds. The larger sample sizes with the LST design provide more data for methods such as signal detection. In addition, the larger number of subjects also increases the probability of picking up adverse events that are less common.[32]

DIETARY SUPPLEMENTS

Dietary supplements including herbs, vitamins, minerals, and other so-called nutraceuticals are regulated much differently than pharmaceuticals. The most striking difference is that these supplements can reach pharmacies and grocery store shelves without FDA approval and without any proof of safety or effectiveness. Until recently, manufacturers of these products were not required to monitor the safety of their products through postmarketing surveillance, and they were not required to share information about safety with the FDA. However, the Dietary Supplement and Nonprescription Drug Consumer Protection Act of 2006 changed this. Manufacturers or marketers of dietary supplements who receive reports or information about severe adverse reactions related to their products are now required to share these reports with the FDA.[33]

Dietary supplements can and do cause ADRs. Many of these products have powerful pharmacological effects, and therefore they can cause ADRs. The medical literature contains many isolated case reports that describe ADRs related to dietary supplements. However, the exact incidence of ADRs with dietary supplements is not known.

An interesting case involves the herb ephedra, also known as *ma huang*. This herb was marketed as a dietary supplement and promoted primarily for weight loss and enhancing athletic performance. It received lots of negative media attention when a Minnesota football player died of heat exhaustion during a training session. It turned out that the football player was using ephedra for weight loss. Over a period of several years, there were well over 100 reports to the FDA of life-threatening ADRs linked to ephedra, including heart attacks, strokes, seizures, and death.

Finally, in March 2004, the FDA banned the sale of dietary supplements containing ephedra,[34] although this ban was lifted by a judge in 2010.[35] Still, the FDA could not prove that ephedra was the cause of these numerous ADRs. The FDA had to act based on the best available evidence. Because there were no reporting standards or requirements for manufacturers to collect data on their products' safety at this time, it would be unlikely that the FDA would ever have enough data to scientifically prove causality. The FDA's actions on ephedra will have long-lasting effects. It will ultimately set the precedent by which other cases against dietary supplements will be decided.

Currently, ADRs related to dietary supplements can be submitted through the FDA MedWatch program using the same approach that is used for prescription drugs. A new system specifically for collecting data about adverse reactions to dietary supplements is also available, called Natural Medicines Watch (http://www.naturalmedicineswatch.com). This system allows any consumer or health professional to complete an electronic form about an adverse event related to any dietary supplement. This system uses a database of over 60,000 commercially available dietary supplements that allows the user to easily select the correct product. Since many commercially available dietary supplements contain multiple ingredients, this system improves the reliability of adverse reaction reporting for supplements. The system is also integrated with drug information resources, such as the Natural Medicines Comprehensive Database (http://www.naturaldatabase.com), which improves accessibility for health care practitioners to the reporting functionality. All reports submitted through Natural Medicines Watch are also simultaneously shared with the FDA's MedWatch program.

IMPLEMENTING A PROGRAM

Prior to implementing an ADR program, the health care facility must educate its staff on the importance and significance of the program. The pharmacy department is in an excellent position to provide this education because of its involvement in the pharmacy and therapeutics (P&T) committee, pharmacokinetic dosing, drug utilization evaluation (DUE), and drug distribution. The pharmacy department can be an excellent resource for developing an ADR program, as well as providing data about ADRs to the P&T committee.

The Joint Commission and ASHP Guidelines

The Joint Commission requires that hospitals have an ADR reporting program. These programs are generally a function of the P&T committee and the department of pharmacy. The Joint Commission encourages the reporting of serious ADRs to the FDA.

ASHP also encourages pharmacists and health care practitioners to take an active role in monitoring adverse events. ASHP has published very specific guidelines as part of its practice standards. The ADR standards can be found on the Internet at http://www.ashp.org/DocLibrary/BestPractices/MedMisGdlADR.aspx.[36]

The Joint Commission and ASHP standards can be used as a basis for starting an ADR monitoring program. In addition to the standards, the pharmacy and medical literature are rich with examples of successful programs, some of which are reviewed in this chapter.

Guidelines for implementing an ADR monitoring program include the following:

1. Develop definitions and classifications for ADRs that work for the institution. The definitions and classifications in this chapter provide a good starting point for discussion.
2. Assign responsibility for the ADR program within the pharmacy and throughout other key departments. A multidisciplinary approach is an essential factor.
3. Develop a program with approval from the pharmacy department, medical staff (P&T committee), and nursing department, as well as other appropriate areas within the facility. Cooperation is essential in the initiation of a successful program.
4. Promote awareness of the program. Newsletters, in-services, grand rounds presentations, and other educational settings are opportunities to increase awareness and garner support for the program.
5. Promote awareness of ADRs and the importance of reporting such events.
6. Develop policies and procedures for handling ADRs being sent to the FDA. Indicate who is responsible for sending them.
7. Establish mechanisms for screening ADRs continuously. These mechanisms should include retrospective reviews and concurrent monitoring, as well as prospective planning for high-risk groups. It is worthwhile to educate pharmacists to check for ADRs when they see orders for certain indicator drugs that are often used in treating an ADR (Table 15–2), orders to discontinue or hold drugs, and orders to decrease the dose or frequency of a drug.[37] Also, electronic screening methods to check for laboratory tests that are indicative of ADRs (e.g., drug levels, *Clostridium difficile* toxin assays, elevated serum potassium, low white blood cell counts) can be helpful.[38] Emergency box

TABLE 15–2. ADR INDICATOR DRUGS

Antidiarrheal agents
Atropine (except preoperatively)
Dextrose 50% (IV push)
Diphenhydramine (except at bedtime)
Epinephrine (IV push)
Flumazenil
Naloxone
Potassium supplement (diuretic or digoxin patients)
Protamine
Sodium polystyrene sulfonate (patients on potassium sparing diuretics or ACE inhibitors)
Topical steroids
Vitamin K

usage is another event that may trigger investigation by the pharmacist to determine if an ADR has occurred (e.g., epinephrine, diphenhydramine).[39]

8. Develop internal forms or other mechanisms for data collection and reporting of ADRs. Some institutions use computer reporting, as well as hotline phone numbers.

9. Establish procedures for evaluating the causality and probability of ADRs.

10. Routinely review ADRs for trends.

11. Develop preventive interventions. This should include identification of patients who are at high risk of developing adverse drug reactions, as well as monitoring the use of drugs that are likely to cause ADRs.

12. Report all findings to the P&T committee.

13. Develop strategies for decreasing the incidence of ADRs, depending on the opportunities presented by the ADRs reported. This vital step has basically been ignored in the literature; however, for an ADR program to be part of the quality assurance process, it must be included wherever possible.

❺ *Communication is a critical component throughout the ADR monitoring process.* To ensure that the suspected drug is not administered again, and that patients receive necessary treatment and monitoring, each ADR should be documented thoroughly in the patient's medical record. However, this action alone is not sufficient, as the information is often poorly visible and may be difficult to access. The Institute for Safe Medication Practices (ISMP) recommends that ADRs be communicated by documenting the reaction on a standardized order form, just as if prescribing drug therapy or ordering lab draws.[40] This increases visibility of the information and facilitates a timely response by all individuals involved in the patient's care. In addition, ASHP recommends that patients and their care-givers be notified when a suspected ADR has occurred.[36] Well-informed patients can help prevent ADRs from recurring in the future.[40] Finally, previously unreported or clinically important ADRs should be disseminated to the medical community by publication and/or presentation in an appropriate forum.[39,40]

TECHNOLOGY

❻ *Information systems and high-end technology play an important role in monitoring, iden-tifying, and minimizing ADRs.* Information systems are available that can identify and alert practitioners to potential ADRs and detect potential drug-drug interactions that may contribute to ADRs. One such system was developed at Brigham and Women's Hospital to detect potential ADRs. The system was programmed to detect a combination of patient-specific factors and medications that may indicate a patient who has the potential to expe-rience an ADR. For example, patients taking medications that require renal-function-based dosing who have elevated serum creatinine may be flagged as patients at risk for the development of an ADR. Various other screening rules were also programmed. This sys-tem was compared to voluntary stimulated reporting and retrospective chart review. The system detected more ADRs than spontaneous reports, but fewer than chart review. Inter-estingly, the errors detected by the computer system were different than those detected by chart review, indicating that a combination of ADR detection systems may provide the best results. As expected, using the computer system saved work time, requiring five times fewer person-hours than the chart review method.[41] In another study, a similar ADE detection system identified potential ADEs in 64 of every 1000 admissions. The prescrib-ing physician did not recognize 44% of the ADEs detected by the system.[42]

Pyxis machines are also being used to help identify potential ADRs. Certain tracer drugs are identified such as flumazenil, protamine, methylprednisolone, and diphenhy-dramine. When a tracer drug is removed from Pyxis, the nurse is asked if this medication is being used to treat an adverse drug reaction. The pharmacy then gets a report indicat-ing the tracer drug removal and for which patient the medication was intended. This allows the pharmacist to follow up and evaluate and report the ADR if necessary.

At LDS Hospital in Salt Lake City, Utah, the HELP (Health Evaluation through Logi-cal Processing) system monitors medical records around the clock and automatically identifies patients who may have experienced an ADR.[43] The system does this by identify-ing certain flags such as stop orders, orders for antidotes, and abnormal laboratory val-ues. The flags or signals are then reported to pharmacy so that pharmacists can follow up to determine if an actual adverse event had occurred.

Because drug-drug interactions may comprise as many as 59% of ADRs,[44] computer systems that detect clinically significant interactions are also important for reducing ADRs. Although software is readily available for this purpose, one survey indicates that only slightly more than half of the hospitals are using drug interaction software integrated with their drug distribution system. Despite this finding, most pharmacists believe that drug interaction software does or would increase their ability to detect clinically significant drug-drug interactions that may contribute to ADRs.[45]

Waller proposed a potentially significant advancement in the use of technology for reporting ADRs. With this system, information regarding ADRs would be automatically captured from the computers of health care professionals.[46] When a trigger event occurred, such as the administration of a drug antidote, reports could be generated and sent to the FDA or other regulatory bodies without any action from the practitioner. This proposal, while not without its challenges for implementation, has the capability to greatly reduce the underreporting of adverse drug reactions.

The health care industry is lagging behind other industries in the implementation of high-end technology information systems.[47] Health care organizations will likely be required to invest in that technology to significantly improve the quality of care and stay competitive in the health care market.[41,47]

Conclusion

Adverse drug reactions are a serious problem in the U.S. health care system, causing significant morbidity and mortality as well as costing billions of dollars annually. The problem is undeniably widespread, with the Food and Drug Administration receiving over 496,000 spontaneous reports of ADRs in 2008 alone.[48] From 1998 to 2005, the number of reports documenting serious ADRs and fatal ADRs increased almost threefold. Astonishingly, during that time, reports related to biological drugs grew almost 16-fold.[49] Because of documented underreporting, these numbers represent only a small fraction of the ADRs occurring annually. Recognition of the problem is an important first step in developing strategies to minimize the occurrence of ADRs. Reporting of these reactions is an absolute necessity to gauge progress and direct our efforts in patient care.

Pharmacists can play a vital role in developing, maintaining, and promoting ADR monitoring programs. These programs provide valuable information about ADRs within the institution as well as information that can be forwarded to the FDA. ADR monitoring programs have been developed that positively impact patient care. These programs have been shown to improve communication channels and provide additional education on adverse events.

An editorial appearing in the *American Journal of Health-System Pharmacy* encourages institutions to recognize the role that pharmacists play in minimizing adverse drug events.[50] Adequate staffing by qualified pharmacists who actively participate in all aspects of the medication use process, including prescribing, dispensing, and administering, has been shown to significantly decrease medication errors, including ADRs.[12] Institutions are urged to use pharmacists to their full potential by more actively employing pharmacists in clinical settings where they can collaborate with other health care professionals so that they may strengthen efforts to reduce adverse drug reactions. Although pharmacists have the responsibility of ensuring the safe and effective use of medications, other health care providers and health care systems must significantly contribute to this effort as well. An ADR program should have a multidisciplinary approach and provide a mechanism to impact the quality of patient care. Only by working together is it possible to decrease the incidence of adverse drug reactions and contribute to improving patient care by actively pursuing improvements in the medication use process.

Study Questions

1. Define adverse drug reaction.
2. List several consequences of adverse drug reactions, including the impact on patient outcomes and on the health care system.
3. List 10 reasons physicians may not report adverse drug reactions.
4. Why is communication important in the prevention and management of adverse drug reactions?
5. Describe a successful adverse drug reaction program.
6. Explain how technology might improve adverse drug reaction monitoring and reporting programs.
7. Does the community pharmacist have a role in the management of adverse drug reactions? Explain why or why not.
8. Why should pharmacists take a leading role in minimizing adverse drug reactions?

Self-Assessment Questions

1. Which of the following refers to an adverse drug reaction (ADR)?
   a. Any iatrogenic hazard or incident associated with a medication
   b. Any injury caused by a medication
   c. Any preventable event that leads to inappropriate medication use or patient harm
   d. Any unexpected, unintended, undesired, or excessive response to a medication
   e. Any reaction related to the intentional or unintentional overdose of a medication

2. Adverse drug reactions account for approximately what percentage of all hospital admissions?
   a. 0.1% to 0.5%
   b. 1% to 5%

   c. 5% to 15%
   d. 15% to 25%
   e. 35%

3. Every year, adverse drug reactions cost the U.S. health care system how much?
   a. $50 to $70 million
   b. $150 million
   c. $5 to $7 billion
   d. $50 to $70 billion
   e. $150 billion

4. Which of the following components are included in the FDA's definition of an adverse drug reaction?
   a. A reaction due to drug abuse
   b. A reaction due to drug withdrawal
   c. Failure of an expected pharmacological action to occur
   d. Drug overdose
   e. All of the above

5. Which of the following definitions of an adverse drug reaction is often excluded by hospitals?
   a. Noxious reaction to a drug given at a normal dose
   b. Reactions due to drug abuse
   c. Excessive pharmacological reaction
   d. Idiosyncratic reactions
   e. None of the above

6. The first step in establishing an institutional adverse drug reaction program is to:
   a. Determine the institution's definition of an adverse drug reaction.
   b. Determine which administrator is responsible for reporting adverse reactions to the FDA.
   c. Develop an adverse reaction reporting form.
   d. Determine drugs most likely to cause adverse reactions.
   e. None of the above.

7. Which of the following factors is *not* used to determine adverse reaction causality?
   a. Dechallenge
   b. Rechallenge
   c. Temporal relationship
   d. Patient gender
   e. Known response pattern

8. Which of the following is the most commonly used algorithm for determining adverse reaction causality?
   a. Bayesian
   b. Kramer method
   c. Naranjo algorithm
   d. Larch algorithm
   e. Probabilistic method

9. Which following is the most universally accepted method for determining adverse reaction causality?
   a. Bayesian
   b. Kramer method
   c. Naranjo algorithm
   d. Karch algorithm
   e. None of the above

10. Who can report adverse drug reactions to the FDA's MedWatch program?
    a. Physicians
    b. Pharmacists
    c. Nurses
    d. Patients
    e. All of the above

11. Which of the following is considered a barrier to reporting an adverse drug reaction?
    a. Fear of litigation
    b. Lack of detection of event
    c. Lack of time
    d. Complacency
    e. All of the above

12. Which of the following statements about reporting adverse reactions related to dietary supplements is *true*?
    a. The FDA's MedWatch system does not accept reports related to dietary supplements.
    b. Manufacturers of dietary supplements are not required to share adverse reaction information with FDA.
    c. Natural Medicines Watch can be used to submit information about adverse reactions to dietary supplements.
    d. There is no system for collecting information about adverse reactions to dietary supplements.
    e. Dietary supplements are natural; therefore, they do not cause adverse reactions.

13. Which of the following is a job responsibility that makes pharmacists well suited to provide education on ADR programs?
    a. Involvement in P&T committee
    b. Pharmacokinetic dosing
    c. Drug utilization review
    d. Drug distribution
    e. All of the above

14. Which of the following is *not* a step in implementing a successful ADR monitoring program?
    a. Develop an institution-wide definition of ADRs.
    b. Obtain approval from the pharmacy, medical, and nursing departments.
    c. Promote awareness of the program.
    d. Screen for ADRs on a retrospective basis only.
    e. Determine who is responsible for sending ADR reports to the FDA.

15. Which of the following best describes the role of technology in the management of ADRs?
    a. Technology can help identify and alert practitioners to potential ADRs.
    b. Technology eliminates the need for pharmacists to get involved in ADR management.
    c. Technology systems have not proven useful in the management of ADRs.
    d. Technology can only be used to report ADRs, not to aid in their detection.
    e. Technology has nearly eliminated fatalities due to ADRs.

REFERENCES

1. American Society of Health-System Pharmacists. Suggested definitions and relationships among medication misadventures, medication errors, adverse drug events, and adverse drug reactions. Am J Health-Syst Pharm. 1998;55:165-6.
2. Rich DS. A process for interpreting data on adverse drug events: determining optimal target levels. Clin Ther. 1998;20(suppl C):C59-C71.
3. Rich DS. The Joint Commission's revised sentinel event policy on medication errors. Hosp Pharm. 1998;33:881-5.
4. Institute of Medicine. To Err Is Human: Building a Safer Health System. Washington, DC: National Academy Press; 1999.
5. White TJ, Arakelian A, Rho JP. Counting the costs of drug-related adverse events. Pharmacoeconomics. 1999;15:445-58.
6. Wong YL. Adverse effect of pharmaceutical recipients in drug therapy. Ann Acad Med. 1993;22:99-102.
7. Classen DC, Pestotnik SL, Evans S, Loyd JF, Burke JP. Adverse drug events in hospitalized patients. JAMA. 1997;277:301-6.

8. Swanson KM, Landry JP, Anderson RP. Pharmacy-coordinated, multidisciplinary adverse drug reaction program. Top Hosp Pharm Manage. 1992;12:49-59.

9. Lazarou J, Pomeranz BM , Corey PN. Incidence of adverse drug reactions in hospitalized patients: a meta-analysis of prospective studies. JAMA. 1998;279:1200-5.

10. Fincham JE. An overview of adverse drug reactions. Am Pharm. 1991;NS31:435-41.

11. Agency for Healthcare Research and Quality. Reducing and preventing adverse drug events to decrease hospital costs. [cited 2010 Feb 19]. Available from: http://www.ahrq.gov/qual/aderia/aderia.htm.

12. Lesar TS, Briceland L, Stein DS. Factors related to errors in medication prescribing. JAMA. 1997;277:312-7.

13. Leape LL, Cullen DJ, Clapp M, Burdick E, Demonaco HJ, Erickson JI, et al. Pharmacist participation on physician rounds and adverse drug events in the intensive care unit. JAMA. 1999;282:267-70.

14. Lamy PP. Adverse drug effects. Clin Ger Med. 1990;6:293-307.

15. Edwards R, Aronson JK. Adverse drug reactions: definitions, diagnosis, and management. Lancet. 2000;356:1212.

16. Karch FE, Lasagna L. Toward the operational identification of adverse drug reactions. Clin Pharmacol Ther. 1977;21:247-54.

17. Agbabiaka TB, Savovic J, Ernst E. Methods for causality assessment of adverse drug reactions: a systematic review. Drug Saf. 2008;31:21-37.

18. Naranjo CA, Busto U, Sellers EM, Sandor P, Ruiz I, Roberts EA, et al. A method of estimating the probability of adverse drug reactions. Clin Pharmacol Ther. 1981;30:239-45.

19. Kramer MS, Leventhal JM, Hutchinson TA, Feinstein AR. An algorithm for the operational assessment of adverse drug reactions: I. Background, description, and instructions for use. JAMA. 1979;242:623-32.

20. Hutchinson TA, Leventhal JM, Kramer MS, Karch FE, Lipman AG, Feinstein AR. An algorithm for the operational assessment of adverse drug reactions: II. Demonstration of reproducibility and validity. JAMA. 1979;242:633-8.

21. Jones JK. Adverse drug reactions in the community health setting: approaches to recognizing, counseling, and reporting. Fam Comm Health. 1982;5(2):58-67.

22. Michel DJ, Knodel LC. Comparison of three algorithms used to evaluate adverse drug reactions. Am J Hosp Pharm. 1986;43:1709-14.

23. Lane DA. The Bayesian approach to causality assessment: an introduction. Drug Info J. 1986;20:455-61.

24. U.S. Food and Drug Administration. What is a serious adverse event? [cited 2010 Aug 25]. Available from: http://www.fda.gov/medwatch/report/desk/advevnt.htm.

25. Faich GA, Dreis M, Tomita D. National adverse drug reaction surveillance: 1986 Arch Intern Med. 1988;148:785-7.

26. Stang PE, Fox JL. Adverse drug events and the Freedom of Information Act: an apple in Eden. Ann Pharmacother. 1992;26:238-43.

27. Rogers AS, Israel E, Smith CR, Levine D, McBean AM, Valente C, et al. Physician knowledge, attitudes, and behaviour related to reporting adverse drug events. Arch Intern Med. 1988;148:1596-600.

28. MedWatch: the FDA Medical Products Reporting Program. FDA Med Bull. 1993; 23:insert.

29. Hoffman RP. Adverse drug reaction reporting—problems and solutions. J Mich Pharm. 1989;27:400-3, 407-8.

30. Van Manen RP, Fram D, DuMouchel W. Signal detection methodologies to support effective safety management. Drug Saf. 2007;6:451-64.

31. Want XY, Hripcsak G, Markatou M, Friedman C. Active computerized pharmacovigilance using natural language processing, statistics, and electronic health records: a feasibility study. J Am Med Inform Assoc. 2009 Mar:16:328-37.

32. Peto R, Collins R, Gray R. Large-scale randomized evidence: large, simple trials and overviews of trials. J Clin Epidemiol. 1995;48:23-40.

33. Food and Drug Administration. Dietary Supplement and Nonprescription Drug Consumer Protection Act. [cited 2010 Sept 27]. Available from: http://www.fda.gov/Regulatory Information/Legislation/FederalFoodDrugandCosmeticActFDCAct/Significant AmendmentstotheFDCAct/ucm148035.htm.

34. Food and Drug Administration. Dietary Supplements Containing Ephedrine Alkaloids Final Rule Summary. [cited 2010 Aug 24]. Available from: http://www.fda.gov/oc/initiatives/ ephedra/february2004/finalsummary.html.

35. Amin RM, Blumenthal M. Federal court overturns FDA ban on ephedra at low doses. 2009. [cited 2010 Aug 25]. Available from: http://cms.herbalgram.org/press/FDAephedra.html.

36. ASHP guidelines on adverse drug reaction monitoring and reporting. Am J Health-Syst Pharm. 1995;52:417-9.

37. Saltiel E, Johnson E, Shane R. A team approach to adverse drug reaction surveillance: success at a tertiary care hospital. Hosp Form. 1995;30:226-32.

38. Classen DC, Pestotnik SL, Evans RS, Burke JP. Computerized surveillance of adverse drug events in hospital patients. JAMA. 1991;266:2847-51.

39. American Society of Consultant Pharmacists. Guidelines of detecting and reporting adverse drug reactions in long-term care environments. [cited 2010 Feb 22]. Available from: http:// www.ascp.com/resources/policy/upload/Gui97-ADRs.pdf.

40. Institute for Safe Medication Practices. Adverse drug reactions: documentation is important but communication is critical. [cited 2010 Feb 17]. Available from: http://www.ismp.org/ Newsletters/acutecare/articles/20000906.asp.

41. Jha AK, Kuperman GJ, Teich JM, Leape L, Shea B, Rittenberg E, et al. Identifying adverse drug events: development of a computer-based monitor and comparison with chart review and stimulated voluntary report. J Am Med Inform Assoc. 1998;5:305-14.

42. Raschke RA, Gollihare B, Wunderlich TA, Guidry JR, Leibowitz AI, Peirce JC, et al. A computer alert system to prevent injury from adverse drug events. JAMA. 1998;280:1317-20.

43. Classen DC, Pestotnik SL, Evans RS, Burke JP. Computerized surveillance if adverse drug events in hospitalized patients. Qual Saf Health Care. 2005;14:221-6.

44. Davies E, Green C, Taylor S, Williamson P, Mottram D, Pirmohamed M. Adverse drug reactions in hospital in-patients: a prospective analysis of 3695 patient-episodes. PLoS ONE. 2009;4:e4439.

45. Dalton M, Chambers G, Halvachs F. Implementing an effective drug interaction reporting program. Hosp Pharm. 1999;34:31-42.
46. Waller P. Making the most of spontaneous adverse drug reaction reporting. Basic Clin Pharmacol Tox. 2006;98:320-3.
47. Felkey BG. Health system informatics. Am J Health-Syst Pharm. 1997;54:274-80.
48. Food and Drug Administration. AERS reporting by healthcare providers and consumers by year. [cited 2010 Feb 22]. Available from: http://www.fda.gov/Drugs/GuidanceCompliance-RegulatoryInformation/Surveillance/AdverseDrugEffects/ucm070456.htm.
49. Moore T, Cohen M, Furberg C. Serious adverse drug events reported to the Food and Drug Administration, 1998-2005. Arch Intern Med. 2007;167:1752-9.
50. Sellers JA. Too many errors, not enough pharmacists. Am J Health-Syst Pharm. 2000;57:337.

SUGGESTED READINGS

1. Naranjo CA, Busto U, Sellers EM, Sandor P, Ruiz I, Roberts EA, et al. A method for estimating the probability of adverse drug reactions. Clin Pharmacol Ther. 1981;30:239-45.
2. U.S. Food and Drug Administration, MedWatch: http://www.fda.gov/Safety/MedWatch/default.htm.

16

Chapter Sixteen

Medication Misadventures II: Medication and Patient Safety

Kathryn A. Crea

Learning Objectives

● *After completing this chapter, the reader will be able to*

- Define and compare the terms medication errors, adverse drug events, and adverse drug reactions.
- Discuss the role of Patient Safety Organizations (PSOs) in health care.
- Assign an event severity rating to reported errors and events.
- Describe reporting systems for medication errors and adverse drug events.
- Discuss two methods of analyzing medication errors and adverse drug events that are utilized to develop action plans for prevention of recurrence.
- Describe examples of skill-based, rule-based, and knowledge-based errors.
- Explain a systems approach to error.
- Determine strategies health care practitioners and health systems can implement to reduce medication errors.
- Reflect on the need for interprofessional education and training on quality and safety principles.
- Compare a Just Culture with a culture of shame and blame.

Key Concepts

❶ The terms medication error, adverse drug event, and adverse drug reaction are similar and often confused. They are interrelated yet distinct occurrences.

❷ Several methods of identifying errors are recommended to gain a more global understanding of the risks and errors occurring within an institution.

❸ Classification of error types is a common method to identify common themes and causes of events. The Common Formats associated with Patient Safety Organizations (PSOs) may become the new standard classification scheme.

❹ Thorough analysis of safety events through root cause analysis (RCA), failure mode and effects analysis (FMEA), or other methods is a key activity to support learning from our mistakes in an effort to prevent recurrence.

❺ Human beings (including health care professionals of all types) have a propensity to commit errors in all aspects of their lives. To err is human.

❻ Understanding human error types (skill-based, rule-based, and knowledge-based errors) is very important to understanding errors and events, and in developing appropriate strategies to reduce the risks of recurrence.

❼ Poorly designed health care systems and processes are a significant contributor to individual human error and subsequent patient harm.

❽ A Just Culture is one in which discipline is applied in a consistent manner based on the intentions of the individual and the situation in which the individual was placed, not on the outcome.

❾ All health professionals should be trained to deliver patient-centered care as members of an interdisciplinary team, emphasizing evidence-based practice, quality improvement approaches, and informatics.

❿ There are many resources available that identify best-practice error prevention strategies.

⓫ Designing with human factor principles in mind is a great way to improve the safety of any process.

Introduction

Much attention has been focused on adverse outcomes in health care in the past decade. Although pockets of research in medical errors were developing prior to 2000, the Institute of Medicine's report, *To Err Is Human: Building a Safer Health System,*[1] released in late 1999, served as a catalyst for additional research in the causes and methods to prevent adverse outcomes in health care. The mortality estimates documented in this report (an estimated 44,000 to 98,000 people die each year as a result of medical errors) were derived from two landmark studies.[1-3] The report notes that medication errors alone (whether occurring within or outside of the hospital) were estimated to account for over 7000 deaths annually. The majority of literature to date has focused on work in the hospital setting, as it is, for the most part, a closed and controlled environment. Other settings are less well researched, although early studies of nursing homes and ambulatory settings have shown significant opportunities for improvement. It is clear that medication safety, and the broader category of patient safety, represent a serious concern for patients and health care providers.

While many health care professionals have roles in the medication use process, pharmacists play a pivotal role in assuring the safe use of medication. Pharmacist provision of accurate drug information and identification of potential medication-related adverse effects to multiple providers is of vital importance. Throughout the medication use process there are many opportunities for unexpected adverse events, including errors in prescribing, dispensing, and administering medications; idiosyncratic reactions; and other adverse effects. These events can all be described as medication misadventures.[4] All pharmacists need a sound understanding of the risks for error and the ability to identify the underlying causes of medication misadventures, as other practitioners tend to focus on other potential causes. Pharmacists are also responsible for taking steps to prevent such occurrences and minimize adverse outcomes. This usually involves collaborative work with other health care team members to ensure optimal outcomes. Pharmacists are well positioned to lead these efforts in reducing harm to patients.

Definitions: Medication Errors, Adverse Drug Events (ADEs), and Adverse Drug Reactions (ADRs)

❶ *The terminology surrounding medication misadventures is often confusing; there are many definitions that are very similar. The term medication misadventure is an overarching term that includes medication errors, adverse drug events (ADEs), and adverse drug reactions (ADRs).* The American Society of Health-System Pharmacists[4] (ASHP) defines a medication misadventure as any iatrogenic hazard or incident:

- That is an inherent risk when medication therapy is indicated.
- That is created through either omission or commission by the administration of a medicine or medicines during which a patient may be harmed, with effects ranging from mild discomfort to fatality.

- Whose outcome may or may not be independent of the preexisting pathology or disease process.
- That may be attributable to error (human or system, or both), immunologic response, or idiosyncratic response.
- That is always unexpected or undesirable to the patient and the health professional.

The National Coordinating Council for Medication Error Reporting and Prevention (NCCMERP), an organization composed of 24 national organizations and individual members, including the Food and Drug Administration (FDA), American Medical Association (AMA), American Pharmacists Association (APhA), United States Pharmacopoeia (USP), and several others (Table 16–1), has developed a detailed definition of what constitutes a medication error:[5]

> Any preventable event that may cause or lead to inappropriate medication use or patient harm while the medication is in the control of the health care professional, patient, or consumer. Such events may be related to professional practice, health care products, procedures, and systems, including prescribing; order communication; product labeling, packaging, and nomenclature; compounding; dispensing; distribution; administration; education; monitoring; and use.

Key points related to medication errors include

- Medication errors are preventable.
- Medication errors can be caused by errors in the planning (deciding what to do—which drug and/or what dose) or execution stages (completing the task that was decided on—administering the drug to the wrong patient).
- Medication errors include errors of omission (missed dose or appropriate medication not prescribed) or commission (wrong drug given).
- Medication errors may or may not cause patient harm.

Based on the NCCMERP definition, an error may occur as a result of not adequately counseling or educating a patient on the proper use of medication. When, for example, a patient inappropriately uses a metered-dose inhaler for asthma and fails to receive the full amount of the medication, a medication error has occurred. The error may be secondary to a lack of education or may have occurred despite adequate counseling and education. Independent of the cause, based on the above definition, a medication error did occur.

Based on this definition, medication errors also occur when a prescriber writes an incorrect dose on a prescription pad. Even if the pharmacist calls the prescriber to clarify and change the order and the patient eventually receives an appropriately dosed medication, an error did occur in the process. An adverse outcome does not necessarily have to occur to classify an event as a medication error.

TABLE 16–1. NATIONAL COORDINATING COUNCIL FOR MEDICATION ERROR REPORTING AND PREVENTION MEMBER ORGANIZATIONS

Founding Members
American Association of Retired Persons
American Hospital Association
American Medical Association
American Nurses Association
American Pharmacists Association
American Society of Health-System Pharmacists
Food and Drug Administration (U.S.)
Generic Pharmaceutical Association
The Joint Commission
National Association of Boards of Pharmacy
National Council of State Boards of Nursing
Pharmaceutical Research and Manufacturers of America
U.S. Pharmacopoeia

Regular Members
American Association of Homes and Services for the Aging
American Society for Healthcare Risk Management
American Society of Consultant Pharmacists
Department of Defense
Department of Veterans Affairs
Institute for Healthcare Improvement
Institute for Safe Medication Practices
National Alliance of State Pharmacy Associations
National Association of Chain Drug Stores
National Council on Patient Information and Education
National Patient Safety Foundation

• An adverse drug event (ADE) involves harm to a patient. An ADE is defined as an injury from a medicine or lack of intended medicine.[6] An ADE refers to all adverse drug reactions (ADRs), including allergic or idiosyncratic reactions, as well as medication errors that result in harm to a patient. It is estimated that 3% to 5% of medication errors result in harm to a patient and can also be classified as an adverse drug event.

• An adverse drug reaction (ADR) is defined by the World Health Organization (WHO) as "any response that is noxious, unintended, or undesired, which occurs at doses normally used in humans for prophylaxis, diagnosis, therapy of disease, or modification of physiological function."[7]

The relationship between the terms is illustrated in Figure 16–1. Although there are standard definitions for medication errors, there may be significant differences

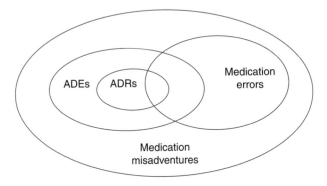

Figure 16–1. Relationship among medication misadventures, adverse drug events, medication errors, and adverse drug reactions. (*Adapted with permission from Bates DW, et al. Relationship between medication and errors and adverse drug events. J Gen Intern Med. 1995;April:10(4):199-205.*)

in the interpretation, reporting rates, and severity ranking between institutions. Common questions that arise are included in Table 16–2. For example, one institution may determine that an error has occurred when a patient does not receive a dose within 30 minutes of the scheduled time, where another may permit 60 minutes before or after the scheduled administration time. Some institutions may not report an inappropriately written prescription if a pharmacist or nurse catches the error before the medication reaches the patient. Instead, a pharmacist or nurse may report it as a professional intervention. According to most definitions, this would count as an error. These variations make it very difficult to compare data from one institution to another. Therefore, it is best for an institution to utilize its own data to monitor improvement.

TABLE 16–2. COMMON QUESTIONS THAT ARISE IN DEFINING MEDICATION ERRORS AND ADVERSE DRUG EVENTS

- Is it an error if it does not reach the patient?
- Is it an error if it doesn't cause harm?
- What constitutes minimal harm? Moderate? Severe?
- Is it an error or event if it's not clinically significant?
- Should pharmacist interventions related to inappropriate physician orders be documented and counted as prescribing errors?
- What is considered preventable?

The Impact of Errors on Patients and Health Care Systems

Patients depend on health systems and health professionals to help them stay healthy. As a result, patients frequently receive drug therapy with the notion that these medications will help them lead a healthier life. The initiation of drug therapy is the most common medical treatment received by patients.[8] In virtually all cases, patients and their health care providers understand that when medications are given, there are some known and some unknown risks. Patients may experience significant unexpected drug-related morbidity and mortality.

Several landmark studies have identified the risk of medication errors and ADEs in varying populations and settings. The Harvard Medical Practice Study I was a landmark study that estimated that 3.7% of hospitalized patients experience adverse events.[2] The findings and extrapolated statistics from this study along with the Harvard Medical Practice Study II served as the grounds for the statement (from *To Err Is Human*) that approximately 44,000 to 98,000 people are killed by medical error every year. Specifically related to medication errors, Bates and associates identified 6.5 ADEs per hospital admission.[6] In the nursing home setting, Gurwitz and associates[9] identified 227 ADEs per 1000 resident-years. Gurwitz and associates[10] also studied the ambulatory patient population, finding 50.1 ADEs per 1000 person-years. Interestingly, the preventability of all ADEs in these studies ranged from 27% to 51%, while the preventability of serious and life-threatening ADEs ranged from 42% to 72%, potentially indicating that improved processes and behaviors should be able to prevent serious harm events.

The economic impact of medication errors and ADEs is staggering and adds to the health care cost burden unnecessarily. Several important studies documented the economic burden of these events.[11-14] A landmark study in 1995 estimated that ADE-related costs were $76.6 billion annually in ambulatory patients alone.[11] Drug expenditures in ambulatory patients at that time were $80 billion per year. This means that for every $1 spent for a drug, almost $1 was also being spent due to a drug-related problem. These costs exceed the total cost of managing patients with diabetes or cardiovascular diseases.[12] A subsequent study demonstrated that the cost of drug-related morbidity and mortality in the ambulatory setting exceeded $177 billion in 2000.[14]

Although it was initially thought that medication misadventures were caused by individual health care practitioners, including pharmacists, physicians, and nurses, now it is clear that our health care systems and processes often are causative or contributing factors in the majority of errors and events. Efforts to decrease adverse outcomes will not be successful if these system and process-related issues are not addressed. Multiple agencies and professional organizations across the country are now contributing efforts to minimize these events (Table 16–3), which are discussed in the section on best practices for error prevention.

TABLE 16–3. ORGANIZATIONS INVOLVED IN PREVENTING ADVERSE DRUG EVENTS

Food and Drug Administration (FDA)	http://www.fda.gov
The Joint Commission (TJC)	http://www.jointcommission.org
World Health Organization (WHO)	http://www.who.int
Institute for Safe Medication Practices (ISMP)	http://www.ismp.org
The United States Pharmacopoeia (USP)	http://www.usp.org
American Society of Health-System Pharmacists (ASHP)	http://www.ashp.org
National Quality Forum (NQF)	http://www.qualityforum.org
Agency for Healthcare Research and Quality (AHRQ)	http://www.ahrq.gov
Patient Safety Network	http://www.psnet.ahrq.gov
Web M&M: Morbidity and Mortality Rounds on the web	http://www.webmm.ahrq.gov
Institute for Healthcare Improvement (IHI)	http://www.ihi.org
Health Resources and Services Administrations (HRSA)	http://www.hrsa.gov
National Patient Safety Foundation	http://www.npsf.org
Centers for Medicaid and Medicare Services (CMS)	http://www.cms.hhs.gov
Centers for Disease Control (CDC)	http://www.cdc.gov
The Leapfrog Group	http://www.leapfroggroup.org

Identification and Reporting of Medication Errors and Adverse Drug Events

❷ *It is important that a systematic approach to the identification and assessment of errors and adverse events be utilized in order to identify trends and opportunities for improvement based on events occurring at a location. This should involve several methods, and include prospective and retrospective methods of identifying errors and risks when possible.* Many methods of identifying errors in health care exist, including voluntary reporting, direct observation, chart review, trigger identification, and computerized monitoring. These methods are described further here.

1. A voluntary reporting system (either paper, telephonic, or online) is the most common method of identification of errors and events. Many institutions include an anonymous option for those who do not feel comfortable providing their name and contact information. Anyone detecting or committing an error

can report it without associating his or her name with the error. It is essentially risk-free for the reporter, and therefore it may increase the likelihood of having an error reported. Although voluntary reporting is the least labor-intensive method, it only identifies approximately 1 out of 20 errors when compared to other identification methods.[15] Therefore, it is important to include other methods of detection.

2. The direct observation method uses trained observers to watch the real-time delivery of medications. Notes from the observations are compared with physicians' orders to determine if an error has occurred. Results with this method are more valid and reliable than with self-reporting, but the impact of the observer on the subject being observed and interobserver agreement has been questioned.[16,17] This method is costly, time-consuming, and limited to the identification of errors that occur during the administration phase of the medication use process. It typically samples a selected time period on a selected unit, limiting the extrapolation to other time periods or patient care areas. On the positive side, errors are often identified that may never be discovered through other methods as they may go unrecognized.

3. Chart review identification of medication errors and ADEs is very labor intensive and is not generally practical outside of the research environment. Various trained staff review charts looking for particular cues or data elements that signify that an error or event has occurred. This method relies on practitioners to document these events when identified, which may lead to an underestimation of the true occurrence.

4. A modified version of manual chart review is the use of the ADE Trigger Tool. This is a tool that is promoted by the Institute for Healthcare Improvement (IHI). It is an augmented chart review method that uses automated systems to identify alerts or triggers that have been shown to efficiently identify patients with potential ADEs.[18-26] The triggers are cues that a patient may have experienced an error and/or adverse event. Example triggers include the use of reversal agents (e.g., flumazenil, naloxone, phytonadione) or abnormal lab values such as partial thromboplastin time (PTT), international normalized ratio (INR), or low glucose value. When these triggers are identified, it is suspected that the patient may have experienced a medication error. The patient's chart is reviewed for evidence of error and/or level or harm and data are collected and collated to determine potential common causes. For example, reviewing the charts of patients who experience hypoglycemia may reveal errors, such as incorrect insulin dosing while patients are receiving nothing by mouth in preparation for a surgical procedure. Upon review of patients requiring the use of naloxone, it may be discovered that the dosing

for hydromorphone and morphine are often confused during the prescribing, administration, and monitoring phases, leading to oversedation. The advantage to using this trigger method is that these types of events are rarely reported as errors. These tools have been used in several ways—as a long-term trend and measure of ADEs and/or in a more focused scope such as triggers related to known high-risk classes of medications.[27–29] Specific information on the use of this tool is available at http://www.ihi.org.

5. Classen[19,20] and Jha[18] developed methods to identify ADEs using an electronic medical record (EMR) with text searching tools and logic-based computer rules. In Classen's model, the text within the computer charting (e.g., lab, nurses' notes, physician progress notes and orders) is searched for defined conditions or cues, such as heparin-induced thrombocytopenia (HIT). When identified, a clinical pharmacist is alerted, reviews the patient record, and relays an appropriate recommendation to the prescribing physician. This serves as a real-time intervention to prevent or mitigate harm to the patient. This seems to be an optimal model, allowing concurrent review of potential harm and intervention to prevent further error or harm. Unfortunately, most institutions do not have an EMR, and if they do, they are often not capable of searching text.

The use of technology has presented new sources of data on potential errors. The increased use of automated distribution machines, smart pumps, computerized physician prescribing, and bar-coding technology provides rich databases. For example, every keystroke a nurse makes in programming a smart infusion pump is recorded. Once an error is identified, it is possible to download the data and review details about the error. The challenge is sorting through the massive volumes of information to derive common themes and strategies to decrease risk and optimize the technology.

The 1999 IOM report spotlighted a serious need to capture data that would help to reduce harm to patients. Congress subsequently passed the Patient Safety and Quality Improvement Act of 2005 (Patient Safety Act). The Act authorized the creation of a nationwide network of Patient Safety Organizations (PSOs) to improve safety and quality through the collection and analysis of data on patient events.[30] The act provides a venue for institutions to report information related to errors and events with the goal of collating the information and learning the underlying risks across similar types of events.

The Act provides confidentiality and privilege protection to organizations. The fear of legal action related to reported event information has prevented many organizations from voluntarily reporting errors and events to external agencies. The confidentiality protections ensure that information about an error that is provided to the authorized PSO is kept confidential. The privilege protections limit or forbid the use of protected information in criminal, civil, and other proceedings. Specifically, the information will not be subject to subpoena, discovery, or disclosure to any federal, state, or local criminal, civil, or administrative proceeding. The information may not be used in a professional disciplinary hearing, nor be admitted as evidence.

One example, the Pennsylvania Patient Safety Reporting System has been collating error data since 2004 and publishes regular advisories with the goal of improving health care delivery systems and educating providers about safe practices. For example, in December 2009,[31] the advisory reviewed errors with neuromuscular blocking agents. In a 5-year span, 154 reports related to neuromuscular blocking agents were submitted. The advisory provides specific information related to the contributing factors (unsafe storage, look-alike drug names, similar packaging, and unlabeled syringes) that increase the risk for a fatal error. Specific risk reduction strategies are outlined. The same errors tend to recur in facilities across the country. Recall the heparin errors in premature infants[32] that have occurred at least three times in different states. It is imperative that health care professionals commit to **learn from others** and critically self-assess the processes within their own institution to ensure that their process is as safe as possible. Being a learning organization is essential to prevent errors within an organization. It is recommended that hospitals, ambulatory centers, and other organizations join a PSO and commit to forwarding data related to adverse outcomes, enabling the collation of larger quantities of data, which the PSO can analyze and use to provide recommendations to member organizations.

CLASSIFICATION OF ERROR TYPES

❸ *The most common way to classify errors is to identify them by type of error. For medications, this classification focuses on whether an error was related to dispensing, administering, prescribing, monitoring, and other reasons. However, it is necessary to understand the underlying causes of the errors to develop effective prevention strategies.* There have been many taxonomies of errors developed by varying groups, including the World Health Organization, The Joint Commission, MEDMARX, and others. The American Society of Health-System Pharmacists' (ASHP) previously designated categories of medication errors are listed here.[33] These are similar to those outlined by NCCMERP.

- Prescribing error
- Omission error
- Wrong time error
- Unauthorized drug error
- Improper dose error
- Wrong dosage form error
- Wrong drug preparation error
- Wrong administration technique

- Deteriorated drug error
- Monitoring error
- Compliance error
- Other medication error

As a result of the development of PSOs, a common taxonomy and language was required to enable health care providers to collect and submit standardized information related to safety events. These standard event-reporting forms are called the Common Formats. The Common Formats define the standardized data elements associated with errors and events that are to be collected and reported to the PSO. The scope of Common Formats applies to all patient safety concerns including events reaching the patient (with or without harm), near-miss events that do not reach the patient, and unsafe conditions that have the potential to cause an error or event.[34] The Common Formats recently updated (V1.1) by the Agency for Healthcare Research and Quality (AHRQ) are likely to become the standard for reporting. The following event types have been defined for medication errors:

- Incorrect patient—An incorrect patient error occurs when a medication is given to the wrong patient, usually caused by an error in patient identification and confirmation. Two identifiers should be used to identify the patient every time a patient is given a medication, and confirming patient identification is necessary whenever a pharmacist writes or enters an order.
- Incorrect medication—This error occurs when a medication is administered that was not ordered for the patient. This may occur when a patient receives a medication intended for another patient due to inadequate patient identification, or when a nurse obtains the incorrect medication for administration, perhaps from floor stock. Barcode scanning is designed to prevent these errors and others.
- Incorrect dose (subcategories of overdose, underdose, omitted dose, extra dose, and unknown)—An incorrect dose error can occur when a prescriber orders an inappropriate dose of a medication or when the dose administered is different than what was prescribed. An omission error occurs when a patient does not receive a scheduled dose of medication. This is considered to be the second most common error in the medication use process.[35]
- Incorrect route of administration (subcategories include the intended route and the actual route).
- Incorrect timing (too early, too late, unknown)—What constitutes a wrong time error may vary considerably among institutions. In general, this type of error occurs when a dose is not administered in accordance with a predetermined administration interval. Most institutions realize that it is often impossible to be totally accurate with the administration interval and typically allow 15 to 60 minutes outside that interval. Institutions must establish a policy to indicate what exactly constitutes an error in this category.

- Incorrect rate (too fast, too slow, unknown)—This category generally applies to intravenous infusions, but can also apply to an intravenous push medication if the drug is pushed too quickly or too slowly.
- Incorrect duration—The patient receives the medication for a shorter or longer time period than prescribed. For example, a patient is prescribed a one-time dose of a medication. The pharmacist must enter the order as daily so it will show up on the medication administration record (MAR) for the nurse to administer and chart; however, the nurse must remember to place "one time" in the correct field so it only appears to the nurse once to administer. If the pharmacist forgets that last step (relying on memory is a poor error-prevention strategy), the medication will appear on the MAR for daily administration.
- Incorrect dosage form (e.g., extended release instead of immediate release)—A wrong dosage form error can occur when the prescriber makes an error or when a patient receives a dosage form different from that prescribed, assuming that the appropriate dosage form was originally ordered.
- Incorrect strength or concentration—This is an error that can occur at several points in the medication use process, from prescribing to administration. The pharmacist may choose the wrong strength when entering the order, or a nurse may choose the wrong drug upon administration. The appropriate use of bar-code administration of medications makes it harder to make these errors as well.
- Incorrect preparation (e.g., splitting tablets, compounding errors)—When medications require some type of preparation, such as reconstitution, this type of error may occur. These kinds of errors may also occur in the compounding of various intravenous admixtures and other products and can occur when nurses, pharmacists, or technicians are preparing medications.
- Expired or deteriorated product—This error occurs when a drug is administered that has expired or has deteriorated prematurely due to improper storage conditions.
- Medication that is a known allergen to the patient.
- Medication known to be contraindicated for the patient because of a drug-drug interaction or drug-food interaction.
- Incorrect patient action (patient taking a dietary supplement that interacted with medication, whether or not the patient was told to avoid taking it)—This type of error occurs when patients use medications inappropriately. Proper patient education and follow-up may play a significant role in minimizing this type of error. This type of error may be a direct result of insufficient patient counseling from a pharmacist, a prescriber, or both. Important components in counseling include consideration of the level of health literacy of patients and methods to gauge their understanding of their medication regimen and information provided.

The second classification section of the medication Common Formats report asks at what stage the incorrect action was discovered (regardless of where or when the incorrect action originated) with the following choices:

- Purchasing
- Storing
- Prescribing
- Transcribing
- Preparing
- Dispensing
- Administering to patient (including verifying medication)
- Monitoring

Prescribing errors generally focus on inappropriate drug selection, dose, dosage form, or route of administration. Examples may include ordering duplicate therapies for a single indication, prescribing a dose that is too high or too low for a patient based on age or organ function, writing a prescription illegibly, prescribing an inappropriate dosage interval, or ordering a drug to which the patient is allergic.

In one study, the most common type of prescribing error (56.1%) was related to an inappropriate dose (either too high or too low). The second most common prescribing error was related to prescribing an agent to which the patient was allergic (14.4%). Prescribing inappropriate dosage forms was the third most common error (11.2%).[8] Other relatively common prescribing errors have included failing to monitor for side effects and serum drug levels, prescribing an inappropriate medication for a particular indication, and inappropriate duration of therapy.

Monitoring errors occur when patients are not monitored appropriately either before or after they have received a drug. For example, if a patient is placed on warfarin therapy and adequate blood tests (baseline and ongoing) are not performed to assess the patient's response, a monitoring error has occurred and has the potential to result in a life-threatening hemorrhage.

These types of medication errors are not mutually exclusive. Multiple types of errors may occur during a single administration of a drug, and a single adverse patient outcome may be the result of more than one type of error.[33]

Additional information is gathered in the PSO reporting process. As the use of Common Formats grows, individual health care organizations will need to adopt these classifications, likely developing a standard taxonomy over time. Visit the PSO Web site for updated versions of the Common Formats at https://www.psoppc.org/web/patientsafety/commonformats.

CLASSIFYING OUTCOME OF THE PATIENT

Although the classification of errors or events frequently is based on type, most are also classified by the patient outcome related to the error or event. When an error occurs, there is not always an adverse outcome. It has been estimated that 3% to 5% of errors result in harm to patients. It is important for institutions to monitor both the types of errors that occur and the outcomes associated with them. Most reporting systems request information regarding the type and outcome of a medication error.

The NCCMERP developed a medication error index that serves to categorize errors based on the severity or outcome of the error. This index is divided into four main categories and nine subcategories as follows.[36] See the index for event classification and corresponding algorithm at http://www.nccmerp.org/medErrorCatIndex.html.

1. No error
   - Category A: Circumstances or events that have the capacity to cause error.
2. Error, no harm
   - Category B: An error occurred, but the medication did not reach the patient.
   - Category C: An error occurred that reached the patient, but did not cause the patient harm.
   - Category D: An error occurred that resulted in the need for increased patient monitoring, but caused no patient harm.
3. Error, harm
   - Category E: An error occurred that resulted in the need for treatment or intervention and caused temporary patient harm.
   - Category F: An error occurred that resulted in initial or prolonged hospitalization and caused temporary patient harm.
   - Category G: An error occurred that resulted in permanent patient harm.
   - Category H: An error occurred that resulted in a near-death event (e.g., anaphylaxis and cardiac arrest).
4. Error, death
   - Category I: An error occurred resulting in patient death.

Oftentimes, the initial staff member(s) reporting the error have an opportunity to indicate their interpretation of the level of harm to the patient. In follow-up, a medication safety pharmacist and the unit/department manager may investigate further details and assign a final severity classification based on the ultimate outcome to the patient.

Institutions may use information about outcomes to focus their error-prevention efforts on the types of errors resulting in the most serious outcomes. It is important to remember that examining near-miss events (those that do not reach the patient) can be as valuable in preventing future errors as focusing on serious outcomes. These near-miss events are often clues to the underlying process issues that require attention before they cause harm to a patient.

NATIONAL REPORTING

Reporting of medication errors is important for every practitioner without regard to his or her practice setting. However, institutional internal reporting is often emphasized (above external reporting) because it is necessary for maintaining the institution's accreditation status. Drug information specialists are in an ideal position to encourage the importance of medication error and adverse drug reaction reporting to all health professionals, especially when they are consulted to answer questions related to potential cases. In an effort to share institutional experiences and avoid the same errors being repeated at several institutions, national reporting systems for institutions have evolved.

- *MedWatch:* This program was developed by the FDA Medical Products Reporting Program for the purpose of monitoring problems with medical products. Med-Watch monitors the quality, performance, and safety of medical products, devices, and medications. This program contributes to the surveillance of medication errors that may be associated with product labeling and names.[37] MedWatch collects reports about faulty products (e.g., improperly functioning devices that led to a medication error). Significant reports may result in the distribution of e-mail and "Dear Doctor" alerts to health care professionals. These announcements can also be viewed on the Internet at http://www.fda.gov/medwatch/safety.htm. Health care professionals and consumers can report ADEs and product problems by completing a MedWatch 3500 form (found on the Web site) and mailing it to the FDA, by calling 1-800-FDA-1088, or reporting online at http://www.fda.gov/medwatch.
- *ISMP Medication Errors Reporting Program (MERP):* This program provides a venue for voluntary medication error reporting to the Institute for Safe Medication Practices (ISMP). Reports can be submitted online at https://www.ismp.org/orderforms/reporterrortoISMP.asp. ISMP is a federally certified Patient Safety Organization that collates errors and provides summary information across multiple cases in an effort to identify risk and support prevention strategies.
- *MEDMARX:* This program is an anonymous, subscription-based, voluntary reporting system that enables facilities to collect and report medication error, ADE, and ADR data. This service allows subscribing organizations to report and monitor organization-specific errors online, and compares their error rates with other subscribing organizations of similar type. Each year data is compiled, summarizes them, and an in-depth annual report is completed. Information in the report includes types of medication errors, causes, contributing factors, products

involved, and actions taken. More information regarding MEDMARX can be found at http://www.medmarx.com. This product differs from the USP-ISMP MERP program in that it is a fee-based service that enables comparison data within the database.

MANAGING AN EVENT-REPORTING SYSTEM

The Joint Commission and ASHP standards can be used as a basis for starting an error-reporting program. In addition to the standards, the pharmacy and medical literature contain abundant examples of successful programs. Guidelines for starting a program include the following:

1. Develop definitions and classifications for errors and events that work for the institution. The definitions and classifications in the literature and this chapter provide a good starting point for discussion. It is anticipated that the Common Formats developed in preparation for external reporting to PSOs will eventually become the standard.

2. Assign responsibility for the program within the pharmacy and throughout other key departments. A multidisciplinary approach is an essential factor. The program needs a leader and an advocate, which often comes from the pharmacy department. It also needs the involvement of nursing, medical, quality, and risk management departments in order to function as a collaborative team to work toward improved processes.

3. Develop forms or online methods for data collection and reporting. (See number 1.) Other mechanisms for reporting (e.g., hotline phone numbers) may be used as well. Electronic reporting can often be designed such that medication errors are reviewed by a medication safety pharmacist to confirm the severity of the event and gather additional information as needed in order to determine whether additional analysis is appropriate. These systems can also forward events based on their severity to other appropriate parties within the institution such as risk management, quality, and safety personnel to ensure the awareness of key staff and leaders. This serves as the voluntary reporting component of the program.

4. Promote awareness of the program and the importance of reporting errors and adverse events. Provide feedback to reporters and individual units that discuss their errors as well as those of others, along with steps taken to prevent them. Providing feedback is very important to ensure that those reporting feel that the identified errors are reviewed and methods to prevent recurrence are developed and implemented.

5. Develop policies and procedures for determining which errors, events, and ADRs are reported to the FDA. The responsibility for this reporting should be defined and usually resides with someone in the pharmacy department.

6. Establish mechanisms for the regular screening and identification of potential medication errors and ADEs to supplement voluntary reporting. These mechanisms should include retrospective reviews and concurrent monitoring, as well as prospective planning for high-risk groups. It is worthwhile to educate pharmacists to check for potential events or reactions when they see orders for certain triggers that are often used to treat an error or event (Table 16–4), orders to discontinue or hold drugs, and orders to decrease the dose or frequency of a drug.[18] Additionally, electronic screening methods to check for laboratory tests that are indicative of potential events (e.g., drug levels, *Clostridium difficile* toxin assays, elevated serum potassium, and low white blood cell counts) can be helpful.[20]

7. Routinely review medication errors, ADEs, and ADRs for trends. Report all findings to the pharmacy and therapeutics committee and other hospital or organization quality and safety committees. It is beneficial to present facility-specific data and nationally reported errors of significance, and to incorporate storytelling into various presentations. Oftentimes, telling a story that engages one's emotions, followed by your own data, reinvigorates the efforts to work toward safer processes.

TABLE 16–4. ADVERSE DRUG EVENT TRIGGERS

Medications	Conditions
Antidiarrheal agents	PTT >100 sec
Atropine (exclude preoperative use)	INR >6
Dextrose 50% (IV push)	WBC <3000
Diphenhydramine (excluding orders for sleep)	Glucose <50 mg/dL
Epinephrine (IV push)	Rising serum creatinine
Flumazenil	*C. difficile*–positive stool
Naloxone	Digoxin level >2
Droperidol	Lidocaine level >5
Sodium polystyrene sulfonate	Gentamicin/tobramycin peak >10 or trough >2
Vitamin K	Amikacin peak >30 or trough >10
D50W	Vancomycin level >26
	Theophylline level >20
	Oversedation, lethargy, fall, rash
	Abrupt medication stop
	Transfer to higher level of care

8. Develop strategies for decreasing the incidence of medication errors and adverse events utilizing the data collected through the various identification and reporting systems. Use caution in aggregating data by error types or other surface-level classifications. The key is getting to the causes of the errors—not just the fact that the majority of errors are omitted doses. Why are the doses omitted? Is the automated dispensing cabinet filled at inappropriate intervals; is there not a clear and standardized process for delivering medications where nurses can easily locate them; do the batteries on the computers-on-wheels drain too quickly and the doses just are not charted? Seek to discover why the doses are omitted, as these are the issues that need to be resolved.

9. Review national resources that identify errors in other institutions such as the ISMP, the FDA, and the USP. It is likely that your institution is experiencing risks similar to other institutions. Learn what risk-reduction strategies are recommended, take a close look at your own processes, and implement additional risk-reduction strategies where warranted. There is no need to repeat errors at every institution to learn what steps need to be taken for prevention.

TYPES OF SAFETY EVENT ANALYSIS

❹ *Thorough analysis of safety events through the use of root cause analysis, failure mode and effects analysis, or other methods is key to learning from our mistakes in an effort to prevent recurrence.*

Analysis of near-miss events (errors that do not reach the patient) and precursors (errors reaching the patient but causing little to no harm) can be very valuable learning experiences. These may be documented in various ways—through interventions or error-reporting systems. These are valuable when reviewed in aggregate to determine if there are common themes or causes that may warrant further investigation and process changes. It is important to remember that the causes of near misses or errors causing minimal harm are often the same errors that lead to serious harm. For example, a nurse administers a dose of cefazolin to the wrong patient. Fortunately, the patient was not allergic and there was no adverse outcome. If the same error occurs with a different drug (e.g., a high-risk drug, such as a paralytic agent), the outcome can be fatal. Precursor events (those causing little to no harm) can be an important learning experience.

Medication errors that are rated severity E through I, using the NCCMERP severity rating system, cause harm to patients, ranging from minor harm to death. Many facilities conduct investigations on these events to better understand the causes.

The Joint Commission (TJC) is an accrediting body that is focused on continuously improving health care for the public by evaluating health care organizations (e.g., hospitals, home care organizations, nursing homes, ambulatory care providers, and clinical laboratories). The goal of TJC is to ensure that each organization meets designated standards for quality and safety. A sentinel event is defined by TJC as "an unexpected occurrence involving death or serious physical or psychological injury, or the risk thereof. Serious injury specifically includes loss of limb or function. The phrase 'or the risk thereof' includes any process variation for which a recurrence would carry a significant chance of a serious adverse outcome."[38] The expectation is that the organization will conduct a timely, thorough, and credible root cause analysis (RCA) in response to a sentinel event, develop and implement an action plan to reduce the risk of recurrence, and monitor the effectiveness of the plan and its implementation. An RCA can also be conducted on events other than sentinel events, such as when a trend of similar precursor or near-miss events is identified.

The goal of the RCA is to investigate the event in such detail that the true root cause(s) of the event are identified. This requires that the team complete a thorough analysis that includes reviewing the human errors and processes that may contribute to the event. An action plan should be developed with the intent of preventing the recurrence with certainty. Risk-reduction strategies such as reeducating the department, asking staff to be more careful, and developing or editing a policy and procedure have been the norm for years. It is now recognized that these are weak action plans that are not able to prevent recurrence without some change to the processes. The concepts of mistake-proofing, standardization, and forcing functions are important considerations in the development of risk-reduction strategies. Taking an action that physically prevents something from happening is the most effective method of preventing an inadvertent action—such as requiring the foot to be pressed on the brake before placing a car in reverse. Another example of a forcing function is when a computer program requires confirmation to delete a file—it prevents inadvertent deletion. An example of a fail-safe is when a garage door will not continue to close if any motion is detected that interferes with the operation of the door.

One of the key challenges in completing a quality RCA is adequate training and coordinating time for front-line staff and management team members (e.g., physicians, vice presidents) to attend the meetings. One strategy is to have predetermined times designated for team-meeting use if and when an RCA is indicated. This ensures that those with busy schedules have adequate time allotted for this most vital activity. A second key in preventing recurrence is monitoring the action plan to ensure that it is implemented in a timely fashion. Measures should be defined as part of the action plan and revisited to assess the implementation and effectiveness of the action plan. Lastly, it is important to the continued development of a safety culture to be transparent within the organization (and between organizations that are a part of a system) about the lessons learned from events. Information about the event and the action plan should be shared within the facility through structured meetings and communications—all the way to the staff level. The last thing anyone wants is to restructure processes in one area of a facility and not translate the lessons learned to other applicable areas of the facility.

While RCA is a retrospective process, the use of failure mode and effects analysis (FMEA) is a prospective process that is required annually by TJC. This type of analysis involves a team that takes an issue that has been identified as a potentially risky process and examines the ways in which the process or product might fail. An FMEA can be done prior to the implementation of a new process or technology in an effort to increase the awareness of how the implementation might fail, before failure occurs. This allows the implementation team to take adequate steps before the new product or process is introduced to avoid failures. In an FMEA, each step of the process is outlined and the team brainstorms all the ways in which the process could fail and defines the effect of each potential failure to the end user (often the patient). An estimation (on a 10-point scale) is made of the likelihood of the failure, the severity of the potential failure, and the probability that the failure will be detected. A criticality index is calculated and those failure modes with the highest scores are prioritized as important steps for which barriers are developed. Generally an action plan to reduce risk within the process is developed, implemented, and monitored.

Case Study 16–1

At your institution, there have been many intravenous (IV) contrast dye extravasation cases. It has been determined that you will combine information from all of the known cases and conduct an aggregate root cause analysis. An aggregate RCA[39,40] provides intense scrutiny of the cases to determine what opportunities exist to decrease the rate of the extravasations.

1. What are the advantages and disadvantages of including multiple cases in the root cause analysis process?

Human Error or System Error?

TO ERR IS HUMAN

As long as human beings are a key component of processes such as the medication use process, errors are inevitable. Therefore, a need exists for redundancies and the incorporation of human factors principles as key elements to more reliable processes to prevent errors from reaching the patient.

When (not if) humans make errors, there are several ways to approach the event. ❺ *Being human, health care professionals of all types have a propensity to commit errors in every area of their professional lives, including the medication use process.* One approach puts emphasis on the individuals involved, which generally implies blame. This approach generally puts the blame on the last person touching the patient and does not usually acknowledge other factors contributing to the error. As a result, people are urged to be more careful, pay more attention, and undergo remedial training. It also results in increased supervision and increased detail within policies and procedures. It is thought that if we are more vigilant, we can reduce our errors.[41] The other approach focuses on how the design of objects (e.g., smart pumps, drug names, labels for medications, connectors for IVs and tube feedings), activities, and procedures (programming a pump that is infrequently used) contributes to the actions and behaviors of individuals. This approach believes that people come to work with good intentions and are skilled and experienced, but may be led to commit errors because of the way in which the design of the system shapes their behaviors.

According to Senders,[42] "An error is a psychological event with psychological causes...." Human error is inevitable—rather, a fact of life. Most human error results in little to no consequence. It occurs regardless of occupation, although the consequences vary significantly depending on the specific occupation. Therefore, an error in medicine can be fatal, as can an error in the airline industry.

To better understand why health care professionals commit errors, it is necessary to look at the cognitive processes that occur at the time of the error. Norman and Reason have written wonderful books reflecting philosophies of human error.[43-45] Humans will most likely commit errors at an unacceptable rate despite best efforts to understand and remedy the occurrence. With this in mind, it is necessary to develop systems of medication use that account for human error and have processes in place to identify and correct human error before medications reach patients.

A key component of analyzing errors is determining why things happened as they did, which requires a basic understanding of human performance. ❻ *There are three modes of human performance: skill based, rule based, and knowledge based.*

- When in skill-based level of performance, humans are doing very routine tasks that are very practiced and automatic. People are very good at these tasks, as they do them all the time. In skill-based mode, a decision has been made on what the intended action is and the individuals are now in the process of executing a task. Activities such as eating or driving a car to work fit into this category. These are effortless and really unconscious activities that do not require much thought or attention. Skill-based errors are termed slips, lapses, or fumbles.[45] They are easily identified. Slips are usually associated with attention or perception failures and lapses generally involve memory failures.

- A slip occurs when a person places the cereal in the refrigerator instead of the milk. This is something people do all the time—perhaps he or she was briefly interrupted by children or the dog and unconsciously reached for the wrong container.
- A lapse occurs when a person walks into a room only to say, "Now why did I come in here?"
- A fumble occurs when the milk is accidentally knocked over while in the process of putting it back into the refrigerator.

- Humans perform in rule-based mode when problem solving or making decisions. Perhaps there has been a change in the situation—like an exit is closed on the usual route to work and it is necessary to choose an alternate route. The person begins to problem solve, realizing that he or she has been in this situation before. People are trained to deal with many situations, perhaps by learning a policy or procedure. It is possible to determine which rule to apply to the situation encountered. This is called an if-then scenario—if this situation, then do this action. Several scenarios can occur:
  - A wrong rule may be chosen because one misperceives the situation and applies the wrong rule.
  - If one misapplies a rule, a rule-based error has occurred. It is possible to unconsciously pull the wrong pattern or rule from memory. Memory may be biased for many reasons: overgeneralization, recent occurrences (causing one to choose the first answer that comes to mind despite available evidence that would lead to another conclusion), or other factors.
  - There is also intentional rule-based noncompliance (with defined policies and procedures) in which an individual chooses an action despite the knowledge that he or she should take a different action (e.g., a nurse administers a medication without checking the patient's armband because he is sleeping soundly or the bar-code reader is not conveniently located).[45]

- The other performance type is knowledge-based mode. Knowledge-based errors occur when the individual is in a situation to which he or she has never been exposed, or has no preprogrammed rules to apply. The person has a lack of required knowledge to complete the task, or has possibly misinterpreted the problem. When in knowledge-based mode, people are much more likely to make an error than when in skill-based or rule-based mode. The best scenario is that the person recognizes that he or she is lacking the information needed and takes the time to consult with other sources (e.g., colleagues, texts, policies, or literature) to determine the next course of action. Oftentimes, humans feel pressured to proceed in the face of uncertainty because of perceived time constraints, to avoid acknowledging their lack of knowledge to complete the task, or because of overconfidence. The worst-case scenario is that an individual does not realize he or she is in knowledge-based mode, has misinterpreted the situation, and proceeds without any question. "You don't know what you don't know" is a representative phrase in this situation.

One very common type of human error is called confirmation bias. Confirmation bias refers to a type of selective thinking where individuals select what is familiar to them or what they expect to see, rather than what is actually there. A similar type of error is inattentional blindness. Inattentional blindness occurs when the person is so focused on performing the assigned task that he or she fails to see an error or change right in front of his or her eyes that should have been plainly visible, and cannot explain the lapse. In many cases, people involved in the errors have been labeled as careless and negligent. It is human nature for people to associate items by certain characteristics, for example, color of vial, cap, or text. It is very important for the health care community to recognize the role that confirmation bias may play in medication errors and to work to develop systems with the understanding that this phenomenon exists and is part of natural human behavior. These types of accidents are common—even with intelligent, vigilant, and attentive people.[46] Attempts to combat these errors are difficult. Saying "pay more attention" is not effective. Bar-coding has increasingly been used to avoid this phenomenon.

SYSTEM ERROR

❼ *Poorly designed health care systems and processes are a significant contributor to individual human error and subsequent patient harm.* Interestingly enough, behind the majority of individual human errors one or more system errors existed that contributed to the human error. Therefore, it is of utmost importance to recognize system errors and gaps when developing prevention strategies. Systems have common characteristics—these generally include technology, tools and machines, interfaces, processes, products, user interaction with the system, and people. The health care system has become, and continues to become, very complex. There are many layers and components to the health care system: individual practitioners, teams working together, policies and procedures (generally for each individual entity), regulations, devices and equipment, communications, leadership, and management. It would be optimal if all of the parts of the system were integrated and had seamless communication and coordination, but that is not the case. They are each managed separately and are likely to have their own culture, that is, common goals, values, beliefs, and behaviors. It is rare that each component of the system has similar cultures, even when speaking of departments or units within an individual entity, such as the patient care areas of a hospital.[41] It is clear that the development and management of systems and processes has a direct link to the actions of individuals. According to The Joint Commission's analysis of multiple sentinel events,[47] ineffective communication contributes to a significant number of adverse outcomes (60% to 70%). The optimization of systems and processes is essential to the optimization of health care safety. This section discusses system failures that contribute to errors that must be identified and corrected to provide safe care.

A latent failure is a weakness that is usually unconsciously built into a system or, more commonly, develops over time. When making decisions about processes, it is not uncommon that the solution to one problem actually creates a problem in another part of the system (i.e., an unanticipated consequence). Here's one example: If bar-coding medication administration technology using computers on wheeled carts is purchased to prevent administration errors, yet there are not adequate outlets or batteries to keep the computer charged, nurses are faced with skipping the scanning step, finding another computer, or rebooting the computer. The latter two options delay the patient's medication—perhaps only 5 to 10 minutes. However, when a patient is in severe pain, the nurse has been placed in a situation where it seems better to give the medication in a timely fashion and then scan once a viable computer is found. These gaps are inevitable and usually lie relatively undetected. They may appear periodically in a near-miss event, where the error slips through several points but is caught by one last stop-gap (a good catch). If organizations do not learn from the near misses, it is quite possible that eventually the same gaps will result in an adverse event.

When an analysis such as an RCA is undertaken, a thorough understanding of how the system is designed (what are the defined policies and procedures) and how it actually functions (include staff in the RCA or go to the location and observe the process) is very important. When designing an action plan, include more than just actions taken with individuals (e.g., peer review, disciplinary action). A good action plan should address the gaps that were found in the system with prevention strategies to prevent the identified causes. If during a code blue (cardiopulmonary arrest), nursing staff pulled the wrong drug from the crash cart and it was determined that not all crash carts had the same contents, the medication labels were not readily visible, the medications were combined with other supplies, and the contents were in different drawers depending on what unit the cart was found, blaming the staff for not reading the label will not effectively prevent the next person from having similar difficulties finding the correct medication. Address the system and process issues that contributed to the human error. Appropriate to the findings of the investigation, the action plan may include standardization of the carts, with the same drugs found in the same place regardless of cart location, placement of dosing charts in the cart to avoid calculation errors, positioning of pharmacists to pull and prepare medications, or other actions to address the true causes of the error.

Discussion Question: Is it possible to eliminate all errors? Think about human nature and system design. Should the goal be no errors or no events of harm?

It is not humanly possible to eliminate all errors. The goal is to work to reduce and eliminate events of harm by instituting adequate barriers to errors that are predictable, improving monitoring strategies (detection of events), and mitigating harm to patients.

Case Study: A pharmacist is staffing the surgery satellite alone, entering postoperative orders for Sue Doe. A nurse who is caring for a different postoperative patient, Janie Snow, from earlier in the day interrupts the pharmacist with a question about her patient's orders. The pharmacist can only view one patient's profile at a time so she pulls up the computer profile to answer a question about Janie Snow. When the pharmacist returned to her original task of entering the orders for Sue Doe, she inadvertently entered them on the wrong patient. It was determined that there is a system that automatically links the scanned order page to the correct patient, but the current version of computer software does not support this process.

1. What questions would you like to ask the pharmacist involved in the error as part of an interview?
2. Would you classify this error as human-error only, system-error only, or a combination of both, and why?

A Just Culture—Not Shame and Blame

In some instances, reporting medication errors, particularly severe or life-threatening errors, have had adverse consequences for both individuals and the organizations involved. Health care professionals have lost their jobs or voluntarily resigned from their jobs and, at times, have left their profession. Consequently, health care professionals and health systems have been reluctant to open themselves up to adverse outcomes associated with reporting medication errors.[48] For example, in one hospital there were only 36 incident reports regarding medication errors over a year-long reporting period. At the same institution, an observational study revealed that as many as 51,200 errors were likely to have actually occurred during that same reporting period.[49]

Hindsight bias often plays a role in the way people react to an error. Hindsight bias is the inclination to see events that have occurred as being more predictable than they were before the event took place. In other words, the person should have known that this would be the outcome. It is very easy to examine the information after the event and conclude that this bad outcome was going to occur. What investigators and facilitators do not have the benefit of is the vast number of exact circumstances and choices that the individuals were facing, along with their thought processes that led them to their conclusions.

In Nevada, a pharmacy was fined 2 weeks' net profit for a dispensing error that resulted from understaffing.[48] A medical center in New Jersey was successfully sued for $12 million and fined by the state board of pharmacy after a medication error killed an infant.[50] In 1996, a medication error occurred in a hospital in Colorado that resulted in the death of a newborn infant. Three nurses involved in the infant's care were indicted on charges of criminally negligent homicide.[51] District attorneys in Colorado pressed criminal charges that could have resulted in 3 to 5 years' imprisonment. A pharmacist in Ohio was more recently indicted and jailed for a chemotherapy error resulting in the death of a young patient.[52]

Learning from errors, events, and near misses is vital to improvement. Despite the negative actions that have been taken against individuals and organizations in the past, the health care culture is evolving toward a culture of safety. Leaders are learning more about Just Culture. Just Culture is a culture in which discipline is applied in a consistent manner based on the intentions of the individual and the circumstances in which he or she was working—not the outcome. One must understand the circumstances (including poorly designed systems) in which errors occur before decisions related to discipline are made. If a system sets up one individual to fail, the next person in the same situation is also likely to fail in the same manner as the first. If the system is not specifically designed to avert likely human errors (no double-check of a high-risk calculation, such as chemotherapy), human errors will continue to reach patients with significant potential for harm.

Action plans to prevent the recurrence of an event should be designed according to the type of error(s) made. It does not make sense to retrain someone in a procedure if the person is very skilled, but was distracted by a colleague and made a skill-based error. Similarly, if a knowledge-based error is identified, working to decrease distractions and interruptions will have little impact on decreasing future repeat errors with the activity. When interviewing individuals involved in errors, be sure to ask them to describe what happened and what else was going on at the time, to ask them to walk through their decision-making process, and to find out why they think the event occurred. Be sure to understand the options presented to them at the time.

Recall those headlines again—"Child Dies from Medication Error";"Journalist Dies of Chemotherapy Error." The rest of the story usually involves details about what happened (on the surface) and who was fired or reprimanded. What disciplinary action should be taken in these cases—if any? It depends on the circumstances entirely. It is important to have a good understanding of exactly what happened and the "whys" behind the decisions and actions taken. If an individual did not consciously make an unsafe decision, how does discipline help one learn from mistakes? Will not staff be less willing to report and discuss them without fear of retribution? Retraining, counseling, and discipline have been hallmark actions taken to prevent error and have failed to substantially improve patient care.

The culture of blame shifted in the 1990s in the health care industry when it was recognized that the punitive nature of discipline was not the best way to encourage staff to talk about risks and errors, and assist in the process of decreasing errors. The culture then shifted to a blame-free culture in an effort to promote reporting. This culture recognized that humans will err, that most unsafe acts are slips or lapses, and that weaknesses in systems and environments contribute significantly to errors in medicine.[53]

What was not recognized at the time was that a solely blame-free culture (also termed nonpunitive) failed to attend to those few who knowingly ignore designated safety procedures and those who are unreasonably reckless or negligent. This undermines those who work hard at providing safe care.

❽ *A Just Culture is one in which discipline is applied in a consistent manner based on the intentions of the individual and the situation in which he or she was working—not the outcome.* A Just Culture is somewhere between the two extremes described previously, with blaming individuals on one end, blame-free culture on the other end, and a Just Culture somewhere in the middle. It is unacceptable to discipline all errors regardless of their circumstances, and is just as unacceptable to be nonpunitive in the face of individuals who are intentionally ignoring safe operating principles.

The hard part is distinguishing between those who make a conscious decision to complete an unsafe action despite knowing that it is unsafe (i.e., at-risk behavior), and those who usually work in a safe manner and experienced a slip or lapse. A substitution test has proven to be useful in these instances.[45] When dealing with a serious event and a person is implicated in an unsafe act, describe the scenario to several other individuals (at least three) of the same qualifications and experience (optimally, who are not aware of the actual incident) and ask them what decisions they would have made in the circumstances at the time. If they would have made the same decision and completed the same actions, then blaming the individual is not likely appropriate, as there is evidence that this issue has a larger scope. Another option is to observe individuals in the same situations, if possible, to determine how others behave in similar instances. This helps one determine whether the problem lies with an individual or an expanded group (perhaps a unit or department), or is a more global problem. This also helps in the development of an action plan. There is no need to reeducate an entire department on a process if there is only one individual that is in need of coaching.

The use of a series of questions helps determine the culpability and accountability of a person's actions and are taken from the Decision Tree for determining the Culpability of Unsafe Acts.[45] It is key that any decisions related to discipline are made not only when there's an adverse outcome. Appropriate discipline, when warranted, should be taken when unsafe behaviors are identified, regardless of outcome.[54]

1. Were the actions as intended?
2. Was the person under the influence of unauthorized substances?
3. Did he or she knowingly violate a safe operating procedure? If so, was the procedure available, workable, intelligible, and correct? This gets at those procedures that staff feel make no sense and are not value-added in their workflow. Perhaps they have a point and there is a component of system-induced error.
4. Does the individual pass the substitution test described previously? Would others have made the same decisions and, if so, is the individidual less likely to be culpable? If not, were there deficiencies in training or experience?
5. Does the individual have a history of unsafe acts? If not, is he or she less likely to be culpable?

The use of these questions and the decision assist in determining the level of culpability of an individual. The actions in the first few questions bear more culpability than those that occur in the last several questions. Therefore, disciplinary actions are more likely to be appropriate for those acts that are intended and/or undertaken while under the influence of unauthorized substances.

There are always a few outliers within any profession—those who intentionally do not follow the processes as designed, feeling that they are immune from human error and/or believing their process is better. There is a difference between unintentional human error, at-risk behavior, and reckless behavior. Intentionally unsafe behavior is identified by the first question and is generally dealt with through disciplinary action. At-risk behavior may be amenable to coaching about the reason for the process as designed and a request for a commitment to better choices.

Case Study 16–3

Patient Samuel Sneer received an overdose of a diltiazem drip and became hypotensive, requiring fluid boluses, but recovered without further effects. After investigation it was discovered that the nurse changed the diltiazem bag as it was nearly empty. The pump required the nurse to enter the concentration (drug in milligrams and then volume of fluid). Instead of entering the drug dose first, she mistakenly entered the fluid volume first. This is the way the concentration information appeared on the labeled bag, which is to what she had referred.

The nurse was under time pressure and was caring for more patients than the usual accepted ratio due to the flu epidemic. The pump has programmed minimum and maximum settings but the rate was just under the maximum setting, meaning she did not receive a warning about the error. This is the first error identified for this nurse who has practiced at the hospital for over a year.

1. What system issues contributed to the error?
2. Walk the error through the culpability decision tree algorithm to determine your reaction as manager of the unit (coaching, consoling, or disciplinary action).
3. What potential system fixes can you identify?

Risk Factors for Errors and Events

The ultimate purpose for defining, classifying, analyzing, and reporting medication errors is to enable individuals and organizations to implement better systems that prevent medication errors. The ASHP has identified a multitude of risk factors associated with the occurrence of medication errors as outlined in the following[33]:

- Shift work—switching from days to nights.
- Inexperienced or inadequately trained staff.
- Medical services with special needs (e.g., pediatrics and oncology).
- Higher number of medications per patient.
- Environmental factors such as high levels of noise, poor lighting, and frequent interruptions.
- High workload for staff.
- Poor communication among health care providers.
- Dosage form—more errors with injectable drugs.
- Drug category—more errors with certain classes of drugs (e.g., antibiotics).
- Type of drug distribution systems—unit dose system is associated with fewer errors; high levels of floor stock are associated with increased errors.
- Improper drug storage.

- Calculations—increased errors with increased complexity and frequency of amount of calculations required.
- Poor handwriting.
- Verbal orders.
- Lack of effective policies and procedures.
- Poorly functioning oversight committees.

Personal and environmental factors are thought to interact to influence cognitive function, which may lead to slips. There are several factors specific to the professionals involved and their working environment that may contribute to their risk of committing an error. Grasha and O'Neill[55] have outlined some of the factors that may affect cognitive processes, resulting in lapses of performance.

1. *Excessive task demand:* Many pharmacists attribute their errors to this situation, complaining that their workload is so heavy and they are overloaded with tasks, making it difficult to work error-free. In one survey, 68% of pharmacists rated work overload as a major contributing factor to the committal of dispensing errors.[56] Most pharmacists and experts in medication errors agree that work overload may be the most significant factor contributing to medication errors. Reevaluation of the workload distribution, with an eye for streamlining processes, may be valuable. Developing a detailed map of all of the steps required to accomplish a task is one way to discover the complexity of a task. This is also called process mapping.

2. *Personal characteristics:* Personal factors, such as age, sensory deficits, or state of health, may contribute to performance lapses. Personal levels of stress or fatigue may also have an impact. Someone who is bored at work may also be more error prone.

3. *Extra-organizational factors:* Factors such as similar product names or packaging from pharmaceutical companies may have an extensive impact on the commission of errors with particular drugs. In one study, look-alike or sound-alike drugs were involved in 37% of medication errors.[57] As an example, this issue is currently being addressed for the sound-alike drugs celecoxib (Celebrex), fosphenytoin (Cerebyx), and citalopram (Celexa). Complex insurance plans are also extra-organizational factors that may serve to complicate the medication use process and contribute to slips. The profession of pharmacy has been referred to as the most heavily regulated of all professions. Legal mandates for policing illegal prescriptions and other regulatory requirements are also good examples of extra-organizational factors.

4. *Work environment:* Poor working conditions may influence the rate of error committal. Poor illumination and high noise levels have been shown to affect

the dispensing error rate in pharmacies.[58] Other factors in this category may include high ambient temperatures and frequent interruptions from the telephone or patients.

5. *Intra-organizational factors:* There is a significant emphasis on other factors besides the quality and safety of medication use within health care systems. Concerns related to finances, throughput, customer service, and quality of employee work life are often competing priorities and major areas of focus in many institutions. Policies and procedures demanding high output or mandating long working hours may significantly affect cognition and the ability to prevent error occurrence.

6. *Interpersonal factors:* Conflicts among coworkers or with patients may distract professionals from the tasks at hand and contribute to error commission. General interruptions from people may also fall into this category.

Some factors that may contribute to cognitive lapses and the commission of medication errors may fall into more than one of these categories. Furthermore, factors from multiple categories may occur simultaneously to contribute to error commission.

Health care professionals have indicated that other factors may also contribute to medication errors. Some of those factors are as follows:

1. *Lack of effective communication:* This factor may also fall under interpersonal factors listed previously. Failure to communicate effectively among fellow employees or among health care professionals has frequently been named as contributing to medical and medication errors. For example, an error may be more likely to occur if a pharmacist chooses not to clarify physician orders or if the pharmacist does not communicate all of the pertinent information so the physician can make an informed decision. Poor physician handwriting and verbal orders are also significant factors.[35]

2. *Failure to comply with policy:* This is a common factor in dispensing and administering drugs. In one survey, 42% to 46% of pharmacists said that failing to check drugs before dispensing was a significant factor in dispensing errors.[56] Noncompliance with policy has also been associated with drug administration errors and is the result of several factors: perceived burden of the task, perceived risk of a bad outcome, and the perceived risk of being observed. Often, nurses develop specific personal routines for the administration of certain agents that they perceive to be an improvement in the medication administration process, despite contrary policy.[35] It is important to understand the challenges that make work difficult. Ensure that processes have been designed with safety in mind.

3. *Lack of knowledge:* This is a frequently cited factor in the committal of medication errors. Mistakes, rather than slips, are typically committed as a result of inadequate knowledge. Placing inexperienced recent graduates in positions where they cannot interact with more experienced practitioners may increase medication errors. Nonspecialists covering a service that is normally staffed by a specialist may also lead to errors.[58] Nurses with less exposure to pharmacology may be less likely to recognize potential inconsistencies in disease state and medication usage and doses, resulting in the possibility of increased medication errors reaching the patient.[35]

4. *Lack of patient counseling:* It has been said that the last safety check prior to dispensing medication should be counseling the patient. Talking to the patient allows the pharmacist to correlate the medication and dose with the patient's condition and helps the pharmacist to detect any errors that may have occurred in the medication use process. In one study, 89% of errors committed in a community pharmacy were detected during patient counseling.[48] However, errors may occur not only from a lack of counseling, but also from providing incorrect information during patient counseling.[59] Providing incorrect information may also fall in the lack of knowledge category. One additional factor that plays a major part in understanding the patient is health care literacy. All professionals should assess the level of patient literacy to ensure that appropriate language and teaching methods are used in their interactions with the patient (see Chapter 20 for more information on this).

These examples are a partial list of contributory factors at the level of the health care practitioner. These factors influence the occurrence of slips or performance lapses and mistakes committed by individuals. They do not address failure of a system or failure of a safety net as a whole process. The medication use process involves multiple health care professionals, nonprofessional staff, patients, and multiple physical environments. To adequately address the causes of errors, failures in the system must also be addressed. Although it is important to address the problem of individuals committing errors (e.g., increasing training if a knowledge deficit was identified and enforcing policy), adequately developed safety systems should be in place to significantly minimize the number of errors reaching patients.

Health Professions Education

Most health care professionals are trained with the thought that individuals cannot make mistakes in health care; when dealing with patients, it is unacceptable to cause an error.

Students as well as practicing professionals (e.g., physicians, nurses, pharmacists, respiratory therapists) learn little about human factors thinking, systems design, quality improvement, and reliability. They do not learn that humans err in many ways. Thus, when they do make an error in practice, many either deny the fact or are jolted into the realization that they should be more careful. Many times, the realization that they have made an error causes physicians, pharmacists, nurses, and other professionals to avoid discussion about errors—with colleagues and patients. When an error or safety event is investigated and analyzed, individuals and/or professions may point fingers at the other, some may avoid telling the whole story, some do not realize the value of the process, and many do not recognize the contribution that processes and systems play in their own errors. Many of the Institute of Medicine reports on quality and safety have referenced the need for changes in health professions education. Pertinent quotes from *To Err Is Human: Building a Safer Health System*[1] (1999) include

> Clinical training and education is a key mechanism for cultural change. Colleges of medicine, nursing, pharmacy, health care administration, and their related associations should build more instruction into their curriculum on patient safety and its relationship to quality improvement.
>
> Many believe that initial exposure to patient safety should occur early in undergraduate and graduate training programs, as well as through continuing education.
>
> The need for more opportunities for interdisciplinary training was also identified. Most care delivered today is done by teams of people, yet training often remains focused on individual responsibilities, leaving practitioners inadequately prepared to enter complex settings.

Another report by the Institute of Medicine, Crossing the Quality Chasm[60] (2001), identifies health professions education as a priority.

❾ *All health professionals should be educated to deliver patient-centered care as members of an interdisciplinary team, emphasizing evidence-based practice, quality improvement approaches, and informatics.*

Subsequently, a summit of over 150 interdisciplinary participants met in 2002 and developed recommendations for reaching this goal. The proceedings and recommendations from the summit are compiled in *Health Professions Education:A Bridge to Quality.*[61] The following strategies are outlined in the book:

- Develop and build consensus around a common language and core competencies.
- Integrate core competencies into oversight processes.

- Motivate and support leaders, and monitor progress of reform effort.
- Develop evidence-based curricula and teaching approaches.
- Develop faculty as teaching and learning experts.

Many teaching institutions (both academic institutions and health care institutions where currently practicing professionals lack this knowledge) struggle with where and how to integrate additional information into either the curriculum or orientation process.

The Institute for Healthcare Improvement (IHI) has developed an interprofessional, international educational online community. The IHI Open School provides a mechanism by which students and their mentors in nursing, medicine, pharmacy, dentistry, health care administration, and other health professions can interact and learn in an interdisciplinary fashion. There are online courses in quality and safety, basic and advanced certifications in quality improvement and patient safety, case studies, podcasts, videos, and feature articles. The IHI's Open School program[62] is one example where online modules on quality and safety can be completed either during professional education or as a part of continuing education and learning for practitioners. See http://www.ihi.org for additional information. This is a great start to providing the types of interdisciplinary learning that will be of great value to the health care community and patients.

Best Practices for Error Prevention

❿ *There are many resources that identify best-practice error prevention strategies.* Listed here are various resources as well as strategies to ensure that medication use processes are as safe as they can be. Remember to be a learning organization by constantly reviewing local and national information and taking proactive steps to prevent error. Do not wait until it happens to you.

The Institute for Safe Medication Practices publishes a "Quarterly Action Agenda" that describes known risks and errors and describes recommendations for risk-reduction strategy implementation. These can be found on their Web site at http://www.ismp.org.

The Institute for Healthcare Improvement (IHI) has sponsored two campaigns (the 100,000 Lives Campaign and the 5 Million Lives Campaign) to save lives and protect patients from harm. At least half of the 12 recommended interventions within the campaigns involve improving the safe use of medications. Pharmacists should be integrally involved in the institution team to ensure successful interventions (Table 16–5). In addition to these two campaigns, the IHI offers many programs, conferences, IMPACT network associations, best-practice postings, the IHI Open School, and much more. Visit http://www.ihi.org for more information.

TABLE 16–5. INTERVENTIONS RECOMMENDED BY THE INSTITUTE FOR HEALTHCARE IMPROVEMENT (IHI) TO SAVE LIVES AND REDUCE PATIENT INJURIES

Strategies from the 100,000 Lives Campaign

- **Deploy Rapid Response Teams...** at the first sign of patient decline
- **Deliver Reliable, Evidence-Based Care for Acute Myocardial Infarction...** to prevent deaths from heart attack
- **Prevent Adverse Drug Events (ADEs)...** by implementing medication reconciliation
- **Prevent Central Line Infections...** by implementing a series of interdependent, scientifically grounded steps
- **Prevent Surgical Site Infections...** by reliably delivering the correct perioperative antibiotics at the proper time
- **Prevent Ventilator-Associated Pneumonia...** by implementing a series of interdependent, scientifically grounded steps

Strategies from the 5 Million Lives Campaign

- **Prevent Harm from High-Alert Medications...** starting with a focus on anticoagulants, sedatives, narcotics, and insulin
- **Reduce Surgical Complications...** by reliably implementing all of the changes recommended by SCIP, the Surgical Care Improvement Project (www.medqic.org/scip)
- **Prevent Pressure Ulcers...** by reliably using science-based guidelines for their prevention
- **Reduce Methicillin-Resistant *Staphylococcus aureus* (MRSA) infection...** by reliably implementing scientifically proven infection control practices
- **Deliver Reliable, Evidence-Based Care for Congestive Heart Failure...** to avoid readmissions
- **Get Boards on Board...** by defining and spreading the best-known leveraged processes for hospital boards of directors, so that they can become far more effective in accelerating organizational progress toward safe care

The Joint Commission's National Patient Safety Goals can serve as guides to improving the safety of health care. Many of The Joint Commission's National Patient Safety Goals released each year are related to safe medication use, and pharmacists should be involved in ensuring that their facility meets these goals. The goals are divided into the type of health care provided—hospital, home care, ambulatory care, behavioral health care, and so forth. There are other goals aside from those listed, some of which indirectly relate to pharmacy. These goals change frequently. A partial list includes

- Accurately and completely reconcile medications during transitions within and across organizations (inpatient to outpatient).
- Improve the effectiveness of communication between caregivers.
  - Write down and read back verbal orders (and critical test results)—The Joint Commission safety goal sets the expectation that for all verbal orders, the receiver of the order must write the order down on the order page and then read the transcribed order back to the practitioner, who then verifies that the order has been transcribed as intended. This prevents transcription errors in

which the receiver may have heard the order correctly and made an error in writing/entering the order after the conversation has ended and prevents errors in which the order was heard and transcribed incorrectly. This is also referred to as closed-loop communication in which the giver and recipient confirm that the information provided and received is accurate.

- ○ Designate unapproved abbreviations and monitor their use.
- Implement a standardized approach to hand-off communications, including an opportunity to ask and respond to questions.
- Improve the safety of using medications.
  - ○ Develop risk-reduction strategies around look-alike and sound-alike medications.
  - ○ Label all medications, medication containers (e.g., syringes, medicine cups, basins), or other solutions on and off the sterile field.
- Reduce the likelihood of patient harm associated with the use of anticoagulant therapy.
  - ○ Includes an anticoagulation management program, approved protocols for initiation and maintenance, individualized care, appropriate baseline and ongoing lab monitoring.
  - ○ Includes notification and involvement of the dietary department, patient education, use of infusion pumps for heparin, and evaluation of anticoagulation safety.
- Implement best practices for preventing surgical site infections. Timely administration of appropriately chosen antibiotics just prior to the surgical procedure is essential to preventing surgical site infections. Most preoperative antibiotics must be given within 1 hour prior to the incision time. There are many errors that may contribute to the development of infection at the surgical site: lack of timely access to the medication, incorrect medication selection, or administration of the drug too early. At one time, the preoperative antibiotic was administered on the patient care unit before transporting the patient to the operating room; however, there are often delays in getting the patient to the operating room.

Consult The Joint Commission Web site for the most up-to-date standards (http://www.jointcommission.org/PatientSafety/NationalPatientSafetyGoals/).

The National Quality Forum (NQF)'s Safe Practices for Better Healthcare identifies 34 practices that have been demonstrated to be effective in reducing the occurrence of adverse events in health care. Although there are two identified best practices identified within a chapter titled "Improving Patient Safety Through Medication Management," many of the other Safe Practices involve medication use. The Safe Practices associated with the medication management chapter are as follows:

- Medication reconciliation—Many adverse events are the result of patients presenting to an acute care facility such as a hospital, identifying a list of the medications that they are taking at home, yet somewhere during the admission, transfer, or discharge process, these medications are inadvertently omitted or duplicate therapy occurs due to therapeutic substitution at discharge. The organization must develop a process to identify, reconcile (compare and confirm which medications are appropriate for the patient to take during the hospitalization or outpatient visit), and communicate an accurate patient medication list throughout the continuum of care (to other primary care and specialist providers).
- Pharmacist leadership structure—Pharmacy leaders should have an active role on the administrative leadership team that identifies their accountability for the performance of the medication management systems across the institution.

Other Safe Practices that relate to medication use include

- Improving patient safety by creating and sustaining a culture of safety.
    - The elements of this safe practice include leadership structures and systems, culture measurement and intervention, teamwork training, and the identification and mitigation of risks and hazards.
- Improving patient safety by facilitating information transfer and clear communication.
    - Elements of this chapter include communication of critical information, order read-back, safe adoption of computerized prescriber order entry (CPOE), and avoiding unapproved abbreviations. Each organization must define a list of unapproved abbreviations, monitor the frequency of use, and develop strategies to reduce the use of these abbreviations. Several high-risk abbreviations have been identified (by ISMP and other organizations) such as MSO_4 and $MgSO_4$, which may be inadvertently misread and administered, causing harm to patients, and U (for units), which has been misinterpreted as a zero, causing 10-fold overdoses of insulin.
- Improving patient safety through the prevention of health care–associated infections.
    - This includes practices around aspiration and ventilator-associated pneumonia (VAP) prevention, surgical site infection prevention, multidrug-resistant organism prevention, hand hygiene, and influenza prevention through the administration of appropriate vaccines to all qualified patients. Administration of appropriate antibiotic prophylaxis in a timely manner is a key prevention strategy for surgical site infections.
- Improving patient safety through condition and site-specific practices.
    - This grouping includes perioperative myocardial infarction and ischemia prevention, venous thromboembolism prevention, anticoagulation therapy, and contrast-media–induced renal failure prevention.

Many of the practices involving medication use and pharmacy should be integrally involved in efforts to meet these goals. Visit the Web site for the latest version (http://www.qualityforum.org/projects/patient_safety_measures.aspx). These two resources combined create a great roadmap for working toward safer medication use systems.

Incorporate human factors principles into the design of processes. ⓫ *Researching, recognizing, and designing with human factors principles in mind is a great way to improve the safety of any process.* Human factors research is a developing type of research in health care; other industries have developed strategies around human factors to successfully improve safety (e.g., nuclear power, air travel). Some of the core principles of human factors design include the following:

- Simplify and standardize—A process that requires a policy and procedure of 10 pages is one that is much too complex.
- Reduce reliance on memory—The human mind can only hold a limited amount of things in short-term memory (four to seven items depending on what source is read). Therefore, formulating other methods of prioritization or reminders is likely to be more effective than relying on the recall of individuals.
- Use constraints and forcing functions—Mistake-proofing is the use of process or design features to prevent errors or the negative impact of errors. Mistake-proofing is also known as *poka-yoke* (pronounced *pokayokay*), which is Japanese slang for avoiding inadvertent errors.[63] One great example is the file cabinet. Tons of papers are stored in file cabinets. An example is when one file drawer and then a second drawer are opened, just to find the entire cabinet falling over. If more than one file drawer is opened at a time, the center of gravity moves, causing the file cabinet to fall. Modern file cabinets are designed to avoid this type of injury, as opening one drawer locks the rest. The design forces correct behavior and only allows for proper use. It takes longer to file, but it prevents injury. Several approaches to mistake-proofing include mistake prevention, mistake detection, and reduction of the effect of user errors.
- Improve information access—Coordination and interfacing computer systems is a huge challenge, but is often the only way to ensure that all information is available to those who need it.
- Decrease reliance on vigilance—Humans will err; therefore, other mechanisms to prevent errors from reaching the patient are much more effective than asking people to be careful. They may be more vigilant for a brief time, and then revert back to previous habits.
- Increase feedback—Feedback (of actions taken and processes improved as a result of reported events) to reporters, end users, and management staff is critical to the development of a safety culture. At times, staff report errors and never see

any changes, which is discouraging and results in staff being less likely to report. If there is never any perceived action taken in response to the report, no review of the reports, no activity to improve the system, or no follow-up or feedback of information back to the reporter, the staff perceive that reporting the known risks they encounter is a waste of time, and they will stop reporting. Completing a report (especially if there is no harm to a patient) takes away time from the bedside or other critical activities.

- o Reduce and/or improve the reliability of handoffs—Handoffs are one of the more common points for error. Oftentimes when contacting a physician, handing off a patient to another caregiver, or during a change of shift report, only portions of the patient's pertinent history are provided. The information provided is often variable and dependent on the person handing off the information and other factors, such as time pressure. There are often gaps when critical information (e.g., allergies, code status, pending physician response to resolve medication-related questions) is not provided, leading to errors and omissions in care.

- A structured handoff process has been incorporated as a National Patient Safety Goal by The Joint Commission as a method of reducing the likelihood that important information is not passed on to the next shift or the next caregiver. The use of SBAR as a communication tool during handoffs of patients or information is one method that has proven successful in reducing the errors introduced during the handoff of patients within or between institutions. SBAR stands for the following:
  - o Situation—Describe the current situation and reason for the call.
  - o Background—Provide pertinent background information (e.g., history, current medications, labs, vital signs) to the situation.
  - o Assessment—Provide your assessment of the situation.
  - o Recommendation/Request—Provide your request or recommendation in succinct terms.

OTHER PRINCIPLES OF ERROR MANAGEMENT

- **Implement new technology and information systems—with caution.** There have been many advances in technology and information systems available within health care: bar-coding technology, smart pumps, CPOE, automated dispensing and distribution technologies, and more. These all have the potential to provide great value; however, one should undertake the implementation of these new technologies carefully. The curse of the unintended consequence is often discovered during or after implementation. Unintended consequences may occur when a new technology is implemented and a new problem develops as a result of the technology. In some cases, a failure mode and effects analysis (FMEA) is used prior to new technology implementation to brainstorm what could go wrong and develop strategies and educational tools to prevent deviations from the desired outcome. Reviewing technology from a human factors perspective early in the process is recommended. For example, placing a computer on top of an automated distribution machine provides great access to information that nursing and pharmacy staff need during the retrieval or refilling of these machines. However, if the font is so small that no one can read it, this technology may actually cause more errors by selecting the wrong patient or wrong drug. It is always recommend that end users be involved in the selection process of these technologies, as they are the ones who interact with the products daily. They can identify potential issues very quickly.

- **Use Quality Improvement Techniques to improve safety. Develop metrics and monitor progress.** Although it is not necessary to conduct a randomized controlled trial with every intervention to improve safety, it is valuable to develop measures, gather baseline data, and remeasure to show improvement. The Plan-Do-Study-Act (PDSA) cycle is one structured method to lead teams through the improvement process. This process involves a planning stage in which a problem statement and implementation strategy are developed based on gaps identified within a process (plan), the strategy is implemented (do), the results are analyzed (study), and any refinements are made to the plan (act).These cycles repeat until a reliable and efficient process is finalized. See Chapter 14 for additional information on this process. Rapid-cycle tests of change are great ways to avoid the full-blown implementation of a poorly designed process. Rapid-cycle testing involves the identification of a new process to be considered or implemented followed by a very brief trial or pilot with just one patient, one physician's patients, or one unit. The learning from this short pilot will be used to edit the new method, allow time to try it again (often several times), gain the input and support of staff in the process, and provide valuable revisions before implementation. Once the cycles have ironed out all of the apparent problems, the process is rolled out on a broader basis.
- **Evaluate areas for environmental contributions to error.** There are numerous workplace factors that may contribute to performance lapses and medication errors. Low lighting, high levels of noise, high temperatures, and stressful work environments are examples. Distractions and interruptions as part of the workflow should also be evaluated and minimized.
- **Involve patients on committees such as the patient safety committee.** Put some thought into who might be chosen to join the team. Use an application process to identify the best people. Ensure that a confidentiality agreement is signed.

Choose someone who will listen to other perspectives, yet provide constructive feedback into how to think from a patient's perspective. It is amazing what changes can result when involving patients and/or family members. The team will alter its thinking and priorities, becoming more patient centered.

- **Establish redundancies around high-risk processes and high-risk medication use.** As humans are susceptible to error, it is recommended that redundancy be a part of processes. This allows an error caused by a slip or lapse to be caught downstream before it reaches a patient. Independent double-checks are recommended for high-risk processes and medications, such as for chemotherapy and neonatal parenteral nutrition. For maximal effectiveness, double-checks should be limited to ensure that they are completed appropriately. It is recommended that double-checks be limited to the following:[64]
  - Situations that involve high-alert medications, such as chemotherapy (including methotrexate), insulin, opiates, and anticoagulants
  - Complex processes (compounding, calculating doses)
  - High-risk patient populations (children and adolescents; elderly or pregnant patients; patients with severe congestive heart failure; and patients with known renal impairment or liver disease)

The average number of errors missed on a check is about 5%. In studies using simulated cart-fills, 93% to 97% of these errors were identified with an independent double-check. Although these numbers seem small, they add up quickly with the number of medications dispensed daily. Be sure to define exactly what is meant by an independent double-check. One person should do the calculations and document the results. Then a second person, without reviewing the work of the first person, should complete the same calculations and then compare the answers for consistency. This is important to avoid confirmation bias. Recall that confirmation bias is a natural tendency to see what we think we see. When glancing at an order to confirm it for another person who has just asked, "Do you think this order says warfarin?" the chance to be biased to see warfarin in the order greatly increases. If the person had just asked what the order appeared to say, there is much less chance for this bias.

Table 16–6 identifies several Web sites that remain sources of updated safe practices and updated news related to safety risks and hazards.

Putting It All Together

Providing safe medication use is paramount to the safety of all patients. Diligent efforts to identify errors (utilizing several methods), understand the human capability and

TABLE 16–6. ORGANIZATIONS PROMOTING BEST PRACTICES IN PATIENT AND MEDICATION SAFETY

Agency for Healthcare Research and Quality	http://www.ahrq.gov
AHRQ Patient Safety Network	http://www.psnet.ahrq.gov
American Society of Health-System Pharmacists	http://www.ashp.org
Centers for Disease Control and Prevention	http://www.cdc.gov
Institute for Healthcare Improvement	http://www.ihi.org
Institute for Safe Medication Practices	http://www.ismp.org
Massachusetts Coalition for the Prevention of Medical Errors	http://www.macoalition.org
National Patient Safety Foundation	http://www.npsf.org
National Quality Forum	http://www.qualityforum.org
Pathways for Medication Safety	http://www.medpathways.info
Patient Safety and Quality Healthcare	http://www.psqh.com/index.html
The Joint Commission	http://www.jointcommission.org
The Joint Commission International	http://www.jointcommissioninternational.org
The Advisory Board	http://www.advisory.com
United States Pharmacopeia (USP)	http://www.usp.org
U.S. Food and Drug Administration (FDA)	http://www.fda.gov

propensity to commit errors in everyday life, analyze and determine the root causes and contributing factors, and devise systems that support humans and prevent expected errors are all a part of developing a culture of safety. Involving staff on the front line when reviewing safety events and developing action plans to prevent recurrence is important—not only to the development of an appropriate action plan, but also to garner support and confidence that once errors are identified, leadership is committed to improving the processes in which staff have to work every day.

Conclusion: Safety as a Priority

In 1998, the IOM formed the Quality of Healthcare in America Committee, which was charged with developing a strategy to improve quality in health care. In their published report, *To Err Is Human: Building a Safer Health System*,[1] the Committee highlighted what was currently known about the extent of medical errors, what contributes to medical errors, and recommendations to minimize errors and improve the quality of health care in the United States. Many of the goals set forth in this report are becoming closer to reality. The many other reports by the IOM have provided additional detail and insight into what is necessary to optimize the safety of the health care system in the United States.

Medication misadventures continue to be a serious problem in the U.S. health care system, both in the hospital and the broader ambulatory scope. Working to provide safe care is a journey, or rather, a marathon. Changing a culture is not something that is accomplished in a few years; it may take 10 or more years. Much of that is dependent on the leadership of executives and staff. Those with a passion for safety may need to help enlighten those in higher leadership positions. Learn from others. It is an important method of preventing errors from occurring within your institution/facility. Take a close look at your own processes when you read a local or national headline about an error. There continues to be ongoing research aimed at increasing the safety and quality of health care. Health care will continue to be complex and require effective coordination and communication. Technology will continue to evolve. Safety truly needs to be a core value that is held by all. Teamwork and mutual respect are vital parts to success. Only through collaboration and a shared, dedicated commitment will patient safety truly become a reality.

Self-Assessment Questions

1. Congress passed the Patient Safety and Quality Improvement Act of 2005, from which Patient Safety Organizations (PSOs) were created. Which of the following is *not* a true statement?
   a. This act provides two types of protections: confidentiality and privilege protections.
   b. One of the goals of the PSOs is to collate and analyze data related to safety errors and events.
   c. PSOs will forward information about facility-specific reported events to The Joint Commission and the media.
   d. PSOs will require the use of Common Formats (standardized reporting and terminology) for reporting errors and events.

2. Patient A is given a dose of penicillin intended for Patient B. The physician was notified when the error was discovered (2 hours after the dose was administered) and no further orders were given. Which of the following NCCMERP classification is *most* appropriate?
   a. Category A
   b. Category B
   c. Category C
   d. Category E
   e. Category F

3. Which national reporting system is intended for problems with medical products and devices?
   a. MedWatch
   b. MEDMARX
   c. USP-ISMP MERP program
   d. All of the above

4. Which of the following action plan items is the *strongest and most likely* to provide sustained reduction in risk?
   a. Reeducate the department about the error and correct process.
   b. Add detail to the very long policy and procedure, spelling out every step that needs to be taken.
   c. Talk to the people involved and ask them to be more careful.
   d. Develop a forcing function such that the human error is not possible.

5. You are an experienced technician delivering a medication to a patient care area on the third floor (as you do every day on this floor) when a colleague stops you to ask a question about a patient's medication. Once the conversation ends, you continue on to the fourth floor, forgetting to leave the medications for the patients on the third floor. What type of human error is this?
   a. Skill-based error
   b. Rule-based error
   c. Knowledge-based error
   d. Interruption-based error

6. A Just Culture exists when there is a nonpunitive environment, where staff are not disciplined based on errors, to ensure that people will report all errors identified.
   a. True
   b. False

7. Which of the following methods utilizes the screening of patients' charts to identify clues (such as an elevated lab value or reversal agent) that a patient may have experienced a medication error or adverse drug event?
   a. ADE trigger tool
   b. Observation method
   c. Voluntary reporting method
   d. None of the above

8. Which of the following is a prospective analysis of a process to determine risk-reduction strategies?
   a. Root cause analysis (RCA)
   b. Interview people involved in previous errors
   c. Failure mode and effects analysis (FMEA)
   d. Trending of error and event reports

9. Which of the following organization(s) provides information related to the prevention of medical and medication error?
   a. Institute for Safe Medication Practice (ISMP)
   b. National Quality Forum (NQF)
   c. Institute for Healthcare Improvement (IHI)
   d. The Joint Commission (TJC)
   e. All of the above

10. Which of the following statements are true?
    a. All medication errors cause harm.
    b. All adverse drug events involve harm.
    c. There is no harm involved in an adverse drug reaction.
    d. All of the above are true.

11. Which of the following are gaps or failures that are designed into or develop within a system, increasing the chance that people working within the system will make an error?
    a. Latent failures
    b. Individual failures
    c. Inevitable failures
    d. Personal failures

12. Which is *not* an example of designing with human factors principles?
    a. Use constraints and forcing functions.
    b. Reduce reliance on memory.
    c. Simplify and standardize.
    d. Reduce handoffs.
    e. All of the above are examples.

13. Which term refers to a type of selective thinking where individuals select out what is familiar to them or what they expect to see, rather than what is actually there?
    a. Hindsight bias
    b. Confirmation bias
    c. System failure
    d. Just Culture

14. A pharmacist is alone in the pharmacy entering a physician order when she receives a call about a patient. In order to answer the question, she must exit the current patient's profile to pull up another patient's profile. Once the question has been answered, she hangs up and proceeds to finish entering the order on the patient's profile (the wrong patient).Which error-prevention strategy would most likely be the *least* effective at preventing a recurrence of this error?
    a. Discipline the pharmacist and remind her to be more careful—do patient identification correctly on every order.
    b. Purchase (or develop) technology that automatically links a physician order to the patient's profile in the pharmacy system—a forcing function.
    c. Alter the practice such that there are minimal to no interruptions for pharmacists entering orders (route calls to one area and responsible staff, segregate order-entry staff to decrease interruptions).
    d. All of the above will be effective and prevent the recurrence.

15. Which of the following is/are risk factors that increase the chance for errors?
    a. Poor lighting
    b. Fatigue or illness
    c. Time pressure
    d. Poor communication with other practitioners or departments
    e. All of the above

REFERENCES

1. Institute of Medicine. To Err Is Human: Building a Safer Health-System. Washington, DC: National Academy Press; 1999.
2. Brennan TA, Leape LL, Laird NM, Hebert L, Localio R, Lawthers AG, et al. Incidence of adverse events and negligence in hospitalized patients: results of the Harvard Medical Practice Study I. N Engl J Med. 1991;324:370-6.
3. Leape LL, Brennan TA, Laird NM, Lawthers AG, Localio AR, Barnes BA, et al. The nature of adverse events in hospitalized patients: results of the Harvard Medical Practice Study II. N Engl J Med. 1991;324(6):377-4.
4. American Society of Health-System Pharmacists. Suggested definitions and relationships among medication misadventures, medication errors, adverse drug events, and adverse drug reactions. Am J Health-Syst Pharm. 1998;55:165-6.
5. National Coordinating Council for Medication Error Reporting and Prevention. Available from: http://www.nccmerp.org. Accessed June 19, 2011.
6. Bates DW, Cullen DJ, Laird N, Peterson LA, Small HD, Servi D, et al. Incidence of adverse drug events and potential adverse drug events. JAMA. 1995;274:29-34.
7. Lamy PP. Adverse drug effects. Clin Ger Med. 1990;6:293-307.

8. Lesar TS, Lomaestro BM, Pohl H. Medication-prescribing errors in a teaching hospital: a 9-year experience. Arch Intern Med. 1997;157:1569-76.

9. Gurwitz JH, Field TS, Avorn J, McCormick D, Jain S, Eckler M, et al. Incidence and preventability of adverse drug events in nursing homes. Am J Med. 2000;109:87-94.

10. Gurwitz JH, Field TS, Harrold LR, Rothschild J, Debellis K, Seger AC, et al. Incidence and preventability of adverse drug events among older persons in the ambulatory setting. JAMA. 2003;289:1107-16.

11. White TJ, Arakelian A, Rho JP. Counting the costs of drug-related adverse events. Pharmacoeconomics. 1999;15:445-58.

12. Johnson JA, Bootman JL. Drug-related morbidity and mortality. Arch Intern Med. 1995; 155:1949-56.

13. Classen DC, Pestotnik SL, Evans S, Loyd JF, Burke JP. Adverse drug events in hospitalized patients. JAMA. 1997;277:301-6.

14. Ernst FR, Grizzle AJ. Drug-related morbidity and mortality: updating the cost-of-illness model. J Am Pharm Assoc. 2001;41:192-9.

15. Phillips MA. Voluntary reporting of medication errors. Am J Health-Syst Pharm. 2002; 59:2326-8.

16. Barker KN, Flynn EA, Pepper GA. Observation method of detecting medication errors. Am J Health-Syst Pharm. 2002;59:2314-6.

17. Barker KN, Mikeal RI, Pearson RE, Illig NA, Morse ML. Medication errors in nursing homes and small hospitals. Am J Hosp Pharm. 1982;39:987-91.

18. Jha AK, Kuperman GJ, Teich JM, Leape L, Shea B, Rittenberg E, et al. Identifying adverse drug events: development of a computer-based monitor and comparison with chart review and stimulated voluntary reporting. J Am Med Inform Assoc. 1998;3:305-14.

19. Classen DC, Pestotnik SL, Evans RS, Burke JP. Description of a computerized adverse drug event monitor using a hospital information system. Hosp Pharm. 1992;27:774, 776-9,783.

20. Classen DC, Pestotnik SL, Evans RS, Burke JP. Computerized surveillance of adverse drug events in hospital patients (published erratum appears in JAMA 1992;267:1992). JAMA. 1991;266:2847-51.

21. Gandhi TK, Bates DW. Chapter 8: Computer adverse drug event (ADE) detection and alerts. [cited 2011 June 19]. Available from: http://archive.ahrq.gov/clinic/ptsafety/chap8.htm.

22. VHA, Inc. Monitoring adverse drug events: finding the needles in the haystack. Vol. 9. VHA 2002 Research Series. Irving (TX): VHA; 2002.

23. Raschke RA, Gollihare B, Wunderlich TA, Guidry J, Leibowitz A, Peirce, J, et al. A computer alert system to prevent injury from adverse drug events: development and evaluation in a community teaching hospital (published erratum appears in JAMA 1999;281:420J). JAMA. 1998;280:1317-20.

24. Bates DW, Evans RS, Murff H, Stetson PD, Pizziferri L, Hripcsak G. Detecting adverse events using information technology. J Am Med Inform Assoc. 2003;10:115-28.

25. Bates DW. Using information technology to screen for adverse drug events. Am J Health-Syst Pharm. 2002;59:2317-9.

26. Schneider PJ. Using technology to enhance measurement of drug-use safety. Am J Health-Syst Pharm. 2002;59:2330-2.

27. Rozich JD, Haraden CR, Resar RK. Adverse drug event trigger tool: a practical methodology for measuring medication related harm. Qual Saf Health Care. 2008;12:194-200.

28. Rozich JD, Resar RK. Medication safety: one organization's approach to the challenge. J Clin Outcomes Manage. 2001;8(10):27-34.

29. Crea KA, Sherrin TP, Morehead D, Snow R. Reducing adverse drug events involving high-risk medications in acute care. J Clin Outcomes Manage. 2004;11(10):640-6.

30. The Patient Safety Act and Quality Improvement Act of 2005. Public Law 109-41, 109th Congress, July 29, 2005.

31. Pennsylvania Patient Safety Authority. Vol. 6(4), December 2009.

32. ISMP Newsletter. Heparin errors continue despite prior, high-profile fatal events. [cited 2011 June 19]. Available from: http://www.ismp.org/newsletters/acutecare/articles/20080717. asp.

33. American Society of Hospital Pharmacists. ASHP guidelines on preventing medication errors in hospitals. Am J Hosp Pharm. 1993;50:305-14.

34. Patient Safety Organization Privacy Protection Center (PSO PPC). [cited 2011 June 19]. Available from: https://www.psoppc.org/web/patientsafety.

35. Pepper GA. Errors in drug administration by nurses. ASHP Online. 1999 [cited 2011 June 19]: [1 screen]. Available from: http://www.ashp.org/public/proad/mederror/pep.html.

36. Dunn EB, Wolfe JJ. Medication error classification and avoidance. Hosp Pharm. 1997;32:860-5.

37. MedWatch: The FDA Medical Products Reporting Program. FDA Med Bull. 1993;23:insert.

38. The Joint Commission Sentinel Event Policy and Procedure. [cited 2011 June 19]. Available from: http://www.jointcommission.org/Sentinel-Events/Policy-andProcedures/.

39. Using aggregate root cause analysis to improve patient safety. JtComm J Qual Patient Saf. 2003 Aug;29(8):434-9.

40. Using aggregate root cause analysis to reduce falls. Jt Comm J Qual Patient Saf. 2005 Jan;31(1):21-31.

41. Bogner MS. Human Error in Medicine. Hillsdale (NJ): Lawrence Erlbaum Associates; 1994.

42. Senders JW. Theory and analysis of typical errors in a medical setting.Hosp Pharm. 1993;28:505-8.

43. Norman DA. The Design of Everyday Things. New York (NY): Basic Book; 1988.

44. Reason J. Human Error. Cambridge, England: Cambridge University Press; 1990.

45. Reason J. Managing the Risks of Organizational Accidents. Burlington (VT): Ashgate; 1997.

46. ISMP Newsletter. Inattentionalblindness: what captures your attention? [cited 2011 June 19]. Available from: www.ismp.org/newsletters/acutecare/articles/20090226.asp.

47. The Joint Commission (TJC). Improving America's hospitals: The Joint Commission annual report on quality and safety, 2007. [cited 2011 June 19]. Available from: http://www.jointcommission.org/assets/1/6/2007_Annual_Report.pdf.

48. Abood RR. Errors in pharmacy practice.US Pharm. 1996;21:122-32.

49. Coleman IC. Medication errors: picking up the pieces. Drug Top. 1999;143:83-92.

50. Glut of medication errors focuses pharmacists on event reporting. Drug Util Rev. 1998:201-6.

51. Cohen MR. ISMP medication error report analysis: the mistake of blaming people and not the process. Hosp Pharm. 1997;32:1106-11.

52. ISMP Newsletter. An injustice has been done: jail time given to pharmacist who made an error. August 21, 2009. [cited 2011 June 19] Available from: http://www.ismp.org/ pressroom/injustice-jailtime-for-pharmacist.asp.

53. ISMP Newsletter.Our long journey towards safety-minded just culture. Part I: Where we've been. Available from: www.ismp.org/newsletters/acutecare/articles/20060907. Accessed June 19, 2011.

54. GAIN Working group E, Flight Ops/ATC Ops Safety Information Sharing. Aroadmap to a Just Culture: enhancing the safety environment. [cited 2011 June 19]. www.flightsafety.org/ files/just_culture.pdf.

55. Grasha AF, O'Neill M. Cognitive processes in medication errors. US Pharm. 1996;21:96-109.

56. Ukens C. Breaking the trust: exclusive survey of dispensing errors. Drug Top. 1992;136:58-69.

57. DeMichele D. Preventing medication errors.US Pharm. 1995;20:69-75.

58. Davis NM. Lack of knowledge as a cause of medication errors. Hosp Pharm. 1997;32:16-25.

59. Fitzgerald WL, Wilson DB. Medication errors: lessons in law. Drug Top. 1998;142:84-93.

60. Institute of Medicine. Crossing the Quality Chasm. Washington, DC: National Academy Press; 2001.

61. Institute of Medicine. Health Professions Education: A Bridge to Quality. Washington, DC: National Academy Press; 2003.

62. Institute for Healthcare Improvement. Open school. [cited 2011 June 19]. Available from: http://www.ihi.org/IHI/Programs/IHIOpenSchool/IHIOpenSchoolforHealthProfessions.htm.

63. Grout J. Mistake-Proofing the Design of Health Care Processes. Rockville (MD). AHRQ Publication No. 07-0020, 2007.

64. Grissinger M. The virtues of independent double checks: they really are worth your time! P&T. 2006;31:9.

Chapter Seventeen

Investigational Drugs

Bambi Grilley

Learning Objectives

● *After completing this chapter, the reader will be able to*

- List the major legislative acts that led to our current system of drug evaluation, approval, and regulation.
- List the steps in the drug approval process.
- List the components of an investigational new drug application (IND).
- Recognize the difference between a commercial IND, a treatment IND, an emergency use IND, and an individual investigator IND.
- List all of the requirements (as specified by the Office of Human Research Protections [OHRP]) for an institutional review board (IRB).
- Define orphan drug status and list the advantages of classifying a drug as an orphan drug.
- Prepare appropriate reviews of protocols for use by the IRB or other review committees when they evaluate new protocols.
- Describe the type of support that is necessary for clinical research, including (but not limited to):
  - o Ordering drug supplies for ongoing clinical trials.
  - o Maintaining drug accountability records as required by the Food and Drug Administration (FDA).
  - o Preparing drug and protocol data sheets for use by health care personnel in the hospital.
  - o Preparing pharmacy budgets for sponsored clinical research.
  - o Aiding investigators in designing and conducting clinical trials in their institution.
  - o Assisting investigators in initiating and conducting clinical trials (including emergency use INDs).

Key Concepts

❶ The Food and Drug Administration (FDA) is the federal agency that decides which drugs, biologics, and medical devices are safe and effective and therefore can be marketed in the United States.

❷ In addition to review by the FDA, research protocols are also reviewed for ethical appropriateness by IRBs.

❸ The drug approval process in the United States is standardized by FDA review. It consists of preclinical testing and Phase I to IV of clinical testing.

❹ The investigational new drug application (IND) is the application by the study sponsor to the FDA to begin clinical trials in humans.

❺ The IND should be amended as necessary. The four types of documents used to amend the IND include
  a. Protocol amendments
  b. Information amendments
  c. IND safety reports
  d. IND annual reports

❻ After Phase III trials have been completed, the sponsor will submit a new drug application/biologics licensing application to the FDA requesting approval of the agent for marketing.

❼ The FDA allows for cost recovery for manufacturers of investigational drugs under certain circumstances.

❽ An orphan drug is one that is used for the treatment of a rare disease affecting fewer than 200,000 people in the United States, or one that will not generate enough revenue to justify the cost of research and development.

❾ Drug accountability records are mandated by law. They can be computerized or in paper form. Necessary components include
  a. Transaction date
  b. Transaction type
  c. The receiving party (for patient dispensing this should include patient initials/identifying number)
  d. The dose/number of units dispensed/received
  e. The lot number dispensed/received
  f. The initials of the person who performed the transaction

Introduction

It is estimated that $802 million is spent to get a new drug product to market in the United States.[1] More recent research indicates that this number may be even higher, costing on average $868 million and ranging from $500 million to more than $2,000 million.[2] Previous data have indicated that for every 4000 products synthesized in the lab, only five will ever be tested in humans, and only one of those will ever reach the market.[3] Currently, the Pharmaceutical Research and Manufacturers of America (PhRMA) database is tracking 23,000 new medicines in development.[4] This should be compared to 24 new drugs and biologics approved by the Food and Drug Administration (FDA) in 2008.[5] ❶ *The Food and Drug Administration (FDA) is the federal agency that decides which drugs, biologics, and medical devices are marketed in the United States.*[6] In fact, FDA-regulated products account for about 20 cents of every consumer dollar spent.[7] The centers of the FDA involved in regulating drugs, biologics, and medical devices used in humans are as follows:

- Center for Biologics Evaluation and Research (CBER)
- Center for Drug Evaluation and Research (CDER)
- Center for Devices and Radiological Health (CDRH)[8]

Because pharmacists are rarely involved in dispensing devices or radiological products, this chapter will concentrate only on the regulations associated with CBER and CDER.

Since 1940, more than 1000 new molecular entities (NMEs) have been approved in the United States.[9] It is very important that the clinical trials upon which the FDA will base its decisions be both scientifically accurate and complete. Pharmacists can play an important role in ensuring that the clinical trials conducted at their institutions meet the goals set forth by the study sponsor, the local investigator, and ultimately the FDA.

Currently, most research conducted on investigational drugs is performed in medical schools, hospitals, and organizations specifically designed to conduct clinical research trials. For this reason, the dispensing of investigational drugs rarely occurs in a community pharmacy setting. In some institutions, a pharmacist will be hired specifically to handle investigational drugs. More frequently, however, this role falls to a specified pharmacist or the drug information pharmacist. To successfully manage investigational drugs, the pharmacist must be a bookkeeper, inventory control manager, and, most importantly, an information disseminator. Before proceeding, it is necessary to define a number of terms that will be used in this chapter.

Definitions

Biologics license application (BLA): A biologics license application is a submission that contains specific information on the manufacturing processes, chemistry, pharmacology, clinical pharmacology, and medical effects of the biologic product. It is a request for permission to introduce, or deliver for introduction, a biologic product into interstate commerce.[10]

Clinical investigation: Any experiment in which a drug is administered or dispensed to one or more human subjects. An experiment is any use of a drug (except for the use of a marketed drug) in the course of medical practice. Although there are many other definitions, this is the FDA's definition and seems the appropriate one to use given the nature of this topic. Please note that the FDA does not regulate the practice of medicine, and prescribers are (as far as the agency is concerned) free to use any marketed drug for off-label use.[11]

Clinical safety officer (CSO): Also known as the regulatory management officer (RMO). This is the sponsor's FDA contact person. Generally, the CSO/RMO assigned to a drug's investigational new drug (IND) application will also be assigned to the new drug application (NDA).

Commercial IND: An IND for which the sponsor is usually either a corporate entity or one of the institutes of the National Institutes of Health (NIH). In addition, CDER may designate other INDs as commercial, if it is clear that the sponsor intends the product to be commercialized at a later date.[12]

Control group: The group of test animals or humans that receive a placebo (a dosage that does not contain active medicine) or active (a dosage that does contain active medicine) treatment. For most preclinical and clinical trials, the FDA will require that this group receive placebo (commonly referred to as the placebo control). However, some studies may have an active control, which generally consists of an available (standard of care) treatment modality. An active control may, with the concurrence of the FDA, be used in studies where it would be considered unethical to use a placebo. A historical control is one in which a group of previous patients is compared to a matched set of patients receiving the new therapy. A historical control might be used in cases where the disease is consistently fatal (e.g., acquired immunodeficiency syndrome [AIDS]). Refer to Chapter 4 for additional information on control groups.

Contract research organization (CRO): An individual or organization that assumes one or more of the obligations of the sponsor through an independent contractual agreement.[11]

Drug master file (DMF): A submission to the FDA that may be used to provide confidential detailed information about facilities, processes, or articles used in the manufacturing, processing, packaging, and storing of one or more human drugs.[13]

Drug product: The final dosage form prepared from the drug substance.[14]

Drug substance: An active ingredient that is intended to furnish pharmacological activity or other direct effect in the diagnosis, cure, mitigation, treatment, or prevention of disease or to affect the structure or any function of the human body.[14]

Food and Drug Administration (FDA): The agency of the U.S. government that is responsible for ensuring the safety and efficacy of all drugs on the market.[11,14]

Institutional review board (IRB): A committee of reviewers that evaluates the ethical implications of a clinical study protocol.[15,16]

Investigational new drug: A drug, antibiotic, or biologic that is used in a clinical investigation. The label of an investigational drug must bear the following statement: "Caution: New Drug—Limited by Federal (or United States) Law to Investigational Use."[11]

Investigational new drug application (IND): A submission to the FDA containing chemical information, preclinical data, and a detailed description of the planned clinical trials. Thirty days after submission of this document to the FDA by the sponsor, clinical trials may be initiated in humans, unless the FDA places a clinical hold. When the FDA allows the studies to proceed, this document allows unapproved drugs to be shipped in interstate commerce.[11]

Investigator: The individual responsible for initiating the clinical trial at the study site. This individual must treat the patients, ensure that the protocol is followed, evaluate responses and adverse reactions, ensure proper conduct of the study, and solve problems as they arise.[11]

New drug application (NDA): The application to the FDA requesting approval to market a new drug for human use. The NDA contains data supporting the safety and efficacy of the drug for its intended use.[14]

New molecular entity (NME): A compound that can be patented that has not been previously approved.

Sponsor: An organization (or individual) that takes responsibility for and initiates a clinical investigation. The sponsor may be an individual or pharmaceutical company, government agency, academic institution, private organization, or other organization.[11]

Sponsor-investigator: An individual who both initiates and conducts a clinical investigation (i.e., submits the IND and directly supervises administration of the drug as well as other investigator responsibilities).[11]

Subject: An individual who participates in a clinical investigation (either as the recipient of the investigational drug or as a member of the control group).[11]

History of Drug Development Regulation in the United States

For more than a century after the Declaration of Independence, drug products were not regulated in the United States. Available drugs were often ineffective, but some were addictive, toxic, or even lethal. During this same period, doctors were not licensed and nearly anyone could practice medicine. The public was, for the most part, responsible for using common sense when evaluating which products they would use.

The evolution of drug regulations in the United States is a study in human tragedy. Crises have instigated the development of many of the laws regulating drug development, preparation, and distribution.

The first federal law developed to deal with drug quality and safety was the Import Drug Act of 1848. This law was passed after it was discovered that American troops involved in the Mexican War had been supplied with substandard imported drugs. The act provided for the inspection, detention, and destruction or reexport of imported drug shipments that failed to meet prescribed standards.

The Pure Food and Drugs Act was passed in 1906. This law required that drugs not be mislabeled or adulterated and stated that they must meet recognized standards for strength and purity. Mislabeling in this context only referred to the identity or composition of drugs (not false therapeutic claims). False therapeutic claims were prohibited with the passing of the Sherley Amendment in 1912.

In 1937, the drug sulfanilamide was released. This drug showed promise as an anti-infective agent and was prepared as an oral liquid. The vehicle used for this preparation was diethylene glycol (a sweet-tasting solvent similar to ethylene glycol, which was used as an automobile antifreeze). A total of 107 people died after taking this preparation. Within 1 year of this tragedy, the Food, Drug and Cosmetic Act of 1938 was enacted. This law required that the safety of drugs, when used in accordance with the labeled instructions, be proven through testing before they could be marketed. It was in this law that the submission of an NDA to the FDA was first described. The NDA was required to list the drug's intended uses and provide scientific evidence that the drug was safe. If after 60 days the FDA had not responded to the manufacturer regarding the NDA, the manufacturer was free to proceed with marketing of the product.

In 1951, the Durham–Humphrey Amendment was passed. This law divided pharmaceuticals into two distinct classes:

1. Over-the-counter (OTC) medications that could be safely self-administered
2. Prescription (R_x) medications that had potentially dangerous side effects and therefore required expert medical supervision

This law required that the following statement be added to the labels for all prescription medications: "Caution: Federal Law prohibits dispensing without a prescription."

In 1962, another drug tragedy occurred that resulted in additional regulations. In that year, an inordinate number of pregnant women in Western Europe gave birth to children with severe deformities. These deformities were related to the use of the drug thalidomide. Although U.S. consumers were not directly affected by this tragedy because thalidomide had not been released in the U.S. market, it was a compelling reason for the legislature to develop stronger laws regarding the testing of new drug products. The Kefauver–Harris Drug Amendment was passed the same year. This law specified that the manufacturer had to demonstrate proof of efficacy, as well as safety, prior to marketing any new drug. Additionally, this law required that drug manufacturers operate in conformity with Current Good Manufacturing Practices (CGMP). Finally, it stated that the FDA had to formally approve an NDA before the drug could be marketed.[17]

There are numerous other laws and regulations that affect drug products in the United States, but those mentioned previously provide the legal foundation for the current regulation of drug products in this country. Based on these laws, the FDA has assumed a large role in assessing the safety and efficacy of drug products prior to their distribution in the United States.

❶ *As stated, the goal of the FDA is to provide American consumers with safe and effective therapy.* Extensive debate regarding the need to reform the FDA has been ongoing in the United States for years. Critics of the FDA have long claimed that the approval process for drugs in this country is too costly and time-consuming.[18,19] Interestingly, a comparison of review times for new drugs approved in the European Union (by the European Medicines Evaluation Agency [EMEA]) and the United States reveals that the average review times are identical. However, there is greater variability in the review times of products reviewed by the FDA.[20] Nevertheless, over the past 15 years, the FDA and the federal government have initiated reforms designed to address criticism.[21] Recent reform acts include the Prescription Drug User Fee Act of 1992 (PDUFA), which was reauthorized in 1997, 2002, and 2007, and the Food and Drug Administration Modernization Act of 1997 (FDAMA). PDUFA redefined the time frames for NDA reviews and established revenues to fund the increased demands created by the new time frames.[22] The FDAMA, which reauthorized PDUFA in 1997, was much broader in scope and impacted not only the drug approval process, but also other aspects of the practices of pharmacy and medicine.[23] The Food and Drug Administration Amendments Act (FDAAA), which was signed into law in 2007, further expanded PDUFA to provide the FDA with additional resources to conduct timely and comprehensive reviews of new drugs in the United States.[24]

Aside from looking at review times, the FDA has also been concerned about the increasing difficulty in drug and biologic development. In an attempt to address this issue, the FDA launched a new initiative in March 2004 called the Critical Path Initiative.

The Critical Path Initiative is the FDA's attempt to facilitate the modernization of the sciences and improve regulatory decision making. The FDA has been working with the public, the pharmaceutical industry, other regulatory agencies, and academia to identify projects it feels are most likely to help the drug development process from test tube to bedside.[25]

The FDA has also undertaken many information technology initiatives to facilitate the regulatory review process. Included in these initiatives is the development of systems allowing for the electronic submission, management, and review of regulatory information.[26] On average, the review time for standard drugs and biologics is 13 months, while the review time for priority drugs and biologics is 6 months.[5] Other attempts by the FDA to increase the availability of investigational drugs and to expedite the drug approval process is discussed later in this chapter.

In order to provide more information to the public regarding ongoing clinical trials, the National Institutes of Health (NIH) has developed a Web-based system that offers information about ongoing clincal trials for a wide range of diseases and conditions. This allows potential study subjects to search for studies for particular diseases and identify treatment centers that offer specific protocols. The site is available at ClinicalTrials.gov (http://www.clinicaltrials.gov). Study sponsors are required to verify that the study is posted on the ClinicalTrials.gov site as part of the IND submission process.

Increasingly, drug companies are involved in global drug development. Historically, the regulatory requirements for drug approval varied from country to country, resulting in a significant amount of time and money being spent to receive multiple approvals. For this reason, the International Conference on Harmonization (ICH) has brought together officials from Europe, the United States, and Japan to develop common guidelines for ensuring the quality, safety, and efficacy of drugs. The FDA has been very involved in the development of the ICH guidelines.[27] The ultimate goal of these guidelines is to provide pharmaceutical firms a method to ensure simultaneous submission and rapid regulatory approval in the world's major markets. This would minimize duplication of effort, improve efficiency, and increase the quality and consistency of medical treatments available to patients worldwide.[28]

For gene therapy products, review and approval by the National Institutes of Health Office of Biotechnology Activities (NIH/OBA) and the Institutional Biosafety Committee are required in addition to review and approval by the FDA and IRB (discussed in the following). Submission requirements for the NIH/OBA are similar to those mandated by the FDA (covered later in this chapter). The review process for gene therapy products is a separate topic that will not be further addressed in this chapter. Individuals interested in the regulatory requirements of gene therapy products can refer to review articles such as "Gene Transfer: Regulatory Issues and Their Impact on the Clinical Investigator and the GMP facility," published in *Cytotherapy* in 2003.[29]

❷ *In addition to the regulatory review of investigational drugs by the FDA, research protocols are also reviewed for ethical appropriateness by IRBs.* The formalized process for protecting human subjects began with the Nuremberg Code. This Code was used to judge the human experimentation conducted by the Nazis around the middle of the twentieth century. The Nuremberg Code states that "the voluntary consent of the human subjects is absolutely essential." The Code goes on to specify that the subject must have the capacity to consent, must be free from coercion, and must comprehend the risks and benefits involved in the research.[30] The Declaration of Helsinki reemphasized these points and distinguished between therapeutic and nontherapeutic research. This document was first developed in 1964 and has been revised multiple times, most recently in 2008.[31]

The NIH, as part of the Department of Health and Human Services (DHHS), used these two documents to develop its own policies for the Protection of Human Subjects in 1966. These policies were raised to regulatory status in 1974 and established the IRB as a mechanism through which human subjects would be protected. The Belmont Report, released in 1978, further delineates the basic ethical principles underlying medical research on human subjects.[32] Title 45 Part 46 of the Code of Federal Regulations (CFR), which was released in 1981, was designed to make uniform the protection of human subjects in all federal agencies.[15] Title 21 Part 50 (approved in 1980) of the CFR sets forth guidelines for appropriate informed consent, and Title 21 Part 56 (approved in 1981) of the CFR sets forth guidelines for the IRB.[16,33] Copies of these regulations can be obtained on the Internet at http://www.gpoaccess.gov/cfr/index.html.

These two documents are used by the FDA and the DHHS to evaluate the ethical conduct of clinical trials in the United States. Further information regarding the role of the IRB is presented later in this chapter.

Case Study 17-1

Company CaCure (not a real company) is doing research with a drug called ALLCure for the treatment of acute lymphocytic leukemia (ALL). The company will need to have regulatory professionals familiar with regulations from the FDA and NIH, which govern both drug approval and human research protections. The regulatory staff at the company will work closely with the staff responsible for developing and implementing the studies at various sites to ensure that the protocols are designed in a way that the product can be approved by the FDA.

The Drug Approval Process

❸ *The first step in the drug approval process is preclinical testing. This testing is either in vitro or in animals.* Before filing an IND, the sponsor must have developed a pharmacologic profile of the drug, and determined its acute and subacute (14 to 90 days) toxicity in at least two species of animals. Chronic toxicity studies in animals can coincide with the use of the drug in clinical trials in humans (although they must be initiated at least 13 weeks in advance). The preclinical chronic toxicity studies must be of at least the same duration as any planned clinical trial (i.e., a 6-month study in humans requires at least 6 months of preclinical data).[17]

After the preclinical testing is completed, the sponsor will file an IND with the FDA. ❹ *The IND is the application by the study sponsor to the FDA to begin clinical trials in humans.* Most often the sponsor is a pharmaceutical company, but occasionally an individual investigator will file an IND and serve as a sponsor-investigator. The investigator IND is submitted when a physician plans to use an approved drug for a new indication (i.e., one that is outside the package labeling) or, on occasion, for an unapproved product or for an NME. The IND requirements for the sponsor-investigator are the same as those for any other sponsor. For that reason, no differentiation will be made in the following discussion of the drug approval process.

The IND can be filed after the study sponsor has identified the pharmacologic profile of the drug and has results from both acute and short-term toxicity studies in animals. An IND is not required if the drug to be studied is marketed in the United States and all of the following requirements are met:

1. The study is not to be reported to the FDA in support of a new indication.
2. The study does not involve a different dose, route, or patient population that increases the risk to patients.
3. IRB approval and informed consent are secured.
4. The study will not be used to promote the drug's effectiveness for a new indication.

In situations where it is unclear whether an IND is required or not, a call to the FDA is the best way to determine the appropriate way to proceed. If an IND is required, the application needs to contain the following information:

1. *Cover sheet*: Form 1571 (available at the FDA Web site under Forms, http://www.fda.gov/AboutFDA/ReportsManualsForms/Forms/default.htm). This form identifies the sponsor, documents that the sponsor agrees to follow appropriate regulations, and identifies any involved CRO. This is a legal document.

2. *Table of contents*: Provides a list of the headings and their page numbers.
3. *Introductory statement*: States the name, structure, pharmacologic class, dosage form, and all active ingredients in the investigational drug; the objectives and planned duration of the investigation should be stated here.
4. *General investigational plan*: Describes the rationale, indications, and general approach for evaluating the drug, the types of trials to be conducted, the projected number of patients that will be treated, and any potential safety concerns; the purpose of this section is to give FDA reviewers a general overview of the plan to study the drug.
5. *Investigator's brochure*: An information packet containing all available information on the drug including its formula, pharmacologic and toxicologic effects, pharmacokinetics, and any information regarding the safety and risks associated with the drug. It is important that this brochure be kept current and comprehensive; therefore, it should be amended as necessary. The investigator's brochure may be used by the investigator or other health care professionals as a reference during the research study.
6. *Clinical protocol*: (In general, Phase I protocols are allowed to be less detailed than Phase II and Phase III protocols.)
   - *Objectives and purpose:* A description of the purpose of the trial (a typical Phase I objective would be to determine the maximum tolerated dose of the investigational drug, whereas a typical Phase III objective would be to compare the safety and efficacy of the investigational drug to placebo or standard therapy).
   - *Investigator data:* Provides qualifications and demographic data of the investigators involved in the clinical trial (may be presented on form 1572—available at the FDA Web site under Forms, http://www.fda.gov/AboutFDA/ReportsManuals Forms/Forms/default.htm).
   - *Patient selection:* Describes the characteristics of patients who are eligible for enrollment in the trial and states factors that would exclude patients.
   - *Study design:* Describes how the study will be completed; if the study is to be randomized, this will be described here with a description of the alternate therapy.
   - *Dose determination:* Describes the dose (with possible adjustments) and route of administration of the investigational drug; if retreatment or maintenance therapy of patients is allowed, it will be detailed in this section.
   - *Observations:* Describes how the objectives stated earlier in the protocol are to be assessed.
   - *Clinical procedures:* Describes all laboratory tests or clinical procedures that will be used to monitor the effects of the drug in the patient; the collection of these data is intended to minimize the risk to the patients.

- *IRB approval for protocol:* Documentation of this approval is not required as part of the IND application process; however, form 1571 does state that an IRB will review and approve each study in the proposed clinical investigation before allowing the initiation of those studies.

7. *Chemistry, manufacturing, and control data*
   - *Drug substance:* Describes the drug substance including its name; its biological, physical, and chemical characteristics; the address of the manufacturer; the method of synthesis or preparation; and the analytical methods used to ensure purity, identity, and the substance's stability.
   - *Drug product:* Describes the drug product including all of its components; the address of the manufacturer; the analytical methods used to ensure identity, quality, purity, and strength of the product; and the product's stability.
   - *Composition, manufacture, and control of any placebo used in the trial:* The FDA does not require that the placebo be identical to the investigational drug; however, it wants to ensure that the lack of similarity does not jeopardize the trial.
   - *Labeling:* Copies of all labels (drug substance, product, and packages).
   - *Environmental assessment:* Presents a claim for categorical exclusion from the requirement for an environmental assessment (a statement that the amount of waste expected to reach the environment may reasonably be expected to be nontoxic).

8. *Pharmacology and toxicology data*
   - *Pharmacology and drug disposition:* Describes the pharmacology, mechanism of action, absorption, distribution, metabolism, and excretion of the drug in animals and *in vitro.*
   - *Toxicology:* Describes the toxicology in animals and *in vitro.*
   - A statement that all nonclinical laboratories involved in the research adhered to Good Laboratory Practice (GLP) regulations.

9. *Previous human experience:* Summary of human experiences, which includes data from the United States and, where applicable, foreign markets. Known safety and efficacy data should be presented (especially if the drug was withdrawn from foreign markets for reasons of safety or efficacy).

10. *Additional information:* Other information that would help the reviewer evaluate the proposed clinical trial should be included here. For example, if a drug has the potential for abuse, data on the drug's dependence and abuse potential should be discussed in this section.[34]

The letter of authorization (LOA) to cross-reference a drug master file, investigational new drug application, or new drug application (referred to in item nine on page one of Form 1571) is required when the investigational product (or some component of the investigational product) being used in the research is being supplied by a manufacturer other than the study sponsor. The original holder of the IND/NDA/DMF prepares the LOA. An LOA is frequently required when two companies are working together toward the development of a product.[13]

⑤ *The IND should be amended as necessary. There are four types of documents that may be used to amend the IND.* They are as follows:

1. *Protocol amendments*: Submitted when a sponsor wants to change a previously submitted protocol or add a new study protocol to an existing IND.[35]

2. *Information amendments*: Submitted when information becomes available that would not be presented using a protocol amendment, IND safety report, or annual report (e.g., new chemistry data).[36]

3. *IND safety reports*: Reports clinical and animal adverse reactions; reporting requirements depend on the nature, severity, and frequency of the experience. The following definitions are used to help evaluate adverse reactions:

   • *Serious adverse drug experience:* Any adverse drug experience occurring at any dose that results in any of the following outcomes: death, a life-threatening adverse drug experience, inpatient hospitalization or prolongation of existing hospitalization, a persistent or significant disability/incapacity, or a congenital anomaly/birth defect. Important medical events that may not result in death, be life threatening, or require hospitalization may be considered a serious adverse drug experience when, based on appropriate medical judgment, they may jeopardize the patient or subject and may require medical or surgical intervention to prevent one of the outcomes listed in this definition.

   • *Unexpected adverse drug experience:* Any adverse drug experience that is not listed in the current labeling for the drug product. This includes events that may be symptomatically and pathophysiologically related to an event listed in the labeling, but differs from the event because of greater severity or specificity.

     For serious and unexpected, fatal, or life-threatening adverse reactions associated with the use of the drug, the sponsor is required to notify the FDA by telephone or fax within 7 calendar days after the sponsor receives the information. The sponsor must also submit a written report within 15 calendar days. For clinical and nonclinical adverse events that are both serious and unexpected, the sponsor must notify the FDA in writing within 15 calendar days. The written reports should describe the current adverse event and identify all previously filed safety reports concerning similar adverse events. The written report may be submitted as a narrative or as Form 3500A.[37]

4. *Annual reports*: Submitted within 60 days of the annual effective date of an IND; it should describe the progress of the investigation including information on the individual studies, summary information of the IND (summary of adverse experiences, IND safety reports, preclinical studies completed in the last year), relevant developments in foreign markets, and changes in the investigator's brochure.[38]

Each submission to a specific IND is required to be numbered sequentially (starting with 000). A total of three sets (the original and two copies) of all submissions to an IND file (whether a new IND or revisions to an existing IND) are sent to the FDA.[34]

Once submitted to the FDA, the IND will be forwarded to the appropriate review division based on the therapeutic category of the product.[17] The FDA has 30 days after receipt of an IND to respond to the sponsor. The sponsor may begin clinical trials if there is no response from the FDA within 30 days.[39] The FDA delays the initiation of a new study or discontinues an ongoing study by issuing a clinical hold. Clinical holds are most often used when the FDA identifies an issue (through initial review or through later submissions) that the agency feels poses a significant risk to the subjects. After this issue has been satisfactorily resolved, the clinical hold can be removed and the investigations can be initiated or resumed.[40]

● ❸ *There are four phases of clinical trials.* Clinical studies generally begin cautiously. As experience with the agent grows, the dose and duration of exposure to the agent may also increase. The number of patients treated at each phase of study and the duration of the studies can vary significantly depending on statistical considerations, the prevalence of patients affected by the disease, and the importance of the new drug. However, some general guidelines regarding the four phases of clinical testing are presented in the following.

● A Phase I trial is the first use of the agent in humans. As such, these studies are usually initiated with cautious (low) doses and in small numbers of subjects. Doses may be increased as safety is established. A Phase I study will usually treat 20 to 80 patients and last an average of 6 months to 1 year. The purpose of a Phase I trial is to determine the safety and toxicity of the agent. Frequently, these trials include a pharmacokinetic portion. These trials assist in identifying the preferred route of administration and a safe dosage range. When possible, these trials are initiated in normal, healthy volunteers. This allows for the evaluation of the effect of the drug on a subject who does not have any preexisting conditions. In situations in which this is not practical, such as with oncology drugs in which the drug itself can be highly toxic, these drugs are usually reserved for patients who have exhausted all conventional options.

● A Phase II trial is one in which the drug is used in a small number of subjects who suffer from the disease or condition that the drug is proposed to treat. The purpose of a

Phase II trial is to evaluate the efficacy of the agent. Data from the Phase I trial, in vitro testing, and animal testing may be used to identify which group of patients is most likely to benefit from therapy with this agent. Phase II trials usually treat between 100 and 200 patients and will average about 2 years in duration.

Phase III trials build on the experience gained during the Phase II trials. The purpose of a Phase III study is to further define the efficacy and safety of the agent. Frequently, in Phase III studies, the new agent is compared to current therapy. These trials are usually multicenter studies, generally treat from 600 to 1000 patients, and usually last about 3 years. Some of the Phase III trials will be pivotal studies and will serve as the basis for the NDA/BLA for a medicinal product's marketing approval.[41]

❻ *After Phase III trials have been completed, the sponsor will submit an NDA/BLA to the FDA requesting approval of the medicinal product for marketing.* The FDA requires the completion of two well-designed, controlled clinical trials prior to submission to the FDA. However, the sponsor will include information gathered from all of the clinical trials to show that the medicinal product is safe and effective and to describe the pharmacology and pharmacokinetics of the drug. The NDA/BLA will include all preclinical data, clinical data, manufacturing methods, product quality assurance, relevant foreign clinical testing (or marketing experience), and all published reports of experience with the medicinal agent (whether sponsored by the company or not). A proposed package insert will be supplied as well.[42]

The NDA/BLA will be distributed to the appropriate FDA review divisions. This is one of the same divisions described earlier in this chapter in the section discussing the IND evaluation process. As noted, these divisions are based on the therapeutic group of the medicinal agent. The same reviewer may be assigned to review the IND and the NDA/BLA.[17]

The speed at which the NDA will be processed is to some extent determined by the classification the drug receives during its initial review. Each agent is rated with a number–letter designation that evaluates two separate aspects of the agent. The number portion of the rating is associated with the uniqueness of the drug product (ranging from 1 for an NME to 7 for a drug that has already been marketed but without an approved NDA/BLA—see Table 13-1 for a detailed list). The letter portion of the rating is associated with the therapeutic potential of the medicinal agent. The P (priority review) designation is given to drugs that represent a therapeutic advance with respect to available therapy, whereas an S (standard review) is given to drugs that have little or no therapeutic gain over previously available drugs). BLA prioritization is slightly simplified but similar.[43]

During the review process, the FDA may utilize one of its prescription drug advisory committees to help review the NDA. These committees are composed of experts. They provide the agency with independent, nonbinding advice and recommendations regarding the NDA.[44] Within 180 days of receipt of an NDA, the FDA will review the application and send the applicant an action letter (stating that the NDA is either approved, approvable, or not approvable). When an approval letter is sent the drug is considered approved as of the date of the letter (this rarely occurs with an original NDA). When an approvable letter is sent it means that the application "substantially meets the requirements for marketing approval and the agency believes that it can approve the application if specific additional information or material is submitted or specific conditions are agreed to by the applicant."[45,46] The sponsor has 10 days to respond to the approvable letter (although an extension is usually granted if requested within the 10-day period).[47] A not-approvable letter is sent when the FDA believes that the NDA is insufficient for approval. The letter will describe the deficiencies in the application. Once again, the sponsor has 10 days to respond to the letter. The sponsor can amend the NDA, withdraw the NDA, or request a hearing with the FDA to clarify whether grounds exist for denying the approval of the application.[48]

After the drug has been approved, Phase IV trials may be initiated. These trials are also referred to as postmarketing studies. They are conducted for the approved indication, but may evaluate different doses, the effects of extended therapy, or the drug's safety in patient populations that were not represented in premarketing clinical trials. These Phase IV trials may be requested by the FDA or they may be initiated by the sponsor in an attempt to gather more data on the safety and efficacy of the drug or to identify a competitive advantage of the drug over other available therapies.[41]

As mentioned previously, the median NDA/BLA review time (from submission to approval) for standard drugs and biologics is 13 months, while the review time for priority drugs and biologics is 6 months.[5] Although there has been a significant decrease in review times since the 1980s, for diseases (e.g., AIDS and cancer) where these investigational drugs may be the only therapy available, this time delay can still be a significant factor.[49] Therefore, in addition to the priority classification assigned at the time of NDA review, the FDA has also developed procedures to expedite the drug development and review process and has established methods for providing promising experimental drugs to desperately ill patients.

The treatment IND is one way the FDA has allowed for the increased accessibility of experimental drugs for desperately ill patients. For a drug to qualify for use under a treatment IND, it must meet the following criteria:

1. The drug must be intended to treat a serious or immediately life-threatening disease.
2. There must be no satisfactory alternative therapy for the patient.
3. The drug must be under investigation in controlled clinical trials.
4. The sponsor must be actively pursuing FDA approval of the drug.

There are two different categories of treatment IND: immediately life-threatening conditions and serious conditions. The FDA defines immediately life-threatening conditions as those where death is likely to occur within a matter of months. In this situation, the FDA would allow treatment with the drug earlier than Phase III, but not earlier than Phase II. Serious conditions are defined as those in which the disease causes major irreversible morbidity (such as Alzheimer disease). For use in treating serious conditions, the drug must meet tougher requirements for safety and efficacy. As a result, treatment INDs for serious illnesses are more likely to be granted during Phase III trials or after all clinical trials have been completed. ❼ *Provisions of the treatment IND regulations permit charging for the investigational drug under certain conditions.* The amount the sponsor may charge for the investigational drug cannot exceed the amount necessary to recover costs associated with drug production, development, and distribution. Both drug sponsors and individual investigators are eligible to request FDA approval of a treatment IND. The drug sponsor may do so via submission of a treatment protocol, which states how and why the drug will be used. If the drug sponsor will not establish a treatment protocol and an investigator feels access to the drug is necessary, the investigator may submit a treatment IND for the drug, assuming the drug is available. The treatment IND that the investigator submits should contain all of the components of a treatment protocol as well as information about the investigator and a description of the steps taken by the investigator to obtain the drug under a treatment protocol from the drug sponsor.[50-52]

Emergency use INDs are another way that the FDA allows access to investigational drugs for desperately ill patients. The emergency use IND allows the shipment of a drug by the sponsor prior to the submission of an IND. This type of IND can only be used to treat individual patients with life-threatening diseases where all other options have been exhausted. The FDA must authorize the emergency use IND; however, prospective IRB approval is not required.[53,54]

The parallel track is a way the FDA has allowed for the increased accessibility of experimental drugs specifically for AIDS patients. Using this mechanism, drugs may be made available after the completion of Phase I studies to patients who are ineligible for enrollment in the clinical trials and are unable to benefit from current therapies. Regular controlled studies for safety and efficacy are still essential, and the sponsors are required to monitor the impact of the parallel track on enrollment in ongoing clinical trials. To date this mechanism has been rarely utilized.[55]

For patients with cancer, increased access to potentially beneficial products was provided through the Cancer Initiative of 1996.[56] The most recent clarification of the initiative was released in 2004.[57] This policy was designed to address the needs of oncology patients. This initiative allows for:

1. Accelerating drug approval by using surrogate endpoints to approve oncology drugs. A surrogate endpoint of a clinical trial is "a laboratory measurement or a physical sign used as a substitute for a clinically meaningful endpoint that measures directly how a patient feels, functions, or survives. Changes induced by a therapy on a surrogate endpoint are expected to reflect changes in a clinically meaningful endpoint."[58]
2. Treating patients in the United States with drugs approved in other countries via expanded access protocols.
3. Expanding the number of consumer members on the advisory committees.
4. Reducing the number of INDs required to conduct studies of marketed oncology drugs.

There has been considerable interest in this program and it has shown promising results.[17]

The FDA has also attempted to expedite the review process for new drugs. Fast Track review is one way that the FDA has tried to speed the development and review of drugs used to treat serious diseases. The Fast Track process allows the sponsor to meet more frequently with the FDA during drug/study development, receive more frequent written correspondence from the FDA regarding the drug/study development, be eligible for accelerated approval based on surrogate endpoints (as discussed previously), and submit NDAs in a modified fashion (called rolling review). In addition, the majority of products that are eligible for Fast Track review would also receive a priority review during the NDA process.[59] This includes a program of meeting with study sponsors to discuss and review the preclinical and clinical studies that will be necessary for drug development and approval. The purpose of these meetings is to help the sponsor minimize wasteful expenditures of time and money while still meeting the scientific objectives necessary for drug approval. For products designed to treat desperately ill patients, these meetings can occur prior to the submission of the initial IND and at the end of Phase I studies. Additionally, the FDA will meet with the sponsor of any IND at the end of Phase II studies and prior to the submission of the NDA.[60-62]

Another such initiative is the accelerated drug approval program. This program can be utilized if the drug is intended for the treatment of a serious or life-threatening condition and it demonstrates the potential to address unmet medication needs for the condition. The application would then be evaluated by weighing the risk/benefit relationship of the severity of the disease and alternatives to the new product. These products could be approved based on surrogate endpoints or on clinical endpoints other than survival or irreversible morbidity if the product can provide a meaningful therapeutic benefit to patients. In some cases, this approval could be given as early as post–Phase II studies. Two pivotal Phase II studies would be required before the NDA could be submitted.

In these situations, the FDA can apply restrictions to the marketing and distribution of such products, and significant postmarketing studies (Phase IV) will be required because they would provide information regarding larger and more diverse patient populations than may be seen in the earlier phases of study.[63]

Case Study 17–2

The ALLCure drug has now completed two positive Phase III studies in ALL. The company can now apply for an NDA to treat ALL. During the review process, an investigator determines that one of his patients would benefit from treatment with this drug, but there are no available open studies for which the patient is eligible. CaCure agrees to provide the drug and support a patient-specific investigator-initiated IND. In a situation where the patient was desperately ill, the FDA and sponsor might agree that this patient could be treated under an emergency use IND.

If during the review process it was determined that other critically ill patients were being denied access to ALLCure in a situation where the patients had no other satisfactory alternatives, CaCure could apply for approval of a treatment IND.

The Orphan Drug Act

Outside of the drug development process described previously, the FDA has developed an incentive program to encourage manufacturers to develop products with limited potential profit. This incentive program is known as the Orphan Drug Act and it was passed in 1983. This Act provides incentives for manufacturers to develop orphan drugs. ❽ *An orphan drug is one used for the treatment of a rare disease (affecting fewer than 200,000 people in the United States) or one that will not generate enough revenue to justify the cost of research and development.* The Orphan Drug Act is administered by the FDA's Office of Orphan Products Development. The orphan drug designation provides the following incentives:

- *Tax incentives*: The sponsor is eligible to receive a tax credit for money spent on research and development of an orphan drug; unfortunately, this is only beneficial to profitable companies as this credit cannot take the form of a tax refund.

- *Protocol assistance*: If a sponsor can show that a drug will be used for a rare disease, the FDA will provide assistance developing the preclinical and clinical plan for the product.
- *Grants and contracts*: The FDA budget may allot money for grants and contracts to be used in developing orphan drugs. In 2006, the FDA allotted $25 million for the development of orphan drugs. Clinical trials are awarded grants from $200,000 to $350,000 per year in direct costs for up to 3 years.
- *Marketing exclusivity*: The first sponsor to obtain marketing approval for a designated orphan drug is allowed 7 years of marketing exclusivity for that indication, but identical versions of the same product marketed by another manufacturer may be approved for other indications.

The Orphan Drug Act does not provide advantages for the drug approval process. Sponsors seeking approval for drugs that will be designated as orphan drugs must still provide the same safety and efficacy data as all other drugs evaluated by the FDA. Exceptions to the rules governing the number of patients that should be treated in the clinical trials may be made based on the scarcity of patients with the condition. Additionally, because in many cases there are no alternative therapies for the disease, the drug may be given a high review priority during the NDA process.[43,64-66]

Case Study 17–3

Based on other studies, CaCure has determined that ALLCure can be useful in treating rare germ cell tumors in children. CaCure could apply for the drug to be designated as an orphan drug for that limited clinical application.

Having discussed the federal infrastructure under which clinical research is conducted, it is now necessary to consider the approvals that need to be obtained locally before research in human subjects can be initiated.

The Institutional Review Board

The IRB is a committee of at least five members formed to review proposed clinical trials and the progress of such studies to ensure that the rights and welfare of human subjects are protected. The IRB must contain at least one member who has specialized in a scientific area (usually this will be a physician) and at least one board member who has a specialty in a nonscientific area such as law, ethics, or religion. Additionally, the IRB must contain at least one individual who is not affiliated with the institution where the research is being conducted. Membership of the IRB varies between institutions. Common members of IRBs include physicians, pharmacists, nurses, lawyers, clergy, and laypeople. The IRB is also responsible for ensuring that the proposed clinical trial is not in conflict with the institution's research policies or philosophy. The IRB and the study sponsor will have little if any direct contact. The primary investigator generally acts as the liaison between these two parties. The IRB should evaluate the research proposal to ensure that the following requirements are met:

- The risks to subjects are minimal.
- The expected risk/anticipated benefit ratio must be reasonable.
- Equitable subject selection is used.
- Informed consent must be received from each participant (or his or her representative).
- Informed consent must be documented in writing.
- Data must be monitored to ensure subject safety.
- Patient confidentiality must be maintained.
- If appropriate, additional safeguards against coercion must be included in studies that include vulnerable subjects (e.g., children, prisoners, pregnant women, mentally disabled people, or economically or educationally disadvantaged persons).

A notable exception to the requirements for written informed consent, as described previously, has been provided for research done in emergency circumstances involving human subjects who cannot give informed consent because of their emerging, life-threatening medical condition (for which available treatments are unproven or unsatisfactory), and where the intervention must be administered before informed consent from the subject's legally authorized representative is feasible. In these situations, the exception from informed consent requirements may proceed only after the sponsor has received prior written permission from the FDA (via IND approval) and from the IRB. In this type of research, both community consultation and public disclosure must be provided for the protocol.[67,68]

The IRB must, at a minimum, perform annual reviews of all ongoing clinical trials and evaluate adverse experiences to ensure that the criteria listed previously continue to be met.[69,70]

The IRB must maintain documentation of all IRB activities including copies of all research proposals reviewed, minutes of IRB meetings, records of continuing review activities, copies of all correspondence between the IRB and the investigators, a list of IRB members, written procedures of the IRB, and statements of significant new findings provided to subjects. This documentation and records that pertain to research should be retained for 3 years after the research is completed.[71-73]

Some institutions divide their review of proposed clinical research into two separate processes. One of these is the review of the protocol for scientific worth (scientific review), and the other is the review of the protocol for ethical considerations (IRB review). For many years, the role of the IRB and the effectiveness of the informed consent process have been questioned.[74-77] Federal officials and regulatory agencies continue to contemplate the reform of the process to better meet the goals of providing study subjects with information from which they can make an educated decision regarding whether or not they wish to participate in a clinical trial. Information regarding the role the pharmacist can assume in both IRB and scientific reviews of protocols is presented later in the chapter.

In some institutions, the IRB is also responsible for evaluating research misconduct. Research misconduct means fabrication, falsification, or plagiarism in proposing, performing, or reviewing research, or in reporting research results.[78] Research misconduct is an issue of increasing concern to study sponsors, institutions, and the government as the pressure on investigators and their associates to produce results has increased. In most institutions, as the emphasis on identifying and handling research misconduct has increased, the institutions have developed separate review processes and policies to deal with the issue.

Case Study 17–4

Some of the studies using ALLCure have indicated that the drug might cause delayed liver damage in the patients who receive it. The lawyers at CaCure do not want this information provided in the consent form as the relationship between the toxicity and the drug is not definite and this information might cause significant concern for the patients. However, it is the responsibility of the IRB to determine if such information is provided to study subjects and how such information is provided. It is interesting to note that in the case of ALLCure, the drug will be used in children. Children are considered a special population in clinical research and review of such studies by the IRB should take this into consideration. In addition, it should be noted that until study subjects reach the age of legal majority (as defined by state law), their parents make health care decisions for them. However, the assent of the child is also sought. If the research is still ongoing at the time the study subject reaches the age of majority, the study subject will need to be re-consented in order to continue on the study.

Role of the Health Care Professional

The health care professional can play a vital role in the clinical research process by

- Being the primary investigator (PI) on a study
- Reporting adverse events
- Preparing the IND
- Serving on the IRB and, where applicable, on the scientific review committee (a separate group that reviews the scientific basis of the study, prior to the time it is reviewed by the IRB)
- Providing financial evaluations of investigational protocols
- Disseminating information regarding both the protocol and the investigational drug to other health care personnel
- Maintaining drug accountability records
- Ordering, maintaining, and, when necessary, returning drug supplies for ongoing clinical trials
- Randomizing and, when necessary, blinding drug supplies for a clinical trial

The health care professional can serve as the PI on clinical research studies. The type of study for which an individual can serve as a PI varies based on his or her expertise and experience. Common types of studies for which nonphysicians serve as PIs include pharmacoeconomic, pharmacology/pharmacokinetic, quality of life, and other noninterventional studies. For some of these trials, a physician must be a coinvestigator.

The health care professional can assist the investigator by reporting clinical trial adverse events to the FDA. A discussion of the types of adverse events and the applicable reporting requirements was presented in the IND section of this chapter. Further information about the concept of adverse drug reaction reporting, including the identification and classification of adverse events, can be found in the adverse drug reaction section of Chapter 15.

The health care professional can assist in preparing the IND by following the guidelines presented earlier in this chapter.

Preferably, health care professionals are voting members of the IRB, and as such they may have some control over clinical trials initiated at the institution. More important, however, is the role they may have in the scientific review of the protocol, whether this occurs as part of the scientific review board review or as part of the IRB review. When reviewing a protocol for scientific purposes, they should help verify that the information in the protocol is complete and that it is logistically possible for the protocol to be conducted as presented. In addition, the health care professional should confirm that any toxicities specified in the protocol are detailed for the patient in the informed consent of the protocol.

Some roles are more specific to the training of the health care professional. Following is a description of the role of the pharmacist in clinical research.

ROLE OF THE PHARMACIST

The pharmacist should verify that the protocol or associated documents such as the investigator's brochure contain the following information:

1. The name and synonyms of the study agent
2. The chemical structure of the study agent
3. The mechanism of action of the study agent
4. The dosage range of the study agent (with appropriate rationale)
5. Animal toxicologic and pharmacologic information (when available, any known human toxicologic and pharmacologic information should also be presented)
6. How the agent will be supplied (dosage form and size)
7. The preparation guidelines for the agent (including stability and compatibility information when appropriate)
8. The storage requirements of the agent (both before and, when appropriate, after preparation)
9. The route of administration (and, if applicable, the rate of administration)

The pharmacist should also review the protocol for other potential problems (such as incompatibilities and inappropriate infusion devices). Frequently, nursing does not have an opportunity to review protocols prior to initiation and it falls to the pharmacist to ensure that the drug can be given as specified in the protocol. For complex protocols, it may be best to request secondary reviews by other specialists such as the nurses who will be giving the doses or the pharmacists who will be preparing the doses. The pharmacist can review the protocol for clinical and scientific issues appropriate to his or her knowledge level and experience. Those pharmacists with research experience or a strong clinical background may, and probably should, comment on the study design or scientific merit of a particular protocol.

With the central role of financial considerations in today's research environment, pharmacists can also provide valuable insight into the costs associated with clinical research. Traditionally, the study sponsors would provide the investigational drug free of charge to the hospital (and to the patient), and the patient (or the third-party payer) would be responsible for paying for all other charges associated with therapy. These charges could include hospitalization charges, laboratory tests, and examinations, to name a few. Increasingly, third-party payers are reluctant to pay for such charges unless they can be considered to be standard of care. This leaves the patient, and subsequently the hospital, in a financially risky situation. ❼ *More recently, some sponsors have started to implement programs for cost recovery for investigational drugs. The FDA allows for the sponsor to charge for the investigational drug only to the extent that such charges cover manufacturing the product.* The sponsor is not allowed to charge for costs that are considered part of doing business, including administrative costs. The sponsor applies to and receives approval from the FDA for a specific dollar amount that can be charged. FDA approval of this charge must be in place before cost recovery can begin.[79] A significant portion of costs associated with clinical research is pharmacy related (e.g., either supportive care medications, or infusion devices or solutions that are used to administer the investigational drug). If, during the review process, the pharmacist can provide the investigator and the scientific review board with information regarding the potential cost of the research (at least as it relates to pharmacy charges), both the investigator and the review board can make a more educated decision regarding the appropriation of resources for research purposes. When preparing an economic review of a protocol, the pharmacist should pay specific attention to the following questions:

1. Can the therapy be converted from inpatient to outpatient?
2. Can the method of infusion or the infusion device be changed to one that is more cost-effective?
3. Does the treatment plan call for the administration of compatible medications that could be mixed in the same container?
4. Is the supportive care adequate and not excessive (this is especially important with high-cost drugs such as antiemetics and growth factors)?
5. Does the protocol have a high risk of reimbursement denial? This can be evaluated by reviewing the package insert, *AHFS Drug Information, USP DI,* and for oncology products, Reimbursement and Patient Assistance Programs: A Guide for Community Cancer Centers (see http://www.accc-cancer.org/publications/publications-PAP.asp). Other factors in reimbursement risk include the cost of the drug and the supportive care or tests associated with the drug. If the protocol does have a high risk of reimbursement denial, can free drug supplies offset part or all of this risk?

Following approval of the research project, the pharmacist can assist in disseminating information regarding both the protocol and the investigational agent by preparing data sheets that may be used by pharmacy and nursing personnel (and in some situations by physicians who may be unfamiliar with the research). This information can be distributed using various methods including hard copy, the hospital mainframe, and the intranet. The investigational agent data sheet should include the following elements:

- Agent name (synonyms)
- Therapeutic classification

- Pharmaceutical data
- Stability and storage data
- Dose preparation guidelines (where applicable)
- Usual dosage range
- Route of administration
- Known side effects and toxicities
- Mechanism of action
- Status (phase of study)
- Study chairperson
- Date effective (and dates of revision)
- References

The protocol data sheet should include the following elements:

- Protocol number (as assigned by the institution)
- Protocol title
- Agent name(s) (synonym[s])
- Protocol description
  1. Objectives
  2. Study design
     a. Registration requirements
     b. Primary location of patients
     c. Type of study
  3. Treatment course (including retreatment criteria)
- Availability
  1. Supplier
  2. Status
  3. How supplied
- Storage, stability, and compatibility
  1. Intact drug
  2. Prepared drug (for injectables this should include both reconstitution and dilution guidelines)
- Dosage range
- Dose preparation guidelines
- Administration guidelines
- Special notes
- Primary investigator
- Research nurse

The primary investigator and study sponsor should approve both the drug data sheet and the protocol data sheet before dissemination. This will help eliminate any potential errors and may reduce the liability the pharmacist assumes in preparing and distributing these documents.

The pharmacist can assume primary responsibility for ordering and maintaining adequate drug supplies for conducting the clinical trial. All investigational drugs should be stored in a locked area, preferably a pharmacy. Usually, ordering can be done via telephone; however, sometimes study sponsors require written drug orders. If the drug under investigation is a controlled substance, a written order will definitely be required. Shipment and receipt of the drug can vary from 1 day to several weeks (or sometimes months for very specialized drug products). The individual responsible for ordering drugs must be sufficiently knowledgeable regarding the rate of patient enrollment in the protocol and subsequent drug usage to ensure that the institution does not run out of drug. The same individual(s) should also assume responsibility for returning unused drug supplies at the completion of the study. The sponsor may authorize the on-site destruction of unused supplies, provided this will not increase the risk to humans (or provide a risk to the environment). Many study sponsors will attempt to have the site save and return all used drug supplies as well. This is not an FDA requirement and for safety and space reasons should be discouraged.

Related to these activities, the same individuals (or team) should assume responsibility for maintaining drug accountability records. ❾ *Maintenance of such records is required by law. Again, it is preferable to have this handled by a pharmacist. These records can be maintained manually or on a computer. The records must document all drug shipments, returns, and dispensing to patients.* At a minimum, these records should document

- The date of the transaction
- The transaction type
- The recipient of the transaction (if this is a drug dispensing, the patient initials and an identifying number are required)
- The number of units being used or received or patient dispensing (this should include the actual dose the patient will receive)
- The lot number of the drug (if multiple lot numbers were used, each one should be documented)
- The initials of the individual who performed the transaction

An audit trail is required. The National Cancer Institute (NCI) has prepared a sample drug accountability form that may be used as a guide. It is available on the Internet at http://ctep.cancer.gov/forms/docs/accountability.pdf.

Computer systems that will maintain drug accountability records are available commercially. Both personal computer (PC)-based, Web-based, and mainframe-based systems exist. Some of these systems will also provide drug labels, drug and protocol information, summaries of investigational drug dispensing (useful in the preparation of productivity reports), and even monthly billing summaries to be used for posting charges to the study budget. One such Web-based system that is currently on the market is IDEA, which is being marketed by DDOTS, Inc.[80] Other commercially available systems include the IDS system, which is being marketed by the Manhatten Group, and WebIDS, which is being marketed by the McCreadie Group.[81,82] Obviously, the development of a personalized system that meets the specific needs of the institution or pharmacy is ideal. However, this can be costly, laborious, and time-consuming. If a personalized system is developed, it is important to remember that the system must be able to maintain the integrity of the records and that a clear audit trail needs to be maintained. Ultimately, the decision to computerize drug accountability records and of which system to use is one that the pharmacist should make only after evaluating the needs of the institution/pharmacy and the available budget.[83-86]

Drug accountability records and drug supplies may be inspected at any time by the sponsor. The frequency of these inspections may vary according to the wishes of the sponsor. They may be monthly, quarterly, or annually. The FDA also has the right to inspect these records. The investigational drug pharmacist should play a key role in providing drug accountability information to either the FDA or the sponsor during an audit. If proper records are not being maintained, the sponsor or the FDA may discontinue the investigator's participation in the clinical investigation.

After the clinical trial is complete, records must be maintained at the study site for the following time periods:

- Two years after approval of the NDA *or*
- Two years after the FDA received notification that the investigation was discontinued[87]

The pharmacist should also assume primary responsibility for randomizing and, where appropriate, blinding clinical trials. These two activities assist the sponsor in reducing or eliminating the bias of the clinical trial. A randomized study is one in which patients are randomly assigned (similar to flipping a coin) to different therapies. Usually, the assignment is done using a computer-generated randomization list; however, a manual list may be used as well. The randomization groups may include a number of different therapy options (e.g., a study may have four different treatment arms with an equal number of patients assigned to each arm). The number of patients assigned to the different groups may vary as well (e.g., a study may have two different treatment regimens where patients will be assigned in a 2:1 ratio to the first treatment option). The investigator should not be aware which arm the patient has been assigned to before randomization. Therefore, the involvement of a third party (such as the pharmacist) is important. A blinded study is one in which, after the patient has been randomized, the drug is masked so that at least one of the involved parties (e.g., physician, nurse, patient, or pharmacist) is not aware of what the patient is to receive. In a single-blind study, the only individual who is not aware of what the patient is receiving is the patient himself. In a double-blind study, the nurse, doctor, and patient are all unaware of what the patient is receiving. The role of a pharmacist in a double-blind study is crucial and sloppy work in this area destroys a clinical investigation. A triple-blind study is one in which the drug arrives at the pharmacy already blinded. In this scenario, the patient, nurse, doctor, and pharmacist are not aware of what drug the patient is to receive. Although this may seem simpler than a double-blind study, it is equally difficult because each patient has his or her own supply of medication and it is important that the supplies be dispensed appropriately. In a triple-blind study, the sponsor supplies the investigator with a mechanism for removing the blind from the patient (in case of emergency). It is critical that the pharmacist keep the master list. The protocol should state who has access to the master list and under what conditions this access should occur. If the FDA discovers that the investigator had access to this list, the study will be considered invalid.

Pharmacists should be willing and able to request reimbursement for the services they provide. Funds for these services are usually negotiated directly with the study sponsor before initiation of the protocol. The majority of pharmacies charge a base fee for each protocol initiated at the institution (these fees generally range from $750 to $1000 per protocol). This base fee may be fixed or it may vary based on the size of the patient population, the complexity of the protocol, or the number of doses to be prepared. Some institutions also charge an annual renewal fee for ongoing clinical trials (ranging from $300 to $1000). Most pharmacies will charge a separate fee for randomizing and blinding a clinical trial. This fee can be a one-time (per-study) fee or it can be a per-patient fee. Some hospitals also charge dispensing fees per dose or per amount of time required to prepare a dose ($15 for oral doses up to $50 for intravenous chemotherapy). Pharmacies can also charge a monthly fee for drug storage and inventory. This fee varies based on the amount of space and type of storage (e.g., freezer, room temperature, or refrigerator) required. The pharmacist can also charge a professional fee for services that exceed the standard services provided for in the base fee. Examples of services that should be charged for separately include monitoring of patients, completing case report forms, special compounding, ordering and handling controlled substances, and completing sponsor-specific drug accountability records. These services are usually charged using an hourly rate.[88–89]

Conclusion

Assisting in the implementation and conduct of clinical trials can be a satisfying role for the health care professional. A large part of the role of the pharmacist will be providing protocol and drug information to the investigators and associated study personnel. An even more satisfying role is that of providing information to the study participants. The laws governing these trials can be complex, but they are understandable once the pharmacist has taken the time to study them. Pharmacists can and should play an integral role in the conduct of clinical trials at their institution.

Self-Assessment Questions

1. What is the role of the FDA related to drugs, biologics, and medical devices in the United States?
   a. Evaluation of safety and efficacy
   b. Evaluation of the informed consent document and ethical appropriateness
   c. Evaluation of research data and marketability
   d. Both a and c

2. For what does the institutional review board (IRB) review research protocols?
   a. Evaluation of safety and efficacy
   b. Determining that the rights and welfare of human subjects are protected
   c. Risk-to-benefit ratio
   d. Both b and c

3. What are the steps of drug approval in the United States?
   a. Phase A, B, C
   b. Phase I, II, III, and IV
   c. IND/NDA
   d. Both b and c

4. What is an IND?
   a. Investigational new data
   b. Institutional novice device
   c. Investigational new drug application
   d. None of the above

5. What are the four types of documents used to amend an IND?
   a. Protocol amendments, product amendments, animal data, annual reports
   b. Manufacturing changes, protocol amendments, consent form changes, annual reports
   c. Protocol amendments, information amendments, IND safety reports, annual reports
   d. Both b and c

6. How and when can cost recovery be used?
   a. Before the product is approved for general marketing.
   b. The amount charged cannot exceed the amount required to produce, develop, and distribute the drug.
   c. Individual investigators can request cost recovery for products developed by a pharmaceutical company.
   d. All of the above.
   e. Both a and b.

7. What is an orphan drug?
   a. A drug used to treat children
   b. A product abandoned by one sponsor and brought to market by another
   c. A drug used in the treatment of a rare disease or one that will not generate enough revenue to justify the cost of research and development
   d. Both a and c

8. What are some of the required components of drug accountability records?
   a. Date of transaction and type of transaction
   b. Number of units being used or received and the initials of the person involved in the transaction
   c. Description of the product
   d. Both a and b
   e. All of the above

9. What does an NDA/BLA allow a sponsor to do?
   a. Market the product
   b. Charge for the product
   c. Advertise the product
   d. All of the above

10. What is the minimum number of members required to constitute an IRB?
    a. 10
    b. 3
    c. 5
    d. 7

11. What does GCP stand for?
    a. Good Clinical Physician
    b. Guide to Clinical Pharmacology
    c. Government Office for Clinical Protocols
    d. Good Clinical Practice

12. Gene Transfer Products are governed by:
    a. FDA
    b. NIH
    c. IRB
    d. Both b and c
    e. All of the above

13. The drug data sheet should include the following elements:
    a. Dose preparation guidelines
    b. Principal investigator name
    c. Agent name
    d. All of the above
    e. Both a and c

14. The protocol data sheet should include the following elements:
    a. Dose preparation guidelines
    b. Principal investigator name
    c. Agent name
    d. All of the above
    e. Both a and c

15. Which of the following must be true for the FDA to grant a Treatment IND?
    a. The sponsor must have already received FDA approval of the drug.
    b. The drug must be intended to treat a serious or immediately life-threatening disease.
    c. The drug must be cheaper than other alternative therapies.
    d. Both a and b.

REFERENCES

1. Tufts Center for the Study of Drug Development. Tufts Center for the Study of Drug Development pegs cost of a new prescription medicine at $802 million. [Article on the Internet] 2000 Mar [cited 2004 Mar]. Available from: http://csdd.tufts.edu/.

2. Adams CP, Brantne VV. Estimating the cost of new drug development: is it really $802 million? Health Affairs. 2006;25(2):420-8.

3. Tufts Center for the Study of Drug Development. How new drugs move through the development and approval process. [Article on the Internet] 2001 Nov 1 [cited 2004 Mar]. Available from: http://csdd.tufts.edu/.

4. Wolters Kluwer Health. Adis R&D Insight Database. [Article on the Internet] 2007 Nov [cited 2009 June]. Available from: www.adisinsight.com/customercommunications/rdi/rdi_landing.htm.

5. Food and Drug Administration. CDER approval times for priority and standard NMEs and new BLAs CY1993-2008. [2008 cited June 2009]. Available from: http://www.fda.gov/downloads/Drugs/DevelopmentApprovalProcess/HowDrugsareDevelopedandApproved/DrugandBiologicApprovalReports/ucm123959.pdf.

6. Food and Drug Administration. Protecting consumers, promoting public health [presentation on the Internet]. Washington, DC; 2004 Aug [cited 2004 Sept 15]. Available from: http://www.fda.gov/oc/opacom/fda101/fda101text.html.

7. Rados C. FDA Law Enforcement: Critical to Product Safety. FDA Consumer Magazine. Food and Drug Administration, Jan/Feb 2006 [Article on the Internet]. Available from: http://www.fda.gov/AboutFDA/WhatWeDo/History/FOrgsHistory/ORA/ucm084102.htm.

8. Food and Drug Administration [homepage on the Internet]. Washington, DC [cited 2009 June] FDA Organization. Available from: http://www.fda.gov/AboutFDA/CentersOffices/OrganizationCharts/default.htm.

9. CDER; Food and Drug Administration. Approval times for priority and standard NMEs calendar years 1993–2003. Washington, DC [updated through 2003 Dec 31; posted 2004 Jan 21; cited 2004 Sept 15]. Available from: www.fda.gov/cder/rdmt/NMEapps93-03.htm.

10. United States Federal Government Code of Federal Regulations. 21CFR601.2 Washington, DC [updated 2008 Apr 1; cited 2009 June]. Available from: http://www.gpoaccess.gov/cfr/index.html.

11. United States Federal Government Code of Federal Regulations. 21CFR312.3 Washington, DC [updated 2008 Apr 1; cited 2009 June]. Available from: http://www.gpoaccess.gov/cfr/index.html.

12. CDER; Food and Drug Administration [procedure on the Internet]. IND process and review procedures [updated 1998 May 1; cited 2004 Sept 15]. Available from: http://www.fda.gov/.

13. CDER; Food and Drug Administration [presentation on the Internet]. Guideline for drug master files [updated 2004 May 26; cited 2004 Sept 15]. Available from: http://www.fda.gov.

14. United States Federal Government Code of Federal Regulations. 21CFR314.3 Washington, DC [updated 2008 Apr 1; cited 2009 June]. Available from: http://www.gpoaccess.gov/cfr/index.html.

15. United States Federal Government Code of Federal Regulations. 45CFR46 Washington, DC [updated 2005 June; cited 2009 June]. Available from: http://www.gpoaccess.gov/cfr/index.html.

16. United States Federal Government Code of Federal Regulations. 21CFR56 Washington, DC [updated 2008 Apr 1; cited 2009 June]. Available from: http://www.gpoaccess.gov/cfr/index.html.

17. Mathieu M. New Drug Development: A Regulatory Overview. 4th ed. Cambridge (MA): PAREXEL International Corporation; 1997.

18. Bruderle TP. Reforming the Food and Drug Administration: legislative solution or self-improvement. Am J Health-Syst Pharm. 1996;53:2083-90.

19. Blum J. Drugs delayed in US as regulators struggle with new duties. Bloomberg.com 2008 Oct 27 [cited 2009 June]. Available from: http://www.bloomberg.com/apps/news?pid=news archive&sid=aC6L0BgriWIw#.

20. Tufts Center for the Study of Drug Development. Impact report 2007: EMEA meets performance goals, but lags US FDA in drug approvals. 2007 [cited 2009 Jun]. Available from: http://csdd.tufts.edu/.

21. Kessler DA, Hass AE, Feidin KL, Lumpkin M, Temple R. Approval of new drugs in the United States. JAMA. 1996; 276:1826-31.

22. Food and Drug Administration. Prescription Drug User Fee Act (amended 2007) [2009 May; cited 2009 June]. Available from: http://www.fda.gov/ForIndustry/UserFees/Prescription-DrugUserFee/default.htm.

23. Food and Drug Administration. Food and Drug Administration Modernization Act of 1997 [1997; cited 2009 June]. Available from: http://www.fda.gov.

24. Food and Drug Administration. Food and Drug Administration Amendments Act of 2007 [2007; cited 2009 June]. Available from: http://www.fda.gov.

25. Food and Drug Administration. Critical Path Initiative [2007 June cited 2009 June]. Available from: http://www.fda.gov/NewsEvents/Testimony/ucm153842.htm.

26. Food and Drug Administration. Electronic regulatory submissions and review helpful links [2009 April; cited 2009 June]. Available from: http://www.fda.gov/Drugs/DevelopmentApprovalProcess/FormsSubmissionRequirements/ElectronicSubmissions/UCM085361.

27. Reynolds T. European Drug Agency promises quicker approvals. JNCI. 1995;87:1050-1.

28. International Conference on Harmonization [Web site on the Internet]. History and future of ICH [revised 2000; cited 2009 June]. Available from: http://www.ich.org.

29. Grilley B, Gee A. Gene transfer: regulatory issues and their impact on the clinical investigator and the GMP facility. Cytotherapy. 2003;5(3):197-207.

30. The Nuremberg Code. Trials of War Criminals before the Nuremberg Military Tribunals under Control Council Law No. 10. Vol. 2. Washington, DC: US Government Printing Office; September 1989:181-2.

31. The World Medical Association. Declaration of Helsinki [amended 2008 Oct; cited 2009 June]. Available from: http://www.wma.net/e/policy/b3.htm.

32. Food and Drug Administration. The Belmont Report: Ethical Principles and Guidelines for the Protection of Human Subjects of Research [updated 1998; cited 2009 June]. Available from: http://www.fda.gov/oc/ohrt/IRBS/belmont.html.

33. United States Federal Government Code of Federal Regulations. 21CFR50 Washington, DC [updated 2008 Apr 1; cited 2009 June]. Available from: http://www.gpoaccess.gov/cfr/index.html.

34. United States Federal Government Code of Federal Regulations. 21CFR312.23 Washington, DC [updated 2008 Apr 1; cited 2009 June]. Available from: http://www.gpoaccess.gov/cfr/index.html.

35. United States Federal Government Code of Federal Regulations. 21CFR312.30 Washington, DC [updated 2008 Apr 1; cited 2009 June]. Available from: http://www.gpoaccess.gov/cfr/index.html.

36. United States Federal Government Code of Federal Regulations. 21CFR312.31 Washington, DC [updated 2008 Apr 1; cited 2009 June]. Available from: http://www.gpoaccess.gov/cfr/index.html.

37. United States Federal Government Code of Federal Regulations. 21CFR312.32 Washington, DC [updated 2008 Apr 1; cited 2009 June]. Available from: http://www.gpoaccess.gov/cfr/index.html.

38. United States Federal Government Code of Federal Regulations. 21CFR312.33 Washington, DC [updated 2008 Apr 1; cited 2009 June]. Available from: http://www.gpoaccess.gov/cfr/index.html.

39. United States Federal Government Code of Federal Regulations. 21CFR312.40 Washington, DC [updated 2008 Apr 1; cited 2009 June]. Available from: http://www.gpoaccess.gov/cfr/index.html.

40. United States Federal Government Code of Federal Regulations. 21CFR312.42 Washington, DC [updated 2008 Apr 1; cited 2009 June]. Available from: http://www.gpoaccess.gov/cfr/index.html.

41. Food and Drug Administration. The FDA's drug review process: ensuring drugs are safe and effective. [updated 2009 May; cited 2009 June]. Available from: http://www.fda.gov/Drugs/ResourcesForYou/Consumers/ucm143534.htm.

42. United States Federal Government Code of Federal Regulations. 21CFR314.50 Washington, DC [updated 2008 Apr 1; cited 2009 June]. Available from: http://www.gpoaccess.gov/cfr/index.html.

43. Food and Drug Administration. Drug approvals for calendar year 2009 [updated 2009 Apr; cited 2009 June]. Available from: http://www.fda.gov/downloads/Drugs/DevelopmentApprovalProcess/HowDrugsareDevelopedandApproved/DrugandBiologicApprovalReports/PriorityNDAandBLAApprovals/UCM090995.pdf.

44. Food and Drug Administration. Advisory Committees [updated 2009 May; cited 2009 June]. Available from: http://www.fda.gov/AdvisoryCommittees/CommitteesMeetingMaterials/Drugs/default.htm.

45. United States Federal Government Code of Federal Regulations. 21CFR314.100 Washington, DC [updated 2008 Apr 1; cited 2009 June]. Available from: http://www.gpoaccess.gov/cfr/index.html.

46. United States Federal Government Code of Federal Regulations. 21CFR314.105 Washington, DC [updated 2008 Apr 1; cited 2009 June]. Available from: http://www.gpoaccess.gov/cfr/index.html.

47. United States Federal Government Code of Federal Regulations. 21CFR314.110 Washington, DC [updated 2008 Apr 1; cited 2009 June]. Available from: http://www.gpoaccess.gov/cfr/index.html.

48. United States Federal Government Code of Federal Regulations. 21CFR314.120 Washington, DC [updated 2008 Apr 1; cited 2009 June]. Available from: http://www.gpoaccess.gov/cfr/index.html.

49. Carpenter D, Chernew M, Smith D, Fedrick AM. Approval times for new drugs: does the source of funding matter? Health Affairs. December 17, 2003:618-24.

50. United States Federal Government Code of Federal Regulations. 21CFR312.34 Washington, DC [updated 2008 Apr 1; cited 2009 June]. Available from: http://www.gpoaccess.gov/cfr/index.html.

51. United States Federal Government Code of Federal Regulations. 21CFR312.35 Washington, DC [updated 2008 Apr 1; cited 2009 June]. Available from: http://www.gpoaccess.gov/cfr/index.html.

52. United States Federal Government Code of Federal Regulations. 21CFR312.7 Washington, DC [updated 2008 Apr 1; cited 2009 June]. Available from: http://www.gpoaccess.gov/cfr/index.html.

53. United States Federal Government Code of Federal Regulations. 21CFR312.36 Washington, DC [updated 2008 Apr 1; cited 2009 June]. Available from: http://www.gpoaccess.gov/cfr/index.html.

54. United States Federal Government Code of Federal Regulations. 21CFR56.104 Washington, DC [updated 2008 Apr 1; cited 2009 June]. Available from: http://www.gpoaccess.gov/cfr/index.html.

55. Food and Drug Administration. Expanded access and expedited approval of new therapies related to HIV/AIDS [updated 2009 Apr; cited 2009 June]. Available from: http://www.fda.gov/ForConsumers/ByAudience/ForPatientAdvocates/HIVandAIDSActivities/ucm134331.htm.

56. CBER; Food and Drug Administration. Reinventing the regulation of cancer drugs: accelerating approval and expanding access [1996 Mar cited; 2004 Mar]. Available from: http://www.fda.gov.

57. CDER/CBER; Food and Drug Administration. Guidance for industry: IND exemptions for studies of lawfully marketed drug or biological products for the treatment of cancer. [2004 January 2004; cited 2004 Mar]. Available from: http://www.fda.gov.

58. Temple RJ. A regulatory authority's opinion about surrogate endpoints. In: Nimmo WS, Tucker GT, editors. Clinical Measurement in Drug Evaluation. New York (NY): Wiley; 1995.

59. Food and Drug Administration. Fast track, accelerated approval and priority review [updated 2009 May cited; 2009 June]. Available from: http://www.fda.gov/ForConsumers/ByAudience/ForPatientAdvocates/SpeedingAccesstoImportantNewTherapies/default.htm.

60. United States Federal Government Code of Federal Regulations. 21CFR312.82 Washington, DC [updated 2008 Apr 1; cited 2009 June]. Available from: http://www.gpoaccess.gov/cfr/index.html.

61. United States Federal Government Code of Federal Regulations. 21CFR312.41 Washington, DC [updated 2008 Apr 1; cited 2009 June]. Available from: http://www.gpoaccess.gov/cfr/index.html.

62. United States Federal Government Code of Federal Regulations. 21CFR312.47 Washington, DC [updated 2008 Apr 1; cited 2009 June]. Available from: http://www.gpoaccess.gov/cfr/index.html.

63. United States Federal Government Code of Federal Regulations. 21CFR314.510-520 (subpart H) Washington, DC [updated 2008 Apr 1; cited 2009 June]. Available from: http://www.gpoaccess.gov/cfr/index.html.

64. United States Federal Government Code of Federal Regulations. 21CFR316 Washington, DC [updated 2008 Apr 1; cited 2009 June]. Available from: http://www.gpoaccess.gov/cfr/index.html.

65. CDER; Food and Drug Administration. OOPD frequently asked questions [updated 2004 Sept 10; cited 2004 Sept 15]. Available from: http://www.fda.gov/orphan/faq/.

66. Food and Drug Administration. Orphan Drug Act: frequently asked questions [updated 2009 May; cited 2009 June]. Available from: http://www.fda.gov/ForIndustry/DevelopingProductsforRareDiseasesConditions/ucm124557.htm.

67. U.S. Government. Department of Health and Human Services. Waiver of Informed Consent Requirements in Certain Emergency Research. Fed Reg. 61:51531-3.

68. Food and Drug Administration. Guidance for Institutional Review Boards, Clinical Investigators, and Sponsors: Exception from Informed Consent Requirements for Emergency Research. March 30, 2000.

69. United States Federal Government Code of Federal Regulations. 45CFR46.108 Washington, DC [updated 2005 June; cited 2009 June]. Available from: http://www.gpoaccess.gov/cfr/index.html.

70. United States Federal Government Code of Federal Regulations. 21CFR56.109 Washington, DC [updated 2008 Apr 1; cited 2009 June]. Available from: http://www.gpoaccess.gov/cfr/index.html.

71. Protecting Human Research Subjects: Institutional Review Board Guidebook [updated 2001 Jun 21; cited 2009 June]. Available from: http://ohrp.osophs.dhhs.gov/irb/irb_guidebook.htm.

72. United States Federal Government Code of Federal Regulations. 21CFR56.115 Washington, DC [updated 2008 Apr 1; cited 2009 June]. Available from: http://www.gpoaccess.gov/cfr/index.html.

73. United States Federal Government Code of Federal Regulations. 21CFR46.115 Washington, DC [updated 2005 June; cited 2009 June]. Available from: http://www.gpoaccess.gov/cfr/index.html.

74. Cho M, Magnus D. Therapeutic misconception and stem cell research. Nature: Reports (Stem Cells) [published online 27 Sept 2007; cited 2009 June]. Available from: www.nature.com/stemcells/2007/0709/070927/full/stemcells.2007.88.html.

75. Davis R. U.S.: human medical tests lack oversight. USA Today. June 8, 1998; ect.A:1, 19-20.

76. Hochhauser M. Is "therapeutic misconception" being used to recruit subjects? ARENA Newsletter. Spring. 2003;16:5-7.

77. Hochhauser M. "Therapeutic misconception" and "recruiting doublespeak" in the informed consent process. IRB: Ethics and Human Research. January-February 2002:240-1.

78. Office of Research Integrity [cited 2010 May]. Available from: http://ori.dhhs.gov/misconduct/definition_misconduct.shtml.

79. Food and Drug Administration. Review of Cost Recovery Regulations and Procedures for Cell and Gene Therapy Products and Medical Devices. Presentation by Tom Finn, PhD. October 2008.

80. DDOTS, Inc. [homepage on the Internet] [cited 2009 June]. Available from: http://www.ddots.com/idea_product_overview.cfm.

81. Manhatten Group: software and solutions [homepage on the Internet] [cited 2009 June]. Available from: http://www.manhattangroup.com/ids.asp.

82. McCreadie Group: innovative solutions for pharmacy [homepage on the Internet] [cited 2009 June]. Available from: http://www.mccreadiegroup.com/home/Products/WebIDS/tabid/62/Default.aspx.

83. Burnham NL, Elcombe SA, Skorlinski CR, Kosanke L, Kovach JS. Computer program for handling investigational oncology drugs. Am J Hosp Pharm. 1989;46:1821-4.

84. Grilley BJ, Trissel LA, Bluml BM. Design and implementation of an electronic investigational drug accountability system. Am J Hosp Pharm. 1991;48:2816.

85. Lakamp JE, Lunik MC, Wilson AL, Armbruster CJ. Using a hospital mainframe computer for pharmacy investigational drug study management. Top Hosp Pharm Manage. 1993;13:37-46.

86. Iteen SE, Cepaglia J. Investigational drug information through a hospital-wide computer system. Am J Hosp Pharm. 1992;49:2746-8.

87. United States Federal Government Code of Federal Regulations. 21CFR312.57 Washington, DC [updated 2008 Apr 1; cited 2009 June]. Available from: http://www.gpoaccess.gov/cfr/index.html.

88. Department of Pharmaceutical Care University of Iowa Hospitals and Clinics. Investigational Drug Study Standard Charge Worksheet for FY 2008-9. [revised 2008 Feb; cited 2009 June]. Available from: http://www.bmc.org/grants/Pre-Award%20Policies/Investigational%20Drug%20Services%20Charge%20Sheet1.doc.

89. Boston Medical Center. Investigational Drug Services Charge Sheet [created 2004 Apr; cited 2009 June]. Available from: http://www.bmc.org/grants/Pre-Award%20Policies/Investigational%20Drug%20Services%20Charge%20Sheet1.doc.

90. Veteran's Medical Research Foundation Pharmacy Service [homepage on the Internet] [cited 2009 June]. Available from: http://www.vmrf.org/researchcenters/pharmacy-service/pharmacy.html.

91. Duke University Hospital Investigational Drug Service: Dispensing Solutions [presentation on the Internet] [presented 2006 Feb; cited 2009 June]. Available from: http://medschool.duke.edu/wysiwyg/downloads/Investigational_Drug_Service.pdf.

SUGGESTED READINGS

1. Archives of the Federal Register: http://www.accessdata.fda.gov/scripts/oc/ohrms/index.cfm
2. CenterWatch: http://www.centerwatch.com/
3. Code of Federal Regulations: http://www.gpoaccess.gov/cfr/index.html
4. FDA: http://www.fda.gov/
5. FDA Dockets Management Page: http://www.fda.gov/ohrms/dockets/default.htm
6. FDA forms: http://www.fda.gov/opacom/morechoices/fdaforms/fdaforms.html
7. ICH: www.ich.org
8. NIH/Office of Biotechnology Activities (OBA): http://oba.od.nih.gov
9. NIH/OHRP: http://www.hhs.gov/ohrp/

18

Chapter Eighteen

Policy Development, Project Design, and Implementation

Stacie Krick Evans

Learning Objectives

● *After completing this chapter, the reader will be able to*

- State reasons for pharmacist involvement in health-system policy development.
- Describe the health-system policy development process.
- List health-system policies that require pharmacy involvement.
- Identify key features of projects.
- Determine strategies for effective project design and implementation.
- Define project management.
- Describe the principles of project management that are applicable to health-system projects involving pharmacy.
- List skills needed to successfully manage a project.

Key Concepts

❶ Use a standardized and systematic approach to develop pharmacy department and health-system policies.

❷ Recognize and use resources including, but not limited to, textbooks, primary literature, and colleagues available to develop the content of policies.

❸ Contact other institutions and make inquiries as to their policies. If a health-system is a member of a group purchasing organization (e.g., Novation), you may have access to policies and procedures that other member organizations have created.

❹ A clear and complete description of a project is necessary prior to the initiation of a project.

❺ Before the initiation of a new program, an analysis of the program's strengths, weaknesses, opportunities, and threats (SWOT analysis) to an organization is needed.

❻ Successful projects are those in which all members of the team actively participate.

❼ Project management is a discipline or science that is goal-oriented, organized, detailed, and has built-in accountability. These characteristics make it an ideal process for use in directing health-system projects.

Introduction

Pharmacists in health systems are often asked to develop policies that not only apply to the pharmacy department, but pertain to other parts of the health system or even the system in its entirety. They are also asked to participate or lead teams that are tasked with a variety of projects, such as creating a process to meet a new regulatory requirement or implementing new technology (e.g., smart pumps). These tasks are unfamiliar to many pharmacists, especially those who may not have had postgraduate residency training or exposure to management or leadership curriculum in pharmacy school. The literature that is available to help the pharmacist is not plentiful and is often directed toward nursing, information technology, or health information management. Much of what the pharmacist is exposed to in these areas is on-the-job training often by individuals who may or may not have received appropriate training themselves. The information presented here is derived from the literature and other available resources and is designed to assist the pharmacist.

Policy Development

Often pharmacists are charged with projects that result in the creation of a policy. The development and creation of policy and procedure documents for health systems requires some training. Most pharmacists are not specifically trained to develop and write policies. However, there are opportunities for on-the-job training and mentoring. Additionally, pharmacists are involved in professional policy development through the American Society of Health-System Pharmacists (ASHP) and state affiliated chapters.[1] The ASHP postgraduate residency program requires that residents either write or review a health-system or pharmacy department policy. Lastly, other postgraduate training experiences also discuss policy development. This discussion will be limited to the role of the pharmacist in the development of health-system policies.

A policy is defined as a deliberate plan or course of action designed to influence and determine decisions and actions.[1] Policies establish the minimum expectations surrounding a particular activity, outline responsibilities of those involved, and set minimum rules for documentation or communication when applicable. Policies in health systems directly or indirectly affect patient care. Those that directly affect patient care give guidance and instruction in the administration of clinical services (e.g., medication administration or wound care) and they are classified as patient-care policies. Those polices that indirectly affect patient care are not inherently clinical in nature but have secondary consequences for clinical outcomes. Examples include policies relating to safety, risk management, and human resources. One example of a classification scheme for all health-system policies is represented in Table 18–1.

Pharmacists are most often involved in department-specific and patient-care polices. As expected, pharmacists create policies that affect the pharmacy department. Pharmacy policies will be written using the same standardized format as a health-system policy (e.g., purpose, definition) and the classification scheme (e.g., administrative, human resources) may be similar. For example, a health system will have a policy on dress code and the pharmacy will have a dress code policy specific to particular pharmacy areas (e.g., clean room). The pharmacists responsible for writing pharmacy department polices should have expertise in the specific area. For example, the supervisor of the sterile products area may be responsible for the development of a sterile compounding policy; the pharmacy manager may develop policies that address human resource issues in the department, such as dress code, absenteeism, and training; and an infectious diseases pharmacy specialist may develop a policy on aminoglycoside and vancomycin dosing.

TABLE 18–1. HEALTH-SYSTEM POLICY CLASSIFICATIONS

Administrative: Policies that address organizational operations

Department Specific: Policies that address an individual department or work area (e.g., pharmacy, nursing, laboratory, food, and nutrition)

Human Resources: Policies that address the work environment and staff rights

Patient Care: Policies that affect patient care directly or indirectly and cross more than one department or work area

Procurement: Policies that address purchasing issues

Safety Policies and Emergency Operations Plan

TABLE 18–2. **MEDICATION USE PATIENT CARE POLICES**

- *High-alert medications*
- *Look-alike/sound-alike medications*
- *Medication administration*
- *Intravenous push medication administration*
- *Medication formulary*
- *Electrolyte infusions*
- *Investigational medications*
- *Medication storage and security*
- *Home medications*
- *Herbal product use*

Other policies that pharmacists are involved with include patient-care policies. These policies cross into several departments (e.g., nursing, radiology) and some are specifically related to medication use and medication management. Some of these policies are required by regulatory agencies such as The Joint Commission and include topics such as high-alert medications, look-alike and sound-alike medications, and medication administration. The pharmacist is often asked to either lead or assist in the development of these policies. Table 18–2 includes a list of policies that are well-suited for pharmacy leadership or input. Some specific examples include policies that address the use of vasoactive medications (e.g., dopamine, norepinephrine), electrolytes, and opioids. Medication use policies benefit from the knowledge of pharmacists, and therefore are often written by pharmacists with review from members of the medical staff and nursing along with other departments affected by the policy. A pharmacist's insight and expertise is crucial for all health-system policies that involve medications. Additionally, there are policies that indirectly affect patient care; these are not inherently clinical in nature but have secondary consequences for clinical outcomes. Examples include policies relating to safety, and admissions and discharges. Pharmacists may or may not be involved in developing these policies. ❶ *When tasked with developing a policy, either health system or departmental, patient care related or not, use a standardized and systematic approach to develop pharmacy department and health-system policies.* There are several steps that can be used to approach and accomplish the assignment successfully. Those steps include gathering background data including the health system's policy formatting requirement; researching the standard of care or best practice; reviewing the evidence using a systematic approach; querying similar health systems for policies; and presenting the draft policy to a multidisciplinary group.

Gathering background data and noting the need for the policy is the initial step. For example, determine if it is mandated by a regulatory agency (e.g., The Joint Commission) or secondary to a new procedure or process. A new policy may be needed as new technology is implemented either in the health system (e.g., smart pumps, automated dispensing cabinets) or pharmacy (e.g., bar coding). The background information can also include such things as the health-system's medication error reports or outside sources such as pharmacy practice journals (e.g., *American Journal of Health-System Pharmacy*) or other publications (e.g., ISMP Medication Safety Alert).

Next, research the standard of care. In medicine, the standard of care is defined as a diagnostic or treatment process that experts agree is appropriate, accepted, and widely used. Sometimes, the standard of care is referred to as best practice. It is based on external clinical information from research, but also includes an individual's practice experiences. Interviewing physicians and others as to what the practice is in the health system is appropriate when researching the standard of care. In pharmacy, the standard of care or best practice is defined as a process or procedure that is widely accepted and routine. The standard of care or best practice can be applied to a disease state or condition and refer to practices in medicine and pharmacy. For example, the standard of care for treatment of a pulmonary embolus includes the use of a weight-based intravenous heparin infusion. Using this same example, in pharmacy the standard of care or best practice for the treatment of a pulmonary embolus includes stocking and dispensing a commercially available, fixed-concentration heparin solution (e.g., 12,500 units/250 mL). Both of these best practices or standards of care are examples of the type of information that is included in a health-system policy on anticoagulant safety. Additionally, pharmacy best practice or standard of care can be related to a pharmacy process or procedure. For example, prior to dispensing a compounded sterile product prepared by a pharmacy technician, both the technician and the pharmacist initial the product label.

❷ *Recognize and use resources including, but not limited to, textbooks, primary literature, and colleagues available to develop the content of policies.* To find information on the standard of care review information in textbooks, including those that provide general product information (e.g., *AHFS Drug Information, DRUGDEX Information*) and pharmacotherapeutic information (e.g., *Applied Therapeutics: The Clinical Use of Drugs, Pharmacotherapy Principles and Practice, Pharmacotherapy: A Pathophysiologic Approach, Harrison's Principles of Internal Medicine*). Next, search the literature; suggested literature search strategies and procedures including useful search engines and databases are discussed in depth in Chapter 3 of this text. However, the most common searchable databases include MEDLINE National Library of Medicine (http://www.nlm.nih.gov) and CINAHL Information Systems (http://www.cinahl.com), or International Pharmaceutical Abstracts for pharmacy-specific topics; see Chapter 3 of this text for a complete description of these and other databases. Contact the medical library at the health system for assistance with literature searches. Often health-system libraries not only assist with the literature search, but are able to obtain articles that may not be part of the library's holdings. Also search for clinical practice guidelines; many guidelines are published in medical journals such as *The New England Journal of Medicine* and therefore can be found using a database such as MEDLINE. A very good place to search is the National Guideline Clearinghouse (http://www.guidelines.gov), which indexes guidelines from many sources. Guidelines can also be found on the Websites of professional organizations such as the American College of Cardiology (http://www.acc.org) or the American Society of Health-System Pharmacy (http://www.ashp.org). The reader is referred to Chapter 7 in this text for a comprehensive overview of clinical practice guidelines including steps to locate guidelines.

Next, the results of the literature search are evaluated. Additionally, clinical practice guidelines and clinical practice statements are also evaluated. There are many methods available that can be used to evaluate the information depending on the type of information (i.e., studies) that is retrieved (e.g., case reports, clinical trials). See Chapters 4 and 5 for methods to evaluate journal articles and Chapter 7 for methods to evaluate clinical practice guidelines.

One method that can be used to evaluate the information retrieved for a patient-care policy is an evidence-based approach. Use of this method has been described in the nursing literature.[2] The evidence-based approach involves finding the best evidence, critically evaluating it, integrating it with clinical expertise and patient preferences, and applying the results to clinical practice.[3] The studies that are retrieved should be grouped according to their design and assigned a weight or level, much the same as is done in preparing a clinical practice guideline. If a health system is going to use an evidence-based approach for policy development, it is useful to employ a tool to complete the process of organizing the literature. The tool should be practical and useful. Currently, there is no standard or accepted tool that is recommended or routinely used. A suggested tool that can be used is presented in Table 18–3.[3,4] For this tool, studies and other information that has been retrieved is assigned a rank according to such characteristics as study design, with a randomized double-blind, placebo-controlled trial receiving the highest rank and a case study or case report the lowest rank.

❸ *The next step is to look to other institutions and make inquiries as to their policies. Many professional organizations (e.g., American Society of Health-System Pharmacists [ASHP], American College of Clinical Pharmacy [ACCP]) have electronic list servers for*

TABLE 18–3. **LEVELS OF EVIDENCE**

Strongest	Level 1	Individual randomized controlled trials
	Level 2	Meta-analysis or systematic review of multiple controlled clinical trials
	Level 3	Nonrandomized controlled trials single-group, pre-post, cohort studies
	Level 4	Uncontrolled studies such as case reports, case series, case studies
Weakest	Level 5	Textbooks

members. Pharmacists often use these list servers for sharing information on policies and other procedures. If your health system is a member of an organization such as the University Health Consortium or other group purchasing organizations (e.g., Novation), you may have access to policies and procedures that other member organizations have created.

Once the information on the background, rationale, and evidence has been gathered and summarized, a draft policy is created and presented to the policy stakeholders and experts for review. Most policies have several individuals responsible for writing a policy. However, there is usually someone who is identified as the lead author. This person serves as the primary contact for comments or questions regarding the policy. Even though several individuals have written the policy, they often will ask for assistance from other colleagues not directly involved in writing the policy to review the draft policy before it is presented to stakeholders or a committee for review. Identification of the appropriate stakeholders is crucial to creating and implementing a successful policy. A stakeholder is anyone who affects or is affected by the problem or issue addressed in the policy. Stakeholders include health-system departments (e.g., nursing, pharmacy, laboratory, radiology) and their personnel who are affected by the policy. Once the stakeholders are identified, individuals, workgroups, or subcommittees that represent the stakeholders are asked to provide comments to the primary author and it is his or her responsibility to revise the policy. At the same time, experts, those who have experience with the information contained in the policy, are asked to review the draft and provide input. After the stakeholders and experts have reviewed the draft policy, it is the lead author's responsibility to review the comments and incorporate them as necessary. Depending on the number of changes or suggestions to the draft, the policy may or may not need to be reviewed once again by the stakeholders or experts. In general, if there are major changes to the policy content (e.g., the stakeholders do not agree with the contents of the policy), a second review is warranted. However, minor changes that do not affect the purpose of the policy can be made and the policy is then ready to be presented to the pertinent health-system committees.

The content of the policy dictates what committees, subcommittees, or workgroups need to approve the policy. For instance, a health-system policy that outlines the process for the timely removal of health care equipment (e.g., infusion devices) that has been recalled will need review and approval from the health-system's engineering and safety workgroups and committees. A policy addressing laboratory specimen collection and labeling will be reviewed and approved by clinical laboratory and nursing workgroups and committees. A policy that outlines the process for administering medications via intravenous (IV) push will need review by nursing, pharmacy, and medical staff.

Policies are presented and approved by the medical staff through the health-system's pharmacy and therapeutics committee. At a minimum, all medication use policies are approved by the pharmacy and therapeutics committee and approved by the chief of the medical staff. The structure of committees, subcommittees, etc. , in a health system is influenced by a number of factors such as regulatory agencies (e.g., The Joint Commission), practice standards particular to a geographical area, or the culture of the health system. The health-system's policy-approval process may be extensive, so investigation of the process prior to developing the policy is essential.

The steps used for developing a pharmacy policy are very similar to those used for developing a health-system policy. For example, the director of pharmacy may ask the IV room manager to develop a policy that addresses admixture compounding for all sterile products prepared by the pharmacy. First, determine the justification of the policy; in this example, the United States Pharmacopeia (USP) recently updated and published standards for preparation of sterile products, Chapter 797 Pharmaceutical Compounding—Sterile Preparations, so the justification for this policy is compliance with regulatory standards and best practice. This policy ultimately affects patient safety. As the process of gathering information continues, use the professional listservers to query colleagues for any existing policies. In this example, it is necessary to obtain the most recent copy of the USP 797 chapter and thoroughly review it. Next, summarize and review the information you have gathered and write the policy draft. In this particular example, the amount of information needed in a policy to address the USP 797 standards is too lengthy for one policy, so five separate policies are written. Each policy contains information on one aspect of sterile compounding. For example, there are policies that outline environmental monitoring, personnel garb, and cleaning and disinfecting the preparation areas. A team of stakeholders including pharmacists, technicians, and supervisors reviews the final policies. Once these stakeholders provide their input and review, the policy is ready for final review and approval by pharmacy management.

Regardless of the type of policy (i.e., health system or department), once the policy information is reviewed and agreed upon, a structured format is used to write the policy. If a pharmacist is not aware of the format at a health system, he or she should ask what is required. Most health systems have a standard format for policies including the required sections. It may be helpful to gather this information when beginning the policy development process. Figure 18–1 contains one example of a health-system policy format including the required sections of the policy. Having a standardized format for policies is important; if different departments in a health system write policies independently and individually, this can create inconsistency and confusion for the health system. Collaboration among departments when developing policies leads to a safer environment for both staff and patients. The information that follows reviews the content of health-system policy sections. Figure 18–1 represents one health system's policy format; it is important to note that the way in which policies are formatted will vary and are dependent on the health system.

The purpose of the policy consists of one or two simple sentences explaining the reason for the policy. The purpose statement must be concise and comprehensive and is included

Type of Policy:	**PATIENT CARE**	Category:

Title:	Policy #:
	Replaces #:
Page: 1 of	Developed By:
Issue Date:	Approved By:
Revision Dates:	

I.   **PURPOSE:**
      This policy
II. **DEFINITIONS:**
      When used in this policy these terms have the following meanings:

III. **POLICY:**
      It is the policy of

IV. **PROCEDURE:**
      A.
      B.
V.   **DOCUMENTATION:**
VI. **REFERENCES:**
VII. **ATTACHMENTS:**

Figure 18–1. Policy template for a patient-care policy.

in nearly all health-system policy formats. For example, a purpose statement for a policy addressing the use of herbal products in a health system may be written as follows: "This policy establishes the position of [health system name] regarding herbal product use."

The definitions section in the policy explains terms such as acronyms and technical or legal terms that may be unfamiliar or that are used with uncommon meanings. Some policy formats do not contain a definitions section, and not all policies need terms defined. However, this section is helpful to the reader especially when a term has a specific meaning related to the policy. If it is necessary to provide definitions for a policy, the definitions section starts with the phrase, *when used in this policy, these terms have the following meanings*. For example, using the previous herbal product use policy example, the definitions section includes the term herbal product so that the reader is clear as to what products are included in policy. Another example is a pharmacy policy on pharmaceutical deterioration that contains not only a definition for expiration date/time, but also states that expiration date/time may be used interchangeably with the term beyond use date.

The next step is the creation of a policy statement, which is a succinct statement of the health-system's position regarding the subject matter. The policy statement is usually only one sentence, but it can be divided into subpoints if there are multiple objectives to the policy. For example, using the herbal product policy, *It is the policy of the [health system name] that: A. [The health system name] does not support the use of herbal products in the acute care setting; B. The pharmacy shall not supply herbal products; C. [The health system name] employees shall not administer herbal products that are not on the hospital formulary to patients.*

- The procedure section contains a description of the steps to take to accomplish the purposes of the policy statement. This section is as detailed as possible, while allowing flexibility to individual departments' operational needs; it is important to remember that the policy needs to be doable within the organization. Using the same herbal product use policy example, the procedure statements are written to clearly delineate nursing and physician responsibilities. For example, the procedure statements for nursing state that the nurse is to collect information from the patient on home herbal use and what form to use for documentation; however, it does not state when in the admission process this is to be completed, so this process can be fit into the admission process on a particular unit. Additionally, the nurse is given clear instructions on how to explain to the patient and family why herbal medications are not allowed in the health system. Each of these procedure statements are detailed; however, they are not so restrictive that they interfere with the admission process on the patient-care unit.

- The documentation section of the policy follows the procedure statement and contains information on what needs to be documented in the medical record or elsewhere. Usually documentation statements are written as follows, as appropriate in the medical record. However, there are some policies that require specific documentation. For example, a pharmacy department policy on staff education may require that attendance at educational sessions be documented on a department-specific roster.

- Policies should be appropriately referenced. A list of related policies and professional, legal, and/or regulatory authorities is included in the references section of the policy along with any references from the literature. A health-system policy on look-alike and sound-alike medications contains references such as The Joint Commission's *Comprehensive Accreditation Manual for Hospitals: The Official Handbook*, ISMP's List of Confused Drug Names, and other health-system policies. Referencing another policy is done when a procedure contained in the policy is explained or contained in another policy. For example, a policy on look-alike and sound-alike medications contains information on storing these products separately in order to avoid selecting the incorrect medication. Therefore, the health-system's policy on medication storage is listed as a reference. Additionally, if information for a policy is obtained from textbooks, clinical practice guidelines, and journal articles, these resources are included in the reference section of the policy.

Policies are designed to equip both the health system and employee with a means to ensure compliance with relevant rules and regulations. All policies must be in compliance with applicable laws and standards of regulatory accrediting agencies including, but not limited to, The Joint Commission and the state licensing boards (e.g., board of pharmacy and board of nursing). A health system will have established standards for policy review, usually every 2 to 3 years and/or as required by changes in processes.

Case Study 18–1

Due to the inherent risks of the incorrect use of concentrated sodium chloride solutions, in particular 3% sodium chloride and 7. 5% sodium chloride, the need for a policy outlining the safe administration of these solutions is requested. The risk management department requests the policy after a serious medication error occurs to a patient in the health system. Additionally, a recent issue of the Institute for Safe Medication Practices (ISMP) Medication Safety Alert newsletter featured a medication error leading to a patient death secondary to a dispensing error involving concentrated sodium chloride solution. The pharmacy department has been asked to author the policy, and the pharmacy manager has selected one of the critical care pharmacists to serve as the lead author for this policy. Because this policy will impact multiple departments (e.g., pharmacy, nursing, medical staff), the decision to create a health-system patient-care policy is made.

■ LIST THE STEPS USED TO APPROACH THIS ASSIGNMENT

- Gather health-system-specific information including the standard policy format.
- Find information on the standard of care including the appropriate dose of concentrated sodium chloride solutions, indication or indications for use, and the necessary monitoring parameters to ensure safe use.
- Review the information that has been gathered using a systematic process.
- Query colleagues using listservers or other professional organizations asking for sample policies.
- Present the draft policy to key stakeholders.

■ DISCUSS THE RESOURCES USED WHEN GATHERING INFORMATION ON THE STANDARD OF CARE

- Textbooks—It is appropriate to review information in textbooks including those that provide general product information (e.g., *AHFS Drug Information, DRUGDEX Information*), therapeutic information (e.g., *Pharmacotherapy Principles and Practice, Pharmacotherapy: A Pathophysiologic Approach, Harrison's Principles of Internal Medicine, Applied Therapeutics: The Clinical Use of Drugs*), and specialty textbooks, such as the nephrology text, *The Kidney*.
- Medical, pharmacy, and nursing literature—Search the literature for information regarding the safe use of concentrated sodium chloride. A database such as CINAHL Information Systems (http://www.cinahl.com) is quite helpful for this example because it contains literature citations from nursing and may contain articles describing nursing practice standards related to the safe administration and monitoring of concentrated sodium chloride solutions. MEDLINE National Library of Medicine (http://www.nlm.nih.gov) will often contain citations from all the clinical disciplines and contains journal citations from some of the leading titles (e.g., *The Journal of the American Medical Association, The New England Journal of Medicine*). MEDLINE also references pharmacy journals that will provide information related to the appropriate preparation and dispensing of concentrated sodium chloride solutions. Also review any evidence-based guidelines or professional association guidelines. The last step in researching the standard of care involves contacting physicians in the health system such as critical care specialists and nephrologists who have experience using concentrated sodium chloride solutions.
- As the literature is being reviewed, contact other health systems asking them for policies they have in place for the use of concentrated sodium chloride solutions. Use the professional list servers available through ASHP and ACCP.

■ EXPLAIN THE PROCESS YOU WOULD USE TO SUMMARIZE THE INFORMATION COLLECTED FOR THE POLICY

- Using an evidence-based approach is helpful for this example. The rating system as described in Table 18–3 can be used to grade the quality of the information gathered.

■ DESCRIBE A STAKEHOLDER AND IDENTIFY THE KEY STAKEHOLDERS FOR THIS POLICY

- Stakeholders are those individuals who are directly affected by the content of the policy; they can include all members of the health care team (e.g., pharmacists, technicians, physicians, nurses, respiratory therapists).

- The stakeholders in this example include the medical staff and the departments of pharmacy, nursing, and laboratory. The impact on the pharmacy department includes ensuring that appropriate procedures for the safe preparation of concentrated sodium chloride solutions are in place and that the pharmacists are competent to review orders for concentrated sodium chloride. For the nursing department, it is necessary to ensure that nurses are competent to correctly assess patients receiving concentrated sodium chloride and administer the solution appropriately (e.g., using a free-flow protected infusion pump). The laboratory department must be able to accurately and rapidly process blood samples sent for serum sodium concentration determinations. All three of these departments are impacted by a policy on the safe administration of concentrated sodium chloride solutions.

■ DESCRIBE HOW THE STAKEHOLDERS ARE INVOLVED IN THE POLICY PROCESS

- Key stakeholders (nurses, physicians) may be part of the team that researches information for the policy and actually assist in writing the policy. Not only can they be involved in the initial stages of policy development, but they also serve as reviewers and presenters of the draft policy. For example, nurses may be asked to present the policy at nursing-specific committees such as a nursing practice committee. Others, such as physicians, may be asked to present the policy to physician groups such as the health-system's department of medicine.

The policy development process can take several weeks to several months for completion. Usually, pharmacy policies can be developed more quickly as there are fewer departments affected, and thus fewer stakeholders who must review the policy. The most time-consuming processes when developing a health-system policy is trying to reach consensus among all stakeholders and experts. Initially, when a pharmacist is asked to develop a health-system policy, the identification of others who will be affected by the policy (e.g., nursing, medicine) and the recruitment of key nurses and physicians to collaborate with and ask for assistance will help facilitate the process.

Project Basics

- A project is defined as a temporary endeavor undertaken to produce a product or service.[5] Health-system projects are diverse and can range from simple projects, such as the implementation of a standard end-of-shift report, to a health-system-wide project, such as implementation of The Joint Commission National Patient Safety Goal (NPSG). Projects can also include the development and implementation of a policy as was just discussed in the previous section of this chapter. Often projects in health systems are initiated to provide a solution to an identified problem, for example, medication dispensing errors originating from poor communication among pharmacy staff at change of shift. In this example, the solution was to create a standardized change-of-shift procedure, which then became a pharmacy department project. Additionally, projects may arise secondary to regulatory requirements (e.g., The Joint Commission standards or National Patient Safety Goals). For example, in 2008, The Joint Commission (TJC) introduced an NPSG recommending practices that health systems implement to reduce the likelihood of patient harm secondary to anticoagulant use. A multidisciplinary project team was assembled to ensure the health-system's compliance with the NPSG.

Projects that involve or are led by pharmacists include those that impact the pharmacy only, the pharmacy and other departments (e.g., nursing, radiology), or the entire health system. Projects may affect pharmacists alone or also other health care professionals (e.g., nurses, physicians, radiology technologists, laboratory technologists). Projects are unique and often involve the creation of a new product or service, and therefore involve uncertainty and change. Because of this, projects may be challenging to implement. Regardless, all projects have similar characteristics by definition. They have a beginning and an end, and therefore are temporary. The project cycle includes project definition, development, implementation, and closeout.[5] Each of the steps in the project cycle will be presented.

Project Definition

Projects can be an original idea or assigned by supervisors or managers. They can also be assigned as part of a workgroup or committee. Regardless of who assigns the project, when it is assigned and prior to the initiation of the project, careful attention must be focused on defining it. If the project is assigned as part of a workgroup or subcommittee, the group that assigned the project may already have defined it. For example, a health-system patient education subcommittee may assign a project to a pharmacist that requires the creation of a comprehensive list of all materials used by health care professionals (e.g., nurses, pharmacists) to teach patients about medications. It is important to note that the pharmacist, the project lead in this example, must have a clear vision or idea of the project outcome or goal before he or she starts the project. In other words, start the project with the end in mind. Is the project outcome to identify outdated patient education materials, to update a list of available educational materials, or decide what patient education resources are to be kept or discarded? It may appear as if the patient education subcommittee has clearly defined the project to the pharmacist and thus the outcome is clear. However, if the project lead, the pharmacist in this example, does not have a clear definition of the project, it is important to seek further clarification or direction from the person who assigned the project. With this same example, does the project include patient medication education tools that are available electronically and in paper format? Does it include educational tools produced by pharmaceutical companies? ❹ *So, before a project can be initiated, the project must be defined and the outcome clear.*

After the project has been clarified, the project lead or manager develops a project description or statement. An example of a project statement for the following project, revision of the health system's patient education system is "to establish a centralized, integrated, state-of-the-art patient education system that will further the corporate mission and strengthen the hospital image as the caregiver of choice."[6] This is an example of a project statement that accurately and concisely describes the project and coincides with the organization's mission statement. Project descriptions are more detailed and usually include the following sections: project title, unit (i.e., the unit or team conducting the project), and purpose statement. The purpose statement is concise and clear and provides the overall objective of the project. It may contain a sentence stating what the project is not addressing as this may help the project team stay focused. Other sections of the project description include terms of reference (i.e., those key personnel assigned to the project), and methodology and milestones.[7] Regardless of what format is chosen, a project description or statement is an important tool for the members of the team, including the project lead, as it helps with communication and keeps team members aligned with the goal of the project. Figure 18–2 contains an example of a project description that can be used for health-system projects.

As the project lead completes the project description or statement, a SWOT (strengths, weaknesses, opportunities, and threats) analysis is developed. This analysis allows the

I.   Project Title—brief and unique

II. Team, department or unit conducting the project

III. Purpose statement—concise and clear; use an action verb in the beginning of the statement

IV. Key personnel assigned to the project—project manager's name is listed first

V.   Methodology and Milestones

Figure 18–2. Project description outline.

Strengths:	Weaknesses:

• Time saver (e.g., no waste therefore no need for witness)
• Needleless system
• Potential decrease for dosing errors, ready-to-use dosage form
	• Time to implement
	  o Update mnemonic codes so that orders can be processed timely
	  o Automated dispensing cabinets must be reconfigured
	  o Education on new device

Opportunities:	Threats:
• Successful implementation may lead to a more timely response from nursing to administer pain medications. This may result in improved pain management for patients and improved patient satisfaction scores.	• Improper usage; the devices are to be used for IV push only • One accessory device must be used for each patient to avoid infection control issues.

Figure 18–3. SWOT analysis.

identification of strengths and weaknesses with respect to the proposed project, what opportunities the proposed project offers, and what threats the project might present to the manager and organization.[7] A SWOT analysis can help the project lead decide whether or not to pursue a project, if the project lead has the authority to do so. Often projects assigned by a supervisor or administrator must be completed. ❺ *Regardless, the SWOT analysis helps to give direction regarding project implementation and identifies areas for project training and education.* Figure 18–3 shows a SWOT analysis for a project involving the use of a new medication administration system (Carpuject) for administering intravenous (IV) morphine.

Whether the project is an original idea or assigned by administration or a committee, once defined, with a project description and SWOT analysis completed, it is helpful to present a summary of the information to gain the support of key stakeholders and others. This is especially true when the project affects department employees, patients, or a budget. The example project, the implementation of the Carpuject system for administration of IV morphine, involves two departments, nursing and pharmacy, and affects patient care. Presenting the project to nursing and asking for their input as to how best to introduce this new device is crucial to the success of the project. This is done by the project lead identifying a nursing group, reviewing the project description and SWOT analysis with it, and asking for its recommendations for the following: nursing education (e.g., vendor-, pharmacist-, or nurse-led education), product labeling, and placement in the automated dispensing cabinets. Additionally, ask the group for any other suggestions of how to introduce and encourage nurses to use the Carpuject device. To proceed without nursing input may make implementation problematic and jeopardize future joint nursing and pharmacy projects. For those projects that need the approval and support of many key stakeholders and others in the health system (e.g., administration) prior to initiation, several customized presentations of the project may be needed. This may be accomplished in different venues ranging from informal discussions (e.g., focus groups) to formal presentations. Projects that impact the health system on many levels (e.g., nursing, pharmacy, medical staff) necessitate a more formal presentation to the groups most affected by the project.

When preparing these communications, it is important to know the audience and develop the presentation accordingly. For example, recently The Joint Commission added an NPSG that directs a health system to have a process that accurately and completely reconciles medications across the continuum of care. In other words, the health system must have a process in place as the patient enters the health system (either as an inpatient or outpatient) to collect a list of medications that the patient uses. The physician reviews that list prior to the initiation of any new medication; additionally, the prescriber selects what medications from the list are to be continued. This process of medication reconciliation continues as the patient is transferred to a different level of care (e.g., from the intensive care unit to an intermediate care unit) or to another facility within the health system (e.g., a rehabilitation unit). Lastly, the medications are reviewed prior to patient discharge from the health system. A list of the medications the patient is to continue at home or in another facility (e.g., a skilled nursing facility) is prepared and is given to the patient and the next health care provider. At many health systems, the task of developing a process that addresses this NPSG is assigned to pharmacy and nursing. Because this is a health system project affecting many different departments, presentations to several groups of key stakeholders are required. Additionally, because this project involves many health care professionals, including physicians and other prescribers, pharmacists, and nurses, several presentations are developed. It is important to prepare these presentations with an understanding of who is the audience and customize them accordingly. One presentation is developed for health-system leadership (e.g., managers, administrators) and another for the staff (e.g., nursing and pharmacy). The health-system leadership or administration is more interested in learning how the proposed medication reconciliation process can improve patient safety and achieve compliance with The Joint Commission accreditation. However, the staff is interested in hearing how performing medication reconciliation will enhance their efficiency and improve patient safety. Managers may be interested in how to educate and motivate staff to carry out the medication reconciliation process. The presentations given to the different groups are not meant to be a comprehensive review of the complete project, but provide enough information to gain approval and support from key stakeholders; the presentations focus on what is important for the particular stakeholders. An added benefit of presentations like this is that they can serve to motivate, and often project team members are chosen from these initial sessions.

Project Development

The next step after support has been gained for the project is to select the project team. In the medication reconciliation example previously mentioned, members of the project team can be identified from the various meetings used to introduce the project. For all projects, large or small, identify project team members from several different groups including those who will be affected by the project (e.g., front-line pharmacists, nurses) and those with particular skills and expertise (e.g., clinical pharmacy specialists, clinical nurse specialists, physicians). Remember, others, such as managers, directors, and administrators, are also needed as project team members. Many projects thought to only affect a pharmacy department impact other departments such as nursing, respiratory care, laboratory, and food and nutrition. Having project team members with diverse backgrounds and experiences is crucial to team success. For that reason, discuss the project with colleagues in other departments, asking for recommendations.

Effective team leadership is challenging in that often project leaders have responsibility for completion of the work, but little authority over the team members, and they may be subordinate to certain project team members. However, project leaders can create effective teams by actively managing expectations. Create a clear and compelling picture of each task's place in the project. Manage accountability, that is, inform project staff of their roles and responsibilities. Play a supportive and facilitating role rather than a directive role as the project lead. Foster ownership and team development by keeping members informed and involving team members in discussions during team meetings.[8] Effective and successful project leaders or project managers create an environment of shared responsibility. Examples of key project management leadership skills are outlined in Table 18–4. Flexibility is a

TABLE 18–4. RECOMMENDED LEADERSHIP SKILLS FOR PROJECT MANAGERS

Ability to work with a variety of team members with different
- Backgrounds (e.g., new employees, long-term employees)
- Disciplines (e.g., nurses, physicians, radiology technologists, laboratory technologists, nutritionists)
- Knowledge levels (e.g., new graduates and nonlicensed personnel)

Ability to translate or bridge the gap among the different team members
- Limit the use of technical jargon

Provide a clear vision, alternative solution, and plan when needed

Build trust and respect among team members
- Make team members decision makers, especially in their specialty areas

Manage conflict or emotional responses
- Be prepared and focus on the facts without blame or emotion

Influential

critical leadership skill, and different leadership styles are needed depending on the type of project and the qualifications and experience of the project team members.[7] For example, the project leader may need to use a more direct style when working with a newly licensed pharmacist, whereas a seasoned pharmacist may need less direction and a hands-off approach would be more effective.

Once the team is assembled, there are several methods that the project lead can use to identify the tasks that must be accomplished in order to the complete the project. One method is to have the project lead develop a task schedule,[9] which is a relatively simple process and does not require the use of project management software. The tasks are listed on a sheet of paper divided into sections (Figure 18–4a). One column prioritizes tasks, another one lists the actual task, and the last two columns are to list who or what resources are needed and the timeframe for completion. Using such a task schedule allows the project lead to identify all the tasks, prioritize them, and assign the tasks to the appropriate person or persons along with a timeframe for completion. Figure 18–4b depicts a task schedule for creating patient education materials for warfarin, an oral anti-coagulant. There are other methods that can be used to develop the project that utilize two key project management tools: the work breakdown structure (WBS) and Gantt chart. These tools are part of project management software packages. Project management and how it can be applied to health care–related projects will be discussed later in the chapter. The WBS is a tool that takes a defined project and groups the project's discrete work elements in a way that helps organize and define the total work scope of the project.[10] It is simply a list of all the individual tasks that must be completed in order to achieve the objective in mind. The WBS structure is a critical first step because it provides a framework for organizing and managing the approved project scope, helps to ensure

Priority	Task	Person responsible	Completion time

Figure 18–4a. Task structure outline.

Priority	Task	Person responsible	Completion time
1	List the requirements for warfarin patient education as stated in TJC* NPSG^ .03.05.01	Pharmacist team member	1 week
2	Gather the current health-system patient education booklet	Nurse team member	1 week
3	Review and edit the general information in the booklet (e.g., INR measurement, follow-up appointments, when to contact 911 or physician office, etc.)	Nurse team member	2 weeks
4	Review and edit the drug interaction information	Pharmacist team member	2 weeks
5	Review and edit the dietary information	Pharmacist and dietician team members	2 weeks
6	Present first draft to team for review	Team	4 weeks
7	Incorporate comments and present to team	Team leader	2 weeks
8	Present edited draft to team for comments	Team leader	1 week
9	Deliver final copy to printer	Team leader/printer	4 weeks
10	Proof the final copy	Team leader	2 weeks
11	Place the final copy on the health-system intranet	Printer and IS team	4 weeks
12	Notify clinical staff (nurses and pharmacists)	Nurse and pharmacist team members	

*The Joint Commission.
^National Patient Safety Goal.

Figure 18–4b. Task structure. Project: warfarin patient education booklet.

that all the work has been defined, and sets the structure for planning and scheduling information. The WBS also will help team members understand all of the project's tasks and how they relate to the project outcome. The concept of the WBS is similar to the task schedule described previously, but the WBS can be completed with the help of project management software such as Microsoft Office Project.

The advantage of using the WBS is that with the help of project management software, it can be converted into a Gantt chart. A Gantt chart is a project management tool used to plan and monitor elements of a project. A Gantt chart takes the task identified in the WBS and represents these as elements of a bar chart.[8] This tool is not commonly

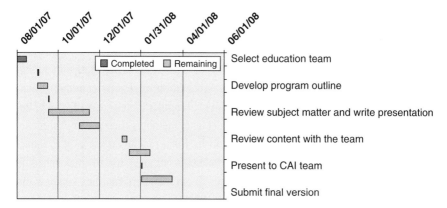

Figure 18–5. Gantt chart for a sample project using Excel software. Project Title: Staff Education for Safe Use of Anticoagulants.

used in pharmacy; however, its use in other health care disciplines (e.g., nursing) has been reviewed.[8] The Gantt chart also guides the execution of the project and serves as a timeline. In the past, Gantt charts were drawn by hand; however, software programs such as Microsoft Office Project can be used to complete a WBS and Gantt chart. A Gantt chart can also be created using Microsoft Word or Excel. A very basic and simple example of a Gantt chart that outlines a project related to The Joint Commission National Patient Safety Goal (NPSG) on anticoagulant safety and staff education is described (Figure 18–5). In order to be in compliance with this NPSG, the health system provides staff education on the safe use of anticoagulants. In this example, a health-system taskforce assigned this project to two nurses and one pharmacist. Figure 18–5 is the Gantt chart created using Excel developed for this project. Notice that the Gantt chart is a visual representation of the project and places each of the elements of a project clearly on a timeline; this is an example of what can be distributed at the first team meeting.

Regardless of what tool is used to identify tasks (e.g., task schedule, WBS), one of the most effective ways to develop project tasks is to bring the project team together for a brainstorming session in which the project lead presents the project and asks the team to identify the tasks that need to be accomplished in order to complete the project. ❻ *When using this structured approach, all team members are required to participate. Unequal participation in project teams not only frustrates team members but also other health care staff and managers and can jeopardize the successful completion of projects. Because the entire team participates in the development of the task schedule and takes ownership in completing the tasks, using this approach fosters cooperative learning and management skills development.*[7] Note that it is not necessary to prioritize the tasks until they have all been identified. When prioritizing tasks, encourage the participation of all team members. Because all the team members have an active role in not only task identification but also task prioritization, there is accountability and the likelihood that all the tasks will be completed and the project outcome will be a success.

- Communication is vital to the success of the team. Regular meetings, including a project kickoff meeting, will help set an expectation of regular communication. Follow-up meetings should be concise and include regular updates and the use of the Gantt chart to track progress. Showing project team members their accomplishments and progress to project completion will motivate them to stay on track up to implementation and project completion. If a Gantt chart is not used, use the task schedule and update it regularly before every meeting. Team members can then see how the project is progressing. Strike through those tasks as they are completed, again to show the team that progress is occurring.

Project Implementation

If a project has been well organized and managed appropriately, implementation will be successful. Once project details have been finalized the team should create an implementation packet. The packet focuses on how the project will be implemented rather than development. A complete implementation packet contains the following: background and rationale for the project, pertinent policies and procedures, educational materials that are created for the specific disciplines involved, and an effective date. For example, if new infusion devices that use smart technology are being introduced into a health system the project implementation phase must be complete in order for the infusion devices to be used correctly and thus improve patient safety. The rationale for why these new devices are being introduced into the health system must be clear. For example, the rationale can include a review of health-system medication errors related to infusion devices and any other local or national medication error data (e.g., ISMP reports). A patient-care policy outlining the procedure for the nursing, pharmacy, and medical staff must be developed, reviewed, and approved by the appropriate committees (e.g., pharmacy and therapeutics) prior to introducing the devices. In this example, an education plan is completed prior to the introduction of the infusion devices to the patient-care unit.

Project Closeout

- Once the project has been completed successfully, the next step is an evaluation of the project.[9] Often, teams are so thankful that a project is completed that they forget to reflect on the project. The team should meet again to discuss if the project goals were met and which processes or steps would be modified if the project were to be done again, for future projects.

Project Management

● Project management is a discipline that combines concepts from a variety of fields, including engineering and construction.[11] It focuses on organizing and managing resources so that the project can be completed within a given time period. ❼ *Using a project management approach offers many strengths. Its strong goal orientation, detailed planning, and accountability help ensure the successful completion of projects. These characteristics make it well suited for health care.* The task schedule, WBS, and Gantt chart previously described are project management tools.

Project management has been applied to large-scale projects (e.g., data systems implementation, large construction projects) in a number of industries other than health care. In health care, the project management methodology has been traditionally associated with information technology (IT) projects (e.g., implementation of a clinical information system). Project management has also been utilized by the pharmaceutical industry to develop new drugs. Additionally, project management techniques have been used to provide care for inpatients[12] and develop patient education materials,[6] and have been suggested as a means to provide health care services and reduce costs with the physician serving as the project manager.[13] However, the principles of project management can be applied to many other and different pharmacy-related projects, both large and small. Project management principles have even been recommended for use in practice-based research (e.g., residency research projects).[11] Some other pharmacy projects that can utilize the project management process include the implementation of a continuing education lecture series or opening an operating room satellite. These projects affect not only personnel but budgets, so they are well suited for a project manager.

● There are a number of tools and processes that need to be in place in order for a project management approach to be used successfully in the pharmacy department. Merely purchasing project management tools such as software without the necessary staff training and development will not create a project-management-savvy department and will not help the pharmacist become an effective project manager. The pharmacy department, including administration and the pharmacy staff (those that lead projects and participate in teams), must be committed to using a project management approach and adopt project management principles as part of their culture. Additionally, senior management must be committed to project management, otherwise staff may not make an effort to use project-planning tools effectively.[7] If a department decides to embrace project management, training of the pharmacists is critical. As mentioned, project management tools and techniques along with leadership skills are used to effectively managed projects. Pharmacists may have some of the basic leadership skills; however, these may need to be enhanced because of the high stress in projects based on time constraints and interpersonal conflicts that may arise among project team members. Additionally, training on the use of the various software tools and other techniques used in project management is essential. There are a variety of organizations and universities that offer project management training. A proposed training program for nursing is described[7] that includes a train-the-trainer format encompassing 3 to 5 days of education. Course content includes a discussion of the tools used in project management and also the essential leadership skills. The Project Management Institute (http://www.pmi.org), a nonprofit professional organization for project management professionals, offers resources such as journals, textbooks, and educational conferences for use. Professionals can also become certified or credentialed in various project management areas. Professional pharmacy associations (e.g., ASHP, ACCP) offer leadership conferences and seminars that provide education on not only leadership styles but also project management.[14] Health systems that have embraced project management may also offer classes or training. These classes, if offered, are coordinated in the organization development department of human resources.

Pharmacists who assume health-system leadership roles in designing, implementing, and evaluating programs that affect patient care can serve as project managers. In order to be effective project managers, pharmacists must possess both management and leadership abilities and skills. A flexible leadership style is essential. Management skills not only include product and technical knowledge, but also knowledge of project management activities and tools. The pharmacist managing the project must be able to define the project and scope, gain approval and support from key stakeholders, establish a team, develop a timeline providing regular updates, allocate resources (e.g., time), direct project activities, manage problems, and ensure quality control. This is a complex task, but there are resources (e.g., textbooks, seminars) available to assist the pharmacist in the successful completion of a project.

Conclusion

Today's health-system pharmacist is recognized as not only a valuable member of the health care team but someone who has an important role in the success of a health system. Pharmacists, with their expertise in pharmacotherapy and medication safety, are uniquely situated to be involved in and lead policy development. They also have skills that allow them to be active participants and leaders on project teams. The tools that pharmacists use for these activities are gradually being introduced via the health care literature and professional societies. The information contained in this chapter is designed to assist pharmacists as they are selected to participate in policy development and project design and implementation.

Self-Assessment Questions

1. The following health-system policies require a pharmacist's participation, *except*:
   a. Herbal product use
   b. High-alert medications
   c. Blood/blood products ordering
   d. Electrolyte infusions

2. When gathering information for inclusion in a health-system policy, what is the initial step?
   a. Conduct a literature search using CINAHL Information Systems.
   b. Ask for a meeting with the director of pharmacy.
   c. Contact colleagues who work at other health systems.
   d. Gather background information including the justification of the policy.

3. Prior to starting a project, a tool that is recommended to use for defining the project is:
   a. Project description
   b. SWOT analysis
   c. Work breakdown structure
   d. Gantt chart

4. Select the skills needed to be an effective project manager.
   a. Technical knowledge of the project components
   b. Ability to work with a multidisciplinary team
   c. Capacity to manage conflicts or emotional responses from project team members
   d. All of the above

5. The components of the project cycle are:
   a. Project definition, development, implementation, and closeout
   b. Project development, justification, implementation, and review
   c. Project strengths, weaknesses, opportunities, and threats
   d. Project identification, justification, implementation, and closeout

REFERENCES

1. Allcock NM. Getting involved in professional policy development. Am J Health-Syst Pharm. 2007;64:1144-46.
2. Oman KS, Duran C, Fink R. Evidence-based policy and procedures. J Nurs Adm. 2008; 38(1):47-51.
3. Sackett DI, Rosenberg WM, Gray JA, Haynes RB, Richardson WS. Evidence-based medicine: what it is and what it isn't. BMJ. 1996;312:71-2.
4. Stetler CB, Brunell M, Giuliano KK, Morsi D, Prince L, Newell-Stokes V. Evidence-based practice and the role of nursing leadership. J Nurs Adm. 1998;28(7):45-53.
5. Doll BA. Project management 101. Skills for leading and working in teams, Part 1. J AHIMA. 2005 (Jan);76(1):50.
6. Patyk M, Gaynor S, Verdin J. Patient education resource assessment: project management. J Nurs Care Qual. 2000;14(2):14-20.
7. Loo R. Project management: a core competency for professional nurses and nurse managers. J Nurse Staff Dev. 2003:19(4):187-93.
8. Doll BA. Project management 101. Skills for leading and working in teams, Part 4. J AHIMA. 2005 (Apr);76(4):48, 50.
9. Berry R. Project management for nurses. J Intraven Nurs. 1994;17(1):28-34.
10. Shirey MR. Project management tools for leaders and entrepreneurs. Clin Nurse Spec. 2008;22(3):129-31.
11. Weber RJ, Corbaugh DJ. Developing and executing an effective research plan. Am J Health-Syst Pharm. 2008;65:2058-65.
12. Kaufman DS. Using project management methodology to plan and track inpatient care. Jt Comm J Qual Patient Saf. 2005;31(8):463-8.
13. Sa Couto J. Project management can help to reduce costs and improve quality in health care services. J Eval Clin Pract. 2008;14:48-52.
14. American Society of Health-System Pharmacists. Proceedings of the ASHP 2007 Conference for Leaders in Health-System Pharmacy. Am J Health-Syst Pharm. 2008;65:e19-e22.

19

Chapter Nineteen

Drug Information in Ambulatory Care

Debra L. Parker

Learning Objectives

● *After completing this chapter, the reader will be able to*

- Describe the importance of drug information provided by the health care professional in the ambulatory care setting.
- Discuss the importance of access to up-to-date formulary information in the provision of care in the ambulatory setting.
- Identify sources with links to full-text evidence-based practice guidelines.
- Describe desired characteristics of drug information resources specific to the ambulatory environment.
- Describe reputable drug information sources geared toward the health care professional that are also useful in providing drug information to patients.
- List ways that practitioners may address concerns regarding access to information.
- Discuss trends in ambulatory practice, including the disposal of unused, unwanted, or expired medications and immunizations.
- Identify resources providing quality-assurance indicators for the optimal provision of ambulatory care.

Key Concepts

❶ The clinician in the ambulatory care setting routinely calls upon many drug information skills on a daily basis to not only provide drug information to patients and other health care providers, but to function competently and efficiently within this practice setting.

❷ The ambulatory care practitioner is the person with the greatest opportunity to fill the role of medication information provider and interpreter.

❸ Knowledge of formulary status of medications is only one part of the prescription decision-making process. Whenever they exist, evidence-based clinical practice guidelines should guide prescriptive decision making.

❹ Ambulatory practitioners have the responsibility to remain up-to-date regarding current practice guidelines.

❺ Electronic or Internet-based databases are attractive to utilize in ambulatory care for multiple reasons.

❻ Ambulatory care clinicians bear a responsibility to educate patients on this topic and should therefore be aware of pertinent sites for information.

❼ While ambulatory clinicians typically recommend and/or dispense most medications, immunizations are medications that are administered in the community setting. Those practitioners immunizing in this setting have the obligation to not only provide these services safely, but to serve as immediate sources of information (i.e., drug information) regarding the medications they are administering.

❽ Health care professionals involved in the provision of care in the ambulatory care setting should familiarize themselves with the pertinent established quality measures.

Introduction

This textbook covers a long list of drug information topics and skills, although not every clinician will use all of these skills on a daily basis. ❶ *The clinician in the ambulatory care setting routinely calls upon many drug information skills on a daily basis to not only provide drug information to patients and other health care providers, but to function competently and efficiently within this practice setting.*

The ambulatory care practitioner is often required to use a variety of drug information skills and resources during routine encounters with patients to provide information at a personalized and appropriate level. Before doing so, the practitioner must know where to look for appropriate information, and how to interpret and practically apply this information to a specific patient or population. This is where many practitioners fall short. This chapter discusses the resources and skills commonly needed by the ambulatory care provider in order to provide appropriate drug information. Topics covered will include commonly used references for (a) prescription formularies; (b) obtaining evidence-based guidelines; (c) desired characteristics of drug information resources and examples of those particularly useful to the ambulatory care clinician; (d) drug information resources pertinent to the current trends in ambulatory care, such as the proper disposal of unused or unwanted or expired medications; (e) preventive health drug information (specifically information regarding immunizations); and (f) quality-assurance considerations in ambulatory care.

Why Focus on Drug Information Specifically in the Ambulatory Care Setting?

Although the provision of health care takes place in a variety of settings ranging from hospital and long-term care facilities to patients' homes, the emphasis in today's patient care environment is to provide as much health care as possible in the outpatient, ambulatory setting. It is also commonly recognized that patients are technologically savvy and utilize the Internet and news media to provide self-care in the outpatient setting. The quality of the medical and drug information patients obtain themselves varies widely, depending on the source (see Chapters 4 and 5 for drug literature evaluation); however, even when quality information is provided, patients still require someone with clinical expertise and drug information training to explain medical information and to provide guidance in the decision-making process.

Applying Drug Information in an Ambulatory Care Setting

Consider the following scenario.

> Ron Spencer, PharmD, is working in a patient care clinic when SG, a Hispanic man who appears to be in his mid-50s, enters with a prescription for esomeprazole (Nexium) and says, "Should I be worried about taking this medication? My doctor says I can just take it as needed, but I'm nervous about any new medication! Do I really need to fill this?" SG says he is not sure what his medication is for and says he doesn't know much about it, but that he was told he could use it as needed.

As a clinician in the ambulatory care setting, being asked a question such as this, with little to no background knowledge, is a familiar situation. Can SG's question be answered? If not, what type of background information would be necessary?

> SG has never filled a prescription at Ron's pharmacy and Ron cannot answer SG's question without gathering more information. After some discussion, Ron discovers that SG has been experiencing a burning feeling in his chest for the last month, saw his family doctor today, and was told it was "just heartburn." SG has no known allergies, and his past medical history includes hypertension and hypercholesterolemia, for which he takes metoprolol succinate 50 mg daily and pravastatin 80 mg daily, respectively. SG was given a prescription for esomeprazole and told he could take it once daily as needed, without any further discussion with his prescriber. What SG really wants to know is whether there are nonprescription treatment options for his symptoms before starting a new medication.

If Ron were not familiar with the appropriate treatment for GERD (gastroesophageal reflux disease), how would he begin to answer SG's question? What type(s) of resources would be easily and quickly accessed in the ambulatory setting to find this type of information?

> Ron, after reviewing current practice guidelines for the treatment of GERD, explains to SG that while his prescription is likely to be effective in relieving his symptoms, there are nonpharmacologic treatments that may also help. SG decides to try the nonprescription options for a few weeks before filling a prescription.
>
> Three weeks later, SG returns to Ron's pharmacy and reports that, while his nonprescription lifestyle modifications have helped, he still has symptoms and wishes to fill his prescription. While filling the prescription, Ron notes that this prescription is third tier in this patient's insurance formulary (i.e., managed care system that results in the highest copayment for the patient). He explains to SG that this means he will pay a higher copayment than if he were to use a medication that is first tier, or preferred on the formulary. SG asks what other prescriptions would work for his condition and cost less.

How should Ron begin to research this information and get an answer in a timely manner? Would your answer change if Ron worked in an environment with limited or no Internet access?

> Ron researches which medications are first tier and contacts SG's prescriber to request a prescription change. Ron counsels SG on signs of worsening disease and when SG should contact his prescriber if symptoms continue or worsen.

In this scenario, the practitioner, in a few routine encounters with the patient, has called upon multiple drug information skills described elsewhere in this text to assist this patient. He has

- Used the modified systematic approach (Chapter 2) and determined the patient's ultimate question.
- Applied evidence-based clinical practice guidelines (Chapter 7), and as a result was able to confirm the appropriateness of the prescribed medication as well as educate the patient regarding appropriate nonpharmacologic approaches he could try to avoid the need for medication.
- Drawn from his knowledge of formulary structures and explained this to the consumer (Chapter 12).

If the scenario were that SG had no prescription insurance, Ron may have also applied practice guidelines (Chapter 7) to recommend a less costly, nonprescription alternative. The scenario exemplifies how frequently, and as a matter of reflex, the ambulatory care clinician applies drug information skills. ❶ *The clinician in the ambulatory care setting routinely calls upon many drug information skills on a daily basis to not only provide drug information to patients and other health care providers, but to function competently and efficiently within this practice setting.*

Providing Drug Information in the Ambulatory Setting

"I CAN JUST GOOGLE IT MYSELF"

In the previous scenario, SG may well have been able to Google the name of the drug he was prescribed, and would likely have found general information regarding its use and side effects. The average patient is able to access a plethora of information via the news media and many Web sites and blogs; however, the reliability, accuracy, and timeliness of this information can vary widely, as discussed in Chapter 3. Although some of these sources of drug information may be reputable, they are impersonal and can only offer general information to the reader. Such sites typically advise patients to talk with their practitioner for specific personal questions.

WHAT SHOULD THE PUBLIC (AND EVEN OTHER HEALTH CARE PROVIDERS) KNOW ABOUT UTILIZING TRAINED CLINICIANS AS A SOURCE OF DRUG INFORMATION VERSUS PERFORMING THEIR OWN DRUG INFORMATION SEARCHES?

Health care providers fill an important role in the provision, interpretation, and practical clinical application of drug information that is often geared toward the layperson. While there is an ever-increasing trend toward providing self-care and self-education, the lay public is often unaware that the health care provider has access not only to the same Web sites as the patient, but also to professional literature and databases (see Chapter 3). The layperson is unable to access and/or interpret such information. Depending on their clinical training, certain health care providers may also lack knowledge regarding available resources and how to best interpret health information data.

Although in some cases, individuals may be able to personally access secondary or even primary literature, interpreting this information and putting it into context with their personal health conditions as well as current evidence-based guidelines (see Chapter 7) requires a health care professional trained in drug information. Interpreting and evaluating primary literature (see Chapters 4 and 5) as well as locating and interpreting evidence-based guidelines are skills that require training and practice. These activities require someone who has been trained in drug information evaluation and has expertise in these areas.

❷ *The ambulatory care practitioner is the person with the greatest opportunity to fill the role of medication information provider and interpreter.* The definition of the ambulatory care practitioner is changing, with a growing number of health care settings lending themselves to providing outpatient care. Any medical care delivered on an outpatient basis is considered ambulatory care. For example, an ambulatory care practitioner may be a clinician who practices in a community pharmacy, a community-based clinic or office, or an outpatient setting of an institutional care facility, or be someone who provides on-site services within an employer-provided wellness and disease management program.

Although, as mentioned previously, proficiently providing drug information is a skill that requires training and practice, often the biggest challenge for ambulatory care practitioners is not providing the needed drug information skills proficiently, but convincing the public that they offer a unique skill in drug information beyond the Internet.

Unfortunately, many practitioners place too little emphasis on the need for their involvement in the interpretation of drug information, assuming that other health care professionals and even the public, with adequate access to information databases, can answer their own questions. In 2001, it was reported that in 1 year, approximately 9 million hospital admissions and over 18 million emergency room visits in the United States were caused by the incorrect use of medications.[1] Although these data were published in 2001, this is an issue that has not been resolved. Consider a study conducted in Vancouver, Canada, published in 2008, which reported that pharmaceuticals were the cause of 12% of emergency room visits and resulted in significantly longer lengths of stay for those patients admitted.[2] Incorrect use of medications includes not only patient non-adherence, but also the use of medications when not clinically appropriate. In today's environment, with direct-to-consumer advertising and increasing numbers of over-the-counter medications that were formerly available only by prescription, the decision to use a medication is not made solely by prescribers, but also by patients themselves. It is evident that these decision makers need guidance. Who guides these decision makers? Unfortunately, the answer is often no one.

There is certainly not a lack of available drug information, nor is there, for most individuals, a lack of accessibility. What is lacking, however, is the provision of quality drug information provided by a practitioner trained to do so for not only patients, but for other health care providers. Until that case is made to the public and other payers for health care, including both employers and legislators, it is likely that pharmaceuticals will continue to have the unintended effect of increasing, rather than decreasing, morbidity and mortality, and contributing to rising health care expenditures.

The following section discusses resources integral to the provision of drug information in ambulatory care.

Drug Information Responsibilities in Ambulatory Care

Integral responsibilities of the ambulatory care clinician are many. Several key responsibilities include (1) assisting prescribers and consumers to find the most cost-effective drug to treat a given condition, (2) ensuring that a prescribed medication is appropriate and follows current treatment guidelines, (3) ensuring patients' understanding of the appropriate use of their medications (Chapter 20), (4) guiding others regarding the proper disposal of unused or unwanted medications, (5) providing preventive health information, and (6) incorporating quality-assurance indicators into daily practice.

DRUG FORMULARY INFORMATION

Whether a clinician is prescribing or filling a prescription order, formulary restrictions increasingly influence medication usage patterns. Several useful tools exist to assist in determining formulary restrictions and then making decisions as to risks versus benefits of abiding by these restrictions.

As a large proportion of health care consumers are Medicare recipients, access to Medicare drug plan (i.e., Medicare Part D) formulary information is paramount. Although many patients may select their own Medicare drug plan, others often look to their ambulatory care clinician to assist them in this decision. Information to guide selection is available at http://plancompare.medicare.gov/pfdn/FormularyFinder/ LocationSearch or by visiting http://www.medicare.gov and clicking on the link for Formulary Finder. Users choose their state of residence and enter their prescription drug profile. The program will then provide a list of Medicare Part D plans that include some or all of the listed drug profile, as well as information regarding the status of each drug in a particular plan and the number of pharmacies that participate with a plan in a given state. Users, including prescribers, can also download complete formularies, as well as appeals and exceptions forms. For practitioners with Internet access, this Web site is extremely useful.

An additional method for obtaining formulary information via the Internet is by typing the name of the prescription insurance provider + formulary in the browser. Most prescription providers will have Web pages including a full formulary guide, a list of covered medications listed by drug or by drug class, a medications tier status in which participants are subject to varying levels of copayment options for a given drug depending on its formulary status, links to suggested alternatives to a medication if it is not covered, and links for forms necessary for prior approval, appeals, and exceptions. An advantage to visiting these sites is immediate access to information and necessary forms. Each prescription provider, however, will have a different Web page design and often there is no consistency as to where the user will find information.

Many clinicians may be familiar with Epocrates, Inc. software programs. Epocrates, Inc. markets programs with a variety of content areas including calculations, continuing medical education, diagnostics, a medical dictionary, disease state information, drugs, medical news, and tables. These content areas are bundled into various versions, some of which are free. All Epocrates programs, including those that are available at no cost, include both national and regional formulary information, including Medicare Part D. Users can access formulary status and restrictions for over 3300 brand and generic medications. Users of these programs select the formulary or formularies they desire to include in their searches. Epocrates, Inc. updates formulary information at least once per week.[3] Epocrates accounts may be established on the Internet, but for those practitioners who work without Internet access, these programs are downloadable to handheld electronic information devices. This program may prove the most practical solution for providers who require timely formulary information and who operate without full Internet access. It is strongly recommended, however, in light of increasing amounts of current drug information available exclusively online, that all providers of drug information and direct patient care insist upon Internet access in order to perform their responsibilities.

Clinicians with prescribing privileges should also note that electronic prescribing (e-prescribing) platforms provide drug and formulary information at the point of care. In a recent study conducted by the Agency for Healthcare Research and Quality (AHRQ) and published in the Archives of Internal Medicine, prescribers utilizing e-prescribing platforms with formulary decision supports (FDS) were significantly more likely to prescribe tier-one medications, with resulting significant potential cost savings.[4] Also, as outlined later in this chapter, Lexicomp online drug information (http://lexi.com) contains useful formulary information.

❸ *It is important to note, however, that knowledge of the formulary status of medications is only one part of the prescription decision-making process. Whenever they exist, evidence-based clinical practice guidelines should guide prescriptive decision making.*

CURRENT PRACTICE GUIDELINE INFORMATION

It is beyond the scope of this chapter to discuss in depth the development and the interpretation of evidence-based clinical practice guideline recommendations (see Chapter 7). ❹ *It is important to note, however, that ambulatory practitioners have the responsibility to remain up-to-date regarding current practice guidelines.* No individual can be expected to know the current treatment guidelines for every condition; however, clinicians can and should be expected to be able to retrieve this information quickly and efficiently. The following outlines several sources for such retrieval.

Clinicians searching for current practice guidelines may wish to visit the National Guideline Clearinghouse (NGC) (http://www.guidelines.gov). This compilation of evidence-based clinical practice guidelines is a project of the American Health Insurance Plan (AHIP) and the Agency for Healthcare Research and Quality (AHRQ). The NGC includes links to full-text current treatment guidelines and guidelines in process, as well as archived guidelines. Side-by-side comparison of two or more treatment guidelines for a given condition is also available. Users may search this site by disease/condition, by treatment/intervention, or by organization.[5] If Internet access is not readily available, users can often download, at no cost, guidelines to their personal handheld devices for quick reference. Clinicians in this situation may wish to consider downloading treatment guidelines that they commonly refer to in their particular practice, checking regularly for updates. For example, a general practitioner may wish to download the current American Diabetes Association (ADA) guidelines, the current National Cholesterol Education Program (NCEP) Adult Treatment Panel for the treatment of hypercholesterolemia, and the current Joint National Committee (JNC) guidelines for the treatment of hypertension. Clinicians who may work primarily with a specialized population may wish to tailor downloads to those pertinent to their area of practice.

The Iowa Drug Information Service (IDIS) database also provides an efficient method for locating treatment guidelines.[6] Users may narrow the type of journal article retrieved through the database by utilizing the descriptor *practice guidelines*, and then typing the disease state they are researching in the appropriate text box. Users have online full-text access to articles published after 1988. This database requires a subscription, however, and is not freely available to the public.

Many additional search engines and Internet sites contain links to current practice guidelines. Those that may be particularly useful to the ambulatory care practitioner because they are available without a subscription and, with the exclusion of PubMed, provide links to full-text guidelines include Heath Services Technology Assessment Texts (HSTAT) http://www.ncbi.nlm.nih.gov/books/bv.fcgi?rid=hstat, the Ontario GAC http://www.gacguidelines.ca, the Turning Research Into Practice (TRIP) Database http://www.tripdatabase.com/, the Combined Health Information Database http://chid.nih.gov, and the Agency for Healthcare Research and Quality (AHRQ) site http://www.ahrq.gov.

The American Society of Health-Systems Pharmacists (ASHP) also provides links to what it has deemed Best Practice policies and treatment guidelines (http://www.ashp.org/bestpractices). The American Pharmacists Association (APhA), although it does not endorse guidelines as ASHP does, also provides links from its Web site to select practice guidelines (http://www.pharmacist.com).

This list is not all-inclusive. For example, MEDLINE and the Cochrane Database of Systematic Reviews indexing systems are excellent resources for retrieving clinical practice guidelines; however, they require subscriptions and familiarity with the search techniques in order to yield optimal results. The reader should refer to Chapters 3, and 7 for a more detailed description of each of these, as well as other databases that may be utilized when searching for clinical practice guidelines. Of note, the most effective search term may be *practice guideline* in the publication type field of various search pages. An additional useful search term may be *treatment guideline* or just *guideline*.

DESIRED CHARACTERISTICS OF DRUG INFORMATION RESOURCES IN THE AMBULATORY SETTING

Please refer to the scenario described at the beginning of this chapter.

> Before leaving the pharmacy, SG asks Ron if he has information in addition to the leaflet stapled to the prescription bag about his medication, and what to expect with GERD. SG further requests that, if possible, he'd like to get information in Spanish, as it is easier for him to read health-related information in his first language.

What resource database(s) could Ron refer to with patient information written at an appropriate level? Are there databases that are useful for traditional drug information geared toward the health care professional and that also have information geared toward patient education? Do any of these databases provide patient information in multiple languages?

⑤ *Increasingly more medical literature, including tertiary references, is being provided in the electronic or Internet-based format, and such databases are attractive to utilize in ambulatory care for multiple reasons.*

- Electronic databases are easily accessible, which is of utmost importance, as ambulatory care may take place in clinics or pharmacies that are part of the same health system but located in multiple locations.
- Electronic databases tend to be updated more easily and frequently, with new drug updates and pertinent changes in patient and disease care, unlike print copies of patient drug information material that may be several years out of date.
- Electronic drug information databases are more quickly and easily searched for specific topics pertinent to a given patient, utilizing hyperlinks or search functions. Recall that, as reviewed in Chapter 3, regardless of the format (electronic versus print), patient education materials should contain language that is directed either toward the patient, parent, or caregiver, and be written at an appropriate reading level. It is recommended that databases specify the reading level of patient education material.

Examples of particularly useful databases are provided in the following.

A REVIEW OF SELECTED DRUG INFORMATION RESOURCES FOR THE AMBULATORY CLINICIAN

Many of the following tertiary resources are also mentioned in Chapter 3; however, rather than focusing solely on the appropriate resource for a specific drug information request, the following is a brief overview of selected resources that (a) are available electronically, (b) are primarily geared toward the health care professional and are useful to the ambulatory care practitioner, (c) may already be utilized in the clinical setting, (d) also provide in-depth drug and alternative product monographs, and (e) provide useful patient-oriented material.

Clinical Pharmacology

Gold Standard (http://www.clinicalpharmacology.com). This database includes Med-Counselor consumer drug information sheets that are available in both English and Spanish, and includes the date of last revision of any given patient education sheet. MedCounselor Sheets are available via hyperlinks from drug monographs or by searching by drug product under a patient education tab within the site. This product includes patient education materials written at a sixth- to eighth-grade reading level regarding prescription, nonprescription, and some herbal medications.

• Drug Facts And Comparisons

WolterKluwer Health, Inc. (http://www.factsandcomparisons.com). The electronic version of this database, http://online.factsandcomparisons.com, utilizes MedFacts Patient Information, which provides customizable patient information in both English and Spanish for over 4000 brand and generic drugs, and includes some herbal medication patient education materials. The reading level is eighth grade or below, with the date of last issue clearly provided on each education sheet.

• Lexicomp Online

Available as an online subscription through Lexicomp, Inc. (http://www.lexi.com), Lexicomp ONLINE incorporates an Internet-based platform to provide not only the electronic version of information found in Lexicomp's Drug Information Handbook, but, depending on the subscription purchased, may also include information from AHFS Drug Information reference and prescription drug plans including information regarding pricing, formulary status, and prior authorization status. Of particular interest to the ambulatory clinician, this resource includes links within drug monographs to Patient Advisory Leaflets (PALS).

PALS delivers patient-specific education regarding a particular medication or a disease, condition, or procedure in up to 18 different languages. PALS are also available for select natural products. Patient information is written at a fifth- to sixth-grade reading level, and may be personalized and printed for distribution to the patient.[7] The practitioner specifies whether a patient advisory leaflet is for an adult or pediatric patient, with pediatric information written toward the parent or caregiver.

• MICROMEDEX Healthcare Series' Detailed Drug Information for the Consumer

Available through Thomson Reuters Healthcare (www.micromedex.com), the MICROMEDEX Healthcare Series includes the educational resource Detailed Drug Information for the Consumer. This database is intended for use by not only retail and hospital pharmacists, physicians, and nurses, but also patient education program coordinators. It provides patient-oriented drug information in lay language, but is written at a 12th-grade reading level, and documents are geared toward patients who desire more in-depth material than what is provided in typical drug information leaflets.[8]

• Carenotes System

Available through Thomson Reuters Healthcare (http://www.micromedex.com), the CareNotes System enables the clinician to provide customizable patient education documents which are written at a sixth- to eighth-grade reading level in 15 languages. These documents may address general health condition information, preprocedure or presurgical information, and information regarding inpatient and discharge care for patients, laboratory test information, and a section titled DrugNotes, which includes patient-directed drug information for both prescription and nonprescription medications.[9]

Natural Medicines Comprehensive Database, Pharmacist's Letter, and Prescriber's Letter

All published by Therapeutic Research Center, subscriptions to each of these publications are available electronically, may be downloaded to electronic handheld devices, and may be of great value, especially in the ambulatory care setting.

- The Natural Medicines Comprehensive Database (NMCD) (http://naturaldatabase. therapeuticresearch.com, log-in required) provides evidence-based information regarding complementary, alternative, and integrative medicine and natural medicines. The database provides full monographs with evidence-based ratings, safety ratings, and interaction ratings based on currently available literature. NMCD includes a useful natural product/drug interaction checker and patient handouts written in both English and Spanish.[10]

- Pharmacist's Letter (http://pharmacistsletter.com) and Prescriber's Letter (http:// prescribersletter.com) contain similar information, with the main difference being the target audience. These publications cover new developments in drug therapy and trends in pharmacy practice, concise updates, and advice regarding current therapeutic issues with links to a detailed document with a more in-depth explanation of the topic. These publications also include useful disease-, medication-, and practice-related charts.

DRUG INFORMATION WEB SITES

Particularly useful Web sites include (1) Food and Drug Administration (http://www.fda. gov), as it provides recent drug-related news; drug approvals; recalls and safety warnings; therapeutic equivalency codes; approved Risk, Evaluation, and Mitigation Strategies (REMS); and MedWatch adverse event reporting data; (2) Centers for Disease Control and Prevention (CDC) (http://www.cdc.gov), as it provides useful information regarding infectious disease treatment and prevention, immunization updates, treatment guidelines for infectious disease, and even travelers' health information, some of which may be available in more than one language; and (3) Medscape from WebMD (http://www.medscape. com), which provides free access to continuing education, select health-related journals, evidence-based information, and pertinent review articles.

ACCESS CONSIDERATIONS

For the reasons outlined previously, the electronic version of each of these databases and publications is the preferred format. Whenever possible, databases that are available for downloading to an electronic handheld device are included; however, even these will require intermittent Internet access for synchronizing and updating information. The responsible provision of up-to-date drug information requires Internet access. Health care providers and employers should ensure that this is available to those providing medical information to others.

Practitioners may also note that by partnering with colleges of pharmacy or medicine to provide experiential education to students, they may expand their access to drug information databases to which the college subscribes, depending on subscription limitations.

• Drug information centers, also referred to as medication information centers, may be a viable source of information, particularly when in-depth research of a topic is not feasible due to a lack of access to appropriate databases, individuals trained in drug information, or time.

Patient Disposal of Unused Medications

Consider the following scenario:

> Ronda, who is working the weekend shift at a community pharmacy, is approached by an elderly man carrying a grocery bag that appears to be full of prescription bottles. "Can you take these, and perhaps give them to someone who could use them? My wife passed away last month, and I probably have hundreds of dollars worth of medication in this bag! If you can't use them, can you tell me where I should take them?"

Although practitioners may be readily able to explain in such a situation that they cannot legally accept medications, they may not be able to answer the following questions. Where can unused, unwanted, or expired medications be taken? If a patient wishes to dispose of medications, are there any legal requirements or guidelines as to how best do so?

More often than in any other setting, ambulatory care practitioners are asked about patient disposal of unused or unwanted medications. Although there no specific laws regarding personal disposal of medications by patients, the disposal of unused or unwanted pharmaceuticals (both prescription and nonprescription) is becoming an emerging and complex environmental issue and is being considered by the government. In a 2006 survey published in the *Journal of the American Board of Family Medicine*, of the 301 patients surveyed at an outpatient pharmacy, 50% reported storing unused or expired medication and another 50% report that they have flushed such medications. Less than 20% of respondents reported having been counseled by a health care provider about the appropriate means of medication disposal.[11] ❻ *Ambulatory care clinicians bear a responsibility to educate patients on this topic and should therefore be aware of pertinent sites for information.* The Pharmaceutical Research and Manufacturers of America (PhRMA), APhA, and the U.S. Fish and Wildlife Service (FWS) have joined forces to begin to educate the public on the importance of appropriate medication disposal via the SMARxT DISPOSAL campaign (http://www.smarxtdisposal.net/). The key message to consumers: do not flush.[12]

The U.S. Food and Drug Administration (http://www.fda.gov) provides consumer health information regarding the disposal of unused medicines, and has worked with the White House Office of National Drug Control Policy (ONDCP) to develop the first consumer guidance regarding this topic. Documents these organizations have developed are available online at the FDA and the ONDCP Web sites.[13,14]

Additional useful online resources with information on the safe disposal of medications include those of the Pharmacist's Letter (http://www.pharmacistsletter.com) and the Institute for Safe Medical Practice (ISMP: http://www.ismp.org).

The Community Medical Foundation for Patient Safety (http://www.community ofcompetence.com) has developed a very useful document, the National Directory of Drug Take-Back and Disposal Programs, which details the rationale, federal laws, state laws, published resources, useful Web sites, and practice guidelines for handling unused and expired medications.[15]

The reader may wish to refer to Appendix 19–1, FDA Guidelines for Proper Medication Disposal, for more information on this topic.

DRUG REPOSITORY PROGRAMS

Drug repository programs (which allow nursing homes, long-term care pharmacies, and wholesalers to donate unused medication for redistribution to those patients who meet prespecified criteria) may exist in certain states. Although patients understandably may be reluctant to throw away their personal unused or unwanted medications, these medications, once dispensed and in patients' homes, are not eligible for donation to drug repository programs, as these drugs have left the custody and controlled environment of a pharmacy or institution. Practitioners should refer to their respective state's Board of Pharmacy Web site for information regarding drug repository programs.

Providing Immunization Information

Formerly provided primarily in the traditional clinician's office or in a county health department, immunizations are increasingly being delivered by pharmacists in ambulatory care settings, including pharmacies and retail groceries. ❼ *As immunizations are considered medications, those practitioners immunizing in the outpatient, ambulatory community have the obligation to not only provide these services safely, but to serve as sources of information (i.e., drug information) regarding the mediations they are administering.*

● SOURCES OF IMMUNIZATION INFORMATION

Centers for Disease Control and Prevention

Although multiple texts exist regarding immunization and vaccine-preventable disease, the Department of Health and Human Services Centers for Disease Control and Prevention (CDC) Web site (http://www.cdc.gov) provides the most comprehensive, regularly updated information regarding immunizations. Links are available from the CDC Web page titled Vaccines and Immunizations (http://www.cdc.gov/vaccines) that provide up-to-date information regarding vaccine-preventable disease, as well as safety, adverse events, administration schedule, and dosing recommendations for immunizations for both the health care provider and for patients. Also available from this site are Vaccine Information Statements (VISs) that must be distributed with their respective immunizations.

Epidemiology and Prevention of Vaccine-Preventable Disease

This textbook, commonly referred to as the Pink Book, is published annually by the National Immunization Program (NIP), Centers for Disease Control and Prevention.[16] It provides physicians, nurses, nurse practitioners, physician assistants, and pharmacists comprehensive information regarding the vaccine-preventable diseases themselves. The textbook is available for purchase in print; however, PDFs of each chapter are available fully formatted for download from the CDC Web site. Although this text does not provide vaccine-specific information, it provides detailed information regarding respective vaccine-preventable diseases, including epidemiology, prevalence, and prevention recommendations.

Immunization Training for the Pharmacist

The prerequisites for pharmacist clinicians to administer immunizations in the community vary from state to state, and pharmacists are advised to refer to their state's laws and confer with their state board of pharmacy regarding specific questions; however, in each state that allows pharmacist immunization, a training program approved by the state pharmacy board is required. The most recognized training program, Pharmacy-Based Immunization Delivery, is offered nationally by the American Pharmacists Association (http://www.pharmacist.com). Other programs exist that may be recognized nationally or within specific states only. The University of Findlay College of Pharmacy, for example, provides a pharmacist immunization-training program that is recognized and approved by all 50 states, while the Ohio Pharmacists Association provides a training program for Ohio pharmacists only. Pharmacists may wish to inquire with their specific state board of pharmacy regarding recognized and approved training programs. Regardless of the training program utilized, it is expected that pharmacists maintain and document appropriate continuing education for the immunizations and the associated drug information they deliver.

Quality-Assurance Considerations in Ambulatory Care

Sam, a recent graduate from pharmacy school, is working in a private practice ambulatory care clinic where; in addition to dispensing responsibilities, he provides medication recommendations to prescribers and counsels patients regarding disease state management. The manager of the clinic approaches Sam and asks him to become involved in measuring quality-assurance indicators for all health care providers in the clinic, including patient satisfaction with the care they have received.

What type of quality-assurance indicators are measured by outside organizations? Is patient satisfaction with care a recognized quality indicator? Are there published guidelines for quality indicators in ambulatory care?

This chapter has thus far covered a variety of drug information topics pertinent to ambulatory care practice, and the case has been made that efficiently accessing and interpreting a variety of types of information is necessary for functional competence in ambulatory care. A final drug information consideration for safe and competent function in the ambulatory setting is quality assurance.

• While departments that are under the umbrella of a health care facility generally consider the standards set forth by The Joint Commission (Chapter 14), as a primary source of quality-assurance guidelines, several other organizations provide quality-assurance guidelines that may be applied to a variety of care settings, and will be discussed in the following paragraphs.

• The Roadmap for Quality Measurement in the Traditional Medicare Fee-for-Service Program, published by the Centers for Medicare and Medicaid Services (CMS), outlines current and proposed initiatives through the Department of Health and Human Services to improve quality assurance in the provision of health care.[17] Via a variety of initiatives, including the Quality Improvement Organization (QIO), CMS has more than 375 established quality measures, which are generally categorized based on practice settings. The settings, with the number of current designated quality measures indicated in parentheses, are hospital inpatient (60), physicians and other designated eligible professionals (153), nursing home (19), home health (12), dialysis or end-stage renal disease (22), the Part D Prescription Drug Benefit administered by private health plans (Part D) (23), and Medicare Advantage (MA) (59).

CMS acknowledges that several of these are not true settings and do not denote a actual physical location in which care is rendered, but are nevertheless used for categorization purposes. Accordingly, the reader should note that although ambulatory care is not designated as a setting, several designated settings are certainly inclusive of ambulatory care.

The quality measures themselves are standards set forth that evaluate efficiency (or resource use), structure, process, intermediate outcome, long-term outcome, and patient centeredness. As noted previously, 153 of the quality measures address physician and other professional behavior where the vast majority of services are provided in the outpatient environment. ❽ *Health care professionals involved in the provision of care in the ambulatory care setting should familiarize themselves with the pertinent established quality measures.* Links to several setting-specific quality initiatives may be found at http://www.cms.hhs.gov/center/quality.asp.

Although CMS provides clinical health care quality standards for designated settings, quality may also be described in light of patients' actual experiences. Launched by AHRQ in the mid-1990s, the Consumer Assessment of Healthcare Providers and Systems (CAHPS) program provides quality information derived from standardized surveys of patient experiences with both ambulatory and facility-level care. The surveys focus on areas of patient care that are important to the consumer, such as accessibility of services and communication skills of the provider(s). Both consumers and health care organizations may use the data to benchmark, report, and compare performance, and to assess and improve quality of care. Further information regarding the CAHPS program may be found at https://www.cahps.ahrq.gov/.[18]

The Patient Safety and Clinical Pharmacy Services (PSPC) Collaborative is one of the newest nationwide initiatives to improve quality of care. Launched in 2008, PSPC is sponsored by the U.S. Health Resources and Service Administration (HRSA). The initiative focuses on cutting medication-related patient errors and improving the quality of health care in America by incorporating clinical pharmacy services into the provision of primary care. Each of the participating organizations in this initiative is focused on incorporating evidence-based clinical pharmacy services into the care of patients with chronic diseases. More information about the PSPC may be found at http://www.hrsa.gov/patientsafety.[19]

Ensuring patient safety is a crucial component of quality care, and the Institute for Safe Medical Practice (ISMP) is an important resource for health care providers in any setting. The ISMP publishes four distinct newsletters, each geared toward practitioners in a different health care setting. The ISMP Medication Safety Alert! Community/ Ambulatory Care edition is targeted toward pharmacists, pharmacy technicians, nurses, physicians, and other community health professionals. This newsletter is sent monthly as an e-mail and provides up-to-date information about medication-related errors, adverse drug reactions, and their implications for community practice sites. The newsletter includes recommendations on how to improve medication safety within the community setting (http://www.ismp.org/Newsletters/default.asp). A subscription to this newsletter is recommended for all ambulatory care providers.

The tracking, reporting, and prevention of not only medication errors, but also of near misses, is paramount to assuring quality in any health care setting, including ambulatory care. ISMP is one organization dedicated to this task. The reader should refer to Chapter 16 for a complete discussion on organizations and programs devoted to assuring quality by the reporting and prevention of medication errors.

The American Pharmacists Association (APhA) Web site (http://www.pharmacist. com) has a Patient Safety and Quality Assurance page that provides links to AHRQ, ISMP, the National Patient Safety Foundation (NPSF), the United States Pharmacopeia (USP) Medication Errors Reporting Form, and the PSPC Collaborative.

Conclusion

As health professionals committed to optimal patient care, the provision of drug information goes far beyond providing patient information leaflets with medications. The application of drug information is performed routinely in the ambulatory care setting in a variety of ways, and it is in this setting that the clinician pulls it all together and takes the most important step—imparting this information not only to patients but to other health care providers in a understandable, personalized, and practical format that will serve to improve health care.

Self-Assessment Questions

1. All of the following statements support the need for the skilled provision of drug information in ambulatory care *except*:
    a. There is not a consistent level of education in the curricula of various health care fields.
    b. There is a lack of high-quality drug information freely available to the public.

c. The ambulatory care clinician is able to access databases that may not be available to the public.

d. A significant number of emergency room visits and hospital admissions each year are attributed to pharmaceuticals.

2. Which of the following statements is true regarding prescription formularies?
   a. Prescription insurance providers often require cardholder identification information in order to gain full access to formulary information.
   b. Clinician use of electronic prescribing has not been shown to affect the likelihood of prescribing tier-1 medications.
   c. Software programs such as Lexicomp and Epocrates include formulary information that can be downloaded to a handheld electronic device.
   d. Medicare Part D participants cannot perform side-by-side comparisons of prescription plans that are available to them and that cover some or all of their medications.

3. Evidence-based clinical practice guidelines:
   a. Are used solely by practitioners who develop formularies
   b. Are accessible without a fee only to practitioners who are members of the organization that developed a given set of guidelines
   c. Are typically too large to download to most handheld devices
   d. Are freely available in full text from a variety of government and public Internet sites

4. All of the following support the desirability of electronic drug information resources in the ambulatory setting *except*:
   a. Ambulatory care may be provided in multiple sites by the same organization.
   b. Internet access is available to all clinicians.
   c. Updates to information are more readily performed.
   d. Electronic databases are conducive to faster and more efficient searches.

5. Which of the following databases provides patient information in languages other than English?
   a. Clinical Pharmacology
   b. Drug Facts and Comparisons
   c. Lexicomp Online
   d. All of the above

6. The Pharmacist's Letter Web site provides all of the following *except*:
   a. Comparison tables for drug classes
   b. Links to medication error reporting databases

    c. Developments in drug therapy

    d. Downloadable documents for handheld devices

7. Which of the following are potential options to increase access to drug information when resources are limited?

    a. Encourage employers to ensure that Internet access is available to all those providing medical information to others.

    b. Consider partnering resources with a local college of medicine or pharmacy.

    c. Utilize the services of a drug information center.

    d. All of the above.

8. All of the following are recommended by the Food and Drug Administration (FDA) as inappropriate in the disposal of unwanted medications except:

    a. Flushing unused liquid medications

    b. Mixing medications with cat litter

    c. Burning with other trash

    d. Using a community dumpster

9. Which of the following organizations have partnered to develop the SMARxT DISPOSAL campaign?

    a. American Pharmacists Association

    b. Pharmaceutical Research and Manufacturers of America (PhRMA)

    c. US Fish and Wildlife Service (FWS)

    d. a and c

    e. a, b, and c

10. Which of the following statements is *false*? Immunizations:

    a. Are not considered medications

    b. May be administered by pharmacists

    c. Must be accompanied by a VIS upon administration

    d. Are becoming increasing available in a variety of community settings including grocery stores and pharmacies

11. Which of the following organizations utilizes reports that include quality indicators as rated by consumers of health care?

    a. The Joint Commission

    b. Centers for Medicare and Medicaid Services (CMS)

    c. Consumer Assessment of Healthcare Providers and Systems (CAHPS)

    d. SMARxT DISPOSAL

12. The PSPC collaborative focuses on:
    a. The safe disposal of unwanted and expired medications
    b. Providing the community with up-to-date immunization information
    c. Cutting medication-related patient errors by incorporating clinical pharmacy services into primary care provision
    d. Creating patient education documents that are written at an appropriate reading level for the target audience

13. Which of the following is *not* a designated setting in which CMS has prescribed quality indicators?
    a. Nursing homes
    b. Pharmacies
    c. Dialysis or end-stage renal disease
    d. Home health

14. Which of the following publishes a monthly newsletter regarding medication safety targeted at pharmacists, pharmacy technicians, and other community health care professionals?
    a. American Pharmacists Association (APhA)
    b. American Health-Systems Pharmacists (ASHP)
    c. Centers for Disease Control and Prevention (CDC)
    d. Institute for Safe Medical Practice (ISMP)

15. Which of the following organizations has a publication that details the rationale, federal laws, state laws, published resources, useful Web sites, and practice guidelines for handling unused and expired medications?
    a. The Community Medical Foundation for Patient Safety
    b. Agency for Healthcare Research and Quality (AHRQ)
    c. American Pharmacists Association (APhA)
    d. Food and Drug Administration (FDA)

REFERENCES

1. Ernst FR, Grizzle AJ. Drug-related morbidity and mortality: updating the cost of illness model. J Am Pharm Assoc. 2001;41:192-9.
2. Zed PJ, Abu-Laban RB, Balen RM, Loewen PS, Hohl CM, Brubacher JR, et al. Incidence, severity and preventability of medication-related visits to the emergency department a prospective study. Can Med Assoc J. 2008;178(12):1563-9.
3. Epocrates. San Mateo, CA: Epocrates, Inc. 2009 [cited 2010 Feb 18]. Available from: http://www.epocrates.com./products/comparison_table.html.
4. Fischer MA, Vogeli C, Stedman M, Ferris T, Brookhart A, Weissman JS. Effect of electronic prescribing with formulary decision support on medication use and cost. Arch Intern Med. 2008;168(22):2433-9.

5. National Guideline Clearinghouse (NGC) [homepage on the Internet]. Rockville (MD) [updated 2009 Sept 7; cited 2010 Feb 18]. Available from: http://www.guidelines.gov.

6. Iowa Drug Information Service [database on the Internet]. Iowa City (IA) [cited 2010 Feb 18]. Available from: http://www.uiowa.edu/~idis/.

7. Lexicomp Online User Guide. Lexicomp, Inc. Hudson (OH) [cited 2010 Feb 18]. Available from: http://online.lexi.com/crlsql/servlet/crlonline.

8. Detailed Drug Information for the Consumer. Thomson Reuters. New York (NY) [2010 Feb 18]. Available from: http://www.micromedex.com/products/ddic/.

9. The CareNotes System. Thomson Reuters. New York (NY) [cited 2010 Feb 18]. Available from: http://www.micromedex.com/products/carenotes/cn_brochure.pdf.

10. Natural Medicines Comprehensive Database. Therapeutic Research. Stockton (CA) [2010 Feb 18]. Available from: http://naturaldatabase.com.

11. Seehusen D, Edwards J. Patient practices and beliefs concerning disposal of medications. J Am Board Fam Med. 2006;19(6):542-7.

12. SMARxT disposal. A prescription for a healthy planet [cited 2010 Feb 18]. Available from: http://www.smarxtdisposal.net.

13. FDA Consumer Health Information. How to dispose of unused medication [cited 2010 Feb 18]. Available from:. http://www.fda.gov/ForConsumers/ConsumerUpdates/ucm101653.htm.

14. Office of National Drug Control Policy. Proper disposal of prescription drugs [cited 2009 Sept 10]. Available from: http://whitehousedrugpolicy.gov/publications/pdf/prescrip_disposal.pdf.

15. Mireles, MC, Miller JA, Smith EA. Directory of drug take-back and disposal programs. Bellaire (TX): Community Medical Foundation for Patient Safety; 2008.

16. Atkinson W, Hamborsky J, McIntyre L, editors. Centers for Disease Control and Prevention. Epidemiology and Prevention of Vaccine-Preventable Diseases. The Pink Book: Course Textbook. 11th ed. Washington, DC: Public Health Foundation; 2009.

17. United States Department of Health and Human Services [cited 2010 Feb 18]. Available from: http://www.cms.hhs.gov/QualityInitiativesGenInfo/downloads/QualityMeasurement Roadmap_OEA1-16_508.pdf.

18. Program brief CAHPS: assessing health care quality from the patient's perspective. AHRQ Pub. No. 08-PB015. Washington, DC. October 2008. [updated 2009 Aug 3; cited 2010 Feb 18]. Available from: https://www.cahps.ahrq.gov/content/cahpsOverview/07-P016.pdf.

19. United States Health Resources and Service Administration. Patient safety and clinical practice services collaborative (PSPC) [updated 2009 July; cited 2010 Feb 18]. Available from: http://www.hrsa.gov/patientsafety/pspc_overview_july2009.pdf.

USEFUL ORGANIZATIONAL HOMEPAGES

Agency for Healthcare Research and Quality: http://www.ahrq.gov
American Health-Systems Pharmacists Best Practices: http://www.ashp.org/bestpractices
American Pharmacists Association (APhA): http://www.pharmacist.com
Centers for Disease Control and Prevention: http://www.cdc.gov
Epocrates: http://www.epocrates.com

Medscape Pharmacists: http://medscape.pharmacists
National Guideline Clearinghouse: http://www.guidelines.gov/
National Heart Lung and Blood Institute: http://www.ncbi.nlm.nih.gov/
SMARxT Disposal Campaign: http://www.smarxtdisposal.net
U.S. Food and Drug Administration: http://www.fda.gov

SUGGESTED READINGS

Atkinson W, Hamborsky J, McIntyre L, editors. Centers for Disease Control and Prevention. Epidemiology and Prevention of Vaccine-Preventable Diseases. The Pink Book: Course Textbook. 11th ed. Washington, DC: Public Health Foundation; 2009.

Mireles MC, Miller JA, Smith EA. Directory of Drug Take-Back and Disposal Programs. Community Medical Foundation for Patient Safety. Bellaire (TX); 2008. Available from: http://www. communityofcompetence.com/.

Chapter Twenty

Drug Information and Contemporary Community Pharmacy Practice

Morgan L. Sperry • Patricia A. Marken

Learning Objectives

● *After completing this chapter, the reader will be able to*

- Discuss limitations of the current approaches pharmacists use to deliver drug information to their patients.
- Compare and contrast patient education and consumer health information (CHI) as drug information sources for patients.
- Define Web 2.0 and social networking and describe how patients use these tools as drug information sources.
- Describe a new model for drug information services delivered by community pharmacists.
- Design three strategies using electronic media to assist patients in receiving and applying high-quality drug information.
- List seven characteristics of a high-quality, health-literate Internet site.
- Define information therapy in the context of pharmacist-delivered drug information services.

Key Concepts

❶ The trend for patients to obtain their health information from sources disconnected from health care professionals is not going away, and it has shifted relationships between patients and their traditional touchstones in health care, physicians, nurses, and pharmacists.

❷ Answering drug information questions is a routine part of a pharmacist's day, but it is too often a passive process that hinges on patients' initiative to ask the important questions regarding their health.

❸ Patient education is a planned activity customized to individual patient needs.

❹ Consumer health information (CHI) is material that is actively sought by the patient and is not tailored to that patient's specific situation.

❺ Social media sites allow patients to create content and share information about their health on the World Wide Web.

❻ Some patients trust the collective wisdom of a group more than the advice of an individual, even if that individual is an expert.

❼ Patients often have difficulty finding appropriate information in response to their specific health concerns on the World Wide Web.

❽ Pharmacists should discuss with their patients why they remain an important source of drug information. Patients should be encouraged not to see CHI as a replacement for actual interaction with a health care provider, but as an extension of care and a way to improve communication.

❾ Health literacy is the capability of patients to read or hear health information, understand it, and then act on it. Once patients acquire quality health information, they may face health literacy barriers when applying that information.

❿ Information therapy elevates the term drug information from a passive-sounding process to an active component of treatment plans by recognizing that accurate and complete drug information proactively relayed to patients is much more effective than just assuming it will be sought out. Information therapy encompasses both the patient and the health care professional, asking both to work together in making the best possible health care decision for the patient.

Introduction

Pharmacist's roles and responsibilities continue to evolve in response to changing practice acts and a dynamic health care environment. One constant is the pharmacist's key function as a provider of quality, evidence-based drug information. However, pharmacists are not the only source of drug information. The Internet has made information from sources other than health professionals more readily available and Web sites devoted to health information are accessible to anyone on the Web. The move toward patient-centered care and consumerism increases the desire for patients to be in control of their health care and be an active part of the decision-making process. ❶ *The trend for patients to obtain their health information from sources disconnected from health care professionals is not going away, and it has shifted relationships between patients and their traditional touchstones in health care, physicians, nurses, and pharmacists.*[1] Recent surveys suggest that 60% to 80% of American consumers use the Internet to search for some type of health or wellness information.[1] The pharmacist's role as drug information expert may also be changing in the eyes of the patient. In January 2008, pharmacists ranked sixth behind the Internet, television, newspapers/magazines, relatives/friends/coworkers, and doctors in terms of sources used to locate or access health information.[1]

Pharmacy practice is moving away from the hands-on drug distribution model toward an emphasis on system management and patient care services.[2,3] It is important for pharmacists to enhance patient care services because of significant expenditures seen with unresolved drug-related problems. For example, the National Council on Patient Information and Education estimated nonadherence to medication therapy to cost $177 billion annually in direct and indirect costs in 2007.[4] A key strategy to improve adherence is to improve patients' understanding of their disease and its management, and include their needs in the treatment planning. Both strategies require individualized care that is not available from the World Wide Web and other information sources. Project Destiny, an initiative between the National Association of Chain Drug Stores(NACDS), the American Pharmacists Association (APhA), and the National Community Pharmacists Association (NCPA) to "embrace community pharmacy health care beyond dispensing," specifically states that there are significant unmet needs for improved medication therapy management.[2] Pharmacists are well positioned to address these needs, as they are the medication experts and trusted professionals. In their model, customers view pharmacists as key medication advisors. For example, patients see results from clinical research on the news or through the Internet. They may not understand how these results relate directly to them and may consider discontinuing their medication. Pharmacists, with their understanding of both the literature and patients' medical histories, can help patients understand whether these new findings are relevant to their individual situation.

Pharmacists can remain a valuable drug information source for patients because they are the most accessible health care practitioners. Pharmacists can help patients customize information they find on the Internet and from other sources. The danger right now for pharmacists is that if they do not step up and add drug information services beyond what patients can find on their own, as well as develop patient demand for these services, they may become less relevant. According to 2008–2009 Chain Pharmacy

Industry Profile, patients select a specific pharmacy based on prescription price, insurance coverage, and convenience. Professional and pharmacy services provided by the pharmacists were cited as a reason for going to a pharmacy only 53% and 56% of the time, respectively, whereas price drove the decision 61% of the time. These results further support the need to develop consumer demand for patient care services.[5] The purpose of this chapter is to demonstrate how patients' increased demand for autonomy and responsibility over their own health care and the use of information sources beyond health professionals impacts community pharmacy. Additionally, new models for community pharmacist-delivered drug information is addressed.

Pharmacists as Drug Information Providers in the Community Setting

Pharmacists are required by the Omnibus Budget Reconciliation Act of 1990 (OBRA 90) to deliver patient education when they dispense a Medicaid prescription.[6] Individual states can and sometimes do mandate that counseling be extended to all patients, irrespective of their insurance. Some pharmacists are very diligent in providing important information to their patients when they pick up a prescription, while others only give information if specifically asked. Patients may be asked by the pharmacy staff to decline counseling by signing a waiver, without being asked whether they want it or not. Some patients do not even know what they are signing. ❷ *Answering drug information questions is a routine part of a pharmacist's day, but it is too often a passive process that hinges on patients' initiative to ask the important questions regarding their health.* A variety of reasons make patients reluctant to use their pharmacist as a primary health information resource. Pharmacists appear too busy and unavailable. Technicians may be the only staff members who speak directly to the patient. Simply asking whether or not a patient has questions is the wrong way to initiate counseling. Patients may not be sure what they need to know in the first place, or feel embarrassed or ashamed to admit their lack of knowledge. In some cases, patients are unaware that they should even have questions. Some simply do not understand the importance of pharmacotherapy to their long-term health and well-being, and are not vested in learning about appropriate medication use.

Patient leaflets are one example why patients may not seek out their pharmacist as a primary health information resource. Instead of direct patient communication, patient leaflets are commonly stapled to the prescription as a substitute for actual patient education. In fact, a 2002 survey of community pharmacies found that while 89% of patients received leaflets from their pharmacy, only 5% were given a verbal explanation along with it, and only 8% of the time did the pharmacist emphasize the important content found within the leaflet.[7] Sixty-six percent of patients were given the document without any further information at all, making it hard for them to establish key points to be taken away from the leaflet. Additionally, many of these leaflets do not adhere to the qualities of good health literacy, making it hard for patients to use as a source of health information. Additional information on the importance of good health literacy is discussed later in the text.

Some pharmacies have developed Web sites to direct patients to quality drug information and offer an additional path for patients to ask questions. Many large chain pharmacies and mail-order pharmacies have begun to post answers to the most frequently asked drug information questions for their consumers on their Web sites. At least one chain allows for even more interaction online by giving patients the opportunity to ask their own questions to a pharmacist. In addition, these Web sites also provide general information regarding medications in the form of patient leaflets. It is important to note that while these pharmacies are headed in the right direction in terms of giving patients more readily available access to quality health information online, these Web sites still have many limitations. In contrast to just providing a Web site for patient information, many disease-state management and medication-therapy management programs require the pharmacist to be engaged in intense and directed patient education as part of a comprehensive treatment plan—something that cannot be done by passive answering of questions or interfacing with a Web site alone.

Current Patient Sources of Drug Information

The practice of providing drug information continues to evolve along with the profession. Drug information can be as simple as obtaining information from references, or it can be an interactive experience between a specific individual and the inquirer.[8] Drug information can be as active as counseling a patient on all of his or her medications and disease states or as passive as a pharmacy technician dispensing a medication leaflet with a prescription. Regardless of how drug information is delivered, patients are in need of a more connected experience when receiving their drug information from health care professionals.

PATIENT EDUCATION VERSUS CONSUMER HEALTH INFORMATION

Patient education and consumer health information are two distinct ways through which patients get information about medications, although the two may merge when pharmacists truly engage their patients. ❸ *Patient education delivers written or verbal drug information through a planned activity initiated by a health care provider. The goal is to change patient behavior, improve adherence, and ultimately improve health.*[9] Pharmacist-driven patient education formats include brief counseling when patients pick up their medication, comprehensive education as a part of medication therapy management, health screenings, and brown bag checkups. A brown bag checkup is when a patient collects all current prescription and nonprescription medications into a brown bag and allows a pharmacist to review them in order to identify any potential problems. Education can be delivered face to face or through other technologies, including the telephone, e-mail, and webcams. The key is that pharmacists interact with individual patients to customize the information to their specific situation.

❹ *Consumer health information (CHI) is material that is actively sought by patients in response to their need for more information about their health. Importantly, CHI is not individualized for a specific patient.* Unlike patient education, which is initiated by the pharmacist, CHI is completely patient driven and has evolved out of the patient's need to be his or her own advocate. CHI has long been available to patients, but the Internet accelerated both access to and the volume of information; the choices are endless for patients seeking their own information. In 2008, the Internet became the number one strategy for patients to locate health and wellness information.[1]

For either patient education or CHI to be of any value to the patient, it is crucial that evidence presented to the patient be of high quality and strength. Controlling quality during a patient education encounter is easier because the health care professional filters information distributed to patients. In contrast, the quality and reliability of consumer health information is variable.[10] CHI may be of excellent quality and beneficial to the patient, or it may be of high quality but dangerous because it lacks relevance to the patient's situation, is incomplete, or simply wrong. Table 20–1 lists examples of popular consumer health information sites.

SOCIAL MEDIA—A NEW FORM OF CONSUMER HEALTH INFORMATION

Patients have long used friends, family, coworkers, and support groups as sources of medical information. The Internet adds to these traditional sources through social media, as described in Table 20–2.[1] ❺ *Web 2.0 is an important concept in understanding the power of social media. Web 2.0 is not new software but a different strategy to use the Web. The Web goes beyond being a search engine and a source of information to include a platform to create, share, and collaborate in developing new knowledge. Social networking is the phenomenon of online communities in which people share interests and/or activities with one another and is an outgrowth of Web 2.0.* With respect to CHI, patients no longer just read about their health information online, but can have an active role controlling content, creating new information, and sharing their experiences with others. For example,

TABLE 20–1. **EXAMPLES OF POPULAR CONSUMER HEALTH INFORMATION AND SOCIAL MEDIA SITES**

Consumer Health Platform	Description
Angie's List (http://www.angieslist.com)	Website tailored to help consumers find high-quality, unbiased reviews and recommendations on a variety of services including contractors, service companies, home repair, and health care providers. Allows patients to seek perspectives and opinions from fellow patients who have previously seen certain health care providers in their area. Angie's List maintains that both patient members and health care providers benefit from feedback given. A fee is required to join Angie's List followed by a 1-year free trial for consumers. At the end of this trial year consumers may choose to pay a monthly or annual fee to maintain their membership.
Consumer Reports (http://www.consumerreportshealth.org)	Requiring a monthly or annual subscription, this online resource provides patients with information and unbiased ratings on topics such as healthy living, conditions and treatments, doctors, insurance companies, natural health, and prescription drugs. Health expert blogs are also provided for subscribers on an array of health topics. The Best Buy Drugs feature of this Web site was created in 2004 to help patients compare brand prescription drugs against generics and provide consumers with the best medicine to treat their disease state for their money.
Google Health (http://www.google.com/health)	Platform established for patients wanting a single place to keep all personal health records and information. Patients are given full control and are allowed to choose what information is accessible to others versus what is kept private. Allows patients to create online health profiles, upload their medical records from hospitals and pharmacies, conduct searches for doctors and hospitals, connect to online health services, and learn more about health issues as well as locate helpful resources.
MicrosoftHealthVault (http://www.healthvault.com)	Offers patients a way to store their personal or family's health information all in one location. Patients are then given the option to make their health information accessible to personal health care providers. HealthVault works with doctors, pharmacies, insurance providers, hospitals, and employers to ensure the ease of adding information electronically to their HealthVault record. The site is also compatible with certain health devices such as blood pressure monitors and heart rate monitors, allowing patients to upload important health data and readings straight to their HealthVault. The goal of this Web site is to provide consumers with a more complete picture of their overall health and give them an opportunity to make the best informed decision.

continued

TABLE 20–1. **EXAMPLES OF POPULAR CONSUMER HEALTH INFORMATION AND SOCIAL MEDIA SITES (*Continued*)**

Consumer Health Platform	Description
PatientsLikeMe.com (http://www.patientslikeme.com)	Privately funded social media site that was founded in 2004 with the intent of positively impacting patients diagnosed with life-changing diseases. This site primarily focuses on neurological, neuroendocrine, psychiatric, and immune conditions and is geared toward developing a new system of healthcare created by patients for patients. Through an online community of doctors, organizations, and patients, patients are encouraged to share information about their disease states, treatments, and overall experiences. The hope is that through this online platform patients will feel more connected to others going through similar circumstances as well as empowered and in more control of their disease state.
Revolution Health (http://www.revolutionhealth.com)	Consumer-centric health company founded to empower and encourage patients to put themselves at the center of their health care. Claims to be a site for comprehensive health and medical information. Free to consumers, the site gears information toward the person they consider the family's chief medical officer (CMO): women or other caregivers. Blogs, forums, and online communities are available so patients can talk to people just like them.
WebMD (http://www.webmd.com)	Health Web site allowing patients to obtain their health information via a variety of different ways. Health information is available on a wealth of different topics such as drugs and treatments, disease states, and prevention. Online communities for patients seeking support or desiring to share their experiences are also set up in the form of blogs, video, and message boards. Additionally, patients have access to slide shows, newsletters, Food and Drug Administration (FDA) consumer updates, symptom checkers, drug identifiers, and an ask-the-expert feature. WebMD has established an Independent Medical Review Board to ensure that all health information made available to the public is accurate and timely. The FDA recently partnered with WebMD to further expand patients' access to reliable and timely health information.

Data from references 11-16.

PatientsLikeMe.com is a privately funded company that was founded in 2004 with the purpose of creating a community of patients with neurological, neuroendocrine, psychiatric, and immune conditions. Site content is posted by actual patients and includes what treatments they have tried, what works and what does not work for them, and what side effects they experience. They often discuss the quality of the care delivered by their providers.

⑥ *Wisdom of crowds is a belief that when patients share information about their common conditions through social networking, their collective wisdom is more beneficial than the*

TABLE 20–2. SOCIAL MEDIA DEFINITIONS AND PLATFORMS USED TO OBTAIN HEALTH INFORMATION

Social Media	Definition	Platform Examples	URLs
Wikis	Allows user editing and adding of content via a collaborative Web site	Wikipedia FluWikie	http://www.wikipedia.org http://www.fluwikie.com
Social networks	A Web site where those with special interests in common can connect and share with one another	Angie's List PatientsLikeMe.com Organized Wisdom Revolution Health Facebook MySpace	http://www.angieslist.com http://www.patientslikeme.com http://www.organizedwisdom.com http://www.revolutionhealth.com http://www.facebook.com http://www.myspace.com
Blogs	An online diary; users can log their personal thoughts on various topics and post to a Web page	WebMD HealthLine Mayo Clinic	http://www.webmd.com http://www.healthmattersblog.com http://www.mayoclinic.com/health/blogs/BlogIndex
Online forums	Thoughts and ideas are shared and open discussion takes place via various mediums such as a Web site, newspaper, or radio	Revolution Health Google Health Groups Yahoo! Groups	http://www.revolutionhealth.com http://groups.google.com http://groups.yahoo.com
Videosharing	A medium where information, ideas, and opinions can be shared via videos accessible to many	YouTube	http://www.youtube.com

Data from reference 17.

expert opinion of just one individual. Patients do not completely resist the advice of health professionals, but are just not as willing to rely on a single expert opinion for their information.[1] Health information received via social media is greatly valued by many consumers, especially the Net generation as described by Don Tapscott in *Grown Up Digital: How the Net Generation Is Changing Your World.*[18] Opinions, stories, successes and failures, treatment options, and adverse effects are just some of what patients share using social media. This feeling of camaraderie and support obtained via these networks is something patients feel they cannot attain from most health care professionals. Some patients may even have issues when it comes to trusting their health care professional. According to the Edelman Trust Barometer conducted in 2008, patients are more inclined to trust a person like them versus an authority figure, including professional organizations, health care professionals, and the media/lay press.[19] The concern is that posts made by patients are a reflection of their unique experience and may be incorrect or inappropriate for another individual. ❼ *Patients often have difficulty finding appropriate information in response to their specific health concerns on the World Wide Web.*

Most social media outlets that give consumers the ability to post opinions, recommendations, and health information state that they are not a substitute for the advice of a qualified health professional. Although the provision of these disclaimers can be a sign of a quality site, unfortunately they are not always posted in the most visible place for many consumers on these Web sites, nor do consumers often heed these warnings.

A New Model of Drug Information in the Community

In order to better serve our constituents, pharmacists must first accept that many patients are likely to seek health information before ever talking to their health care provider. This can be a dangerous practice as many patients are ill equipped to find and understand all the information they need to address their health care situation. Pharmacists have an option to either ignore the fact that patients will continue to seek health information elsewhere, or embrace the opportunity to collaborate with their patients as they seek and use information to improve their health and quality of life. Pharmacists should simply ask their patients where they get health information besides a health care provider and their preferred method to obtain such information. The answer to these simple questions can open the door to more specific education about how the patient can obtain useful, quality health information. Pharmacists must become familiar with the range of consumer health information sources and how and why their patients use them. ❽ *Pharmacists should discuss with their patients why they remain an important source of drug information. Patients can be encouraged not to see CHI as a replacement for actual interaction with a health care provider, but as an extension of care and a way to improve communication.*

Patients need to know the differences between patient education and CHI. Pharmacists can direct patients to quality CHI sites tailored to their situation and teach them how to seek information from the Web. This skill is important because 75% of patients report that they do not consistently check the source of information they find on the Web.[20] Pharmacists may consider developing a list of online resources that have their seal of approval as providing high-quality information. Pharmacist-recommended Web sites can be shared in a variety of different ways ranging from pamphlets, bulletin boards, and space provided on the pharmacy Web site. Such service is something relatively easy and quick to do and goes a long way toward helping patients avoid low-quality or risky information. When providing resources such as these, it is imperative that they are monitored and updated on a consistent basis; otherwise, potential exists for these same resources to become yet another avenue by which low-quality CHI reaches patients. Patients will also need tips on how to navigate the information sources, as well as helping them understand what information is relevant to their individual situation. Not only does this include providing aid in navigating health information found on the Web, but also in other resources, such as brochures and patient leaflets given out with prescriptions. The success of a Web site in delivering meaningful information is heavily reliant upon the consumers' ability to identify, interpret, and apply information that is relevant to their situation. If patients do not understand their health condition, they may use the wrong information for their situation, even if it is of good quality. A 2008 study in the *Journal of the American Medical Informatics Association* gave patients a scenario that described angina symptoms, but not the actual diagnosis. They used MedlinePlus to find information on the condition. The authors found that searches yielded information that led patients to draw incorrect conclusions 70% of the time. The authors concluded that patients and/or family and friends of patients searching the Web for information without a diagnosis most likely are confronted with a wealth of information and are unable to sift through what is relevant versus what is irrelevant.[21]

Additionally, pharmacists may offer classes to teach patients how to use CHI to their advantage. Patients can be taught about the Health on the Net Foundation (HON). This nonprofit, nongovernmental organization's mission is to assess and stringently review Internet sites offering health information. Sites passing inspection receive HON certification and are given the HON symbol to place in a visible area of their Web site for patients to see, giving assurance that the Web site provides reliable and appropriate information. Unfortunately, as the number of health Internet sites increases, there are more and more places patients will find their health information, and they may not all have the HON seal of approval. Patients can also be referred to the National Library of Medicine's tutorial through MedlinePlus. It is specifically dedicated to giving patients instruction on how to evaluate health information they find on the Web and is located at http://www.nlm.nih.gov/medlineplus/webeval/webeval.html.[22] Pharmacists can function as rumor control for misinformation on the Web, mainstream media, or from family and friends. A paper by IBM Global Business Services, titled "Healthcare 2015 and Care Delivery: Delivery Models Refined, Competencies Defined," discussed the need for health coaches who support citizens in their lifestyle decisions and proactively help them understand the risks and outcomes of their choices.[23] Providing quality drug information is clearly a role for a health coach.

An additional motivation for pharmacists to be responsive to patients' information needs is the emerging Pharmacy Quality Alliance (PQA) measures on consumer feedback and assessment. The PQA is a joint project created in conjunction with the Centers for Medicare and Medicaid Services (CMS), America's Health Insurance Plans, the National Community Pharmacists Association (NCPA), and the National Association of Chain Drug Stores (NACDS). With the primary goal being to develop strategies for defining and measuring pharmacy performance, the PQA also hopes to create new pharmacy payment models as well. These measures are in development, but may eventually be part of the pay for performance for providing Medication Therapy Management (MTM) services.[24,25]

EVALUATING THE QUALITY OF HEALTH INTERNET WEB SITES

Questions have been raised about current standards for evaluating the quality of health and medical information on the Internet; many health care professionals feel that proxy measures for evaluating the quality of such Web sites are less than ideal. One study suggests that even sites certified with the HON code may be questionable, with little correlation seen between certification and the accuracy or completeness of information.[10] Although this study questions the reliability of HON certification, it is still considered a useful system for assessing and stringently reviewing Internet sites offering health information. Table 20–3 is an example of the aforementioned current standards in health Internet evaluation.

A great deal of focus is put on the structural design of a Web site, who the site sponsor is (government, non-for-profit, academic institution), and whether or not the site lists its sources, but little emphasis is placed on actual content made available to consumers. In fact, when actual health information content has been reviewed in terms of a specific disease state across many different Web sites, Web site sponsorship has been a very poor predictor of quality.[26] This suggests that there is no efficient and effective method in place to evaluate the quality of health information online. The only real way is for the pharmacist

TABLE 20–3. EXAMPLE OF CURRENT STANDARDS USED TO EVALUATE THE QUALITY OF HEALTH INFORMATION ON THE INTERNET

Considerations When Determining Whether or Not a Web Site Is Reliable and/or Trustworthy
Who is responsible for the Web site? Does the Web site provide this information? Is information provided on how to contact the site?
Is the only purpose of the Web site to provide information, or is the Web site trying to sell something?
If the Web site inquires about personal information, does it offer a reason why and give an explanation about what it will do with that information once collected?
Is health information provided on the Web site backed up with evidence? Are there references to support recommendations being made, etc.?
Does the Web site give the source of its health information? Does the Web site provide an explanation about whether or not health information is reviewed and by whom?
Is health information provided in an unbiased and objective manner? Is material written in a way that would be understandable to most patients no matter their health literacy level?
Does health information on the Web site get updated regularly?
Does health information on the Web site seem reasonable and credible overall?

Data from reference 27.

to individually review each Web site or resource and evaluate actual health information content provided before recommending the sites to patients. Sites devoted to a particular disease state tend to be much more complete and accurate than sites that attempt to cover multiple health topics, but there are still no guarantees. Strict regulation of health content on the Internet is improbable, but health care providers can attempt to help their patients by selecting and evaluating a handful of sites that they would recommend for patients.[26]

HEALTH LITERACY—THE FINAL KEY TO THE PATIENT'S SUCCESSFUL USE OF INFORMATION

❾ *Health literacy is the capability of patients to read or hear health information, understand it, and then act on it.*[28] *Once patients identify or are given quality health information, they still may face barriers in being able to use it to improve their health.* The Institute of Medicine estimates that nearly 90 million adults lack the ability to use the U.S. health system sufficiently due to poor literacy skills. Patients with poor health literacy may have trouble recognizing when health information is even needed, identifying or obtaining health information resources, determining the quality of health information resources or acknowledging that quality is even an issue, and finally analyzing and understanding information found. Pharmacists must consider patients' health literacy when providing information and education. Studies show that most health-related materials, whether on the Web or given out in the pharmacy, surpass most U.S. adults' average reading ability.[29] Table 20–4 describes the qualities of health literate Web sites and can be used as a screen for pharmacists as they identify Web sites for their patients. Visit Pfizer Clear Health Communication at http://www.pfizerhealthliteracy.com/ for additional details about health literacy standards and the role health care professionals can play in helping patients.

INFORMATION THERAPY

The term *information therapy* has recently appeared as an organizing principle for the new model of drug information. In 2009, the Argus Commission, a committee of past

TABLE 20–4. GUIDELINES FOR HIGH-QUALITY HEALTH-LITERATE INTERNET SITES

• Designed for old hardware and software	• Links clearly defined
• Simple home page	• Printer-friendly option
• Information prioritized	• Audio option
• Minimal text per screen	• Site map easy to find
• Navigation simple and consistent	• Contact information easy to find
• Searching simplified	• Content uses other principles of health literacy
• Scrolling need minimized	

Data from reference 30.

presidents of the American Association of Colleges of Pharmacy who offer analysis on contemporary education issues in pharmacy, included information therapy, a term coined by the Center for Information Therapy, as a new way to think about the pharmacist's role in patient care. The Argus Commission recognized that health care is in the midst of an information technology revolution in which the availability of health information is accelerating at an extraordinary rate. They raised questions about the pharmacist's role in this revolution.[31] Information therapy provides patients with evidence-based patient education and/or medical information at just the right time to most effectively assist patients in making a specific health decision or change in their behavior.[10,32] Although an initial counseling session can be very effective for patients, oftentimes reminders or a reiteration of concepts will do more to help the patient if provided at a later time in the form of an information prescription. Information prescriptions are delivered to patients via technology when certain key points between a health care professional and patient need to be reemphasized, a very exciting and practical approach to patient education for community pharmacists. For example, every counseling session could include a follow-up information prescription given at just the right time to effectively reinforce any important late-onset adverse drug reactions (ADRs), adherence strategies, or administration techniques. Adherence to preventative health measures could be improved with information prescriptions if patients receive reminders to seek such care that are individualized to their health status. Pharmacy-based examples include flu shots for people over 50 years of age or a bone density measure for postmenopausal women. These reminders, along with simply written evidence-based information on why the procedure is important, increase awareness and increase demand for important pharmacy-delivered preventative services.[33] ❿ *Information therapy elevates the term drug information from a passive-sounding process to an active component of treatment plans by recognizing that accurate and complete drug information proactively relayed to patients is much more effective than just assuming it will be sought out. Information therapy encompasses both the patient and the health care professional, asking both to work together in making the best possible health care decision for the patient.* From asking more useful questions of doctors and other health care providers to more effectively managing conditions and participating in their own treatment, information therapy has helped patients take back some control over their lives in terms of their health.

PHARMACISTS' PAYMENT FOR PROGRESSIVE DRUG INFORMATION SERVICES

In order for pharmacists to evolve into progressive drug information practitioners, a sustainable business model that includes reimbursement must be designed. The need for reimbursement is key in light of declining revenues from the dispensing operation. MTM is reimbursable through Medicare Part D, and MTM requires patient education as part of the service. Pharmacists should include the strategies described in this chapter in their MTM patient education approaches to begin to get reimbursed for these services. Additionally, some patients are willing to pay directly for care that they cannot receive from other sources. Initiatives such as Project Destiny and the Joint Commission of Pharmacy Practitioners' (JCPP's) Pharmacy 2015 Vision understand the key role reimbursement plays in the sustainability of new practice models, including financial models for how pharmacists can get paid for these services.[2,3] The business case for reimbursement cannot rest solely on financial models alone, though; it is imperative that the establishment of patient and consumer demand for these services is also built into business plans and future visions for pharmacy practice.

Conclusion

A brand new frontier exists for both patients and pharmacists when it comes to obtaining and using health information. It is vital that pharmacists are positioned to be an integral part of their patients' approach to gaining an understanding of their health. As traditional pharmacist roles change, new opportunities to get involved in managing patients' health care present themselves. A lot is at stake if pharmacists do not move toward these new roles, as someone else will step in. It has been the job of pharmacists for decades to educate and provide patients with quality drug information. In the end, it is up to pharmacists to design this new role and demonstrate value to the patient so that they continue to be used as a key ally in health care.

Case Study 20–1

You are the only pharmacist on duty at a local community pharmacy. You are short staffed, the phone is ringing, and you have 50-plus prescriptions yet to verify. You are doing your best to make the wait as short as possible. In the midst of all this, one of your regular patients comes up to the counter and announces that she will no longer be taking her antidepressant. She describes how lately she has been feeling "strange" and feels fairly certain it is due to the antidepressant. She then explains to you how she has recently gone online to find more information about the specific medication she is taking. "You wouldn't believe all the good information that is out there," she says, "I was able to talk to other patients and they were so helpful!" She then goes on to talk about the many patient testimonials she read telling her to discontinue her medication.

Although your patient potentially discontinuing her medication concerns you, she seems adamant that she is going to stop taking it. The pharmacy technician calls you to resume verifying prescriptions because the pharmacy is quickly getting out of control.

Questions:

1. Do you take the time to counsel this patient or do you get back to filling prescriptions before patients start complaining about the wait time?
2. If you decide to counsel this patient, how would you educate her on the appropriate use of online resources to find health information?
3. After counseling your patient she still is determined to stop her antidepressant. What is the most important advice you can give her at this point?

Self-Assessment Questions

1. Which of the following is/are limitation(s) a pharmacist faces when delivering drug information to their patients?
   a. Lack of readability of most patient leaflets given with prescriptions.
   b. Pharmacists appear too busy and unavailable.
   c. Counseling has become a passive process where patient education is only given if requested.
   d. Pharmacists' lack of understanding in regard to patients' desire to take control of their own health.
   e. All of the above.

2. Patient education is best described by the following:
   a. Delivered by health care professional verbally only
   b. Occurs with the pickup of new prescriptions only
   c. Unplanned activity
   d. b and c only
   e. None of the above

3. Consumer Health Information (CHI) is best described by the following:
   a. Tailored to a patient's specific situation
   b. Actively sought by patients

    c. Created in response to patients' need for more information about their health

    d. b and c only

    e. None of the above

4. Which of the following site(s) is considered a social media or social networking site?

    a. PatientsLikeMe.com

    b. Revolution Health

    c. Lexicomp

    d. a and b only

    e. a and c only

5. Through social media sites, patients share a wealth of personal information regarding their disease states and conditions. Examples of personal information shared includes all of the following *except*:

    a. Treatment successes

    b. Treatment failures

    c. Adverse effects

    d. Opinions

    e. None of the above

6. All of the following are reasons why some patients prefer the collective wisdom of a group over the advice of an expert individual *except*:

    a. Patients are provided with a feeling of camaraderie and support.

    b. Patients may not trust their health care professional.

    c. Patients are more inclined to trust a person like themselves.

    d. Patients are not as willing to rely on a single expert for their information.

    e. None of the above.

7. Which of the following is *not* a useful strategy for community pharmacists to employ when helping patients to empower themselves and effectively use consumer health information (CHI)?

    a. Ask patients where else they get health information besides their health care professional.

    b. Become familiar with the range of CHI resources available.

    c. Encourage patients to quit seeking information online regardless of the source.

    d. Develop a list of CHI resources that are pharmacist recommended.

    e. Discuss with patients why pharmacists still remain an important drug information source.

8. Which of the follow are characteristics of a high-quality health-literate Internet site?
   a. Simple homepage.
   b. Information is prioritized.
   c. Designed for newest hardware and software.
   d. a and b only.
   e. All of the above.

9. Which of the following questions are considered standard for evaluating the quality of a consumer health information site?
   a. Is health information provided on the Web site backed up with evidence?
   b. Is health information provided in an unbiased and objective manner?
   c. Is health information provided on a wide variety of disease states and/or conditions?
   d. a and b only
   e. All of the above

10. Which social media site primarily provides consumers with high-quality, unbiased reviews and recommendations on a variety of services including health care providers?
   a. WebMD
   b. Google Health
   c. PatientsLikeMe.com
   d. Revolution Health
   e. Angie's List

11. Which social media site primarily focuses on consumer sharing of information in regard to their disease states, treatments, and overall experiences with, in particular, neurological, neuroendocrine, psychiatric, and immune conditions?
   a. WebMD
   b. Google Health
   c. PatientsLikeMe.com
   d. Revolution Health
   e. Angie's List

12. Which social media site is partnered with the Food and Drug Administration (FDA) to further expand patients' access to reliable and timely health information?
   a. WebMD
   b. Google Health
   c. PatientsLikeMe.com
   d. Revolution Health
   e. Angie's List

13. Which type of social media is best defined as a Web site where those with special interests in common can connect and share with one another?
    a. Wiki
    b. Blog
    c. Social network
    d. b and c only
    e. None of the above

14. Which of the following are issues patients with poor health literacy may face?
    a. Trouble recognizing when health information is needed
    b. Trouble identifying or getting a hold of health information resources
    c. Trouble analyzing and understanding information found
    d. a and b only
    e. All of the above

15. Information therapy can best be described as a/an:
    a. Passive process providing patients with evidence-based drug information at just the right time to most effectively assist the patient
    b. Passive process providing health care professionals with evidence-based drug information at just the right time to most effectively assist the patient
    c. Active process providing health care professionals with evidence-based drug information at just the right time to most effectively assist the patient
    d. Active process providing patients with evidence-based drug information at just the right time to most effectively assist the patient
    e. None of the above

REFERENCES

1. California HealthCare Foundation [Internet]. Oakland (CA): California HealthCare Foundation; 2009. The wisdom of patients: health care meets online social media; 2008 Apr [cited 2009 Oct 31]. Available from: http://www.chcf.org/.
2. American Pharmacists Association, National Association of Chain Drug Stores, National Community Pharmacists Association. Project Destiny executive summary. 2008 Feb. p. 5.
3. Joint Commission of Pharmacy Practitioners. Executive summary: an action plan for implementation of the JCPP future vision of pharmacy practice. 2008 Jan. p. 19.
4. National Council on Patient Information and Education. Enhancing prescription medicine adherence: a national action plan. Bethesda (MD). 2007 Aug. p. 38.
5. Miller L. 2008-2009 Chain Pharmacy Industry Profile. Alexandria (VA): National Association of Chain Drug Stores (US); 2008.
6. Omnibus Budget Reconciliation Act of 1990, Pub. L. 101-508, 104 Stat.1388 (Nov. 5, 1990).

7. Svarstad BL, Bultman DC, Mount JK. Patient counseling provided in community pharmacies: effects of state regulation, pharmacist age, and busyness. J Am Pharm Assoc. 2004;44(1):22-9.

8. Malone PM, Kier KL, Stanovich JE. Drug Information: A Guide for Pharmacists. 3rd ed. New York (NY): McGraw-Hill; 2006.

9. Massengale L. Resources for Quality Health Information Online. Proceedings of the 119th Annual Meeting of the American Association of Colleges of Pharmacy. 2008 July 19-23. Chicago (IL).

10. Felkey BG, Fox BI, Thrower MR. Health Care Informatics: A Skills-Based Resource. Washington, DC: American Pharmacists Association; 2006.

11. Angie's List [homepage on the Internet]. Indianapolis (IN): Angie's List; c1995-2009 [cited 2009 Dec 2]. Available from: http://www.angieslist.com/.

12. Consumer Reports Health [homepage on the Internet]; c2004-2009 [cited 2009 Dec 2]. Available from: http://www.consumerreportshealth.org/.

13. Google Health [homepage on the Internet]; c2008 [cited 2009 Dec 2]. Available from: http://www.google.com/health/.

14. PatientsLikeMe.com [homepage on the Internet]; c2005-2009 [cited 2009 Dec 2]. Available from: http://www.patientslikeme.com/.

15. Revolution Health Group, LLC [homepage on the Internet]; c2009 [cited 2009 Dec 2]. Available from: http://www.revolutionhealth.com/.

16. WebMD [homepage on the Internet]; c2005-2009 [cited 2009 Dec 2]. Available from: http://www.webmd.com/.

17. California HealthCare Foundation. The Wisdom of Patients: Health Care Meets Online Social Media. Oakland (CA): California HealthCare Foundation; 2008.

18. Tapscott D. Grown Up Digital: How the Net Generation Is Changing Your World. New York (NY): McGraw-Hill; 2009.

19. Edelman. 2008 Edelman Trust Barometer [Internet].2008 Jan 22 [cited 2009 Oct 21]. Available from: http://www.edelman.com/trust/2008/.

20. Centers for Disease Control and Prevention [Internet] [cited 2009 Oct 21]. Atlanta (GA): National Center for Health Marketing. Online health information seekers: e Health marketing. Dec 5, 2007. [cited 2009 Oct 31]. Available from: http://www.cdc.gov/healthmarketing/ehm/databriefs/healthseekers.pdf.

21. Keselman A, Browne AC, Kaufman DR. Consumer health information seeking as hypothesis testing. J Am Med Inform Assoc. 2008;15(4):484-95.

22. Medline Plus [Internet]. Bethesda (MD): National Library of Medicine. 2007. Evaluating Internet health information: a tutorial from the national library of medicine [cited 2009 Nov 1]. Available from: http://www.nlm.nih.gov/medlineplus/webeval/webeval.html/.

23. Adams J, Bakalar R, Boroch M, Knecht K, Mounib EL, Stuart N. Healthcare 2015 and Care Delivery: Delivery Models Refined, Competencies Defined. Somers (NY): IBM Institute for Business Value; 2008. p. 2.

24. Sheffer J. Shifting the focus to quality of care: PQA forges path toward improved quality. Pharmacy Today. 2008;14(7):37.

25. Pharmacy Quality Alliance [Internet][cited 2009 Nov 1]. Available from: http://www.pqaalliance.org/.

26. Center for Information Therapy [Internet]. Bethesda (MD): Center for Information Therapy, Inc. Seidman J, Steinwachs D, Rubin HR. The mysterious maze of the World Wide Web: what makes Internet health information high quality; 2004 July 6 [cited 2009 Oct 10]. Available from: http://www.ixcenter.org/publications/documents/e0035.pdf.

27. National Business Group on Health. Health information on the Internet: a checklist to help you judge which websites to trust. 2008 [cited 2009 Oct 21]. Available from: http://www.businessgrouphealth.org/benefitstopics/communications/topic4.cfm.

28. Kutner M, Greenberg E, Jin Y, Paulsen C. The Health Literacy of America's Adults: Results From the 2003 National Assessment of Adult Literacy. Washington, DC: National Center for Education Statistics; 2003. Report No.: NCES 2006-483. Supported by the U.S. Department of Education.

29. Nielsen-Bohlman L, Panzer AM, Kindig DA. Health Literacy: A Prescription to End Confusion. Committee on Health Literacy, Board on Neuroscience and Behavioral Health. Institute of Medicine. Washington, DC: The National Academies Press; 2004.

30. Agency for Healthcare Research and Quality. Accessible health information technology (IT) for populations with limited literacy: a guide for developers and purchasers of health IT. 2007 Oct [cited 2009 Dec 2]. Available from: http://healthit.ahrq.gov/portal/server.pt/gateway/PTARGS_0_1248_803031_0_0_18/LiteracyGuide.pdf.

31. Wells BG, Beck DE, Draugalis JR, Kerr RA, Maine LL, Plaza CM, et al. Report of the 2007-2008 Argus Commission: what future awaits beyond pharmaceutical care? Am J Pharm Educ. 2008 Nov 15;72(Supp):S08.

32. Center for Information Therapy. [Internet]. Bethesda (MD): Center for Information Therapy, Inc.; c2006 [cited 2009 Oct 21]. Available from: http://www.ixcenter.org/.

33. Center for Information Therapy [Internet]. Bethesda (MD): Center for Information Therapy, Inc. Kemper DW. The business case for information therapy in hospitals; 2006 [cited 2009 Oct 21]. Available from: http://www.ixcenter.org/publications/documents/e0678.pdf.

SUGGESTED READINGS AND WEB SITES

Center for Information Therapy	http://www.informationtherapy.org/
Joint Commission of Pharmacy Practitioners' (JCPP's) Future Vision of Pharmacy Practice 2015	Visithttp://www.ascp.com/advocacy/coalitions/upload/JCPP-ExecSummary.pdf for an executive summary of the action plan for implementation of the JCPP Future Vision of Pharmacy Practice.
National Business Group on Health	http://www.businessgrouphealth.org/
Pfizer Clear Health Communication Initiative	http://www.pfizerhealthliteracy.com
Project Destiny (APhA, NACDS, NCPA)	More information on this joint initiative and future vision of the profession of pharmacy can be found at any of the following organizations' Web sites: APhA, NACDS, NCPA.

21

Chapter Twenty-One

Drug Information Education and Training

Kelly M. Smith

Learning Objectives

● *After completing this chapter, the reader will be able to*

- Determine fundamental drug information skills that should be developed in pharmacy students.
- Identify settings in which student drug information skills can be developed and refined.
- Describe the recommended training path for drug information specialists.

Key Concepts

❶ Information retrieval, evaluation, and application skills represent a significant component of the core skill set each pharmacist must possess.

❷ Drug information skills are core concepts that must be incorporated in pharmacy curricula.

❸ The majority of foundational skill development should occur prior to student participation in advanced pharmacy practice experiences (APPEs).

❹ Drug information rotations may also occur in nontraditional settings (e.g., pharmaceutical industry, group purchasing organization), which is a reflection of the expanding role of drug information in contemporary pharmacy practice.

5 Activities in which students should engage to foster their skill development, ranging from responding to drug information requests to preparing materials for consideration by a pharmacy and therapeutics committee, have been identified by the Accreditation Council for Pharmaceutical Education (ACPE).

6 Pharmacy residency training standards include core drug information retrieval and evaluation skills for both postgraduate year one (PGY1) and postgraduate year two (PGY2) programs.

7 Consistent with the profession-wide model for specialist training, the preferred training model for a drug information specialist is a postgraduate year one (PGY1) residency program, followed by completion of a postgraduate year two (PGY2) residency in drug information.

8 The American Society of Health-System Pharmacists (ASHP), the organization charged with accrediting pharmacy residency programs, outlines areas in which PGY2 programs should prepare pharmacists for specialized practice.

9 PGY2 programs in drug information are not limited to health system sites, as many have extended to academic, industrial, and medical writing, managed care, and policy settings.

10 Cultivating research skills beyond those built during residency training is accomplished through fellowship programs.

Introduction

1 *Information retrieval, evaluation, and application skills represent a significant component of the core skill set each pharmacist must possess.* Combined with other practice responsibilities that have traditionally been linked to the practice of drug information (e.g., medication use policy), developing and maintaining a cadre of practitioners with an expertise in such activities is also important. This chapter focuses on key models of education and training for all pharmacists, as well as those that specialize in the practice of drug information.

Foundational Skill Development

Building basic drug information skills, a signature feature of early doctor of pharmacy degree programs, remains an essential component of contemporary entry-level pharmacy education. Skills are cultivated through both didactic and experiential methods. Although instruction has traditionally been provided in courses dedicated to the topic area, nearly 30% of colleges of pharmacy integrate drug information content into other coursework, as noted in a 2006 publication.[1]

❷ *Regardless of the delivery method, drug information skills are core concepts that must be incorporated in pharmacy curricula.* To meet the profession's broader needs, the scope of drug information practice has evolved beyond a focus on literature retrieval, evaluation, and application to a patient care situation. Pharmacy curricula should incorporate drug-information-related topic areas, accordingly. The accreditation standards for professional degree programs include the broad set of related concepts that must be taught and evaluated (e.g., communication skills, practice management, biostatistics).[2] Those that are readily identifiable as connected to drug information are broadly categorized as drug information, literature evaluation and research design, biostatistics, economics/pharmacoeconomics, pharmacoepidemiology, and patient safety. However, a number of foundational elements relevant to drug information practice are integrated into other categories of the Accreditation Council for Pharmacy Education (ACPE) accreditation standard.[2] Those elements include:

- Interpretation of drug screens (e.g., urine toxicology)
- Pharmacists' role in poison control centers
- Dietary Health Supplement and Education Act and impact on regulation of dietary supplements and herbal products
- Incidence of and problems associated with drug overuse, underuse, and misuse in the health care system
- Managing and improving the medication use process
- Ethical issues related to the development, promotion, sales, prescription, and use of drugs
- Effective verbal and written interpersonal communication
- Health literacy
- Evidence-based practice and decisions
- Assurance of safety in the medication use process
- Medication error reduction programs
- Continuous quality improvement programs
- Evaluation of clinical trials that validate treatment usefulness

Beyond the accrediting body, drug information specialist members of the American College of Clinical Pharmacy (ACCP) have identified key drug information elements for inclusion in doctor of pharmacy curricula (Table 21–1).[3] Other topic areas closely aligned with drug information practice include alternative medicine, adverse drug reaction surveillance, safety monitoring during clinical trials, and managing investigational drug services.

TABLE 21–1. ESSENTIAL DRUG INFORMATION CONCEPTS FOR PROFESSIONAL DEGREE CURRICULA

- Applying medical information to specific patient situations
- Counter-detailing and appropriate interactions with the pharmaceutical industry
- Creating effective and efficient literature searching strategies
- Critically evaluating marketing and promotional materials and advertisements
- Critically evaluating medical literature
- Describing the process of drug regulation in the United States
- Distinguishing statistical versus clinical significance
- Discerning and communicating appropriate health information for patient education
- Evaluating medication use policies and procedures
- Identifying, evaluating, and utilizing key print (text) sources of medical information
- Identifying, managing, reporting, and preventing adverse drug events
- Incorporating principles and practices of evidence-based medicine (EBM) into pharmaceutical care
- Locating and critically evaluating medical information on the Internet
- Preparing, presenting, and participating in journal clubs
- Providing verbal and written responses to drug information requests
- Summarizing basic biostatistics and research design methods
- Understanding the creation, maintenance, and management of a medication formulary
- Using electronic medical information databases and other technologically enhanced references and resources in an effective and efficient manner to advance pharmaceutical care

Data from reference 7.

A number of pedagogical approaches may be used to build skills in the didactic setting. The growing availability of instructional technologies, coupled with a focus on active learning components that colleges of pharmacy must implement in the professional program, afford instructors the opportunity to bring practical, practice-oriented scenarios to students prior to the experiential portion of the curriculum. For example, drug information requests can be directly posed in the classroom setting, with the expectation that students seek an appropriate response using mobile computing and the broad array of electronic references and databases available. Students can be asked to locate and quickly assess the validity and utility of a consumer medical Web site. Student-created web logs that critique the merits of a clinical trial can support the application of literature evaluation skills in a dynamic medium.

❸ *The majority of foundational skill development should occur prior to student participation in advanced pharmacy practice experiences (APPEs).* Yet, integration of practice-related activities in the introductory pharmacy practice experiences (IPPEs) are also important activities and are supported by the ACPE.[2] Once a student reaches the final year in the professional curriculum, he or she can benefit greatly from a practice experience devoted to drug information practice. Having the opportunity to provide responses to drug information requests following the completion of didactic coursework gives students even greater opportunities to apply pharmacotherapeutic, pharmacokinetic, legal, and ethical principles to their approach to providing drug information. Drug information historically was a required learning experience for each doctor of pharmacy student. However, the growth in the number of colleges of pharmacy and pharmacy student population, coupled with a somewhat diminishing number of drug information centers, has yielded an inadequate number of teaching sites to support a required drug information APPE for every student.[4] While some colleges develop their own formalized centers to overcome this imbalance, others provide only elective drug information practice experiences.[1,5] ❹ *Drug information rotations may also occur in nontraditional settings (e.g., pharmaceutical industry, managed care, group purchasing organization), which is a reflection of the expanding role of drug information in contemporary pharmacy practice.*

❺ *Activities in which students should engage to foster their skill development, ranging from responding to drug information requests to preparing materials for consideration by a pharmacy and therapeutics committee, have been identified by the ACPE* (Table 21–2).[2]

TABLE 21–2. SUGGESTED DRUG INFORMATION ACTIVITIES FOR INCORPORATION IN ADVANCED PHARMACY PRACTICE EXPERIENCES

- Accessing, evaluating, and applying information to promote optimal health care
- Conducting a drug use review
- Developing and analyzing clinical drug guidelines
- Educating the public and health care professionals regarding medical conditions, wellness, dietary supplements, durable medical equipment, and medical and drug devices
- Identifying and reporting medication errors and adverse drug reactions
- Managing the medication use system and applying the systems approach to medication safety
- Participating in discussions and assignments concerning key health care policy matters that may affect pharmacy
- Participating in discussions and assignments regarding compliance with accreditation, legal, regulatory/legislative, and safety requirements
- Participating in discussions and assignments regarding the drug approval process and the role of key organizations in public safety and standards setting
- Participating in the health system's formulary process
- Participating in the pharmacy's quality improvement program
- Participating in therapeutic protocol development
- Performing prospective and retrospective financial and clinical outcomes analysis to support formulary recommendations and therapeutic guideline development
- Retrieving, evaluating, managing, and using clinical and scientific publications in the decision-making process
- Working with the technology used in pharmacy practice

Data from reference 2.

Students do require adequate supervision and oversight to ensure the quality of service they provide, as well as to provide them valuable feedback to subsequently improve their performance. However, the site may realize a return on investment in preceptors, as students may be able to expand the capacity of services the center provides, including responding to more drug information requests, preparing analyses of drug policy issues for consideration by the pharmacy and therapeutics committee, and conducting retrospective reviews of medical records for medication use evaluations or adverse drug reaction surveillance.

Specialized Skill Development

Drug information skills are a core skill set for all pharmacists, regardless of their practice setting, area of therapeutic focus, or declared area of specialty. ❻ *In fact, pharmacy residency training standards include core drug information retrieval and evaluation skills for both postgraduate year one (PGY1) and postgraduate year two (PGY2) programs.* As early as 1972, pharmacists recognized the need for a cadre of individuals with specialized skills in drug information.[6] What began as specialized internships and later the focus of degree programs has evolved to the current model of postgraduate training, specifically through residency programs, to train drug information specialists. ❼ *Consistent with the profession-wide model for specialist training, the preferred training model for a drug information specialist is a postgraduate year one (PGY1) residency program, followed by completion of a postgraduate year two (PGY2) residency in drug information.*[7] Such a model is also supported by drug information specialist members of the ACCP.[3]

Despite the long-standing recognition of the importance of advanced training in cultivating specialized skills, the number of drug information pharmacists who have completed such training does not exceed 40%.[8] This may reflect an imbalance in advanced trained pharmacists and job openings. A relative lack of popularity or desirability of the specialty to students and new trainees, or pressures on employers to fill positions with applicants who lack the desired formal training, may have contributed to this imbalance; no formal assessment of these or other factors has been conducted. Nonetheless, specialized training can be critical for preparation for practice. Training paths and their connections to practice activities and preparedness were assessed in a 2006 U.S. survey of pharmacists with presumed drug information practices. The most common primary job responsibilities of those surveyed were instructing pharmacy students and staff (64%), maintaining formal drug information center operations (63%), responding to drug information queries (59%), providing pharmacy and therapeutics committee support (46%), publishing pharmacy-related newsletters (38%), and developing medication use policy (35%). Respondents generally felt prepared to undertake their responsibilities in relation to the extent of postgraduate training they received. However, areas in which pharmacists felt less prepared included information systems support (41%), pharmacoeconomic evaluations (32%), and clinical outcomes research (19%). Approximately 80% of those who had completed postgraduate training felt adequately prepared overall for their job roles. Preparing for practice changes and innovations is a focus of residency training, and perhaps that was reflected in the greater sense of preparedness residency-trained pharmacists reported.

❽ *The American Society of Health-System Pharmacists (ASHP), the organization charged with accrediting pharmacy residency programs, outlines areas in which PGY2 programs should prepare pharmacists for specialized practice.* PGY2 drug information residents should focus on cultivating their abilities to provide drug-related information, develop and support an organized drug information service, lead drug use policy decision-making processes (e.g., making formulary recommendations), and maintain knowledge of and contribute to biomedical literature.[9] These skill sets should exceed those of a PGY1 resident, who should be capable of fulfilling patient-specific drug information needs, creating drug policy tools, and ensuring safety and efficacy in the medication use process. As noted in the 2006 survey, contemporary drug information specialists should be prepared to use technology (e.g., clinical decision support) and advanced population-based approaches (e.g., data mining, pharmacoepidemiology) to support a safe and effective medication use process.[10] These tools and approaches include clinical decision support, informatics, data mining, and other such techniques that are consistent with the Institute of Medicine's (IOM) focus on evidence-based medicine, technology, and quality assurance as core competencies for health care practitioners.[10]

❾ *PGY2 programs in drug information are not limited to health system sites, as many have extended to academic, industrial, and medical writing, managed care, and policy settings.* Engaging residents in the practice environment can yield a number of benefits to the site, from building its capacity to fulfill its mission, to serving as a potential pipeline for the recruitment of new specialists. Individuals who have trained in these areas but subsequently become employed in different environments may have a greater understanding of the operations of the other settings that can improve their decision making. For instance, a rotation in the pharmaceutical industry can better inform a pharmacist of the FDA regulations and internal policies that may shape the manner in which a manufacturer can provide information about an investigational drug or suspected adverse effects of a marketed drug.

❿ *Cultivating research skills beyond those built during residency training is the niche filled by fellowship programs.* As with therapeutic specialties, fellowship training in drug information should focus on expanding the fellow's research abilities. There are no accreditation standards for fellowship programs, so their structure, duration, and delivery are guided by the program director. Given the growing complexity and cost of health care, the need for a cadre of practice-grounded researchers has grown more vital. Drug information fellowships that focus on research skills in pharmacoepidemiology, pharmacoeconomics, and comparative effectiveness, or the role of informatics to support a safe and effective medication use system, would be well suited to fill this need.

Pursuing Specialty Training

Identifying potential residency or fellowship programs that may meet an individual's training needs should begin with a directory search. Factors that may be important to individual candidates include the ability to gain experience working with students or PGY1 residents, performing contract work, extensive opportunities to manage drug policy across a health system, and intensive training in medical writing. Regardless of the special features or characteristics, there should be opportunities that will prepare individuals for the type of practice they envision. A directory of accredited, or accreditation-pending, residency programs can easily be accessed from the ASHP Online Residency Directory.[11] In addition to employment (e.g., salary, benefits) and contact (e.g., program director) information, each program's listing includes a description of the practice site, key program features, and application information. Residency programs, including those that are not accredited, may also be identified through a review of the Directory of Residencies, Fellowships, and Graduate Programs hosted on the ACCP Web site.[12] This directory is also the primary catalog of possible fellowship options. Fellowship programs are generally listed under the heading of the research focus (e.g., pharmacoeconomics), rather than by the term drug information.

Conclusion

All pharmacists, regardless of practice setting, require drug information skills in order to provide adequate patient care and appropriate support to other health care professionals. Equipping pharmacists with those skills begins in professional degree programs, continues into residency training, and often extends into research-based fellowship programs. Each of these important elements of the education and training continuum should continue to evolve to meet contemporary practice and research needs, and to prepare future practitioners to integrate technologic and therapeutic advances to provide innovative services.

Self-Assessment Questions

1. As a faculty member at a new college of pharmacy, you have been asked to assist your colleagues in integrating drug information concepts into their coursework. Which pharmacotherapeutic content area is suitable for integration with drug information skill development?
   a. Cardiology
   b. Neurology
   c. Pediatrics
   d. All of the above
   e. None of the above

2. A drug information APPE can be conducted in which of the following settings?
   a. College-based drug information center
   b. Hospital-based drug information center
   c. State Medicaid formulary management group
   d. All of the above
   e. None of the above

Questions 3 through 5 relate to your role as a faculty member of the curriculum committee at a college of pharmacy.

3. The committee is identifying points in the professional degree program in which students are instructed in various content areas (i.e., conducting curricular mapping). The process entails the listing of various topic areas in broad categories, with a corresponding listing of the courses in which each topic is taught. One broad content category is drug information. The committee has been struggling with this element, as it realizes that there are a number of concepts commonly related to drug information that may be integrated into several courses. Which of the following course(s) are likely to include drug information-related concepts?
   a. Drug dosage form design (pharmaceutics)
   b. Physiology
   c. Complementary and alternative medication use
   d. All of the above
   e. None of the above

4. The committee is reviewing a proposal to create an elective professional degree course entitled "Foundations of Medical Writing." Which of the following potential course concepts(s) are relevant to drug information practice?
   a. Critiquing the research design of a recently published clinical trial
   b. The process of assigning a corresponding editor to each manuscript submitted to a medical journal

c. Both of the above
d. Neither of the above

5. During your college's review of its professional degree program, a committee member recommends the elimination of a course entitled "Drug Information Skill Development." When asked to justify the recommendation, the faculty member replies, "The accreditation standards don't require a drug information course." What is a factual response to the statement?
   a. The standards *do not* prescribe specific concepts that must be taught in professional degree curricula.
   b. The standards *do* require the inclusion of concepts directly categorized as drug information, in addition to related concepts.
   c. Drug information concepts *are* required to be taught only during advanced pharmacy practice experiences (APPEs).
   d. All of the above.
   e. None of the above.

Questions 6 through 8 relate to your role as the instructor of a drug information course in a professional degree program at a college of pharmacy.

6. In which activity can you engage the students to demonstrate the broad applicability of drug information skills, using an example from the popular media?
   a. Critiquing the accuracy of a local television news reporter's segment about a newly approved prescription drug
   b. Crafting a letter to the editor describing the role pharmacists play in preventing medication errors, in response to an article about the national impact of medication errors published in the local newspaper
   c. Both of the above
   d. Neither of the above

7. Potential sources of actual drug information requests that you can adapt for use as a student assignment include:
   a. Drug information requests that have been posed to the college's drug information center
   b. Drug information requests posed during medical rounds to APPE students during the previous academic year, which are documented in each student's portfolio
   c. Questions posted on a patient information Web site
   d. All of the above
   e. None of the above

8. Analyzing the contents of a direct-to-consumer advertisement for a newly approved prescription drug is an activity that can illustrate which drug information-related concept?

   a. Regulation of dietary supplements and herbal products

   b. Incidence of drug overuse, underuse, and misuse in the U.S. health care system

   c. Ethical issues related to the promotion of drugs

   d. All of the above

   e. None of the above

9. In which APPE(s) can students continue to develop their ability to evaluate the biomedical literature?

   a. Internal medicine

   b. Pediatrics

   c. Hospital pharmacy

   d. All of the above

   e. None of the above

10. The preferred credentials for a drug information specialist practicing in a drug information center are:

    a. Doctor of Pharmacy

    b. Doctor of Pharmacy + PGY1 Pharmacy Residency

    c. Doctor of Pharmacy + Pharmacoeconomics Fellowship

    d. All of the above

    e. None of the above

11. The organization responsible for conducting the accreditation process for drug information residencies is:

    a. American Society of Health-System Pharmacists

    b. American College of Clinical Pharmacy

    c. Accreditation Council for Pharmacy Education

    d. All of the above

    e. None of the above

12. What role(s) can PGY2 drug information residents play in the education of Doctor of Pharmacy students?

    a. Review a student's assessment of the causality of a suspected adverse drug reaction.

    b. Provide classroom instruction about literature evaluation skills.

    c. Edit a student-authored drug monograph.

    d. All of the above.

    e. None of the above.

13. The preferred training path for a drug information pharmacist faculty member capable of supporting a federally funded research program is:
    a. Doctor of Pharmacy + PGY1 Residency
    b. Doctor of Pharmacy + PGY2 Drug Information Residency
    c. Doctor of Pharmacy + Pharmacoeconomics Residency
    d. All of the above
    e. None of the above

14. You wish to determine the employment paths graduates of Postgraduate PGY2 drug information residencies have pursued over the last 5 years. Which of the following is/are true?
    a. The ACPE Online Residency Directory lists the current employment of program graduates.
    b. The ACCP Online Residency Directory lists the current employment of program graduates.
    c. The ASHP Online Residency Directory lists the current employment of program graduates.
    d. All of the above.
    e. None of the above.

15. You are conducting a national survey of drug information residency programs to assess their program size, affiliation with a college of pharmacy, role in the APPE training environment, and funding sources. The demographics section of your questionnaire includes a question about the setting in which the residency program is conducted. Your coinvestigator insists that you should only provide a text box for the response, "because I bet 99% of the programs are in hospitals, anyway." You disagree and suggest that a variety of settings need to be provided as options. Which of the following is the best answer?
    a. Hospital, college of pharmacy
    b. Hospital, college of pharmacy, managed care
    c. Hospital, college of pharmacy, managed care, industry, medical communications company
    d. None of the above

REFERENCES

1. Wang F, Troutman WG, Seo T, Peak AS, Rosenberg JM. Drug information education in doctor of pharmacy programs. Am J Pharm Educ. 2006;70(3): Article 51.
2. Accreditation Council for Pharmacy Education. Accreditation standards and guidelines for the professional program in pharmacy leading to the doctor of pharmacy degree. [cited 2009 July 25].

Available from: http://www.acpe-accredit.org/pdf/ACPE_Revised_PharmD_Standards_Adopted_Jan152006.pdf.

3. Rosenberg JM, Koumis T, Nathan JP, Cicero LA, McGuire H.Current status of pharmacist-operated drug information centers in the United States. Am J Health-Syst Pharm. 2004;61:2023-32.

4. Cole SW, Berensen NM. Comparison of drug information practice curriculum components in US colleges of pharmacy. Am J Pharm Educ. 2005;69(2):Article 34.

5. Hirschman JL. Building a clinically orientated drug information service. In: Francke DE, Whitney HAK, editors. Perspectives in Clinical Pharmacy. Hamilton (IL): Drug Intelligence Publications; 1972. p. 150-77.

6. American Society of Health-System Pharmacists. Pharmacy residency training in the future: a stakeholders' roundtable discussion. Am J Health-Syst Pharm. 2005;62:1817-20.

7. Bernknopf AC, Karpinski JP, McKeever AL, Peak AS, Smith KM, Smith WD, et al. Drug information: from education to practice. Pharmacotherapy. 2009;29(3):331-46.

8. Gettig JP, Jordan JK, Sheehan AH. A survey of current perceptions of drug information practice and training. Hosp Pharm. 2009;44:325-31.

9. American Society of Health-System Pharmacists. ASHP accreditation standards for post-graduate year two (PGY2) pharmacy residency programs. [cited 2011 June 17]. Available from: http://www.ashp.org/DocLibrary/Accreditation/ASD-PGY2-Standard.aspx.

10. Institute of Medicine: executive summary. In: Greiner AC, Knebel E, editors. Health professions education: a bridge to quality. Washington, DC: National Academy Press; 2003. p. 1-18.

11. American Society of Health-System Pharmacists. Residency Directory. [cited 2009 July 25]. Available from: http://accred.ashp.org/aps/pages/directory/residencyProgramSearch.aspx.

12. American College of Clinical Pharmacy. Directory of Residencies, Fellowships, and Graduate Programs. [cited 2009 July 25]. Available from: http://www.accp.com/resandfel/index.aspx.

SUGGESTED READINGS

1. Accreditation Council for Pharmacy Education. Accreditation standards and guidelines for the professional program in pharmacy leading to the doctor of pharmacy degree. [cited 2009 July 25]. Available from: http://www.acpe-accredit.org/pdf/ACPE_Revised_PharmD_Standards_Adopted_Jan152006.pdf.

2. Bernknopf AC, Karpinski JP, McKeever AL, Peak AS, Smith KM, Smith WD, et al. Drug information: from education to practice. Pharmacotherapy. 2009;29(3):331-46.

3. Cole SW, Berensen NM. Comparison of drug information practice curriculum components in US colleges of pharmacy. Am J Pharm Educ. 2005;69(2):Article 34.

Chapter Twenty-Two

Pharmaceutical Industry and Regulatory Affairs

Opportunities for Drug Information Specialists

Jean E. Cunningham • Lindsay E. Davison

Learning Objectives

● *After completing this chapter, the reader will be able to*

- Describe the organization of a pharmaceutical company.
- Discuss opportunities for health care professionals (HCPs) within the pharmaceutical industry.
- Describe how HCPs are regulated in the pharmaceutical industry.
- Determine acceptable interactions between pharmaceutical companies and HCPs.
- List the components of a clinical response and personalized letter.
- Explain the importance of collecting adverse event information.
- Recommend methods for communicating safety information to consumers.
- Identify industry-associated organizations.
- Describe the role of the Division of Drug Information (DDI) at the Food and Drug Administration (FDA).
- List the main differences between the DDI and a typical drug information center.
- Illustrate the different types of drug information services provided by the FDA.
- Identify factors that guide the selection of a specific FDA-sponsored resource/Web site.
- Discuss student and professional opportunities within the FDA.

Key Concepts

1 Pharmaceutical companies' scientific or medical divisions are filled with highly trained HCPs working in a variety of specialized fields.

2 The goal of the Pharmaceutical Research and Manufacturers of America's (PhRMA) *Code on Interactions With Health Care Professionals* (HCPs) is to provide transparency to HCPs and patients alike as to the motives and channels through which industry conducts business with external customers and business partners.

3 Clinical response letters are written correspondences that contain company-approved content in response to an unsolicited request for medical information.

4 Postmarketing surveillance allows companies and the Food and Drug Administration (FDA) to continually review the recorded adverse events with a medication to evaluate the safety profile and continued use of the medicine by patients exposed to its risks.

5 The best way to communicate risk is still being decided by the FDA, and many programs are already in place such as Risk Evaluation and Mitigation Strategies (REMS), Risk Minimization Action Plans (RiskMAPs), patient package inserts, medication guides, and others.

6 The FDA strives to advance public health by setting standards for the efficient approval of new products that are safe, effective, and helpful to the U.S. public in combination with serving as a source of reputable and fair science-based information for consumers to effectively use these products.

7 The FDA has several proactive mechanisms to communicate information about human drug products to the public through Web sites, listservers, CDERLearn programs, continuing education, and drug safety podcasts.

Introduction

There are many roles available to health care professionals (HCPs) within the pharmaceutical industry and regulating agencies. In industry, these roles span medical education, publications, marketing, medical information, and more. In regulatory affairs, the roles are usually separate functions supporting the organizational mission statement and generally pertain to ensuring the safe and effective use of medications available to the public. Job titles and descriptions may vary slightly from company to company or agency to agency, but the importance of HCPs within each area is constant across organizations.

Throughout this chapter the reader will become familiar with the organization of a pharmaceutical company, professional mentoring relationships, industry's regulated interactions with outside health care professionals, the fulfillment of a medical information request and responses to unsolicited inquiries, the many roles and career paths available to HCPs in the industry, and the importance and requirements of adverse event reporting and postmarketing surveillance. Information surrounding the role of medical information within regulatory agencies, specifically the Food and Drug Administration (FDA), is then presented. At the end, the reader should have a general knowledge of the roles and responsibilities of health care professionals employed in the pharmaceutical industry or regulating agencies, the expectations HCPs may have of receiving medical information from a pharmaceutical company or regulating agency, and how to pursue opportunities and careers within the pharmaceutical industry or regulating agencies.

Opportunities for HCPs Within Industry

❶ *Pharmaceutical companies' scientific or medical divisions are staffed with highly trained HCPs working in a multitude of specialized fields* (Figure 22–1).[1] The following section highlights specific opportunities within the pharmaceutical industry for HCPs.

CUSTOMER RESPONSE CENTER

Customer response center representatives are the first-line response team for unsolicited requests (unsolicited requests must be created by the requester free from influence by the pharmaceutical company or its representatives) for medical information. HCPs are well trained for customer response center representative positions. Customer response center HCPs are faced with a variety of responsibilities as the first-line of communication with patients and providers, including capturing adverse events (AEs) and product quality

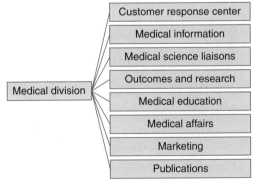

Figure 22–1. Organization of pharmaceutical companies' medical division. (This figure is based on information from reference 1.)

complaints (PQCs), and triaging medical information requests (MIRs) and nonmedical information requests. Customer response center HCPs are provided with a variety of tools, including but not limited to, product labeling (or package inserts), response letters, question and answer (Q&A) documents, and clinical topic overviews, typically drafted by peers in medical information to assist in answering unsolicited requests for product information. Customer response center HCPs use product labeling, response letters, and literature searches to assist them in responding to MIRs. HCPs serving in this capacity must have excellent verbal communication skills and are highly trained in effectively searching for information. Some MIRs may require additional research or analysis resulting in the customer response center HCP escalating the inquiry to a medical information specialist for further investigation.[1]

MEDICAL INFORMATION

Medical information specialists are HCPs who respond to unsolicited medical information requests, write and update response letters, conduct scientific analyses of medical literature topics, review promotional materials, develop dossiers for formulary consideration, and train company staff (e.g., sales force, peers, account managers, and others) (Figure 22–2).[2] Medical information specialists also respond to MIRs that are escalated to them by customer response center representatives. Escalation, or the transfer of MIRs,

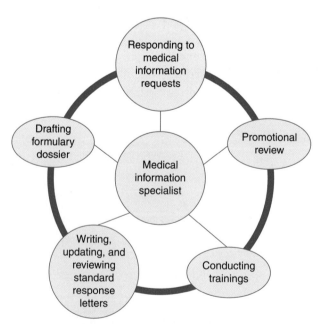

Figure 22–2. Responsibilities of medical information specialists. (This figure is based on information from reference 2.)

occurs frequently when the customer response center representatives do not have the resources necessary to formulate a response. Medical information specialists may have access to additional resources, such as comprehensive reports from clinical trials, information provided to study investigators, marketing materials, posters and abstracts, and contacts in other departments, which makes them invaluable resources for analyzing and synthesizing information.

MEDICAL SCIENCE LIAISONS

Medical science liaisons (MSLs) originated as highly specialized customer response center representatives. A MSL supports, and is supported by, the scientific affairs and medical information team. MSLs have a close working relationship with key opinion leaders (key opinion leaders are HCPs considered to be experts in their area by their peers and are often highly regarded for their expertise in publications, speaking engagements, and influential value in the medical community) and are expected to engage in clinical conversations ranging from broad clinical guidelines to patient-specific care (Table 22–1).[3] MSLs are expected to attend national meetings and to provide comprehensive clinical presentations. MSLs may focus on one product or therapeutic area, so there may be overlapping MSLs working for the same company in one location supporting different products and specialty areas, or there may be one MSL in a remote location responsible for multiple products and therapeutic areas.

OUTCOMES RESEARCH

Outcomes research specialists are known in some companies as field-based outcomes liaisons FBOLs. This position is similar to that of a MSL, except the focus of FBOLs may be to demonstrate the value of a product to managed care organizations, pharmacy

TABLE 22–1. **RESPONSIBILITIES OF MEDICAL SCIENCE LIAISONS**

Responsibilities of medical science liaisons may include the following
Building and maintaining relationships with key opinion leaders
Recruiting interested investigators for clinical trial research
Supporting advisory boards
Assisting with company projects
Providing peer-to-peer exchange of information
Presenting at meetings with formulary decision makers
Conducting training sessions for branded product speakers, medical residents, and/or sales representatives
Performing and overseeing clinical trial and health outcomes research
Providing continuing education and branded product presentations

This table is based on information from reference 3.

benefit managers (PBMs), or other HCPs in similar decision-making roles through the generation of outcomes data. Outcomes data typically provides studies focused on identifying, measuring, and evaluating the end result of a health care service or treatment. For example, a company that is marketing an antiplatelet medication might request that their FBOLs demonstrate to customers the value of the product through quality-life years gained or may request that the FBOLs create a risk stratification tool (e.g., stratification of risk for patients with cardiovascular disease) to assist clinicians in determining appropriate therapy options for their patients.[1]

MEDICAL EDUCATION

HCPs in medical education evaluate funding requests for continuing medical education (CME), continuing education (CE) for other health care practitioners, and other programs submitted by qualified organizations. Grants are reviewed by medical education HCPs to ensure that the program outlined in the grant addresses the specific needs of HCPs in clinical practice and is consistent with the company's educational goals and objectives for a specific therapeutic area.[1] CME and CE programs must meet standards set by the corresponding accrediting body for the audience and must also abide by guidance provided by the FDA.[4,5]

MEDICAL AFFAIRS

Medical affairs HCPs typically oversee Phase IV clinical trial programs and may also be involved with Phase III and postmarketing research as well. These HCPs primarily conduct research on marketed pharmaceuticals in areas of high therapeutic demand or information need. In addition, medical affairs HCPs are involved in a variety of tasks with peers in medical information, marketing, and with key opinion leaders in the field. These tasks include reviewing promotional and marketing materials, supporting Phase IV clinical trial sites, and maintaining communication with trial investigators; reviewing product labeling, formulary dossiers, and training materials for promotional and educational purposes; and developing and presenting original research in the form of posters, abstracts, and manuscripts. Medical affairs HCPs are responsible for reviewing these materials for the accuracy of the medical information and to ensure that the final products (e.g., promotional materials and package inserts) are unbiased, fair-balanced, and not misleading.[1]

MARKETING

HCPs in the marketing division of a pharmaceutical company are responsible for developing the branded messages for a product. The tag lines and main selling points seen in journal advertisements, on Web pages, and on printed materials are created by the marketing division. It is important for HCPs in marketing to understand the clinical practice environment of their peers so they can provide valuable tools and materials. Marketing drafts a plethora of promotional materials such as journal and television advertisements, and functional educational tools (e.g., dose conversion guides). Peers in medical information and medical affairs, and other internal business partners in regulatory and legal departments then review all of these materials.[1]

PUBLICATIONS

The team of HCPs in the publications department has the important task of ensuring that the appropriate information reaches the appropriate audience. For example, a company coming to market with a new hypertension medication would want its publications department to create a plan that would publish trial data (preclinical through *post hoc* and review data) concurrently with major meetings of physicians treating hypertension. Similarly, posters and abstracts would need to be submitted to these organizations for presentation at their meetings, rather than to be presented at a meeting of orthopedic surgeons or any other group with little use for information on a antihypertensive product. The publications department ensures that reprints of posters, abstracts, and manuscripts are readily available for dissemination to HCPs in the field. HCPs in this department are also responsible for reviewing the final content of publications and drafting comments if necessary, often through a partnered review process with medical affairs and medical information, to make certain that accurate information is available for HCPs in clinical practice.[1]

As outlined in this section, HCPs have many varied opportunities within the industry. Each of the functions described previously abide by a set of rules and regulations. Understanding and complying with these rules and regulations helps ensure the success of industry-employed HCPs.

Regulation of HCPs in Industry

Pharmaceutical companies are regulated both externally by the FDA and internally by standard operating procedures (SOPs).[6-23] To help internal HCPs to understand the regulations governing their department's duties and to establish an efficient methodological approach to the business, SOPs are developed internally by companies.[23] Although HCPs in clinical practice may not be governed by the same regulations as industry, having a basic understanding of the company's regulations will help align the external HCPs' expectations with what can be provided by internal industry HCPs.

CODE OF FEDERAL REGULATIONS

●The Code of Federal Regulations (CFR) Title 21 regulates the U.S. pharmaceutical industry throughout the life cycle of a product, from Phase I through Phase IV clinical trials, including postmarketing data collection.[6,7,12,19,20,24,25] HCPs working for a U.S. pharmaceutical company must achieve a thorough understanding of these regulations to ensure compliance with the regulations that pertain to their daily duties.

STANDARD OPERATING PROCEDURES

SOPs provide additional guidance to employees, supplementing regulations from federal and state government agencies. A SOP allows a company to digest regulations from the federal government, making them applicable to employees and their everyday job functions.[23] The pharmaceutical industry employs health care professionals and lawyers in regulatory affairs to ensure that SOPs are up-to-date and provide employees proper guidance for complying with all applicable regulations.

_____ Case Study 22–1

■ DRUG A

The pharmaceutical company, Awesome Drug, Inc. is planning to file a new drug application (NDA) for DRUG A, its new medication to treat moderate to severe hiccups. Awesome Drug, Inc. is a small startup company and has never launched a marketed product prior to DRUG A. The company currently employs a small number of HCPs in medical affairs and marketing. It is expected that DRUG A will be approved in 10 months following NDA filing.

Discussion questions:

1. What internal documents should Awesome Drug, Inc. prepare so its employees are aware of the regulations governing their job functions?
2. What external regulations should Awesome Drug, Inc. include in education for their HCPs?
3. Discuss the job responsibilities in the present medical departments at Awesome Drug, Inc.
4. What are some other departments Awesome Drug, Inc. should consider developing in the future? What are some of the job responsibilities of these departments?

PhRMA and the Code on Interactions With Health Care Professionals

HCPs within the pharmaceutical industry hold themselves to a high standard when it comes to providing accurate, concise, and timely information. Interactions between pharmaceutical companies and HCPs are defined but not regulated by a code of conduct established by PhRMA (Pharmaceutical Research and Manufacturers of America), through the revised version of the *Code on Interactions With Health Care Professionals.*[26] The prior edition, from 2002, primarily addressed products being marketed and activities prior to the launch of a medication. The updated version released in January 2009 included more specific guidance regarding the interactions between pharmaceutical industry representatives and health care professionals. ❷*The goal of these regulations is to provide transparency to health care professionals and patients alike as to the motives and channels through which industry conducts business with external customers and business partners.*[26]

Case Study 22–1 Continued

Discussion questions:

5. What department(s) would review grants for educational programming for DRUG A?
6. What department(s) may be involved in approving marketing materials for DRUG A?

Fulfillment of Medical Information Requests

HCPs and patients may contact a pharmaceutical company with questions regarding a medication when an answer is not readily available. A typical process for responding to these questions is described in Figure 22–3.

RESPONSE LETTERS

❸ *Clinical response letters are written correspondences that contain company-approved* (may be approved by any or all of the following departments: medical affairs, medical information, legal, and regulatory) *content in response to an unsolicited request for medical*

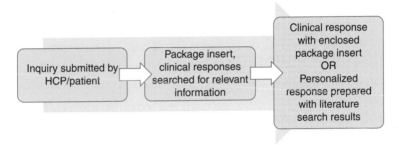

Figure 22–3. Medical information request receipt and fulfillment process.

information. The use of evidence-based medicine in response letters allows consumers and health care professionals to be confident that they are receiving fair-balanced, unbiased, and not misleading information.[27] Response letters are usually created according to a template for consistency (Table 22–2) and are drafted in anticipation of, or in response to, frequently asked questions.[28] One paper described how Solvay Pharmaceuticals determined that prior to the launch of a product, response letters took 4 to 8 hours each to create. The time spent by Solvay HCPs to create a response letter following launch significantly increased, taking 4 to 7 days to create. This was directly related to the increased workload and the continuous arrival of new MIRs.[29] Once a product is available on the market, the number and complexity of MIRs is likely to increase. This increases HCPs' total workload and therefore increases the time it takes to complete individual tasks, such as creating response letters. Because of this, the time to create a response letter and respond to an MIR may differ from Solvay's results.

Pharmaceutical companies' response letters are created from source documents in response to frequently asked questions and are peer-reviewed internally.[30] Clinical response letters developed by companies may be either proactive or reactive. For example, if the evening news reports that STRIPES causes yellow stripes to appear on patients' skin, the company that makes STRIPES should react immediately by developing a response letter to address questions from HCPs and patients on this adverse event (i.e., reactive). In another

TABLE 22–2. **COMPONENTS OF A CLINICAL RESPONSE LETTER**

1. Opening
2. Indication(s)
3. Disclaimer
4. Body
5. Closing
6. Adverse Event Reporting
7. Signature and Contact Information
8. Enclosure(s)
9. References

This table is based on information from reference 27.

example, a company launching DRUG A, a drug with a similar mechanism of action to STRIPES, may wish to proactively develop a response letter in anticipation that the likelihood of experiencing yellow stripes with DRUG A will be frequently asked about, based on the report of this reaction with STRIPES. Using this example, the company that manufactures DRUG A may need more than 1 day to prepare a complete, concise response, and thus in the meantime may tell customers that they are currently researching the issue in question. When this response is provided, the requestor should expect a complete response to be delivered in a timely manner (see Appendix 22-1 for an example of a response letter).

UNIQUE RESPONSES FOR NON-FREQUENTLY ASKED QUESTIONS

Patient variability, clinician experience, and previously unaddressed questions require personalized responses that cannot be fulfilled with a clinical response letter. HCPs in the customer response center and medical information department then use literature search and evaluation skills to determine if relevant information has been published or is available through internal company data (also known as data on file) that addresses the inquiry.[30] If no information is found, the requestor is contacted with the results and a statement that the company cannot provide any information. If relevant publications are found, a response is drafted that includes the citations or reprints (when copyright allows) of the information, and this is provided to the requestor along with a verbal conversation (if possible) to discuss the findings and applicability to the requestor's situation.[30] Requestors expect their inquiry to be addressed in a timely manner and often prefer a verbal answer, allowing for a peer-to-peer discussion and the option to request written information.[30] All medical information requests are valuable and provide timely information to the company regarding the current state of the product in clinical practice. MIRs are typically compiled and analyzed periodically to identify trends and patterns. These trends are published internally in the form of periodic reports; this may signal to a company that a response letter is needed on a particular topic that is reported frequently, to identify new educational gaps, or to lead to the development of new product formulations. Periodic reports may alternatively signal to a company that previous hot topics, or frequently asked questions, are no longer of interest to practitioners in clinical practice, often identifying new areas of interest that practitioners need to have addressed.

_____ Case Study 22–1 Continued

DRUG A received approval by the FDA to be marketed and has quickly become very successful. Awesome Drug, Inc. has expanded the number of HCPs on staff and now employs HCPs in multiple departments within the medical division. Due to the media coverage of

DRUG A's success, other companies are investigating similar compounds. One company has manufactured the product STRIPES for the treatment of mild to moderate hiccups in another country for many years and is looking to enter the U.S. market. It is suspected that STRIPES labeling will include a boxed warning if it is approved because it is well known to occasionally cause yellow stripes to appear on the skin.

Discussion questions:

7. What should Awesome Drug, Inc. do to prepare for inquiries regarding product comparisons to STRIPES and other investigational compounds?
8. What questions should Awesome Drug, Inc. anticipate receiving due to their similar indication to STRIPES?

Adverse Event Reporting

The approval of a medication to the market by the FDA does not automatically denote the complete safety of the product. It is important to keep in mind that any medicine capable of curing or treating a disease may also cause serious adverse events. An adverse drug experience is defined by the FDA *CFR Title 21, Section 314.80—Postmarketing reporting of adverse drug experiences* as "any adverse event associated with the use of a drug in humans, whether or not considered drug related, including the following: an adverse event occurring in the course of the use of a drug product in professional practice; an adverse event occurring from drug overdose whether accidental or intentional; an adverse event occurring from drug abuse; an adverse event occurring from drug withdrawal; and any failure of expected pharmacological action."[21] Adverse drug experiences, or adverse events, are required to be reported to the FDA by pharmaceutical companies. It is the charge of the pharmaceutical company to monitor these risks once the drug is on the market, also known as the postmarketing phase of the drug's life cycle.[21,32]

Pharmaceutical companies learn of adverse events in a variety of ways, including postmarketing trials, publications, customer calls, health care practitioner reports, and in some cases, even by being in close proximity to a personal conversation. The reporting process may vary from company to company as long as the information required by the FDA is reported with each adverse event through completion of FDA Form 3500A. FDA Form 3500A requests such information as patient demographics, medication identifiers, and a description of the adverse event (see http://www.fda.gov/Safety/MedWatch/HowToReport/DownloadForms/default.htm).[24] Postmarketing surveillance allows companies and the

FDA to review suspected adverse events associated with a medication once it reaches the public.[21] This is important because the number of patients enrolled in clinical trials is much smaller than the number of patients who use the medication when it reaches the market.[25] It has been reported that medication clinical trials typically enroll around 10,000 patients, which can often provide enough efficacy and safety information to warrant approval by the FDA.[33] Rare AEs may occur in only 1 out of every 10,000 or 100,000 people, and therefore may go undetected during clinical trials. ❹ *Thus, postmarketing surveillance of adverse events is entrusted with ensuring the safety of the medication for each and every patient exposed to its risks and benefits.* The FDA uses adverse event reports to determine if updates and changes need to be made to the product labeling or package insert of a medication. The strongest labeling change the FDA can require also comes from postmarketing reports of adverse events: the addition of a boxed warning to a medication's labeling. ❺ *The best way to communicate these risks is still being decided by the FDA, and many programs are already in place to communicate safety information to consumers such as Risk Evaluation and Mitigation Strategies (REMS), RiskMAPs, and medication guides, which will be explained in further detail in the next section.*[12,21,24]

COMMUNICATING SAFETY INFORMATION TO CONSUMERS

Risk Evaluation and Mitigation Strategies

The creation of the REMS program is one of the newest methods of communicating safety information to patients and HCPs.[24] REMS were enacted on September 27, 2007, as part of the Food and Drug Administration Amendments Act (FDAAA). REMS provide information specifically regarding the risks of a medication in an effort to ensure that the benefits will outweigh the risks for a potential patient, mitigating the likelihood of a negative outcome with the product's use. Following the enactment of FDAAA, REMS may be requested by the FDA as part of the new drug application (NDA) for initial approval, may be submitted voluntarily as part of the NDA prior to receiving a request from the FDA, or may be requested after drug approval; regardless, REMS content requirements outlined by the FDA, are subject to the FDA's approval, and are enforceable through penalties.[24]

Assessment of REMS

REMS requirements for industry include assessment of the REMS by the company at 18 months, 3 years, and 7 years following approval of the REMS.[24] REMS are assessed by the company to ensure that all appropriate risk information is conveyed and that no changes to the labeling (e.g., new indications) have occurred. As outlined in the current *Guidance for Industry Format and Content of Proposed Risk Evaluation and Mitigation Strategies (REMS), REMS Assessments, and Proposed REMS Modifications*, REMS are required by the FDA to ensure that the benefit-to-risk ratio of a drug is favorable for patients.[24]

REMS Are Enforceable

As previously mentioned, REMS are enforced by the FDA. Failure to comply with the REMS requirements subjects a company to penalties of misbranding. In addition, a responsible person who is found to have violated the requirements of the REMS is subject to civil and federal penalties of fines up to $250,000 per violation ($1 million total per incident). REMS not rectified within 30 days receive double penalties for every 30-day period that passes from the notification date; and the cap becomes $1 million per violation, $10 million per incident.[24]

Medication Guides and More

Medication guides, patient package inserts (PPI), and RiskMAPs are examples of safety measures required by the FDA prior to FDAAA and REMS, compared to communication plans and elements to assure safe use (ETASU), which are additional components that may be included with a REMS.[12,24] Medication guides are paper handouts that are required by the FDA to be issued with certain prescription medications to address issues specific to that drug or drug class in an effort to reduce adverse events.[34] Patient package inserts are required to be issued with oral contraceptive and hormone products to satisfy the requirement that patients using these products are fully informed of all the potential risks and benefits.[19] Manufacturers of oral contraceptives may request informal guidance text from the FDA to help them create a patient package insert. RiskMAPs are safety plans that are designed to achieve prespecified goals and objectives.[35] RiskMAPs are intended to minimize the known safety risks of a medication while concomitantly maintaining the benefits. RiskMAPs can employ one or more tools to achieve their set goals and objectives. REMS present information regarding the risks and benefits of a medication through required content outlined by the FDA. Additional components of REMS may include communication plans and ETASU. Communication plans include detailed information on how the company plans to educate HCPs about its REMS. ETASU are in place in case the previously described components of REMS are not sufficient in explaining the risks and benefits to the patient. In this case, ETASU will be put in place with specific goals to minimize the serious risks associated with the medication (see Table 22–3 for details).

Case Study 22–1 Continued

DRUG A begins receiving reports of patients noting yellow stripes on their skin.

Discussion questions:

9. How must Awesome Drug, Inc. document patient reports of yellow stripes?
10. Does Awesome Drug, Inc. need to send the reports of yellow stripes to any other agency or organization?

DRUG A and STRIPES are found to have a high incidence of causing yellow stripes on the skin. The FDA believes this adverse event warrants additional communication to patients regarding safety information.

Discussion questions:

11. What are some examples of ways safety information is communicated to patients?

SPOTS, a drug with a similar mechanism of action to DRUG A and STRIPES, is preparing its NDA for submission to the FDA for approval to market its product for the treatment of mild to severe hiccups.

Discussion questions:

12. What might the SPOTS manufacturer want to submit voluntarily with its NDA package given the known risks associated with DRUG A and STRIPES?

TABLE 22–3. OTHER METHODS OF COMMUNICATING SAFETY INFORMATION TO CONSUMERS[12,24]

1. Medication Guides	Medication guides may be required: • If patient labeling could mitigate serious adverse events • If the product has serious adverse events relative to benefits that may cause patients to reconsider their use of the product • If patient adherence can seriously alter the drug's effectiveness
2. Patient Package Inserts	Patient package inserts may be required if the FDA believes the package insert will help mitigate a serious risk. Usually either a medication guide or patient package insert exists for a product, not both.
3. RiskMAPs	RiskMAPs are designed to maintain a product's benefits while minimizing its risks through educational materials and prespecified monitoring parameters for HCPs and their patients. RiskMAPs may remain in place indefinitely as a separate entity from REMS, as they often require specific monitoring beyond risk/benefit information.
4. Communication Plan	A communication plan may be requested in which a company submits its plan to educate HCPs about its strategy for minimizing risk/maintaining benefit as outlined in its REMS.
5. Elements to Assure Safe Use (ETASU)	In certain cases, if these previously described measures are not sufficient to mitigate the risks associated with the medication, additional ETASU may be implemented. ETASU include specific goals to minimize serious risk. If a REMS program includes ETASU, the REMS must also include a specific implementation plan and education for the patient to be able to monitor and evaluate the risks of the medication and to recommend improvements to the ETASU.

This table is based on information from reference 12 and 24.

TABLE 22–4. PHARMACEUTICAL INDUSTRY ORGANIZATIONS

Organization	Web Site
American Association of Pharmaceutical Scientists (AAPS)	http://www.aapspharmaceutica.org/
Association of Clinical Research Professionals (ACRP)	http://www.acrpnet.org/default.aspx
Drug Information Association (DIA)	http://www.diahome.org/DIAHome/Home.aspx
Generic Pharmaceutical Association (GPhA)	http://www.gphaonline.org/
Health Industry Representatives Association (HIRA)	http://www.hira.org
Institute for Safe Medication Practices (ISMP)	http://www.ismp.org/
National Association of Pharmaceutical Representatives (NAPRx)	http://www.napsronline.org/
Pharmaceutical Research and Manufacturers of America (PhRMA)	http://www.phrma.org/
Regulatory Affairs Professionals Society (RAPS)	http://www.raps.org/

Staying Connected With the Pharmaceutical Industry

Pharmaceutical companies are dynamic entities that are constantly evolving. In today's media, it is possible to keep up-to-date with new information from industry including drug approvals, publications, and presentations, as well as safety alerts and labeling changes. The Drug Information Association (DIA) and other industry-associated organizations (Table 22–4) are the best resources for pharmaceutical company information. HCPs in clinical practice should familiarize themselves with these reliable sources for industry news so that they can share current industry information with their patients and other HCPs.

Anatomy of Regulatory Agencies

The U.S. Department of Health and Human Services (HHS) is made up of 11 agencies working to promote public health.[36,37] The Office of the Secretary of the HHS also works with the 11 agencies to conduct the work and support the mission of the HHS. These agencies and offices are responsible for a variety of tasks and services that include research, public health, food and drug safety, grants and other funding, and health insurance. Table 22–5 describes each agency and office and provides the mission statement for each. This information shows how the organizations under the HHS have their own goals and objectives. Each organization is further divided into groups depending on the roles and responsibilities assigned to the agency. The anatomy of each regulatory agency or office under the HHS varies. Ultimately, a common theme can be applied to these agencies. The HHS creates

TABLE 22–5. LIST OF HEALTH AND HUMAN SERVICES AGENCIES AND OFFICES

Agency or Office	Purpose
Office of the Secretary (OS)[38]	"To help provide the building blocks that Americans need to live healthy, successful lives."
Administration for Children and Families (ACF)[39]	". . . to provide family assistance (welfare), child support, child care, Head Start, child welfare, and other programs relating to children and families."
Administration on Aging (AoA)[40]	". . . to develop a comprehensive, coordinated, and cost-effective system of home and community-based services that help elderly individuals maintain their health and independence in their homes and communities."
Agency for Healthcare Research and Quality (AHRQ)[41]	". . . to improve the quality, safety, efficiency, and effectiveness of health care for all Americans. Information from AHRQ's research helps people make more informed decisions and improve the quality of health care services."
Agency for Toxic Substances and Disease (ATSDR)[42]	". . . serves the public by using the best science, taking responsive public health actions, and providing trusted health information to prevent harmful exposures and diseases related to toxic substances."
Centers for Disease Control and Prevention (CDC)[43]	". . . to collaborate to create the expertise, information, and tools that people and communities need to protect their health—through health promotion, prevention of disease, injury, and disability, and preparedness for new health threats."
Centers for Medicare and Medicaid Services (CMS)[44]	". . . to ensure effective, up-to-date health care coverage and to promote quality care for beneficiaries."
Food and Drug Administration (FDA)[45]	. . . to protect "the public health by assuring the safety, efficacy, and security of human and veterinary drugs, biological products, medical devices, our nation's food supply, cosmetics, and products that emit radiation."
Health Resources and Services Administration (HRSA)[46]	". . . to improve health and achieve health equity through access to quality services, a skilled health workforce, and innovative programs."
Indian Health Service (IHS)[47]	". . . to raise the physical, mental, social, and spiritual health of American Indians and Alaska Natives to the highest level."
National Institutes of Health (NIH)[48]	". . . to seek fundamental knowledge about the nature and behavior of living systems and the application of that knowledge to enhance health, lengthen life, and reduce the burdens of illness and disability."
Office of Inspector General (OIG)[49]	". . . to protect the integrity of Department of Health and Human Services (HHS) programs, as well as the health and welfare of the beneficiaries of those programs."
Substance Abuse and Mental Health Services Administration (SAMHSA)[50]	". . . to reduce the impact of substance abuse and mental illness on America's communities."

agencies to address specific areas of public health. These agencies are further divided into centers or offices supporting the roles assigned to the agencies. For every aspect of health care (and this is in addition to food and cosmetics, just to name a few) in the United States, there is a center or office that provides regulatory guidance. These centers and offices report to the overarching agency that is a division of the HHS.

MISSION OF REGULATORY AGENCIES

The mission of HHS is to promote and protect the health of all Americans. The mission of the FDA is to protect "the public health by assuring the safety, efficacy, and security of human and veterinary drugs, biological products, medical devices, our nation's food supply, cosmetics, and products that emit radiation."[51] ❻ *The FDA also strives to advance public health by setting standards for the efficient approval of new products that are safe, effective, and helpful to the U.S. public in combination with serving as a source of reputable and fair science-based information for consumers to effectively use these products.*

REGULATORY AGENCY SPOTLIGHT—FOOD AND DRUG ADMINISTRATION

In order to support the missions of the HHS and the FDA, the FDA is made up of six centers, two offices, and one research center. Figure 22–4 depicts the organization of centers and offices at the FDA. One center of particular interest to pharmacists and other HCPs is the Center for Drug Evaluation and Research (CDER). The CDER is the center responsible for evaluating new drugs and also focuses on helping the public access accurate, science-based information needed to use medicines to improve their health. The CDER strives to provide information to the public from all of the FDA published guidance, compliance, and regulatory documents. One way the FDA and CDER provide information to the public is through maintaining and updating the FDA's Web site, http://www.fda.gov. The FDA works to ensure that the Web site allows for easy retrieval and navigation of information, as it is a starting place for most inquiries relating to the FDA. Due to the vast amount of information maintained by the FDA, consumers, health professionals, and industry representatives sometimes have a difficult time accessing and finding the information they need. If the public is unable to find information about human drug products and regulations, these inquiries are sent to the CDER and then are handled by the Division of Drug Information (DDI) in the Office of Communications.

Division of Drug Information at the FDA

The DDI is the CDER's main starting point for general inquiries regarding regulations and human drug products.[52] The Division exists to serve the global community by assisting all inquirers and providing useful, accurate information in a timely manner. The staff

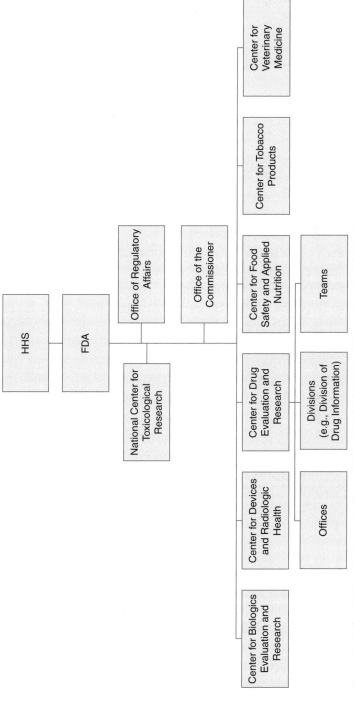

Figure 22–4. Organization of centers and offices within the FDA. HHS, Health and Human Services; FDA, Food and Drug Administration. (This figure represents an overview of how the FDA is organized. Every center and organization under the FDA has its own organization chart. The Center for Drug Evaluation and Research is further broken down into its organizational parts as an example.)

TABLE 22–6. DDI REQUESTORS

Consumers	Industry
Health Care Professionals	Consultants
Academia	Attorneys
Federal/State Agencies	Insurance Providers
Investment Brokers	Special Interest Groups
Clinical Investigators	Law Enforcement
Correctional Facilities	International Government Agencies

at the DDI is mainly made up of pharmacists serving as consumer safety officers (CSOs), but other health care professionals also are part of the DDI. The main role of the CSO is to serve as an expert and give guidance on all aspects of CDER activities. This requires the CSO to have a wide knowledge base on not only human drug products, but also on the regulations surrounding these drug products.

The division has several unique characteristics that differentiate it from the typical drug information center; mainly the customers, the resources used, and the role of the DDI. First, the DDI has a very unique customer makeup. The majority of requests that come from within the United States to the FDA are from consumers, then industry and HCPs. However, it is not uncommon for the DDI to prepare responses for a wide variety of requestors (Table 22–6). The DDI also responds to several international inquirers, with the majority of requests coming from international industry, then consumers, then HCPs. Second, although the DDI will use traditional drug information resources when needed, the majority of the information provided to requestors comes directly from the FDA's Web site. CSOs are trained to utilize publically available information first and then, if needed, also rely on an internal database that serves as a repository for previously researched and answered inquires. Finally, the role of the DDI is unique because not only does it serve the general public, but similar to medical information in the industry, the DDI also works internally to support the Center, often by collaborating with CDER scientists to create consistent overviews of important and emerging topics.

Drug Information Services Provided by the FDA

Drug information services provided by the DDI fit into one of three categories: correspondence, dissemination, and other (Table 22–7). Correspondence represents a majority of the contact made by the public with the Division. In an average month, the DDI handles 3000 e-mails, 4000 telephone calls, and about 600 letters. Each contact made with DDI will

TABLE 22–7. DRUG INFORMATION SERVICES PROVIDED BY THE DDI

CORRESPONDENCE
- Phone calls 1-888-INFO-FDA)
- E-mails (druginfo@fda.hhs.gov)
- Mail (Division of Drug Information [CDER], Office of Communication, HILL 4th Fl, 10001 New Hampshire Avenue, Silver Spring, MD 20903)
- MedWatch (1-800-FDA-1088)

DISSEMINATION
- DDI Web site
- DDI Listserv
- Twitter @FDA_Drug_Info
  Facebook
  RSS Feeds
- Podcasts, Publications, Posters, Presentations, FDA Drug Info Rounds videos
- Exhibits

OTHER
- Imprint Identification
- International Visitations
- FDA Pharmacy Student Program
- FDA Regulatory Pharmaceutical Fellowship
- CDERLearn Continuing Education
- FDA Liaisons
- Enterprise Database

receive a response. In the past, the most common inquiries related to regulatory issues, such as the drug review process (Table 22–8). Many times the same question will be asked in a different way by a different requestor. For example, a consumer might call the FDA wanting to know when a generic for a certain drug will be available. The same question might be addressed when industry contacts the FDA wanting to know when it can manufacture the generic version of a certain drug, or HCPs call wanting to know when the generic version will be available to prescribe/dispense or to update formulary recommendations.

TABLE 22–8. CLASSIFICATION OF COMMON DDI INQUIRIES

Drug review process
Generic drugs
Specific drug safety issues
Investigational new drugs
New drug approvals
Importation of drugs
Adverse reactions
Nonprescription drugs
Drug identification
Recalls and shortages

■ ALBUTEROL

The FDA announced a final rule to amend regulations (21 CFR 2.125) on the use of ozone-depleting substances (ODSs) in medical products. This rule established December 31, 2008, as the date by which production and sale of single-ingredient albuterol chlorofluorocarbon (CFC) metered-dose inhalers (MDIs) had to stop, by removing the essential-use designation for albuterol MDIs under 2.125. Many consumers contacted the DDI with several questions and concerns regarding the discontinuation of single-ingredient albuterol CFC MDIs.

Discussion questions:

1. Because the rules stated that production had to stop by December 31, 2008, a pharmacist wanted to know if he could dispense the remaining CFC MDIs he has in stock after December 31, 2008, until he runs out. Can he do this? What information can you find on the FDA's Web site to support your answer?
2. A pharmacist wanted to know if he could automatically switch patients from an albuterol CFC to an HFA inhaler. Can he do this? What rules and regulations support your answer?
3. A patient contacted the DDI to report that the new HFA inhalers do not work for her and she cannot feel any effect after using the inhaler. What do you tell her? Where can you refer her to report this problem?
4. An activist group sent hundreds of letters to the FDA regarding the new co-pays averaging $125.00 for the HFA inhalers (previously $10.00 with CFC inhalers). What type of role does the FDA have in regulating the price of medications? What impact can the FDA have on the pricing of medications? Based on the information you find, do you feel it is right that the FDA can mandate changes that will impact the price of medications to consumers?
5. A mother of an asthmatic child called the FDA to express that the government cares more about the ozone than the health of her child. What potential responses can you develop that support both arguments?

New Food and Drug Administration Amendments Act (FDAAA) requirements encouraging the public to report any suspected adverse drug events to the FDA as part of its MedWatch program (see Chapter 15) has drastically changed the DDI's scope and workload.[53] Recent estimates show that almost 80% of phone calls made to the DDI are generated from the new MedWatch program initiative. As part of the MedWatch program (under FDAAA), the following statement is now required on all published direct-to-consumer advertisements and is even being printed on many over-the-counter medication and dietary supplement labels: "You are encouraged to report negative side effects of prescription drugs to the FDA. Visit www.fda.gov/medwatch, or call 1-800-FDA-1088." Now that consumers are readily exposed and have access to a toll-free number, the DDI has had a drastic increase in adverse event reporting. Consumer safety officers in the DDI will respond to all calls from those who are simply looking to report to those who are looking for more information about a drug or other product regulated by the FDA. For those who are looking to report, consumers are referred to the MedWatch Web site (http://www.fda.gov/Safety/MedWatch/HowToReport/default.htm), mailed a MedWatch form (MedWatch form can be found at http://www.fda.gov/Safety/MedWatch/HowToReport/DownloadForms/default.htm), or their report is taken orally over the phone. If consumers are looking for more information about a drug, then the consumer safety officer will assist them as appropriate.

Many may assume that the FDA only reacts to public concerns or requests, but in truth ❼ *the DDI has several proactive mechanisms to communicate information about human drug products to the public.* Much of this proactive information is available to the public through the DDI's Web site, listserver, CDERLearn programs, continuing education, drug safety podcasts, videos, Twitter updates, RSS feeds and Facebook page. All of these examples represent new ways to promote the safe and effective use of human drug products.

FDA-Sponsored Drug Information Resources

Like many drug information centers, the DDI utilizes traditional drug information resources and databases when needed to respond to inquiries. However, the first place consumer safety officers visit when preparing their response will be the FDA's Web site. The FDA's Web site contains valuable information and strives to make the most frequently requested information readily available. However, with an organization as large as the FDA, consumers are often daunted by the sheer amount of material readily available on the Web site. Table 22–9 lists commonly used FDA Web sites and the intended purpose for each page. In order to select the most appropriate FDA-sponsored resource/Web site, practitioners must have a basic understanding of what Web sites are available and what information is provided. Table 22–9 provides a brief overview of these Web sites, and practitioners are strongly encouraged to visit these Web sites on their own and view for themselves the variety of information available to the public.

TABLE 22–9. **FDA-SPONSORED DRUG INFORMATION LINKS**

Web Site	Purpose
http://www.fda.gov/ AboutFDA/ CentersOffices/CDER/ ucm082585.htm	Division of Drug Information (DDI). Provides background and purpose of DDI. Also maintains several helpful links for finding information relating to: • Student and fellowship opportunities • Frequently asked questions about drugs • Continuing education • Drug identification
http://www.fda.gov/drugs	CDER. The DDI's first resource for responding to questions from the public and where most questions pertaining to regulations can be answered. Site maintains sections dedicated to the following topics: • Emergency preparedness • Drug approvals and databases • Drug safety and availability • Drug development and approval process • Guidance, compliance, and regulatory information • Drug science and research • Consumer, health professional, and industry resources • Recalls and alerts • Approvals and clearances
http://www.fda.gov/Drugs/ DrugSafety/default.htm	Drug safety communications. This page provides a list of drugs that have been the subject of postmarketing drug safety communication efforts.
http://www.fda.gov/ AboutFDA/ContactFDA/ StayInformed/GetEmail Updates/default.htm	Email Updates. This page allows users to sign up for the FDA e-mail listserver that distributes important FDA news and information as it is available.
http://www.accessdata. fda.gov/scripts/cder/ drugsatfda/index.cfm	Drugs@FDA. Searchable FDA database containing official information about FDA-approved brand and generic drugs and therapeutic biological products. This database also contains: • Labels for approved drug products • Consumer information for drugs approved after 1998 • Approval history for drug products (including FDA review documents)
http://www.accessdata. fda.gov/scripts/cder/ ob/default.cfm	Orange Book: Approved Drug Products With Therapeutic Equivalence Evaluations. Free electronic access to the Approved Drug Products With Therapeutic Equivalence Evaluations list. Can search by active ingredient, proprietary name, patent, applicant holder, or application number.
http://www.accessdata. fda.gov/scripts/cder/ ndc/default.cfm	National Drug Code Directory Searchable list of universal product identifier for approved and unapproved human drugs.

continued

TABLE 22–9. FDA-SPONSORED DRUG INFORMATION LINKS (*Continued*)

Web Site	Purpose
http://www.fda.gov/ Training/ForHealth Professionals/default.htm	CDERLearn. Web page for CDER-sponsored educational tutorials, some with CE credit
http://www.fda.gov/Safety/ MedWatch/ default.htm	MedWatch for the FDA's safety information and adverse event reporting program. Contains a searchable list of safety labeling changes and updated safety information. Also, it contains links to online and downloadable forms to report serious problems to the FDA.
http://www.fda.gov/Drugs/ DrugSafety/ DrugSafetyPodcasts/ default.htm	Drug Safety Podcasts prepared in order to address frequently asked questions from consumers and HCPs.
http://www.fda.gov/Drugs/ ResourcesForYou/ HealthProfessionals/ ucm211957.htm	FDA Drug Info Rounds videos are training videos offered to pharmacist covering drug information topics to help improve patient outcomes.
http://twitter.com/#!/FDA_ Drug_Info	FDA Drug Information Twitter account.

Opportunities Within the FDA

There are several opportunities for both current and future health professionals within the FDA.

FOR THE STUDENT

The FDA offers many opportunities for health professional students. One of the most popular programs is the FDA Pharmacy Student Experiential Program.[54] This program provides an opportunity for students to gain experience working within various divisions of the FDA. Depending on where the student is placed, he or she will have the chance to learn about the FDA's multidisciplinary processes for addressing public health issues involving drugs, biologics, or medical devices. Pharmacy students who complete the FDA Pharmacy Student Experiential Program will gain unique experience in regulatory affairs that will prove beneficial to their future careers.

Student opportunities are also available within the U.S. Public Health Service (USPHS) Commissioned Corps.[55] The Commissioned Corps created the Commissioned Corps Officer Student Training and Extern Program (COSTEP) for students studying in the health professions field. There are two programs: the Junior COSTEP and Senior COSTEP. Students in selected health fields can apply to the Junior COSTEP program if they have completed at least 1 to 2 years of their professional program. The Junior COSTEP program takes place during school breaks, and most assignments last anywhere from 1 to 4 months. There is no obligation to commit or work for the Commissioned Corps after graduation, as this opportunity is focused on allowing students to experience the program before joining.

Full-time health professional students having 8 months of education or less left in their final year are eligible to join the Senior COSTEP program. SRCOSTEP participants sign a contract to work for the Commissioned Corps after graduation and receive financial assistance in return. In general, the service obligation is equal to twice the time the Corps sponsors the student.

One major benefit for those students enrolled in the COSTEP programs is the diverse opportunities available after completion of the program. Some have gone on to work in labs at the National Institutes of Health, provide care to patients in the Bureau of Prisons, or join agencies within the FDA or Centers for Disease Control and Prevention, to name a few.

Those students who wish to find out more information or apply are encouraged to visit the U.S. Public Service Web site at http://www.usphs.gov/student/.

Postgraduate opportunities for students are also available with the FDA. One opportunity is the Regulatory Pharmaceutical Fellowship.[56] The purpose of this fellowship is to develop candidates with advanced experience in the medical and regulatory aspects of drug information dissemination or marketing. The program exposes fellows to three areas of regulatory pharmaceutical experience: FDA, academia, and pharmaceutical industry.

Only a few of the potential opportunities for health professional students are described in this chapter. There are several opportunities for students interested in regulatory affairs beyond what is described here, and students are encouraged to research and contact those programs directly for further information.

FOR THE PROFESSIONAL

Opportunities for health care professionals to join the FDA are growing. One opportunity is the FDA/CDER Academic Collaboration Program.[20] This unique opportunity will allow 15 to 20 recent graduates from a health-related field to begin work for the Commissioned Corps and obtain a Masters or Doctor of Philosophy degree in Pharmaceutical Outcomes and Policy. The goal of this program will be to develop health professionals with advanced experience in regulatory science.

Another opportunity for current health professionals is to join an Agency under HHS, like the FDA, directly.[57] Due to new legislation, the CDER has an ongoing need to recruit qualified health professionals in order to carry on the mission of the Agency. Health professionals have several opportunities to serve either as civil servants or join the U.S. Commissioned Corps. Physicians are needed to help evaluate submitted clinical trial data of new drugs for safety and efficacy concerns. Scientists are utilized to help evaluate the technical portions of investigational new drug (IND) or NDA. CSOs are vital to managing and monitoring regulatory teams in certain divisions. The CSO is sometimes referred to as a project manager or division liaison, and often these roles are filled with biologists, chemists, pharmacists, physicians, engineers, etc. Statisticians and computer specialists are also hired for statistical and technical support of human drug product reviews. The team of health professionals working at the FDA is diverse, and so are the opportunities to help fulfill the mission of ensuring the safety and efficacy of drugs available to the American public.

Conclusion

Pharmaceutical companies and regulatory agencies provide many services to and have many opportunities for HCPs. Pharmaceutical companies' scientific or medical divisions are filled with highly trained HCPs working in a variety of specialized fields in order to provide medical information and support for various brands marketed by the company. Efforts are currently ongoing to make the pharmaceutical industry more transparent in the way it conducts the business of drug development and product marketing. In addition, regulatory agencies are also focusing on ways to monitor and improve the communication of risk information from industry to the general public. Not only are regulatory agencies, like the FDA, striving to hold the pharmaceutical industry to higher standards, but efforts to improve transparency and communication from the regulatory agencies to the general public are being made as well. Most pharmaceutical companies have detailed and structured processes for responding to HCP questions. Regulatory agencies also have various methods of disseminating information relating to public health to HCPs. An informed HCP is a professional who is aware of the valuable information and roles that pharmaceutical companies and regulatory agencies can provide.

Self-Assessment Questions

1. Which of the following is a department within the medical division that employs health care professionals (HCPs)?
   a. Research and Development
   b. Medical Information
   c. Epidemiology
   d. Biometrics

2. Which of the following best describes an appropriate lifecycle of a medical information request?
   a. Inquiry solicited by representative, standard response letter verbally communicated.
   b. Inquiry solicited by representative, package insert information verbally communicated.
   c. Inquiry submitted by HCP, package insert information verbally communicated.
   d. Inquiry submitted by representative, opinion of industry HCP verbally communicated.

3. Identify which of the following is *not* a typical component of a clinical response letter.
   a. Outline
   b. Opening
   c. Signature
   d. Closing

4. Which of the following departments may be involved in approving a clinical response letter?
   a. Medical Publications
   b. Marketing
   c. Medical Information
   d. Metrics

5. HCPs are regulated in industry in which of the following ways?
   a. Externally by the FDA
   b. Externally by FDAAA
   c. Internally by SOPs
   d. All of the above

6. Identify which interaction between pharmaceutical industry and HCPs is unacceptable according to PhRMA's *Code on Interactions With Health Care Professionals*.
   a. An industry representative stops by an HCP's office to invite him or her to an upcoming industry-sponsored continuing medical education event.
   b. An industry representative makes an appointment with an HCP to discuss a newly approved indication for BESTDRUGEVER.
   c. An industry representative drops off a basket of BESTDRUGEVER pens, mugs, and coffee to an HCP's office.
   d. An industry representative refers an HCP to contact his or her medical information department to discuss an off-label use.

7. What is the purpose of the FDA mandating that the pharmaceutical industry collect adverse event information?
   a. The FDA wants to ensure that the pharmaceutical industry captures all post-marketing adverse effects (AEs).
   b. The FDA wants to ensure that the pharmaceutical industry HCPs are busy at their desks.
   c. The FDA wants to ensure that the pharmaceutical industry is burdened by AE paperwork.
   d. The FDA wants to ensure that the pharmaceutical industry captures all bad doctors causing AEs.

8. Which of the following is *not* a valid method for communicating safety information to consumers?
   a. Elements to assure safe use
   b. Risk minimization action plans
   c. Risk mitigation and evaluation strategies
   d. Risk minimization television advertisements

9. Identify which of the following is an organization associated with the pharmacy industry.
   a. American Pharmacists Association
   b. Drug Information Association
   c. American Medical Association
   d. Parenteral Drug Association

10. The role of the Division of Drug Information (DDI) at the Food and Drug Administration (FDA) is best described by which of the following?
    a. The CDER's last option for unanswered general inquires regarding regulations and human drug products.
    b. The division exists as a traditional drug information center responding to calls and questions from the general consumer.
    c. The CDER's main starting point for specific inquiries regarding minute details of interdivision decision-making processes.
    d. The division exists to serve the global community by assisting all inquirers and providing useful, accurate information in a timely manner.
    e. Answers b and d only.

11. Which of the following is *not* a main difference between the DDI and a typical drug information center?
    a. The customers
    b. The resources used
    c. The role of the DDI

    d. None of the above

    e. All of the above

12. An FDA consumer safety officer prepares a podcast updating health profession-als about a new safety concern with a marketed human drug product. This activ-ity would best be categorized by which of the following?

    a. Correspondence of information by the FDA

    b. Dissemination of information by the FDA

    c. Development of a standard response

    d. Reactive responses by the FDA

13. An international manufacturer e-mails the DDI with questions regarding the regulations for selling a new herbal product containing toothpaste in the United States. When the DDI responds, this activity would best be categorized by which of the following?

    a. Correspondence of information by the FDA

    b. Dissemination of information by the FDA

    c. Development of a standard response

    d. Reactive responses by the FDA

14. A researcher contacts the DDI wanting to know about the approval process for a marketed human drug process. Which Web site would be the best place to refer the requestor for this information?

    a. CDER homepage

    b. Drugs@FDA database

    c. Orange Book online

    d. National Drug Code Directory online

    e. Index to drug-specific information page

15. Which of the following is *not* a student opportunity within the FDA?

    a. Junior COSTEP Program

    b. Senior COSTEP Program

    c. FDA Pharmacy Student Experiential Program

    d. FDA/CDER Academic Collaboration Program

    e. Commissioned Corps Officer Student Training and Extern Program

REFERENCES

1. Cadogan AA, Fung SM. The changing roles of medical communications professionals: evolu-tion of the core curriculum. Drug Inf J. 2009 Nov;43(6):673-84.

2. Soares SC, March C. Metrics implementation in an industry-based medical information department and comparison to metrics tracked within other industry-based medical infor-mation departments. Drug Inf J. 2008 Mar;42(2):175-82.

3. Marrone CM, Bass JL, Klinger CJ. Survey of medical liaison practices across the pharmaceutical industry. Drug Inf J. 2007 Jul;41(4):457-70.

4. Department of Health and Human Services (U.S.). FDA guidance for industry: industry-supported scientific and educational activities. Final rules. Fed Regist. 1997 Nov;62(232):64093.

5. ACCME standards for commercial support: standards to ensure the independence of CME activities. Chicago (IL): Accreditation Council for Continuing Medical Education (U.S.); 2007. p. 3.

6. Electronic records; electronic signatures, 21 C.F.R. Sect. 11 (2009).

7. Good laboratory practice for nonclinical laboratory studies, 21 C.F.R. Sect. 58 (2009).

8. General, 21 C.F.R. Sect. 200 (2009).

9. Labeling, 21 C.F.R. Sect. 201 (2009).

10. Prescription Drug Advertising, 21 C.F.R. Sect. 202 (2009).

11. Prescription Drug Marketing, 21 C.F.R. Sect. 203 (2009).

12. Medication Guides for Prescription Drug Products, 21 C.F.R. Sect. 208 (2009).

13. Requirement for Authorized Dispensers and Pharmacies to Distribute a Side Effects Statement, 21 C.F.R. Sect. 209 (2009).

14. Current Good Manufacturing Practice in Manufacturing, Packing, or Holding of Drugs; General, 21 C.F.R. Sect. 210 (2009).

15. Current Good Manufacturing Practice for Finished Pharmaceuticals, 21 C.F.R. Sect. 211 (2009).

16. Special Requirements for Specific Human Drugs, 21 C.F.R. Sect. 250 (2009).

17. Controlled Drugs, 21 C.F.R. Sect. 290 (2009).

18. Drugs; Official Names and Established Names, 21 C.F.R. Sect. 299 (2009).

19. New Drugs, 21 C.F.R. Sect. 310 (2009).

20. Investigational New Drug Application, 21 C.F.R. Sect. 312 (2009).

21. Applications for FDA Approval to Market a New Drug, 21 C.F.R. Sect. 314 (2009).

22. Bioavailability and Bioequivalence Requirements, 21 C.F.R. Sect. 320 (2009).

23. Gough J, Hamrell M. Standard operating procedures (SOPs): how companies can determine which documents they must put in place. Drug Inf J. 2010 Jan;44(1):49-54.

24. U.S. Food and Drug Administration [Internet]. Silver Spring (MD): U.S. Department of Health and Human Services; c2010. MedWatch Form FDA 3500A; [cited 2010 Mar 4]; [2 screens]. Available from: http://www.fda.gov/Safety/MedWatch/HowToReport/Download-Forms/ucm149238.htm.

25. Stegarchis A, Boudrea D, Hazlet TK. Pharmacotherapy: A Pathophysiologic Approach. 7th ed. New York (NY): McGraw Hill; c2008:67-9. Chapter 9, Pharmacoepidemiology.

26. PhRMA: New Medicines. New Hope. [Internet]. Washington, DC: Pharmaceutical Researchers and Manufacturers of America; c2010. Code on interactions with healthcare professionals; 2009 Jan [cited 2010 Mar 10]; [about 3 screens]. Available from: http://www.phrma.org/code_on_interactions_with_healthcare_professionals.

27. Bryant PJ, Steinberg MJ, Marrone CM. A practical approach to evidence-based medicine for the medical communications professional. Drug Inf J. 2009 Nov;43(6):663-72.

28. Gazo A, Wyble C, Schiappacasse H, Petses J, Toscano M, El-Toukhy N, et al. Mega mergers: a systematic approach to the integration of two medical information departments. Drug Inf J. 2008 Mar;42(2):183-91.

29. Donald T, Marsh C, Ashworth L. An assessment of preparation methods and personnel requirements in a medical information department during product launch. Drug Inf J. 2007 Mar;41(2):241-9.

30. Black P, March C, Ashworth L. Assessment of customer satisfaction with verbal responses provided by a pharmaceutical company's third-party medical information call center. Drug Inf J. 2009 May;43(3):263-71.

31. Fett R, Bruns K, Lischka-Wittmann S. Results of a qualitative market research study evaluating the quality of medical letters. Drug Inf J. 2009;43(6):697-703.

32. U.S. Food and Drug Administration [Internet]. Silver Spring (MD): U.S. Department of Health and Human Services; c2010. FDA guidance for industry: format and content of proposed risk evaluation and mitigation strategies (REMS): REMS assessments, and proposed REMS modifications. Draft Guidance; [cited 2010 Mar 9]; [38 screens]. Available from: http://www.fda.gov/downloads/Drugs/GuidanceComplianceRegulatoryInformation/Guidances/UCM184128.pdf/.

33. Dieck GS, Berger S, Kracov DA, Manion D, Tanner A. Constant vigilance: the role of pharmaceutical companies in medicine safety. Drug Inf J. 2009 Sep;43(5):603-16.

34. U.S. Food and Drug Administration[Internet]. Silver Spring (MD): U.S. Department of Health and Human Services; c2010. Medication guides; [cited 2010 Sept 15]; [1 screen]. Available from:http://www.fda.gov/Drugs/DrugSafety/UCM085729.

35. U.S. Food and Drug Administration [Internet]. Silver Spring (MD): U.S. Department of Health and Human Services; c2010. FDA guidance for industry: development and use of risk minimization action plans; [cited 2010 Sept 15]; [27 screens]. Available from: http://www.fda.gov/downloads/RegulatoryInformation/Guidances/UCM126830.pdf.

36. U.S. Department of Health and Human Services [Internet]. Washington, DC: U.S. Department of Health and Human Services; c2010. About HHS; [cited 2010 May 1]; [about 1 screen]. Available from: http://www.hhs.gov/about/.

37. U.S. Department of Health and Human Services [Internet]. Washington, DC: U.S. Department of Health and Human Services; c2010. About HHS; [cited 2010 May 1]; [about 1 screen]. Available from: http://www.hhs.gov/about/.

38. U.S. Department of Health and Human Services [Internet]. Washington, DC: U.S. Department of Health and Human Services; c2010. HHS secretary; [cited 2010 Sept 20]; [about 1 screen]. Available from: http://www.hhs.gov/secretary/.

39. Administration for Children and Families [homepage on the Internet]. Washington, DC: U.S. Department of Health and Human Services; c2010 [cited 2010 Sept 20]. Available from: http://www.acf.hhs.gov/index.html.

40. Administration on Aging [Internet]. Washington, DC: U.S. Department of Health and Human Services; c2010. About AoA; [updated 2010 Feb 1; cited 2010 Sept 20]; [about 1 screen]. Available from: http://www.aoa.gov/AoARoot/About/index.aspx.

41. Agency for Healthcare Research and Quality [Internet]. Rockville (MD): U.S. Department of Health and Human Services; c2010. Health Care: AHRQ Mission and Budget Subdirectory Page; [cited 2010 Sept 20]; [about 2 screens]. Available from: http://www.ahrq.gov/about/budgtix.htm.

42. Agency for Toxic Substances and Disease Registry [homepage on the Internet]. Atlanta (GA): Centers for Disease Control and Prevention; c2010 [updated 2010 Sept 20; cited 2010 Sep 20]; [about 2 screens]. Available from: http://www.atsdr.cdc.gov/.

43. Centers for Disease Control and Prevention [Internet]. Atlanta (GA): Centers for Disease Control and Prevention; c2010. About CDC organization; [updated 2010 Sept 20; cited 2010 Sep 20]; [about 2 screens]. Available from: http://www.cdc.gov/about/organization/cio.htm.

44. Centers for Medicare and Medicaid Services [Internet]. Baltimore (MD): U.S. Department of Health and Human Services; c2010. Overview mission, vision, and goals; [updated 2010 Jun 1; cited 2010 Sept 20]; [about 2 screens]. Available from: http://www.cms.gov/MissionVisionGoals/.

45. U.S. Department of Health and Human Services [Internet]. Washington, DC: U.S. Department of Health and Human Services; c2010. About HHS; [cited 2010 May 1]; [about 1 screen]. Available from: http://www.hhs.gov/about/.

46. U.S. Department of Health and Human Services Health Resources and Services Administration [Internet]. Washington, DC: U.S. Department of Health and Human Services; c2010. About HRSA; [cited 2010 Sept 20]; [about 1 screen]. Available from: http://www.hrsa.gov/about/index.html.

47. Indian Health Service [Internet]. Rockville (MD): U.S. Department of Health and Human Services; c2010. Introduction to HIS by Dr. Yvette Roubideaux; [cited 2010 Sept 20]; [about 2 screens]. Available from: http://www.ihs.gov/PublicInfo/PublicAffairs/Welcome_Info/IHSintro.asp.

48. National Institutes of Health [Internet]. Bethesda (MD): U.S. Department of Health and Human Services; c2010. About the National Institutes of Health; [updated 2010 May 18; cited 2010 Sept 20]; [about 2 screens]. Available from: http://www.nih.gov/about/mission.htm.

49. Office of Inspector General [homepage on the Internet]. Washington, DC: U.S. Department of Health and Human Services; [cited 2010 Sept 20]. Available from: http://www.oig.hhs.gov/.

50. Substance Abuse and Mental Health Services Administration [Internet]. Rockville (MD): U.S. Department of Health and Human Services; c2010. Agency overview; [updated 2010 Aug 13; cited 2010 Sept 20]; [about 2 screens]. Available from: http://www.samhsa.gov/About/background.aspx.

51. U.S. Food and Drug Administration [Internet]. Silver Spring (MD): U.S. Department of Health and Human Services; c2010. What we do; 2009 May 22 [cited 2010 May 1]; [about 1 screen]. Available from: http://www.fda.gov/AboutFDA/WhatWeDo/default.htm.

52. U.S. Food and Drug Administration [Internet]. Silver Spring (MD): U.S. Department of Health and Human Services; c2010. Division of Drug Information; 2009 Nov 3 [cited 2010 May 1]; [about 3 screens]. Available from: http://www.fda.gov/AboutFDA/CentersOffices/CDER/ucm082585.htm.

53. U.S. Food and Drug Administration [Internet]. Silver Spring (MD): U.S. Department of Health and Human Services; c2010. Division of Drug Marketing, Advertising, and Communications (DDMAC); 2010 Mar 1 [cited 2010 May 1]; [about 2 screens]. Available from: http://www.fda.gov/AboutFDA/CentersOffices/CDER/ucm090142.htm.

54. U.S. Food and Drug Administration [Internet]. Silver Spring (MD): U.S. Department of Health and Human Services; c2010. FDA Pharmacy Student Experiential Program; 2010 Mar 23 [cited 2010 May 3]; [about 3 screens]. Available from: http://www.fda.gov/AboutFDA/WorkingatFDA/FellowshipInternshipGraduateFacultyPrograms/PharmacyStudentExperientialProgramCDER/default.htm.

55. U.S. Public Health Service Commissioned Corps [Internet]. Rockville (MD): U.S. Department of Health and Human Services; c2010.Student opportunities; 2010 Jan 4 [cited 2010 May 3]; [about 4 screens]. Available from: http://www.usphs.gov/student/.

56. U.S. Food and Drug Administration [Internet]. Silver Spring (MD): U.S. Department of Health and Human Services; c2010. Regulatory Pharmaceutical Fellowship; 2009 Nov 3 [cited 2010 May 3]; [about 2 screens]. Available from: http://www.fda.gov/AboutFDA/CentersOffices/CDER/ucm188804.htm.

57. U.S. Food and Drug Administration [Internet]. Silver Spring (MD): U.S. Department of Health and Human Services; c2010. Jobs at the Center for Drug Evaluation and Research; 2010 Jan 22 [cited 2010 May 4]; [about 6 screens]. Available from: http://www.fda.gov/AboutFDA/CentersOffices/CDER/ucm081244.htm.

Appendices

Appendix 2-1

Drug Consultation Request Form

☐ Completed (Review Pending)   **DRUG CONSULTATION REQUEST FORM**   LOG# _____
☐ Reviewed   DRUG INFORMATION SERVICE   Final QA Check _____
☐ Communicated   NATIONAL INSTITUTES OF HEALTH

REQUESTER INFORMATION

Date Received _____   Time Received _____ AM / PM *(circle one)*
Name _____   Phone# _____   FAX# _____
Pager# _____   e-mail _____

INTERNAL:	EXTERNAL:	AFFILIATION CATEGORY:
☐ MD ☐ DDS	☐ Pharmacist	☐ Institute _____
☐ RN	☐ Physician	☐ Clinic _____
☐ Pharmacist	☐ General Public	☐ Pt Care Unit _____
☐ Other Professional _____	☐ Other Healthcare Professional _____	☐ Other _____
☐ NIH Patient	☐ Other Professional/Organization _____	
☐ Other _____		

HOW RECEIVED: ☐ Phone   ☐ Voice Mail   ☐ E-Mail   ☐ Mail   ☐ FAX   ☐ In Person   ☐ Referred by : _____
PRIORITY: ☐ Urgent   ☐ High Priority   ☐ Routine   ☐ Low Priority

ORIGINAL QUESTION / REQUEST

CLEAR STATEMENT(S) OF ACTUAL DRUG INFORMATION NEED

PERTINENT PATIENT DATA / BACKGROUND INFORMATION

Name _____   Pt Care Unit/Clinic _____   ☐ Inpatient ☐ Outpatient
Age _____ Race _____ ☐ Male ☐ Female   Height _____ cm _____ ft _____ in   Weight _____ lb _____ kg
Primary Diagnosis _____   Allergies/Intolerances _____
End-Organ Function _____   Special Circumstances _____

CC:
HPI:
PMH:
FH:
SH:
ROS:
Meds:
PE:
Labs:
Diagnostics:
Problem List:

LOG# _____

CLASSIFICATION(S) OF REQUEST

☐ Administration (Routes/Methods)
☐ Adverse Effects/Intolerances
☐ Allergy/Cross Reactivity
☐ Alternative Medicine
☐ Biotechnology/Gene Therapy
☐ Clinical Nutrition/Metabolic Support
☐ Compatibility/Stability/Storage
☐ Contraindications/Precautions
☐ Cost/Pharmacoeconomics
☐ Dose/Schedule
☐ Drug Delivery Devices/Systems/Forms
☐ Drug Interactions (Drug-Drug, Drug-Food)
☐ Drug of choice/Therapeutic Alternatives/Therapeutic Use
☐ Drug Standards/Legal/Regulatory
☐ Drug Use in Special Populations
  (Effects of Age, Organ System Function, Disease,
  Extracorporeal Circulation, etc.)
☐ Excipients/Compounding/Formulations

☐ Investigational Products (Pre-Clinical and Clinical)
☐ Lab Test Interferences (Drug-Lab Interactions)
☐ Monitoring Parameters
☐ Nonprescription Products
☐ Patient Information/Education
☐ Pharmacokinetics (LADME/TDM)
☐ Pharmacology/Mechanisms/Pharmacodynamics
☐ Physicochemical Properties
☐ Poisoning/Toxicology (Environmental/Occupational Exposure,
  Mutagenicity, Carcinogenicity)
☐ Pregnancy/Lactation/Teratogenicity/Fertility
☐ Product Availability/Status
☐ Product Identification (Tablet/Capsule)
☐ Product Identification (Generic, Brand, Orphan,
  Foreign, Chemical Substances, Discontinued Products, etc.)
☐ Product Information
☐ Study Design/Protocol Development/Research Support
☐ Other _____

REQUEST CATEGORY

☐ Patient Care   ☐ Research   ☐ Other _____

RESPONSE (Referenced)

REFERENCES (Numbered)

TRACKING / FOLLOW-UP

Request Received By_____   Reviewed By_____
Response Formulated By_____   Response Communicated By_____
                                                                Time Required to Answer_____

☐ Documents/Literature Provided   ☐ Verbal Response   ☐ E-Mail   ☐ Written Response/Consult

OUTCOME / FOLLOW-UP

Appendix 2-2

Sample Questions for Obtaining Background Information From Requestors[*]

Regardless of the type or classification of the question, the following information should be obtained:

1. The requestor's name
2. The requestor's location and/or page number
3. The requestor's affiliation (institution or practice), if a health care professional
4. The requestor's frame of reference (i.e., title, profession/occupation, rank)
5. The resources the requestor has already consulted
6. If the request is patient specific or academic
7. The patient's diagnosis and other medications
8. The urgency of the request (negotiate time of response)

The following questions could be asked when appropriate for calls of the following classes[a]:

Availability of Dosage Forms

1. What is the dosage form desired?
2. What administration routes are feasible with this patient?
3. Is this patient alert and oriented?
4. Does the patient have a water or sodium restriction?
5. What other special factors regarding drug administration should be considered?

Identification of Product

1. What is the generic or trade name of the product?
2. Who is the manufacturer? What is the country of origin?
3. What is the suspected use of this product?
4. Under what circumstances was this product found? Who found the product?
5. What is the dosage form, color markings, size, etc.?
6. What was your source of information? Was it reliable?

---

[a]Question for only selected types of requests presented; other questions would be appropriate for other types of requests.
[*]Originally prepared by Craig Kirkwood.

General Product Information

1. Why is there a particular concern for this product?
2. Is written patient information required?
3. What type of information do you need?
4. Is this for an inpatient, outpatient, or private patient?

Foreign Drug Identification

1. What is the drug's generic name, trade name, manufacturer, and/or country of origin?
2. What is the dosage form, markings, color, strength, or size?
3. What is the suspected use of the drug? How often is the patient taking it? What is the patient's response to the drug? Is the patient male or female?
4. If the medication was found, what were the circumstances/conditions at the time of discovery?
5. Is the patient just visiting, or are they planning on staying?

Investigational Drug Information

1. Why do you need this information? Is the patient in need of the drug or currently enrolled in a protocol?
2. If a drug is to be identified, what is the dosage form, markings, color, strength, or size of the product?
3. Why was the patient receiving the drug? What is the response when the patient was on the drug? What are the patient's pathological conditions?
4. If a drug is desired, what approved or accepted therapies have been tried? Was therapy maximized before discontinued?

Method and Rate of Administration

1. What dosage form or preparation is being used (if multiple salts available)?
2. What is the dose ordered? Is the drug a one-time dose or standing orders?
3. What is the clinical status of the patients? Could the patient tolerate a fluid push of [ ] mL? Is the patient fluid or sodium restricted? Does the patient have congestive heart failure (CHF) or edema?
4. What possible delivery routes are available?
5. What other drugs is the patient receiving currently? Are any by the same route?

Incompatibility and Stability

1. What are the routes for the patient's medications?
2. What are the doses (in mg), concentrations, and volumes for all pertinent medications?
3. What are the infusion times/rates expected or desired?
4. What is the base solution or diluent used?
5. Was the product stored in a refrigerator or at room temperature? For how long?
6. Was the product exposed to sunlight? For how long?
7. Was the product frozen? For how long?
8. When was the product compounded/prepared?

Drug Interactions

1. What event(s) suggest that an interaction occurred? Please describe.
2. For the drugs in question, what are the doses, volumes, concentrations, rate of administration, administration schedules, and length of therapies?
3. What is the temporal relationship between the drugs in question?
4. Has the patient received this combination or a similar combination in the past?
5. Other than the drugs in question, what other drugs is the patient receiving currently? When were these started?

Drug-Laboratory Test Interference

1. What event(s) suggest that an interaction occurred? Please describe.
2. For the drug in question, what is the dose, volume, concentration, rate of administration, administration schedule, and length of therapy?
3. What is the temporal relationship between drug administration and laboratory test sampling?
4. What other drugs is the patient receiving?
5. Has clinical chemistry (or the appropriate laboratory) been contacted? Are they aware of any known interference similar to this event?
6. Was this one isolated test or a trend in results?

Pharmacokinetics

1. What are the generic name, dose, and route of the drug?
2. What are the patient's age, sex, height, and weight?
3. What are the disease being treated and the severity of the illness?
4. What is the patient's hepatic and renal function?
5. What other medications is the patient receiving?
6. What physiologic conditions exist (e.g., pneumonia, severe burns, or obesity)?
7. What are the patient's dietary and ethanol habits?

Serum or Urine Therapeutic Levels

1. Is the patient currently receiving the drug? Have samples already been drawn? At what time?
2. What is the disease or underlying pathology being treated? If infectious in nature, what is the organism suspected/cultured?
3. If not stated in the question, what was the source of the sample (blood, urine, saliva; venous or arterial blood)?
4. What was the timing of the samples relative to drug administration? Over what period of time was the drug administered and by what route?
5. What were the previous concentrations for this patient? Was the patient receiving the same dose then?
6. How long has the patient received the drug? Is the patient at steady state?

Therapy Evaluation/Drug of Choice

1. What medications, including doses and routes of administration, is the patient receiving?
2. What are the patient's pathology(ies) and disease(s) severity?
3. What are the patient's specifics: age, weight, height, gender, organ function/dysfunction?

4. Has the patient received the drug previously? Was the response similar?
5. Has the patient been compliant?
6. What alternative therapies has the patient received? Was therapy maximized for each of these before discontinuation? What other therapies are being considered?
7. What monitoring parameters have been followed (serum concentrations/levels, clinical status, other clinical lab results, objective measurements, and subjective assessment).
8. What is the patient's name and location?

Dosage Recommendations (Normal and Compromised)

1. What disease is being treated? What is the extent/severity of the illness?
2. What are the drugs (all) being prescribed? Has the patient been receiving either to date?
3. Does the patient have any insufficiency of the renal, hepatic, or cardiac system?
4. For drugs with renal elimination, what are the serum creatinine/creatinine clearance, BUN, and/or urine output? Is the patient receiving peritoneal dialysis or hemodialysis?
5. For drugs with hepatic elimination, what are the liver function tests, bilirubin (direct and indirect), and/or albumin?
6. For drugs with serum level monitoring utility, characterize the most recent levels per timing relative to dose and results.
7. Are these lab values recent? Is the patient's condition stable?
8. Does this patient have a known factor that could affect drug metabolism (ethnic background such as Oriental, or acetylator status)?

Adverse Effects

1. What are the name, dosage, and route for all drugs currently and recently prescribed?
2. What are the patient's specifics (age, sex, height, weight, organ dysfunction, and indication for drug use)?
3. What is the temporal relationship with the drug?
4. Has the patient experienced this adverse relationship (or a similar event) with this drug (or similar agent) previously?
5. Was the suspected drug ever administered before? Why was it discontinued then?
6. What were the events/findings that characterize this adverse drug reaction (ADR) (include onset and duration)?
7. Has any intervention been initiated at this time?
8. Does the patient have any food intolerance?
9. Is there a family history for this ADR and/or drug allergy?

Toxicology Information

1. What is your name, relationship to the victim, and telephone number?
2. What are the patient specifics (age, sex, height, weight, organ dysfunction, and indication for drug use)?
3. Is this a suspected ingestion or exposure?
4. When is it suspected the product was ingested? What is the strength of the product and the possible quantity ingested (e.g., how much was in the bottle)?

5. How long ago did the ingestion occur?
6. How much is on the patient or surrounding floor?
7. How much was removed from the patient's hands and mouth? Was the ingestion in the same room where the product was stored?
8. What has been done for the patient already? Has the Poison Control Center or ER been called?
9. Do you have syrup of ipecac available? Do you know how to give it properly?
10. What is the patient's condition (sensorium, heart rate, respiratory rate, temperature, skin color/turgor, pupils, sweating/salivation, etc.)?
11. Does the patient have any known illnesses or organ dysfunction?

Teratogenicity

1. What is the drug the patient received and what was the dose? What was the duration of therapy?
2. Is the patient's pregnant or planning to become pregnant?
3. When during pregnancy was the exposure (trimester or weeks)?
4. What are the patient specifics (age, height, weight, sex)?
5. What is the source of the case information?
6. Was the patient compliant?
7. For what indication was the drug being prescribed?

Drugs in Breast Milk

1. What is the drug the patient received and what was the dose? What was the duration of therapy?
2. How long has the infant been breast-feeding?
3. Has the infant ever received nonmaternal nutrition? Is bottle-feeding a plausible alternative?
4. What is the frequency of the breast feeds? What is the milk volume?
5. How old is the infant?
6. Does the mother have hepatic or renal insufficiency?
7. What was the indication for prescribing the drug? Was this initial or alternate therapy?
8. Has the mother breast-fed previously while on the drug?

3-1

Performing a PubMed Search

PubMed Search

PubMed is a database which is maintained by the National Library of Medicine and is available to the public at no charge. This database is available online at: http://www.ncbi.nlm.nih.gov/PubMed. The information indexed by PubMed includes Medline, OldMedline (articles from the 1950's to the mid 1960's), as well as citations for additional life science journals.

This database is especially helpful when looking for off-label uses of medications. For example, if a prescriber contacts you asking for information about the efficacy of fluoxetine in treatment of anorexia nervosa, it may be appropriate to seek information from the primary literature. A PubMed search might be a good place to start this search. When performing a search using PubMed one can begin with just a key word, for example fluoxetine. As Figure 1 shows, just using the term fluoxetine yields in 8953 results. The results can be narrowed by entering a second key word, such as anorexia nervosa, and combining the two terms with the BOOLEAN operator AND.

While the addition of a second search term (Figure 2) did narrow the results, there are still 77 results that match these two terms. At this time it may be wise to explore the limit option (Figure 3) provided by the database. Limits allow the user to restrict the number of results returned for a search. Some databases allow searches to be limited by a variety of factors, including: language of publication, year of publication, type of article (e.g., human study, review, case report) or by type of journal where publication is found. Since the requestor is seeking efficacy data it is appropriate to limit these search results to just clinical trials.

By limiting the results to only human clinical trials published in English, 22 citations of possible interest have been identified (Figure 4). It is now necessary to look at the abstracts for these citations (Figure 5) and determine if these are helpful to provide a response to the query. By clicking on the blue hyperlink an abstract is displayed; this abstract summarizes the information in the article, as well as providing complete citation information for that specific article. If the publisher's Web site offers full-text of an article, a link is provided at the top of the page to the journal Web site. Some journals charge a fee for access to the full-text article while others do not. Those journals not charging for an article are clearly marked as "free full text." You can then select that icon and go directly to a full-text PDF or html of the desired article.

One additional helpful feature offered by PubMed is the "Related citations" link. The database will first identify the key words or Medical Subject Headings (MeSH) associated with the article selected and then identify secondary words and terms. The database will then compare these terms (both primary and secondary terms) with other articles indexed in PubMed to determine which other articles include similarly ranked terms and therefore might be of interest.

The best way to effectively search this database is by experience. However, PubMed offers a tutorial to gain additional experience in how to most effectively conduct literature searches. This interactive tutorial session is available at http://www.nlm.nih.gov/bsd/disted/pubmedtutorial/.

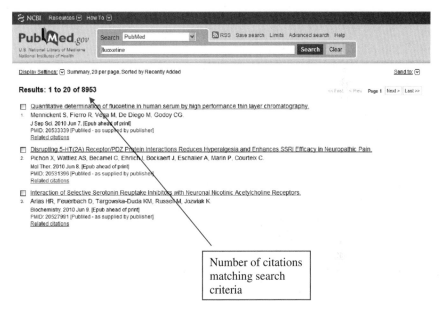

Figure 1. Key word search.

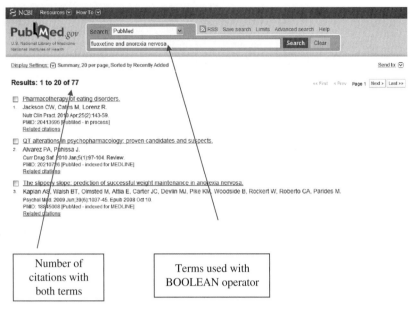

Figure 2. Multiple key word search.

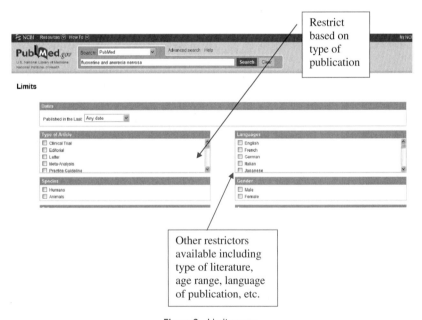

Figure 3. Limit screen.

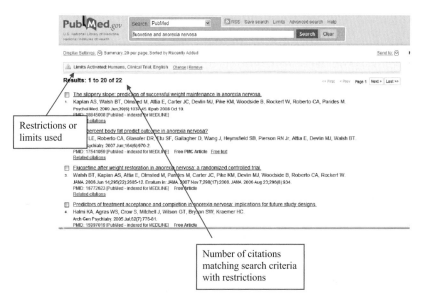

Figure 4. Results of search with restrictions.

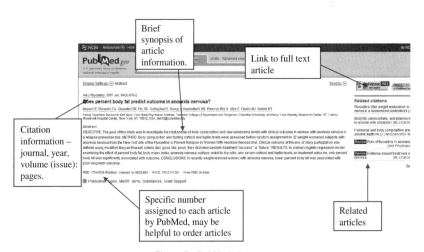

Figure 5. PubMed abstract.

Appendix 3-2

Selected Primary Literatures Sources

Journal Title	Publisher	ISSN	Areas covered
American Journal of Health-System Pharmacy: AJHP	American Society of Health-System Pharmacy	1079-2082	Clinical and managerial areas of pharmacy practice in health systems
American Journal of Pharmacy Education	American Association of Colleges of Pharmacy	0002-9459	Scholarship and advancement of pharmacy education
Annals of Internal Medicine	American College of Physicians	0003-4819	Internal medicine, including management of disease states
Annals of Pharmacotherapy	Harvey Whitney Books Company	1060-0280	Safe, effective, and economical use of drugs
Antimicrobial Agents and Chemotherapy	American Society for Microbiology	0066-4804	Information regarding the use of antimicrobial agents
Archives of Internal Medicine	American Medical Association	0003-9926	Focus on the diagnosis and treatment of disease states
Clinical Pharmacokinetics	Adis International Limited	0312-5963	Focus on pharmacokinetic and pharmacodynamic properties of drugs
Clinical Pharmacology and Therapeutics	Mosby Year Book Incorporated	0009-9236	The effect of drugs on the human body
Drug Information Journal	Drug Information Association	0092-8615	Technology related to disseminating drug information
Drug Topics	Thomson Healthcare	0012-6616	Focus on issues impacting community pharmacy and on new drug therapies
Drugs	Adis International Limited	0012-6667	Pharmacotherapeutic aspects of both new and established drugs
Formulary	Advanstar Communications Incorporated	1082-801X	Contemporary issues in drug policy management and pharmacotherapy
Hospital Pharmacy	Facts & Comparisons Incorporated	0018-5787	Issues related to pharmacy in institutional settings
JAMA (the Journal of the American Medical Association)	American Medical Association	0098-7484	New research and review information that impacts health care

continued

Journal Title	Publisher	ISSN	Areas covered
Journal of Cardiovascular Pharmacology	Lippincott Williams & Wilkins	0160-2446	New information about the treatment of cardiovascular disease.
The Journal of Clinical Pharmacology	Lippincott, Williams & Wilkins	0091-2700	Clinical information about the safety, tolerability, efficacy, therapeutic use, and toxicology of drugs
Journal of Pharmaceutical Sciences	Wiley	0022-3549	Application of physical and analytical chemistry to pharmaceutical sciences
Journal of Pharmacology and Experimental Therapeutics	American Society for Experimental Pharmacology and Therapeutics	0022-3565	Covers interaction between chemicals and biological systems as well as metabolism, distribution and toxicology.
Journal of Pharmacy and Pharmacology	Pharmaceutical Press	0022-3573	Addresses a variety of practice areas including: drug delivery systems, biomaterials and polymers, and implications of human genome on drug therapies.
Journal of The American Pharmacists Association	American Pharmacists Association	1544-3191	News, information and research in the area of pharmacotherapeutic management
Medical Letter on Drugs and Therapeutics	Medical Letter, Inc.	0025-732X	Provides information on new drug therapies and drugs of choice for disease management
New England Journal of Medicine	Massachusetts Medical Society	0028-646X	Results of recent research considered important to the practice of medicine
Pharmaceutical Research	Plenum Press	0724-8741	Emphasis on drug delivery, drug formulation, pharmacokinetics, pharmacodynamics and drug disposition
PharmacoEconomics	Adis International Limited	1170-7690	Information regarding the economical use of drug therapies
Pharmacological Reviews	American Society of Pharmacology and Experimental Therapeutics	0031-6997	Current topics of interest including: cellular pharmacology, drug metabolism and disposition, renal pharmacology and neuropharmacology.
Pharmacotherapy	IOS Press	0277-0008	Published by American College of Clinical pharmacy and focused on original research in clinical practice
Pharmacy Times	Romaine Pierson Publishing Incorporated	0003-0627	Focus on new drug therapies and patient counseling as it relates to community pharmacy
Therapeutic Drug Monitoring	Lippincott Williams & Wilkins	0163-4356	Fosters exchange of knowledge between fields of pharmacology, pathology, toxicology and analytical.
U.S. Pharmacist	Jobson Publishing Corporation	0148-4818	Information regarding the practice of community pharmacy

4-1

Questions for Assessing Clinical Trials

OVERALL ASSESSMENT

- Was the article published in a reputable, peer-reviewed journal?
- Are the investigator's training/education/practice sites adequate for the study objective?
- Can the funding source bias the study?

TITLE / ABSTRACT

- Was the title unbiased?
- Did the abstract contain information not found within the study?
- Did the abstract provide a clear overview of the purpose, methods, results, and conclusions of the study?

INTRODUCTION

- Did the authors provide sufficient background information to demonstrate the rationale for the study?
- Were the study objectives clearly identified?
- What were the major null hypothesis and alternate hypothesis?

METHODS

- Was an appropriate study design used to answer the question?
- Were reasonable inclusion/exclusion criteria presented to represent an appropriate patient population?
- Was a selection bias present?
- Was subject recruitment described? If so, how were subjects recruited? Was the method appropriate?
- Was IRB approval obtained?
- Was subject informed consent obtained?
- Were the intervention and control regimens appropriate?
- What type of blinding was used? Was this type appropriate?

- Was randomization included? If so, what type was used? Was this appropriate?
- Who generated the allocation sequence, enrolled participants, and assigned participants to groups? Was this appropriate?
- Which ancillary treatments were permitted? Would they have affected the outcome?
- Was a run-in period included? How does this affect the results?
- Did the investigators measure compliance? How was compliance measured? Was compliance adequate?
- Was the primary endpoint appropriate for the study objective?
- Were secondary endpoints measured? If so, were they adequate for what was being studied?
- Were planned subgroup analyses planned? If so, were they appropriate?
- Was the method used to measure the primary endpoint appropriate?
- What type of data best describes the primary endpoint?
- Were data collected appropriately?
- What number of patients was needed for the primary endpoint to detect a difference between groups (power analysis)? Was the necessary sample size calculated? Were there enough patients enrolled to reach this endpoint?
- What were the alpha (α) and beta (β) values? Were these appropriate?
- Were the statistical tests used appropriate?

RESULTS

- Were the numbers of patients screened, enrolled, administered treatment, completing, and withdrawing from the study reported? Were reasons for subject discontinuations reported? Were withdrawals handled appropriately?
- Was the trial adequately powered?
- Were the subject demographics between groups similar at baseline? If not, were the differences likely to have an affect on the outcome data?
- Were data presented clearly?
- Were the results adjusted to take into account confounding variables?
- Was intention-to-treat analysis used? Was this appropriate?
- Were estimated effect size, p-values, and confidence intervals reported?
- Were the results statistically significant? Clinically different?
- Was the null hypothesis accepted or rejected?
- Can the trial results be extrapolated to the population?
- Based on the results, could a Type I or Type II error have occurred?
- Are subgroup analysis presented? Are these appropriate?
- Was ancillary therapy included? Did this affect the study results?
- Were therapy adverse effects included?

CONCLUSIONS/DISCUSSION

- Did the information appear biased, and did the trial results support the conclusions?
- Were trial limitations described?
- Did the investigators explain unexpected results?
- Are the results able to be extrapolated to the population?
- Were the study results clinically meaningful?

REFERENCES

- Were the references listed well represented (e.g., current, well-representing the literature)?
- Is a comprehensive list of published articles related to the trial objective presented?

5-1

Beyond the Basics: Questions to Consider for Critique of Primary Literature

RANDOMIZED CONTROLLED TRIAL

- Refer to Chapter 4, Literature Evaluation I: Controlled Clinical Trial Evaluation

PHARMACOECONOMIC ANALYSIS

- Refer to Chapter 6, Pharmacoeconomics

NON-INFERIORITY TRIAL

- Is the reference drug's efficacy established using adequate historical data and/or addition of a placebo arm?
- Are the participants and outcome measures for the non-inferiority similar compared to previous studies that confirmed the efficacy of the reference drug (e.g., constancy assumption)?
- Is the method used to determine the Non-inferiority Margin predetermined before the study, both clinically and statistically sound, and the reasoning clearly stated in the article?
- Was a per-protocol analysis used? If so, did they also perform an intention-to-treat analysis?
- Was the sample size modified as the study progressed? If so, was a clear explanation of how the blinded information was handled and by what method these modifications were determined provided?
- Was this study an attempt to rescue a failed superiority trial?

N-OF-1 TRIAL

- Was assignment of active and control treatment to study periods randomized?
- Was the study blinded?
- Were multiple observation periods used?
- Were study endpoints clearly defined?

ADAPTIVE CLINICAL TRIAL (ACT)

- Are the methodologies used to make adaptive changes in the trial adequately described?
- What logistical issues exist, and have they been adequately addressed?

- Are the adaptive changes based on evidence and good clinical judgment?
- Did extensive adaptation to the protocol occur during the study?
- To what extent is intrusion of bias noted?
- Who has access to the information created from interim analyses?
- If the study was stopped early, is the totality of evidence adequate?

STABILITY STUDY

- Were study methodologies and test conditions clearly defined?
- Were validated assays used?
- Were assays validated using time-zero measurements and an adequate number of test samples taken?

BIOEQUIVALENCY STUDY

- Did the protocol define the characteristics of the subjects?
- Were confounding factors (e.g., smoking, alcohol use) identified and controlled?
- Was a crossover design used?
- Was the study randomized and blinded?

PROGRAMMATIC RESEARCH

- Were one of two options used for subject comparison: (1) comparison of subjects to those not using the program or service, (2) comparison of subjects before or after initiation of the program or service?
- Was the program or service clearly defined?
- Did the authors specify from whose perspective (e.g., patient, provider, physician, third-party payer) the study was undertaken?
- If costs were analyzed, were all costs associated with provision of the program or service included in the analysis, including personnel, inflationary changes, and cost-savings had the intervention not occurred?
- Were clinically important outcome parameters used to assess effectiveness of the program or service?

COHORT STUDY

- Was the research question clearly stated?
- Were inclusion and exclusion criteria described in detail?
- Were exposed and unexposed subjects similar in terms of demographic characteristics and susceptibility to disease states?
- Was selection bias obviously present?
- Were confounding factors obviously present?
- Were the same efforts to measure outcomes made in each group?

- Were 95% confidence intervals calculated?
- Were follow-up rates the same for the exposed and unexposed groups?

CASE-CONTROL STUDY

- Was predisposition of disease similar in cases and controls except for exposure to the risk factor?
- Were cases and controls matched?
- Was exposure to the risk factor similar to that which would occur in the general population?
- Did cases and controls undergo similar diagnostic evaluations?
- Were investigators who assessed patients or collected data blinded to the status of the subject as a case or control?
- Did the investigators compare cases with several different control groups?
- Were 95% confidence intervals calculated?

CROSS-SECTIONAL STUDY

- Did investigators ensure accuracy in data collection?
- If a survey or questionnaire was used, was it validated?
- Were the inclusion and exclusion criteria clearly defined and stated?
- Was selection of cases clearly described?

CASE STUDY, CASE REPORT, OR CASE SERIES

- Did the authors recognize the preliminary nature of the results (e.g., recommendations for clinical application of the results should be guarded)?

SURVEY STUDY

- Was the survey instrument valid and reliable? Was a pretest or pilot test conducted on the survey instrument?
- Was the sample size large enough to detect a difference between groups?
- Was the survey objective and carefully planned?
- Were data quantifiable?
- Was the sample representative of the target population?
- Was response rate high enough to reflect results that would be expected of the target population?
- Did the investigators determine whether nonresponders differed from responders?

POSTMARKETING SURVEILLANCE STUDY

- Was a large enough sample studied to reflect current uses of and side effects associated with the new drug therapy?
- Were appropriate methods used to measure clearly defined endpoints?

NARRATIVE (NON-SYSTEMATIC) REVIEWS—QUALITATIVE

- Was an extensive search for available studies undertaken?
- Did the authors use a variety of resources to identify studies for inclusion in the review article?
- Was the review article focused on a clearly defined population?
- Did the studies included in the review article use valid research methods?
- Did the author examine reasons for differences in study results and conclusions?
- Were outcomes of the studies clinically important?
- Did the author consider benefits and risks of the drug therapy?

SYSTEMATIC REVIEWS—QUALITATIVE

- Did the authors clearly define the research question?
- Was the review article focused on a clearly defined patient population?
- Was an extensive search for available studies undertaken?
- Did the authors consider using results from both published and unpublished studies in the analysis?
- Did the authors clearly define criteria for study inclusion in the analysis?
- Did the authors list studies that were included in and excluded from the analysis?
- Did the authors provide details concerning methodologies of studies used in the analysis?
  - Were included studies addressing the same clinical question(s)?
  - Did all included studies use appropriate doses, regimens, and routes of administrations for both treatments and comparators?
  - Were all included studies of appropriate duration?
- Were tests of homogeneity performed and results reported?
- Were those who selected studies for inclusion in the analysis blinded to the names of the original authors, place of publication of the study, and final study results?

META ANALYSIS—QUANTITATIVE

- Did the authors clearly define the research question?
- Was the review article focused on a clearly defined patient population?
- Was an extensive search for available studies undertaken?
- Did the authors consider using results from both published and unpublished studies in the analysis?
- Did the authors clearly define criteria for study inclusion in the analysis?
- Did the authors list studies that were included in and excluded from the analysis?
- Did the authors include gray literature in the analysis?
- Did the authors provide details concerning methodologies of studies used in the analysis?
  - Were included studies addressing the same clinical question(s)?
  - Did all included studies use appropriate doses, regimens, and routes of administrations for both treatments and comparators?
  - Were all included studies of appropriate duration?

- Was a funnel plot provided to determine if publication bias was potentially present?
- Were tests of homogeneity performed and results reported?
- Were those who selected studies for inclusion in the analysis blinded to the names of the original authors, place of publication of the study, and final study results?
- Were appropriate statistical tests used (usually Mantel-Haenszel test) and the probability of type I and type II errors considered?
- Were 95 percent confidence intervals calculated?
- Were results presented in a forest plot?

PRACTICE GUIDELINES

- Is there an explicit description of the procedures used to identify, select, and combine evidence?
- Are the recommendations valid?
- Are the guidelines regularly reviewed and updated to incorporate new evidence as it becomes available?
- Was the guideline peer-reviewed?
- Can the recommendations be generalized to a larger population?
- Was the source of funding for the development of the guideline provided, and could it bias the conclusions?
- If another group of experts were to independently develop a guideline on the same clinical situation, would the recommendations be the same (are the recommendations reliable)?

QUALITY OF LIFE STUDIES

- Are Health-Related Quality of Life (HR-QOL) instruments validated?
- If a series of HR-QOL measurements are used, does this result in a valid HR-QOL battery?
- Are HR-QOL instruments sensitive to changes in the patients' status as the trial progresses?
- Are important aspects of patients' lives measured, as determined by patients themselves?
- Is timing of HR-QOL measurements to answer the research questions appropriately related to anticipated timing of the clinical effects?
- Were sequences of HR-QOL assessments conducted in the same order for all patients?
- Was mode of data collection (self-report versus trained interviewer) appropriate for type of questions being asked?
  - If mode of data collection was a trained interviewer, could the interview location lead to biased answers?
- Were response rates to questionnaires reported?
- Is there missing data?
  - If missing data exists, is there a specific pattern that suggests author manipulation providing desired results (missing data could have countered author's hypothesis)?

- If a multicenter trial, did all sites evaluate HR-QOL?
- Is the QOL instrument valid for examining the specific disease in question?
- Are both positive and negative findings reported?
- Are adverse drug events and HR-QOL measurements considered separately?
- Is impact of treatment effects included with HR-QOL measurements?
- Is there evidence of culturally defined factors that may have impacted patient HR-QOL measurements and/or the assessment of these measurements?
- Does there appear to be a bias on the part of the study researchers?
- Were general measures of QOL evaluated?

DIETARY SUPPLEMENT MEDICAL LITERATURE

- Which plant part was utilized?
- Was a standardized botanical extract utilized?
- Was the study product standardization appropriate?
- Was a specific plant species or specific salt form utilized?
- Was the study dose appropriate?
- Was trial length appropriate to perceive treatment effects or differences?
- Was sample size sufficient to detect a difference between groups if one exists?

7-1

Appendix 7-1

New Zealand Guidelines Group (NZGG)

Steps in Guideline Development

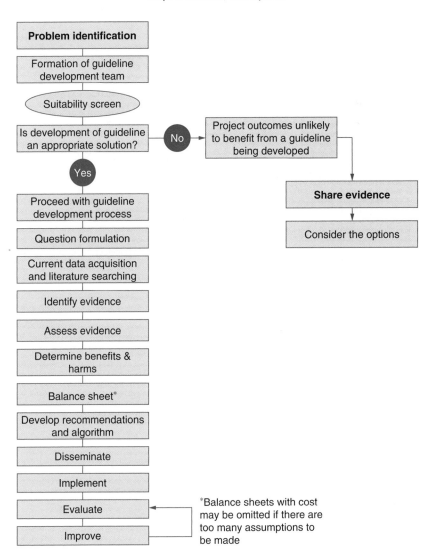

Problem identification

Formation of guideline development team

Suitability screen

Is development of guideline an appropriate solution? — No → Project outcomes unlikely to benefit from a guideline being developed

Yes

Proceed with guideline development process

Question formulation

Current data acquisition and literature searching

Identify evidence

Assess evidence

Determine benefits & harms

Balance sheet*

Develop recommendations and algorithm

Disseminate

Implement

Evaluate

Improve

Share evidence

Consider the options

*Balance sheets with cost may be omitted if there are too many assumptions to be made

7-2

Appendix 7-2

National Institute for Clinical Excellence (NICE)

A summary of key stages of NICE guideline developement (for developers)

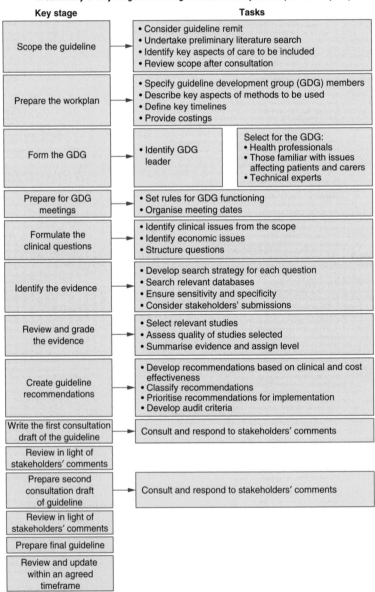

Key stage	Tasks
Scope the guideline	• Consider guideline remit • Undertake preliminary literature search • Identify key aspects of care to be included • Review scope after consultation
Prepare the workplan	• Specify guideline development group (GDG) members • Describe key aspects of methods to be used • Define key timelines • Provide costings
Form the GDG	• Identify GDG leader Select for the GDG: • Health professionals • Those familiar with issues affecting patients and carers • Technical experts
Prepare for GDG meetings	• Set rules for GDG functioning • Organise meeting dates
Formulate the clinical questions	• Identify clinical issues from the scope • Identify economic issues • Structure questions
Identify the evidence	• Develop search strategy for each question • Search relevant databases • Ensure sensitivity and specificity • Consider stakeholders' submissions
Review and grade the evidence	• Select relevant studies • Assess quality of studies selected • Summarise evidence and assign level
Create guideline recommendations	• Develop recommendations based on clinical and cost effectiveness • Classify recommendations • Prioritise recommendations for implementation • Develop audit criteria
Write the first consultation draft of the guideline	Consult and respond to stakeholders' comments
Review in light of stakeholders' comments	
Prepare second consultation draft of guideline	Consult and respond to stakeholders' comments
Review in light of stakeholders' comments	
Prepare final guideline	
Review and update within an agreed timeframe	

Appendix 7-3

National Institute for Clinical Excellence (NICE) Topic Selection Criteria

NATIONAL INSTITUTE FOR CLINICAL EXCELLENCE

Topic suggestion and selection

Criteria for selecting topics for the advisory committee on topic selection

The Department of Health and the Welsh Assembly Government are responsible for selecting topics for the NICE technology appraisal and clinical guidelines work programmes. As part of the process of selecting topics to refer to NICE, the Advisory Committee on Topic Selection (ACTS) uses the criteria below to assess the suggestions put forward.

We recommend that health care professionals, patients and carers, and the general public who suggest topics read these criteria before submitting their suggestion.

1. *Would guidance promote the best possible improvement in patient care given available resources? In particular, are one or more of the following criteria satisfied:*

   a. does the proposed guidance relate to one of the NHS clinical priority areas , or to other government health-related priorities such as reducing health inequalities
   b. does the proposed guidance address a condition which is associated with significant disability, morbidity, or mortality in the population as a whole or in particular subgroups
   c. does the proposed guidance relate to one or more interventions that could significantly improve patients' or carers' quality of life and/or reduce avoidable morbidity or avoidable premature mortality, relative to current standard practice, or if used more extensively or more appropriately would do so
   d. does the proposed guidance relate to one or more interventions which if more extensively used would impact significantly on NHS or other societal resources (financial and other)
   e. does the proposed guidance relate to one or more interventions which could without detriment to patient care be used more selectively, thus freeing up resources for use elsewhere in the NHS?

2. *Will NICE be able to add value by issuing guidance, taking into account the following factors:*

NATIONAL INSTITUTE FOR CLINICAL EXCELLENCE
Topic suggestion and selection
Criteria for selecting topics for the advisory committee on topic selection

a. is the evidence base sufficient to develop robust guidance across most or all of the interventions to be covered by the proposed guidance

b. is there evidence and/or reason to believe that there is or will be inappropriate practice and/or significant variation in clinical practice and/or variation in access to treatment (between geographical areas or social groups) in the absence of guidance?

3. *Would the most appropriate form of guidance consist of an appraisal, a clinical guideline, or a combination of the two, taking into account:*

a. the availability of an existing clinical guideline from NICE or from another authoritative source for the condition in question

b. the degree of urgency for guidance on any specific intervention for the condition in question

c. the possible complexity of the proposed guidance if formulated as an appraisal?

In general, the presumption is that guidance will take the form of a clinical guideline if no suitable guidance relating to the condition as a whole is available or in preparation. An appraisal should be considered if the perceived need relates to a particular intervention for a particular condition, and if either (a) there is an urgent need for guidance or (b) a clinical guideline for that condition is already available or in preparation.

4. *For new interventions, does the balance of advantage for patient care lie with appraisal at time of launch or at some specified future date, taking account of the following factors and the attached checklist:*

a. the possible impact on uptake or equity of access in the absence of guidance at time of launch

b. the likely robustness of the evidence base at time of launch;

c. the prospect of relevant additional data becoming available in the period immediately after launch

d. for surgical and related interventions, whether safety and efficacy have already been assessed (or will be assessed in the near future) by the Interventional Procedures Advisory Committee?

NATIONAL INSTITUTE FOR CLINICAL EXCELLENCE
Topic suggestion and selection
Criteria for selecting topics for the advisory committee on topic selection

Appendix 7-4

Study Selection Process—Centre for Reviews and Dissemination (CRD)*

Flow Diagram of Study Selection Process

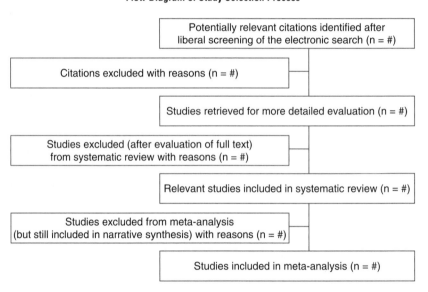

*Khan KS, ter Riet G, Glanville J, Showden AJ, Kleijnen J, editors. Undertaking systematic reviews of research on effectiveness CRD's guidance for those carrying out or commissioning reviews. 4th ed. CRD Report Number 4. University of York, York (UK): Centre for Reviews and Dissemination; 2001.

Appendix 7-5

Study Selection Points—Centre for Reviews and Dissemination (CRD)

KEY POINTS ABOUT STUDY SELECTION

- Studies should be selected in an unbiased way, based on selection criteria that flow directly from the review questions, and that have been piloted to check that they can be reliably applied.
- Study selection is a staged process involving sifting through the citations located by the search, retrieving full reports of potentially relevant citations and, from their assessment, identifying those studies that fulfill the inclusion criteria.
- Parallel independent assessments should be conducted to minimize the risk of errors of judgment. If disagreements occur between reviewers, they should be resolved according to a predefined strategy using consensus and arbitration as appropriate.
- The study selection process should be documented, detailing reasons for inclusion and exclusion.

Study selection criteria (example)

Review question
In patients undergoing hip replacement, to what extent is the risk of postoperative infection reduced by antimicrobial prophylaxis?

Selection criteria	Inclusion criteria	Exclusion criteria
Population	• Patients undergoing hip replacement (primary or revision procedure)	Other operations
Interventions	• Antimicrobial prophylaxis compared to placebo or no prophylaxis • Comparison of different antimicrobials	Lack of comparison
Outcome	• Surgical wound infection confirmed by appropriate microbiologic techniques	Infection not confirmed
Study design	• Randomised controlled trials	Non-randomised studies

Source: Khan KS, ter Riet G, Glanville J, Sowden AJ, Kleijnen J, editors. Undertaking systematic reviews of research on effectiveness CRD's guidance for those carrying out or commissioning reviews. 4th ed. CRD Report Number 4. University of York, York (UK): Centre for Reviews and Dissemination; 2001.

Appendix 7-6

Data Synthesis—Centre for Reviews and Dissemination (CRD)*

Key Concepts in Data Synthesis for Systematic Reviews

DESCRIPTIVE DATA SYNTHESIS

A nonquantitative synthesis of the collated evidence to assess the extent of the evidence and to plan the quantitative synthesis. It allows a qualitative assessment of variation in study characteristics, quality, and results (heterogeneity). In some situations where there are numerous studies with consistent and large effects, it may be possible to discern effects solely from this synthesis.

QUANTITATIVE DATA SYNTHESIS

A synthesis using a group of statistical techniques to combine the results of the included studies (meta-analysis), to assess heterogeneity, and to quantitatively evaluate other aspects like publication bias. Meta-analysis is used to calculate a pooled estimate of effect and its confidence interval.

HETEROGENEITY

The variability or differences between studies in terms of key characteristics (clinical heterogeneity), quality (methodological heterogeneity), and effects (heterogeneity of results). Statistical tests of heterogeneity may be used to assess whether the observed variability in study results (effect sizes) is greater than that expected to occur by chance.

---

*Khan KS, ter Riet G, Glanville J, Sowden AJ, Kleijnen J, editors. Undertaking systematic reviews of research on effectiveness CRD's guidance for those carrying out or commissioning Reviews. 4th ed. CRD Report Number 4. University of York, York (UK): Centre for Reviews and Dissemination; 2001.

HOMOGENEITY

The degree to which the studies included in a review are similar. Studies are considered statistically homogeneous if their results vary no more than might be expected by the chance.

SENSITIVITY ANALYSIS

An analysis used to determine how the results of a systematic review change due to variations arising from uncertain decisions or assumptions about the data and the methods that were used.

PUBLICATION BIAS

A bias in the research literature where the likelihood of publication of a study is influenced by the significance of its results. For example, studies in which an intervention is not found to be effective may be less likely to be published. Systematic reviews that fail to identify such studies may overestimate the true effect of an intervention. In some subject areas (e.g., in alternative medicine), studies showing effectiveness may also suffer from publication bias.

7-7

National Institute for Clinical Excellence (NICE)—Evidence Table Format for Intervention Studies

Bibliographic Reference	Study Type	Evidence Level	Number of Patients	Patient Characteristics	Intervention	Comparison	Length of Follow-up	Outcome Measures	Effect Size	Source of Funding	Additional Comments
Author, title, journal, volume, year, pages	Observational, cohort, case studies, and so forth	Report the classification with the SIGN or NICE systems	Total number of patients included in the study, including number of patients in each arm; with inclusion/exclusion criteria, number of patients who started and completed	Relevant characteristics to the area of interest: age, gender, ethnic origin, comorbidity, disease status, community/hospital-based	Intervention (treatment, procedure) studied. If important for the study, specify length of treatment. *Note: for diagnostic studies the intervention is the diagnostic test studied*	Placebo, alternative treatment. *Note: for diagnostic studies comparison of the test is with another test*	The length of time patients take part in the study, from first staging treatment until either a prespecified end-point (for example, death, specified length of disease-free remission) or the end of the data-gathering phase is reached. If the study is halted earlier than originally planned for any reason, this should also be noted here	All outcome measures, including associated harms. For studies with a diagnostic component there will be two interventions to consider—the diagnostic test used and the associated treatment. *Note: separate line for each outcome*	Absolute risk reduction and relative risk (reduction), number needed to treat, number needed to harm, odds ratios, as required. p values and confidence intervals whenever possible	Government funding (for example, National Health Service), voluntary charity (for example, Wellcome Trust), pharmaceutical company	Additional characteristics/interpretations of the studies that the reviewer wishes to record. Important flaws in the study not identifiable from other data in the table. A range of additional questions or issues that will need to be considered, but do not figure in the results table

NOTE: An evidence table is a table summarizing the results of a collection of studies which, taken together, represent the evidence supporting a particular recommendation or series of recommendations in a guideline. Evidence table for intervention studies, National Institute for Clinical Excellence, February 2004.

7-8

New Zealand Guidelines Group (NZGG)— Considered Judgment

CONSIDERED JUDGMENT FORM

Key Question	Evidence Table Ref.

1. Volume of evidence
Comment here on any issues concerning the quantity of evidence available on this topic and its methodological quality.

2. Consistency
Comment here on the degree of consistency demonstrated by the available evidence. Where there are conflicting results, indicate how the group formed a judgment as to the overall direction of the evidence.

3. Applicability
Comment here on the extent to which the evidence is directly applicable in the New Zealand setting. Comment here on how reasonable it is to generalize from the results of the studies used as evidence to the target population for this guideline.

4. Clinical impact
Comment here on the potential clinical impact that the intervention in question might have, e.g., size of patient population; magnitude of effect; relative benefit over other management options; resource implications; and balance of risk and benefit.

5. Other factors
Indicate here any other factors that you took into account when assessing the evidence base.

	Evidence level
6. Evidence statement *Please summarize the development group's synthesis of the evidence relating to this key question, taking all the above factors into account, and indicate the evidence level which applies.*	
7. Recommendation *What recommendation(s) does the guideline development group draw from this evidence? Please indicate the grade of recommendation(s) and any dissenting opinion within the group.*	**Grade of recommendation**

SOURCE: New Zealand Guidelines Group. Handbook for the Preparation of Explicit Evidence-based Clinical Practice Guidelines; 2001. Available from: www.nzgg.org.nz/development/documents/nzgg_guideline_handbook.pdf.

Appendix 7-9

Guidelines Advisory Committee (GAC) Levels of Evidence and Grades of Recommendation

Levels of Evidence and Grades of Recommendation:
A Guidelines Advisory Committee (GAC) Comparison of Guideline Developer's Evidence Taxonomies

GAC Level of Evidence to Recommend	ACC/AHA	AHCPR	AHRQ	CTFPHC	CCOPGI	CPSO	ICSI	SIGN	USPTF
Excellent/Good Evidence to Recommend	Class I Class III	Grade A	Class I	Level I	Grade EV*	Level I Level II	Class A Class M*	1++/A 1+/A	Grade A
Fair Evidence to Recommend	Class II a	Grade B	Class II	Level II-1 Level II-2	Grade PE*	Level III	Class B Class C Class D*	1– 2++/B 2+/C	Grade B Grade D
Insufficient (Poor) Evidence to Recommend	Class II b	Grade C	Class III*	Level II-3	Grade O	Level IV	Class D**	2-3/D	Grade C Grade I
Consensus Opinion		Grade D	Class III**	Level III	Grade C Grade E Grade X	Level V	Class R Class X	4/D	

Notes:
M*: variable depending on study design. For example, meta-analysis or systematic reviews based on randomized trials yield stronger evidence than other study designs.

Class D*: ICSI groups cross-sectional studies, case series, and case reports as Class D evidence. The GAC considers cross-sectional studies to be fair evidence to recommend.

Class D**: ICSI groups cross-sectional studies, case series, and case reports as Class D evidence. The GAC considers case series and case reports to be insufficient (Poor) evidence to recommend.

EV*: CCOPGI considers a comprehensive systematic review of the best available evidence to be evidence-based. The GAC considers systematic reviews excellent/good evidence, unless the systematic review is based on case series or case reports only. In the event that a systematic review was based on case series and case reports only, the GAC would consider the level of evidence to be insufficient (Poor).

PE*: CCOPGI considers a partially evidence-based recommendation to be based on a comprehensive review, but the method of selecting and evaluating evidence is less systematic or unspecified. The GAC considers partially evidence-based recommendations to be fair evidence, unless the partial review is based on case series or case reports only. In the event that a partial review was based on case series and case reports only, the GAC would consider the level of evidence to be insufficient (Poor).

Class III*: AHRQ groups case reports, uncontrolled case series and expert or consensus opinion as Class III evidence. The GAC considers case reports and uncontrolled case series as insufficient (Poor) evidence to recommend.

Class III**: AHRQ groups case reports, uncontrolled case series and expert or consensus opinion as Class III evidence. The GAC considers consensus opinion as its own category under "consensus".

(Continued)

Acronyms:

ACC/AHA: American College of Cardiology and the American Heart Association, Recommendations and Level of Evidence

AHCPR: Agency for Healthcare Policy and Research: Evidence Grading System

AHRQ: Agency for Healthcare Research and Quality: Strength of Evidence Rating

CCOPGI: Cancer Care Ontario Practice Guidelines Initiative: Evidence-Based Categorization Scheme

CPSO: College of Physicians and Surgeons of Ontario

CTFPHC: Canadian Task Force on the Periodic Health Examination: Quality of Guidelines

ICSI: Institute for Clinical Systems Improvement: Evidence Grading System

SIGN: Scottish Intercollegiate Guidelines Network: Levels of Evidence

USPTF: U.S. Preventive Services Task Force: Classifications

From the Ontario Guidelines Advisory Committee. Available from: http://gacguidelines.ca/pdfs/LevelsOfEvidenceChart.pdf.

Appendix 7-10

National Institute for Clinical Excellence (NICE) Guideline Structure

GUIDELINE STRUCTURE

The full guideline contains all the recommendations, plus details of the methods used and the underpinning evidence. The structure and format of the full guideline are at the discretion of the National Collaborating Centre (NCC), but core elements should be as follows:

- Summary of recommendations and algorithm
- Introduction
  - Responsibility and support for guideline development
  - Funding
  - Guideline Developement Group membership
  - Patient and carer involvement
  - Epidemiologic data
  - Experience of those receiving care, or service use
  - Outcomes
  - Clinical issues
  - Aim and scope of the guideline
- Methods
  - Literature search strategy
  - Sifting and reviewing the literature
  - Synthesizing the evidence
  - Economic analysis
  - Assigning levels to the evidence
  - Areas without evidence and consensus methodology
  - Forming recommendations
  - Consultation
  - Related guidance: details of related NICE technology appraisals or clinical guidelines that are published or in preparation

- Guideline recommendations
  - Evidence statements
  - Recommendations
  - Audit criteria
  - Scheduled review of the guideline
  - Recommendations for research
- References
- Appendices, which may include:
  - Evidence tables (preferably on a CD-ROM)–details of search strategies

For examples of published guidelines refer to the NICE Web site: <<http://www.nice. org.uk/>>

Appendix 7-11

Scottish Intercollegiate Guidelines Network (SIGN) Consultation and Peer-Review

Scottish Intercollegiate Guidelines Network March 2004

Systematic literature review and draft recommendations

Draft guideline available on SIGN Web site for limited period

Draft guideline presented and discussed at national open meeting

Feedback incorporated and draft guideline submitted to SIGN

In-house editing and methodological checks

Peer-review reports obtained

Draft circulated for information to various health service organizations

Comments compiled and discussed with development group chairman, in consultation with group

SIGN editorial group review guideline and peer review comments

Guideline development group members sign off final draft

Dissemination and implementation

Appendix 7-12

Grades of Recommendation Assessment Development and Evaluation (GRADE) System Advantages

COMPARISON OF GRADE AND OTHER SYSTEMS

Factor	Other Systems	GRADE	Advantages of GRADE System*
Definitions	Implicit definitions of quality (level) of evidence and strength of recommendation	Explicit definitions	Makes clear what grades indicate and what should be considered in making these judgments
Judgments	Implicit judgments regarding which outcomes are important, quality of evidence for each important outcome, overall quality of evidence, balance between benefits and harms, and value of incremental benefits	Sequential, explicit judgments	Clarifies each of these judgments and reduces risks of introducing errors or bias that can arise when they are made implicitly
Key components of quality of evidence	Not considered for each important outcome. Judgments about quality of evidence are often based on study design alone	Systematic and explicit consideration of study design, study quality, consistency, and directness of evidence in judgments about quality of evidence	Ensures these factors are considered appropriately
Other factors that can affect quality of evidence	Not explicitly taken into account	Explicit consideration of imprecise or sparse data, reporting bias, strength of association, evidence of a dose-response gradient, and plausible confounding	Ensures consideration of other factors

continued

COMPARISON OF GRADE AND OTHER SYSTEMS

Factor	Other Systems	GRADE	Advantages of GRADE System*
Overall quality of evidence	Implicitly based on the quality of evidence for benefits	Based on the lowest quality of evidence for any of the outcomes that are critical to making a decision	Reduces likelihood of mislabeling overall quality of evidence when evidence for a critical outcome is lacking
Relative importance of outcomes	Considered implicitly	Explicit judgments about which outcomes are critical, which ones are important but not critical, and which ones are unimportant and can be ignored	Ensures appropriate consideration of each outcome when grading overall quality of evidence and strength of recommendations
Balance between health benefits and harms	Not explicitly considered	Explicit consideration of trade-offs between important benefits and harms, the quality of evidence for these, translation of evidence into specific circumstances, and certainty of baseline risks	Clarifies and improves transparency of judgments on harms and benefits
Whether incremental health benefits are worth the costs	Not explicitly considered	Explicit consideration after first considering whether there are net health benefits	Ensures that judgments about value of net health benefits are transparent
Summaries of evidence and findings	Inconsistent presentation	Consistent GRADE evidence profiles, including quality assessment and summary of findings	Ensures that all panel members base their judgments on same information and that this information is available to others
Extent of use	Seldom used by more than one organization and little, if any empirical evaluation	International collaboration across wide range of organizations in development and evaluation	Builds on previous experience to achieve a system that is more sensible, reliable, and widely applicable

*Most other approaches do not include any of these advantages, although some may incorporate some of these advantages.
Source: Reproduced from: Atkins D, Best D, Briss PA, Eccles M, Falck-Ytter Y, Flottorp S, et al., for the GRADE Working Group. Grading quality of evidence and strength of recommendations. BMJ. 2004;328:1490.

Appendix 7-13

Appraisal of Guidelines Research & Evaluation (AGREE) Instrument

AGREE INSTRUMENT ITEMS FOR EVALUATION[*]

Domain 1	Scope and Purpose
Item 1	The overall objective(s) of the guideline is (are) specifically described
Item 2	The clinical question(s) covered by the guideline is (are) specifically described
Item 3	The patients to whom the guideline is meant to apply are specifically described
Domain 2	**Stakeholder Involvement**
Item 4	The guideline development group includes individuals from all relevant professional groups
Item 5	The patients' views and preferences have been sought
Item 6	The target users of the guideline are clearly defined
Item 7	The guideline has been piloted among target users
Domain 3	**Rigor of Development**
Item 8	Systematic methods were used to search for evidence
Item 9	The criteria for selecting the evidence are clearly described
Item 10	The methods used for formulating the recommendations are clearly described
Item 11	The health benefits, side effects, and risks have been considered in formulating the recommendations
Item 12	There is an explicit link between the recommendations and the supporting evidence
Item 13	The guideline has been externally reviewed by experts prior to its publication
Item 14	A procedure for updating the guideline is provided
Domain 4	**Clarity and Presentation**
Item 15	The recommendations are specific and unambiguous
Item 16	The different options for management of the condition are clearly presented
Item 17	The key recommendations are easily identifiable
Item 18	The guideline is supported with tools for application
Domain 5	**Application**
Item 19	The potential organizational barriers in applying the recommendations have been discussed
Item 20	The possible cost implications of applying the recommendations have been considered
Item 21	The guideline presents key review criteria for monitoring and/or audit purposes
Domain 6	**Editorial Independence**
Item 22	The guideline is editorially independent from the funding body
Item 23	Conflicts of interest of guideline development members have been recorded

*This is a list of the 23 items used by the AGREE instrument. A more detailed description of each item and scoring instructions for use of this instrument is provided at the AGREE collaboration Web site: http://www.agreecollaboration.org. Each item is scored on a four point scale: 1 = strongly disagree, 2 = disagree, 3 = agree, and 4 = strongly agree. In addition, the AGREE instrument includes an "overall assessment" regarding a recommendation to use the guideline in practice. The overall assessment uses a three point scale: 1= not recommended, 2 = recommended with provisos or modifications, 3 = strongly recommended.

7-14

Appendix 7-14

Conference on Guideline Standardization (COGS) Checklist

THE COGS CHECKLIST FOR REPORTING CLINICAL PRACTICE GUIDELINES

Topic	Description
1. Overview material	Provide a structured abstract that includes the guideline's release date, status (original, revised, updated), and print and electronic sources.
2. Focus	Describe the primary disease/condition and intervention/service/technology that the guideline addresses. Indicate any alternative preventive, diagnostic, or therapeutic interventions that were considered during development.
3. Goal	Describe the goal that following the guideline is expected to achieve, including the rationale for development of a guideline on this topic.
4. Users/setting	Describe the intended users of the guideline (e.g., provider types and patients) and the settings in which the guideline is intended to be used.
5. Target population	Describe the patient population eligible for guideline recommendations and list any exclusion criteria.
6. Developer	Identify the organization(s) responsible for guideline development and the names/credentials/potential conflicts of interest of individuals involved in the guideline's development.
7. Funding source/ sponsor	Identify the funding source/sponsor and describe its role in developing and/or reporting the guideline. Disclose potential conflict of interest.
8. Evidence collection	Describe the methods used to search the scientific literature, including the range of dates and databases searched, and criteria applied to filter the retrieved evidence.
9. Recommendation grading criteria	Describe the criteria used to rate the quality of evidence that supports the recommendations and the system for describing the strength of the recommendations. Recommendation strength communicates the importance of adherence to a recommendation and is based on both the quality of the evidence and the magnitude of anticipated benefits or harms.
10. Method for synthesizing evidence	Describe how evidence was used to create recommendations, e.g., evidence tables, meta-analysis, and decision analysis.
11. Prerelease review	Describe how the guideline developer reviewed and/or tested the guidelines prior to release.
12. Update plan	State whether or not there is a plan to update the guideline and, if applicable, an expiration date for this version of the guideline.
13. Definitions	Define unfamiliar terms and those critical to correct application of the guideline that might be subject to misinterpretation.

continued

14. Recommendations and rationale	State the recommended action precisely and the specific circumstances under which to perform it. Justify each recommendation by describing the linkage between the recommendation and its supporting evidence. Indicate the quality of evidence and the recommendation strength, based on the criteria described in 9.
15. Potential benefits and harms	Describe anticipated benefits and potential risks associated with implementation of guideline recommendations.
16. Patient preferences	Describe the role of patient preferences when a recommendation involves a substantial element of personal choice or values.
17. Algorithm	Provide (when appropriate) a graphical description of the stages and decisions in clinical care described by the guideline.
18. Implementation considerations	Describe anticipated barriers to application of the recommendations. Provide reference to any auxiliary documents for providers or patients that are intended to facilitate implementation. Suggest review criteria for measuring changes in care when the guideline is implemented.

SOURCE: Shiffman RN, Shekelle P, Overhage M, Slutsky J, Grimshaw J, Deshpande AM. Standardized reporting of clinical practice guidelines: a proposal from the conference on guideline standardization. Ann Intern Med. 2003;139:493-8.

Appendix 7-15

Implementation Strategies

CLASSIFICATION OF PROFESSIONAL INTERVENTIONS FOR GUIDELINE IMPLEMENTATION[*]

- *Distribution of educational materials*: Distribution of published or printed recommendations for clinical care, including clinical practice guidelines, audiovisual materials, and electronic publications. The materials may have been delivered personally or through mass mailings.
- *Educational meetings*: Health care providers who have participated in conferences, lectures, workshops, or traineeships.
- *Local consensus processes*: Inclusion of participating providers in discussion to ensure that they agreed that the chosen clinical problem was important and the approach to managing the problem was appropriate.
- *Educational outreach visits*: Use of a trained person who met with providers in their practice settings to give information with the intent of changing the provider's practice. The information given may have included feedback on the performance of the provider(s).
- *Local opinion leaders*: Use of providers nominated by their colleagues as "educationally influential." The investigators must have explicitly stated that their colleagues identified the opinion leaders.
- *Patient-mediated interventions*: New clinical information (not previously available) collected directly from patients and given to the provider, e.g., depression scores from an instrument.
- *Audit and feedback*: Any summary of clinical performance of health care over a specified period. The summary may also have included recommendations for clinical action. The information may have been obtained from medical records, computerized databases, or observations from patients.

The following interventions are excluded:

- Provision of new clinical information not directly reflecting provider performance which was collected from patients, e.g., scores on a depression instrument and abnormal test results. These interventions should be described as patient mediated.

[*]Reproduced from: Grimshaw JM, Thomas RE, MacLennan G, Fraser C, Ramsay CR, Vale L, et al. Effectiveness and efficiency of guideline dissemination and implementation strategies. Health Technol Assess. 2004;8(6):iii-iv, 1-72.

- Feedback of individual patients' health record information in an alternative format (e.g., computerized). These interventions should be described as organizational.
- *Reminders*: Patient- or encounter-specific information, provided verbally, on paper or on a computer screen, which is designed or intended to prompt a health professional to recall information. This would usually be encountered through their general education, in the medical records or through interactions with peers, and so remind them to perform or avoid some action to aid individual patient care. Computer-aided decision support and drugs dosage are included.
- *Marketing*: Use of personal interviewing, group discussion (focus groups), or a survey of targeted providers to identify barriers to change and subsequent design of an intervention that addresses identified barriers.
- *Mass media*: (1) Varied use of communication that reached great numbers of people including television, radio, newspapers, posters, leaflets and booklets, alone or in conjunction with other interventions; (2) targeted at the population level.

9-1

Appendix 9-1

Question Example

DRUG INFORMATICS CENTER

St. Anywhere Hospital

Name of Inquirer:	Dr. Meghan J. Malone	Date: XX/XX/XX
Address	2184 Fall St.	Time Received: XX:XX am/pm
	Seneca Falls, NY 13148	Time Required: 5 hours
		Nature of Request: Therapeutics
Telephone Number:	(315)555-1212	Type of Inquirer: Pharmacist

QUESTION

A young, adult male patient recently arrived from Japan and presented to the physician sparse medical records indicating he is suffering from tsutsugamushi disease. Because of the language difficulties, not much is known about the patient, other than that he is taking drug X for the illness. Physical exam reveals a patient in some discomfort with elevated temperature, swollen lymph glands, and red rash. All other findings appear to be normal. (*Note:* the person answering this question obtained as much background as possible about the patient.) The physician has little information on the disease and would like to know if that drug X is the most appropriate treatment.

ANSWER

Tsutsugamushi disease is an acute infectious disease seen in harvesters of hemp in Japan.[1] It is caused by *Rickettsia tsutsugamushi*. Common symptoms of the disease include fever, painful swelling of the lymph glands, a small black scab in the genital region, neck or axilla, and large dark-red papules. The disease is known by a number of other names, including akamushi disease, flood fever, inundation fever, island disease, Japanese river fever, and scrub typhus.[2,4] (*Note:* background information presented.) The standard treatment of the disease includes either drug X or drug Y, although there are several other less effective treatments.[5-7] In the remainder of this paper, a comparison of the two major drugs will be presented. (*Note:* clear objective for paper is presented.)

A thorough search of the available literature was conducted. Unfortunately, there were few textbooks available on this disease. A search of MEDLINE (1966 to present) and EMBASE's *Drugs and Pharmacology* (1980 to present) produced a number of articles that were obtained and are reviewed below. (*Note:* This documents the type of search and acts as a lead-in to the remainder of the body of the paper.)

Smith and Jones[8] performed a double-blind, randomized comparison of the effects of drug X and drug Y in patients with tsutsugamushi fever. Patients were required to be between 18 and 70 years old, and could not have any concurrent infection or disorder that would affect the immune response to the disease (e.g., neutropenia, AIDS). Twenty patients received 10 mg of drug X three times a day for 15 days. Eighteen patients received 250 mg of drug Y twice a day for 10 days. The two groups were comparable, except that the patients receiving drug X were an average of 5 years younger ($p < .05$). Drug X was shown to produce a cure, both in terms of symptoms and cultures in 85% of patients, whereas drug Y only produced a cure in 55.5% of patients. The difference was statistically significant ($p < .01\%$). No significant adverse effects were seen in either group. Although it appears that drug X was the better agent, it should be noted that drug Y was given in its minimally effective dose, and might have performed better in a somewhat higher or longer regimen. (*Note:* evaluative comments made about article.)

(*Note:* Other articles would be described at this point.)

Based on the literature found, it appears that drug Y is generally accepted as the better agent, except in those patients with severe renal insufficiency. Because this patient does not appear to be suffering from that problem, it is recommended that he receive a 3-week course of drug Y in a dose of 500 mg three times a day. Renal function should be monitored weekly. The patient should receive an additional week of therapy, if the symptoms have not gone for the final week of therapy. (*Note:* This patient's situation was specifically addressed, rather than just presenting a general conclusion.)

Signature: _____ Date: March 20, 2011

      Sandy Q. Pharmacist, PharmD

REFERENCES

(Present references here.)

Appendix 9-2

Abstracts

Abstracts are a synopsis (usually of 250 words or less) of the most important aspect of an article. They should be clear, concise, and complete enough for readers to have a reasonable understanding of the important portions of the article.[1] Since they are the most commonly read as part of an article, they must be accurate and avoid the three most common errors: differences in information presented in the abstract and in the body of the article, information given in the abstract that was not presented in the article, and conclusions presented in the abstract that are not supported by information in the abstract.[2–4]

There are basically three types of abstracts that are seen in the literature. The first two (descriptive and informational) are somewhat traditional; however, they do not convey as much information as structured abstracts. Structured abstracts were originally designed to convey more information, and have been in use since the 1980s. The type of abstract to be used depends on the type of information and the requirements of the particular place the work is being submitted or used.

In addition to writing an abstract, some journals ask that indexing terms be submitted. Whenever possible, Medical Subject Headings (MeSH) from the National Library of Medicine should be used for the indexing terms. Each of the abstracts will be discussed in more detail in the following sections.

DESCRIPTIVE ABSTRACTS

A descriptive abstract, as its name implies, simply describes the information found in an article. Few specific details are given and it would mostly be used in a review article. An example of this type of abstract is as follows:

> Lists of references that should be available, depending on location of the drug information service, are presented. These lists are specific to community, hospital, long-term care facility, and academic sites. Included are general references, indexing and abstracting services, and journals. Specialty references that would be useful in specific circumstances are also presented. In addition, the equipment necessary to access the computerized resources is shown for the individual references.

INFORMATIONAL ABSTRACTS

Informational abstracts concisely summarize the factual information presented in a study. This type of abstract is more applicable to clinical studies.

Key points to include in an informational abstract include:

- Study design (e.g., double-blind, crossover)
- Purpose
- Number of patients
- Dosages
- Results
- Conclusions

An example of this type of abstract is as follows:

A double-blind, randomized comparison of the effects of drug X and drug Y was performed in patients with tsutsugamushi fever, in order to determine whether either drug was superior in efficacy or safety. Twenty patients received 10 mg of drug X three times a day for 15 days. Eighteen patients received 250 mg of drug Y twice a day for 10 days. The two groups were comparable, except that the patients receiving drug X were an average of 5 years younger ($p < 0.05$%). Drug X was shown to produce a cure, both in terms of symptoms and cultures in 85% of patients, whereas drug Y only produced a cure in 55.5% of patients. The difference was statistically significant ($p < 0.01$%). No significant adverse effects were seen in either group. Drug X was shown to be significantly better than drug Y in the treatment of tsutsugamushi fever.

STRUCTURED ABSTRACTS

Due to perceived deficiencies in abstracts,[5] including lack of sufficient information,[6] a new type of abstract was presented in 1987[7] and later updated in 1990.[8] This structured abstract was designed to present more information about clinical studies and possibly laboratory studies, as compared to the informational abstract presented earlier.[9,10] This type of abstract is not meant for case reports, studies of tissues or animals, opinion articles, and position papers.[7] Abstracts following this standard seem to be gaining in popularity and have been mandated by an influential group of journals (e.g., *New England Journal of Medicine,[11] Annals of Internal Medicine,[7] JAMA: Journal of the American Medical Association,[8] British Medical Journal,[12] Canadian Medical Association Journal,[13] Chest[14]*), sometimes in a somewhat modified form. This type of abstract has also been suggested in the pharmacy literature.[15] Although the overall acceptance and approval of this format of abstract appears to be good, there are some who disapprove.[16–18] Also, there is at least some data suggesting that structured abstracts do not always contain as much information as they should, if the published rules were followed,[19] and that they do not necessarily contain any more useful information than traditional abstracts.[20]

It is worth noting that articles with structured abstracts are indexed with a greater number of terms in MEDLINE, which may lead to ease of finding such articles on computer search.[21]

An abstract following this procedure would contain the following subheadings and information:

- *Objective*—The main objective and key secondary objectives.
- *Design*—The basic design of the study (e.g., randomized, double-blind, crossover, placebo-controlled) and duration of any follow-up.

- *Setting*—The location and level of clinical care available at that location (e.g., tertiary care hospital, ambulatory clinic).
- *Patients or other participants*—Description of the patients, including illnesses and key socio-demographic features and how they were selected for the study (including whether it was a random, volunteer, etc. sample); it should also include number of patients that refused to enroll in the study, proportion of the patients completing the study, and the number of patients withdrawn due to adverse effects.
- *Intervention(s)*—A brief description of any treatment(s) or intervention(s).
- *Main outcome measure(s)*—The main study outcome measurements, as planned before data collection was begun; if most of the article covers other material (e.g., data or hypotheses not planned to be observed before the study was started), that should be made clear.
- *Results*—The method(s) by which patients were assessed and the main results of the study, including any blinding. Statistical significance (particularly confidence intervals, odds ratios, numerators, and denominators) and levels of significance should be mentioned. Absolute, rather than relative, differences are presented (e.g., "adverse effects were seen in 5% of patients in group A and 10% of patients in group B," rather than "Group B had twice as many adverse effects"). Provide response rate in survey articles.
- *Conclusion(s)*—The key conclusion(s) directly supported by the evidence presented in the study and their clinical application(s). Should also include whether further study is necessary.

An example of this type of abstract is as follows:

Study Objective—To compare the safety and efficacy of drug X and drug Y in the treatment of tsutsugamushi fever.

Design—Randomized, double-blind trial.

Setting—Tertiary care, military hospital located on Guam.

Patients—Sequential sample of 40 young (age 20 to 37), otherwise healthy male patients with tsutsugamushi fever. Patients randomly divided into two equal groups. Two patients were removed from the group receiving drug Y, due to transfer to U.S. mainland hospitals. The two groups were comparable, except that the patients receiving drug X were an average of 5 years younger ($p < .05\%$).

Interventions—Twenty patients received 10 mg of drug X three times a day for 15 days. Eighteen patients received 250 mg of drug Y twice a day for 10 days.

Main Outcome Measures—Physician and patients' global assessment of disease activity; five point scale from 0 (no symptoms) to 5 (severe disability). Presence or absence of organism on laboratory specimens.

Results—Drug X was shown to produce a cure, both in terms of symptoms and cultures in 85% of patients, whereas drug Y only produced a cure in 55.5% of patients. The difference was statistically significant ($p < 0.01\%$). No significant adverse effects were seen in either group.

Conclusions—Drug X was shown to produce significantly higher cure rates than drug Y in the treatment of tsutsugamushi fever, with no difference in adverse effects. Additional trials at different doses and lengths of therapy should be performed.

A method to prepare a structured abstract for a review article differs from the first example.[146] This method would only be applicable in specific situations, where a number of similar studies were evaluated together. It would not be useful in a situation where a number of dissimilar articles dealing with the same topic were discussed (e.g., a review of all therapies for a particular disease). Such an abstract would consist of the following items:

- *Purpose*—The main objective of the review article, including information about the population tested, how they were tested, and the outcome
- *Data sources*—A brief summary of data sources and the time periods covered
- *Study selection*—The number of studies covered in the article and how they were selected for inclusion
- *Data extraction*—A description of the guidelines for abstracting data and how those guidelines were applied
- *Data synthesis*—The main results of the review and the method to obtain the results are outlined
- *Conclusions*—Important conclusions, including applications and need for further study

An example of this type of abstract would be as follows:

Purpose—To evaluate the effect of the antihistamine, drug X, on symptoms of allergy, as determined by physicians' and patients' global symptom assessment.

Data sources—Studies published from January 1980 to December 2004 were identified by computer searches of MEDLINE and Embase—*Drugs and Pharmacology* and hand searching of bibliographies of the articles identified via the computer search.

Study selection—Fifty-three studies evaluating the effects of drug X in the treatment of allergy were located.

Data extraction—Descriptive data regarding the population, dosing, effects, and adverse effects were assessed, along with the study's quality.

Results of data analysis—Subjective and objective measures of effectiveness demonstrated that drug X decreased or eliminated allergic symptoms approximately 80% of the time in a variety of patient types (e.g., seasonal allergic rhinitis, perennial allergic rhinitis, anaphylaxis). The only adverse effects seen were dryness of mucous membranes and sedation, seen in approximately 5% and 2% of patients, respectively.

Conclusions—Drug X is an effective agent for the treatment of allergic reactions. It has a low incidence of typical antihistamine adverse effects. Further studies should be performed to verify the effectiveness of Drug X in comparison to other drugs commonly used for anaphylaxis.

9-3

Appendix 9-3

Bibliography

Meghan J. Malone, Patrick M. Malone

Although there seems to be a different method to prepare a bibliography for every English class ever given, there is fortunately a standardized method to prepare a bibliography in medical writing. This method is used by the National Library of Medicine and has been incorporated into the *Uniform Requirements for Manuscripts Submitted to Biomedical Journals* and published in *Citing Medicine* [23,24,25]; it has been used widely since the 1970s in both journals and other medical writing. This method will be presented here.

References in the bibliography are placed in the order they are first cited in the text of a document, and each reference is assigned a consecutive Arabic number. Those cited only in tables or figures are numbered according to the place the table or figure is identified in the text. References are not listed multiple times in the bibliography, if they are cited more than once in the text of the document. Instead, subsequent citations to the same reference use the original reference number. It should also be noted that *Ibid.* is not used. The reference number in the text will be the Arabic number in parenthesis or, commonly, superscript. This number is often cited after the sentence that contains the fact being referenced. If there are several references used to prepare a specific sentence, they may be listed at the end of the sentence or throughout the sentence. Also, if the sentence is a lead-in to an abstract, the authors' names are commonly listed followed by the reference number. See the sentences below for examples.

- Drug X has been shown to cause green rash with purple spots.[2,3]
- Drug Y is useful in the treatment of hypertension,[4] congestive heart failure,[5] and arrhythmias.[6]
- Smith and Jones[7] studied the effects of....
- Brown *et al.*[9] treated... (please notice on this example, *al.* is followed by a period since it is an abbreviation, whereas *et* is a full Latin word, and there is no need for a comma after the first author's name)
- Brown and associates[9] treated... (this is used the same way as the previous example, but is preferred by some people over the use of et al.)

Before getting into the method for listing references and examples, it should be mentioned that there are a number of general rules to be followed. They are:

- Citations are often not found in conclusions of documents. The conclusions are based on the information presented, and cited, earlier in the article.

- Avoid using abstracts as references, if at all possible. Sometimes, however, the information is only published as an abstract, so it is necessary to cite the abstract in this situation.
- Avoid using unpublished observations or personal communications as references. In the latter case, it is proper to insert references to written, but not oral, communications in parentheses in the text only and indicate it will not be formally referenced at the end of publication. Permission must be obtained from the author for the use of this material and this should only be used if the material is not available from a public source of information. A note should be made at the end of the publication stating that permission was given.
- If reference is made to an article that has been accepted by a journal, but not yet published, the phrase *Forthcoming* should be inserted where the year, volume, and page numbers would normally be listed. It is usually necessary to get permission to cite this type of article, since the publisher may have strict confidentiality rules, and verification of acceptance by the journal should be obtained if that is the case.
- The use of the Internet has increased substantially, so it is important to use the correct citation based on which medium is used.
- Only place a period at the end of a web address if a back slash is the last character in the address.
- For items such as wikis, blogs, databases, when they are still open (people can still add something), use a hyphen with three spaces following it for date of publication. If they are closed (people can no longer add something), list the range of dates when it was open.

Examples of the aforementioned references used in a bibliography are provided in the balance of this appendix. Please note, these should provide adequate direction in how to cite most publications. However, if detailed directions and further examples are needed, the reader is referred to *Citing Medicine*, which is available free on the Internet at http://nlm.nih.gov/citingmedicine.[25]

JOURNAL ARTICLES

To cite a journal article, the following information should be given:

- Last name of author(s) and initials each separated by commas, with a period at the end. Please note that some publications will list only three or six authors followed by the phrase *et al.*
- Title of article (do not use quotation marks, capitalize only the initial word of sentences and proper nouns in English) followed by a period with the exception when punctuation is already at the end of the title—for example, if a title ends with a question mark or exclamation point, use that instead of the period.
- Journal Title (abbreviated as found in the list of journals at http://www.nlm.nih.gov/tsd/serials/lji.html) followed by a period.
- Date of Publication: Year, month (three letter abbreviation), and day of month (if available) followed by a semicolon.
- Volume number (listing the issue number in parenthesis) followed by a colon.
- Page numbers (if continuous, use first and last pages separated by a hyphen. If separate pages, list the pages separated by a comma. If a combination of continuous and separate

pages, use both (e.g., 18-29,33,40) followed by a period. If an Internet article does not have page numbers, put the actual number of pages in square brackets, followed by p. (e.g., [20 p.]). If the article is in unpaginated format (e.g., html, xml), precede the number with the word about (e.g., [about 10 screens], [about 15 p.]).

A condensed version of the above information is as follows:

Author(s). Title of Article. Journal Title. Date of Publication;Volume (Issue): Page Number(s).

Journal Article on the Internet

Author(s). Title of Article. Journal Title [Internet]. Date of Publication [Date of Update; Date of Citation]; Volume (Issue): Page Number(s) or [Length of Article]. Available from: Web Address.

Example Journal Citations

Standard Journal Article

Smythe M, Hoffman J, Kizy K, Dmuchowski C. Estimating creatinine clearance in elderly patients with low serum creatinine concentrations. *Am J Hosp Pharm*. 1994 Jan 15;51:198-204.

Beck DE, Aceves-Blumenthal C, Carson R, Culley J, Noguchi J, Dawson K, Hotchkiss G. Factors contributing to volunteer practitioner-faculty vitality. *Am J Pharm Ed*. 1993 Apr;57:305-12.

Journal Article on the Internet

Robinson ET. The pharmacists as educator: implications for practice and education. *Am J Pharm Ed* [Internet]. 2004 [cited 2010 Jun 17];68(3):[4 p.]. Available from: http://www.ajpe.org/aj6803/aj680372/aj680372.pdf/.

Nemecz G. Evening primrose. *US Pharmacist* [Internet]. 1998 Nov [cited 1998 Dec 10];23:[about 1 p.]. Available from: http://www.uspharmacist.com/NewLook/Docs/1998/Nov1998/EveningPrimrose.htm/.

Organization as Author

Task Force on Specialty Recognition of Oncology Pharmacy Practice. Executive summary of petition requesting specialty recognition of oncology pharmacy practice. *Am J Hosp Pharm*. 1994 Jan 15;51:219-24.

Personal Authors and Organization as Author

Wiencke K, Louka AS, Spurkland A, Vatn M, The IBSEN Study Group, Schrumpf E. Association of matrix metalloproteinase-1 and -3 promoter polymorphisms with clinical subsets of Norwegian primary sclerosing cholangitis patients. *J Hepatol*. 2004 Aug;41(2):209-14.

No Author Given

N.Y. court rules against Medicaid co-pay. *Drug Topics*. 1994 Mar;138(3):6.

Article not in English (note that the language is stated at the end)

Antoni N. Zur kritik der irrtümlich sogenannten sehnen- und periostreflexe. *Acta Psychiatrica Neurologica*. 1932;VII:9-19. German.

Volume with Supplement

Nayler WG. Pharmacological aspects of calcium antagonism. Short term and long term benefits. *Drugs*. 1993 Apr;46(Suppl 2):40-7.

Issue with Supplement

Graves NM. Pharmacokinetics and interactions of antiepileptic drugs. *Am J Hosp Pharm*. 1993 Dec;50(12 SupplA):S23-S29.

Volume with Part

Katchen MS, Lyons TJ, Gillingham KK, Schlegel W. A case of left hypoglossal neurapraxia following G exposure in a centrifuge. *Aviat Space Environ Med*. 1990 Sep;61(Pt 2):837-9.

Issue with Part

Dudley MN. Maximizing patient outcomes of antiinfective therapy. *Pharmacotherapy*. 1993 Mar-Apr;13(2 Pt 2):29S-33S.

Issue with no Volume

Slaga TJ, Gimenez-Conti IB. An animal model for oral cancer. *Monogr J Nat Cancer Instit*. 1992;(13):55-60.

No Issue or Volume

Payne R. Acute exacerbation of chronic cancer pain: basic assessment and treatments of breakthrough pain. *Acute Pain Sympt Manage*. 1998:4-5.

Pagination in Roman Numerals

Koretz RL. Clinical nutrition. *Gastroenterol Clin North Am*. 1998 Jun;27(2):xi-xiii.

Expressing Type of Article (as needed)

Goldwater SH, Chatelain F. Taking time to communicate [letter]. *Am J Hosp Pharm*. 1994 Feb 1;51: 232,234.

Talley CR. Reducing demand through preventive care [editorial]. *Am J Hosp Pharm*. 1994 Jan 1; 51:55.

Saritas A, Cakir Z, Emet M, Uzkeser M, Akoz A, Acemoglu F. Factors affecting the b-type natriuretic peptide levels in stroke patients [abstract]. *Ann Acad Med Singapore*. 2010 May;39(5):385.

Article Containing a Retraction

Brown MD. Retraction. *Am Heart J*. 1986;111:623. Retraction of: Slutsky RA, Olson LK. *Am Heart J*. 1984;108:543-7.

Article Retracted

Slutsky RA, Olson LK. Intravascular and extravascular pulmonary fluid volumes during chronic experimental left ventricular dysfunction. *Am Heart J*. 1984 Sep;108:543-7. Retraction in: *Am Heart J*. 1986 Mar;111:623.

Article with Published Erratum

Reitz MS Jr, Juo HG, Oleske J, Hoxie J, Popovic M, Read-Connole E. On the historical origins of HIV-1 (MN) and (RF) [letter]. *AIDS Res Hum Retroviruses*. 1992 Aug;8:1539-41. Erratum in: *AIDS Res Hum Retroviruses*. 1992 Aug;8:1731.

Item (e.g., Table or Figure) in Article

Hohnloser SH, Pajitnev D, Pogue J, Healey JS, Pfeffer MA, Yusuf S, Connolly SJ. Incidence of stroke in paroxysmal versus sustained atrial fibrillation in patients taking oral anticoagulation or combined antiplatelet therapy: an ACTIVE W substudy. *J Am Coll Cardiol*. 2007 Nov 22;50(22): 2156-61. Table 4, Incidence of stoke or non-CNS systemic embolism in patients with paroxysmal versus persistent/permanent AF treated with aspirin plus clopidogrel or OAC; p. 2159.

Unpublished Article

Malone PM. Topics in informatics. *Adv Pharm*. Forthcoming 2004.

BOOKS

To cite a book, the following information should be given:

- Last name of author(s) and initials each separated by a comma and followed by a period. Some publications will list only three authors followed by the phrase *et al.*
- Title of book (capitalize only the initial word of sentences and proper nouns in English) followed by a period with the exception that punctuation is already at the end of the title—for example, if a title ends with a question mark or exclamation point, use that instead of the period.
- Edition, other than first followed by period (e.g. 5th ed.).
- Place of publication (city) followed by colon (if the location is not clear with just a city name, the state or country abbreviation may be placed in parenthesis after the city name and before the colon).
- Name of publisher followed by semicolon.
- Year of publication followed by period.

A condensed version of the above information is as follows:

Author(s). Title of Book. Edition. Place of Publication: Publisher; Date of Publication.

Example Book Citations

Book on the Internet

Author(s). Title of Book [Internet]. Place of Publication: Publisher; Date of Publication [Date of Update; Date of Citation]. Available from: Web Address.

Standard Book

Albright RG. A basic guide to online information systems for health care professionals. Arlington (VA): Information Resource Press; 1988.

Book on the Internet

DiPiro JT, Talbert RL, Yee GC, Matzke GR, Wells BG, Posey LM, editors. Pharmacotherapy: a pathophysiologic approach [Internet]. 7th ed. New York: McGraw-Hill; 2008 [cited 2010 Jun 15]. Available from: http://www.accesspharmacy.com/resourceToc.aspx?resourceID=406/.

Lacy CF, Armstrong LL, Goldman MP, et al, editors. Lexi-comp online [Internet]. Hudson (OH): Lexi-Comp, Inc.; c1978-2010 [cited 2010 Jun 16]. Available from: http://online.lexi.com/crlsql/servlet/crlonline/.

Editor(s) as Author

Chisholm-Burns MA, Schwinghammer TL, Wells BG, Malone PM, Kolesar JM, Dipiro JT, editors. Pharmacotherapy principles and practice. 2nd ed. New York: McGraw Hill; 2010.

No Specific Editor(s), Compiler, or Author Identified

Drug facts and comparisons 1999. St. Louis: Facts and Comparisons; 1998.

Organization as Author and Publisher

United States Pharmacopeial Convention, Inc. USAN and the USP dictionary of drug names. Rockville: United States Pharmacopeial Convention, Inc.; 1993.

Volumes (Same Author(s)/Editor(s))

United States Pharmacopeial Convention, Inc. USP dispensing information. 22nd ed. Vol. 2, Advice for the patient: drug information in lay language. Greenwood Village (CO): Micromedex; 2002.

If on the Internet use the following format:

Author(s). Title of Book. Volume Number, Volume Title [Internet]. Place of Publication: Publisher; Date of Publication [Date of Update; Date of Citation]. Available from: Web Address.

Ross IA. Medicinal plants of the world. Vol. 3, Chemical constituents, traditional and modern medicinal uses [Internet]. Totowa (NJ): Humana Press, Inc.; 2005 [cited 2010 Jun 23]. Available from: http://metis.findlay.edu:2080/xtf-ebc/search?keyword=pharmacy/.

Portion of a Book (e.g., Chapter, Table, Figure, or Appendix) With Author(s) Writing Entire Book

Bauer LA. Applied clinical pharmacokinetics. 2nd ed. New York: McGraw Hill; 2008. Chapter 6, Digoxin; p. 301-55.

If on the Internet use the following format:

Author(s). Title of Book [Internet]. Place of Publication: Publisher; Date of Publication [Date of Update of Book]. Portion Number, Portion Title; [Date of Update of Portion; Date of Citation]; Page Number(s) or [Length of Portion]. Available from: Web Address.

Bauer LA. Applied clinical pharmacokinetics [Internet]. 2nd ed. New York: McGraw Hill; 2008. Chapter 6, Digoxin; [cited 2010 Jun 23]; [about 20 screens]. Available from: http://metis.findlay.edu:2209/content.aspx?aID=3519569/.

Contribution to Book (Portions of Book Written by Different Authors)

Malesker MA, Morrow LE. Fluids and electrolytes. In: Chisholm-Burns MA, Schwinghammer TL, Wells BG, Malone PM, Kolesar JM, Dipiro JT, editors. Pharmacotherapy principles and practice. 2nd ed. New York: McGraw Hill; 2010. p. 479-94.

If on the Internet use the following format:

Chapter Author(s). Chapter Title. In: Author(s)/Editor(s). Title of Book [Internet]. Place of Publication: Publisher; Date of Publication [Date of Citation]. Available from: Web address.

Malone PM. Professional writing. In: Malone PM, Kier KL, Stanovich JE, editors. Drug information: a guide for pharmacists [Internet]. 3rd ed. New York: McGraw-Hill; 2006 [cited 2010 Jun 23]. Available from: http://metis.findlay.edu:2209/content.aspx?aid=2465415/.

Book on CD-ROM or DVD

Haux R, Kulikowski C. Yearbook 04 of medical informatics—towards clinical bioinformatics [CD-ROM]. Stuttgart (Germany): Schatteuer; 2004.

Video Clip, Videocast, or Podcast Associated with Book

Author(s). Title of Book [Internet]. Place of Publication: Publisher; Date of Publication. [Video or Videocast or Podcast], Title of Video; [Date of Citation]; [Length of Video]. Available from: Web Address.

Brunton LL, Parker KL, Murri N, Blumenthal DK, Knollmann BC, editors. Goodman and Gilman's: the pharmacological basis of therapeutics [Internet]. 11th ed. New York: McGraw-Hill; 2006 [Video], Adrenergic neuroeffector junction; [cited 2010 Jun 23]; [5 min.]. Available from: http://metis.findlay.edu:2209/video.aspx?file=anj_01/anj_01/.

OTHER MATERIAL

Format and Example Citations

Conference Paper

Author(s) of Conference Paper. Title of Paper. In: Editors of Conference Proceedings. Conference Title; Date(s) of Conference; Conference Location. Place of Publication: Publisher; Date of Publication. Pages Number(s).

Keyserlingk E. Ethical guidelines and codes—can they be universally applicable in a multi-cultural world? In: Allebeck P, Jansson B, editors. Ethics in medicine. Individual integrity versus demands of society. Karolinska Institute Novel Conference Series. Proceedings of the 3rd International Congress on Ethics in Medicine; 1989 Sep 13-15; Stockholm. New York: Raven Press; 1990. p. 137-49.

If on the Internet use the following format:

Author(s) of Conference Paper. Title of Paper. In: Conference Title [Internet]; Date(s) of Conference; Conference Location. Place of Publication: Publisher; Date of Publication [Date of Citation]. [Length of Paper]. Available from: Web Address.

Keyserlingk E. Ethical guidelines and codes—can they be universally applicable in a multi-cultural world? In: Allebeck P, Jansson B, editors. Ethics in medicine. Individual integrity versus demands of society. Karolinska Institute Novel Conference Series. Proceedings of the 3rd International Congress on Ethics in Medicine [Internet]; 1989 Sep 13-15; Stockholm. New York: Raven Press; 1990 [cited 2010 Jun 23]. [about 2 p.]. Available from: http://jmp.oxfordjournals.org/cgi/issue_pdf/backmatter_pdf/13/4.pdf

Conference Proceedings

Editor(s). Conference Title; Date(s) of Conference; Conference Location. Place of Publication: Publisher; Date of Publication.

Allebeck P, Jansson B, editors. Ethics in medicine. Individual integrity versus demands of society. Karolinska Institute Novel Conference Series. Proceedings of the 3rd International Congress on Ethics in Medicine; 1989 Sep 13-15; Stockholm. New York: Raven Press; 1990.

If on the Internet use the following format:

Editor(s). Conference Title [Internet]; Date(s) of Conference; Conference Location. Place of Publication: Publisher; [Date of Citation]. [Length of Publication]. Available from: Web Address.

Allebeck P, Jansson B, editors. Ethics in medicine. Individual integrity versus demands of society. Karolinska Institute Novel Conference Series. Proceedings of the 3rd International Congress on Ethics in Medicine [Internet]; 1989 Sep 13-15; Stockholm. New York: Raven Press; [cited 2010 Jun 23]. 8 p. Available from: http://jmp.oxfordjournals.org/cgi/issue_pdf/backmatter_pdf/13/4.pdf

Dictionary Definition

Dictionary Name. Place of Publication: Publisher; Date of Publication. Word Being Defined; Page Number.

Stedman's medical dictionary. 27th ed. New York: Lippincott Williams & Wilkins; 2000. Asthenia; p. 158.

If on the Internet use the following format:

Dictionary Name [Internet]. Place of Publication: Publisher; Date of Publication. Term Being Defined; [Date of Citation]. Available from: Web Address.

Merriam-Webster Online [Internet]. Springfield (MA): Merriam-Webster, Inc.; c2010. Blood pressure; [cited 2010 Jun 23]. Available from: http://www.merriam-webster.com/dictionary/blood%20pressure.

Dissertation/Thesis

Author(s). Title[dissertation or master's thesis]. Place of Publication: Publisher; Date of Publication.

Wellman CO. Pain perceptions and coping strategies of school-age children and their parents: a descriptive-correlational study [dissertation]. Omaha (NE): Creighton University; 1985.

If on the Internet use the following format:

Author(s). Title[dissertation or master's thesis on the Internet]. Place of Publication: Publisher; Date of Publication [Date of Update; Date of Citation]. Available from: Web Address.

Mil JW. Pharmaceutical care, the future of pharmacy: theory, research, and practice [dissertation on the Internet]. Groningen (Netherlands): University of Groningen; 2000 Feb 1 [updated 2009 Sept 8; cited 2010 Jun 23]. Available from: http://dissertations.ub.rug.nl/faculties/science/2000/j.w.f.van.mil/?pLanguage=en&pFullItemRecord=ON/.

Legal Documents

Please consult: The bluebook: a uniform system of citation. 19th ed. Cambridge (MA): Harvard Law Review Association; 2010.

Newspaper Article

Author(s). Title of Article. Newspaper Title (Edition). Date of Publication; Section: Page Number (Column Number).

Fein EB. Rise in fetal tests prompts ethical debate. The New York Times (National Ed.). 1994 Feb 5; Sect. A:1(col. 2).

If on the Internet use the following format:

Author(s). Title of Article. Newspaper Title [Internet]. Date of Publication [Date of Update; Date of Citation]; Section: Page Number or [Length of Article]. Available from: Web Address.

Painter K. Your health: feet bear the strain of extra weight. USA Today [Internet]. 2010 Jun 20 [cited 2010 Jun 23]; Health and Behavior:[about 2 screens]. Available from: http://www.usatoday.com/news/health/painter/2010-06-21-yourhealth21_ST_N.htm/.

Package Insert

Package inserts are commonly cited in professional writing, however, the Uniform Requirements do not address the format to use. The following is a common format that is similar to those presented in this appendix:

Medication Name [package insert]. Place of Publication: Publisher; Date of Publication.

Prilosec (omeprazole) delayed-release capsules [package insert]. Wayne, PA: Astra Merck; 1998 Jun.

If on the Internet use the following format:

Medication Name [package insert on the Internet]. Place of Publication: Publisher; Date of Publication [Date of Update; Date of Citation]. Available from: Web Address.

Omeprazole [package insert on the Internet]. Bethesda (MD): U.S. National Library of Medicine; 2009 Aug [updated 2009 Dec; cited 2010 Jun 23]. Available from: http://dailymed.nlm.nih.gov/dailymed/drugInfo.cfm?id=14749.

Meeting Presentations of Paper and Poster Sessions

Author(s). Title of Paper or Poster. Paper or Poster session presented at: Conference Title; Date(s) of Conference; Conference Location.

Ciaccia V, Hinders C, Malone M, Morales R, Sanchez A. Comparison of evidence based hypertension guideline model to an alternative model. Poster session presented at: The University of Findlay Symposium for Scholarship and Creativity; 2010 Apr 13; Findlay, OH.

Patent

Inventor(s); Assignee(Applicant). Title. Patent Country patent Country Code Patent Number. Date patent issued.

Schwartz B, inventor; New England Medical Center Hospital, Inc., assignee. Method of and solution for treating glaucoma. United States patent US 5,212,168. 1993 May 18.

Personal Communication

In text citation only (e.g. Letter from or Conversation with; unreferenced, see Notes Section) In Notes Section state that permission was given to reference the letter or conversation.

(Letter from Max Jones to Charlie Smith on June 23, 2010; unreferenced, see Notes Section)

Scientific or Technical Report

Author(s). Title. Place of Publication: Publisher; Date of Publication. Report Number.:
Issued by funding/sponsoring agency:

Shekelle P, Morton S, Maglione M (Southern California Evidence-Based Practice Center/RAND, Santa Monica, CA). Ephedra and ephedrine for weight loss and athletic performance enhancement: clinical efficacy and side effects. Vol 1, Evidence report and evidence tables. Rockville (MD): Agency for Healthcare Research and Quality; 2003 Mar. (Evidence report/technology assessment; no. 78). Report No.: AHRQPUB03E022. Contract No.: AHRQ-290-97-001.

Issued by performing agency:

Shekelle P, Morton S, Maglione M. Ephedra and ephedrine for weight loss and athletic performance enhancement: clinical efficacy and side effects. Vol. 1, Evidence report and evidence tables. Santa Monica: Southern California Evidence-Based Practice Center/RAND; 2003 Mar. (Evidence report/technology assessment; no. 78). Report No.: AHRQPUB03E022. Contract No.: AHRQ-290-97-001. Sponsored by the Agency for Healthcare Research and Quality.

If on the Internet use the following format:

Author(s). Title [Internet]. Place of Publication: Publisher; Date of Publication [Date of Citation]. Report Number.: Available from: Web Address.

Qureshi N, Wilson B, Santaguida P, Carroll J, Allanson J, Culebro CR, Brouwers M, Raina P. Collection and use of cancer family history in primary care [Internet]. Rockville (MD): Agency for Healthcare Research and Quality; 2007 Oct [cited 2010 Jun 23]. (Evidence reports/technology assessments no. 159) Report No.: AHRQPUB08E001. Contract No.: 290- 02-0020. Available from: http://www.ncbi.nlm.nih.gov/bookshelf/br.fcgi?book=erta159/.

OTHER ELECTRONIC MATERIAL PART OF A BLOG (ONLY ONE AUTHOR)

Since this is personal communication, as above, it usually is done as an in-text citation only (posting on given date from author on given blog; unreferenced, see Notes Section). In Notes Section state that permission was given to reference the blog post. Otherwise can follow format below:

Author of Blog. Title of Blog [blog on the Internet]. Place of Publication: Publisher. [Start Date of Blog]. Title of Part; Date of Publication [Date of Citation]; [Length of Part]. Available from: Web Address.

Daria. Living with Cancer [blog on the Internet]. Edmonton (AB): Daria. [2008 Aug]. Chemo went well; 2010 Jun 12 [cited 2010 Jun 16]; [about 1 screen]. Available from: http://daria-livingwith-cancer.blogspot.com/.

Part of a Blog (Multiple Authors)

Since this is personal communication, as above, it usually is done as an in-text citation only (posting on given date from author on given blog; unreferenced, see Notes Section). In Notes Section state that permission was given to reference the blog post. Otherwise can follow format below:

Author of Comment. Title of Blog Comment. Date of Publication of Comment [Date of Citation]. In: Author of Blog. Name of Blog [blog on the Internet]. Place of Publication: Publisher. Date of Publication. [Length of Comment]. Available from: Web Address.

Smith J. Dialysis. 2010 Jun 16 [cited 2010 Jun 16]. In: Kidney Coaching Foundation, Inc. KCF Blog and News [blog on the Internet]. Raleigh (NC): Kidney Coaching Foundation, Inc. c2005-2010-. [about 1 paragraph]. Available from: http://www.thekcf.org/bn/.

Computer Program on CD-ROM or DVD

Author(s). Title [Medium]. Version. Place of Publication: Publisher; Date of Publication.

A.D.A.M. animated dissection of anatomy for medicine [CD-ROM]. Version 2.2. for Windows. Marietta (GA): A.D.A.M. Software, Inc.; 1993.

Database on the Internet

Title of Database [Internet]. Place of Publication: Publisher. Date of Publication [Date of Update; Date of Citation]. Available from: Web Address.

PubMed [Internet]. Bethesda (MD): National Library of Medicine. 2004- [cited 2004 Aug 18]. Available from: http://www.ncbi.nlm.nih.gov/entrez/query.fcgi.

DRUGDEX [Internet]. Greenwood Village (CO): Thomson Reuters Inc. c1974-2010 [cited 2010 Jun 16]. Available from: http://www.micromedex.com/products/drugdex/.

Part of a Database on the Internet (e.g., a single drug monograph out of a publication)

Title of Database [Internet]. Place of Publication: Publisher. Date of Publication. Record Identifier, Title of Part; [Date of Update; Date of Citation]; [Length of Part]. Available from: Web Address.

MeSH Browser [Internet]. Bethesda (MD): National Library of Medicine. 2004. unique ID: D015201, Phenytoin; [cited 2004 Aug 18]; [about 670 p.]. Available from: http://www.nlm.nih.gov/mesh/MBrowser.html.

DRUGDEX [Internet]. Greenwood Village (CO): Thomson Reuters Inc. c1974-2010. Amiodarone; [updated 2010 Apr 23]; [about 8 screens]. Available from: http://www.micromedex.com/products/drugdex/.

Electronic Mail

Since this is personal communication, as above, it usually is done as an in-text citation only (e-mail on given date from sender to recipient; unreferenced, see Notes Section). In Notes Section state that permission was given to reference the e-mail. Otherwise can follow format below:

Author. Title of Email [Internet]. Message to: Recipient(s). Date of Message [Date of Citation]. [Length of Email].

Malone, Patrick. Drug information textbook [Internet]. Message to: John Stanovich; Mark Malesker. 2010 Jun 14 [2010 Jun 16]. [3 paragraphs].

Encyclopedia Entry

Name of Encyclopedia [Internet]. Place of Publication: Publisher; Date of Publication. Name of Entry; [Date of Update; Date of Citation]; [Length of Entry]. Available from: Web Address.

Encyclopedia Britannica Online [Internet]. Chicago: Britannica; 2010. Stroke; [cited 2010 Jun 23]; [about 5 screens]. Available from: http://www.britannica.com/EBchecked/topic/569347/stroke/.

LISTSERV

Since this is personal communication, as above, it usually is done as an in-text citation only (posting on given date from sender to given LISTSERV; unreferenced, see Notes Section). In Notes Section state that permission was given from the sender to reference the e-mail. Otherwise can follow format below:

Author. Title of Message. In: Name of LISTSERV [Internet]. Place of Publication: Publisher; Date of Message [Date of Citation]. [Length of Message].

Malone PM. CAMIPR—discussion forum for medication information specialists. In: CAMIPR [Internet]. Iowa City: Consortium for the Advancement of Medication Policy and Research; 2010 May 6 [cited 2010 June 18]. [about 1 p.].

Video Clip, Videocast, or Podcast

Title of Homepage [Internet]. Place of Publication: Publisher; Date of Publication of Homepage. [Video or Videocast or Podcast], Title of Video; Date of Publication of Video (if different from Homepage) [Date of Update; Date of Citation]; [Length of Video]. Available from: Web Address.

American Society of Health-System Pharmacists [Internet]. Bethesda (MD): ASHP Advantage; c2010. [Podcast], Multidisciplinary approach to identifying patients at risk for VTE; 2010 May 4 [cited 2010 Jun 23]; [45 min.]. Available from: http://www.ashpadvantage.com/podcasts/.

Web site Homepage

Author(s). Title of Homepage [Internet]. Place of Publication: Publisher; Date of Publication [Date of Update; Date of Citation]. Available from: Web Address.

American Society of Health-System Pharmacists [Internet]. Bethesda (MD): American Society of Health-System Pharmacists; c1997-2004 [updated 2004 Aug 18; cited 2004 Aug 18]. Available from: http://www.ashp.org/.

Part of a Web site

Title of Homepage [Internet]. Place of Publication: Publisher; Date of Publication of Homepage. Title of Part; Date of Publication of Part (if different from Homepage) [Date of Update; Date of Citation]; [Length of Part]. Available from: Web Address.

American Society of Health-System Pharmacists [Internet]. Bethesda (MD): American Society of Health-System Pharmacists; c1997-2004. Compounding Resource Center; [updated 2004 Aug 18; cited 2004 Aug 18]; [about 1 screen]. Available from: http://www.ashp.org/compounding/.

Wiki

Since this is personal communication, as above, it usually is done as an in-text citation only (posting on given date from author on given wiki; unreferenced, see Notes Section). In Notes Section state that permission was given from the author to reference the wiki. Otherwise follow format below:

Author of Part. Title of Part of Wiki. Date of Posting [Date of Update; Date of Citation]. In: Title of Wiki [Internet]. Place of Publication: Publisher. Start Date of Wiki- . [Length of Part]. Available from: Web Address.

If no author for part.

Title of Wiki [Internet]. Place of Publication: Publisher. Start Date of Wiki- . Title of Part of Wiki; [Date of Update; Date of Citation]; [Length of Part]. Available from: Web Address.

Wiki Public Health [Internet]. [place unknown]: WikiPH. [date unknown]- . Health care; [updated 2007 Mar 27; cited 2010 Jun 16]; [about 2 screens]. Available from: http://wikiph.org/index. php?title=Health_care.

REFERENCES

1. Staub NC. On writing abstracts. Physiologist. 1991;34:276-7.
2. Pitkin RM, Branagan MA. Can the accuracy of abstracts be improved by providing specific instructions? A randomized controlled trial. JAMA. 1998;280:267-9.
3. Pitkin RM, Branagan MA, Burmeister LF. Accuracy of data in abstracts of published research articles. JAMA. 1999;281:1110-11.
4. Winker MA. The need for concrete improvement in abstract quality. JAMA. 1999;281:1129-30.
5. Huth EJ. Structured abstracts for papers reporting clinical trials. Ann Intern Med. 1987; 106:626-7.
6. Narine L, Yee DS, Einarson TR, Ilersich AL. Quality of abstracts of original research articles in CMAJ in 1989. CMAJ. 1991;144:449-53.
7. Ad Hoc Working Group for Critical Appraisal of the Medical Literature. A proposal for more informative abstracts of clinical articles. Ann Intern Med. 1987;106:598-604.
8. Haynes RB, Mulrow CD, Huth EJ, Altman DG, Gardner MJ. More informative abstracts revisited. Ann Intern Med. 1990;113:69-76.
9. Rennie D, Glass RM. Structuring abstracts to make them more informative. JAMA. 1991;266:116-17.
10. Haynes RB. Dissent. More informative abstracts: current status and evaluation. J Clin Epidemiol. 1993;46:595-7.

11. Relman AS. New "Information for Authors"—and readers. NEJM. 1990;323:56.

12. Lock S. Structure abstracts. Now required for all papers reporting clinical trials. BMJ. 1988;297:156.

13. Squires BP. Structured abstracts of original research and review articles. CMAJ. 1990;143:619-22.

14. Soffer A. Abstracts of clinical investigations. A new and standardized format. Chest. 1987;92:389-90.

15. Kane-Gill S, Olsen KM. How to write an abstract suitable for publication. Hosp Pharm. 2004;39:289-92.

16. Spitzer WO. Second thoughts. The structured sonnet. J Clin Epidemiol. 1991;44:729.

17. Heller MB. Dissent. Structured abstracts: a modest dissent. J Clin Epidemiol. 1991;44:739-40.

18. Heller MB. Structured abstracts. [letter] Ann Intern Med. 1990;113:722.

19. Froom P, Froom J. Variance and dissent. presentation. Deficiencies in structured medical abstracts. J Clin Epidemiol. 1993;46:591-4.

20. Scherer RW, Crawley B. Reporting of randomized clinical trial descriptors and use of structured abstracts. JAMA. 1998;280:269-72.

21. Harbourt AM, Knecht LS, Humphreys BL. Structured abstracts in MEDLINE, 1989-1991. Bull Med Libr Assoc. 1995;83(2):190-5.

22. Mulrow CD, Thacker SB, Pugh JA. A proposal for more informative abstracts of review articles. Ann Intern Med. 1988;108:613-15.

23. International Committee of Medical Journal Editors. Uniform requirements for manuscripts submitted to biomedical journals [Internet]. Philadelphia: International Committee of Medical Journal Editors;2009 [cited 2010 Jun 13]. Available from: http://www.icmje.org.

24. International Committee of Medical Journal Editors. Uniform requirements for manuscripts submitted to biomedical journals: sample references [Internet]. Philadelphia (PA): International Committee of Medical Journal Editors;2003 [updated 2009 Aug 28; cited 2010 Jun 13]. Available from: http://www.nlm.nih.gov/bsd/uniform_requirements.html/.

25. Patrias K. Citing medicine: the NLM style guide for authors, editors, and publishers [Internet]. 2nd ed. Wendling DL, technical editor. Bethesda (MD): National Library of Medicine (US); 2007 [updated 2009 Oct 21; cited 2010 June 11] Available from: http://nlm.nih.gov/ citingmedicine/.

Appendix 11-1

Code of Ethics for Pharmacists[1]

Pharmacists are health professionals who assist individuals in making the best use of medications. This Code, prepared and supported by pharmacists, is intended to state publicly the principles that form the fundamental basis of the roles and responsibilities of pharmacists. These principles, based on moral obligations and virtues, are established to guide pharmacists in relationships with patients, health professionals, and society.

I. A pharmacist respects the covenantal relationship between the patient and pharmacist.

Considering the patient-pharmacist relationship as a covenant means that a pharmacist has moral obligations in response to the gift of trust received from society. In return for this gift, a pharmacist promises to help individuals achieve optimum benefit from their medications, to be committed to their welfare, and to maintain their trust.

II. A pharmacist promotes the good of every patient in a caring, compassionate, and confidential manner.

A pharmacist places concern for the well-being of the patient at the center of professional practice. In doing so, a pharmacist considers needs stated by the patient as well as those defined by health science. A pharmacist is dedicated to protecting the dignity of the patient. With a caring attitude and a compassionate spirit, a pharmacist focuses on serving the patient in a private and confidential manner.

III. A pharmacist respects the autonomy and dignity of each patient.

A pharmacist promotes the right of self-determination and recognizes individual self-worth by encouraging patients to participate in decisions about their health. A pharmacist communicates with patients in terms that are understandable. In all cases, a pharmacist respects personal and cultural differences among patients.

IV. A pharmacist acts with honesty and integrity in professional relationships.

A pharmacist has a duty to tell the truth and to act with conviction of conscience. A pharmacist avoids discriminatory practices, behavior or work conditions that impair professional judgment, and actions that compromise dedication to the best interests of patients.

V. A pharmacist maintains professional competence.

A pharmacist has a duty to maintain knowledge and abilities as new medications, devices, and technologies become available and as health information advances.

VI. A pharmacist respects the values and abilities of colleagues and other health professionals.

When appropriate, a pharmacist asks for the consultation of colleagues or other health professionals or refers the patient. A pharmacist acknowledges that colleagues and other health professionals may differ in the beliefs and values they apply to the care of the patient.

VII. A pharmacist serves individual, community, and societal needs.

The primary obligation of a pharmacist is to individual patients. However, the obligations of a pharmacist may at times extend beyond the individual to the community and society. In these situations, the pharmacist recognizes the responsibilities that accompany these obligations and acts accordingly.

VIII. A pharmacist seeks justice in the distribution of health resources.

When health resources are allocated, a pharmacist is fair and equitable, balancing the needs of patients and society.

Adopted by the membership of the American Pharmacists Association, October 27, 1994.[1]

REFERENCE

1. American Pharmacists Association. Code of ethics for pharmacists. [Internet]. Washington: American Pharmacists Association. [cited 2010 March 26]. Available from: http://www.pharmacist.com/AM/Template.cfm?Section=Search1&template=/CM/HTMLDisplay.cfm&ContentID=2903.

Pharmacy and Therapeutics Committee Procedure

This appendix includes two policy and procedure operational statements. The first is specifically written to centralize the formulary decision process for a multihospital health system: a Formulary Committee. The second, and closely related, operational statement is written as a model to function as the traditional Pharmacy and Therapeutics Committee for a Hospital's Medical Staff. Both operational statements describe the functions of their related committees based on a certain degree of autonomy. Their membership is ultimately chosen by an administrative leader as a means to best isolate the committee from organizational as well as economic influences. The decision process for each operational statement is intended to create predictability and transparency. To implement this set of operational statements, each Executive Committee of the hospitals in a multihospital system would pass the following resolution:

> The Medical Staff of Alpha Hospital agrees to delegate its Pharmacy and Therapeutic Committee responsibilities to ALPHAOMEGA HEALTH based on the policy and procedures for a "Hospital Formulary System" and a "Hospital Pharmacy and Therapeutics Committee."

The two operational statements can also be combined to reflect the traditional functions of a single-hospital, medical-staff-based pharmacy and therapeutics committee. Also, there may be other arrangements where the two operational statements could provide the organizational environment for a closed health system, a pharmacy benefits manager, or one of the new organizational structures created by federal legislation in 2004 for the new financing of drug coverage in the United States.

POLICY TITLE: HOSPITAL FORMULARY SYSTEM

I. Purpose

To maintain a **HOSPITAL FORMULARY** and a Formulary Committee for all ALPHAOMEGA HEALTH Hospitals as a means to enhance the quality of health care for all patients served by ALPHAOMEGA HEALTH

II. Policy

A. The Formulary Committee of ALPHAOMEGA HEALTH will periodically evaluate its performance as a means to improve its ability to support the Vision and Mission of ALPHAOMEGA HEALTH.

B. ALPHAOMEGA HEALTH will maintain one Formulary Committee and a Pharmacy and Therapeutics Committee (P&T COMMITTEE) at each ALPHAOMEGA HEALTH Hospital to implement this POLICY in accord with the applicable Medical Staff Bylaws and this POLICY.

C. The Formulary Committee of ALPHAOMEGA HEALTH will maintain a standard format for a **HOSPITAL FORMULARY** that is based on the provisions of this POLICY.

D. The Formulary Committee will develop and continually revise a list of therapeutic products, a **HOSPITAL FORMULARY**, which reflects the current clinical judgment of the Medical Staff of ALPHAOMEGA HEALTH Hospitals regarding the selection of the best therapeutic products for the health care of hospitalized patients. The Formulary Committee will evaluate the various alternative therapeutic products available and develop the **HOSPITAL FORMULARY** based on an evaluation of each therapeutic product's indications, effectiveness, risks, patient safety, and overall impact on health care costs.

E. The Formulary Committee will collaborate with the P&T Committee at each ALPHAOMEGA HEALTH Hospital to monitor compliance with the provisions of the **HOSPITAL FORMULARY**.

F. The Formulary Committee will support the quality improvement functions of ALPHAOMEGA HEALTH where necessary to improve the use of the **HOSPITAL FORMULARY**.

III. Procedure

A. FORMULARY COMMITTEE DEVELOPMENT

1. The Formulary Committee will recommend, when appropriate, amendments to this POLICY AND PROCEDURE to the Chief Medical Officer of ALPHAOMEGA HEALTH. After revisions to any of these proposed amendments by the Chief Medical Officer, in collaboration with the Formulary Committee, the Chief Medical Officer will submit the amendments to the Executive Committee of the Medical Staff at each ALPHAOMEGA HEALTH Hospital for final approval.

2. The Officers of the Formulary Committee will prepare an Annual Membership Report to the Chief Medical Officer of ALPHAOMEGA HEALTH regarding participation of its Members and any recommendations that may be important to maintain the expertise necessary for the affairs of the Formulary Committee.

3. The Officers of the Formulary Committee will prepare an Annual Report and submit it to the Professional Affairs Committee of ALPHAOMEGA HEALTH for approval. As a result of this review, the Professional Affairs Committee may make recommendations to the Formulary Committee for consideration regarding its affairs or to the Chief Medical Officer regarding amendments to this POLICY AND PROCEDURE.

B. FORMULARY COMMITTEE ORGANIZATION

1. REGULAR MEMBERS

a. MEDICAL STAFF MEMBERS

i. There may be up to 16 Medical Staff members nominated annually by the Chief Medical Officer of ALPHAOMEGA HEALTH, each President or Chief of Staff from the Medical Staff of an ALPHAOMEGA HEALTH Hospital, or the Officers of the Formulary Committee. Any Medical Staff nominee must have demonstrated an active interest in evidence-based therapeutics, a willingness to be an active participant in the affairs of the Formulary Committee, and represent as a group, whenever possible, the specialties of: Family Practice, Internal Medicine, Pediatrics, Obstetrics and Gynecology, Hematology and Oncology, Cardiology, Infectious Disease, Pulmonology, and General Surgery.

ii. From any Nominees, 12-16 will be selected by the Chief Medical Officer of ALPHAOMEGA HEALTH on the basis of maintaining a reasonable balance among the following factors: hospital and outpatient-based physicians, primary care and disease focused physicians, physician liaison to the Medical Staff Executive Committee or P&T Committee of each ALPHAOMEGA HEALTH Hospital, and a balanced representation from the Medical Staffs of the ALPHAOMEGA HEALTH Hospitals.

b. ADMINISTRATION MEMBER—The Chief Medical Officer of ALPHAOMEGA HEALTH, or designee who is a Medical Staff Member of an ALPHAOMEGA HEALTH Hospital, will be a Member of the Formulary Committee.

2. SPECIAL MEMBERS AND SOURCE OF SELECTION

a. The Chief Medical Officer of ALPHAOMEGA HEALTH will select Special Members as may be needed to provide administrative or technical support for the affairs of the Formulary Committee. The Special Members will include, at a minimum:

i. any pharmacist recommended by the Pharmacist in charge at a Hospital Pharmacy of ALPHAOMEGA HEALTH and

ii. at least one Registered Nurse from among the Nursing Staff of an ALPHAOMEGA HEALTH Hospital.

b. The Chairperson of the Formulary Committee may select one or more Special Members from the personnel of ALPHAOMEGA HEALTH or the Medical Staff of any ALPHAOMEGA HEALTH Hospital on a temporary basis as may be necessary for:

i. technical support for the activities of the Formulary Committee or any Ad Hoc Subcommittee of the Formulary Committee or

ii. information for the deliberations of the Formulary Committee regarding a proposal to add or delete an individual therapeutic product listed on the **HOSPITAL FORMULARY**.

3. FORMULARY COMMITTEE OFFICERS

a. The CHAIRPERSON will be selected by the Chief Medical Officer of ALPHAOMEGA HEALTH from among the Regular Members of the Formulary Committee. The Chairperson will:

i. manage the affairs of the Formulary Committee in a manner to

I) support the active, positive involvement of each Regular and Special Member,

II) acknowledge any conflict of interests,

III) initiate a replacement appointment of any Officer, Regular Member, or Special Member becoming inactive during a calendar year,

IV) appoint temporary Special Members, and

V) select the location for Meetings of the Formulary Committee;

ii. prepare the Annual Membership and Self-Evaluation reports; and

iii. appoint an Ad Hoc Committee when necessary to study decisions in greater depth or to arrive at consensus recommendations for consideration by the Formulary Committee whose membership will be

    I) six or fewer members from the Medical Staffs of the ALPHAOMEGA HEALTH Hospitals,

    II) at least one member who is a Regular Member of the Formulary Committee, and

    III) the Secretary, or designee, of the Formulary Committee.

b. The VICE CHAIRPERSON will be selected by the Chief Medical Officer of ALPHAO-MEGA HEALTH from the Regular Members of the Formulary Committee. The Vice-Chairperson will assume the duties of the Chairperson during his or her absence.

c. The SECRETARY will be selected by the Chief Medical Officer of ALPHAOMEGA HEALTH from among the Regular or Special Members of the Formulary Committee. The Secretary will assist the Chairperson in managing the affairs of the Formulary Committee by:

  i. preparing the minutes for each meeting of the Formulary Committee or any of its Ad Hoc Committees,

  ii. sending an Agenda to the Members prior to each meeting of the Formulary Committee,

  iii. maintaining a schedule for the annual regular review by the Formulary Committee of all therapeutic products listed on the **HOSPITAL FORMULARY**, and

  iv. coordinating the preparation of any Drug Monograph or any other report necessary for a meeting of the Formulary Committee by a Pharmacist In Charge, or designee, at an ALPHAOMEGA HEALTH Hospital.

4. TERM OF APPOINTMENT

a. The Regular and Special Members will be appointed or reappointed each January for 1 year.

b. Each Officer will be appointed or reappointed each January for 1 year.

5. VOTING

a. Each Regular Member will have one vote, and each Special Member will have not have a vote.

b. Any two Regular Members present during a Meeting of the Formulary Committee will constitute a quorum.

c. The Regular Members present at a meeting of the Formulary Committee should recognize that a decision regarding a special issue may not be appropriate if certain Regular or Special Members having expertise related to the issue are not present. Based on attendance or any other pertinent reason, the Regular Members present at a meeting of the Formulary Committee should delay making any permanent decision when the appropriate expertise is not available during a meeting of the Formulary Committee.

    d. A simple majority of Regular Members voting will be required for any action of the Formulary Committee. Any abstention on the basis of a conflict of interests will be noted in the minutes for the meeting.

6. LIAISON—A Regular or Special Member may be appointed by the Chief Medical Officer of ALPHAOMEGA HEALTH to report on the affairs of the Formulary Committee during the deliberations of any other Committee of ALPHAOMEGA HEALTH.

7. MEETINGS—The meetings of the Formulary Committee will be:
   a. scheduled once a month for 1 hour or as may be planned by the Members of the Formulary Committee,
   b. attended by Regular and Special Members only, and
   c. convened at a location arranged by the Chairperson.

8. COMMITTEE PROTOCOLS—The Formulary Committee may also arrange for the:
   a. definitions applicable to the resignation and replacement of any Regular Member, Special Member, or Officer during a calendar year;
   b. management of any potential or actual conflict of interests affecting the participation of a Regular or Special Member during a meeting of the Formulary Committee;
   c. use of ALTERNATIVE MEDICATION for the health care of a patient at any ALPHA-OMEGA HEALTH Hospital;
   d. information necessary to request a change in the list of therapeutic products or other information described in the **HOSPITAL FORMULARY**;
   e. contents of a DRUG MONOGRAPH that must be prepared before a therapeutic product not listed on the **HOSPITAL FORMULARY** is administered to a patient or before a therapeutic product is added to the **HOSPITAL FORMULARY**; and
   f. management of any shortage of a therapeutic product listed in the **HOSPITAL FORMULARY** by the:
      i. timely notification of the Medical Staff at each ALPHAOMEGA HEALTH Hospital listing the specific dosage forms in limited or unavailable supply,
      ii. development of alternative strategies for a patient's health care using therapeutic products currently available on the **HOSPITAL FORMULARY** when a therapeutic product becomes either not available or in limited supply,
      iii. collaboration with the appropriate expertise within the Medical Staff of ALPHAO-MEGA HEALTH Hospitals when a rationing protocol is necessary for a critical therapeutic product in limited supply, and
      iv. review of any proposal for a rationing protocol by the Ethics Council of ALPHAO-MEGA HEALTH when the Formulary Committee requests assistance before final approval to ensure that the appropriate ethical standards have been considered.

C. **HOSPITAL FORMULARY** FORMAT
   1. Any therapeutic product used in the health care of a patient will be eligible for the **HOSPITAL FORMULARY**. This includes samples, prescription drugs as defined by the Food and Drug Administration, herbal or other alternative therapies administered topically or enterally, nutraceuticals, over-the-counter drugs, vaccines, diagnostic or contrast agents, radioactive agents, respiratory products, parenteral or enteral nutrients, blood

products, intravenous solutions, and anesthetic gases. A therapeutic product may not be considered for the **HOSPITAL FORMULARY** if it would normally be considered a medical device, durable medical equipment, or implant.

2. The **HOSPITAL FORMULARY** will list the therapeutic products approved by the Formulary Committee in a format approved by the Formulary Committee. The format for the **HOSPITAL FORMULARY** will reflect the recommendations of nationally recognized organizations and include certain attributes, where appropriate, as described in the following.

   a. Any restricted use provision will be defined by credentialing categories in use by the Medical Staffs of ALPHAOMEGA HEALTH Hospitals and be implemented when necessary to monitor or limit the use of a **HOSPITAL FORMULARY** therapeutic product known to be associated with:

      i. an increased risk of a substantial adverse patient reaction,

      ii. a highly specific therapeutic indication, or

      iii. an unusual impact on the overall cost of health care.

   b. Specific patient education provisions will be added for any **HOSPITAL FORMULARY** therapeutic product known to require:

      i. special nutritional adjustments,

      ii. prevention of substantial adverse effects or noncompliance, or

      iii. unique requirements for informed consent.

   c. Continuing education provisions will be added when a Medical Staff Member or qualified Hospital employee requires specialized knowledge prior to or during the administration of a given **HOSPITAL FORMULARY** therapeutic product. This is particularly applicable in the professional areas of oncology and cardiology.

   d. Special information may be added to assist the Medical Staff at each ALPHAOMEGA HEALTH HOSPITAL when necessary to improve the:

      i. level of compliance with prescribing only therapeutic products listed on the **HOSPITAL FORMULARY**,

      ii. acceptance of rational therapeutic concepts as a basis for planning health care intervention strategies, and

      iii. acceptance of therapeutic interchange strategies involving therapeutic products not listed on the **HOSPITAL FORMULARY**.

3. Each therapeutic product listed in the **HOSPITAL FORMULARY** will normally be stocked in each ALPHAOMEGA HEALTH Hospital's Pharmacy. The Formulary Committee may establish an alternative provision for inventory control of a **HOSPITAL FORMULARY** therapeutic product when the alternative provision will not interfere with the health care of an individual patient hospitalized at an ALPHAOMEGA HEALTH Hospital.

   D. **HOSPITAL FORMULARY** MAINTENANCE

1. A proposal for a change in a single therapeutic product listed on the **HOSPITAL FORMULARY** will require a specific set of steps before final approval by the Formulary Committee. These steps are defined below. The Formulary Committee may make a temporary

exception to this provision when necessary to improve the quality of health care to patients at an ALPHAOMEGA HEALTH Hospital.

   a. timely submission of a completed Formulary Request form to any pharmacist at an ALPHAOMEGA HEALTH Hospital by a Medical Staff member of an ALPHAOMEGA HEALTH Hospital or other professional employee of ALPHAOMEGA HEALTH,

   b. review of the Formulary Request by a pharmacist in charge, or designee, of an ALPHAOMEGA HEALTH Hospital's Pharmacy to be sure that it has been fully completed,

   c. preparation of a Drug Monograph, as may be arranged by the Secretary of the Formulary Committee if a new therapeutic product has been proposed by the Formulary Request for the **HOSPITAL FORMULARY**,

   d. preliminary review of the Formulary Request and any associated Drug Monograph by representative specialists affected by any proposed change in the **HOSPITAL FORMULARY**,

   e. initial approval or disapproval of the Formulary Request at one meeting of the Formulary Committee, followed by review for comments at each ALPHAOMEGA HEALTH Hospital's P&T Committee, before final approval or disapproval including any amendments to the Formulary Request at a subsequent meeting of the Formulary Committee.

2. The Formulary Committee will annually review all therapeutic products listed on the **HOSPITAL FORMULARY** according to a schedule of therapeutic classes as may be arranged throughout a calendar year by the Secretary of the Formulary Committee. The review of each class of therapeutic products will require a specific set of events before final approval. These steps are defined in the following:

   a. review of a class of therapeutic products preliminarily by the pharmacists in charge, or designees, of the ALPHAOMEGA HEALTH Hospital Pharmacies prior to a meeting of the Formulary Committee regarding the possible need to:

      i. initiate a Formulary Request for a new addition to the **HOSPITAL FORMULARY**,

      ii. deletion of a therapeutic product because of production defects, nonuse, nonavailability, recall, or replacement by another therapeutic product, or

      iii. a need to change information included in the **HOSPITAL FORMULARY** such as patient education, professional education, therapeutic interchange, or a restricted use provision;

   b. preliminary review of the proposed revisions to the **HOSPITAL FORMULARY** by representative specialists affected by the proposed revisions;

   c. initial approval or disapproval of the therapeutic product class review at one meeting of the Formulary Committee, followed by review for comments at each ALPHAOMEGA HEALTH Hospital's P&T Committee, before final approval or disapproval including amendments to the class review at a subsequent meeting of the Formulary Committee.

3. The Formulary Committee may authorize certain strategies by the ALPHAOMEGA HEALTH Hospital pharmacies that are necessary to offer the most appropriate therapeutic

products for hospitalized patients. The Formulary Committee may authorize these special strategies when supported by its own decision and the support of each ALPHAOMEGA HEALTH Hospital's P&T Committee. Certain specific strategies to be authorized by this POLICY AND PROCEDURE are listed in the following.

    a. A class review of **HOSPITAL FORMULARY** therapeutic products as described previously may also be initiated when there is a Formulary Request for a therapeutic product that substantially affects the inclusion or supplementary information of other therapeutic products currently listed in the **HOSPITAL FORMULARY**.

    b. The pharmacist in charge, or designee, at all ALPHAOMEGA HEALTH Hospital Pharmacies will arrange to prepare a preliminary or full Drug Monograph before any therapeutic product is dispensed that has not previously been ordered for a hospitalized patient at any ALPHAOMEGA HEALTH Hospital.

    c. The Formulary Committee may provide for automatic therapeutic interchange between a therapeutic product that is not listed for another therapeutic product that is listed on the **HOSPITAL FORMULARY** when supported by appropriate scientific evidence and appropriately considered standards of practice.

    d. The Formulary Committee may also select certain therapeutic products for the **HOSPITAL FORMULARY** that will be dispensed for certain indications or any indication even if prescribed with a "Do Not Substitute" designation. The Formulary Committee will use the same process for this designation as defined previously for a new change in the **HOSPITAL FORMULARY**.

E. **HOSPITAL FORMULARY** COMPLIANCE

   1. The P&T Committee of each ALPHAOMEGA HEALTH Hospital will be responsible for monitoring each Medical Staff physician's orders for a therapeutic product that is:

    a. not listed or does not have an automatic therapeutic interchange with a therapeutic product listed on the current **HOSPITAL FORMULARY**,

    b. for an indication not permitted by the **HOSPITAL FORMULARY**, or

    c. for an indication having a restricted use provision.

   2. Any ALPHAOMEGA HEALTH Hospital's P&T Committee may establish a Special Formulary as a means to temporarily support the efforts of its Medical Staff in the health care of hospitalized patients having special requirements that are unique to that Hospital. The Special Formulary therapeutic products will be selected using the same process defined previously for a change in the **HOSPITAL FORMULARY**. For a Special Formulary, the other Committees of the Hospital's Medical Staff will provide the advise and consent process. For any therapeutic product listed on an ALPHAOMEGA HEALTH Hospital's Special Formulary for 1 year or more, continued use of the Special Formulary status for the therapeutic product will require the approval of the Formulary Committee.

   3. If a P&T Committee votes to not accept a decision of the Formulary Committee, the Chairperson, or designee, of the P&T Committee will be invited to a subsequent meeting of the Formulary Committee. At this Formulary Meeting, the Formulary Committee will attempt to develop a strategy for resolving the conflict between the original decision of the Formulary Committee and the respective P&T Committee. In the event that a

resolution is not achieved, the issue may be appealed by either Committee to the Professional Affairs Committee for a final decision within 3 months of the appeal.

F. QUALITY IMPROVEMENT

1. The Formulary Committee will maintain access to the decisions of other hospitals' Formulary or P&T Committees as a resource for the basis in managing difficult decisions regarding the **HOSPITAL FORMULARY**. The hospitals chosen should reflect regional as well as national locations.

2. The Formulary Committee will regularly assess the pending availability of new therapeutic products in the future that will likely require the preparation of a Formulary Request and Drug Monograph.

3. The Formulary Committee will regularly monitor the possible evolution of a shortage involving the availability of a therapeutic product listed on the **HOSPITAL FORMULARY**.

4. The Formulary Committee may recommend to each P&T Committee certain quality improvement projects, such as a Drug Use Evaluations for a certain product that would reflect the health care at all ALPHAOMEGA HEALTH Hospitals.

5. The Formulary Committee will monitor all black box warnings or other Advisories issued by the Food and Drug Administration or pharmaceutical manufacturing company. The Formulary Committee will use the monitoring process as a basis to collaborate with each ALPHAOMEGA HEALTH Hospital's P&T Committee as a means to promote patient safety.

6. The Formulary Committee will maintain a newsletter regarding its decisions and distribute it to each member of the Medical Staff of all ALPHAOMEGA HEALTH Hospitals.

7. The Formulary Committee will collaborate with the P&T Committee at each ALPHAOMEGA HEALTH Hospital to develop educational strategies for the ALPHAOMEGA HEALTH professional employees and each Hospital's Medical Staff that builds support for the principles and priorities used to maintain the **HOSPITAL FORMULARY**.

8. The Formulary Committee will offer consultation when requested or directed by the Board of Directors of ALPHAOMEGA HEALTH, its Committees, or any other ALPHAOMEGA HEALTH Committee regarding therapeutic products in the investigation, protocols, standard order sets, or quality assessment of health care.

9. The Formulary Committee will offer a means to coordinate the standardization of POLICY AND PROCEDUREs for the Pharmacy Departments of ALPHAOMEGA HEALTH Hospitals.

POLICY TITLE: HOSPITAL PHARMACY AND THERAPEUTICS COMMITTEE

I. Purpose

To maintain a Pharmacy and Therapeutics Committee as a means to enhance the quality of health care for all patients served by the Alpha Medical Center.

II. Policy

A. The Pharmacy and Therapeutics Committee of Alpha Medical Center will periodically evaluate its performance as a means to improve its ability to support the Vision and Mission of ALPHAOMEGA HEALTH.

B. The Alpha Medical Center will maintain a Pharmacy and Therapeutics Committee (P&T committee) to implement this POLICY in accord with the applicable Medical Staff By-Laws and this POLICY.

C. The P&T Committee may maintain a SPECIAL FORMULARY at the Alpha Medical Center based on the provisions of the Hospital Formulary System POLICY AND PROCEDURE of ALPHAOMEGA HEALTH.

D. The P&T Committee will monitor compliance with the provisions of the **HOSPITAL FORMULARY**.

E. The P&T Committee will support the quality improvement functions of ALPHAOMEGA HEALTH where necessary to improve the use of the **HOSPITAL FORMULARY**.

F. The P&T Committee will review and approve any POLICY AND PROCEDURE of the Alpha Medical Center Pharmacy.

III. Procedure

A. PHARMACY AND THERAPEUTICS COMMITTEE DEVELOPMENT

   1. The P&T Committee will recommend, when appropriate, amendments to this POLICY AND PROCEDURE to the Administrator of Alpha Medical Center. After revisions to any of these proposed amendments by the Administrator, in collaboration with the P&T Committee, the Administrator will submit the amendments to the Executive Committee of the Alpha Medical Center Medical Staff for final approval.

   2. The Officers of the P&T Committee will prepare an Annual Membership Report to the Administrator of the Alpha Medical Center regarding participation of its Members and any recommendations for changes in its membership that may be important to maintain the expertise necessary for the affairs of the P&T Committee.

   3. The Officers of the P&T Committee will prepare an Annual Report and submit it to the Executive Committee of the Alpha Medical Center Medical Staff for approval. As a result of this review, the Executive Committee may make recommendations to the P&T Committee for consideration regarding its affairs or to the Administrator regarding amendments to this POLICY AND PROCEDURE.

B. FORMULARY COMMITTEE ORGANIZATION

   1. REGULAR MEMBERS AND SOURCE OF SELECTION

      a. MEDICAL STAFF MEMBERS

         i. There may be up to eight Medical Staff members nominated annually by the Administrator, or designee, of Alpha Medical Center, the President of the Medical Staff of the Alpha Medical Center, or the Officers of the P&T Committee. Any Medical Staff nominee must have demonstrated an active interest in evidence-based therapeutics, a willingness to be an active participant in the affairs of the P&T Committee, and represent as a group, whenever possible, the specialties of:

Family Practice, Internal Medicine, Pediatrics, Obstetrics and Gynecology, Hematology and Oncology, Cardiology, Infectious Disease, Pulmonology, and General Surgery.

ii. From any nominees, eight will be selected by the Administrator, or designee, of Alpha Medical Center on the basis of maintaining a reasonable balance among the following factors: hospital and outpatient-based physicians, primary care and disease focused physicians, physician continuity from year to year, and physician liaison to the Medical Staff Executive Committee of the Alpha Medical Center or the Formulary Committee of ALPHAOMEGA HEALTH.

b. PHARMACY MEMBERS—The Administrator, or designee, of Alpha Medical Center will select two pharmacists that will include the Pharmacist In Charge of the Hospital's Pharmacy.

c. NURSING SERVICE MEMBER—The Administrator, or designee, of Alpha Medical Center will select one registered nurse from the Nursing Service.

2. SPECIAL MEMBERS AND SOURCE OF SELECTION

a. The Administrator, or designee, of Alpha Medical Center may select Special Members as needed to provide administrative or technical support for the affairs of the P&T Committee.

b. The Chairperson of the Formulary Committee may select one or more Special Members from the personnel of the Alpha Medical Center or its Medical Staff on a temporary basis as may be necessary for:

i. technical support for the activities of the P&T Committee or any Ad Hoc Subcommittee or

ii. information for the deliberations of the P&T Committee regarding a proposal to add or delete an individual therapeutic product listed on the **HOSPITAL FORMULARY**.

3. P&T COMMITTEE OFFICERS AND SOURCE OF SELECTION

a. The CHAIRPERSON will be selected by the Administrator, or designee, of the Alpha Medical Center from the physician Regular Members of the P&T Committee. The Chairperson will:

i. manage the affairs of the P&T Committee in a manner to:

I) support the active, positive involvement of each Regular and Special Member,

II) acknowledge any conflicts of interest,

III) initiate a replacement appointment of any Officer, Regular Member, or Special Member becoming inactive during a calendar year,

IV) appoint temporary Special Members,

V) select the location for Meetings of the P&T Committee;

ii. prepare the Annual Membership and Self-Evaluation reports; and

iii. appoint an Ad Hoc Committee when necessary to study decisions in greater depth or to arrive at consensus recommendations for consideration by the P&T Committee whose membership will be

      I)   six or fewer members from the Medical Staff of the Alpha Medical Center,

      II) at least one member who is a physician Regular Member of the P&T Committee, and

      III) the Secretary, or designee, of the P&T Committee.

  b. The VICE-CHAIRPERSON will be selected by the Administrator of the Alpha Medical Center from among the physician Regular Members of the P&T Committee. The Vice-Chairperson will assume the duties of the Chairperson during his or her absence.

  c. The SECRETARY will be selected by the Administrator of the Alpha Medical Center from among the Regular or Special Members of the P&T Committee. The Secretary will assist the Chairperson in managing the affairs of the P&T Committee by:

    i. preparing the minutes for each meeting of the P&T Committee or any of its Ad Hoc Committees,

    ii. sending an Agenda to the Members prior to each meeting of the P&T Committee,

    iii. maintaining liaison with the other Committees of the Medical Staff,

    iv. maintaining a schedule for the annual Quality Assurance activities of the P&T Committee, and

    v. assisting in the preparation of any Drug Monograph or any other report necessary for a meeting of the Formulary Committee of ALPHAOMEGA HEALTH.

4. TERM OF APPOINTMENT

  a. The Regular and Special Members will be appointed or reappointed each January for 1 year.

  b. Each Officer will be appointed or reappointed each January for 1 year.

5. VOTING

  a. Each Regular Member will have one vote, and each Special Member will have not have a vote.

  b. Any two physician Regular Members present during a Meeting of the Formulary Committee will constitute a quorum.

  c. The Regular Members present at a meeting of the P&T Committee should recognize that a decision regarding a special issue may not be appropriate if certain Regular or Special Members having expertise related to the issue are not present. Based on attendance or any other pertinent reason, the Regular Members present at a meeting of the P&T Committee should delay making any permanent decision when the appropriate expertise is not available during a meeting of the P&T Committee.

  d. A simple majority of Regular Members voting will be required for any action of the P&T Committee. Any abstention on the basis of a conflict of interests will be noted in the Minutes for the meeting.

6. LIAISON— A Regular or Special Member may be appointed by the Administrator to report on the affairs of the P&T Committee during the deliberations of any other Committee of the Alpha Medical Center.

7. MEETINGS—The meetings of the P&T Committee will be:

  a. scheduled once a month for 1 hour or as may be planned by the Members of the P&T Committee,

    b. attended by Regular and Special Members only,

    c. convened at a location arranged by the Chairperson.

  8. COMMITTEE PROTOCOLS—The P&T Committee may also arrange for the:

    a. use of definitions applicable to the resignation and replacement of any Regular Member, Special Member, or Officer during a calendar year as may be established by the Formulary Committee of ALPHAOMEGA HEALTH and

    b. management of any potential or actual conflict of interests affecting the participation of a Regular or Special Member during a meeting of the P&T Committee as may be determined by the Formulary Committee of ALPHAOMEGA HEALTH.

C. HOSPITAL FORMULARY DEVELOPMENT

  1. The P&T Committee will review for comment at each meeting any therapeutic product recommended for addition or deletion to the **HOSPITAL FORMULARY** by the Formulary Committee of ALPHAOMEGA HEALTH.

  2. The P&T Committee will review for comment at each meeting any class review of therapeutic products by the Formulary Committee of ALPHAOMEGA HEALTH and its recommendations for changes in the **HOSPITAL FORMULARY**.

D. HOSPITAL FORMULARY COMPLIANCE

  1. The P&T Committee will monitor each Medical Staff physician's orders for a therapeutic product that is:

    a. not listed or does not have an automatic therapeutic interchange with a therapeutic product listed on the current **HOSPITAL FORMULARY**,

    b. for an indication not permitted by the **HOSPITAL FORMULARY**, or

    c. for an indication having a restricted use provision.

  2. The P&T Committee may establish a Special Formulary for therapeutic products not listed on the **HOSPITAL FORMULARY** as a means to temporarily support the efforts of the Medical Staff for hospitalized patients having special requirements that are unique to Alpha Medical Center. The Special Formulary therapeutic products will be selected using the same process defined by the ALPHAOMEGA HEALTH Formulary Committee for the **HOSPITAL FORMULARY**. For a Special Formulary, the other Committees of the Alpha Medical Center's Medical Staff will provide the advise and consent process. For any therapeutic product listed on the Special Formulary for 1 year or more, continued use of the Special Formulary status for the therapeutic product will require the approval of the Formulary Committee.

  3. If the Alpha Medical Center P&T Committee votes to not accept a decision of the Formulary Committee, the Chairperson, or designee, of the P&T Committee will attend a subsequent meeting of the Formulary Committee. At this Formulary Meeting, the Formulary Committee will attempt to develop a strategy for resolving the conflict between the original decision of the Formulary Committee and the P&T Committee of the Alpha Medical Center. In the event that a resolution is not achieved, the issue may be appealed by either the Formulary Committee or the Alpha Medical Center P&T Committee to the Professional Affairs Committee for a final decision within 3 months of the appeal.

E. QUALITY IMPROVEMENT

1. The P&T Committee will regularly review the decisions of the ALPHAOMEGA HEALTH Formulary Committee as a means to evaluate any issues requiring the development of carefully considered implementation requirements at the Alpha Medical Center, such as the shortage of a therapeutic product.

2. The P&T Committee will maintain an annually revised schedule for Drug Use Evaluations as may be established through consultation with other Medical Staff Committees.

3. The P&T Committee or an Ad Hoc Committee will review all Medication Error Reports.

4. The P&T Committee will quarterly review all Adverse Medication Reaction Reports.

5. The P&T Committee will participate in the development of standard order sets as may be requested by a Member, a group of Members, or a Committee of the Medical Staff. Generally, the P&T Committee will not have primary responsibility of a standard order set unless specifically requested by the Executive Committee of the Medical Staff.

6. The P&T Committee will prepare an annual report to the Executive Committee regarding the overall level of prescribing compliance with the **HOSPITAL FORMULARY**.

7. The P&T Committee in collaboration with the Formulary Committee will monitor all black box warnings or other advisories issued by the Food and Drug Administration or pharmaceutical manufacturing company. The Formulary Committee will use the monitoring process as a basis to collaborate with each P&T Committee of ALPHAOMEGA HEALTH as a means to promote patient safety.

8. The P&T Committee will suggest information to the Formulary Committee for inclusion in the **HOSPITAL FORMULARY** newsletter.

9. The P&T Committee may make recommendations to the Medical Staff of Alpha Medical Center regarding the health care of hospitalized patients regarding the use of the **HOSPITAL FORMULARY** based on the outcome of certain studies undertaken by the P&T Committee. These studies will exclude any direct identification of patient names or medical records.

F. PHARMACY DEPARTMENT POLICY AND PROCEDURE

1. The P&T Committee will periodically review and approve the POLICY AND PROCEDURES of the Alpha Medical Center Pharmacy Department.

2. The review and approval will be, whenever possible, coordinated with the operational statements of the other Pharmacy Departments of ALPHAOMEGA HEALTH Hospitals.

12-2

Formulary Request Form

PHARMACY AND THERAPEUTICS COMMITTEE
FORMULARY ADDITION REQUEST

NOTE: Both sides of this form must be completed in order for consideration by the **Formulary Committee** at its next regularly scheduled meeting. You may submit additional information based on the outline of this **request** if more space is required. If you are not a member of the committee, you must also complete a Conflict of Interest Statement and attach it to this request.

Generic Name _____ **Brand Name** _____

Indications - Describe the FDA-approved or potential off-label uses that have prompted this **request.** _____

Dosing - Describe the specific strength and administration form of this product necessary for this **request.** _____

Comparative Efficacy - Describe how this agent relates to other products in terms of effectiveness. _____

Contraindications and Warnings - Describe any substantial issues related to this product. _____

Adverse Effects - List any substantial issues related to this product. _____

Expected Outcomes - Describe how this product would substitute or add to the current **Formulary** products. _____

Cost of Therapy - Describe how this product would change the overall cost of medical care. _____

Impact on Inpatient Care Processes - Describe any special requirements on the hospital for use of this product such as nursing/medical staff education, standards of care, discharge planning, certification, or standard order sets. _____

Impact on Outpatient Care Processes - Describe any special requirements on ambulatory care for use of this product such as compliance, follow-up, or monitoring. _____

Other Considerations - Describe any information not applicable to the above categories. _____

Requested By - Must be a **Formulary Committee Member** or **Hospital Medical Staff Member.** _____

Printed Name _____

Signature _____

Response - For record keeping by the **Formulary Committee**.

   Received by a **Formulary Committee Member** date   _____

   Initial **Formulary Committee** consideration date   _____

   Final **Formulary Committee** consideration date   _____

Action Taken

Notification of Medical Staff Member submitting **request** date _____

P&T Committee Meeting Attributes[1-3]

I. TIMING

    A. Regular—The choice is often between monthly or bimonthly. Overall, a long-term commitment to one schedule that does not vary is ideal. An atypical but practical variation might include monthly meetings except August and December, in order to adjust for times when it is difficult to get quorum because of vacations and holidays. To support a regular meeting cycle, any cancellation on a sudden, unexpected basis must be avoided virtually without exception. Finally, a 2- to 3-year experience with a given schedule would be necessary to permit members an opportunity to work a membership commitment into their own schedule.

    B. Monthly work cycle—Virtually all holidays occur in association with the first or last week of any month during the calendar year. Similarly, Mondays and Fridays frequently have distractions caused by these associated weekend demands. Thus, the second or third Tuesday-Wednesday-Thursday of the calendar month is often the best choice for a regular meeting.

    C. Daily work cycle—Given the character of the previous discussion, the start of the morning or afternoon would be ideal for a meeting. The afternoon timing could be associated with a light lunch prior to starting the meeting.

II. MEETING ROOM CHARACTER

    A. Location—A location that minimizes the travel barriers encountered by all the members of the committee is best. In a multihospital organization, this choice may not be ideal if a perception of interhospital territoriality would create a perception of bias in the decisions of the committee. There have also been suggestions regarding the use of teleconferencing.[4] As this becomes a more widely accepted professional tool in the future, the barriers of travel time could be eliminated as a means to incorporate a higher degree of expertise within the members of the committee.

    B. Size —The room should have a rectangular table, or tables set up in a U shape if there are too many members for a single table, with chairs on all sides and enough room for additional chairs next to the walls for guests who might be attending a meeting. The room should allow a comfortable fit for a table that is large enough for the usual attendance as well as appropriate audiovisual equipment. Overall, the room or table should not be so large that the usual attendees might feel isolated and thus less engaged in the agenda of any meeting. Similarly, a full turnout would crowd the room, giving greater emphasis to the character of the deliberations.

C. Seating—This can be highly defined as seen in cases with assigned seats having a name card displayed on the table for each member. The benefits of universal identity of the members would thus be enhanced, especially if they are generally unknown to each other because of the size of an institution or hospital group. More commonly, there could be no fixed seating arrangements for a more informal tradition that could better support collaboration and open discussion. A decision by the chairperson to sit in different locations would further emphasize this approach to a seating tradition. It is also often good for pharmacy personnel to disperse themselves throughout the room to avoid a feeling of us/them in discussions.

REFERENCES

1. Doyle M, Straus D. How to Make Meetings Work: The New Interaction Method. New York, NY: Berkeley Publishing Group; 1993.
2. Nair KV, Coombs JH, Ascione FJ. Assessing the structure, activities, and functioning of P&T committees: a multisite case study. P&T. 2000;25(10):516-28.
3. Balu S, O'Connor P, Vogenberg FR. Contemporary issues affecting P&T committees. Part 2: beyond managed care. P&T. 2004;29:780-3.
4. Boedeker B. Virtual Pharmacy and Therapeutics Meetings. The Harry S. Truman VA Hospital Experience. Columbia (MO): Harry S. Truman Memorial Veteran's Hospital; 1999 Mar [cited 2004 Jan 27]. Available from: http://www.gasnet.org/esia/1999/march/virtual.html.

12-4

Example P&T Committee Minutes

ORGANIZATION, INC.

PHARMACY AND THERAPEUTICS COMMITTEE MEETING

January 21, 2011

SCHEDULED AT 0700

THESE MINUTES ARE PRIVILEGED AND NOT SUBJECT TO DISCLOSURE OR LEGAL DISCOVERY PROCEEDINGS UNDER (STATUTE NUMBER)

I. **Call to order**. The members or Guests present or members absent are indicated below: (legal names, usually with degrees)

The meeting was called to order by the chairperson at 7:00AM. The physician members present represented a quorum. The minutes for the previous meeting were presented to the members. The section regarding a report of the chairperson from a discussion with the executive committee about illegible handwriting and unapproved abbreviations was specifically reviewed by the chairperson. The minutes did not describe the executive committee's request that the P&T committee quarterly forward five to eight examples of physician progress notes that reflect these two issues. The executive committee decided to have the president of the medical staff have individual contact with the medical staff members involved. A motion was made to approve the amended minutes and seconded. There being no further discussion, the motion was approved unanimously. After the vote, there was a brief discussion of the impending transition to a total electronic medical record with physician order entry and its ability to reduce transcribing errors. The physician members expressed concern regarding the ease of order entry. No further action was taken.

II. PHARMACY AND THERAPEUTICS COMMITTEE ORGANIZATIONAL AFFAIRS

A. Policy and Procedure Amendments—The chairperson submitted a draft revision of the entire policy and procedure for the P&T committee in response to new standards of TJC and previously discussed requirements for the functions of the committee. The committee reviewed the proposed draft and agreed informally to reconsider it at the next meeting after the chairperson has had a chance to meet with the Chief Medical Officer regarding any other amendments that may be necessary.

B. Committee Procedures
1. Conflict of Interest Disclosure—The chairperson gave the Members the forms necessary to declare any potential or actual conflicts of interest according to the procedure established previously by the committee. The chairperson briefly reviewed this process and emphasized that conflicts of interest were only unacceptable when not acknowledged or no action is take to resolve them during a meeting of the committee.
2. Formulary Request format—no change
3. Alternate Medication Use—no change
4. Drug Monograph—no change
C. Committee membership—no action; end of year report due December 31st
D. Annual Report—Draft Report due January 5th
E. Ad hoc committees—none currently
F. Budget—reports due February, May, August, November
III. Formulary System
A. Formulary Maintenance
1. Formulary additions/deletions
   a. IV lansoprazole (Protonix)
   b. fondaparinux (Arixtra)
   c. escitalopram (Lexapro)
2. Formulary Class Reviews
   28:04 General anesthetic agents
   72:00 Local anesthetic agent
   86:00 Smooth muscle relaxants
   24:00 Cardiovascular agents
3. Nonformulary usage report
4. Review of standard order sets/guidelines
   TPN order sheet
IV. Drug Use and Quality Improvement
A. Medication error report—no report
B. Adverse medication reaction report—no report
C. Drug Usage Evaluation report—no report
D. Medication recall—no report
V. Hospital Pharmacy Policies—no report
VI. Current Medication Shortages

Chairperson Skills

I. Experience

A. KNOWLEDGE OF FORMULARY ISSUES

This occurs ideally as a result of prior experience on the committee for several years. P&T committee meetings are often associated with an individual hospital, group of hospitals, a staff model health maintenance organization, or an insurance related pharmacy benefit management (PBM) process. A chairperson having experience in each of these areas would be ideal.

B. PROFESSIONAL PRACTICE

It could be suggested that at least 10 years is required for a pharmacist, nurse, administrator, or physician to have a sense of the overall trends evolving within health care. Within a P&T committee, the chairperson would need this background to best respond to the biases that each member might bring to the deliberations. It is beneficial if the members have had mutual experience with the chairperson at a direct patient care level.

C. LEADERSHIP

The chairperson is likely to be the most essential person for the overall success of a P&T committee. This is most directly related to the organization truism that it is nearly impossible to hold a committee responsible for anything except when a committee is acting as the ultimate authority for an organization. Thus, the value of a P&T committee is related to its ability to the serve the common interests of the entire organization affected by its actions. If the costs of the P&T committee members' time are considered, the committee's activities are the result of a very expensive effort. To best utilize this expertise, the chairperson must be skilled at mobilizing these resources in a manner that best supports the overall efforts of the organization to which it is attached. A previously demonstrated ability to create this role for a committee is the most valuable attribute in choosing a committee's chairperson.

II. Meeting Strategies

A. PUNCTUALITY

Given the busy schedules of the members, it is necessary to start and end on time. To open a meeting, it is best to lay out the agenda including any new additions and briefly discuss any items that will require a special discussion. Within 2 to 3 minutes, the chairperson and each member should have an understanding of the scope of the meeting ahead.

B. FAIRNESS

Often the health care process vacillates unpredictably between deductive and inductive reasoning processes. External observers are often baffled by this interplay. Related to this, it is suggested that a strict use of the *Robert's Rules of Order* for a meeting agenda may not facilitate the spontaneity for a committee's members that usually underlies their involvement in the character of health care. It is the responsibility of the chairperson to guide this process and seek out the opinions that the members have for a given issue. Also, if the knowledge necessary to make the best judgment for a given issue does not exist for a decision on the issue, it is important that the chairperson be able to facilitate a consensus that develops a means to rectify the deficiency.

C. INVOLVEMENT

Some members may not normally wish to participate spontaneously during a meeting. It is up to the chairperson to ask these members a specific question that would allow them a meaningful opportunity to participate in a given discussion. Occasionally, the chairperson might ask each member present about his or her opinion for a final decision being faced by the committee. This strategy should begin at one place around the table moving to each member present clockwise around the meeting room.

12-6

Appendix 12-6

Conflict-of-Interest Declaration

Formulary Addition Request Conflict-of-Interest Statement

Generic Name _____ Trade Name _____

Substantial Involvement with a Competing Organization - ▫ Yes ▫ No

Please describe if:

1) A member of a health insurance company or another health system Pharmacy and Therapeutics Committee.
2) Another health system medical staff officer.
3) A member of a group practice primarily affiliated with another health system.

Substantial Involvement with a Company that Manufactures the Product or Competes with the Product's Company - ▫ Yes ▫ No

Please describe if:

1) Receiving financial income or support in the last 12 months of more than $100 for research, attendance at a company supported seminar, travel to an out-of-town meeting, or participation in a company-sponsored speaker's bureau.
2) Receiving pharmaceutical products from the company in the last 12 months for personal or family use, gifts for family or personal use, or samples for use other than as a courtesy for patients.
3) Maintaining in the last 12 months a substantial ownership of stock (>10% of outstanding shares) in the company having >30% of its revenue from sales to this organization, its affiliated organizations, or another local health system.

Substantial Inside Information - ▫Yes ▫No

Please describe if there are other outside relationships for which involvement in this **request** may be actually or potentially perceived as affecting the decision of the committee such as:

NOTE: This must be submitted along with the actual Request Form if the person submitting the Request is not a member of the Formulary Committee. A copy of the Formulary Committee's Policy on Conflict-of-Interest Management is attached.

1) Having a substantial position of authority in another organization that might affect a member of the committee for employment or medical staff privileges.

2) Disclosing information about this request to another organization directly or indirectly, which might give this organization, the other organization, or the requester an unfair advantage.

3) Receiving substantial assistance from the company or its representative that manufactures the requested product in the preparation of this Formulary Addition Request.

13-1

Format for Drug Monograph

INSTITUTION NAME HEADING

Generic Name: Can include other common, nonofficial names, e.g., TPA for alteplase.

Trade Brand Name: If more than one, indicate company for each.

Manufacturer (or source of supply): Include Web site address.

Therapeutic Category: For example, Thromobolytic Agent for alteplase

Classification: Note—other classifications, such as the VA Class, can also be used.
  - AHFS Number and Classification: If not in the book yet, see the list in the front of the *American Hospital Formulary Service—Drug Information* book and determine the most appropriate classification.
  - FDA Classification: Include specific FDA Web site URL concerning approval.
  - Status—Prescription, Nonprescription, and/or Controlled Substance Schedule (if applicable)

Similar agents: A list of common treatments used for the same indication(s).

Summary: Includes a short summary of advantages and disadvantages of the drug, particularly in relation to other drugs or treatments used for each major indication, and any other significant information.

Recommendations: Indicate whether or not the drug should be added to the Drug Formulary of an institution, including specifying the indications for which it is approved for use in the institution, assuming the institution would have patients who would be treated for illnesses for which this drug might be used. Also indicate the specific formulary status for the drug (i.e., uncontrolled, monitored, restricted, conditional—see ASHP guidelines) and whether the drug will replace any other product that might already be on the formulary. In addition, include any information on how the drug is to be placed in any clinical guidelines. For third-party payer monographs, information will need to be included on the payment tier.

Page one consists of the above information

Pharmacological Data
  - Mechanism of Action (usually brief)
  - Bacterial Spectrum (if applicable)

Therapeutic Indications

- FDA-Approved Indications (see package insert)—Clearly indicate which indications are FDA approved.
- Potential unlabeled uses (List only if they are considered to be acceptable medical practice, although it is allowable to mention others that are early in investigation with a statement that the drug should not be used for them or that they require more study.)—Clearly indicate they are not FDA approved.
- How the drug, and similar drugs, fit into clinical guidelines.
- Clinical Comparison (Include abstracts for at least two studies; see Professional Writing Appendix 9-2 for more guidelines. Include human efficacy studies and, where available, studies comparing the product to standard therapy. Note: if there are other supportive studies for an indication, they can be covered briefly, if you desire, along with the major study covered in detail. Be sure to note any deficiencies in the studies). Also, pharmacogenomic information may need to be included here and elsewhere.

Bioavailability/Pharmacokinetics

A table summarizing the following, in comparison to the gold standard, can be very useful.

- Absorption
- Distribution
- Metabolism
- Excretion

Dosage Forms

- Forms and Strengths—Compare to other agents (consider a table), because new products often have a limited number of dosage forms/routes as compared to established products. Purity and composition information should be included for herbal and alternative medications.
- Explain any special information needed for preparation and storage, in comparison to other products. Sometimes a product will be so difficult to prepare or have such a limited shelf life after preparation that it is not worth stocking.

Dosage Range

- Adults
- Children
- Elderly
- Renal or Hepatic Failure
- Special Administration Requirements
- Any anticipated problems in supplies (i.e., shortages) or restrictions in distribution (e.g., physician needs to be certified to prescribe)

Known Adverse Effects/Toxicities

- Frequency and Type (A table comparing the drug to others can be a clear and concise way of expressing this information.)

- Prevention of Toxicity
- Risk and Benefit Data

Special Precautions: Usually includes pregnancy and lactation.

Contraindications

Drug Interactions

A simple one or two sentence statement for each—usually various interactions are separated into short paragraphs and compared to other drugs.

- Drug-Drug
- Drug-Food
- Drug-Laboratory

Patient Safety Information

Includes medication error information and product safety information from outside sources (e.g., Institute for Safe Medication Practices, MedWatch, FDA Patient Safety News, United States Pharmacopeia Patient Safety Program)

Patient Monitoring Guidelines

Include effectiveness, adverse effects, compliance, and other appropriate items.

Patient Information

- Name and description of the medication
- Dosage form
- Route of administration
- Duration of therapy
- Special directions and precautions
- Side effects
- Techniques for self-monitoring
- Proper storage
- Refill information
- What to do if dose is missed

Cost Comparison

Use AWP and institutional prices, and make sure there are comparisons with any similar products at equivalent doses—a pharmacoeconomic analysis (see Chapter 6: Pharmacoeconomics) is the best method of comparing drugs in this section; remember to include any required concomitant therapy. Providing a spreadsheet file with information to consider different circumstances may be helpful.

Date Presented to Pharmacy and Therapeutics Committee, and name and title of the person preparing the document

References

Follow the guidelines as described in Appendix 9-3.

Appendix 13-2

Example Drug Monograph

Note: This example is based on fictional products and is condensed. It shows examples of most sections in a real drug monograph, but often does not go into all of the details (e.g., a table of adverse effects is shown, but only a couple items are listed, whereas a full drug monograph would list at least all common and/or serious reactions).

St. Anywhere Medical Center
Pharmacy and Therapeutics Committee
Drug Evaluation Monograph

Recommendations

It is recommended that artiblood be added to the Drug Formulary for use restricted to those who cannot use natural blood replacement products because of religious reasons or because suitable blood types are not available, including for use in cardiac catheterization procedures. It is not approved for use as a volume expander, except when in conjunction with the previous indications.

Generic Name:	artiblood	**Therapeutic Category:**	Blood substitute
Brand Name:	MegaBlood	**Classification:**	AHFS 16:00 Blood Derivatives
			FDA Classification: 1A
			Status: Prescription Only
Manufacturer:	MegaPharmics	**Similar Agents:**	fakered

Summary

Artiblood is a new perfluorocarbon that has many similarities to the only other product in its class, fakered. Both products have the ability to temporarily replace the oxygen-carrying function of red blood cells in patients in whom the use of whole blood or packed red blood cells is impossible due to medical or religious reasons. In general, artiblood was found to be more efficacious than fakered; however, it also has been shown to produce a greater number of adverse effects. The adverse effects are mostly gastrointestinal in nature; however, the increased international normalized ratio (INR) can be a problem in some patients. Artiblood is not metabolized in the body, whereas fakered is approximately 50% metabolized to inactive components. These differences are generally not clinically significant, because the dose of either product is unlikely to need adjustment. Fakered is available in several different volume bags, allowing the dose to be matched more closely to the anticipated patient need. Although the cost of fakered appears to be lower, a pharmacoeconomic analysis shows that artiblood would produce the greatest cost savings for the institution.

Pharmacological Data

Artiblood is a type of perfluorocarbon, similar to fakered. These products have the unique ability to freely bind with or give up oxygen, depending on the partial pressures of the gas where the product is located (i.e., in the lungs there is an abundance of oxygen, so the product adsorbs oxygen; in the tissues there is a relative deficiency of oxygen, so the product gives up the gas).[1,2] The products do not have direct immunologic properties, nor do they have the ability to aid in blood clotting, although there may be some effect on blood clotting (either interference by coating platelets or precipitation of the clotting pathway mechanism).[3]

In addition to oxygen-carrying capabilities, the products have some plasma volume expansion properties. Artiblood has a similar effect to Dextran 40,[1] whereas fakered's properties are relatively insignificant.[4] Maximum plasma volume expansion occurs within several minutes of administration and lasts for approximately one day in normal patients. This results in increased central venous pressure, cardiac output, stroke volume, blood pressure, urinary output, capillary perfusion, and pulse pressure. Microcirculation is improved.

Therapeutic Indications

Indications

Artiblood is FDA approved for the short-term replacement of the oxygen-carrying capabilities of blood in patients who cannot use normal whole blood.[1] In addition, the product has been used successfully in cardiac catheter procedures, although this use is not FDA approved.[5] There is some early research into the use of the product as a plasma expansion product, but there is not enough information to support this use.[6]

Fakered is approved only for use in cardiac catheterization,[2] although it is commonly used as a blood replacement product in patients who cannot or will not use whole-blood products.[7]

Evidence-Based Clinical Guidelines

A search of the literature was performed to identify evidence-based clinical guidelines. This included Medline, Embase Drugs and Pharmacology, the National Guideline Clearinghouse Web site, the American College of Cardiology Web site, and approximately a dozen Internet search engines; however, no applicable guidelines were identified.

Clinical Studies

Max and Sugar[6] conducted a comparison trial of artiblood (500 mL/day administered once daily over 1 hour to 80 patients) and fakered (750 mL administered once over 90 minutes to 82 patients) in patients (18 to 80 years of age) suffering from massive blood loss (>1 L), who could not use whole blood due to religious beliefs (e.g., Jehovah's Witnesses). In the artiblood group, all patients were undergoing open-heart surgery, as were 78 of the patients in the fakered group. The remainder of the fakered group consisted of gunshot patients. Patients with renal insufficiency (creatinine clearance < 50 mL/min) or diagnosed with liver dysfunction were eliminated from consideration. Both groups were similar, except that the artiblood group had more smokers, which may have had an effect on oxygen requirements. Withdrawals from the artiblood group were for the following reasons: death due to failure of heart-lung machine (1 patient), noncompliance with protocol (10 patients), worsening symptoms (3 patients), and side effects (1 patient, vomiting). The authors noted that protocol compliance problems were due to inappropriate staff education and were not related to the drug itself. In the fakered group, withdrawals were due to side effects (1 patient, diarrhea; 1 patient, nausea; 1 patient, abdominal cramps) and noncompliance with protocol (2 patients). The patients were assessed on the following items: oxygen and carbon dioxide content of the blood (samples drawn immediately before and after administration, and every 4 hours for 24 hours), coagulation profile of patient (drawn within 2 hours before and after administration), affect on normal blood chemistry profiles (SMA-20) (drawn within 2 hours before and after administration), and time to discontinuation of supplemental oxygen to the patient. Adverse effects were also noted. Results were analyzed using appropriate statistical methods. Artiblood was found to increase the oxygen-carrying capabilities of the blood in comparison to fakered ($p < 0.01$), although fakered did significantly improve oxygen-carrying capabilities over baseline ($p < 0.05$). Although fakered had a minimal effect on blood chemistry and coagulation profile, it was noted that INRs were increased in patients receiving artiblood ($p < 0.001$). Other adverse effects, mostly gastrointestinal in nature, were more common with fakered, although the symptoms typically disappeared within 2 hours of administration. Other measured characteristics seemed similar between the two groups. The authors concluded that artiblood was the superior agent, due to increased oxygen-carrying capabilities. The authors downplayed adverse effects, although the effects on INRs do appear worrisome.

[Other studies would be covered here for all likely uses within an institution.]

There were no studies found that demonstrated any affects of genome on either artiblood or fakered therapy.

Bioavailability/Pharmacokinetics[16-18]

Absorption

Absorption is not applicable, because these agents are administered by IV infusion.

Distribution

Artiblood is found in the blood stream, with little being distributed to the tissues. Approximately 5% of fakered is found in the liver, with the rest being in the bloodstream.

Metabolism

Artiblood is not metabolized in the body, whereas approximately 50% of fakered is broken down to inactive components and is excreted in the bile.

Elimination

Artiblood has a half-life of 5 to 15 hours. It is excreted unchanged in the urine. The longer half-life is seen in patients with renal insufficiency. Because the drug is usually given as a single dose, renal insufficiency does not pose a significant problem. Fakered has a half-life of 4 to 7 hours in normal patients. Significant renal or hepatic impairment may double the half-life.

Dosage Forms

Large Volume Parenteral

- Artiblood—500 mL IV bags
- Fakered—500, 750, and 1000 mL IV bags

No other forms or strengths are available. This product will have limited availability for the next 6 months due to the ability of the manufacturer to produce an adequate amount to satisfy demands. No problems in availability are expected after that point. Due to the restrictions on indicated uses in the institution, this is not expected to cause any difficulties, and therefore no specific procedures are being mandated to address a possible shortage.

Dosage Range

The normal dose of artiblood for blood replacement is 500 mL, which may be repeated once after 4 hours. Doses may be cut in half for patients weighing less than 50 Kg. No dosage adjustments are necessary in renal or hepatic impairment. The product has not been tested in patients younger than 12 years of age and is not recommended in that population. No dosage adjustment is necessary in the elderly.[1]

Fakered is given in doses of 500 mL to 1 L, with a maximum daily dose of 1.5 L. The dose is adjusted based on the clinical response of the patient. The product can be used in patients as young as 6 years of age; however, the initial dose is 250 mL.[2]

Known Adverse Effects/Toxicities

The two agents are compared in the following table:

Adverse Effect	Artiblood (% of patients)	Fakered (% of patients)
Gastrointestinal		
Nausea	20	7
...	...	...

Special Precautions

Neither drug has been studied long term; therefore, the effects are not known.

Both products are considered Pregnancy Category C. Tests in pregnant animals have shown adverse effects and no adequate, well-controlled studies have been conducted in humans. There is no information available on the excretion of the drug in human milk. Overall, when considering use in pregnant or lactating women, the physician must consider the benefits versus the risks.

Safety and effectiveness of artiblood in children have not been established, although fakered may be used in children at least 6 years old.

Contraindications

Both agents are contraindicated in patients with hypersensitivities to the drug or any component of the dosage form.

Drug Interactions

Drug-Drug Interactions

Heparin—Effects of heparin or low-molecular-weight heparins may be significantly increased by either artificial blood replacement agent, although the effect by artiblood tends to be greater. There is no effect on either artiblood or fakered, although the heparin may improve circulation of the products to underperfused tissues. (Other interactions for both drugs would be listed and compared.)

Drug-Food Interactions

None are known or expected, because these agents are given intravenously and do not undergo enterohepatic recirculation.

Drug-Laboratory Test Interactions

INR - INRs can be increased by both agents, although the effect is more noticeable with artiblood.
(Other interactions for both drugs would be listed and compared.)

Patient Safety

This product has a good patient safety profile, with relatively minor adverse effects (e.g., nausea). Because the product has no coagulation or immunologic activity, health care providers must be aware that it is only used for temporary help in oxygen-carrying capabilities. Other specific safety concerns include

- Patients on warfarin must have a baseline INR and one each day for the 2 days following administration.
- The product has been on the market less than 6 months and information is limited.
- The product must be refrigerated until approximately 30 minutes prior to infusion.

Patient Monitoring Guidelines

Monitor patient for objective evidence of effectiveness (e.g., oxygen content of blood and clinical effects). Obtain baseline INR and normal chemistry values, and monitor regularly. Monitor for adverse effects.

Patient Information

In a patient receiving the product due to trauma, it is likely that he or she will not be able to be given information. In that case, provide the information to the next of kin or guardian. Inform patients that the product is an intravenous product that does not contain any blood products. The patient or family should know that the patient might receive this product once or more during the first day after surgery. The patient or family should be informed that the drug has few noticeable adverse effects other than some gastrointestinal upset; however, the physician or pharmacist should be consulted if anything unusual occurs. The patient or family should know that some blood tests would be regularly performed to exclude the possibility of adverse effects. The nurse will keep the drug refrigerated until approximately 30 minutes before infusion. Warnings about missed doses are irrelevant.

Cost Comparison

General Pricing Information

	AWP	Daily Dose[a]	St. AMC	Daily Dose[a]
Artiblood 500 mL	$2500/bag	$2500	$2310/bag	$2310
Fakered 500 mL	$1000/bag	$1000	$800/bag	$800
Fakered 750 mL	$1500/bag	$1500	$1200/bag	$1200
Fakered 1000 mL	$2000/bag	$2000	$1600/bag	$1600

[a]Assume use of one bag of each strength.

Pharmacoeconomic Analysis

- Problem Definition—The objective of this analysis is to determine which artificial blood product should be included on our Drug Formulary.
- Perspective—This will be from the perspective of the institution.
- Specific Treatment Alternatives and Outcomes—There are two drugs to be compared: artiblood and fakered. It will be assumed that natural blood products are not an alternative, because the ability to use natural products would preclude consideration of the artificial products. The outcomes to be measured are hospital costs.
- Pharmacoeconomic Model—A cost-benefit analysis will be performed. A cost-utility analysis would be desirable, but insufficient information is available. Note: no published pharmacoeconomic analysis is available. The following is based on information obtained from the literature concerning efficacy, adverse effects, monitoring, etc., and uses St. AMC costs, because outside prices would be irrelevant.

	Cost per Patient	Benefit-to-Cost Ratio	Net Benefit
Cost of artiblood (including administration, monitoring, adverse reactions, etc.)	$5120	$7430/$5120 = 1.45:1	$7430 - $5120 = $2310
Benefits of artiblood (money saved by early patient discharge from ICU)	$7430		
Cost of fakered (including administration, monitoring, adverse reactions, etc.)	$4000	$4500/$4000 = 1.125:1	$4500 - $4000 = $500
Benefits of fakered (money saved by early patient discharge from ICU)	$4500		

Note to reader: The previous information is a summary of information, including averages, decision analysis, and sensitivity analysis, that would be used in a pharmacoeconomic evaluation. Although the details could be presented here, it may be distracting and confusing to some readers—a decision must be made as to whether all of the details will be presented. See Chapter 6 (Pharmacoeconomics) for details on how to prepare a pharmacoeconomic analysis of a drug being evaluated by the P&T Committee.]

Presented by John Q. Doe, PharmD to the Pharmacy and Therapeutics Committee on February 30, 20XX.

References

References would be listed in the order in which they are cited in the text—see Appendix 9–3 in the Chapter 9: Professional Writing for format and details.

Appendix 14-1

Comparison of Quality Assurance and Total Quality Management in Health Care

Comparison	TQM Approach	QA Approach
Purpose	Improve quality of all services/products for all patients and customers	Improve quality of patient care
Scope	All systems and processes (clinical and nonclinical)	Clinical systems and processes
	Actions directed toward improving processes	Actions directed toward improving people
Leadership	All clinical and nonclinical leadership	Physicians and clinical leadership
Aims	Continuous improvements if no problems are identified	Problem solving
	Focus on common causes of failed quality	Identify individuals whose performance or outcomes are outside expectations
Focus	Process improvement and people	Individuals (peer review)
	Improve performance of everyone	Training or elimination of unacceptable few
	Prevention and process design	Inspection
	Customers are everyone involved in the system	Customers are patients, professionals, and review organizations
Customers and requirements	Measures based on customers and professionals	Measures established by health professionals
Methods	Brainstorming	Audits
	Nominal group technique	Nominal group technique
	Force field analysis	Hypothesis testing
	Coaching/mentoring	
	Flow charts	
	Pareto charts	
	Cause-and-effect diagrams	
	Run chart	
	Control chart	
	Histogram	
	Scatter diagram	
	Stratification	
	Quality function deployment	

continued

Comparison	TQM Approach	QA Approach
People involved	Everyone Actions are decided by a team with no time constraints	Quality assurance committee/staff Actions are decided by committees appointed for a specified time period
Outcomes	Improves performance for everyone involved in the process Reduces threats Promotes team effort and eliminates territoriality	Improves individual performance Creates defensiveness
Continuing activities	Continual process improvement through monitoring	Monitors deviations; actions are taken when deviations occur

14-2

Tools Used in Quality Improvement

FLOW CHARTS

Flow charts illustrate the steps of a process and how the steps are related to each other. They can be used to describe the process, to increase a team's knowledge of the entire process, to identify weaknesses or breakdown points in the current process, or to design a new process. An example of a flow chart outlining how adverse drug reactions might be addressed within an organization is provided.

Flowchart: suspected adverse drug reactions

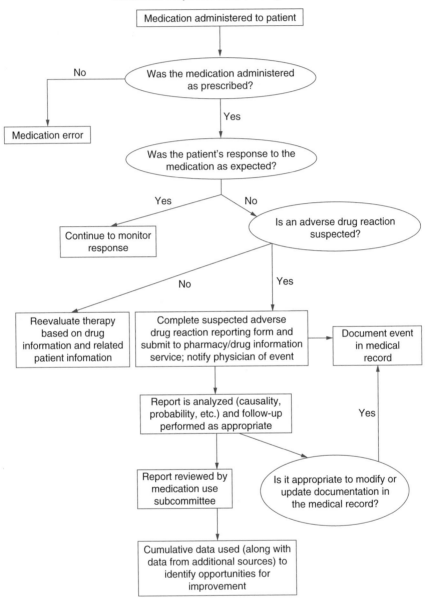

PARETO CHART

Pareto charts are vertical bar graphs with the data presented so that the bars are arranged from left to right on the horizontal axis in their order of decreasing frequency. This arrangement helps to identify which problems to address in what order. By addressing the data represented in the tallest bars (e.g., the most frequently occurring problems or contributing factors), efforts can be focused on areas where the most gain can be realized. Pareto charts are commonly used to identify issues to address, to delineate potential causes of a problem, and to monitor improvements in processes. An example of a Pareto chart is provided. This example illustrates frequently occurring factors contributing to improper dose medication errors. By focusing on transcription errors as a contributing factor on which to focus quality improvement efforts, the quality improvement team will generally gain more than by tackling the smaller bars.

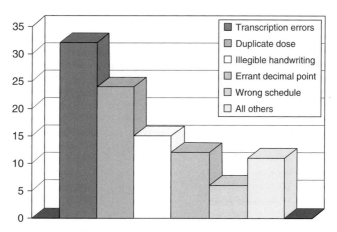

Pareto chart: factors contributing to improper dose errors.

FISHBONE OR CAUSE-AND-EFFECT DIAGRAM

Fishbone or cause-and-effect diagrams represent the relationship between an outcome (represented at the head of the fish) and the possible causes of the outcome (represented as the bones of the fish). The bones of the fish should represent causes and not symptoms of the issue. Fishbone diagrams are commonly used to identify components of a process to address, to delineate potential causes of a problem, or to identify practitioner groups that participate in producing an outcome, and should be represented in the group addressing quality issues in the process(es). An example of a Fishbone diagram is provided.

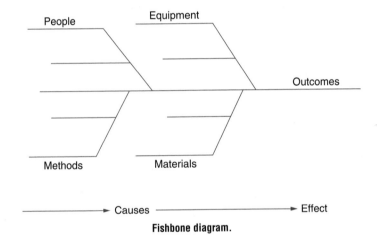

Fishbone diagram.

CONTROL CHARTS

Control charts are run charts or line graphs with defined allowable limits of variation. Data are plotted on the graph as they become available with new data points connected to older data by a continuous line. The x-axis is usually a measure of time. The control limits help to identify which variations in data are important. Control limits are statistically determined based on average ranges and sample size. Fluctuation in data points above and below the average is expected and is referred to as common variation or common cause as long as they remain between the control limits. Data points above the upper control limit or below the lower control limit are referred to as "special variation" or "special cause." Special cause variation indicates that something different is going on outside the normal operation of the process. Also, a series of data points above or below average may indicate a trend in performance that may need to be addressed. As variability in a process is reduced by quality improvement efforts, control limits should be recalculated (and narrowed) based on ongoing data. An example of a control chart is provided. Calls from pharmacists to prescribers in response to questions or issues related to new medication orders are represented over a 6-month period. Data from the month of July indicates a significant increase in the number of calls made. A quality improvement team evaluating these data would then attempt to identify what contributed to this increase. A potential cause in many institutions might be the influx of new medical house staff into the organization each July. One potential intervention to reduce this special cause is to improve the orientation of new practitioners to the medication use process within the organization.

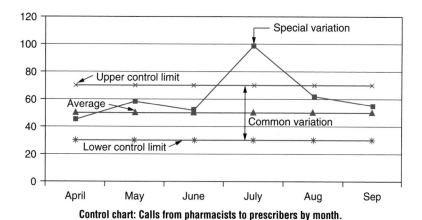

Control chart: Calls from pharmacists to prescribers by month.

Appendix 14-3

Examples of Approaches to Quality Improvement

SMART PROBLEM-SOLVING PROCESS

Statement: Written statement outlining problem or opportunity for improvement.
Selection of problem.
Definition of problem in measurable terms.

Measurement: Collection of baseline data based on most influential factors.
Determine what needs to be known about the problem.
Develop data collection method; compile data.

Analysis: Analyze data and identify causes.
Outline root causes of problems.
Evaluate collected data to identify causes of specific outcomes.

Remedy: Generate solutions and implement action.
Identify action(s) needed to address root causes and implement.

Test: Assess impact of corrective action(s).
Reassess (collect data) to determine if improvement has occurred.

FOCUS-PDCA

Find a Process to Improve

Review of data, brainstorming a list of processes, and/or customer feedback can be used to identify processes in need of improvement.

Organize the Team

Team membership should include those who participate in the process and who are most familiar with its day-to-day function.

Clarify the Current Process

It is essential that team members understand how the process currently works. Flow charts are useful tools to achieve this objective.

Understand the Current Process

Once the process is understood, causes of variation are identified. These could also be described as breakdowns of flaws in the process. Fishbone diagrams are useful tools to identify causes of variation.

This step also includes data collection on the process and, more specifically, the variations identified. Check sheets, Pareto charts, histograms, and control charts are useful to display data.

Solution

Possible improvement solutions are then identified. Brainstorming and nominal group technique can be useful in this step.

Plan the Improvement

Plan who, what, when, where, and how solutions will be implemented. Also, determine what data will be needed to verify that the improvement has occurred.

Do the Improvement

Following appropriate coordination and training, implement the improvement solution.

Check the Results

Collect data to evaluate the effectiveness of the solution. These results should be compared to baseline data (obtained in the Understand the Current Process step). The same tools mentioned previously can be useful in displaying these data.

Act on Results

If results were as expected, the new process should be standardized. If the results were not as expected, return to the Solution step to select an alternative solution and continue through the remaining steps. This cycle is repeated until the process improvement is achieved.

TEN-STEP PROCESS

1. Assign responsibility for monitoring and evaluation.
2. Delineate scope of care and service provided by the organization.
3. Identify important aspects of care and service provided by the organization.
4. Identify indicators, data sources, and collection methods to monitoring important aspects of care.
5. Establish means to trigger evaluation (e.g., trends or patterns of use, thresholds).
6. Collect and organize data.
7. Initiate evaluation of care (as indicated by triggers set in step 5).
8. Take actions to improve care and service.
9. Assess the effectiveness of actions and maintain the improvement, document improvements in care.
10. Communicate results to relevant individuals and groups.

14-4

Appendix 14-4

Example of a Quality Improvement Activity Plan

The following components should be included in the presentation of a proposal:

1. A description of the aspect of care to be assessed including historical background if appropriate (e.g., if this is a follow-up to a previous evaluation)
2. A description of the group responsible for developing the criteria, indicators, guidelines, etc., to be used in the evaluation
3. The proposed criteria or indicators and performance expectations
4. A summary of the data collection methods, case identification methods, time frame for data collection, minimal cases to be evaluated
5. The proposed reporting channels and frequency of reports

EXAMPLE OF CRITERIA AND REQUEST FOR APPROVAL

Medication Use Evaluation Criteria

Antiemetic Use in the Prophylaxis of Chemotherapy-Induced Nausea and Vomiting

Request for Approval by Medication Use Evaluation Committee

Purpose of Evaluation: The purpose of this Medication Use Evaluation (MUE) is to evaluate the use of antiemetic therapy in the prevention of chemotherapy-induced nausea and vomiting. This agent was selected for evaluation based on its essential role in the management of this patient population, potential inappropriate use, and increased cost relative to other antiemetic agents. This class of medications has not been evaluated within the organization for at least 5 years.

Criteria: A multidisciplinary group including physicians, clinical nurse specialists, staff nurses from the oncology unit, and pharmacists developed the attached criteria. They are submitted for approval by the MUE Committee.

Data Collection: Data will be collected on all patients with orders for this agent written throughout a period of approximately 30 days beginning in mid-January 2010. A minimum of 50 cases will be reviewed. Pharmacists and clinical nurse specialists will collect data concurrently from the medical record. Patients will be identified by means of the clinical information system.

Results: Results will be presented to this Committee. Information will also be shared with the Cancer Care Committee and Hospital Performance Improvement Council. Prescriber-specific results will be confidentially provided to Medical Staff Support for use in the reappointment/recredentialing process.

MEDICATION USE EVALUATION CRITERIA

ANTIEMETIC USE IN THE PROPHYLAXIS OF CHEMOTHERAPY-INDUCED NAUSEA AND VOMITING

Name _____ **Rm** _____ **Age** _____ **Sex** _____ **Wt** ____ **Ht** _____

Allergies _____ **Service** _____

Chemo/Dose/Date/Time _____ **Attending MD:** _____

Medication Use Process Elements	S(%)	Exceptions
Prescribing		
A. Indication—antiemetic (IV or PO)		
1. No other drug and nondrug causes of preexisting nausea and vomiting identified	95	(A2a) Pt receiving other less emetic cancer chemotherapy regimen and not responsive to other antiemetics
2. Prevention of acute nausea and vomiting during the first 24 hours following the initiation of highly or moderately highly emetogenic cancer chemotherapy regimens: (a) Highly emetogenic (>90%): cisplatin, dacarbazine, mechlorethamine, streptozocin, cytarabine (>500 mg/m^2); (b) Moderately high (60 to 90%): carmustine, lomustine, cyclophosphamide, dactinomycin, plicamycin, procarbazine, methotrexate (>200 mg/m^2)	95	Chemo/dose: Other antiemetic/dose: (A2b) Pt has had significant documented adverse reactions to alternative antiemetics and is receiving a regimen with a lesser emetogenic potential
3. Prevention of anticipatory nausea and vomiting associated with any chemotherapy regimen		
Dispensing/Administering		
A. Dosage—IV antiemetic		
1. 0.4 mg/kg infused over 15 minutes begun 30 minutes prior to initiation of chemotherapy regimen; then two additional doses given 4 and 8 hours after first dose of therapy, or	95	Dosage reduced by 50% in patients with significant renal dysfunction (i.e., measured or estimated creatinine clearance < 25 mL/min)
2. A single 85 mg dose infused over 15 minutes begun 30 minutes prior to initiation of chemotherapy regimen		
B. Dosage—oral antiemetic 20 mg administered 30 minutes before chemotherapy is initiated, second dose 8 hours after first dose. Continue therapy twice a day for 1 to 2 days after completion of therapy	95	
Monitoring		
Adverse Effects		Preventive and/or responsive management:
1. Headache	< 15	Identify other drug and nondrug causes
2. Diarrhea	< 15	Provide supportive and symptomatic
3. Constipation	< 10	therapy
4. Sedation	< 10	
Outcome Measures		
1. Prevention of nausea and emesis	95	(2) Medical contraindications:
2. Cancer chemotherapy course not interrupted by nausea and vomiting	95	(a) to continuation of chemotherapy. (b) patient expired. (c) lost to follow-up.

Appendix 14-5

Example Report—Prescriber-Specific Results

Prescriber-specific reports from medication use evaluation activities should be provided for use in the reappointment/recredentialing process. It is important that these reports contain sufficient information to facilitate peer review. A summary of all cases involving the prescriber should be included in the report including a brief description of cases in which criteria were not met. A mechanism to access the medical record (e.g., a medical record number) should be provided to allow chart review, if needed. An example follows.

PRESCRIBER-SPECIFIC INFORMATION FOR USE IN REAPPOINTMENT/RECREDENTIALING

Source: Medication Use Evaluation (MUE) Committee

Evaluation Topic: Antiemetic Medication Use Evaluation

Dates of Evaluation: January-February 2010

Data Enclosed:

    a. Summary of overall results reviewed by MUE Committee and actions taken by the Committee (see attached)

    b. Criteria used in evaluation (see attached, approved by MUE Committee prior to data collection)

    c. Prescriber-specific results (following)

       1. Table outlining patient case number, medical record number, diagnosis, attending physician (by first letters of last name followed by identification number), and criteria not met (when applicable) for all patients managed by this attending during the evaluation period.

       2. Any other prescriber-specific correspondence, etc., from the Committee.

Results for Attending Physician #12345

ATTENDING #	CASE #	MEDREC #	DIAGNOSIS	CRITERIA NOT MET
12345	43	54321	OVARIAN CANCER	
12345	44	43215	BREAST CANCER	Dosing
12345	55	32154	SMALL CELL CANCER/ LIVER METASTESES	Dosing
12345	58	15432	METASTATIC BREAST CANCER	Outcome
12345	59	53215	METASTATIC BREAST CANCER	
12345	71	42153	ACUTE MYELOGENOUS LEUKEMIA	Outcome
12345	121	15342	OVARIAN CANCER	

Summary of cases where dosing criteria are not met

- Case #44 did not meet dosing criteria. Patient received 85 mg IV antiemetic on chemotherapy day 1 (cisplatinum and etoposide) then 85 mg in 24 hours on day 2 (etoposide only).
- Case #55 did not meet dosing criteria. Patient received 85 mg IV antiemetic on chemotherapy day 1 (cisplatinum and etoposide) then 85 mg in 24 hours on day 2 (etoposide only).

MUE Committee action taken (specific to this prescriber): letter written to prescriber (copy attached).

Summary of cases where outcome criteria are not met

- Case #58 did not meet outcome criteria (i.e., prevention of nausea and vomiting). Patient experienced nausea/vomiting×1 less than 24 hours following antiemetic dose (85 mg IV × 1).
- Case #71 did not meet outcome criteria (i.e., prevention of nausea and vomiting). Patient received 85 mg IV antiemetic daily×6 days. On sixth day had one episode of nausea.

MUE Committee action taken (specific to this prescriber): none.

Appendix 14-6

Example of MUE Results

MEDICATION USE EVALUATION

Summary of Overall Results

Antiemetic: January-February 2010

Background: This topic was selected based on the high use, potential misuse, and high cost of these agents. Criteria for this evaluation were approved at the MUE Committee's December 2009 meeting. Please refer to attached criteria for additional information.

Total Patients Evaluated (All Indications for Use) = 52

Element	Standard	Results	Compliance
Prescribing			

Indication for use	95%	OVERALL RESULTS
		  Treatment/prevention of nausea/
		    vomiting associated with
		    chemotherapy
			100%
			(52/52)

		Highly emetogenic chemotherapy	46/46
		Anticipatory N/V associated with chemotherapy	6/6
Dispensing/Administering			
Dosing	95%	OVERALL RESULTS	71% (37/52)
		Highly emetogenic chemotherapy	31/46
		Anticipatory N/V associated with chemotherapy	6/6
Monitoring			

Adverse Drug Reaction(s)	≤10%-25%
	(varies with
	ADR)
		OVERALL RESULTS:
		  Headache: 1 patient
		  Constipation: 1 patient
			4% (2/52)

Outcome			
Prevention of nausea and emesis	95%	OVERALL RESULTS	92% (46/50)[a]
		Highly emetogenic chemotherapy	41/44
		Anticipatory N/V associated with chemotherapy	5/6

Element	Standard	Results	Compliance
Chemotherapy course not interrupted	95%	OVERALL RESULTS (ALL INDICATIONS)	100% (52/52)

[a]Includes only patients in whom outcome was documented. Outcome was not assessed in two patients who were discharged immediately following administration of chemotherapy.

Summary of Results

Prescribing: Criteria for indication for use were met in all cases.

Dispensing/Administering: Criteria for dosing was met in 37 of 52 cases with all cases involving anticipatory nausea and vomiting meeting criteria.

In 15 cases, patients receiving the antiemetic prior to highly emetogenic chemotherapy received doses not included in the approved criteria. Five of these patients received doses based on an investigational protocol. This dose is now under consideration by the FDA for approval, and preliminary results (available only in abstract form) were recently presented at the American Society of Clinical Oncology meeting. Results with the new dosing regimen have been comparable to those with the currently approved doses.

In seven cases not meeting dosing criteria, patients received a single dose prior to chemotherapy consistent with the criteria. However, an additional dose was administered 24 hours after the first dose. These orders were written by two prescribers.

Two cases did not meet dosing criteria because the dose was not adjusted based on renal dysfunction. In both cases, the estimated creatinine clearance was between 20 and 25 mL/min and nephrotoxic drugs were not being administered concurrently. In both cases, the estimated creatinine clearance increased to 30 mL/min or more by day 2 of the admission (probably due to rehydration of the patient). Neither patient experienced adverse effects.

One dose was not administered within the appropriate time frame. In this case, the antiemetic dose was administered just 5 minutes prior to the initiation of chemotherapy administration. The nurse administering the antiemetic documented its administration on the way to the patient's room. When she arrived, the patient was not in the room. The dose was administered after he was located, approximately 25 minutes later. The nurse did not correct the actual administration time until after a second nurse administered the chemotherapy.

Recommendations:

1. Add new dosing regimen to dosing criteria.
2. Send letters to prescribers giving extra dose.
3. Renal dosing was not significantly outside guidelines. Mention findings in report to be published in quality improvement newsletter but do not take prescriber-specific action.
4. The dose administered late was reported via an incident report; no further action by this group is required at this time.

Monitoring: The rate of adverse drug reactions was less than that reported in the literature. This might be reflective of underreporting and under-documenting of adverse drug events.

Recommendations:

1. The Adverse Drug Event Task Force is currently implementing a new process to improve reporting and documentation. No specific action by this group is required at this time.

Outcome: Ninety-two percent of patients did not experience nausea or vomiting. Outcome was assessable in 50 patients; two patients were discharged immediately following the administration of chemotherapy.

The patient who received his antiemetic dose just 5 minutes prior to chemotherapy experienced moderate nausea and no vomiting. Otherwise, the occurrence of nausea and vomiting was not related to problems with administration or dosing.

Recommendations:

1. Ninety-two percent success rate is acceptable based on literature; no action is necessary.

General Recommendations:

1. After approval, implement recommendations presented previously.
2. Publish results in the Quality Improvement Newsletter following review by the Cancer Care Committee and the Quality Improvement Committee.
3. Perform a follow-up evaluation focusing on dosing issues.
4. Initiate planned assessment of this agent's use in postoperative nausea and vomiting as soon as possible.

Note to reader: An example of a prescriber-specific report for appointment/recredentialing appears in Appendix 14-5.

Appendix 14-7

Quality Evaluation: Response to Drug Information Request

Request #	Date of Request			
Response by (circle one):	DI Staff	Resident	Student	
Caller (circle type):	MD	RPh	Nurse	Other:

Assessment of Search and Response to Request				
	Yes	No	NA	Standard %[a]
1. Is requestor's demographic information complete?				100%
2. Background information is: 　A. Thorough 　B. Appropriate to request				100%
3. Is the question clearly stated?				100%
4. Search Strategy/References: 　A. Appropriate references were used 　B. Search was sufficiently comprehensive 　C. Is search strategy clearly documented				100%
5. Response was 　A. Appropriate for the situation 　B. Sufficient to answer the question 　C. Provided in a timely manner 　D. Integrated with available patient data 　E. Supported by appropriate materials supplied to 　　requestor				100%
6. If complete response could not be provided within time frame requested, was requestor advised as to the status of their request and the anticipated delivery of the final response?				100%

[a]If performance falls below 90% in any category during any month, the service director will coordinate an assessment of the process and report findings and actions will be reported to the P&T committee.

Comments:

Reviewed By:_____

15-1

Appendix 15-1

Kramer Questionnaire*

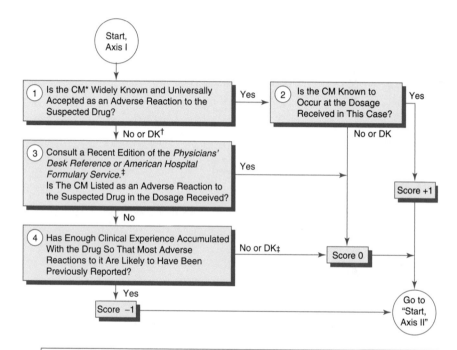

*Abbreviation CM indicates clinical manifestation, the abnormal sign, symptom, or laboratory test, or cluster of abnormal signs, symptoms, and tests, that is being considered as a possible adverse drug reaction.

†Abbreviation DK indicates do not know. This answer should be given when no data are available for the question being answered or when the quality of the data does not allow a firm "Yes" or "No" response.

‡When these are not available, an equivalent reference source may be used.

Figure 1. Axis I. Previous general experience with drug.

*Kramer MS, Leventhal JM, Hutchinson TA, Feinstein AR. An algorithm for the operational assessment of adverse drug reaction: I. background, descriptions, and instructions for use. JAMA 1979; 242(7):623-32.

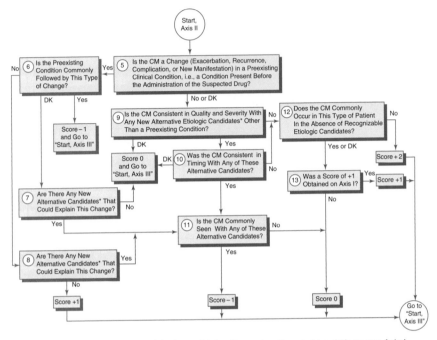

Figure 2. Axis II. Alternative etiologic candidates. For explanation of abbreviations, see Axis I.

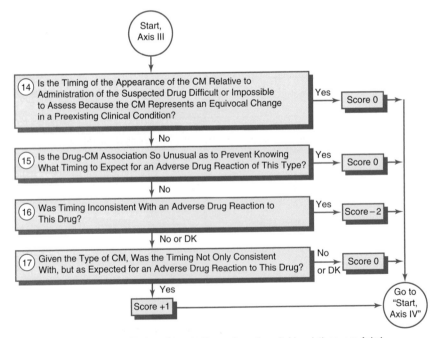

Figure 3. Axis III. Timing of events. For explanantion of abbreviations, see Axis I.

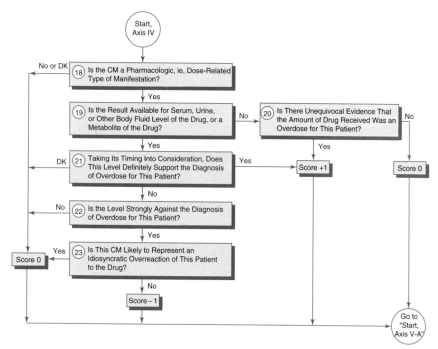

Figure 4. Axis IV. Drug levels and evidence of overdose. For explanantion of abbreviations, see Axis I.

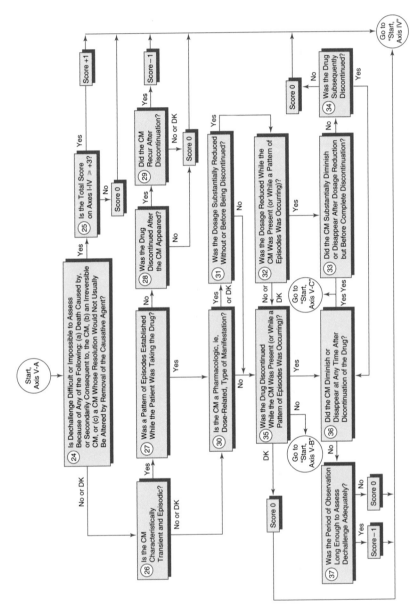

Figure 5A. Axis V-A. Dechallenge: Difficult assessments. For explanation of abbreviations, see Axis I.

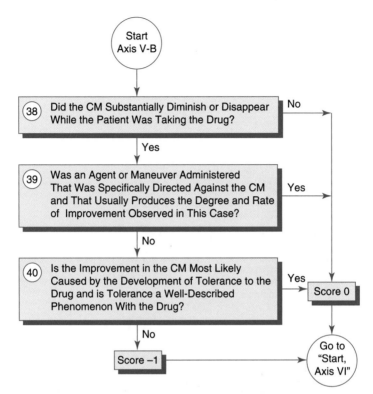

Figure 5B. Axis V-B. Dechallenge: Absence of dechallenge. For explanation of abbreviation, see Axis I.

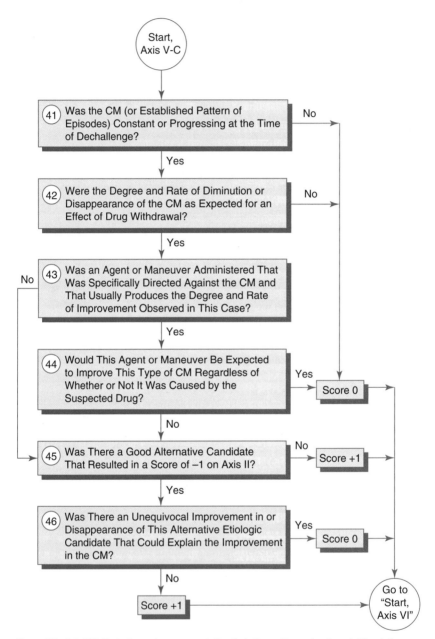

Figure 5C. Axis V-C. Dechallenge: Improvement after dechallenge. For explanation of abbreviation, see Axis I.

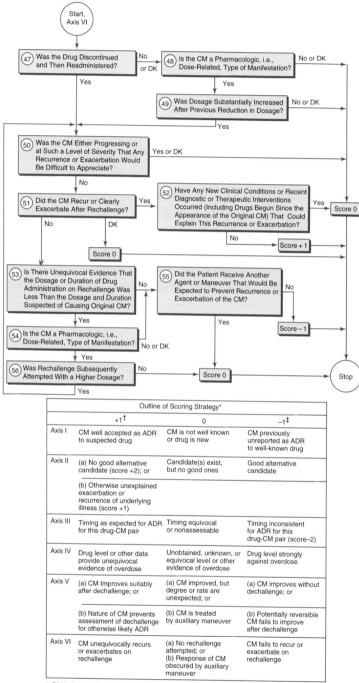

Figure 6. Axis VI. Rechallenge. For explanation of abbreviation, see Axis I.

Appendix 15-2

Naranjo Algorithm[*]

To assess the adverse drug reaction, please answer the following questionnaire and give the pertinent score.

	Yes	No	Don't know	Score
1. Are there previous conclusive reports on this reaction?	+1	0	0	
2. Did the adverse event appear after the suspected drug was administered?	+2	−1	0	
3. Did the adverse reaction improve when the drug was discontinued or a specific antagonist was administered?	+1	0	0	
4. Did the adverse reaction reappear when the drug was readministered?	+2	−1	0	
5. Are there alternative causes (other than the drug) that could on their own have caused the reaction?	−1	+2	0	
6. Did the reaction reappear when a placebo was given?	−1	+1	0	
7. Was the drug detected in the blood (or other fluids) in concentrations known to be toxic?	+1	0	0	
8. Was the reaction more severe when the dose was increased, or less severe when the dose was decreased?	+1	0	0	
9. Did the patient have a similar reaction to the same or similar drugs in any previous exposure?	+1	0	0	
10. Was the adverse event confirmed by any objective evidence?	+1	0	0	

Total Score_____

Score Interpretation

___Definite: ≥9
___Probable: 5 to 8
___Possible: 1 to 4
___Doubtful: ≤0

---

*Naranjo CA, Busto U, Sellers EM, Sandor P, Ruiz I, Roberts EA, et al. A method of estimating the probability of adverse drug reactions. Clin Pharmacol Ther. 1981;30(2):239-45.

Appendix 15-3

Jones Algorithm*

START HERE:**

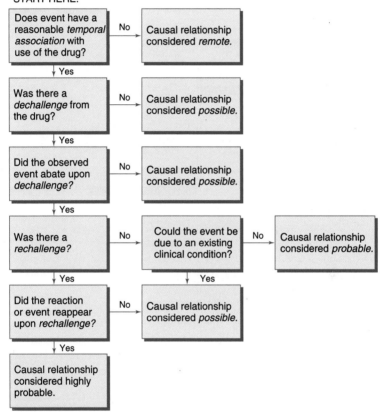

**Each drug is carried through independently; if > 1 drug was dechallenged or rechallenged simultaneously causality for all is ≤ possible.

QUESTIONS:

1. Did the reaction follow a reasonable temporal sequence?
2. Did the patient improve after stopping the drug?
3. Did the reaction reappear on repeated exposure (rechallenge)?
4. Could the reaction be reasonably explained by the known characteristics of the patient's clinical *state?*

---

*Jones JK. Adverse drug reactions in the community health setting: approaches to recognizing, counseling, and reporting. Clin Comm Health. 1982;5(2):58-67.

Appendix 15-4

| Next Page | Reset Form | Delete Page | Delete Multiple Pages |

U.S. Department of Health and Human Services

Form Approved: OMB No. 0910-0291, Expires: 12/31/2011
See OMB statement on reverse.

MEDWATCH

The FDA Safety Information and
Adverse Event Reporting Program

For VOLUNTARY reporting of
adverse events, product problems and
product use errors

General Instructions   Page 1 of ____

FDA USE ONLY

Triage unit
sequence #

A. PATIENT INFORMATION   Section A - Help

1. Patient Identifier	2. Age at Time of Event or Date of Birth:	3. Sex	4. Weight
		☐ Female	lb
In confidence		☐ Male	or ___ kg

B. ADVERSE EVENT, PRODUCT PROBLEM OR ERROR

Check all that apply: Section B - Help

1. ☐ **Adverse Event**   ☐ **Product Problem** (e.g., defects/malfunctions)
☐ **Product Use Error**   ☐ **Problem with Different Manufacturer of Same Medicine**

2. Outcomes Attributed to Adverse Event
(Check all that apply)

☐ Death: _____ (mm/dd/yyyy)
☐ Life-threatening
☐ Hospitalization - initial or prolonged
☐ Required Intervention to Prevent Permanent Impairment/Damage (Devices)
☐ Disability or Permanent Damage
☐ Congenital Anomaly/Birth Defect
☐ Other Serious (Important Medical Events)

3. Date of Event (mm/dd/yyyy)	4. Date of this Report (mm/dd/yyyy)

5. Describe Event, Problem or Product Use Error

(Continue on page 3)

6. Relevant Tests/Laboratory Data, Including Dates

(Continue on page 3)

7. Other Relevant History, Including Preexisting Medical Conditions (e.g., allergies, race, pregnancy, smoking and alcohol use, liver/kidney problems, etc.)

(Continue on page 3)

PLEASE TYPE OR USE BLACK INK

C. PRODUCT AVAILABILITY   Section C - Help

Product Available for Evaluation? (Do not send product to FDA)

☐ Yes   ☐ No   ☐ Returned to Manufacturer on: _____ (mm/dd/yyyy)

D. SUSPECT PRODUCT(S)   Section D - Help

1. Name, Strength, Manufacturer (from product label)
#1 Name:
Strength:
Manufacturer:
#2 Name:
Strength:
Manufacturer:

2. Dose or Amount	Frequency	Route
#1		
#2		

3. Dates of Use (If unknown, give duration) from/to (or best estimate)	5. Event Abated After Use Stopped or Dose Reduced?
#1	#1 ☐ Yes ☐ No ☐ Doesn't Apply
#2	#2 ☐ Yes ☐ No ☐ Doesn't Apply

4. Diagnosis or Reason for Use (Indication)	8. Event Reappeared After Reintroduction?
#1	#1 ☐ Yes ☐ No ☐ Doesn't Apply
#2	#2 ☐ Yes ☐ No ☐ Doesn't Apply

6. Lot #	7. Expiration Date	9. NDC # or Unique ID
#1	#1	
#2	#2	

E. SUSPECT MEDICAL DEVICE   Section E - Help

1. Brand Name

2. Common Device Name

3. Manufacturer Name, City and State

4. Model #	Lot #	5. Operator of Device
		☐ Health Professional
Catalog #	Expiration Date (mm/dd/yyyy)	☐ Lay User/Patient
Serial #	Other #	☐ Other:

6. If Implanted, Give Date (mm/dd/yyyy)	7. If Explanted, Give Date (mm/dd/yyyy)

8. Is this a Single-use Device that was Reprocessed and Reused on a Patient?
☐ Yes   ☐ No

9. If Yes to Item No. 8, Enter Name and Address of Reprocessor

F. OTHER (CONCOMITANT) MEDICAL PRODUCTS

Product names and therapy dates (exclude treatment of event)   Section F - Help

(Continue on page 3)

G. REPORTER (See confidentiality section on back)

1. Name and Address   Section G - Help
Name:
Address:
City: State: ZIP:

Phone #	E-mail

2. Health Professional?	3. Occupation	4. Also Reported to:
☐ Yes ☐ No		☐ Manufacturer

5. If you do NOT want your identity disclosed to the manufacturer, place an "X" in this box: ☐
☐ User Facility
☐ Distributor/Importer

FORM FDA 3500 (1/09)   Submission of a report does not constitute an admission that medical personnel or the product caused or contributed to the event.

| Next Page | Previous Page | Delete Page | Delete Multiple Pages |

ADVICE ABOUT VOLUNTARY REPORTING
Detailed instructions available at: http://www.fda.gov/medwatch/report/consumer/instruct.htm

Report adverse events, product problems or product use errors with:

- Medications *(drugs or biologics)*
- Medical devices *(including in-vitro diagnostics)*
- Combination products *(medication & medical devices)*
- Human cells, tissues, and cellular and tissue-based products
- Special nutritional products *(dietary supplements, medical foods, infant formulas)*
- Cosmetics

Report product problems - quality, performance or safety concerns such as:

- Suspected counterfeit product
- Suspected contamination
- Questionable stability
- Defective components
- Poor packaging or labeling
- Therapeutic failures (product didn't work)

Report SERIOUS adverse events. An event is serious when the patient outcome is:

- Death
- Life-threatening
- Hospitalization - initial or prolonged
- Disability or permanent damage
- Congenital anomaly/birth defect
- Required intervention to prevent permanent impairment or damage (devices)
- Other serious (important medical events)

Report even if:

- You're not certain the product caused the event
- You don't have all the details

How to report:

- Just fill in the sections that apply to your report
- Use section D for all products except medical devices
- Attach additional pages if needed
- Use a separate form for each patient
- Report either to FDA or the manufacturer *(or both)*

Other methods of reporting:

- 1-800-FDA-0178 - To FAX report
- 1-800-FDA-1088 - To report by phone
- www.fda.gov/medwatch/report.htm - To report online

If your report involves a serious adverse event with a device and it occurred in a facility outside a doctor's office, that facility may be legally required to report to FDA and/or the manufacturer. Please notify the person in that facility who would handle such reporting.

If your report involves a serious adverse event with a vaccine, call 1-800-822-7967 to report.

Confidentiality: The patient's identity is held in strict confidence by FDA and protected to the fullest extent of the law. FDA will not disclose the reporter's identity in response to a request from the public, pursuant to the Freedom of Information Act. The reporter's identity, including the identity of a self-reporter, may be shared with the manufacturer unless requested otherwise.

-Fold Here-

The public reporting burden for this collection of information has been estimated to average 36 minutes per response, including the time for reviewing instructions, searching existing data sources, gathering and maintaining the data needed, and completing and reviewing the collection of information. Send comments regarding this burden estimate or any other aspect of this collection of information, including suggestions for reducing this burden to:

Department of Health and Human Services	*Please DO NOT*	*OMB statement:*
Food and Drug Administration	*RETURN this form*	*"An agency may not conduct or sponsor, and a*
Office of Chief Information Officer	*to this address.*	*person is not required to respond to, a collection of*
1350 Piccard Drive, Room 400		*information unless it displays a currently valid*
Rockville, MD 20850		*OMB control number."*

U.S. DEPARTMENT OF HEALTH AND HUMAN SERVICES
Food and Drug Administration

FORM FDA 3500 (1/09) (Back)   Please Use Address Provided Below -- Fold in Thirds, Tape and Mail

DEPARTMENT OF
HEALTH & HUMAN SERVICES

Public Health Service
Food and Drug Administration
Rockville, MD 20857

Official Business
Penalty for Private Use $300

BUSINESS REPLY MAIL
FIRST CLASS MAIL PERMIT NO. 946 ROCKVILLE MD

POSTAGE WILL BE PAID BY FOOD AND DRUG ADMINISTRATION

MEDWATCH
The FDA Safety Information and Adverse Event Reporting Program
Food and Drug Administration
5600 Fishers Lane
Rockville, MD 20852-9787

| Next Page | Previous Page | Reset Form | Delete Page | Delete Multiple Pages |

U.S. Department of Health and Human Services

MEDWATCH

The FDA Safety Information and
Adverse Event Reporting Program

(CONTINUATION PAGE)

**For VOLUNTARY reporting of
adverse events and product problems**

Page 3 of ▢

Back to Form

B.5. **Describe Event or Problem** *(continued)*

Back to Form

B.6. **Relevant Tests/Laboratory Data, Including Dates** *(continued)*

Back to Form

B.7. **Other Relevant History, Including Preexisting Medical Conditions** *(e.g., allergies, race, pregnancy, smoking and alcohol use, hepatic/renal dysfunction, etc.) (continued)*

Back to Form

F. **Concomitant Medical Products and Therapy Dates** *(Exclude treatment of event) (continued)*

Appendix 17–1

Investigational New Drug Application

DEPARTMENT OF HEALTH AND HUMAN SERVICES
FOOD AND DRUG ADMINISTRATION

Form Approved: OMB No. 0910-0014.
Expiration Date: January 31, 2006
See OMB Statement on Reverse.

INVESTIGATIONAL NEW DRUG APPLICATION (IND)
(TITLE 21, CODE OF FEDERAL REGULATIONS (CFR) PART 312)

NOTE: No drug may be shipped or clinical investigation begun until an IND for that investigation is in effect (21 CFR 312.40).

1. NAME OF SPONSOR

2. DATE OF SUBMISSION

3. ADDRESS *(Number, Street, City, State and Zip Code)*

4. TELEPHONE NUMBER *(Include Area Code)*

5. NAME(S) OF DRUG *(Include all available names; Trade, Generic, Chemical, Code)*

6. IND NUMBER *(If previously assigned)*

7. INDICATION(S) *(Covered by this submission)*

8. PHASE(S) OF CLINICAL INVESTIGATION TO BE CONDUCTED:
☐ PHASE 1 ☐ PHASE 2 ☐ PHASE 3 ☐ OTHER _____ *(Specify)*

9. LIST NUMBERS OF ALL INVESTIGATIONAL NEW DRUG APPLICATIONS (21 CFR Part 312), NEW DRUG OR ANTIBIOTIC APPLICATIONS (21 CFR Part 314), DRUG MASTER FILES (21 CFR Part 314.420), AND PRODUCT LICENSE APPLICATIONS (21 CFR Part 601) REFERRED TO IN THIS APPLICATION.

10. **IND submission should be consecutively numbered. The initial IND should be numbered "Serial number: 0000." The next submission (e.g., amendment, report, or correspondence) should be numbered "Serial Number: 0001." Subsequent submissions should be numbered consecutively in the order in which they are submitted.**

SERIAL NUMBER

11. THIS SUBMISSION CONTAINS THE FOLLOWING: *(Check all that apply)*
☐ INITIAL INVESTIGATIONAL NEW DRUG APPLICATION (IND) ☐ RESPONSE TO CLINICAL HOLD

PROTOCOL AMENDMENT(S):
☐ NEW PROTOCOL
☐ CHANGE IN PROTOCOL
☐ NEW INVESTIGATOR

INFORMATION AMENDMENT(S):
☐ CHEMISTRY/MICROBIOLOGY
☐ PHARMACOLOGY/TOXICOLOGY
☐ CLINICAL

IND SAFETY REPORT(S):
☐ INITIAL WRITTEN REPORT
☐ FOLLOW-UP TO A WRITTEN REPORT

☐ RESPONSE TO FDA REQUEST FOR INFORMATION ☐ ANNUAL REPORT ☐ GENERAL CORRESPONDENCE
☐ REQUEST FOR REINSTATEMENT OF IND THAT IS WITHDRAWN, INACTIVATED, TERMINATED OR DISCONTINUED ☐ OTHER _____ *(Specify)*

CHECK ONLY IF APPLICABLE

JUSTIFICATION STATEMENT MUST BE SUBMITTED WITH APPLICATION FOR ANY CHECKED BELOW. REFER TO THE CITED CFR SECTION FOR FURTHER INFORMATION.

☐ TREATMENT IND 21 CFR 312.35(b) ☐ TREATMENT PROTOCOL 21 CFR 312.35(a) ☐ CHARGE REQUEST/NOTIFICATION 21 CFR312.7(d)

FOR FDA USE ONLY

CDR/DBIND/DGD RECEIPT STAMP	DDR RECEIPT STAMP	DIVISION ASSIGNMENT:
		IND NUMBER ASSIGNED:

FORM FDA 1571 (3/05) PREVIOUS EDITION IS OBSOLETE. PAGE 1 OF 2

PSC Media Arts (301) 443-1090 EF

12.

CONTENTS OF APPLICATION
This application contains the following items: *(Check all that apply)*

☐ 1. Form FDA 1571 *[21 CFR 312.23(a)(1)]*

☐ 2. Table of Contents *[21 CFR 312.23(a)(2)]*

☐ 3. Introductory statement *[21 CFR 312.23(a)(3)]*

☐ 4. General Investigational plan *[21 CFR 312.23(a)(3)]*

☐ 5. Investigator's brochure *[21 CFR 312.23(a)(5)]*

☐ 6. Protocol(s) *[21 CFR 312.23(a)(6)]*

    ☐ a. Study protocol(s) *[21 CFR 312.23(a)(6)]*

    ☐ b. Investigator data *[21 CFR 312.23(a)(6)(iii)(b)]* or completed Form(s) FDA 1572

    ☐ c. Facilities data *[21 CFR 312.23(a)(6)(iii)(b)]* or completed Form(s) FDA 1572

    ☐ d. Institutional Review Board data *[21 CFR 312.23(a)(6)(iii)(b)]* or completed Form(s) FDA 1572

☐ 7. Chemistry, manufacturing, and control data *[21 CFR 312.23(a)(7)]*

    ☐ Environmental assessment or claim for exclusion *[21 CFR 312.23(a)(7)(iv)(e)]*

☐ 8. Pharmacology and toxicology data *[21 CFR 312.23(a)(8)]*

☐ 9. Previous human experience *[21 CFR 312.23(a)(9)]*

☐ 10. Additional information *[21 CFR 312.23(a)(10)]*

---

13. IS ANY PART OF THE CLINICAL STUDY TO BE CONDUCTED BY A CONTRACT RESEARCH ORGANIZATION? ☐ YES ☐ NO

IF YES, WILL ANY SPONSOR OBLIGATIONS BE TRANSFERRED TO THE CONTRACT RESEARCH ORGANIZATION? ☐ YES ☐ NO

IF YES, ATTACH A STATEMENT CONTAINING THE NAME AND ADDRESS OF THE CONTRACT RESEARCH ORGANIZATION, IDENTIFICATION OF THE CLINICAL STUDY, AND A LISTING OF THE OBLIGATIONS TRANSFERRED.

14. NAME AND TITLE OF THE PERSON RESPONSIBLE FOR MONITORING THE CONDUCT AND PROGRESS OF THE CLINICAL INVESTIGATIONS

15. NAME(S) AND TITLE(S) OF THE PERSON(S) RESPONSIBLE FOR REVIEW AND EVALUATION OF INFORMATION RELEVANT TO THE SAFETY OF THE DRUG

I agree not to begin clinical investigations until 30 days after FDA's receipt of the IND unless I receive earlier notification by FDA that the studies may begin. I also agree not to begin or continue clinical investigations covered by the IND if those studies are placed on clinical hold. I agree that an Institutional Review Board (IRB) that complies with the requirements set fourth in 21 CFR Part 56 will be responsible for initial and continuing review and approval of each of the studies in the proposed clinical investigation. I agree to conduct the investigation in accordance with all other applicable regulatory requirements.

16. NAME OF SPONSOR OR SPONSOR'S AUTHORIZED REPRESENTATIVE

17. SIGNATURE OF SPONSOR OR SPONSOR'S AUTHORIZED REPRESENTATIVE

18. ADDRESS *(Number, Street, City, State and Zip Code)*

19. TELEPHONE NUMBER *(Include Area Code)*

20. DATE

(WARNING: A willfully false statement is a criminal offense. U.S.C. Title 18, Sec. 1001.)

Public reporting burden for this collection of information is estimated to average 100 hours per response, including the time for reviewing instructions, searching existing data sources, gathering and maintaining the data needed, and completing reviewing the collection of information. Send comments regarding this burden estimate or any other aspect of this collection of information, including suggestions for reducing this burden to:

Department of Health and Human Services
Food and Drug Administration
Center for Drug Evaluation and Research
Central Document Room
5901-B Ammendale Road
Beltsville, MD 20705-1266

Department of Health and Human Services
Food and Drug Administration
Center for Biologics Evaluation and Research (HFM-99)
1401 Rockville Pike
Rockville, MD 20852-1448

Please DO NOT RETURN this application to this address.

"An agency may not conduct or sponsor, and a person is not required to respond to, a collection of information unless it displays a currently valid OMB control number."

Appendix 17–2

Statement of Investigator

DEPARTMENT OF HEALTH AND HUMAN SERVICES
FOOD AND DRUG ADMINISTRATION

Form Approved: OMB No. 0910-0014.
Expiration Date: January 31, 2006.
See OMB Statement on Reverse.

STATEMENT OF INVESTIGATOR
(TITLE 21, CODE OF FEDERAL REGULATIONS (CFR) PART 312)
(See instructions on reverse side.)

NOTE: No investigator may participate in an investigation until he/she provides the sponsor with a completed, signed Statement of Investigator, Form FDA 1572 (21 CFR 312.53(c)).

1. NAME AND ADDRESS OF INVESTIGATOR

2. EDUCATION, TRAINING, AND EXPERIENCE THAT QUALIFIES THE INVESTIGATOR AS AN EXPERT IN THE CLINICAL INVESTIGATION OF THE DRUG FOR THE USE UNDER INVESTIGATION. ONE OF THE FOLLOWING IS ATTACHED.

☐ CURRICULUM VITAE   ☐ OTHER STATEMENT OF QUALIFICATIONS

3. NAME AND ADDRESS OF ANY MEDICAL SCHOOL, HOSPITAL OR OTHER RESEARCH FACILITY WHERE THE CLINICAL INVESTIGATION(S) WILL BE CONDUCTED.

4. NAME AND ADDRESS OF ANY CLINICAL LABORATORY FACILITIES TO BE USED IN THE STUDY.

5. NAME AND ADDRESS OF THE INSTITUTIONAL REVIEW BOARD (IRB) THAT IS RESPONSIBLE FOR REVIEW AND APPROVAL OF THE STUDY(IES).

6. NAMES OF THE SUBINVESTIGATORS *(e.g., research fellows, residents, associates)* WHO WILL BE ASSISTING THE INVESTIGATOR IN THE CONDUCT OF THE INVESTIGATION(S).

7. NAME AND CODE NUMBER, IF ANY, OF THE PROTOCOL(S) IN THE IND FOR THE STUDY(IES) TO BE CONDUCTED BY THE INVESTIGATOR.

FORM FDA 1572 (3/05)   PREVIOUS EDITION IS OBSOLETE.   PAGE 1 OF 2

PSC Media Arts (301) 443-1090   EF

8. ATTACH THE FOLLOWING CLINICAL PROTOCOL INFORMATION:

☐ FOR PHASE 1 INVESTIGATIONS, A GENERAL OUTLINE OF THE PLANNED INVESTIGATION INCLUDING THE ESTIMATED DURATION OF THE STUDY AND THE MAXIMUM NUMBER OF SUBJECTS THAT WILL BE INVOLVED.

☐ FOR PHASE 2 OR 3 INVESTIGATIONS, AN OUTLINE OF THE STUDY PROTOCOL INCLUDING AN APPROXIMATION OF THE NUMBER OF SUBJECTS TO BE TREATED WITH THE DRUG AND THE NUMBER TO BE EMPLOYED AS CONTROLS, IF ANY; THE CLINICAL USES TO BE INVESTIGATED; CHARACTERISTICS OF SUBJECTS BY AGE, SEX, AND CONDITION; THE KIND OF CLINICAL OBSERVATIONS AND LABORATORY TESTS TO BE CONDUCTED; THE ESTIMATED DURATION OF THE STUDY; AND COPIES OR A DESCRIPTION OF CASE REPORT FORMS TO BE USED.

9. COMMITMENTS:

I agree to conduct the study(ies) in accordance with the relevant, current protocol(s) and will only make changes in a protocol after notifying the sponsor, except when necessary to protect the safety, rights, or welfare of subjects.

I agree to personally conduct or supervise the described investigation(s).

I agree to inform any patients, or any persons used as controls, that the drugs are being used for investigational purposes and I will ensure that the requirements relating to obtaining informed consent in 21 CFR Part 50 and institutional review board (IRB) review and approval in 21 CFR Part 56 are met.

I agree to report to the sponsor adverse experiences that occur in the course of the investigation(s) in accordance with 21 CFR 312.64.

I have read and understand the information in the investigator's brochure, including the potential risks and side effects of the drug.

I agree to ensure that all associates, colleagues, and employees assisting in the conduct of the study(ies) are informed about their obligations in meeting the above commitments.

I agree to maintain adequate and accurate records in accordance with 21 CFR 312.62 and to make those records available for inspection in accordance with 21 CFR 312.68.

I will ensure that an IRB that complies with the requirements of 21 CFR Part 56 will be responsible for the initial and continuing review and approval of the clinical investigation. I also agree to promptly report to the IRB all changes in the research activity and all unanticipated problems involving risks to human subjects or others. Additionally, I will not make any changes in the research without IRB approval, except where necessary to eliminate apparent immediate hazards to human subjects.

I agree to comply with all other requirements regarding the obligations of clinical investigators and all other pertinent requirements in 21 CFR Part 312.

INSTRUCTIONS FOR COMPLETING FORM FDA 1572
STATEMENT OF INVESTIGATOR:

1. Complete all sections. Attach a separate page if additional space is needed.

2. Attach curriculum vitae or other statement of qualifications as described in Section 2.

3. Attach protocol outline as described in Section 8.

4. Sign and date below.

5. FORWARD THE COMPLETED FORM AND ATTACHMENTS TO THE SPONSOR. The sponsor will incorporate this information along with other technical data into an Investigational New Drug Application (IND).

10. SIGNATURE OF INVESTIGATOR	11. DATE

(**WARNING:** A willfully false statement is a criminal offense. U.S.C. Title 18, Sec. 1001.)

Public reporting burden for this collection of information is estimated to average 100 hours per response, including the time for reviewing instructions, searching existing data sources, gathering and maintaining the data needed, and completing reviewing the collection of information. Send comments regarding this burden estimate or any other aspect of this collection of information, including suggestions for reducing this burden to:

Department of Health and Human Services
Food and Drug Administration
Center for Drug Evaluation and Research
Central Document Room
5901-B Ammendale Road
Beltsville, MD 20705-1266

Department of Health and Human Services
Food and Drug Administration
Center for Biologics Evaluation and Research (HFM-99)
1401 Rockville Pike
Rockville, MD 20852-1448

"An agency may not conduct or sponsor, and a person is not required to respond to, a collection of information unless it displays a currently valid OMB control number."

Please DO NOT RETURN this application to this address.

FORM FDA 1572 (3/05)   PAGE 2 OF 2

Appendix 17–3

Protocol Medication Economic Analysis

Date:
Protocol title:
Study chairperson:

Hospital Cost Analysis

Drug	Hospital Cost per Cycle*	Number of Cycles	Total Cost per Patient	Number of Patients	Total Protocol Cost	Annual Cost
Primary Therapy						
Supportive Care						

*When applicable, doses calculated on 1.7 m^2 or 70 kg at initial dose level and costs include infusion fluids, administration sets, and tubing.

Patient Charge Analysis

Drug	Patient Charge per Cycle*	Number of Cycles	Total Charge per Patient	Number of Patients	Total Patient Billing
Primary Therapy					
Supportive Care					

*When applicable, charges include infusion fluids, administration sets, and tubing.

Reimbursement Risk

Drug	FDA Labeled	Compendium

Comments

Summary

Appendix 17–4

Investigational Drug Accountability Record

Form approved
OMB No. 0925-0240
Expires: 6/30/91

National Institutes of Health National Cancer Institute **Investigational Drug Accountability Record**	PAGE NO. _____ CONTROL RECORD ☐ SATELLITE RECORD ☐

Name of Institution	Protocol No. (NCI)

Drug Name, Dose Form and Strength

Protocol Title	Dispensing Area

Investigatior

Line No.	Date	Patient's Initials	Patient's I.D. Number	Dose	Quantity Dispensed or Received	Balance Forward Balance	Manufacturer and Lot No.	Recorder's Initials
1.								
2.								
3.								
4.								
5.								
6.								
7.								
8.								
9.								
10.								
11.								
12.								
13.								
14.								
15.								
16.								
17.								
18.								
19.								
20.								
21.								
22.								
23.								
24.								

NIH-2564
9-85

Appendix 18–1

High-Alert Medications

1. PURPOSE

This policy outlines the process for the safe use of high-alert medications.

II. DEFINITIONS

When used in this policy these terms have the following meaning:

A. High-alert medications: Medications that have a higher risk of causing harm when an error occurs.

B. Independent double verification (IDV):

1. Is performed by two staff members (as appropriate to the task, e.g., blood administration, breast milk retrieval) in the same proximity but separately, without prompting by another, as an independent cognitive task.

2. Both professionals will dialog to confirm what was checked independently prior to administration.

3. IDV of a medication also includes the following steps in addition to the two steps above:

   a. Performed by two professionals (e.g., RN/GN/RPh,/MD/LPN [within the approved LPN scope of practice]) in the same proximity but separately, without prompting by another, as an independent cognitive task.

   b. Each professional must check: the actual prescriber's order, the drug, the calculation, the concentration and other information specific to the medication.

   c. Each professional performing the verification performs all calculations independently without knowledge of any prior calculations and documents the verification in the medical record.

III. POLICY

It is the policy of the health system that:

A. All systems and data repositories relating to medication use (medication error reports, adverse drug event reports, etc.) shall be systematically evaluated on an ongoing basis to identify those medications in the hospital formulary determined to be high-alert medications.

B. Medications being added to the hospital formulary shall be evaluated for their high-alert potential.

C. Medications identified as high-alert shall be targeted for specific error reduction interventions.

D. The following three principles shall be followed to safeguard the use of high-alert medications:

1. Reduce or eliminate the possibility of error (e.g., limit the number of high-alert medications on the hospital formulary; remove high-alert medications from the clinical areas).

2. Make errors visible by detecting serious events before they reach the patient (e.g., follow the five rights and when appropriate utilize the independent double verification process).

3. Minimize the consequences of errors (e.g., stock high-alert medications in smaller volume units of use minimizing the error effect if the medication was administered in error).

E. Engineering safety controls shall be used as appropriate.

IV. PROCEDURE

A. The Pharmacy and Therapeutics Committee will approve all medications added to the formulary.

B. The following processes for safeguarding high-alert medication use have been implemented:

1. Build in system redundancies (e.g., unit dose drug distribution).

2. Use fail-safes (e.g., pumps with locking mechanisms).

3. Reduce options (e.g., limit concentration available).

4. Utilize engineering safety controls (e.g., oral syringes that will not fit IV tubing, computer systems that force the order of standardized products).

5. Externalize or centralize error-prone processes (e.g., centralize IV solution preparations).

6. Use differentiation (e.g., identify and isolate look alike and sound alike products, use generic names).

7. Store medications appropriately (e.g., separate potentially dangerous drugs with similar names or similar packaging).

8. Screen new products (e.g., inspect all new drugs and drug delivery devices for poor labeling and/or packaging).

9. Standardize and simplify order communication (e.g., only approved abbreviations will be used, all verbal orders will be read back verbatim to the ordering physician).

10. Limit access (e.g., high-alert medications will be securely stored).

11. Use of constraints (e.g., Pharmacy will screen all medication orders, automatic stop orders or duration limits).

12. Standardize or automate dosing procedures (e.g., use of standard dosing charts rather than calculating doses based upon weight or renal function when appropriate).

C. When initiating any high-alert medication by any route, and for those high-alert medications administered via pump, and with all subsequent bag/syringe changes and with dose changes requiring pump adjustment, the following must occur:

1. Independent double verification, each professional will independently:

a. Review/verify the physician order in the medical record (i.e. on the physician's order sheet or in the clinical information system).

    b. Verify the correct medication, dose (all required dosage calculations must be done independently by each nurse), frequency/rate/titration and route against the order.

        1) Note: After the initial IDV, ongoing titration in Level I areas is exempt from the IDV process for each continuing adjustment.

        2) Some medications require IDV of pump settings at change of shift (e.g., insulin).

        3) Additional information regarding medication-specific IDV requirements is available in the Independent Double Verification Policy and Procedure.

  2. The nurse administering the medication will:

    a. Identify the patient using two acceptable identifiers.

    b. Verify the correct connection/patient access when administering the medication via an intravenous drip, trace the flow of the medication from the bag > to the pump > to the patient access, prior to hanging the medication.

    c. Document the verification.

D. When an infusion device with pre-built infusion parameters is used (e.g., Alaris Medley Pump with Guardrails or Medfusion Syringe Pump with PharmGuard) and pre-set infusion parameters are not available for a high alert medication (e.g., when the medication is new and not yet added to the library), independent double verification of the medication parameters programmed into the pump must occur prior to initiation of the infusion.

V. DOCUMENTATION

As appropriate in the medical record or clinical information system.

VI. REFERENCES

  A. Institute for Safe Medication Practices (ISMP); *ISMP's list of high-alert medications.* 2008.

  B. Patient Care Policy and Procedure #0282, *Independent Double Verification.*

  C. Patient Care Policy and Procedure #0500, *Verbal Orders.*

  D. Patient Care Policy and Procedure #0700, *Abbreviations.*

  E. Patient Care Policy and Procedure #0282, *Independent Double Verification.*

  F. Patient Care Policy and Procedure #5010, *Anticoagulant Safety.*

  G. Patient Care Policy and Procedure #5020, *Chemotherapy: Oncology/Hematology.*

  H. Patient Care Policy and Procedure #5070, *Electrolyte Infusions.*

  I. Patient Care Policy and Procedure #5117, *Insulin Intravenous Infusions.*

  J. Patient Care Policy and Procedure #5130, *Medication Administration.*

  K. Patient Care Policy and Procedure #5131, *Medfusion Syringe Infusion Pump.*

  L. Patient Care Policy and Procedure #5140, *Medication Use Analysis/Error Prevention.*

  M. Patient Care Policy and Procedure #5150, *Moderate/Deep Sedation/Analgesia.*

VII. ATTACHMENTS

High-Alert Medications/Classes, one page.

High Alert Medications/Classes	Safeguards, Etc.
Chemotherapy agents (all routes, includes antineoplastic, biological, immunological agents used for malignant oncology and hematology diagnoses)	Chemotherapy Policy and Procedure outlines requirements for independent double verification of order, laboratory parameters, BSA, medication, dose, route, frequency etc. Chemotherapy Order form (or electronic equivalent) required Only attending physicians with chemotherapy privileges may write orders No verbal or telephone orders allowed (except to clarify as outlined in policy) Only Chemo-verified RN's may administer (exceptions are made for some oral agents, refer to the Chemotherapy Policy and Procedure for details)
IV Electrolytes (i.e., potassium chloride and phosphate, concentrated sodium chloride, magnesium sulfate, calcium chloride and calcium gluconate)	Independent double verification required. (IDV not required for 1000 mL pre-mixed IV solutions.) No concentrated products outside Pharmacy (*Rare exceptions exist, but only with specific safeguards.*) Electrolyte policy provides specific administration parameters and limits Electrolyte replacement protocol includes dosing and monitoring parameters. Standard concentrations/premixes and use of Bristojects for calcium chloride injection.
IV/SQ anticoagulants (i.e., heparin, lepirudin, enoxaparin, argatroban, bivalirudin – excluding flushes)	Independent double verification required. Weight-based protocol for heparin. The prescriber must designate the specific protocol (e.g., Cardiac, Non-Cardiac) to be implemented. Duplication warning in Clinical Information System Standardized order review requirements for enoxaparin and fondaparinux. Standardized laboratory assessments for heparin, enoxaparin and fondaparinux for treatment of deep vein thrombosis/pulmonary embolism, Premixed heparin solutions in standard concentrations
Neuromuscular blocking agents	Independent double verification required. Availability limited to specific units and access limited on these units (e.g., ED, OR, ICU) Special labeling of packages/baggies Standard concentrations established
Insulin	Independent double verification required. (Note: verification of the insulin product is not required when insulin is supplied directly from Pharmacy in patient-specific units of use (e.g., pre-filled syringes vs. vials.) Floor stock limited to specific agents and Pharmacy removes unused patient-specific vials from patient care units daily Resources include the Insulin Infusion Policy and the IV push insulin parameters defined within policy. Sliding scale order sets create a consistent process
Anesthetic agents used outside the OR (e.g., propofol, ketamine, methohexital, etomidate, dexmedetomidine)	Independent double verification required. Guidelines for use and administration of propofol These agents have been added to the Moderate-Deep Sedation Policy with defined safeguards for use.

continued

Warfarin	Independent double verification required.
	Standard administration time to allow access to INR results prior to daily dosing
	Laboratory monitoring standards and standardized order review processes.
	Critical value—Clinical Laboratory calls with INR results > 5
	Automated dispensing cabinet (ADC) inquiry—nurse is asked if he/she knows the patient's current INR as warfarin is being taken from ADC for administration to the patient.
	Pharmacy monitoring of at risk patients.

Appendix 18–2

Medication Shortages and Backorders

I. PURPOSE

The purpose of this policy is to outline an appropriate response to current or impending medication shortages in order to provide patients appropriate alternative therapy. In addition, the policy will ensure proper communications among the health system facilities to develop a unified action plan in addressing medication shortages.

II. DEFINITIONS

When used in this policy these terms have the following meanings:
- A. Shortage: A drug product shortage is a supply issue that affects how the pharmacy prepares or dispenses a drug product or influences patient care when prescribers must use an alternative agent.
- B. Backorder: A short-term and/or long-term unavailability of drug products

III. POLICY

- A. It is the policy of the health system that medication shortages and/or backorders shall be handled in an efficient, consistent, and timely manner.
- B. Pharmacy Services shall gather information and work collaboratively to assess alternatives, develop communication plans, and ensure safety when handling medication shortages or backorders.

IV. PROCEDURE

- A. The individual aware of the shortage or backorder will notify the Corporate Pharmacy Contracting Coordinator as soon as it has been identified.
- B. Upon identification of a medication shortage the Corporate Pharmacy Contracting Coordinator or designee will activate the communications with the Pharmacy Buyers to obtain an accurate inventory count and site based utilization data.
- C. The Pharmacy Buyers will also proceed with the following steps:

1. Sending a completed Medication Shortage Form (Attachment A) to the site based Pharmacy Management Team and the Corporate Pharmacy Contracting Coordinator. The entire form must be completed to the extent possible. Any information not readily available may be left blank.

2. Conduct an accurate and complete inventory inclusive of medication supply in satellite pharmacies, automated dispensing cabinets, storage, main pharmacy, code carts, medication kits, and other procedural areas.

3. During severe shortages (less than 2 week supply) the decentralized medication stock (ADM, satellite pharmacy, etc.) will be quarantined to the main pharmacy with the approval of the Pharmacy Manager or designee. The Pharmacy Manager or designee must communicate this decision with the Pharmacy Staff.

4. Maximize purchasing according to allocation at each site

5. Transfer and balance the utilization of the remaining supply with facilities in greatest need and inform site based Pharmacy Management Team.

D. For severe and acute shortages a group (Backorder Action Team) will convene under the direction of the Corporate Pharmacy Contracting Coordinator. The group will be responsible for developing a detailed backorder/shortage action plan for alternatives, communications, and a monitoring of the backorder for updates. The group may be inclusive of, but not limited to the Drug Information Coordinator, Pharmacy Managers, Operations Coordinators, Clinical Coordinators, and when applicable Clinical Specialist, Pyxis System Specialist, Pharmacy Information Systems Coordinator, Pharmacy Buyer, Pharmacy Educator, and Risk Management.

E. The Drug Information Coordinator will assist with developing a list of alternatives and a plan for substitution in the event the medication supply becomes depleted. This plan must be forwarded to the site based Pharmacy Manager or designee. Therapeutic substitutions must receive the approval of the Pharmacy and Therapeutics Committee Chair or designee prior to implementation.

F. The organizational backorder/shortage action plan should include the following information: current supply and utilization, how long will current supplies last, anticipated duration of the shortage/backorder, plan to conserve current supply [assessment of medical necessity (patient prioritization)], development of therapeutic alternatives and dosing when all supplies are depleted.

G. With a clear operational assessment of impact and a clinical impact on patient care, the group will develop a communication plan when appropriate (for pharmacists, nurses, physicians, respiratory therapists or other health care professionals as needed). The Pharmacy Manager or designee will implement the communication plan for each site respectively.

1. Plans to address a corporate shortage will include notification of at least the following groups and individuals:

    a. Chief Nursing Officer, Clinical Unit Educators and Nurse Managers

    b. Chief of Staff, Chief Medical Officers, and Medical Department Chairpersons. Notices to the Clinical Information System and faxes can be facilitated via Medical Staff Support and Information Services.

    c. Managers of other departments impacted by the shortage/backorder (such as the clinical laboratory, respiratory therapy, radiology, infection control, and others.

    d. Information Services should be notified if clinical information systems are impacted (e.g., if an alternative medication must be added to the system, if an interchange must be implemented, etc.)

  2. Committees with oversight for the clinical area should also be notified as appropriate, such as the Corporate Code Blue Committee, Critical Care Committee, Surgical Issues, and others.

  3. Plans may be site-specific as appropriate

V. DOCUMENTATION

None.

VI. REFERENCES

ASHP Guidelines on Managing Drug Product Shortages. *Am J Health-Syst Pharm.* 2009; 66. 1399-1406.

VII. ATTACHMENTS

  A. Medication Shortage/Backorder Form, one page

  B. Decision Flow Diagram

Medication Shortage/Backorder Form

Pharmacy: _____

Drug Name: Generic:_____   Brand:_____

Drug formulation(s) and/or strength(s) affected: _____

_____

Therapeutic interchanges affected: _____

Backorder or Discontinuation. If backorder, anticipated duration/resupply date: _____

Current Supply: _____

Current Usage: _____

How much additional supply can be obtained: _____

Cost concerns related to obtaining product from outside sources: _____

Reason for shortage/backorder (if known):

- Raw and bulk material unavailability
- Manufacturing difficulties
- Voluntary recalls_
- Manufacturer production decisions (e.g. discontinuation of product)
- Orphan drug products
- Restricted drug distribution
- Industry consolidations
- Market shifts
- Unexpected increases in demand
- Nontraditional distributors (e.g. international)
- Natural disasters
- Other: _____

Other comments: _____

Threat to Patient Care and Cost Assessments:
Assessment by Pharmacy Contracting Coordinator:
- Alternative sources (other wholesalers, direct purchases, etc.): _____
Assessment by Drug Information Coordinator:
- Alternative therapies: _____
- Medical necessity: _____

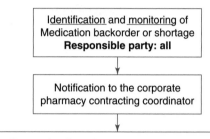

Identification and monitoring of
Medication backorder or shortage
Responsible party: all

Notification to the corporate
pharmacy contracting coordinator

Corporate Contracting Coordinator will inform ALL Pharmacy Buyers

Pharmacy Buyers will proceed with following steps once notified:
• Conduct an accurate and complete inventory (ADM, main pharmacy,
  satellite, code carts etc.)
• Complete Medication Shortage Form (Attachment A) and send to
  Pharmacy Management Team and Corporate Contracting Coordinator
• Quarantine decentralized supply when applicable for severe shortages
  (with approval from Pharmacy Manager or designee)
• Maximize purchasing according to allocation
  Transfer supplies to sites in greatest needs (inform Pharmacy Manager)

The health system is experiencing
severe or acute shortage

Corporate Contracting Coordinator:
• Pursue alternative sources for securing additional supply
Corporate Pharmacy Contracting Coordinator or Site-based Pharmacy Manager:
• Convenes a call or a meeting with the Backorder Action Team to develop a
  backorder/shortage action plan
• Backorder Action Team to develop a communication plan for the health care team as
  appropriate
• Pharmacy Manager or designee must implement plan at their individual sites
• Plan must be revised and redistributed as the situation evolves
Drug Information Coordinator
• Develop a list of alternatives and a plan for therapeutic substitution when necessary
• Receive endorsement/approval from Pharmacotherapy Committee Chair or designee
• Pharmacy Manager or designee must implement plan at their individual sites

Appendix 19-1

FDA Guidelines for Proper Medication Disposal

This set of guidelines was released in February 2007 and provides guidelines for drug disposal, the reasons for precaution, and current environmental concerns. The following guidelines are recommended:

- Patients should follow specific disposal instructions if they are provided with the medication. If none are provided, throw the medication in the trash after doing the following:
  - Mark out the patient's name and number for safety.
  - Remove medications from original containers.
  - To make medications less recognizable, less appealing, and less susceptible to diversion
    - Mix liquid medications with undesirable substance (e.g., cat litter, coffee grounds).
    - Add liquid to solid medications to start dissolving them.
  - Place medication bottle inside sealable, opaque, nondescript containers to prevent leaking and avoid diversion.
- Take advantage of community drug take-back programs (contact city or county government's household trash and recycling services to check on availability).
- Consider saving old or unwanted medications for hazardous waste collection (patients should be advised to check with their state Environmental Protection Agency [EPA] office regarding the availability of these in their area), also known as community take-back programs.
- Other good general practice may include wrapping medications with masking or duct tape to hide blister packs, and only placing medications in the trash just prior to pickup.
- Patients should NOT burn pharmaceuticals or personal care items, as doing so may create dioxins and other air pollutants.
- Patients should NOT routinely flush medications down the toilet. Although this prevents accidental ingestion in the home, it can cause water contamination that water treatment plants may not be able to filter. This is considered to be the least desirable method of pharmaceutical waste disposal, and should be done ONLY if the label or accompanying patient information specifically instructs doing so.

The following is a list of the limited number of medications the FDA advises be flushed rather than thrown in the trash.[1] (From Office of National Drug Control Policy. Proper disposal of prescription drugs. http://whitehousedrugpolicy.gov/drugfact/factsht/proper_disposal.html. (Accessed January 6, 2009.)

FDA List of Medications That Should Be Flushed (and Not Placed in Trash)
Fentanyl citrate (Actiq)
Methylphenidate (Daytrana Transdermal Patch)
Fentanyl (Duragesic Transdermal System)
Oxycodone (OxyContin)
Morphine sulfate (Avinza capsules)
Entecavir (Baraclude tablets)
Atazanavir sulfate (Reyataz capsules)
Gatifloxacin (Tequin tablets)
Stavudine (Zerit for oral solution)
Meperidine HCl tablets
Oxycodone and acetaminophen (Percocet)
Sodium oxybate (Xyrem)
Fentanyl buccal tablet (Fentora)

REFERENCE

1. Mireles, MC, Miller JA, Smith EA. Directory of drug take-back and disposal programs. Bellaire (TX): Community Medical Foundation for Patient Safety; 2008.

Appendix 22-1

Response Letter Drug A—*Incidence of Yellow Stripes*

DRUG A—Adverse Event—Yellow Stripes

Dear Dr. Smith,

Thank you for your inquiry. The following information is provided in response to your question regarding the use of DRUG A and the incidence of yellow stripes appearing on the skin.

Please note that the information provided is not intended to advocate the use of our product in any manner other than as described in the enclosed full prescribing information.

INDICATION(S)

DRUG A is indicated for the relief of moderate to severe hiccups in patients 18 years of age or older.[1]

PRESCRIBING INFORMATION

Please refer to the following sections of the enclosed Full Prescribing Information that are relevant to your inquiry: ADVERSE REACTIONS, WARNINGS, PRECAUTIONS.[1]

LITERATURE SEARCH RESULTS

A literature search of MEDLINE databases (and other resources) pertaining to the incidence of yellow stripes appearing on the skin associated with the use of DRUG A was conducted through May 2010.

CLINICAL STUDIES

In Phase III efficacy and safety studies of DRUG A for the relief of moderate to severe hiccups, yellow stripes appearing on patients' skin was reported in 7% of patients (see Table: Incidence of Yellow Stripes Appearing on Skin).[2]

TABLE   **INCIDENCE OF YELLOW STRIPES APPEARING ON SKIN[2]**

Adverse Event	DRUG A	Placebo
Yellow Stripes on Skin	7%	7%

In a 12-month long-term safety study, the incidence of yellow stripes appearing on the skin was evaluated. DRUG A users reported yellow stripes on their skin with an incidence rate of 9% (see Table: Incidence of Yellow Stripes Appearing on Skin—Long-Term Study).[3]

TABLE   **INCIDENCE OF YELLOW STRIPES APPEARING ON SKIN—LONG-TERM STUDY[3]**

Adverse Event	DRUG A	Placebo
Yellow Stripes on Skin	9%	8%

Multiple case reports were identified reporting yellow stripes appearing on patients' skin.

In a report by Jones A and associates,[4] a 90-year-old woman suffering from severe hiccups reported yellow stripes appearing on the skin within four days of starting treatment. She was treated with DRUG FIX-IT and her yellow stripes resolved immediately.

In a report by Jones B and associates,[5] a 20-year-old man suffering from moderate hiccups reported yellow stripes on his skin within 2 minutes of starting treatment. The patient did not seek treatment, continued taking DRUG A, and the yellow stripes resolved.

ADVERSE EVENT REPORTING

Please see the enclosed Prescribing Information for the complete safety and drug interaction information on our product. In order to monitor the safety of our products, we encourage clinicians to report adverse events by calling 1-800-555-9999 from 9 AM to 9 PM Mountain time, Monday through Sunday. Adverse events may also be reported to the FDA MedWatch program by phone (1-800-FDA-1088), by fax (1-800-FDA-0178), or by email (www.fda.gov/medwatch). To view a description of ongoing clinical trials for our products, please visit www.clinicaltrials.gov.

REFERENCES

1. DRUG A® (hiccaflixamab) tablets, 50 mg [package insert]. Any Town (OW): Awesome Drug, Inc.; 2010 Feb. Distributed by Awesome Drugs Pharmaceuticals.
2. Jones Z. Efficacy and safety of DRUG A® in the treatment of hiccups. JAHA. 2009 Feb;65(42): 735-746.
3. Jones Y. Long-term safety of the use of DRUG A® in severe hiccups. JAHA. 2009 Apr;65(43): 887-896.
4. Jones A. 90-year old woman with yellow stripes. Hiccup Central. 2009 Jul;78(4):232-235.
5. Jones B. 20-year old male with resolved yellow stripes. Hiccup Central. 2010 Jan;83(3):196-199.

Glossary

A priori In reference to clinical trials, to do something prior to initiation of the study.

Absolute risk reduction The difference in the percentage of subjects developing the adverse event in the control group versus subjects in the intervention group. Also refers to the number of subjects spared the adverse event by taking the intervention compared to the control.

Abstracting service A database that provides abstracts and citations for journal articles.

Abstracts A synopsis (usually of 250 words or less) of the most important aspect(s) of an article.

Academic detailing Process by which a health care educator visits a physician to provide a 15 to 20 minute educational intervention on a specific topic. Information provided is based on the physician's prescribing patterns and evidence-based medicine.

Action-guides A term coined by Beauchamp and Childress to refer to a hierarchical approach to the analysis of an ethical issue when forming particular judgments about the issue.

Adjunctive therapy Inclusion of a treatment that can affect the study outcome, but is equally distributed between both the intervention and control groups (e.g., controlled diet in a study measure lipid reduction therapy).

Adverse drug event (ADE) Any injury caused by a medicine. This includes adverse drug reactions and medication errors.

Adverse drug reaction (ADR) The Food and Drug Administration's (FDA) definition of ADRs is "any adverse event associated with the use of a drug in humans, whether or not considered drug related, including the following: adverse event occurring in the course of the use of a drug product in professional practice; an adverse event occurring from drug overdose, whether accidental or intentional; an adverse event occurring from drug abuse; an adverse event occurring from drug withdrawal; and any significant failure of expected pharmacologic action." Adverse drug reactions also include drug interactions. Several other definitions are available, many of which are discussed in Chapter 15.

Agenda for Change An initiative adopted by the JCAHO in 1986 intended to improve standards by focusing on key functions of quality of care, to monitor the performance of health care organizations using indicators, to improve the relevance and quality of the survey process, and to enhance the accuracy and value of JCAHO accreditation.

Aggregator A piece of software that is used to automatically collect information from RSS and weblog sites, which allows the user to look at material from many of those sites at one time and in one place.

Alpha (level of significance) The probability of a false-positive result in a study.

Analytic research   Quantitative research conducted in a controlled environment to determine cause-and-effect relationships.

Ancillary therapy   Inclusion of a treatment, which can directly affect the study outcome, that is not equally distributed between the intervention and control groups (e.g., antacid use in a study measuring reduction of heartburn symptoms between two acid-suppressive agents).

Article proposal   A letter asking the publisher whether he or she would be interested in possibly publishing something on a particular topic written by the person(s) who is inquiring.

Aspect of care   A term used in quality assurance programs to indicate the title that describes the area being evaluated.

Attributable risk   A statistical technique used in follow-up studies to determine the risk associated with exposure to a certain factor on disease state development. Attributable risk estimates the number of disease cases per number of exposures to the factor.

Beta   The probability of a false-negative result in a study.

Bibliography   A list of references, usually seen at the end of a piece of professional writing.

Bioequivalence studies   Research that evaluates whether products are similar in rate and extent of absorption.

"Black Letter Rules"   Principles of law that are known generally to all and are free from doubt and ambiguity. Also known as hornbook law, because they are in a format that would probably be enunciated in a hornbook.

Blinding   The procedures used in a clinical study to ensure that the investigator, subject, or both are unaware of which treatment is being administered. In a single-blind study either the investigator or the subject does not know the treatment being received, and in a double-blind study both the investigator and the subject are unaware of the treatment being received. Triple-blinding refers to the subjects, investigators, and the investigators analyzing the study results (either interim or final) being unaware of the treatment being received.

Blog   See Weblog.

Body area network (BAN)   A multidevice, interconnected computer system carried on a person. Sometimes referred to as a wearable computer.

Boolean operators (logical operators)   Words used to combine search terms (i.e., AND, OR, NOT) when using computerized databases.

Case-control study   A retrospective study where a group of subjects (i.e., cases) with a particular characteristic (e.g., disease) is compared to a group (i.e., controls) without the characteristic to determine the influence of certain factors on the development of the characteristic. Also called a trohoc study.

Case law   The aggregate of reported cases; the law pertaining to a particular subject as formed by adjudged cases.

CD-ROM   See Compact Disc–Read Only Memory.

Clinical investigation   Any experiment in which a drug is administered or dispensed to one or more human subjects. Relating to investigational drugs, an experiment is any use of a drug (except for the use of a marketed drug) in the course of medical practice. Although there are many other definitions, this is the Food and Drug Administration's definition and would seem the appropriate one to use given the nature of this topic. Please note that the Food and Drug Administration does not regulate the practice of medicine, and prescribers are (as far as the agency is concerned) free to use any marketed drug for "off-label use."

Clinical practice guidelines The U.S. Department of Health and Human Services, Public Health Service, Agency for Health Care Policy and Research (AHCPR) defines clinical practice guidelines as "systematically developed statements to assist practitioner and patient decisions about appropriate health care for specific clinical circumstances."

Clinical safety officer (CSO) Also known as the regulatory management officer (RMO). This will be the sponsor's Food and Drug Administration contact person. Generally the CSO/RMO assigned to a drug's Investigational New Drug Application will also be assigned to the New Drug Application.

Clinical significance The clinical importance of data generated in a study, irrespective of statistical results. Usually refers to the application of study results into clinical practice. Also can be called clinical meaningfulness.

Closed formulary A drug formulary that restricts the drugs available within an institution or available under a third-party plan.

Coauthor Any individual who writes a portion of an article, chapter, book, etc. This includes individuals other than the primary author, whose name is normally listed first on a publication.

Cohort study See Follow-up study.

Community rule See Locality rule.

Compact Disc–Read Only Memory (CD-ROM) A storage and retrieval system for large quantities of computerized data. Modern computers usually cannot only read the data on these disks, but usually can write new data to disks designed to accept that new data.

Comparative negligence The allocation of responsibility for damages incurred between the plaintiff and defendant, based on relative negligence of the two; the reduction of the damages to be recovered by the negligent plaintiff in proportion to his or her fault.

Compliance A measure of how well instructions are followed. In a study, compliance refers to how well a patient follows instructions for medication administration and how well the investigator follows the study protocol.

Computer network An interconnection of computers and computer-related devices (e.g., printers, modems) that allows the devices to interchange data, electronic mail, programs, and other files. In addition, a network allows sharing of peripheral devices, such as printers, modems, fax boards, etc. Normally, this interconnection is via a dedicated wiring system (other than telephone/modem communication); however, wireless connections are becoming common.

Concurrent indicator An indicator used in any quality assurance program that determines whether quality is acceptable while an action is being taken or care is being given.

Confidence intervals A measurement of the variability of study data. A 95% confidence interval is a numerical range that contains the true value for the population 95% of the time.

Consequentialist theories Moral theories that describe actions or decisions as morally right or wrong based on their consequences.

Continuous quality improvement (CQI) The term given to the methodologies used in the process of Total Quality Management. Efforts to improve quality are part of each participant's responsibilities on an ongoing basis.

Contract research organization (CRO) An individual or organization that is a sponsor of an investigational new drug (IND) or new drug application (NDA) that assumes one or more of the obligations of the sponsor through an independent contractual agreement.

Control group   The group of test animals or humans that receives a placebo or active control. For most preclinical and clinical trials, the Food and Drug Administration will require that this group receive placebo (commonly referred to as the placebo control). However, some studies may have an "active" control that generally consists of an available (standard of care) treatment modality. An active control may, with the concurrence of the Food and Drug Administration, be used in studies where it would be considered unethical to use a placebo. A historical control is one in which a group of previous patients is compared to a "matched" set of patients receiving the new therapy. A historical control might be used in cases where the disease is consistently fatal (e.g., AIDS).

Controlled clinical trial   A prospective study that directly compares an intervention to a control to measure a difference in effect (outcome); the best study design to measure a cause-and-effect relationship between the intervention and outcome.

Controls   A treatment (placebo, active, historical) used for comparison in a study to measure a difference in effect against an investigational agent. The investigator usually wishes to determine the superiority of a new treatment over the control in terms of efficacy and safety.

Copayment   Payment made by an individual who has health insurance at the time the service is received to offset the cost of care. Copayments may vary depending on the service rendered.

Cost-benefit study   A study where monetary value is given for both costs and benefits associated with a drug or service. The results are expressed as a ratio (benefit-to-cost), and the ratio is used to determine the economic value of the drug or service.

Cost-effectiveness study   A study where the cost of a drug or service is compared to its therapeutic impact. Cost-effectiveness studies determine the relative efficiency of various drugs or services in achieving desired therapeutic outcomes.

Cost-minimization study   A study that compares costs of drugs or services that have been determined to have equivalent therapeutic outcomes.

Cost-utility study   A study that relates therapeutic outcomes to both costs of drugs or services and patient preferences, and measures cost per unit of utility. Utility is the amount of satisfaction obtained from a drug or service.

Coverage error   See Sampling error.

Coverage rules   Criteria for specific drugs determined by the health plan in conjunction with the Pharmacy and Therapeutics Committee that is used to determine if a prescription is covered. Criteria are based on evidence-based medicine.

CQI   See Continuous quality improvement.

Criteria   A statement of the activity to be measured and evaluated. Also see Indicator.

Cross-sectional study   A study where measurements are taken at a single point in time.

Crossover study   A study where each subject receives all study treatments, and endpoints during the various treatments are compared.

Dechallenge   In relation to adverse drug reactions, this occurs when the drug is taken away and the patient is monitored to determine if the ADR abates or decreases in intensity.

Deep pocket   Practical consideration that involves the naming of additional codefendants in personal injury lawsuits to provide assurance to the plaintiff that there will be sufficient assets to pay the judgment.

Delta   The amount of difference that the investigators wish to detect between intervention and control groups in a study.

Deontological theories   Propose that intrinsic qualities of an act or decision assert its moral rightness or wrongness rather than consequences.

Descriptive research   Quantitative research that describes naturally occurring events.

Descriptive statistics   Statistics that describe data such as medians, modes, and standard deviations.

DIC   See Drug information center.

Digital video disk (DVD)   Also known as digital versatile disk. A disk that physically resembles a CD-ROM, but allows the storage of much larger amounts of data. It requires a special reading/writing device in a computer, although this device may also be combined with that used for CD-ROMs. DVDs have been used to a large extent to store and replay movies; however, they are now being used on computers to store large amounts of computer data, particularly large multimedia files.

DIS   See Drug information service.

Drug formularies   See Formulary.

Drug formulary system   See Formulary system.

Drug informatics   A technologically advanced version of drug information. This often denotes the electronic management of drug information.

Drug information   The provision of unbiased, well-referenced, and critically evaluated information on any aspect of pharmacy practice.

Drug information center (DIC)   A physical location where pharmacists have the resources (e.g., books, journals, computer systems, etc.) to provide drug information. This area is generally staffed by a pharmacist specializing in drug information, but may be used by a variety of the pharmacy staff or other individuals.

Drug information service   A professional service providing drug information. This service is normally located in a drug information center.

Drug interaction   The Food and Drug Administration defines this as "a pharmacologic response that cannot be explained by the action of a simple drug, but is due to two or more drugs acting simultaneously."

Drug master file (DMF)   Reference on file with the Food and Drug Administration that contains information regarding the drug. There are five different types of DMFs. The one that is most commonly used when filing an IND is the CMC-DMF (chemistry, manufacturing, and controls–drug master file), which contains information regarding the chemistry, manufacturing, and controls of the drug.

Drug product   The final dosage form; prepared from the drug substance.

Drug regimen review (DRR)   The monthly evaluation of nursing home charts by pharmacists.

Drug substance   Bulk compound from which the drug product is prepared.

Drug use/usage evaluation (DUE)   See Medication use evaluation.

Drug utilization review (DUR)   A program related to outpatient pharmacy services designed to educate physicians and pharmacists in identifying and reducing the frequency and patterns of fraud, abuse, gross overuse, or inappropriate or medically unnecessary care. DUR is typically retrospective in nature and utilizes claims data as its primary source of information.

Duty   A moral or legal obligation.

Editorial   Commentary, usually prepared by an expert identifying the strengths and limitations plus application of the results of a clinical trial, which is published in the same journal issue as the study.

E-mail   See Electronic mail.

Electronic mail (e-mail)   Brief messages sent from one computer to another, similar in use to interoffice memos. This serves as a quick, informal method of written communication. Also, e-mail may be used to send other items, such as word processing files, graphics, video, etc. to others.

Endpoint   A parameter measured in a clinical study. The primary endpoint is the major variable analyzed and reflects the main objective of the study. Secondary endpoints are additional variables of interest monitored during clinical studies.

Ethical theories   Integrated bodies of principles and rules that may include mediating rules that govern cases of conflicts.

Ethics (defined by AACP)   Philosophical inquiry into the moral dimensions of human conduct.

Ethics (defined by Beauchamp and Childress)   A generic term for several ways of examining the moral life.

Exclusion criteria   Characteristics of subjects that prohibit entrance into the study, if present.

Exploratory research   Research of a qualitative nature in which the investigators examine an unknown area to generate hypotheses.

Extemporaneous compounding   The practice of compounding prescriptions from a list of several ingredients—usually performed by a pharmacist.

False negatives   Individuals with the disease that were incorrectly identified as being disease-free by the test.

False positives   Individuals without the disease that were incorrectly identified as having the disease by the test.

File transfer protocol (FTP)   A method to transfer of files from one computer to another.

Follow-up study   A study where subjects exposed to a factor and those not exposed to the factor are followed forward in time and compared to determine the factor's influence on disease state development. Also called a cohort study.

Food and Drug Administration (FDA)   The agency of the U.S. government that is responsible for ensuring the safety and efficacy of all drugs on the market. This agency will approve drugs for marketing.

Formulary   A continually revised list of medications that are readily available for use within an institution or from a third-party payer (e.g., insurance company, government) that reflects the current clinical judgment of the medical staff or the payer.

Formulary system   A method used to develop a drug formulary. It is sometimes even thought of as a philosophy.

Galley proofs   A copy of a written work as it is to be published. The purpose of this document is to allow the author(s) to make a final check to ensure that everything is correct before actual publication.

Gray literature   Documents provided in limited numbers outside the formal channels of publication and distribution.

Health Insurance Portability and Accountability Act of 1996   Commonly referred to as HIPAA, this act includes privacy restrictions for electronic health records.

Health maintenance organization (HMO)   Form of health insurance whereby the member prepays a premium for the HMO's health services, which generally include inpatient and outpatient care.

Health Plan Employer Data and Information Set (HEDIS)   A set of performance measures used to compare managed health care plans.

Health-related quality of life (HR-QOL)   A general term for the impact of many dimensions of health status (such as physical, social, and cognitive functioning; mental health; symptom tolerance; overall well-being, etc.) on quality of life.

HIPAA   See Health Insurance Portability and Accountability Act of 1996.

Historical data   Data used in research that was collected prior to the decision to conduct the study (e.g., medical records, insurance information, MEDICAID databases).

HMO   See Health Maintenance Organization.

Homogenicity tests   Tests used when conducting a meta-analysis to determine the similarity of studies whose results were combined for the analysis.

http (hypertext transfer protocol)   A method by which information is encoded and transmitted on the World Wide Web.

https   A secure form of http used to transmit confidential information, such as credit card numbers.

Hypothesis   The researchers' assumptions regarding probable study results. The research hypothesis or alternative hypothesis (H_A) is the expectations of the researchers in terms of study results. The null hypothesis (H_0) is the no difference hypothesis, which assumes equality among study treatments. The null hypothesis is the basis for all statistical tests and must be rejected in order to accept the research hypothesis.

Incidence rate   Measures the probability that a healthy person will develop a disease within a specified period of time. It is the number of new cases of disease in the population over a specific time period.

Inclusion criteria   Characteristics of subjects that must be present in order for subjects to be entered into the study

Indexing service   A searchable database of biomedical journal citations.

Indicator   A statement of a measurable item in the area being evaluated that signals whether the area being evaluated is or is not of sufficient quality.

Indicator drug   A drug that, when prescribed, may offer evidence that an adverse effect to a drug may have occurred. Pharmacists can then investigate further to determine whether there really was an adverse effect. Examples are found in Chapter 15.

Inferential statistics   Statistics (i.e., parametric and nonparametric tests) that determine the statistical importance of differences between groups and allow conclusions to be drawn from the data.

Informed consent   The document signed by a subject, or the subject's representative, entering into a trial that informs the subject of his or her rights as a research subject, plus potential benefits and risks of the trial. This document indicates that the person is willing to participate in the study.

Inherent drug risks   Are unique to the drug and usually identified in the package insert, but do not include probable or common side effects.

Institutional review board (IRB)   A group of individuals from various disciplines (e.g., laypeople, physicians, pharmacists, nurses, clergy) who evaluate protocols for clinical studies to assess risks to the research participants and benefits to society. Approval of a local IRB (i.e., an IRB located in the community in which the study is to be conducted) is necessary prior to initiation of a clinical study involving patients.

Intention-to-treat analysis   Analysis of all subject results randomized in a clinical trial regardless of whether they completed or dropped out of the study.

Interim analysis   Evaluation of data at specified time points before the scheduled termination or completion of a study.

Internet   A worldwide computer network.

Interval data   Data in which each measurement has an equal distance between points, but an arbitrary zero (e.g., temperature in Fahrenheit).

Interventional study   A study where the investigator introduces a factor and examines the factor's influence on certain variables or outcomes.

Investigational new drug   A drug, antibiotic, or biological that is used in a clinical investigation. The label of an investigational drug must bear the statement, "Caution: New Drug-Limited by Federal (or United States) law to investigational use."

Investigational new drug application (IND)   A submission to the FDA containing chemical information, preclinical data, and a detailed description of the planned clinical trials. Thirty days after submission of this document to the FDA by the sponsor, clinical trials may be initiated in humans (unless a clinical hold is placed by the FDA). When the FDA allows the studies to proceed, this document allows unapproved drugs to be shipped in interstate commerce.

Investigator   The individual responsible for initiating the clinical trial at the study site. This individual must treat the patients, ensure that the protocol is followed, evaluate responses and adverse reactions, solve problems as they arise, and ensure the proper conduct of the study.

JCAHO   Joint Commission on Accreditation of Healthcare Organizations.

Joint and several liability   Refers to the sharing of liabilities among a group of people collectively and also individually. If the defendants are "jointly and severally" liable, the injured party may sue some or all of the defendants together, or each one separately, and may collect equal or unequal amounts from each.

Kurtosis   Refers to how flat or peaked the curve appears. A curve with a flat or board top is referred to as platykurtic, while a peaked distribution is described as leptokurtic.

Law   Involves written rules set by the whole society, or its representatives, that address the responsibilities of that society's members.

Letter to the editor   Comments from readers of a study or other article published in a journal. These are published in a later issue of the same journal and usually have a reply from the original study/article author(s). Occasionally, short reports of a case or small study may be reported this way.

Listserver   A service offered by some e-mail systems that allows a member of the listserver to send an e-mail message to one particular Internet address where it will be sent to all members of the listserver. This acts as a dynamic distribution list for e-mail messages.

Local area network (LAN)   A group of computers connected in a way that they may share data, programs, and/or equipment over a small geographic area (e.g., building, department).

Locality rule   Legal doctrine created in the latter part of the nineteenth century that stated that the local defendant practitioner would have his or her standard of performance evaluated in light of the performance of other peers in the same or similar communities. Also known as community rule.

Logical operator   A term such as AND, OR, NOT, NEAR, or WITH that can be used in searching a computer database. See the chapter on Electronic Information Management for more detailed information.

Mail service drug program   Program that provides free home delivery for up to a 90-day supply of maintenance prescription drugs.

Mainframe computer   A large, centralized computer that is used via computer terminals or other devices. This term is becoming blurred as smaller computer systems gain greater capabilities.

Managed care organization (MCO)   Health care provider that contracts with participating providers to provide a variety of services to enrolled members.

MCO   See Managed care organization.

Mean (arithmetic mean)   The most common measure of central tendency for data measured on an interval or ratio scale, best described as the average numerical value for the data set. Calculated as the sum of the observations divided by the number of observations.

Measurement error   Error that occurs when the interviewer influences the collection of data or when the survey item itself is unclear from the respondent's point of view. Also called response bias.

Measures of association   Calculation and interpretation of nominal study results using relative risk (RR), relative risk reduction (RRR), absolute risk reduction (ARR), and numbers needed to treat (NNT).

Median   The middle value in a set of ranked data. In other words, the value such that half of the data points fall above it and half fall below it. In terms of percentiles, it is the value at the fiftieth percentile.

Medical executive committee   A committee that acts as the administrative body of a medical staff in an institution. It is responsible for overseeing all aspects of care within the institution. This committee may be known by other names at specific institutions.

Medical Literature Analysis and Retrieval System (MedLARS)   The computerized information retrieval system at the National Library of Medicine.

Medical Subject Headings (MeSH terms)   A thesaurus of official indexing terms used when searching some of the databases of the National Library of Medicine (e.g., MEDLINE, TOXLINE).

Medication error   Any preventable event that has the potential to lead to inappropriate medication use or patient harm.

Medication misadventure   Any iatrogenic hazard or incident associated with medications. It includes adverse drug events (ADEs), adverse drug reactions (ADRs), and medication errors.

Medication use evaluation (MUE)   The component of a health care organization's quality improvement program that should examine all aspects of medication use including prescribing, dispensing, administration, and monitoring of medication use. Prior to 1986, this function was commonly referred to as drug use (or usage) evaluation (DUE).

MedLARS   See Medical Literature Analysis and Retrieval System.

MedWatch   The FDA Medical Products Reporting Program that monitors clinically significant adverse drug events and problems with medical products. Information is found at http://www.fda.gov/medwatch.

Meta-analysis   A type of review where conclusions are based on the summarization of results obtained from combining and statistically evaluating data from previously conducted studies. Also called a quantitative systematic review.

Middle technical style   A writing style used by professionals addressing professionals in other fields. It tends to be formal and avoids the use of the first person (e.g., I, us). Technical jargon is avoided in this writing style.

Mode   The most frequently occurring value or category in the set of data. A data set can have more than one mode.

Modified systematic approach   A seven-step approach to answering drug information requests that includes the following: (1) secure demographics of requestor; (2) obtain background information; (3) determine and categorize ultimate question; (4) develop strategy and conduct search; (5) perform evaluation, analysis, and synthesis; (6) formulate and provide response; and (7) conduct follow-up and documentation.

Morbidity   Detrimental consequences (other than death) related to a treatment, exposure, or disease state.

MUE   See Medication-use evaluation.

Narrative review   See Nonsystematic review.

National Committee for Quality Assurance (NCQA)   An organization dedicated to assessing and reporting on the quality of managed care plans; it surveys and accredits managed care organizations much like the JCAHO accredits hospitals.

NCQA   See National Committee for Quality Assurance.

Negative formulary   A drug formulary that starts out with every marketed drug product and specifically eliminates products that are considered inferior, unnecessary, unsafe, too expensive, etc.

Negligence   Failure to exercise that degree of care that a person of ordinary prudence or a reasonable person would exercise under the same circumstances. Elements of a negligence case include (1) duty breached, (2) damages, (3) direct causation, and (4) defenses absent.

New drug application (NDA)   The application to the FDA requesting approval to market a new drug for human use. The NDA contains data supporting the safety and efficacy of the drug for its intended use.

N-of-1 study   A controlled study conducted in a single subject where periods of exposure to a treatment are compared to periods of exposure to a placebo to determine the effects of the treatment on various variables and outcomes in the subject.

NNT   See Number needed to treat.

Nominal data   Data that is categorical (e.g., yes/no; male/female).

Noninherent drug risks   Are created by the particular drug in combination with some extrinsic factor that the pharmacist should reasonably know about.

Nonparametric statistics   Statistical tests used to analyze data that is not normally distributed such as nominal and ordinal data.

Nonresponse bias   See Nonresponse error.

Nonresponse error   Error that occurs when a significant number of subjects in the sample do not respond to the survey and when responders differ from nonresponders in a way that influences, or could influence, the results. Also called nonresponse bias.

Nonsystematic review   A review article that summarizes previously conducted research, but does not provide a description of the systematic methods used to identify the research included in the article. Also called a narrative review.

Null hypothesis   See Hypothesis.

Number needed to treat (NNT)   The number of patients who need to be treated for every one patient who benefits from a treatment. NNT is calculated as the reciprocal of absolute risk reduction.

OBRA '90   See Omnibus Reconciliation Act of 1990.

Observational study   A study where the investigator analyzes naturally occurring events.

Odds ratios   A statistical technique used in case-control studies to determine the risk of exposure to a factor on the development of a certain characteristic or disease state. Odds ratios estimate relative risk.

Omnibus Reconciliation Act of 1990 (OBRA '90)   A statute (Public Law 101-508) focused on drug benefits provided under Medicaid. The statute requires pharmacists to conduct a drug utilization review (DUR) including prescription screening, patient counseling, and documentation of interventions.

Online   The process of connecting to a remote computer via a modem or network.

Open formulary   A formulary that allows any marketed drug to be ordered in an institution or under a third-party plan. Can be considered an oxymoron.

Ordinal data   Data measured on an arbitrary scale that reflects a ranking (e.g., 1+, 2+ edema).

ORYX   A JCAHO initiative to mandate the use of performance-measurement tools to monitor outcomes and integrate this data into the accreditation process.

Outcome indicators   Quality assurance indicators that review whether the final desired result was obtained from whatever action was being reviewed.

Overview   A general term for a summary of the literature. Includes nonsystematic (narrative), systematic (qualitative), and qualitative (meta-analyses) reviews.

p **value**   A number (probability) that is generated during the use of inferential statistics. The *p* value indicates whether a statistical difference exists between groups. If the *p* value is less than or equal to alpha or the level of significance, the difference is statistically significant. If the *p* value is greater than alpha, the difference is not statistically significant. Also refers to the probability of rejecting a true null hypothesis.

P&T committee   See Pharmacy and therapeutics committee.

Parallel study   A study where two or more groups receive different treatments and the outcomes are compared.

Parameter   A measurement that describes part of the population.

Parametric statistics   Statistical tests used to analyze data with a normal (e.g., bell-shaped) distribution. Commonly used to analyze ratio and interval data.

Parenteral admixtures   Solutions containing drug products for intravenous administration.

Patient pocket formulary   A pocket-sized drug formulary listing top therapeutic drug classes, preferred products within those classes, cost index for the products, and other pertinent information.

PBM   See Pharmacy benefit management companies.

Peer review   A quality assurance program that centers on the evaluation of specific individuals by other similar professionals. Also, the process by which a group of experts review a manuscript for accuracy and appropriateness for publication in a biomedical journal.

Per protocol analysis   Assessment of the study results in only those subjects completing the entire study duration.

Pharmaceutical care   The responsible provision of drug therapy for the purpose of achieving definite outcomes that improve a patient's quality of life.

Pharmacoeconomics   The study of the economic impact of drug therapies or services.

Pharmacy and therapeutics (P&T) committee   A group in an institution or company that oversees any and/or all aspects of drug therapy for that institution or company. In hospitals, it is usually a subcommittee of the medical staff. May be known by a variety of similar names, such as pharmacy and formulary committee, drug and therapeutics committee (DTC), or formulary committee.

Pharmacy benefit design   Contract that specifies the level of coverage and types of pharmaceutical services available to the health plan member.

Pharmacy benefit management (PBM) companies   Organizations that manage pharmaceutical benefits for managed care organizations, medical providers, or employers.

Pharmacy network   Select pharmacies and pharmacy chains where members of a health plan have to go to get their prescriptions filled usually at a lower cost.

Placebo   A pharmaceutical preparation that does not contain a pharmacologically active ingredient, but is otherwise identical to the active drug preparation in terms of appearance, taste, and smell.

Poison information   A specialized area of drug information. By definition, it is the provision of information on the toxic effects of an extensive range of chemicals, as well as plant and animal exposures.

Poison information center   A place that specializes in the research, management, and dissemination of toxicity information. A physician usually directs it, although a pharmacist directs many on a day-to-day basis. Often, pharmacists and nurses provide the staffing of these centers.

Policy   A broad, general statement that takes into consideration and describes the goals and purposes of a policy and procedure document.

Popular technical style   A writing style used by professionals addressing laypeople. This is less formal than writing addressed to professionals.

Population Every individual in the entire universe with the characteristics or disease states under investigation. Because entire populations are generally very large, a sample representative of the population is usually selected for an investigation.

Positive formulary A drug formulary that starts out with no drug products and specifically adds products, after appropriate evaluation, that are needed by the institution or company.

Postmarketing surveillance study A study designed to examine drug use and the frequency of side effects following approval by the Food and Drug Administration (FDA).

Power The ability to detect a statistical difference between study groups. Power is dependent on sample size and mathematically is calculated as 1-beta.

Preferred drug product Specific drug product within a specific therapeutic class selected as the most appropriate to treat a specific disease or condition as determined by the pharmacy and therapeutics committee.

Preferred therapeutic class Specific drug class selected as the most appropriate to treat a specific disease or condition as determined by the pharmacy and therapeutics committee.

Prescribability The ability of a drug to be prescribed for the first time.

Prevalence Measures the number of people in the population who have a disease at a given time.

Primary author The author listed first on a publication. Sometimes referred to as the "first author."

Primary literature Original research published in biomedical journals.

Principles In ethical analysis, a principle is relatively broad and fundamental in scope, and guides ethical decision making or actions.

Prior authorization Authorization from the health plan or pharmacy benefit manager in conjunction with the pharmacy and therapeutics committee for specified medications or specified quantities of medications. The request is reviewed against preestablished criteria that are based on evidence-based medicine.

Procedures Specific actions to be taken.

Process indicators Quality assurance indicators based on the presence or absence of policies and procedures. These assume that if policies and procedures are appropriate they will be effective and be properly performed.

Professional ethics Rules of conduct or standards by which a particular group in society regulates its actions and sets standards for its members.

Professional writing Any written communication prepared in the fulfillment of the practice of a profession.

Programmatic research Research focused on the impact and economic value of programs and services provided by pharmacists in community and institutional settings.

Prospective indicator An indicator used in any quality assurance program that determines whether quality is acceptable before an action is taken or care is given.

Prospective study A study where data are collected forward in time from the date of study initiation.

Publication bias The situation where research demonstrating favorable results is more likely to be published than that showing negative results.

Pure technical style   A writing style used by professionals addressing other professionals in the same field. It tends to be formal and avoids the use of the first person (e.g., I, us). Technical jargon can be used in this writing style.

Push technology   A method by which information is actively sent to users' computers with little, if any, effort required by the user. The information may be displayed as a screen saver, or the computer may in some way let the user know that the information is available to be displayed (e.g., pop-up notification).

Qualitative systematic review   See Systematic review.

Quality   A degree or grade of excellence that and can be applied to goods, services, processes, or even people.

Quality assessment and assurance committee   A committee found in long-term care facilities to evaluate the quality of care, including drug usage evaluation.

Quality assurance   A process used to ensure that something is done or made well enough. It is usually retrospective and focuses only on a particular component within a process, not the entire process.

Quality of life   This is an evaluation of a patient's living situation based on the patient's environment, family life, financial situation, education, and health. It is used in quality assurance programs when developing indicators. In some cases, quality-of-life aspects will take precedence over the absolute best treatment. For example, a quick cure to a disease state may not be desirable when it costs so much that a family is bankrupted in the process.

Quantitative systematic review   See Meta-analysis.

Quantity limits   Set quantity of drug that can be prescribed that is set by the health plan in conjunction with the pharmacy and therapeutics committee that is usually based on FDA prescribing guidelines.

Random error   See Sampling error.

Randomization   The process used to ensure that subjects in a study have an equal and independent chance of being assigned to the intervention or control groups in a study.

Randomized clinical trial   See Controlled clinical trial.

Range   The difference between the highest data value and the lowest data value.

Ratio data   Data in which each measurement has an equal distance between points and also an absolute zero (e.g., temperature in Kelvin).

Rechallenge   In relation to adverse drug reactions, this indicates that the drug was taken away and, after the ADR abated, the patient was given the same medication in an attempt to elicit the same response a second time.

Referee   An expert in a particular area who reviews a written document to determine whether it is appropriate for publication.

Refereed publication   A publication in which the editors have experts in the appropriate field review items submitted for possible publication to determine whether those items are of suitable quality.

Relative risk   A statistical technique used in follow-up studies to determine the risk associated with exposure to a certain factor on disease state development. Relative risk estimates how many times greater the risk of disease state development is in patients exposed to a certain factor compared to those who are not exposed.

Research hypothesis See Hypothesis.

Respondeat Superior Refers to the proposition that the employer is responsible for the negligent acts of its agents or employees.

Response bias See Measurement error.

Restatement (Second) of Torts "An attempt by the American Law Institute to present an orderly statement of the general common law of the United States, including in that term not only the law developed solely by judicial decision, but also the law that has grown from the application by the courts of statutes..." It takes into account other factors, such as the modern trend of the law according to influential jurisdictions and well-thought-out opinions.

Retrospective indicator An indicator used in any quality assurance program that determines whether quality was acceptable after an action was taken or care was given.

Retrospective study A study that analyzes historical data (e.g., previously collected data such as medical records or insurance information).

RSS This acronym has multiple meanings, but is usually defined as Really Simple Syndication. It is a method by which an aggregator program collects information from Web sites and weblogs (blogs), which is then displayed as a collation. This allows individuals to monitor new or additional information on the Internet without having to use a browser to go to multiple Web sites.

Rule In ethical analysis, a rule guides ethical decision making or actions, but is relatively specific in context and restricted in scope.

Run-in phase A phase of a clinical trial prior to randomization in which all subject complete to determine the incidence of a prespecified outcome determined by the investigators (e.g., medication compliance, adverse effects).

Sample A group of subjects chosen as representatives of a population to participate in a study.

Sample frame Describes the population that will actually be drawn from to make up the survey sample.

Sample size The number of subjects in a study.

Sampling bias See Sampling error.

Sampling error Error that occurs when the research surveys only a subset (sample) of all possible subjects within the population of interest.

Secondary literature Resources that index and/or abstract literature from biomedical journals.

Selection bias A problem with the way subjects are entered into a study. It can be of two primary types. In the first, subjects meeting the inclusion and exclusion criteria are not randomized into the study. The other type is the recruiting of unique subjects not completely representative of the population (i.e., those with a GI bleed with aspirin).

SEM See Standard error of the mean.

Sensitivity The probability that a diseased individual will have a positive test result. It is the true positive rate of the test; the ability of a test to correctly identify those with the disease.

Sensitivity analysis Tests that are undertaken to determine the influence of various criteria or conditions on study results. Sensitivity analyses are commonly used in meta-analyses and pharmacoeconomic research.

Skewness The measure of symmetry of a curve.

Specificity   The probability that a disease-free individual will have a negative test result. Specificity is the true negative rate of the test; the ability of a test to correctly identify those without the disease.

Sponsor   An organization (or individual) that takes responsibility for and initiates a clinical investigation. The sponsor may be an individual or pharmaceutical company, government agency, academic institution, private organization, or other organization.

Sponsor-investigator   An individual who both initiates and conducts a clinical investigation (i.e., submits the IND and directly supervises administration of the drug), as well as performing other investigator responsibilities.

Stability study   A study designed to determine the stability of drugs in various preparations.

Standard   A term used in quality assurance programs that indicates how often an indicator must be complied with. The level of compliance will be set at either 0% (i.e., never done) or 100% (i.e., always done). A threshold, which allows compliance of between 0% and 100%, has sometimes been used instead of a standard.

Standard deviation   (1) A measurement of the range of data values (i.e., variability) around the mean. (2) The measure of the average amount by which each observation in a series of data points differs from the mean. In other words, the distance each data point is from the mean (dispersion or variability) or the average deviation from the mean.

Standard error of the mean (SEM)   An estimate of the true mean of the population from the mean of the sample. Mathematically, SEM is calculated as the standard deviation divided by the square root of the sample size. Ninety-five percent of the time, the true mean of the population lies within ±2 standard errors of the sample mean.

Statistic   A measurement that describes part of a sample.

Statistical significance   The impact of a study in terms of the outcome of statistical tests conducted on the data. A study is said to be statistically significant when statistical tests demonstrate a difference between treatment groups.

Statute   Written law enacted by a legislature other than that of a municipality.

Step therapy   Prescribing guidelines set by the health plan in conjunction with the pharmacy and therapeutics committee that specify which drugs should be prescribed first before more expensive drugs will be covered. Guidelines are based on evidence-based medicine.

Strict liability   Liability without fault. Defendant is liable even though not lacking in care. Negligence despite proof of prudence.

Structure indicators   Quality assurance indicators based on the presence or absence of items, such as staffing patterns, available space, equipment, resources, or administrative organization.

Study objective   A brief statement of the goals and purpose of a research study.

Subgroup analysis   Evaluation of study results within a subset of subjects enrolled in the study according to specific demographics (e.g., age, gender, disease state).

Subject   An individual who participates in a clinical investigation (either as the recipient of the investigational drug or as a member of the control group).

Surrogate endpoint   A study measurement that serves as a substitute for a clinical outcome.

Survey research Research where responses to questions asked of subjects are analyzed to determine the incidence, distribution, and relationships of sociological and psychological variables.

Switchability The ability to exchange one drug for another.

Symposium A meeting focused on a particular topic.

Systematic review A summary of previously conducted studies where the research to be included in the review is systematically identified; however, the results are not statistically combined as would occur with a quantitative systematic review or meta-analysis. Also called a qualitative systematic review.

Target drug program A program that evaluates the use of a medication or group of medications on an ongoing basis. Within these programs, interventions are usually made at the time of discovery based on established criteria or guidelines.

Telnet A program for microcomputers that causes the computer to mimic a dumb terminal, so that it can run programs on other computers (usually minicomputers or mainframes) over the Internet or other computer networks.

Teratogenicity Toxicity of drugs to an unborn fetus.

Tertiary literature Textbooks and drug compendia (includes full-text computer databases) that consist of established knowledge.

Third-party payer Organization that pays for or underwrites coverage for health care expenses for another entity.

Third-party plan A method of reimbursement for medical care in which neither the care provider nor patient is charged. Third-party payers include insurance companies, health maintenance organizations, and government entities.

Threshold A term used in quality assurance programs that indicates how often an indicator must be complied with. Unlike standards, thresholds can be set at any level of compliance, from 0% to 100%.

Tiered copayment benefit A pharmacy benefit design that encourages patients to use generic and formulary drugs by requiring the patient to pay progressively higher copayments for brand-name and nonformulary drugs.

Total quality management (TQM) A management concept dealing with the implementation of continuous quality improvement.

TQM See Total quality management.

Trohoc study See Case-control study.

True experiment A study where researchers apply a treatment and determine its effects on subjects.

True negatives Individuals without the disease who were correctly identified as being disease-free by the test.

True positives Individuals with the disease who were correctly identified as diseased by the test.

Type I error The probability of a false-positive result. The probability of a type I error is equal to alpha and occurs when the null hypothesis is rejected when it is in fact true.

Type II error The probability of a false-negative result. The probability of a type II error is equal to beta and occurs when the null hypothesis is accepted when it is in fact false.

Unexpected drug reaction   The Food and Drug Administration defines this as "one that is not listed in the current labeling for the drug as having been reported or associated with the use of the drug. This includes an ADR that may be symptomatically or pathophysiologically related to an ADR listed in the labeling but may differ from the labeled ADR because of greater severity or specificity (e.g., abnormal liver function vs. hepatic necrosis)."

Uniform resource locator (URL)   An Internet address (e.g., http://druginfo.creighton.edu).

USENET news   A large number of discussion groups that are replicated in numerous places on the Internet. Users can read items posted on a topic and can contribute their own items to be posted.

Validity   The truthfulness of study results. Internal validity refers to the extent to which the study results reflect what actually happened in the study (i.e., appropriate and sound study methods). External validity is the degree to which the study results can be applied to patients routinely encountered in clinical practice.

Variables   Factors (characteristics that are being observed or measured) that are the focus of a study. The independent variable (e.g., treatment) causes change in the dependent variable (e.g., outcome).

Variance   A measurement of the range of data values (i.e., variability) about the mean. Variance is the square of the standard deviation.

Virtual private network (VPN)   A method to connect computers over a distance, for example, over the Internet, that allows the secure transmission of confidential data.

Warranty   An assurance by one party to a contract of the existence of a fact upon which the other party may rely, intended to relieve the promisee of any duty to ascertain the fact for him or herself. Amounts to a promise to indemnify the promisee for any loss if the fact warranted proves untrue. Warranties may be express (made overtly) or implied (by implication).

Web browser   A computer program used to access information on the World Wide Web. Common programs include Microsoft Internet Explorer, Mozilla Firefox and Google Chrome.

Web portal   A Web site that acts as an interface to the Internet for users. Many Internet search engines are considered to be Web portals. A variation on this, the enterprise portal, can also be used by an institution to help guide employees to necessary information within the institution or out on the Internet.

Web site   A group of Web pages that will provide information to the person requesting that information. These pages are generally grouped under one main Internet address (URL).

Weblog   (also known as blog) This is a public Web site where a person maintains a journal that is open to viewers.

Wide area network (WAN)   A group of computers connected in a way that they may share data, programs, and/or equipment over a distance (e.g., connection between computers owned by an institution that are scattered in clinics around a city).

World Wide Web (WWW)   Computers connected to the Internet that provide a graphical interface to a variety of information that is available as text, pictures, sounds, databases, and other electronic files. Generally accessed using a Web browser, such as Internet Explorer.

XHTML (Extensible HTML)   A combination of HTML and Extensible Markup Language.

XML (Extensible Markup Language)   A superset of HTML that provides information on the content of a Web page, presentation of the information (how it looks), and semantics (what it means). This is designed to make it easier to find more relevant information using search engines.

Answers for Case Studies

Chapter 4

CASE STUDY 4–1

1. Yes, any study enrolling human subjects requires IRB approval. Even though the EPE product is a nonprescription agent, the subjects may still be at risk while partaking in this study. The IRB approval is needed to protect the patient.

2. Placebo being selected as the control for this controlled clinical trial is appropriate. The purpose of this study is to measure and quantify the LDL-C lowering effects produced by EPE. This is the first clinical trial published evaluating EPE. The differences in the LDL-C change between the two groups can document whether EPE has a pharmacological effect. This study was designed with a small sample size to measure changes in LDL-C levels but not place too many subjects at risk. After LDL-C lowering by EPE is documented by this study, using an active control (e.g., statin) would be appropriate as the control for future studies. Historical controls would not be appropriate to measure changes in LDL-C level since this outcome is not a significant risk to the subjects; many therapies are available that are considered safe to reduce LDL-C levels.

3. This indicates that 68% (one standard deviation from the mean) of the LDL-C values collected from the patients taking EPE were measured to be between 128 and 184 mg/dL.

4. Since all patients were to follow the same diet, this would be classified as adjunctive therapy. The diet should not interfere with measuring a difference in LDL-C lowering between EPE and placebo since both groups are following the same diet.

5. The probability of rejecting a true Ho is < 4.5%. Since this p-value is less than the stated alpha value, the Ho would be rejected and H_1 accepted. The probability of a Type I error is less than 4.5%, which could be due to chance. In addition, the probability of chance being the reason a difference was calculated between EPE and placebo would be less than 4.5%.

6. The use of the EPE product would not be recommended to the patient at this time. Primary reasons include:
   - Only one clinical trial published evaluating the efficacy and safety of EPE;
   - The clinical trial included a small sample size (< 75 total patients) and had a duration of only 12 weeks;
   - The p-value is less than the established alpha value (5%), but this does not automatically indicate a clinical difference between EPE and placebo;
   - Although the mean LDL-C level increased by 6 mg/dL (~4%), the mean LDL-C level decreased only 8 mg/dL (< 5%) with the EPE product;
   - A body of reliable evidence that documents significant mean LDL-C level reductions is lacking.

- The EPE product does not have evidence of reduction in clinical outcomes, such as MIs or stroke, whereas, other FDA-approved cholesterol medications do have this data.

CASE STUDY 4–2

1. Double-blinding is the most appropriate blinding type. The primary and secondary endpoints are subjective in nature. Thus, neither the patients nor investigators should know who is taking which therapy. Reduction in pain is not going to be reported by patients knowing they are taking placebo. In addition, the probability is highly likely that changes in pain scores reported by both patients and investigators are biased if the therapy is known.

2. Ordinal. This type of data is classified as ranked or scaled. Patients rated their pain during this trial using a scale. Rating pain on a scale is not dichotomous (e.g., yes/no data) nor has equal intervals (as does continuous data).

3. Mode and median are the appropriate measures of central tendency to present ordinal data. The mode is the most frequently occurring observation of the data set. The median is the point in which 50% (or middle) of the data in the set are above and 50% of the data below.

4. A selection bias may be present. Patients who met the inclusion and exclusion criteria may have not been randomized to one of the active therapies or placebo. Patients may be selected out of the study if they do not meet the run-in phase criteria. The exclusion of these patients may bias the results (e.g., eliminating patients experiencing side effects or not responding to therapy during the run-in phase).

5. Tapentadol appears to be efficacious in reducing pain; the primary endpoint result was lower than placebo and the results were statistically significant. However, this study only evaluated pain score changes in patients with OA who were candidates for THR or TKR. This study does not support the use of tapentadol to treat other types of pain. In addition, tapentadol was no different in reducing pain scores compared to the commonly prescribed analgesic oxycodone (p-value was > 0.05 thus not statistically nor clinically different). This study does not provided the evidence that tapentadol is more efficacious than oxycodone in reducing pain scores.

CASE STUDY 4–3

1. RRR = 20%
   RRR = 1 − RR. RR = $(139/2626)/(170/2575)$ = 0.053/0.066 OR 5.3%/6.6% = 0.80
   The calcium plus vitamin D combination reduced the baseline risk of a stress fracture by 20%. This result indicates that the calcium plus vitamin D combination reduces stress fracture risk versus placebo.

2. ARR = 1.3%
   ARR = $(170/2575)$ − $(139/2626)$ = 0.066 − 0.053 OR 6.6% − 5.3% = 1.3%
   A total of 1.3% (or 34) patients were spared a stress fracture by taking the calcium plus vitamin D combination compared to placebo. This result indicates that the calcium plus vitamin D combination reduces stress fracture risk versus placebo.

3. If the study was repeated, 95% confident that the calculated RR would be between 0.64 and 0.97. Since the value of equality (one) is not within the range, 9% confident that the calcium plus vitamin D combination reduces the risk of stress fracture compared to placebo. The RR can be as low as 0.64 but as high as 0.97. Both of these range limits are below one, the point in which the incidence of stress fracture is no different between Calcium plus vitamin D combination and placebo.

4. The analysis of results with the data from only the patients who completed the study (n = 3700) is called per-protocol (PP). This differs from the ITT analysis, which the data from all of the patients enrolled in the study and taking at least one dose of the intervention

or control are included in the study result analyses. Calculating and reporting the results using PP in conjunction with the ITT results is not inappropriate. The PP results provide data regarding the results if all patients are compliant and complete the study while the ITT results usually are not biased by those patients who do not complete the study.

5. The use of the calcium plus vitamin D supplement would be recommended to this female university soccer player. Although only one study has been published evaluating a reduction in stress fractures, the study was well designed and reported favorable results. Study strengths included controlled clinical trial design, appropriate primary endpoint and assessment, large sample size, double-blinding, randomization, placebo-control, ITT, appropriate alpha value, and statistically significant p-value for the primary endpoint. The results can be extrapolated to the female soccer player even though not a Navy recruit (similar age, stressful exercise, healthy). Also, few side effects were reported, which was a concern of the patient questioning this therapy. Intense training for young athletes can maximize bone strength and resist fractures but intense training increases calcium demands for bone formation and increases cutaneous calcium losses. Typically, females should have sufficient daily calcium and vitamin D intake. The doses in this study do not exceed daily intake recommendations.

Chapter 5

CASE STUDY 5–1

1. Null hypothesis: The treatment difference (mean and 95%CI) between dronedarone and amiodarone demonstrates dronedarone is not non-inferior to amiodarone and possibly inferior.

   Alternative hypothesis: The treatment difference (mean and 95% CI) between dronedarone and amiodarone shows dronedarone is non-inferior to amiodarone in maintaining sinus rhythm.

2. How was the NI margin was determined? Did the investigators set the NI margin prior to the study being conducted? Did the investigators confirm amiodarone's efficacy against placebo, which is referred to as assay sensitivity? Were historical trials and this NI study identical as possible regarding important characteristics (referred to as "constancy assumption")?

3. No, an intention-to-treat (ITT) analysis includes all patients randomized to treatment regardless of whether they completed the study duration. Smaller observed treatment effects can result with an ITT analysis since patients did not necessarily complete the duration of the trial and experience the maximum effect of dronedarone. Using an ITT analysis with a NI trial design can significantly increase the risk of falsely claiming non-inferiority. For this reason, a per protocol (PP) analysis is preferred. The FDA recommends performing both ITT and PP analyses and checking to see if there are significant differences in the results. An explanation as to why there was a significant difference is expected.

4. See Figure 5–1. Non-Inferiority Trial Design. The conclusion would be that dronedarone is non-inferior to amiodarone in maintaining sinus rhythm.

5. See Figure 5–1. Non-Inferiority Trial Design. The conclusion would be that dronedarone is not non-inferior to amiodarone in maintaining sinus rhythm.

6. Performing a superiority analysis after non-inferiority has been established is acceptable and appropriate. It is generally not acceptable or appropriate to seek the conclusion of non-inferiority from a failed superiority trial.

CASE STUDY 5–2

1. Investigator is picking study subjects based on a private interview that as far as we know has no clear-cut criteria for choosing subjects and putting them in one or the other group. Also, this being an observation study, there is no guarantee that the two groups have similar characteristics with the exception of being in the same observational cohort study. The bottled water group may be made up of healthier subjects than the tap water group.

2. Not all subjects are from the same local area; they could be passing through New York City on vacation or for business and thus be more susceptible to local organisms in the tap water. Age is a confounding factor in that the older the subject, the more susceptible they are to infections since their immune system is less effective in defending off germs and viruses. There are many other confounding factors that can be identified.

3. The outcome should be measured the same way and at the same frequency for both groups. Adequate follow-up should be determined.

4. No cause-effect relationship can be determined with an observational study such as this cohort study.

CASE STUDY 5–3

1. The quality of the meta-analysis depends on the quality of the studies used to develop the meta- analysis.

2. Publication bias is a form of selection bias where publication of studies is based on the magnitude, direction, or statistical significance of the results. It is documented that researchers are more likely to publish studies that demonstrate positive effects of drugs. A technique often used to identify the potential existence of publication bias is called the "funnel plot." A funnel plot is a scatter plot of treatment effect versus study size. If this plot shows an inverted symmetrical funnel, publication bias is probably not present. An asymmetrical funnel plot indicates the possibility that publication bias is present. (See Figure 5–4. Symmetrical versus Asymmetrical Funnel Plots.)

3. Factors that preclude pooling of results include discrepancies and low quality of studies in general, inconsistencies in methods, improper conduct of the trials, and reporting of data and widely disparate findings. For this particular meta-analysis, low quality of study design in two trials and inconsistencies in methods between all five studies would suggest a heterogeneity with these studies that prevents pooling of the data.

4. The authors should have used a Forest plot to provide the results of this meta-analysis because the reader can easily visualize the similarities and differences noted between studies and a confidence interval is included, which provides additional information about the variability of the results for individual studies.

CASE STUDY 5–4

1. Specific plant parts utilized in a study are important to consider. If a trial evaluated the use of an herb's root, but the product about which a practitioner is searching for information contains the herb's leaves and flowers, the results cannot be extrapolated. In this case, we know the physician is interested specifically in echinacea extract, and the study is utilizing echinacea root so the results cannot be extrapolated.

2. The majority of dietary supplement trials are conducted in Europe and Asia. Appropriateness of generalizability of results to a practitioner's own patient population must always be considered, just as with standard drug trials.

3. As with prescription drug clinical trials, duration of therapy is important. Inadequate duration for appropriate assessment is a common flaw in dietary supplement trials. In this trial, the echinacea is not being used for the same length of time the prophylactic

antibiotic therapy is being continued. This could be one reason there was no difference noted between treatment and placebo groups.

4. Small subject population is another common flaw with dietary supplement trials. Small-sized groups may not have adequate statistical power to reveal a potential difference between a dietary supplement and a placebo. In this case, power is not met since it takes 30 patients per group to meet power and only 20 patients per group were entered into the trial. In addition, adverse reactions or drug interactions can be overlooked in smaller groups versus a larger one. A small subject population can limit trial generalizability to a broader patient population.

Chapter 7

CASE STUDY 7–1

Select a topic for guideline development   This first step is similar to selecting topics for a medication use evaluation program. There are specific disease conditions that possess the maximum potential for benefit from guideline development and implementation. These disease conditions share common characteristics such as high prevalence, high frequency/severity, availability of high-quality evidence supporting reduction in morbidity and mortality with treatment, feasibility of guideline implementation, potential cost-effectiveness, evidence that current practice is not optimal, evidence of practice variation, and the availability of personnel, expertise, and resources to implement a practice guideline if one is developed.

Recruit appropriate multidisciplinary membership for a panel to be involved in development of guidelines   Developing a clinical practice guideline should be considered a multidisciplinary process involving groups that have a stake in the development and implementation of the guideline. Conflicts of interest should be identified. Anyone with expertise in guideline development would be valuable to the panel.

Define the clinical questions to be addressed   This step is critical to be successful in searching for the necessary evidence and providing useful valid conclusions. Many guideline development groups use the PICO format for framing the question. The "P" stands for patients who are being considered for the question. Which treatment intervention to be considered is represented by the "I" and the "C" stands for comparison of main alternatives that should be compared to the intervention. Finally, the "O" stands for what outcome is most important to the patient such as mortality, morbidity, treatment complications, rates of relapse, physical function, quality of life, and costs.

Determine the criteria for evidence   This step defines the admissible evidence. The admissible evidence includes the types of published or unpublished research to -be considered so that appropriate literature searches may be performed. The panel needs to decide if they will accept evidence from previous guidelines, meta-analyses, systematic reviews, randomized, controlled trials, observational studies, diagnostic studies, economic studies, and qualitative studies. This process may be revisited at various stages of guideline development depending on the results of the original search.

CASE STUDY 7–2

Conduct a systematic search for the qualifying evidence   Typically, a search is first conducted to identify previously completed guidelines and systematic reviews that involve related questions. The actual retrieval process should include a search of available bibliographic resources. Next a search of any specialized databases related to the subject of the guideline should be performed. Citations listed in published bibliographies, textbooks, and identified literature should be reviewed to identify other evidence not produced from database searches. Search terms can be identified from the clinical questions developed earlier by the panel.

Perform a systematic evaluation and grading of the evidence   Several different methods exist for evaluating studies identified in the literature. The primary purpose of the systematic evaluation is to identify issues with trial design or any potential biases that would affect internal or external validity. Some issues to consider include basic trial design, sample size, statistical power, selection bias, inclusion/exclusion criteria, choice of control group, randomization methods, comparability of groups, definition of exposure or intervention, definition of outcome measures, accuracy and appropriateness of outcome measures, attrition rates, data collection methods, methods of statistical analysis confounding variables, unique study population characteristics, and adequacy of blinding. Formal methods also exist to assign a quality score to each study evaluated. Note that other factors are considered in the overall body of evidence such as the consistency of results between studies, amount of evidence available, safety of treatments studied, and serious adverse events that occur infrequently.

Prepare a synthesis of the evidence   Evidence represented by selected studies should be summarized in a format that allows the panel to begin developing conclusions. Best formats facilitate consideration of the characteristics and quality of individual studies, consistency of the results between studies, overall size of the evidence database, and size of treatment effects for benefits and harms. In the absence of high levels of evidence, guideline development groups have elected to state that the evidence of developing a recommendation is inconclusive and, in place of a recommendation, a summary of the available evidence is provided. Other guideline groups will consider a variety of consensus methods to develop a recommendation.

CASE STUDY 7–3

Formulate and grade recommendations based on the grade of evidence and the balance of benefits, harms, and costs of treatment options.   Recommendations in a guideline must be worded carefully and clearly communicate that the expected outcomes will be achieved if the recommendations are followed. These recommendations should be written to stand alone since users may not read the full guideline document. Confusion exists for the end user because a variety of grading systems are currently used by different guideline development groups. For each guideline that is used, practitioners are required to read the grading scheme description so they will correctly interpret the strength of the recommendations, quality of the evidence, and the balance between benefits and harms of the interventions considered. To minimize this confusion and potential for misinterpretation, a standardized system such as the Grades of Recommendation Assessment Development and Evaluation (GRADE) should be used by the panel to grade recommendations in the practice guideline being developed.

Draft the guideline document.   Using the evidence tables compiled in the synthesis step and the graded recommendations developed above, a draft guideline document can be created. A formal narrative summary should be included with all relevant details of decisions made in the development of the guideline captured. Detail of the scope of the guideline including target patient population, restrictions on the population, interventions considered, specific outcomes or performance measures, intended users of the guideline, and overall objective of the guideline should be provided. Authorship, sponsorship, and any potential conflicts of interest should be identified, in addition to a detailed description of all production methods used, decision-making methods, recommendations of how to apply the guidelines to practice, comments about ongoing studies that may affect recommendations, and any plans for updating the guideline. The guideline should be written in a way that reflects the thought process used in evaluating and applying the information.

Conduct peer-review and pilot testing of the guideline. The methods to obtain peer-review and feedback on the draft guideline are dependent upon the scope deemed necessary by the panel. The peer-review can be confined within that organization, focused on target organizations, or obtained by open input from any interested party via a public notice. Participation by feedback on the draft can provide a sense of ownership to a broader audience and be a positive factor in the guideline implementation phase. A pretesting of the guideline in practice settings can provide additional feedback to the panel. From peer-review and feedback, revisions can be made to ensure that the guideline meets intended goals. These revisions or decisions to reject specific feedback should be documented.

Create tools for implementation of the guideline. A variety of tools may be used including preparing various formats of the guideline that will facilitate implementation in specific practice setting, creating guidelines that facilitate automated implementation, algorithms, or flow charts that facilitate understanding of the use of the guideline, or educational programs.

Establish a plan for follow-up and periodic updating of the guideline. A review interval to update the guideline should be established by the panel. The duration of the interval is dependent upon the topic and knowledge of ongoing studies.

CASE STUDY 7–4

The seven categories of guideline implementation barriers that limit or restrict complete physician adherence include: lack of awareness, lack of familiarization, lack of agreement, lack of self-efficacy (disbelief they could perform the behavior or activity recommended by the guideline), lack of outcome expectancy (disbelief that expected outcome would occur by following guideline), inertia of present practice (lack of motivation to change current practice), and a host of external barriers such as patient resistance, patient embarrassment, lack of reminder system, cost to patient, and lack of time.

Chapter 8

CASE STUDY 8–1

1. The population of interest is all individuals recently discharged with heart failure diagnosis.
2. This will most likely require a convenience sample because the patients need to be identified within the specific hospital where the intervention is occurring. It could be argued that anyone could randomly need the hospital, but at the very least, the sample is a convenience on a regional level. The randomness of the convenience sample is determined by the demographics of the patients, where hospitals in bigger cites may have a more generalizable sample.
3. The DV is 30-day hospital readmission. There are two levels—30-day readmit versus no 30-day readmit. The scale of measurement is nominal or dichotomous.
4. The appropriate measure of central tendency is the mode because the data are nominal. This data should be presented as frequency count and percentage.
5. The IV is treatment group. There are two levels—treatment versus control. The scale of measurement is nominal or dichotomous.

6. Confounding variables are considered as sources of error. There are numerous sources of error applicable to the patient, hospitalist, pharmacist, or nurse.
   - Patient—length of stay prior to discharge, severity of disease state, comorbid disorders, concomitant medications, demographic characteristics (e.g., age, gender, race, family history, support system), among others.
   - Healthcare practitioners—years of experience, number of patient seen daily, demographic characteristics, among others.
7. The control group can be matched based on various variables described above, but this may reduce generalization and sample size. Thus, by controlling for various sources of error (confounding variables) the control group can include any patient discharged with a heart failure diagnosis who will not receive the intervention.
8. The binomial distribution should be used, because there is one mutually exclusive outcome and the study is analyzed retrospectively (i.e., although the study was conducted prospectively, the analysis assesses the overall occurrence of 30-day readmits retrospectively). You may think the Poisson distribution can be used, and this would have been correct if the study had been interested in the rate of 30-day readmissions.
9. An odds ratio is the most appropriate epidemiological statistic, as this is essentially a case-control study.

CASE STUDY 8–2

1. The DV is percent platelet inhibition. The DV is a continuous variable measured on an interval scale.
2. No. An independent samples t test is inappropriate because the participants are measured repeatedly. Thus, the two measurements are related, violating the assumption of the independent samples t test.
3. No. The authors should have tested for differences following random assignment because random assignment to groups does not ensure homogenous groups.
4. Yes. With a two-way mixed ANOVA, the statistical significance of the interaction effect indicates the presence or absence of an order effect.
5. A statistically significant interaction indicates that order affected the effectiveness of the medication. No further analysis can be conducted.
6. This depends on the distribution of the DV. If the DV is normally distributed, then the paired samples-test test is appropriate. However, if the distribution is skewed, the nonparametric signed-rank test is more appropriate.
7. You would use the signed ranks test or sign test because they are most appropriate when skewed distributions are observed and the DV was measured repeatedly.
8. No. Because the groups did not differ at baseline, there was nothing to adjust and the covariate will not increase statistical power enough to be useful.

CASE STUDY 8–3

1. Theoretically, multiple linear regression is the correct analysis because the researcher wanted to predict the effect of hospital cost (a continuous DV measured on a ratio scale) resulting from nicardipine versus other antihypertensive medications after controlling for a number of covariates.
2. Yes. One of the primary assumptions of multiple linear regression is that the DV is distributed normally. If the variable is not transformed, the results are significantly biased, and the study is rendered useless.

3. No. Transforming systolic and diastolic blood pressure is not required because the distribution of the IVs is not nearly as important as transforming the DV. However, normalizing these variables will increase the statistical power of the analysis. If the analysis was run with the variables untransformed, results can still be interpreted appropriately.

4. The omnibus F test indicates that all the variables included in the analysis (i.e., IV and covariates) significantly predict hospital cost. Yes, the overall regression model is statistically significant at $p < 0.05$.

5. Yes, because the omnibus F test was statistically significant.

6. The adjusted R^2 value indicates that 14.6% of the variance in the hospital cost was explain by treatment modality (i.e., nicardipine versus other) as well as age, gender, race, concomitant antihypertensive agents, inpatient complications, systolic and diastolic blood pressure, coronary artery disease, and diagnosis of a noncardiac event. That is, 14.6% of the reason a patient had a specific hospital cost was due to the treatment modality and covariates.

7. The slope of –5.29 indicates that when compared to patients taking any other antihypertensive medications, using nicardipine in the ICU decreased hospital cost by $5.29. Although this was statistically significant finding at $p < 0.05$, a $5.29 decrease is by no means substantial. Thus, results are not important clinically.

Chapter 9

CASE STUDY 9–1

1. Since the topic is known and the boss informed you that you are the sole author, it is possible to skip some of the first steps listed in the book. Also, it is known where it will be published—in the policy and procedure section of the institutional intranet. So, the first thing to do is probably review the format of policies and procedures in the institution, to determine what needs to be written. As a part of this, determine that it needs to be written in the middle technical style, since it is being aimed at a variety of health care practitioners (e.g., pharmacist, physician, nurse). Then, it is necessary to do research into the topic.

2. First, organize the material. This can be done in conjunction with preparation of an outline of the order in which the material needs to be covered. That outline can done on a word processor and serve as the template for the document. In many cases, the way the institution lays out its policy and procedure documents can serve as a good part of the outline. Then proceed to write the material. At this stage, simply make sure everything necessary is recorded in the document. The document can be written in order of the topics, or each individual section may be written separately, in whatever order is easiest. Also, remember to cite material as the document is written. Besides being appropriate to give credit, it is also useful for the future when someone may have to come back to revise the document after several years and may not otherwise be able to tell the origin of some of the information.

3. Some would say to just present it to the pharmacy and therapeutics committee, but there are a couple of things that need to be done first. To start, the author should reread and edit the document. Then, get others who have expertise in the area to read and edit it. These others should include one or more representatives from each group affected by the document (e.g., pharmacist, physician, nurse). An effort must be made to make sure the

document is in a logical order, covers all aspects of the topic and is understandable. Then incorporate any necessary revisions. This process may need to be done several times (e.g., some chapters in this book went through a dozen versions before being submitted to the publisher).

CASE STUDY 9–2

1. First, clarify whom the Web site is addressing—its audience. It will be different for patients versus other health care practitioners. Sometimes it will be both groups. Then, in relationship to the above, determine what information or features need to be on the Web site. Then determine what equipment (e.g., computer hardware and software) and budget are available to prepare the Web site.

CASE STUDY 9–3

1. First, be sure to prepare slides on something that is compatible with the program used at the meeting. Then determine what information needs to be on the slides. Generally, assume that each slide should be shown for a minute or two. Each slide should be kept simple, with a maximum of five bullet points and five words per bullet point, so that attendees can concentrate on the message. Also, remember that the speaker is not to read directly from the slides, but use them just as a jumping off spot for the presentation and to organize thoughts.

Chapter 14

CASE STUDY 14–1

Possible responses include:
- Staff does not know that the medication should be infused over 60 minutes.
- The medication label does not provide infusion-time directions to the nurse administering the medication.
- Nurses are not using the "smart" features of the infusion pumps that would default to the appropriate infusion rate for a 60-minute infusion.
- Staff are rushed and opt to infuse medications more rapidly in order to get everything done.

CASE STUDY 14–2

Possible responses include:
- Physicians (surgeons, medicine/family medicine, infectious disease specialists)
- Nurses from the perioperative areas, inpatient units and home care areas
- Pharmacists
- Discharge planners/case managers who help to plan for discharge and arrange home care

CASE STUDY 14–3

Existing guidelines or standards for warfarin use to assist in drafting criteria for MUE:
- Search the medical literature.
- Ask practitioners with experience/expertise in this area.
- Professional organizations (pharmacy, nursing, medical).
- Identify any prior evaluations of this topic with the organization.
- Post an inquiry on professional-list serves.

Chapter 16

CASE STUDY 16–1

1. Advantages and disadvantages of including multiple cases in the Root Cause Analysis process:
   - Combining cases of similar types provides a larger volume of information from which to extract potential causes common to many events. For example, reviewing one case and making major system changes may in fact miss the most common factor that is causing the events. The power of multiple cases increases the chance that the frequent causative reasons are identified, which can then be addressed.
   - One disadvantage is that each case that is included in an aggregate RCA requires adequate investigation in order to understand the causes and therefore takes more time. All the cases are then reviewed in aggregate to determine those most common causes.

CASE STUDY 16–2

1. Questions you would like to ask the pharmacist involved in the error as part of an interview:
   - It is important to ask staff to provide a description of the situation as they remember it, without leading questions. It is also very important to interview staff early to prevent unintentional alterations to the story based on fading memory or hearing other discussions related to the event.
   - Ask the pharmacist to describe what happened and what they remember.
   - Ask the pharmacist what they do if/when they realize an error has occurred. What resources are they aware of to identify what patient they may have entered the orders on in error—many computer systems have a searching function that enables a report that identifies all patients on a given drug.
   - Ask other pharmacists what their process is when interrupted to assure they are entering orders on the correct patient.
2. Reason for classifying this error as human-error only, system-error only, or a combination of both:
   - It depends on the information that is gathered during interviews and observation of the usual process. If there exists the opportunity to devise a no-interruption zone for order entry (in which telephone calls are received by other staff), then this is a system opportunity. It is a human error in that it was not an intentional action and the system set up the pharmacist to potentially fail. It is likely considered a combination of both human error and system contributing cause.

CASE STUDY 16–3

1. System issues which contributed to the error:
   - The nurse had more patients than the recommended nurse to patient ratio.
   - The drug label had the volume first and the drug listed second, yet the infusion pump requires programming the drug first and the volume second, setting up the nurse to program it incorrectly.
2. Your reaction as manager of the unit:
   - Were the actions as intended? Did the nurse intentionally program the pump incorrectly? No.
   - Was the person under the influence of unauthorized substances? No
   - Did he or she knowingly violate a safe operating procedure? There was not a required double-check and pump programming was taught to all staff upon institution of the new pumps. She did not make a conscious choice to skip steps within the process or subvert the process.
   - Do they pass the substitution test described above? When this was discussed with several other nurses, two of the three noted that they had made a similar error and/or caught a similar error. This appears to be a skill-based error in which the nurse has done it many times and this time there was a slip. Would others have made the same decisions and, if so, less likely to be culpable? If not, were there deficiencies in training or experience? The training must be carefully considered. Providing didactic information without practice or competency testing is not the most appropriate method of teaching staff. Adequate practice is needed to develop good habits and skill-based actions.
   - Does the individual have a history of unsafe acts? This is the first error of this type that has been identified for this nurse. If not, again less likely to be culpable.
3. Identifying potential system fixes:
   - The label design should match the entry in the pump if at all possible. Rearranging or increasing the visibility of the required information for programming is another option.
   - Providing adequate staffing ratios to decrease the risk of competing priorities with multiple patients is appropriate.

Chapter 20

CASE STUDY 20–1

1. As a pharmacist in a busy pharmacy, it is important to triage the problems in front of you. In this situation you have multiple things going on and you are the only pharmacist on duty. It is up to you to decide what takes priority. This patient may be making decisions about her health based solely on information found online. If the patient follows through on her plan to stop taking the antidepressant she will be at risk of being harmed. This should make her your top priority.

   The patient in this particular case is actually seeking input from the pharmacist in her attempt to have a dialogue about quitting her antidepressant. The pharmacist would be negligent in their duties if they do not to counsel the patient on the pros and cons of obtaining health information online, the danger of stopping an antidepressant abruptly and the risk of recurrence of her depression.

Pharmacists have a professional obligation to engage with their patients and provide them the education and tools to obtain the best healthcare possible. Patients are increasingly using alternative sources beyond health care providers for advice and/or counseling, which makes it vital that pharmacists initiate even difficult conversations.

2. First, the patient should be encouraged to continue to take an active role in her own health care. Patient empowerment has many positives for their health outcomes. On the flipside, it is important to make the patient aware that when taking their healthcare into their own hands there can be negative consequences as well. It is crucial that they involve a health care practitioner if they decide to change their therapy in anyway.

   Second, agree with your patient that there are a lot of good places to find health information out there but what is really important is that they identify quality web sites to obtain the required information from. Even then, every individual is different and the information they find on these web sites may not necessarily be patient-specific or applicable to their situation. For example, the patient in this case is making a decision to discontinue her antidepressant based on other patient's opinions of the medication. These other patients quite possibly have an entirely different health situation. Encourage the patient to take these concerns to her primary care practitioner so that they may have a discussion on whether or not what she's found online is relevant to her situation.

   Third, you review suggestions for determining a quality health information web site, thereby ensuring patients are obtaining information from reputable sources and bringing information to discuss with their health care practitioner that has value. In this specific case, the pharmacist is unable to meet now so they should arrange a time to call the patient or make an appointment for the patient to come back in to discuss her plans.

   Our role is to support the patient and their beliefs. Show respect and the desire to collaborate with them and you'll gain their trust. Trivialize what they bring to you and insist that the health care practitioner is the expert and the one who knows best and you may damage the relationship beyond repair.

3. Safety first. If the patient has made up her mind that there is no stopping her from discontinuing her antidepressant immediately, advising her how to do so safely becomes your number one priority. First, direct the patient to see her primary care practitioner as soon as possible. Together they can work out a plan of action to taper her off the medication and possibly get her started on something she feels more comfortable taking. The practitioner may also establish a plan in order to monitor the patient for signs of relapse into depression.

   If you sense the patient will not consult her doctor; it is important to counsel her on possible withdrawal symptoms she may experience as well as the consequences of quitting her medication all at once without tapering. Also arrange a follow up time after your initial discussion to evaluate the control of her depression and how well she tolerated stopping the medication. At follow-up, if the patient is suicidal or at imminent risk of harming herself or someone else it is imperative you seek immediate assistance.

Answers for Self-Assessment Questions

Chapter 1

1. e	6. c	11. b
2. c	7. e	12. d
3. a	8. e	13. c
4. b	9. b	14. e
5. d	10. a	15. a

Chapter 3

1. a	5. b	9. e
2. c	6. c	10. d
3. c	7. d	11. e
4. a	8. e	

Chapter 4

1. a	6. e	11. b
2. c	7. b	12. d
3. b	8. c	13. a
4. d	9. d	14. e
5. a	10. e	15. c

Chapter 5

1. a	6. d	11. d
2. b	7. d	12. a
3. c	8. b	13. d
4. c	9. d	14. d
5. b	10. c	15. a

Chapter 6

1. d	6. d	11. d
2. a	7. a	12. a
3. c	8. d	13. b
4. b	9. c	14. a
5. a	10. c	15. c

Chapter 7

1. e	6. e	11. a
2. c	7. d	12. c
3. e	8. b	13. d
4. a	9. e	14. c
5. e	10. e	15. a

Chapter 8

1. c	6. b	11. b
2. a	7. b	12. a
3. c	8. a	13. c
4. d	9. d	14. b
5. a	10. c	15. a

Chapter 9

1. e	6. b	11. b
2. b	7. b	12. b
3. b	8. a	13. b
4. e	9. a	14. d
5. b	10. a	15. b

Chapter 11

1. b	6. a	11. d
2. a	7. c	12. d
3. a	8. a	13. c
4. b	9. c	14. a
5. d	10. c	15. c

Chapter 12

1. a	6. d	11. d
2. a	7. d	12. d
3. d	8. a	13. b
4. c	9. a	14. a
5. a	10. a	15. a

Chapter 13

1. a	6. d	11. d
2. a	7. e	12. a
3. b	8. b	13. a
4. a	9. a	14. a
5. a	10. d	15. a

Chapter 14

1. c	6. d	11. e
2. d	7. a	12. d
3. b	8. b	13. b
4. f	9. a	14. c
5. e	10. c	15. a

Chapter 15

1. d	6. a	11. e
2. c	7. d	12. c
3. c	8. c	13. e
4. d	9. e	14. d
5. b	10. e	15. a

Chapter 16

1. c	6. b	11. a
2. c	7. a	12. e
3. a	8. c	13. b
4. d	9. e	14. a
5. a	10. b	15. e

Chapter 17

1. a	6. e	11. d
2. d	7. c	12. e
3. d	8. e	13. e
4. c	9. d	14. d
5. c	10. c	15. b

Chapter 18

1. c	3. a	5. a
2. d	4. d	

Chapter 19

1. b	6. b	11. c
2. c	7. d	12. c
3. d	8. b	13. b
4. b	9. e	14. d
5. d	10. a	15. a

Chapter 20

1. e	6. e	11. c
2. e	7. c	12. a
3. d	8. d	13. c
4. d	9. d	14. e
5. e	10. e	15. d

Chapter 21

1. d	6. c	11. a
2. d	7. d	12. d
3. c	8. c	13. e
4. a	9. d	14. e
5. b	10. e	15. c

Chapter 22

1. b	6. d	11. c
2. a	7. a	12. b
3. a	8. d	13. a
4. c	9. b	14. b
5. d	10. c	15. d

Index

Page numbers followed by italic f or t indicate figures or tables, respectively.